76.50

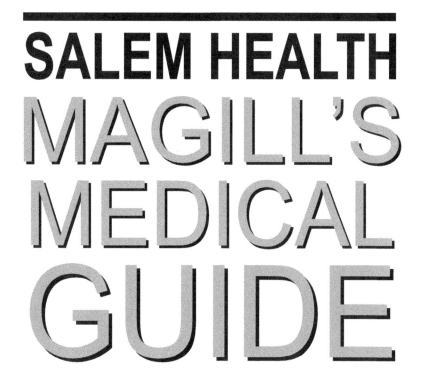

SALEM HEALTH

MAGILL'S
MEDICAL
GUIDE

SALEM HEALTH

MAGILL'S MEDICAL GUIDE

Seventh Edition

Volume V

Shock – Zoonoses
Appendixes
Indexes

Medical Editors

Bryan C. Auday, Ph.D.
Gordon College

Michael A. Buratovich, Ph.D.
Spring Arbor University

Geraldine F. Marrocco, Ed.D., APRN, CNS, ANP-BC
Yale University School of Nursing

Paul Moglia, Ph.D.
South Nassau Communities Hospital

SALEM PRESS
A Division of EBSCO Information Services, Inc.
Ipswich, Massachusetts

GREY HOUSE PUBLISHING

Magill's Medical Guide: Health and Illness, 1995
Supplement, 1996
Magill's Medical Guide, revised edition, 1998
Second revised edition, 2002
Third revised edition, 2005
Fourth revised edition, 2008
Sixth edition, 2011
Seventh edition, 2014

∞ The paper used in these volumes conforms to the American National Standard for Permanence of Paper for Printed Library Materials, Z39.48-1992 (R1997).

Note to Readers

The material presented in *Magill's Medical Guide* is intended for broad informational and educational purposes. Readers who suspect that they suffer from any of the physical or psychological disorders, diseases, or conditions described in this set should contact a physician without delay; this work should not be used as a substitute for professional medical diagnosis or treatment. This set is not to be considered definitive on the covered topics, and readers should remember that the field of health care is characterized by a diversity of medical opinions and constant expansion in knowledge and understanding.

Library of Congress Cataloging-in-Publication Data

Magill's medical guide / medical editors: Bryan C. Auday, Ph.D., Gordon College [and three others].
    — Seventh Edition.

5 volumes : illustrations ; cm. — (Salem health)

Title page verso indicates: Seventh Revised Edition, 2014.
Includes bibliographical references and index.
ISBN: 978-1-61925-214-1 (set)
ISBN: 978-1-61925-503-6 (v.1)
ISBN: 978-1-61925-504-3 (v.2)
ISBN: 978-1-61925-505-0 (v.3)
ISBN: 978-1-61925-506-7 (v.4)
ISBN: 978-1-61925-507-4 (v.5)

1. Medicine--Encyclopedias. I. Auday, Bryan C., editor. II. Series: Salem health (Pasadena, Calif.)

RC41 .M345 2014
610.3

First Printing

COMPLETE TABLE OF CONTENTS

VOLUME I

Publisher's Note v
The Patient Protection and Affordable
   Health Care Act ix
List of Contributors xxiii

Abdomen. 1
Abdominal disorders 4
Abortion 7
Abscess drainage 11
Abscesses 11
Abuse of the elderly 13
Accidents. 15
Achalasia. 19
Acid-base chemistry 20
Acid reflux disease 23
Acidosis. 24
Acne 26
Acquired immunodeficiency syndrome (AIDS) 30
Acupressure. 34
Acupuncture 35
Acute respiratory distress syndrome (ARDS) 39
Addiction. 41
Addison's disease 46
Adenoid removal. *See* Tonsillectomy and
   adenoid removal.
Adenoids. 47
Adenoviruses. 48
Adolescence. *See* Puberty and adolescence.
Adrenal disorders. *See* Addison's disease;
   Cushing's syndrome.
Adrenal glands 50
Adrenalectomy 51
Adrenoleukodystrophy 52
Advance directives 53
Aging 54
Aging: Extended care 58
Agnosia 62
AIDS. *See* Acquired immunodeficiency
   syndrome (AIDS).
Alcoholism 63
Allergies 67
Allied health 73
Alopecia 77
Alternative medicine 80

Altitude sickness 84
Alzheimer's disease. 85
Amebiasis 90
Amenorrhea. 91
American Medical Association (AMA) 92
Amnesia 93
Amniocentesis 95
Amputation 98
Amyotrophic lateral sclerosis 101
Anal cancer 103
Anatomy 104
Anemia 108
Anesthesia 111
Anesthesiology 114
Aneurysmectomy. 118
Aneurysms. 119
Angelman syndrome 119
Angina. 121
Angiography 121
Angioplasty 122
Animal rights vs. research. 123
Ankylosing spondylitis 127
Anorexia nervosa 129
Anosmia 131
Anthrax 132
Antianxiety drugs 134
Antibiotic resistance 135
Antibiotics. 140
Antibodies 144
Antidepressants 145
Antihistamines. 147
Antihypertensives 148
Anti-inflammatory drugs. 152
Antioxidants 154
Anus 155
Anxiety 156
Aortic aneurysm 159
Aortic stenosis. 161
Apgar score 163
Aphasia and dysphasia 164
Aphrodisiacs 166
Apnea 167
Appendectomy 167
Appendicitis 169

Aromatherapy 170
Arrhythmias 171
Arteriosclerosis 172
Arthritis 176
Arthroplasty 181
Arthroscopy 182
Asbestos exposure 183
Asperger's syndrome 185
Aspergillosis 186
Asphyxiation 187
Assisted living facilities 189
Assisted reproductive technologies 191
Assisted suicide 195
Asthma 195
Astigmatism 200
Ataxia 201
Athlete's foot 202
Atrial fibrillation 203
Atrophy 204
Attention-deficit disorder (ADD) 205
Audiology 208
Auras 211
Autism 212
Autoimmune disorders 216
Autopsy 220
Avian influenza 223

Babesiosis 228
Bacillus Calmette-Guérin (BCG) 228
Back disorders. *See* Back pain; Spinal cord
  disorders.
Back pain 230
Bacterial infections 231
Bacteriology 235
Balance disorders 238
Baldness. *See* Hair.
Bariatric surgery 239
Basal cell carcinoma. *See* Skin cancer.
Batten's disease 240
Bed-wetting 241
Bedsores 243
Behçet's disease 244
Bell's palsy 245
Benign prostatic hyperplasia. *See* Prostate
  enlargement.
Beriberi 246
Bile 246
Biofeedback 247
Bioinformatics 251
Biological therapies 252
Bionics and biotechnology 254
Biopsy 259

Biostatistics 263
Biotechnology. *See* Bionics and biotechnology.
Bipolar disorders 266
Birth. *See* Childbirth; Childbirth complications.
Birth defects 270
Bites and stings 274
Bladder cancer 275
Bladder infections. *See* Urinary disorders.
Bladder removal 277
Bladder stones. *See* Stone removal; Stones.
Bleeding 278
Blepharoplasty. *See* Face lift and blepharoplasty.
Blindness 283
Blindsight 285
Blisters 286
Blood and blood disorders 287
Blood banks 291
Blood poisoning. *See* Septicemia.
Blood pressure 295
Blood testing 297
Blood transfusion. *See* Transfusion.
Blood vessels 299
Blue baby syndrome 300
Blurred vision 301
Body dysmorphic disorder 302
Bonding 303
Bone cancer 305
Bone disorders 307
Bone fractures. *See* Fracture and dislocation.
Bone grafting 310
Bone marrow transplantation 310
Bones and the skeleton 312
Botox 316
Botulism 317
Bowlegs 318
Braces, orthodontic 319
Braces, orthopedic 320
Brain 322
Brain banks 326
Brain damage 327
Brain disorders 329
Brain tumors 332
Breast biopsy 333
Breast cancer 334
Breast disorders 338
Breast-feeding 340
Breast surgery 344
Breasts, female 346
Breathing difficulty. *See* Pulmonary diseases;
  Respiration; Respiratory distress syndrome.
Bronchi 350
Bronchiolitis 350

Bronchitis 351
Brucellosis. 352
Bruises. 355
Bulimia 355
Bunions 356
Burkitt's lymphoma. 357
Burns and scalds 358
Bursitis 362
Bypass surgery 363

Caffeine. 366
Calculi. *See* Stones.
Campylobacter infections 366
Cancer 367
Candidiasis 372
Canker sores 375
Capgras syndrome. 376
Carbohydrates 377
Carcinogens. 378
Carcinoma. 379
Cardiac arrest 379
Cardiac rehabilitation 380
Cardiac surgery 385
Cardiology. 387
Cardiopulmonary resuscitation (CPR) 391
Carotid arteries 393
Carpal tunnel syndrome 393
Cartilage 396
Casts and splints 398
CAT scans. *See* Computed tomography (CT)
   scanning.
Cataract surgery 399
Cataracts 401
Catheterization 404
Cavities 406

Celiac sprue. 407
Cells 408
Centers for Disease Control and Prevention (CDC) . . 412
Cerebral palsy 415
Cervical, ovarian, and uterine cancers. 417
Cervical procedures. 421
Cesarean section 423
Chagas' disease 424
Charcot-Marie-Tooth Disease 425
Chemotherapy 427
Chest 432
Chest pain. *See* Angina; Heart attack; Pain.
Chiari malformations. 436
Chickenpox 437
Childbirth 439
Childbirth complications. 444
Childhood infectious diseases 445
Chiropractic. 449
Chlamydia. 452
Choking. 454
Cholecystectomy. 454
Cholecystitis 455
Cholera 456
Cholesterol 458
Chorionic villus sampling 462
Chromosomal abnormalities. *See* Birth defects;
   Genetic diseases.
Chronic fatigue syndrome 463
Chronic granulomatous disease. 467
Chronic obstructive pulmonary disease (COPD) . . . 468
Chronic wasting disease (CWD) 470

Entries by Anatomy or System Affected. A-1
Entries by Specialties and Related Fields A-27

VOLUME II

Chyme............................... 471
Circulation........................... 471
Circumcision, female, and genital mutilation 474
Circumcision, male 476
Cirrhosis 479
Claudication 480
Cleft lip and palate 481
Cleft lip and palate repair 484
Clinical trials........................ 485
Clinics 487
Cloning 489
Clostridium difficile infection 493
Club drugs........................... 494
Cluster headaches 495
Coccidioidomycosis 497
Cockayne Disease 498
Cognitive development 499
Cognitive enhancement.................. 503
Cold agglutinin disease 504
Cold sores 506
Colic 507
Colitis 509
Collagen 512
Collodion baby 513
Colon............................... 513
Colon therapy 515
Colonoscopy and sigmoidoscopy 515
Color blindness 517
Colorectal cancer...................... 517
Colorectal polyp removal 520
Colorectal surgery 521
Coma. *See* Minimally conscious state.
Common cold 522
Computed tomography (CT) scanning 526
Conception 528
Concussion 532
Congenital adrenal hyperplasia.............. 534
Congenital disorders 536
Congenital heart disease 538
Congenital hypothyroidism............... 542
Congestive heart failure. *See* Heart failure.
Conjunctivitis 543
Connective tissue 544
Constipation 545
Contraception 546
Corneal transplantation 550
Cornelia de Lange syndrome............... 551
Corns and calluses..................... 552
Coronary artery bypass graft.............. 553
Coronaviruses 554

Corticosteroids 556
Cosmetic surgery. *See* Plastic surgery.
Coughing............................ 557
Craniosynostosis 558
Craniotomy 559
Cretinism. *See* Congenital hypothyroidism.
Creutzfeldt-Jakob disease (CJD)............. 560
Critical care.......................... 562
Crohn's disease 566
Crossed eyes. *See* Strabismus.
Croup............................... 568
Crowns and bridges..................... 569
Cryosurgery.......................... 570
CT scanning. *See* Computed tomography (CT)
    scanning.
Culdocentesis 572
Cushing's syndrome 573
Cutis marmorata telangiectatica congenita 574
Cyanosis 575
Cyst removal 577
Cystic fibrosis 578
Cystitis 582
Cystoscopy 585
Cysts 586
Cytology 587
Cytomegalovirus (CMV)................. 591
Cytopathology........................ 592

Deafness 594
Death and dying 595
Decongestants 599
Deep vein thrombosis 600
Defibrillation......................... 601
Dehydration.......................... 602
Delirium 604
Dementias 605
Dengue fever......................... 608
Dental diseases 610
Dentistry 613
Dentures 616
Department of Health and
    Human Services...................... 617
Depression........................... 619
Dermatitis 623
Dermatology 627
Dermatopathology..................... 630
Developmental disorders................. 632
Developmental stages 634
Diabetes mellitus...................... 638
Diagnosis............................ 644

Dialysis 645
Diaphragm. 649
Diarrhea and dysentery 650
Diet. *See* Nutrition.
Dietary deficiencies. *See* Malnutrition;
   Nutrition; Vitamins and minerals.
Dietary reference intakes (DRIs). 654
DiGeorge syndrome 655
Digestion. 656
Diphtheria 659
Disease 660
Disk removal. 663
Dislocation. *See* Fracture and dislocation.
Disseminated intravascular coagulation (DIC) 665
Diuretics 666
Diverticulitis and diverticulosis. 668
Dizziness and fainting. 672
Down syndrome 675
Drowning 680
Drug addiction. *See* Addiction.
Dry eye 682
Dwarfism. 683
Dysentery. *See* Diarrhea and dysentery.
Dyskinesia. 687
Dyslexia 688
Dysmenorrhea. 691
Dysphasia. *See* Aphasia and dysphasia.
Dystonia 692

E. coli infection. 695
Ear infections and disorders 696
Ear, nose, and throat medicine. *See*
   Otorhinolaryngology.
Ear surgery 700
Ears. 701
Earwax 705
Eating disorders. 706
Ebola virus 710
ECG or EKG. *See* Electrocardiography (ECG or
   EKG).
Echocardiography 713
Eclampsia. *See* Preeclampsia and eclampsia.
Ectopic pregnancy. 714
Eczema 715
Edema 716
EEG. *See* Electroencephalography (EEG).
Ehrlichiosis 720
Electrical shock. 720
Electrocardiography (ECG or EKG) 722
Electrocauterization. 724
Electroencephalography (EEG). 724
Electrolytes. *See* Fluids and electrolytes.

Electromyography. 726
Elephantiasis 728
Embolism 731
Embolization. 732
Embryology. 733
Emergency medicine. 737
Emergency rooms 741
Emerging infectious diseases 743
Emphysema. 744
Encephalitis. 748
End-stage renal disease 749
Endarterectomy 751
Endocarditis 752
Endocrine disorders. 753
Endocrine glands. 756
Endocrinology. 758
Endocrinology, pediatric 761
Endodontic disease 763
Endometrial biopsy 764
Endometriosis 765
Endoscopic retrograde cholangiopancreatography
   (ERCP) 769
Endoscopy. 770
Enemas 773
Enterocolitis 773
Enteroviruses. 774
Enuresis. *See* Bed-wetting.
Environmental diseases. 775
Enzyme therapy. 779
Epidemics and pandemics 780
Epidemiology 783
Epidermal nevus syndromes 786
Epiglottitis. 788
Epilepsy. 789
Episiotomy 793
Epstein-Barr virus 793
Erectile dysfunction 795
Ergogenic aids. 797
Esophageal cancer. *See* Mouth and throat cancer.
Esophagus 799
Estrogen replacement therapy. *See* Hormone
   therapy.
Ethics. 799
Euthanasia 803
Ewing's sarcoma 807
Exercise physiology 808
Extended care for the aging. *See* Aging:
   Extended care.
Extended care for the terminally ill. *See*
   Terminally ill: Extended care.
Extremities. *See* Feet; Foot disorders; Lower
   extremities; Upper extremities.

Eye infections and disorders 813
Eye surgery 817
Eyes. 820

Face lift and blepharoplasty 825
Facial palsy. *See* Bell's palsy.
Facial transplantation 826
Factitious disorders 828
Failure to thrive. 829
Fainting. *See* Dizziness and fainting.
Family medicine 830
Fascia 834
Fatigue. 835
Fatty acid oxidation disorders 839
Feet 840
Fetal alcohol syndrome 843
Fetal surgery 844
Fetal tissue transplantation 847
Fever 851
Fiber 854
Fibrocystic breast condition 855
Fibromyalgia. 856
Fifth disease 858
Fingernail removal. *See* Nail removal.
First aid 859
First responder. 861
Fistula repair 862
Flat feet 864
Fluids and electrolytes. 864
Fluoride treatments 868
Fluoroscopy. *See* Imaging and radiology.
Food allergies 869
Food and Drug Administration (FDA) 871
Food biochemistry. 874
Food guide plate 877
Food poisoning 879
Foot disorders 882
Forensic pathology 884
Fracture and dislocation 886
Fracture repair. 891
Fragile X syndrome. 893
Frontal lobe syndrome. 893
Frontotemporal dementia (FTD) 895
Frostbite 896
Fructosemia. 900
Fungal infections. 900

Galactosemia. 905
Gallbladder 905
Gallbladder cancer 907
Gallbladder diseases 908

Gallbladder removal. *See* Cholecystectomy.
Gallstones. *See* Gallbladder diseases; Stone
    removal; Stones.
Gamete intrafallopian transfer (GIFT) 911
Ganglion removal 913
Ganglions. *See* Cysts; Ganglion removal.
Gangrene. 913
Gastrectomy 915
Gastric bypass. *See* Bariatric surgery.
Gastritis. *See* Abdominal disorders;
    Gastroenteritis; Gastrointestinal disorders.
Gastroenteritis. 916
Gastroenterology. 918
Gastrointestinal disorders 921
Gastrointestinal system 924
Gastrostomy 928
Gaucher's disease 929
Gender identity disorder 930
Gender reassignment surgery 932
Gene therapy 933
Genetic counseling 936
Genetic diseases 940
Genetic engineering 944
Genetic Imprinting 948
Genetic sequencing. *See* Genomics.
Genetics and inheritance 952
Genital disorders, female. 956
Genital disorders, male 959
Genomics 962
Geriatric assessment 965
Geriatrics and gerontology 966
Gestational diabetes 970
Giardiasis 972
Gigantism 972
Gingivitis. 974
Glands 976
Glasgow coma scale 980
Glaucoma 981
Glomerulonephritis. *See* Nephritis.
Glioma. 985
Gluten intolerance 986
Glycogen storage diseases. 988
Glycolysis 990
Goiter 994
Gonorrhea 995
Gout 997
Grafts and grafting 1000
Gram staining 1003

Entries by Anatomy or System Affected. A-1
Entries by Specialties and Related Fields A-27

VOLUME III

Growth 1007
Guillain-Barré syndrome.................. 1010
Gulf War syndrome..................... 1013
Gum disease 1015
Gynecology.......................... 1017
Gynecomastia 1020

Hair............................... 1022
Hair transplantation.................... 1024
Hammertoe correction................... 1025
Hammertoes 1025
Hand-foot-and-mouth disease 1026
Hantavirus.......................... 1027
Harelip. See Cleft lip and palate.
Hashimoto's thyroiditis.................. 1028
Havening touch....................... 1028
Hay fever........................... 1031
Head and neck disorders 1031
Headaches 1033
Healing 1036
Health care reform..................... 1040
Health maintenance organizations (HMOs) 1042
Hearing 1045
Hearing aids 1047
Hearing loss......................... 1049
Hearing tests 1052
Heart 1054
Heart attack......................... 1058
Heart disease 1061
Heart failure 1065
Heart transplantation 1069
Heart valve replacement 1071
Heat exhaustion and heatstroke............. 1073
Heel spur removal 1075
Heimlich maneuver..................... 1075
Hematology.......................... 1076
Hematomas 1080
Hematuria 1081
Hemiplegia 1082
Hemochromatosis 1083
Hemolytic disease of the newborn 1084
Hemolytic uremic syndrome................ 1085
Hemophilia 1086
Hemorrhage. See Bleeding.
Hemorrhoid banding and removal............ 1089
Hemorrhoids 1090
Hepatitis 1094
Herbal medicine 1098
Hermaphroditism and pseudohermaphroditism.... 1101
Hernia 1102

Hernia repair 1105
Herniated disk. See Slipped disk.
Herpes 1107
Hiccups 1108
Hip fracture repair..................... 1109
Hip replacement 1109
Hippocratic oath 1111
Hirschsprung's disease 1115
Histiocytosis 1116
Histology........................... 1116
HIV. See Human immunodeficiency virus (HIV).
Hives 1120
Hodgkin's disease 1121
Home care........................... 1124
Homeopathy 1126
H1N1 influenza....................... 1130
Hormone therapy...................... 1132
Hormones 1135
Hospice 1138
Host-defense mechanisms 1141
Human Genome Project. See Genomics.
Human immunodeficiency virus (HIV).......... 1145
Human papillomavirus (HPV)............... 1147
Huntington's disease 1148
Hydroceles........................... 1149
Hydrocephalus........................ 1150
Hydrotherapy......................... 1152
Hyperadiposis 1153
Hyperbaric oxygen therapy 1154
Hypercholesterolemia 1156
Hyperhidrosis 1156
Hyperlipidemia 1157
Hyperparathyroidism and hypoparathyroidism 1159
Hyperplasia 1161
Hypertension......................... 1162
Hyperthermia and hypothermia.............. 1166
Hypertrophy 1171
Hyperventilation 1174
Hypnosis 1175
Hypochondriasis 1178
Hypoglycemia 1182
Hypoparathyroidism. See Hyperparathyroidism
    and hypoparathyroidism.
Hypospadias repair and urethroplasty 1185
Hypotension 1186
Hypothalamus 1187
Hypothermia. See Hyperthermia and
    hypothermia.
Hypothyroidism. See Congenital
    hypothyroidism.

Hypoxia. 1188
Hysterectomy 1188

Iatrogenic disorders. 1193
Ileostomy and colostomy. 1194
Imaging and radiology. 1198
Immune system 1202
Immunization and vaccination 1206
Immunodeficiency disorders. 1212
Immunopathology. 1215
Impetigo 1216
Impotence. *See* Sexual dysfunction.
In vitro fertilization 1217
Incontinence 1221
Infarction. 1225
Infarction, myocardial. *See* Heart attack.
Infection 1225
Infertility, female. 1229
Infertility, male 1233
Inflammation. 1237
Influenza 1238
Informed consent. 1242
Insect-borne diseases. 1242
Insomnia. *See* Sleep disorders.
The Institute of Medicine 1248
Intensive care. *See* Critical care.
Intensive care unit (ICU). 1248
Internal medicine. 1251
Internet medicine. 1255
Interpartner violence 1258
Interstitial pulmonary fibrosis (IPF) 1259
Intestinal cancer. *See* Stomach, intestinal, and
   pancreatic cancers.
Intestinal disorders 1260
Intestines. 1263
Intoxication. *See* Alcoholism; Poisoning.
Intravenous (IV) therapy. 1266
Intraventricular hemorrhage 1267
Invasive tests. 1268
Irritable bowel syndrome (IBS). 1269
Ischemia 1272

Jaundice. 1274
Jaw wiring. 1274
Joint diseases. *See* Arthritis.
Joint replacement. *See* Arthroplasty; Hip
   replacement.
Joints. 1277
Juvenile rheumatoid arthritis. 1279

Kaposi's sarcoma. 1281
Karyotyping 1282

Kawasaki disease 1283
Keratitis. 1284
Kidney cancer. 1285
Kidney disorders. 1286
Kidney removal. *See* Nephrectomy.
Kidney stones. *See* Kidney disorders; Stone
   removal; Stones.
Kidney transplantation 1289
Kidneys. 1291
Kinesiology. 1295
Klinefelter syndrome. 1295
Klippel-Trenaunay syndrome 1296
Kluver-Bucy syndrome 1297
Kneecap removal. 1298
Knock-knees 1299
Korsakoff's syndrome. 1300
Kwashiorkor 1301
Kyphosis. 1302

Laboratory tests. 1304
Laceration repair. 1308
Lactose intolerance 1309
Laminectomy and spinal fusion. 1310
Laparoscopy 1310
Laryngectomy 1312
Laryngitis 1313
Laser use in surgery. 1314
Law and medicine. 1318
Lead poisoning 1322
Learning disabilities 1324
Legionnaires' disease 1328
Leishmaniasis 1332
Leprosy 1333
Leptin 1336
Leptospirosis. 1337
Lesions 1339
Leukemia. 1340
Leukodystrophy 1344
Lice, mites, and ticks. 1345
Ligaments 1348
Light therapy. 1349
Lipids 1350
Liposuction 1354
Lisping 1356
Listeria infections 1356
Lithotripsy. 1357
Liver 1359
Liver cancer. 1362
Liver disorders 1364
Liver transplantation 1368
Local anesthesia 1370
Lockjaw. *See* Tetanus.

Lou Gehrig's disease. *See* Amyotrophic lateral sclerosis.
Longevity 1371
Lower extremities 1372
Lumbar puncture........................ 1375
Lumpectomy. *See* Mastectomy and lumpectomy.
Lumps, breast. *See* Breast cancer; Breast disorders; Breasts, female.
Lung cancer........................... 1377
Lung diseases. *See* Pulmonary diseases.
Lung surgery 1379
Lungs................................ 1381
Lupus. *See* Systemic lupus erythematosus (SLE).
Lyme disease........................... 1384
Lymph................................ 1385
Lymphadenopathy and lymphoma 1386
Lymphatic disorders. *See* Lymphadenopathy and lymphoma.
Lymphatic system 1390
Lymphoma. *See* Lymphadenopathy and lymphoma.

Macronutrients 1395
Macular degeneration 1397
Magnetic field therapy 1399
Magnetic resonance imaging (MRI) 1399
Malabsorption.......................... 1401
Malaria 1402
Malignancy and metastasis 1405
Malnutrition 1409
Mammography 1413
Managed care 1416
Manic-depressive disorder. *See* Bipolar disorders.
Maple syrup urine disease (MSUD) 1417
Marburg virus 1418
Marfan syndrome 1419
Marijuana 1421
Massage............................... 1422
Mastectomy and lumpectomy 1422
Mastitis 1426
Masturbation 1427
Measles 1427
Meckel's diverticulum..................... 1430
Medical home 1432
Medicare.............................. 1433
Meditation............................ 1435
Melanoma............................. 1436
Melatonin 1438
Memory loss 1439
Ménière's disease 1441
Meningitis............................. 1442

Menopause 1444
Menorrhagia 1447
Men's health 1448
Menstruation 1454
Mental retardation....................... 1459
Mental illness. *See* Psychiatric disorders; specific diseases.
Mental status exam 1463
Mercury poisoning 1464
Mesenchymal stem cells 1465
Mesothelioma 1467
Metabolic disorders...................... 1469
Metabolic syndrome 1472
Metabolism 1475
Metastasis. *See* Cancer; Malignancy and metastasis.
Methicillin-resistant *staphylococcus aureus* (MRSA) infections 1479
Microbiology........................... 1480
Microscopy 1484
Microscopy, slitlamp...................... 1485
Minimally conscious state.................. 1485
Mirror neurons 1487
Miscarriage 1488
Mites. *See* Bites and stings; Lice, mites, and ticks; Parasitic diseases.
Mitral valve prolapse...................... 1490
Mold and mildew 1491
Moles................................ 1492
Monkeypox............................ 1493
Mononucleosis 1494
Morgellons disease 1495
Mosquito bites. *See* Bites and stings; Insect-borne diseases
Motion sickness......................... 1496
Motor neuron diseases..................... 1498
Motor skill development 1500
Mouth and throat cancer 1504
MRI. *See* Magnetic resonance imaging (MRI).
MRSA infections. *See* Methicillin-resistant *staphylococcus aureus* (MRSA) infections
MSUD. *See* Maple syrup urine disease (MSUD)
Mucopolysaccharidosis (MPS) 1505
Multiple births......................... 1506
Multiple chemical sensitivity syndrome 1511
Multiple sclerosis 1512
Mumps 1516
Münchausen syndrome by proxy 1518
Muscle sprains, spasms, and disorders 1520
Muscles............................... 1522
Muscular dystrophy....................... 1526
Mutation 1529

Myasthenia gravis 1533
Myocardial infarction. *See* Heart attack.
Myomectomy 1535
Myopia 1536
Myringotomy 1537

Nail removal 1538
Nails 1538
Narcolepsy 1541
Narcotics 1545
Nasal polyp removal 1548
Nasopharyngeal disorders 1549
National Cancer Institute (NCI) 1553
National Institutes of Health (NIH) 1555

Nausea and vomiting 1558
Neck injuries and disorders. *See* Head and neck
   disorders.
Necrosis 1562
Necrotizing fasciitis 1562
Neonatal brachial plexus palsy 1563
Neonatology 1566
Nephrectomy 1571
Nephritis 1573
Nephrology 1575
Nervous system 1579

Entries by Anatomy or System Affected A-1
Entries by Specialties and Related Fields A-27

VOLUME IV

Neuralgia, neuritis, and neuropathy 1583
Neuroethics 1586
Neurofibromatosis 1587
Neuroimaging 1588
Neurology 1590
Neurology, pediatric 1594
Neuropsychology 1596
Neuroscience 1597
Neurosis 1598
Neurosurgery 1599
Niemann-Pick disease 1602
Nonalcoholic steatohepatitis (NASH) 1604
Noninvasive tests 1605
Noroviruses 1608
Nuclear medicine 1609
Nuclear radiology 1613
Numbness and tingling 1615
Nursing 1616
Nutrition 1620

Obesity 1625
Obesity, childhood 1628
Obsessive-compulsive disorder 1631
Obstetrics 1635
Occupational health 1638
Oncology 1639
Ophthalmology 1642
Opportunistic infections 1645
Optometry 1648
Oral and maxillofacial surgery 1651
Orchiectomy 1653
Orchitis 1654
Organs. See Systems and organs.
Orthodontics 1655
Orthopedic braces. See Braces, orthopedic.
Orthopedic surgery 1658
Orthopedics 1659
Osgood-Schlatter disease 1663
Osteoarthritis 1664
Osteochondritis juvenilis 1666
Osteogenesis imperfecta 1666
Osteomyelitis 1668
Osteonecrosis 1669
Osteopathic medicine 1670
Osteoporosis 1673
Otoplasty 1678
Otorhinolaryngology 1678
Ovarian cancer. See Cervical, ovarian, and
    uterine cancers.
Ovarian cysts 1682

Ovaries 1683
Over-the-counter medications 1685
Overtraining syndrome 1688
Oxygen therapy 1689

Pacemaker implantation 1690
Paget's disease 1694
Pain 1696
Pain management 1699
Palliative care 1700
Palliative medicine 1702
Palpitations 1704
Palsy 1705
Pancreas 1709
Pancreatic cancer. See Stomach, intestinal, and
    pancreatic cancers.
Pancreatitis 1712
Panic attacks. See Anxiety.
Pap test 1714
Paralysis 1715
Paramedics 1719
Paranoia 1723
Paraplegia 1725
Parasitic diseases 1726
Parathyroidectomy 1730
Parkinson's disease 1730
Pathology 1735
Pediatrics 1738
Pelvic inflammatory disease (PID) 1743
Penile implant surgery 1744
Peptic ulcers. See Ulcers.
Perinatology 1746
Periodontal surgery 1747
Periodontitis 1748
Peristalsis 1749
Peritonitis 1754
Pertussis. See Whooping cough.
PET scanning. See Positron emission
    tomography (PET) scanning.
Pharmacology 1754
Pharyngitis 1758
Pharynx 1759
Phenylketonuria (PKU) 1759
Phlebitis 1761
Phlebotomy 1764
Phobias 1764
Phrenology 1766
Physical examination 1767
Physical rehabilitation 1771
Physician assistants 1776

Physiology 1779
Phytochemicals 1782
Pick's disease 1783
PID. *See* Pelvic inflammatory disease (PID).
Pigeon toes 1785
Pigmentation 1786
Pimples. *See* Acne.
Pinworms 1789
Pituitary gland 1790
Pityriasis alba 1791
Pityriasis rosea 1792
PKU. *See* Phenylketonuria (PKU)
Placenta 1793
Plague 1794
Plaque, arterial 1795
Plaque, dental 1796
Plasma 1797
Plastic surgery 1798
Pleurisy 1801
Pneumocystis jirovecii 1802
Pneumonia 1803
Pneumothorax 1807
Podiatry 1808
Poisoning 1811
Poliomyelitis 1814
Polycystic kidney disease 1819
Polycystic ovary syndrome 1820
Polydactyly and syndactyly 1821
Polyp removal. *See* Colorectal polyp removal;
    Nasal polyp removal.
Polymyalgia rheumatica 1823
Polyps 1824
Porphyria 1825
Positron emission tomography (PET) scanning . . . 1826
Postherpetic neuralgia 1828
Postpartum depression 1829
Post-traumatic stress disorder 1830
Prader-Willi syndrome 1832
Precocious puberty 1833
Preeclampsia and eclampsia 1834
Pregnancy and gestation 1836
Premature birth 1840
Premenstrual syndrome (PMS) 1843
Preventive medicine 1845
Prion diseases 1848
Proctology 1850
Progeria 1853
Prognosis 1854
Prostate cancer 1855
Prostate enlargement 1857
Prostate gland 1859
Prostate gland removal 1863

Prostheses 1864
Protein 1867
Proteinuria 1868
Proteomics 1869
Protozoan diseases 1870
Psoriasis 1872
Psychiatric disorders 1875
Psychiatry 1879
Psychiatry, geriatric 1881
Psychoanalysis 1882
Psychosis 1885
Psychosomatic disorders 1887
Pterygium/Pinguecula 1888
Ptosis 1889
Puberty and adolescence 1890
Public health. *See* Occupational health.
Pulmonary diseases 1894
Pulmonary edema 1898
Pulmonary hypertension 1899
Pulmonary medicine 1900
Pulse rate 1903
Pyelonephritis 1904
Pyloric stenosis 1905

Quadriplegia 1907
Quinsy 1908

Rabies 1909
Radiation sickness 1912
Radiation therapy 1913
Radiculopathy 1917
Radiology. *See* Imaging and radiology; Nuclear
    radiology.
Radiopharmaceuticals 1918
Rape and sexual assault 1922
Reconstructive surgery. *See* Plastic surgery.
Rectal polyp removal. *See* Colorectal polyp
    removal.
Rectal surgery. *See* Colorectal surgery.
Raynaud's Phenomenon 1925
Rectum 1925
Reflexes, primitive 1926
Refractive eye surgery 1928
Reiter's syndrome 1929
Renal failure 1930
Reproductive system 1931
Research vs. animal rights. *See* Animal rights vs.
    research.
Respiration 1935
Respiratory diseases. *See* Pulmonary diseases;
    Respiration; specific diseases.
Respiratory distress syndrome 1938

Restless legs syndrome 1939
Resuscitation 1942
Retroviruses 1945
Reye's syndrome 1947
Rh factor 1947
Rheumatic fever 1951
Rheumatoid arthritis 1952
Rheumatology 1954
Rhinitis 1958
Rhinoplasty and submucous resection. 1959
Rhinoviruses 1960
Rickets. 1962
Ringworm 1963
Rocky Mountain spotted fever 1964
Root canal treatment 1964
Rosacea 1965
Roseola 1966
Rotator cuff surgery 1967
Rotavirus. 1968
Roundworms 1969
Rubella 1970
Rubinstein-Taybi syndrome 1972

Safety issues for children 1973
Safety issues for the elderly 1978
Salmonella infection 1981
Sarcoidosis 1983
Sarcoma. 1985
SARS. *See* Severe acute respiratory syndrome
    (SARS).
Scabies 1986
Scalds. *See* Burns and scalds.

Scarlet fever 1986
Schistosomiasis. 1987
Schizophrenia 1989
Sciatica 1992
SCID. *See* Severe combined immunodeficiency
    syndrome (SCID).
Scleroderma 1993
Scoliosis 1994
Screening. 1998
Scurvy 2002
Seasonal affective disorder 2002
Seizures. 2004
Self-medication. 2007
Semen 2008
Sense organs 2009
Separation anxiety. 2012
Septicemia. 2013
Serology 2015
Severe acute respiratory syndrome (SARS) 2018
Severe combined immunodeficiency
    syndrome (SCID) 2020
Sexual differentiation 2022
Sexual dysfunction 2025
Sexuality 2029
Sexually transmitted diseases (STDs) 2033
Shaking. *See* Tremors.
Shigellosis. 2037
Shingles. 2038

Entries by Anatomy or System Affected. A-1
Entries by Specialties and Related Fields A-27

VOLUME V

Shock. 2039
Shock therapy 2042
Shunts 2046
Sickle cell disease 2047
SIDS. *See* Sudden infant death syndrome
   (SIDS).
Signs and symptoms 2050
Single photon emission computed
   tomography (SPECT) 2051
Sinusitis. 2053
Sjögren's syndrome. 2055
Skeletal disorders and diseases. *See* Bone
   disorders.
Skeleton. *See* Bones and the skeleton.
Skin. 2056
Skin cancer 2060
Skin disorders 2061
Skin grafting. *See* Grafts and grafting.
Skin lesion removal. 2064
Sleep 2065
Sleep apnea 2068
Sleep disorders 2070
Sleeping sickness 2074
Sleepwalking. 2076
Slipped disk. 2077
Small intestine. 2078
Smallpox. 2080
Smell. 2082
Smoking 2086
Snakebites 2088
Soiling. 2090
Sore throat. 2092
Speech disorders 2094
Sperm banks 2096
Sphincterectomy 2098
Spider bites. *See* Bites and stings.
Spina bifida. 2099
Spinal cord disorders. 2101
Spinal fusion. *See* Laminectomy and spinal
   fusion.
Spinal tap. *See* Lumbar puncture.
Spine, vertebrae, and disks 2104
Spinocerebellar ataxia. 2109
Splenectomy 2109
Split-brain 2110
Spondylitis. 2112
Sports medicine. 2113
Sprains. *See* Muscle sprains, spasms, and
   disorders.
Squamous cell carcinoma. *See* Skin cancer.

Staphylococcal infections 2117
Stem cells 2118
Stenosis. 2122
Stents. 2123
Sterilization. 2124
Steroid abuse. 2127
Steroids 2128
Stevens-Johnson syndrome 2132
Stillbirth 2133
Stings. *See* Bites and stings.
Stomach, intestinal, and pancreatic cancers 2134
Stomach removal. *See* Gastrectomy.
Stone removal 2137
Stones 2140
Strabismus. 2142
Streptococcal infections 2143
Stress. 2143
Stress reduction 2147
Strokes. 2148
Sturge-Weber syndrome 2153
Stuttering. 2154
Styes 2155
Subdural hematoma. 2155
Substance abuse 2157
Sudden infant death syndrome (SIDS) 2159
Suffocation. *See* Asphyxiation.
Suicide. 2161
Supplements 2165
Surgery, general. 2167
Surgery, pediatric 2170
Surgical procedures. 2172
Surgical technologists 2173
Sweating 2177
Sympathectomy. 2177
Syndrome 2178
Synesthesia 2180
Syphilis. 2181
Systemic lupus erythematosus (SLE) 2182
Systemic sclerosis 2185
Systems and organs. 2187

Tapeworms 2192
Tardive dyskinesia. 2193
Taste 2194
Tattoo removal 2199
Tattoos and body piercing. 2200
Tay-Sachs disease 2201
Tears and tear ducts. 2202
Teeth 2203
Teething. 2207

Shading indicates current volume.

Telemedicine. *See* Internet medicine.
Temporal arteritis 2208
Temporomandibular joint (TMJ) syndrome 2209
Tendinitis. 2209
Tendon disorders 2211
Tendon repair 2212
Teratogens 2213
Terminally ill: Extended care 2214
Testicles, undescended 2217
Testicular cancer 2218
Testicular surgery 2219
Testicular torsion. 2221
Tests. *See* Invasive tests; Laboratory tests;
    Noninvasive tests.
Tetanus 2221
Thalassemia. 2225
Thalidomide 2226
Thoracic surgery 2227
Throat. *See* Esophagus; Pharynx.
Throat, sore. *See* Sore throat.
Thrombocytopenia 2229
Thrombolytic therapy and TPA. 2230
Thrombosis and thrombus. 2234
Thumb sucking 2237
Thymus gland 2238
Thyroid disorders 2239
Thyroid gland 2241
Thyroidectomy 2243
TIAs. *See* Transient ischemic attacks (TIAs).
Ticks. *See* Lice, mites, and ticks.
Tics 2244
Tingling. *See* Numbness and tingling.
Tinnitus 2248
Tiredness. *See* Fatigue.
Toenail removal. *See* Nail removal.
Toilet training 2249
Tonsillectomy and adenoid removal 2251
Tonsillitis. 2252
Tonsils. 2253
Tooth decay. *See* Cavities.
Tooth extraction 2254
Torticollis 2255
Touch. 2256
Tourette's syndrome 2260
Toxemia. 2262
Toxic shock syndrome. 2263
Toxicology 2264
Toxoplasmosis. 2266
Trachea 2267
Tracheostomy 2269
Trachoma. 2270
Transfusion 2271

Transient ischemic attacks (TIAs). 2278
Transitional care 2279
Transplantation 2279
Traumatic brain injury. 2283
Tremors. 2285
Trichinosis. 2286
Trichomoniasis 2287
Tubal ligation 2288
Tuberculosis 2289
Tularemia 2293
Tumor removal 2293
Tumors 2296
Turner syndrome 2299
Twins. *See* Multiple births.
Typhoid fever 2300
Typhus. 2301

Ulcer surgery. 2303
Ulcerative colitis 2304
Ulcers 2306
Ultrasonography 2309
Umbilical cord. 2313
Undescended testicles. *See* Testicles,
    undescended.
Upper extremities 2314
Uremia. 2318
Urethritis 2319
Urethroplasty. *See* Hypospadias repair and
    urethroplasty.
Urinalysis 2320
Urinary disorders. 2322
Urinary system 2325
Urology 2328
Uterine cancer. *See* Cervical, ovarian, and
    uterine cancers.
Uterus 2332

Vaccination. *See* Immunization and vaccination.
Vagotomy 2333
Vagus nerve. 2334
Varicose vein removal 2335
Varicose veins 2336
Vas deferens 2338
Vascular medicine 2339
Vascular system. 2342
Vasculitis. 2345
Vasectomy. 2347
Venereal diseases. *See* Sexually transmitted
    diseases (STDs).
Venous insufficiency. 2350
Vertigo. 2351
Viral hemorrhagic fevers. 2352

Shading indicates current volume.

Viral infections 2354
Vision 2358
Vision correction. *See* Refractive eye surgery.
Vision disorders. 2361
Vitamin D deficiency 2363
Vitamins and minerals. 2364
Vitiligo 2368
Voice and vocal cord disorders 2369
Vomiting. *See* Nausea and vomiting.
Von Willebrand's disease 2371

Weaning 2373
Weight loss and gain 2374
Weight loss medications 2377
Well-baby examinations 2377
Wernicke's aphasia 2379
West Nile virus 2380
Whiplash 2383
Whooping cough 2384
Williams syndrome 2385
Wilson's disease 2387
Wisdom teeth. 2388
Wiskott-Aldrich syndrome 2389

World Health Organization 2390
Wounds 2393

X rays. *See* Imaging and radiology.
Xenotransplantation 2396

Yeast infections. *See* Candidiasis.
Yellow fever 2398
Yoga 2399

Zoonoses 2402

Glossary 2407
Symptoms and Warning Signs. 2457
Diseases and Other Medical Conditions 2461
Pharmaceutical List. 2481
Types of Health Care Providers. 2491
General Bibliography 2495
Resources 2511

Entries by Anatomy or System Affected. A-1
Entries by Specialties and Related Fields A-27
Index. A-57

Shading indicates current volume.

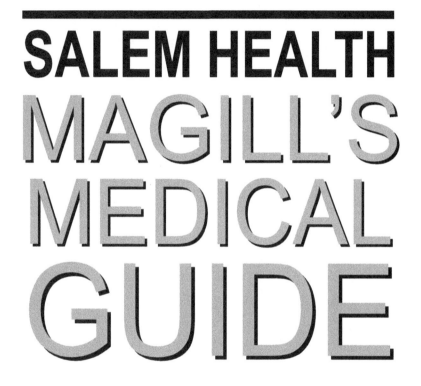

SALEM HEALTH

MAGILL'S MEDICAL GUIDE

SHOCK

Disease/Disorder

Anatomy or system affected: All

Specialties and related fields: Critical care, emergency medicine, family medicine, internal medicine

Definition: Shock is a life-threatening condition that may occur in response to a variety of circumstances (allergic reaction, infection, injury, blood loss, heart attack, toxic substances in the blood) which causes the heart to be unable to pump enough blood to supply the vital organs, which are therefore deprived of oxygen and nutrients and lose normal function; symptoms include rapid and shallow breathing, clammy skin, low blood pressure, rapid and weak pulse, and dizziness and if untreated will progress to unconsciousness and death.

Key terms:

blood pressure: the amount of pressure on blood vessel walls when the heart contracts and relaxes

cardiovascular system: the organ system consisting of the heart and all blood vessels (vasculature)

vasculature: all the blood vessels, including the arteries (blood vessels carrying blood away from the heart), the capillaries (the smallest blood vessels, where fluid and nutrients are exchanged), and the veins (blood vessels that return blood to the heart)

vital organs: organs of the body essential to life; the brain, heart, lungs, and sometimes the kidneys

Causes and Symptoms

The primary goal of the cardiovascular system is to provide blood flow, carrying oxygen and other nutrients to all tissues to meet their requirements. The cardiovascular system performs this function by maintaining a blood pressure high enough to push sufficient blood flow throughout the body, especially the vital organs. To keep the blood pressure up, the heart must pump sufficient amounts of blood even when the demand for increased blood flow to some tissues occurs. The blood vessels also play an important role in maintaining blood pressure. The heart and the blood vessels work in a coordinated manner to maintain blood pressure and blood flow.

A healthy heart is capable of adjusting the strength of its beats and the rate of its beats (the heart rate) to produce enough flow to match the demands placed on it by the tissues of the body. For example, during exercise, the exercising muscles require greater blood flow. If the heart does not pump the increased amount of blood that is necessary, then the blood pressure will fall. Hormones such as adrenaline help the heart beat faster and harder to meet the increased demand for blood by the muscles.

The blood vessels (vasculature) have a special structure and function to help maintain blood pressure. The arteries and veins are elastic in nature and squeeze on the blood like an inflated balloon does to the air inside it. In addition, the walls of blood vessels have special muscle tissue, called smooth muscle, that can contract to make the vessels' internal diameter smaller, which helps keep pressure up. If the vessels' internal

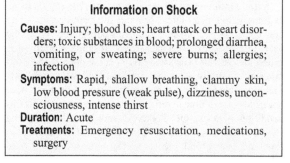

Information on Shock

Causes: Injury; blood loss; heart attack or heart disorders; toxic substances in blood; prolonged diarrhea, vomiting, or sweating; severe burns; allergies; infection

Symptoms: Rapid, shallow breathing, clammy skin, low blood pressure (weak pulse), dizziness, unconsciousness, intense thirst

Duration: Acute

Treatments: Emergency resuscitation, medications, surgery

diameter becomes too small, however, then the blood flow through them will decrease. The concept of blood vessels getting narrow and making it more difficult to push blood through is termed resistance to flow or vascular resistance. The balance of blood flow produced by the heart (cardiac output) and vascular resistance keeps blood pressure at the proper level. When one or both of these components falter, cardiac output and blood pressure fall, which, if untreated, leads to shock.

When the cardiovascular system cannot supply blood flow to the essential organs that is adequate to sustain their function, the body is said to be in shock. A reduction in cardiac output is the primary problem in shock. There are two major ways in which cardiac output can decrease enough to cause shock. When the ability of the heart to pump falls to about 40 percent of its normal capacity, it is termed cardiogenic shock. Cardiogenic shock may occur after a heart attack, heart valve disease, lung collapse, and other disorders.

Cardiogenic shock may occur in several ways. The most common cause is a myocardial infarction (heart attack). During a heart attack, the heart is damaged, and like any other muscle when injured, does not have the strength to pump much blood. Thus, cardiac output goes down and a fall in blood pressure will follow. Cardiogenic shock will progress to death if medical treatment is not rapidly obtained. After a myocardial infarction, while the heart is still healing, it has a reduced ability to pump blood. Exercise, even light exercise such as walking, must be resumed gradually. If it is not, the heart may not be able to pump enough blood to supply muscles even though demand for more flow is only slightly increased. This inability to meet the oxygen demand of the heart will cause further damage to the heart.

In cardiac tamponade, a type of obstructive circulatory shock, the stiff but pliable sac surrounding the heart (pericardium) fills with fluid or swells. This takes up room in the sac, squeezing the heart and prohibiting it from filling adequately from beat to beat. Therefore, the amount of blood pumped decreases, and a drop in blood pressure occurs. Cardiac tamponade can occur for several reasons. It can occur rapidly after trauma or heart surgery if the heart is punctured and bleeds into the pericardial sac. Cardiac tamponade occurs much more slowly when excess fluid is produced by the pericardium or when the pericardium becomes swollen. Both of these conditions can be caused by an infection.

A less common form of cardiogenic shock is caused by an extremely high heart rate. Normally, the heart beats at a rate between sixty and one hundred beats per minute. When the heart rate exceeds one hundred, the resulting condition is called tachycardia. Occasionally, in some people, the heart rate can go rapidly up to near two hundred beats per minute. The time between beats becomes so short that the heart does not have enough time to refill and cardiac output falls. If this condition persists, the blood pressure may fall, causing shock. When this occurs, the combination of the rapid heart rate and low blood pressure may cause a myocardial infarction.

Shock caused by a problem in the vascular system, not by a primary decrease in heart function, is generally termed hypovolemic shock. It is characterized by a lack of sufficient blood volume returned to the heart by the vascular system. Hypovolemic shock can be caused by a decrease in the body's total blood volume.

Excessive bleeding (hemorrhage) is the most common form of hypovolemic shock. The blood vessels are elastic in nature, and they must remain filled with blood for arterial pressure to be maintained. In addition, enough blood must be in the veins to push it back to the heart, to be pumped through the lungs and back out into the arteries. When blood loss is slight, the body attempts to compensate by contracting the veins and arteries, thereby maintaining enough pressure and sufficient cardiac output. When enough circulating blood volume is lost, approximately 15 percent to 20 percent, hypovolemic shock occurs.

There are other ways in which blood volume may decrease. When a person is burned severely, plasma (the fluid in which blood cells are suspended) is lost through the burn sites. Enough can be lost to cause hypovolemic shock. Different forms of dehydration can also result in shock. Prolonged diarrhea, vomiting, and sweating can ultimately result in shock if the person does not drink enough liquids to replace fluid lost. All these conditions lead to a loss in the circulating blood volume and subnormal return of blood to the heart, and thus reduced cardiac output.

A virtual loss in blood volume may also occur, resulting in neurogenic shock. Sometimes anesthesia, hypoxia (inadequate oxygen), low blood sugar, spinal cord injuries, or damage to the brain stem can cause the vascular smooth muscle around the arteries and veins to relax. This results in a loss of arterial and venous pressure. Blood tends to accumulate in the veins and is not returned to the heart, and cardiac output falls. A systemic (entire body) allergic reaction can cause a similar response, called anaphylactic shock. Severe infections, usually bacterial, can cause septic shock, which has a death rate of approximately 40 percent. In this type of shock, the immune system of the body responds to the infection. However, this response can cause damage to blood vessels or cause a release of chemicals that cause the vessels to dilate (expand). All types of shock can be deadly if they are not promptly treated.

Applications

In spite of the different causes of circulatory shock, the symptoms are quite common in nearly all cases of shock. The pulse (heart rate) is usually rapid and feeble. Breathing is generally rapid and shallow. The skin is pale, cool, and sometimes moist. The mouth is dry, and thirst is intense. Blood pressure is decreased. Some of these signs are attributable to the body's attempt to alleviate the problem.

The body has several defense mechanisms to help avoid circulatory shock. Several reflex systems function to maintain cardiac output and blood pressure. The body has sensors in the cardiovascular system that tell the brain what the pressure is in the arteries and the veins. When the brain senses a change in either or both of these pressures, it calls on its defenses.

When the arterial pressure sensors tell the brain that blood pressure is falling, the brain produces several responses. Through the nerves, the brain can make the heart beat faster and with greater force. In addition, the nerves can cause vascular smooth muscle to contract, making the vessels squeeze against the blood and increasing pressure. When the smooth muscle contracts, the veins squeeze blood back to the heart to enable it to pump more. The brain can also cause the release of adrenaline into the blood. This hormone can also cause the heart to beat harder and faster. The combined actions of this reflex mechanism attempt to compensate for the decreased cardiac output and blood pressure; however, these responses are only temporary before the person progresses to decompensation and death.

The sensors in the large veins and atria of the heart can cause a different response. Since most (75 percent) of the blood in the body is in the veins at any point in time, a 10 percent to 15 percent decrease in volume triggers the release of a hormone called vasopressin into the blood, which constricts the blood vessels to increase both arterial and venous pressure. The increase in venous pressure squeezes more blood back to the heart to improve cardiac output. The squeeze on the arteries raises blood pressure. Vasopressin also causes the kidneys to retain water. This fluid retained by the kidney is returned to the blood to keep up the vascular volume.

Specialized blood vessels in the kidneys can also initiate a reflex response to a decrease in blood pressure. The kidneys release a hormone called renin into the blood. Renin activates another hormone, angiotensin, which is a powerful constrictor of blood vessels. Angiotensin increases the release of yet another hormone, aldosterone, which helps the kidneys to reabsorb more fluid. All the above reflexes work together to increase blood volume, cardiac output, and blood pressure, in an attempt to alleviate shock. Despite these mechanisms to prevent shock, however, the by-products of these reflexes actually produce negative effects in the body that eventually lead to more damage.

When average arterial blood pressure falls below 60 millimeters of mercury (mmHg), the blood flow to the blood vessels supplying the heart (coronary vessels) cannot be maintained. When this occurs in shock, it happens at a time when the heart needs its critical supply of oxygen. In fact, the heart is trying to beat harder and faster, which increases its need for oxygen. As a result, the heart can weaken. When weakened, it pumps less and thus cannot bring the pressure back to normal. The heart becomes weaker and weaker. This condition is termed cardiac failure. In addition to cardiac failure caused by reduced coronary blood flow, the body can produce a hormone called myocardial depressant factor (MDF). This hormone directly causes a weakening of the heart that is independent of coronary blood flow. MDF also causes the body's bacterial defense system to function poorly. The maintenance of heart function is important to defend against shock.

Because the blood vessels contract in most of the body during shock, blood flow to nonessential tissues such as skin, muscle, bone, and the intestines is reduced, depriving these tissues of oxygen. These tissues can tolerate short periods of low oxygen supply, but if shock persists for more than a few minutes, these tissues revert to other energy sources. The end products of these alternative energy sources are acids, which can begin a process of tissue damage. If this process is not controlled or reversed, tissues can die. If a critical amount of tissue in an organ dies, the organ cannot function and may fail. Acid produced by other tissues gets into the blood and can directly decrease the function of the heart and its ability to respond to beneficial reflex signals. Acid production makes it more difficult for the body to fight shock.

Derangements in blood clotting can occur during shock. Blood clots can form in the early stages of shock, blocking small vessels. This causes a loss of oxygen that results in acid production. Increased acid in the blood can increase the rate of formation of blood clots. Thus, the clotting system can start a vicious cycle that increases the severity of shock.

Even when shock is not bacterial in origin, the body needs its bacteria-fighting systems. During shock, the bacterial defenses are weakened. Normally, bacteria from the intestines constantly enter the blood and are rapidly neutralized. If this does not occur, endotoxic shock can intensify the already existing shock. Therefore, a capable bacteria-fighting system is important in defending against shock.

In shock, the blood vessels of the heart and brain are spared the constriction experienced by all other tissue blood vessels. In fact, arteries in these organs relax to permit as much blood flow as possible, maintaining oxygen supply to these vital organs. Even so, when very low blood pressure persists (less than 50 mmHg), the brain's function decreases. At this point, the brain sends fewer of the beneficial reflex signals to the heart and blood vessels. The final result is a continuous decline in blood pressure and death. Maintenance of brain blood flow is a very important factor in surviving shock.

Treatment and Therapy

Emergency procedures in response to circulatory shock entail contacting emergency service providers such as paramedics and keeping the victim warm and flat on his or her back, with slightly elevated legs. The victim must get medical attention immediately.

Treatment of shock can vary depending on the cause. In many cases, shock can be effectively treated with intravenous

(IV) fluids and medication. Some cases require surgical intervention. In all cases, the status of body fluids must be monitored and treated. The body's blood volume is one of the most important things to maintain.

It is particularly important to optimize blood volume in forms of hypovolemic shock. With hemorrhagic shock, whole blood is given intravenously to replace lost blood. In other forms of hypovolemic shock, different intravenous fluids are usually given. In burn shock, when the blood's plasma weeps from the burn sites, blood plasma is the medicine of choice to restore lost volume. IV fluids are immediately started to restore lost volume until the needed blood products can be acquired. When hypovolemia is caused by excessive diarrhea, vomiting, or sweating, IV fluids are given to replenish lost volume.

In other cases of shock, special drugs are needed to alleviate the symptoms. Shock caused rapidly by a myocardial infarction, with cardiac arrest, can be immediately supported by cardiopulmonary resuscitation (CPR), provided by a trained individual. After resumption of the heartbeat, the heart can be helped with several types of drugs. In the case of sustained tachycardia, a drug such as amiodarone can lower the very rapid heart rate to normal, allowing the heart to fill properly and pump adequate blood. Cardiac tamponade must be corrected to allow the heart to pump usual amounts. If the onset is rapid, as when it is caused by chest trauma, then the fluid in the pericardial sac may need to be removed immediately. A needle is placed into the sac, and the excess fluid is removed to alleviate the pressure around the heart. If fluid accumulates slowly as with an infection and is recognized early, appropriate drug treatment for the infection (antibiotics) may resolve the problem. In cases of shock in which acidosis is a complication or even a potential complication, sodium bicarbonate, a chemical that can reduce the acidity of the blood, may be given. There is no universal treatment for the complex process of shock. For example, hemorrhage may become complicated by heart failure and/or septic shock. Each case must be treated in accordance with the patient's existing conditions.

Perspective and Prospects

Chinese writings of more than three thousand years ago indicate that a connection existed between the heart and the blood. Until the second century, it was thought that arteries carried air, not blood. Through the Middle Ages, it was believed that "spirits" were the essence of life or "vitality." This belief encouraged "bloodletting" as a treatment for many ailments, including shock. Leeches were applied to remove the "evil spirit" causing the sickness. This was not a very successful mode of therapy.

It was not until the seventeenth century that blood transfusions were tried, with the first experiments conducted by Richard Lower. In the 1660s, Jean-Baptiste Denis administered lamb's blood to a sixteen-year-old boy who was very weak and who had a high fever. The condition of the boy, who had been bled several times, improved for a short period of time. Others continued to experiment with transfusion as the remedy for loss of blood, but until the discovery of blood typing at the turn of the twentieth century, most attempts were of limited success.

The practice of giving transfusions greatly increased after the discovery of blood types in 1901 by Karl Landsteiner, who won the 1930 Nobel Prize in Physiology or Medicine for his work. By 1920, blood could be transfused from a bottle, since Luis Agote had discovered that citrated blood would not clot after being removed from the body. Blood banking was established in the 1920s by Russian scientists who discovered that citrated blood could be stored at 40 degrees Fahrenheit.

All types of shock are treated by determining and correcting the underlying cause. Oxygen is given in shock to improve the amount of circulating oxygen to the tissues. In hypovolemic shock, the goal is to improve the amount of circulating volume. This volume is replaced by intravenous fluids until blood products are available. Potent intravenous cardiac drugs that improve the contractions of the heart, improve blood pressure, or cause vasoconstriction may be used in cardiogenic and other types of shock. Mechanical devices have been developed (an intra-aortic balloon pump and a ventricular assist device) to use in severe cardiogenic shock that has not responded to traditional therapy. Synthetic epinephrine (adrenalin) is the first-line treatment for anaphylactic (allergic reaction) shock. It causes the smooth muscle in the bronchioles (tubes into the lungs) to relax and constricts blood vessels. Other treatments may include oxygen, antihistamines and corticosteroids. Septic shock is treated with IV antibiotics and fluids. Shock is a dangerous process that can occur for a variety of reasons. Quick detection and medical treatment are required to prevent negative outcomes.

—J. Timothy O'Neill, Ph.D.;
updated by Amy Webb Bull, D.S.N., A.P.N.

See also Allergies; Bites and stings; Bleeding; Blood and blood disorders; Blood pressure; Blood vessels; Burns and scalds; Cardiac arrest; Cardiopulmonary resuscitation (CPR); Critical care; Critical care, pediatric; Electrical shock; Emergency medicine; First aid; Heart attack; Heart failure; Hemophilia; Hemorrhage; Hypotension; Necrotizing fasciitis; Resuscitation; Septicemia; Transfusion; Unconsciousness; Vascular system.

For Further Information:

American College of Emergency Physicians. *Pocket First Aid*. New York: DK, 2003. An excellent reference guide illustrated with photographs and written in a clear, step-by-step format. Covers many first aid methods, from resuscitation of conscious and unconscious choking victims, to how to deal with bleeding, shock, spinal injuries, poisoning, seizures, fractures, and bandages.

Avraham, Regina. *The Circulatory System*. Philadelphia: Chelsea House, 2000. This text explains the function of the circulatory system in reasonably simple terms. Provides historical development of knowledge about the heart and blood vessels.

Holcomb, Susan Simmons. "Helping Your Patient Conquer Cardiogenic Shock." *Nursing* 32, no. 9 (September, 2002). 32cc1-32cc6. Reference for nurses who work in the intensive care unit.

Klein, Deborah G. "Shock and Sepsis." In *Introduction to Critical Care Nursing*, edited by Mary Lou Sole, Deborah G. Klein, and Marthe J. Moseley. 5th ed. St. Louis, Mo.: Saunders/Elsevier, 2009. A chapter in a critical-care nursing textbook.

Marx, John A., et al., eds. *Rosen's Emergency Medicine: Concepts and Clinical Practice*. 7th ed. Philadelphia: Mosby/Elsevier, 2010. A logical and straightforward presentation of current standards of emergency medicine. Intended to be a reference in busy emergency rooms. The writing is clear and to the point.

Porth, Carol M., and Glenn Matfin. "Heart Failure and Circulatory Shock." In *Essentials of Pathophysiology*, edited by Carol M. Porth. 2d ed. Philadelphia: Lippincott Williams & Wilkins, 2007. A chapter in a textbook on pathophysiology. Offers a detailed explanation of various types of shock.

SHOCK THERAPY

Treatment

Also known as: Electroshock, shock treatment, electroconvulsive therapy (ECT)

Anatomy or system affected: Brain, nerves, nervous system, psychic-emotional system

Specialties and related fields: Neurology, psychiatry

Definition: A psychiatric treatment in which chemical, electrical, or other measures are used to induce a coma, convulsions, or seizure in the brain, altering its chemistry and relieving psychiatric distress.

Key terms:

anesthetic: any of a variety of drugs used to cause a patient to become unconscious and amnesiac for a brief period of time; very short-acting anesthetics, such as methohexital, thiamylal sodium, thiopental sodium, and etomidate, are often used in conjunction with electroconvulsive therapy

convulsion: an instance of high-frequency and amplitude-random electrical activity in the brain; electroconvulsive therapy causes a convulsion in the brain, which is believed to be related to its mechanism of action

electrocardiogram: a recording of the electrical activity of the heart; used during electroconvulsive therapy to monitor changes in heart rate, rhythm, and conduction, any or all of which may be temporarily affected by this procedure

electroencephalogram: a brain wave trace used to monitor the onset, termination, and duration of the convulsion or seizure

mood disorders: any of a number of mental conditions characterized by a primary disturbance of mood as distinct from thinking or behavior

muscle relaxant: any of a number of medications used to paralyze the muscles of the patient temporarily before delivering the electrical stimulus; the main medication used for this purpose is succinylcholine

organic brain syndrome (organicity): changes in memory, orientation, and perception that occur as a side effect of electroconvulsive therapy

psychotic disorder: a psychiatric condition in which an individual's mental state is out of touch with reality, as displayed by abnormal and bizarre perceptions, thoughts, behavior, judgment, and reasoning

seizure: used interchangeably with the term "convulsion"

Indications and Procedures

Shock therapy, also known as shock treatment, is an intervention that has been used for many years to treat severe

SHOCK THERAPY • 2043

psychiatric conditions, such as life-threatening depression and psychotic disorders. Many methods of shock treatment exist, ranging from chemically induced shock (via substances such as insulin) to electrically induced shock (from an electrical current). What all the methods share is the purpose of inducing a temporary loss of consciousness, convulsions, and/or seizure in an effort to disrupt brain activity and reset it to a healthier state.

Insulin shock therapy was developed in 1933 by Manfred Sakel. He found that intramuscular administrations of insulin were able to induce a coma that appeared effective for treating severe cases of schizophrenia. By and large, this approach was replaced with other methods of shock therapy, predominantly electroconvulsive therapy (ECT); however, it is still used today when other methods of shock therapy or intervention are judged to be less appropriate. Modern-day procedures are superior to what was originally done. The impact of the shock on the body is better controlled, and the shock treatment itself is more refined in its application.

Historically shock therapy is equated with ECT. Formerly called electroshock therapy, it is a very powerful treatment for psychiatric conditions such as mood disorders and psychotic disorders. It is based on the idea that electrically induced convulsions change the chemistry of the brain in a way that relieves the symptoms of severe mental illness, in which depression, mania, or both become debilitating.

In most situations, electroconvulsive therapy involves the participation of the psychiatrist providing the treatment and an anesthesiologist, who anesthetizes the patient for the procedure. The patient is instructed to take nothing by mouth for eight hours prior to the treatment, so that the stomach is empty for the induction of general anesthesia. The danger of having food or liquid in the stomach is that it might be aspirated into the lungs, where it could cause pneumonia, respiratory obstruction, or death. An intravenous needle is placed in an arm vein. The patient is then connected to a number of monitors, including a blood pressure cuff, electrocardiogram, and pulse oximeter (to measure the level of tissue oxygenation). The patient is then anesthetized with a short-acting intravenous drug (usually methohexital, also known as Brevital). This is followed by the administration of a short-acting muscle relaxant (usually succinylcholine). Ventilation is controlled by mask, using 100 percent oxygen. As soon as it is determined that the muscles are paralyzed, a mild electrical current is administered to the patient's brain. The duration of the stimulus is two seconds or less. There is a brief contraction of the muscles of the face, followed by a generalized seizure, which is monitored on the electroencephalogram. Small amounts of physical movement may be seen in the face, feet, or hands. These movements are not nearly as severe as those that occurred before the advent of muscle relaxants. The anesthesiologist continues to ventilate the patient until the effects of the muscle relaxant have worn off and spontaneous respiration is reestablished (three to five minutes). There is a period of confusion and disorientation that rapidly follows the treatment; it clears quickly. With each successive treatment, the patient is left with an ongoing loss of memory

which will gradually clear after the course of therapy is finished. The average patient requires between six and twelve treatments. They are administered two or three times per week.

The decision to conduct electroconvulsive therapy usually comes after there has been failure in other forms of treatment, including medication and psychotherapy. Since there are so many medications and combinations of medication that can be used, however, ECT arguably cannot be thought of as a treatment of last resort, as it was in earlier decades. The idea of administering ECT generally arises when it is critical that the patient improve as rapidly as possible. This consideration is often punctuated by frustration on the part of the patient, the family, and/or the psychiatrist with the slowness of response to current therapeutic modalities. In the 1980s, ECT began to be considered earlier rather than later in the course of treatment. It is realistic to say that if one or two medications are not successful, it is unlikely that others will be successful. Yet there are always those cases in which a sudden and complete remission in mood and psychotic disorders occurs without the use of ECT.

Mood and psychotic disorders tend to recur. When treating a patient for the first time, the doctor cannot know whether the effect of ECT will last for a week, months, or years. Some people need only one course of ECT in a lifetime; others will respond well and remain symptom-free for many years, requiring further ECT when symptoms recur. For many patients who develop devastating symptoms with their illnesses, the early initiation of a course of ECT is warranted. Those who have responded well to ECT in the past will forgo medication trials in favor of starting ECT as soon as the symptoms reappear. For those patients who respond well to ECT but who have recurrences within weeks or months, maintenance ECT may be a reasonable option. With this regimen, a single treatment is given every four to twelve weeks in order to prevent a recurrence of psychiatric distress. The actual frequency of treatment is based on each patient's particular clinical course and history. For many patients, maintenance ECT has been a way of preventing multiple and frequent hospitalizations. Very little cognitive impairment is associated with low-frequency maintenance ECT, and patients go on to live very productive lives while being maintained in this way.

The following case is an example of the uses of electroconvulsive therapy in clinical practice: A seventy-five-year-old white, widowed female was referred by her psychiatrist for evaluation for electroconvulsive therapy. She had been well until two years prior to this evaluation. At that time, a month following the death of her husband, she began to experience a variety of symptoms, including loss of appetite with a ten-pound weight loss, decreased interest in her friends and the ordinary activities of life which she had found enjoyable, and sleep disturbance characterized by difficulty falling asleep and early morning awakening. The sleep difficulty was responsive to the use of triazolam, a sleep-inducing drug. Additionally, she began to experience episodes of dizziness that were made worse by antidepressant medications. She was not actively suicidal, but she did experience a wish to die and join her husband, whom she believed was waiting for her. She had been treated with tricyclic antidepressants (nortriptyline and desipramine) with lithium augmentation, but the side effects of constipation and dizziness made these medications intolerable. Her depression did not improve, and she began to exhibit medical signs of dehydration and malnutrition. The treating psychiatrist believed that electroconvulsive therapy was indicated and that it should be instituted as rapidly as possible as a lifesaving measure.

The patient was given a course of seven unilateral ECT treatments over the period of a month. She responded to the treatments with an elevation in her mood, an improvement in sleep and appetite, and increasing engagement with hospital staff and family. When she was discharged from the hospital, she showed evidence of mild memory impairment. In the weeks following her treatment, her memory improved, and she became brighter and resumed her normal activities with vigor. She was started on a small dose of fluoxetine (Prozac), an antidepressant known to have a milder side effect profile than the medications she had taken previously. After one year of follow-up, she was still doing well.

Electroconvulsive therapy continues to be widely practiced in the United States and abroad. There is consensus within the field of psychiatry that it is a valuable tool in the psychiatric armamentarium. Patients, patient advocates, and clinicians alike, however, continue to be concerned about its ethical and appropriate use. Practitioners support efforts of the lay community to ensure the proper and ethical use of ECT as long as it does not obstruct access to the treatment for those who require it.

Uses and Complications

Electroconvulsive therapy is used for a variety of psychiatric conditions, including major depressive disorder, depressed bipolar disorder, manic bipolar disorder, mixed bipolar disorder, schizophrenia, manic excitement, and catatonia. Before starting electroconvulsive therapy, all patients are screened for medical illnesses, for two reasons. First, a variety of medical illnesses are associated with depression or mania; the list is long and includes occult cancer, hypothyroidism, vitamin deficiencies, endocrine abnormalities, and brain tumors or infections, among many others. If there is a treatable cause for depression, it must be found and treated before the decision to perform electroconvulsive therapy is made. Once it is clear that the psychiatric illness is not being caused by something else, ECT may be used. It is important to note that there are certain untreatable medical causes for depression or mania in which the disorder may respond to ECT. For example, depressed patients with Alzheimer's disease may respond to ECT, showing significant improvements in mood. Brain-injured patients with depression may, in some circumstances, respond to electroconvulsive therapy.

The second reason for screening the patient is to establish that it is safe to proceed with ECT. A routine evaluation should include a medical history and physical examination, psychiatric history, mental status examination, blood count, blood chemistries, urinalysis, and electrocardiogram. Other tests may be done if they seem important to rule out other possible illnesses. Such tests might include a computed tomography (CT) scan, a magnetic resonance imaging (MRI) scan, an electroencephalogram (EEG, or brain wave study), or tests for antidepressant drug levels.

There are no absolute reasons not to perform electroconvulsive therapy. There are certain conditions, however, that produce a significant increase in risk with ECT. Cerebral aneurysm may increase the danger of electroconvulsive therapy. An aneurysm is a balloonlike swelling of an artery, which may cause severe brain damage if it bursts. The high blood pressure associated with ECT may cause a cerebral aneurysm to burst. Patients who have recently experienced a heart attack are at increased risk of dying with ECT. Electroconvulsive therapy should be delayed for six months, if possible, following a heart attack. Other illnesses that increase risk include emphysema, multiple sclerosis, and muscular dystrophy.

Despite these risks, electroconvulsive therapy is considered by many to be the safest of the somatic treatments available in psychiatry. The death rate from ECT itself is one patient in ten thousand-much lower, for example, than the death rate for patients taking antidepressant medications; the death rate from suicide in depressed people is much higher. Electroconvulsive therapy may be done safely with patients representing a broad range of age and physical condition. For the elderly, malnourished patient, it is clearly safer and more effective than medication. Prior to the use of muscle relaxants, broken bones and vertebrae were a considerable problem with ECT. This is no longer the case. Complications such as uncontrolled hypertension, stroke, and heart attack rarely occur; they are extremely unlikely, because the patients are medically screened prior to beginning the treatment.

In each situation, the risk of doing ECT must be weighed against the risk of not doing the treatment. If the patient is imminently suicidal-so that he or she cannot be left alone-ECT may be indicated even though the risk is high. Similarly, patients who are starving to death as a result of their illness may require immediate treatment. Patients with manic excitement or delirium, who are completely out of control and require seclusion, may require ECT despite increased risk. For individuals who cannot tolerate or effectively process antidepressant medications, as a result of a compromised liver or other health conditions, ECT may the most effective choice to save their lives.

The most disturbing and severe side effect of ECT is memory loss. It is believed that this side effect is attributable to the electricity that is passed through the brain. The postseizure state may also have some effect. What seems to be clear is that this memory deficit is not the result of physical damage to the brain. Some memories, especially those of events that occur around the time of the treatment, may be permanently lost. Many patients will lose their memory of the periods of most severe depression or mania. The ability to learn new information may be temporarily lost. Most people return to reasonable function within the first month and to complete function after six months.

There are a number of ways to gauge the response of a patient to ECT. It is a complicated process that has to take into account and weigh three factors: the improvement of the mood of the patient, the number of treatments or total seizure seconds, and the amount of confusion and/or memory loss that is produced. Additionally, it is important to gauge the emotional response of the patient and the family to the changes being brought about by the treatment.

With each successive treatment, the patient's mood should get better. If the patient has been depressed, there should be a decrease of the depressive symptoms. Appetite and sleep patterns should improve. There should be an increased level of activity, and social engagement should get better. These changes may first be noticeable to the family and hospital staff. Very often, the improvement becomes apparent to the patient later. Occasionally, the improvement will not be obvious until there has been a chance for the confusion and memory loss to resolve. If the patient is manic, there should be an improvement in symptoms of hyperactivity, grandiosity, irritability, and inability to organize activity and behavior. The response of mania to ECT is often very rapid, and the results may be quite gratifying.

If confusion occurs too early in the course of ECT and it is clear that more treatment needs to be done, decreasing the frequency of treatment from three times a week to once or twice a week may be indicated. Ultimately the decision to stop ECT is based on balancing the above-mentioned factors in an optimal way. This determination is made by the clinician with the input of the patient and all the others (psychiatrist, family, and staff) who know the patient best. If the patient does not seem to be improving and is not having memory difficulty, ECT should be continued. Some patients may need as many as twenty treatments to achieve resolution of psychiatric distress.

Electroconvulsive therapy is the most effective treatment for major mood disorders and for psychotic disorders with a mood component. The likelihood of success depends on the specific diagnosis as well as the accuracy of the diagnostic assessment. Patients who have not responded to adequate trials of medication are less likely to respond to ECT than are those who have not been treated with medication. This would seem to reflect the idea that treatment-resistant psychiatric distress is less likely to respond to any form of treatment.

Perspective and Prospects

Electroconvulsive therapy was discovered as a therapy of mental illness in 1938. It was first used by Ugo Cerletti and Lucio Bini in Italy. The basis of its use was the observation that patients with epilepsy did not suffer from schizophrenia. It was believed that there was something about brain seizures that either prevented or was protective against schizophrenia. While that clinical observation was not accurate, it became the impetus for research into the curative effects of electrically induced seizures.

The first electrical convulsions were induced without the benefit of general anesthesia. Patients had violent seizures and often suffered broken bones and teeth. They were held down in order to keep the seizures from causing excessive physical harm. The responses to ECT in certain patients were quite dramatic. Symptoms such as depression and mania could often be eliminated. Agitated behavior associated with schizophrenia could be mitigated, and patients suffering from catatonia would often become animated as a result of a course of electroconvulsive therapy. The therapy was soon brought to the United States, where it enjoyed frequent use until the early 1950s.

At that time, antipsychotic and antidepressant medications for the treatment of psychiatric illnesses became available. The drugs chlorpromazine and imipramine were shown to be effective in managing the symptoms of schizophrenia and mood disorders. As a result, electroconvulsive therapy was used less frequently and then only in severe, treatment-refractory cases. The political climate of the 1960s and 1970s and films such as *One Flew over the Cuckoo's Nest* (1975) portrayed ECT as a tool of the repressive and oppressing psychiatric establishment to exert behavioral and mind control over an unwitting public. Laws were passed in many jurisdictions making it more difficult for patients to obtain ECT. There were efforts to outlaw ECT. Now, however, even the most powerful patient advocacy groups accept the appropriate use of this treatment.

Electroconvulsive therapy has been utilized with increasing frequency for a number of reasons: recognition of its efficacy, the safety of electroconvulsive therapy in medically ill patients, the increased safety of anesthetic techniques, improved diagnostic criteria, an improved process of informed consent, and disappointing efficacy and side effects of medication in certain patients.

During the 1990s, an alternative stimulatory procedure to the use of ECT as a standard treatment for severe depression was developed. Transcranial magnetic stimulation (TMS) is able to provide a similar adjustment to brain activity without the use of electric current or chemically induced shock. The procedure uses a magnetic coil to deliver a pulse to specified areas of the brain, generally in the region of the prefrontal cortex above the temple. The stimulating coil is held close to the scalp so that the field is focused and can pass through the skull. Rapid-rate TMS can deliver up to fifty stimuli per second. When stimulation is delivered at regular intervals, it is termed repetitive TMS (rTMS). TMS therapy can be used on an outpatient basis, reducing the necessity to hospitalize the patient. Unlike ECT, no side effects such as vomiting, fatigue, or memory loss are typically seen with TMS. The use of TMS is also being studied in connection with movement disorders, epilepsy, bipolar disorders, anxiety disorders, developmental stuttering, Tourette's syndrome, and schizophrenia.

One of the reasons for the renewed interest in ECT is the improvement in informed consent procedures. Physicians no longer adopt as authoritative an attitude toward patients as they did in the past. In the early years of ECT, patients were not informed of all the potential side effects of the treatment. They were often not told that they had alternatives and what the risks and side effects of the alternatives were. The result was that they experienced complications and side effects for which they were not prepared. They became disappointed and angry. Modern informed consent procedures allow the patient to participate as fully as possible in the decision to take any particular form of therapy. The patient is cognizant of the fact that there are choices and alternatives. The patient is also aware that he or she may decide to discontinue treatment at any time if there is no benefit and the side effects are intolerable. Accurate descriptions of side effects and complications are given to the patient. The patient is apprised of the fact that the treatment may fail and that the treatment is being done this time because it is the one that is most likely to help at this juncture. The patient learns that the choice is simply the best choice, not the only one. Both patients and doctors have benefited from such an enlightened approach to informed consent.

—*Frank Guerra, M.D.;*
updated by Nancy A. Piotrowski, Ph.D.

See also Bipolar disorders; Brain; Depression; Emotions: Biomedical causes and effects; Epilepsy; Memory loss; Nervous system; Neurology; Psychiatric disorders; Psychiatry; Psychiatry, child and adolescent; Psychiatry, geriatric; Schizophrenia; Seizures; Sleep disorders.

For Further Information:
Abrams, Richard. *Electroconvulsive Therapy.* 4th ed. New York: Oxford University Press, 2002. A textbook on electroconvulsive therapy that presents a complete picture of all aspects of treatment, from the scientific to the clinical.

American Psychiatric Association. *The Practice of Electroconvulsive Therapy: Recommendations for Treatment, Training, and Privileging.* 2d ed. Washington, D.C.: American Psychiatric Press, 2001. This book is the result of the work of a task force on electroconvulsive therapy in the American Psychiatric Association. It shows how psychiatrists have worked to make the practice of ECT as ethical and safe as possible. Argues for the importance of this form of treatment to psychiatric patients.

Endler, Norman S. *Holiday of Darkness.* Rev. ed. New York: John Wiley & Sons, 1990. This book documents the clinical depression of the author, a psychologist, who responded well to electroconvulsive therapy. A very important work that many patients who are contemplating the possibility of ECT may find comforting and useful.

Endler, Norman S., and Emmanuel Persad. *Electroconvulsive Therapy: The Myths and the Realities.* Toronto, Ont.: Hans Huber, 1988. Another good text on electroconvulsive therapy, written by a psychologist who experienced the treatment for his own depression. He has gone on to become a much-honored and internationally recognized teacher and researcher in the field of psychology.

Fink, Max. *Convulsive Therapy: Theory and Practice.* New York: Raven Press, 1979. This book continues to be an excellent introduction to electroconvulsive therapy by the leading practitioner and researcher in the United States. A classic text.

George, Mark S., and Robert H. Belmaker, eds. *Transcranial Magnetic Stimulation in Neuropsychiatry.* Blackwood, N.J.: American Psychiatric Press, 2000. Compares the effects of transcranial magnetic stimulation (TMS) and ECT in animal models of depression, showing that their similarities may further support the potential role of TMS as an antidepressant treatment.

Kellner, Charles H., et al. *Handbook of ECT.* Washington, D.C.: American Psychiatric Press, 1997. This source describes the procedure, its pros and cons, and how it works and is used in contemporary medicine.

Manning, Martha. *Undercurrents: A Therapist's Reckoning with Depression.* New York: HarperCollins, 1995. A memoir written by a therapist about her experience with depression and shock therapy.

Shunts
Procedure
Anatomy or system affected: Abdomen, brain, circulatory system, gastrointestinal system, head, liver, nervous system

Specialties and related fields: General surgery, neonatology, perinatology, vascular medicine

Definition: Surgically inserted tubes that are used to bypass blocked vessels that normally allow fluid to move from one region of the body to another.

Key terms:

anesthesia: the use of drugs to inhibit pain and alter consciousness

catheter: a tube passed into the body for fluid transport

incision: a cut made with a scalpel

portacaval: referring to a type of shunt used to carry blood from the portal vein to the inferior vena cava, allowing blood to bypass the liver

ventriculoperitoneal: referring to a type of shunt used to carry cerebrospinal fluid from the brain to the abdominal cavity

Indications and Procedures
The surgical placement of shunts is performed to reduce fluid pressures when the vessel that normally carries the fluid is blocked. Two major types of shunts are ventriculoperitoneal and portacaval. Ventriculoperitoneal shunts are used to remove excess fluid from the brain in hydrocephalus. Shunts used to decrease blood pressure in the portal veins are known as portacaval shunts.

Hydrocephalus is a condition characterized by an excessive amount of cerebrospinal fluid in the brain caused either by too much cerebrospinal fluid production or by the blockage of its flow. Hydrocephalus can occur at birth or be caused by head trauma, infection, or brain hemorrhage. If it occurs at birth, the main signs are an enlarged head that continues to grow more rapidly than normal. An infant's skull bones have yet to fuse, and the fluid pressure causes them to expand. The infant may have seizures, vomiting, abnormal reflexes, and other neurological signs. If hydrocephalus occurs in an adult, when the skull bones cannot expand, the pressure on the brain causes headaches, mental deterioration, loss of consciousness, and, if not treated, death.

Physicians use computed tomography (CT) scanning or magnetic resonance imaging (MRI) to find the blockage. The patient is then prepared for surgery to have a shunt inserted to drain the accumulating fluid. After the individual is anesthetized, the head is prepared for the operation. An incision is made through the skin of the head and a hole drilled into the skull, a procedure called craniotomy. A catheter that is part of the ventriculoperitoneal shunt is inserted into the ventricles of the brain and passed under the skin into the abdominal cavity, which is lined by the peritoneum. The peritoneum is a large membrane capable of absorbing the excess cerebrospinal fluid.

Portacaval shunts are used to reduce the blood pressure in the veins carrying blood from the digestive tract to the liver. Patients with abnormally elevated blood pressure in these veins have portal hypertension. This pressure reduces blood flow from the esophagus, stomach, and intestines, which leads to a pooling of blood and an engorgement of these vessels that may lead to their rupturing. Fluid leaking from the portal vein accumulates in the abdominal cavity, a condition known as ascites.

The most common cause of portal hypertension is cirrhosis of the liver, in which the liver is diseased and scar tissue forms. This scar tissue can block blood entering the liver from the portal vein and lead to portal hypertension. Occasionally, a thrombus (blood clot) will form in the portal vein and cause portal hypertension when the liver is not diseased. The patient may have ruptured vessels that bleed into the digestive tract, causing the feces to appear black. If the physician suspects portal hypertension, he or she will perform an ultrasound and arteriography to view the vessels.

A portacaval shunt operation may be necessary to reduce the pressure in the portal vein if other treatments have failed. In this surgical procedure, the patient is anesthetized and prepared for a major abdominal surgery called a laparotomy. An incision is made into the abdominal cavity, and the portal vein is exposed. The surgeon must then carefully place a catheter between the portal vein and another large abdominal vein. The latter vein is the inferior vena cava, which helps return blood to the heart from the lower body and the abdominal cavity. Another surgical option is for the surgeon to connect part of the portal vein to the inferior vena cava directly without the use of a catheter. The portacaval shunt diverts some of the blood that normally goes to the liver directly into the inferior vena cava, thus reducing the pressure within the portal vein.

Uses and Complications

The major problem associated with the ventriculoperitoneal shunt is the fact that it will need to be replaced as the infant grows. It is also possible for this tube to become blocked or infected. If the shunt remains in place for a long period of time, it may spontaneously penetrate an abdominal organ.

Portacaval shunt operations reduce the high blood pressure in the portal vein and help prevent bleeding. Unfortunately, they do not significantly improve liver function in most patients and may even cause further liver damage.

Perspective and Prospects

Early detection and treatment of increased intracranial pressure (pressure on the brain) in hydrocephalus and increased blood pressure in portal hypertension are important to the long-term health and survival of the patient.

Early treatment of hydrocephalus with shunt placement prevents further neurological damage and, if the increase in brain pressure is rapid, may even be necessary to prevent death. Drugs such as acetazolamide that inhibit the formation

of cerebrospinal fluid may, in certain cases, prevent the need for shunt operations. These agents will likely prove most effective in patients with mild disease.

Physicians may try to stop bleeding from ruptured vessels that is caused by portal hypertension by injecting a solution into the veins to seal them (sclerotherapy). Dietary restriction of salt (sodium) and diuretic drugs may be tried to reduce blood pressure, vessel engorgement, and ascites fluid accumulation.

—Matthew Berria, Ph.D.,
and Douglas Reinhart, M.D.

See also Abdomen; Blood vessels; Brain; Brain disorders; Bypass surgery; Catheterization; Cirrhosis; Craniotomy; Fluids and electrolytes; Hydrocephalus; Hypertension; Liver; Liver disorders; Vascular system.

For Further Information:

Brunicardi, F. Charles, et al., eds. *Schwartz's Principles of Surgery.* 9th ed. New York: McGraw-Hill, 2010. A standard textbook on the topic. Intended for practicing surgeons, but valuable to general readers for its details.

Leikin, Jerrold B., and Martin S. Lipsky, eds. *American Medical Association Complete Medical Encyclopedia.* New York: Random House Reference, 2003. A concise presentation of numerous medical terms and illnesses. A good general reference.

Parker, James N., and Philip M. Parker, eds. *The Official Parent's Sourcebook on Hydrocephalus.* San Diego, Calif.: Icon Health, 2002. Guides patients in using the Web to educate themselves about hydrocephalus and draws from public, academic, government, and peer-reviewed research to provide comprehensive information on a range of topics related to the condition.

Toporek, Chuck, and Kellie Robinson. *Hydrocephalus: A Guide for Patients, Families, and Friends.* Sebastopol, Calif.: O'Reilly, 1999. Covers a range of topics related to the condition, including detailed discussion of shunt revision surgery.

SICKLE CELL DISEASE
Disease/Disorder

Anatomy or system affected: Blood, cells, kidneys, lungs, spleen

Specialties and related fields: Genetics, hematology

Definition: Genetic disorders of the hemoglobin molecule.

Key terms:

anemia: the pathologic state of decreased concentration of hemoglobin

aplastic crisis: a sudden decrease in the bone marrow release of red blood cells, associated with very severe anemia

hemoglobin: the substance within red blood cells that transports oxygen and carbon dioxide

infarction: death in a tissue or organ caused by the obstruction of blood flow

Causes and Symptoms

Sickle cell disease is a genetic disorder of hemoglobin, which gives the red color to blood. The hemoglobin molecule is made up of two pairs of globin polypeptide chains (two α chains and two β chains) and four heme molecules containing iron. Normal hemoglobin (hemoglobin A) is a remarkable protein that changes the biophysical configuration of its amino acid chains so that it can deliver oxygen safely to the tissues without oxidizing iron. Oxygen removal occurs during each cycle of blood flow from the lungs to the tissues. Sickle hemoglobin has a single amino acid substitution of valine for glutamic acid at the sixth position from the end of the β chain. Sickle hemoglobin has the unfortunate propensity to condense as rods in red blood cells when the oxygen is removed during the normal circulation of the blood. These rods distort the cells, making them stiff and rigid and unable to transverse the smaller blood vessels rapidly. The result is vasocclusion (obstruction) of the small and medium-sized blood vessels, damaging the endothelial inner lining of the blood vessel and thereby resulting in tissue necrosis (ischemia).

The most common genotypes of sickle cell disease are sickle cell anemia-homozygous sickle cell disease (SS disease), sickle cell hemoglobin C disease (SC disease), sickle cell $β^0$ thalassemia ($Sβ^0$ thalassemia), and sickle cell $β^+$ thalassemia ($Sβ^+$ thalassemia). Less common genotypes include sickle cell hemoglobin E disease (SE disease), sickle cell hemoglobin D Los Angeles (SD Los Angeles), and sickle cell hemoglobin O Arab (SO Arab). In addition to these conditions, more than four hundred other abnormal human hemoglobins can combine with sickle hemoglobin. This genetic heterogeneity accounts for the wide spectrum of clinical severity in patients with sickle cell disease, with some forms essentially asymptomatic, such as Hβ SE or S deer lodge.

Sickle cell anemia (SS disease) is the most common and the most severe form of sickle cell disease. It results from the inheritance of the sickle cell gene from both parents. Its hallmark clinical manifestations are anemia and severe episodes of pain; similar but less frequent manifestations are seen with other forms of sickle cell disease. In sickle cell anemia, anemia is caused by the rapid destruction of the red blood cells as they circulate because of a shortened peripheral survival time of less than 30 days (normal is 120 days).

Acute painful episodes-particularly in the older child, adolescent, or adult-are characteristic of sickle cell anemia. Sickle cell crisis often begins with pain in the abdomen or extremities and joints. Painful sickle crisis in the young child is usually precipitated by an acute fever, with excruciatingly tender swelling of the hands and feet (dactylitis) caused by small infarctions of the small growing bones of the hands and feet. Approximately 25 percent of SS patients have endless and repeated painful episodes throughout life requiring frequent hospital care.

The clinical course of sickle cell anemia involves intermittent episodes of acute painful illnesses interspersed with periods of clinical quiescence and relative well-being. Commonly occurring acute complications necessitating intensive medical care are septicemia and meningitis during childhood, recurrent sickle cell pain crises, cerebral infarction with stroke, acute chest syndrome (often termed pneumonia), severe upper respiratory tract infections, gallbladder disease with gallstones, aplastic crisis, hypersplenism with splenic sequestration crisis, bone infarctions, priapism (a painful erection of the penis not associated with sexual desire), and pyelonephritis (infection of the kidney).

Information on Sickle Cell Disease

Causes: Genetic disorder
Symptoms: Severe anemia, episodes of acute pain; complications may include septicemia, meningitis, pneumonia, severe upper respiratory tract infections, bone infarctions, kidney infections
Duration: Chronic with acute recurrent episodes
Treatments: Prophylactic antibiotics, hospitalization, analgesics

---

An increased incidence of invasive infections caused by the bacteria *Streptococcus pneumoniae* is found in children with SS disease who are between the ages of four months and five years; this is thirty to one hundred times that which would be expected in a healthy population of the same race and age. Blood infections in SS infants and young children are associated with a rapid elevation of temperature, often to 104 degrees Fahrenheit, and the patient becomes even more anemic. In the untreated patient, death occurs within eight to twelve hours.

Chronic major organ failure in SS disease is the direct consequence of irreversible and ongoing damage to the endothelial lining of the small blood vessels as a result of sickle cells (sickle vasculopathy). Vascular damage begins years before the overt clinical symptoms are apparent. The spleen is the first organ to be destroyed, usually by five years of age. During childhood (three to ten years of age), 10 percent of children with this disease will have strokes, with resulting severe brain damage. Strokes cause paralysis and weakness of the extremities and difficulties in learning. This devastating complication in young children often makes functioning in school or living as self-sustaining adults difficult. Brain infarction can be accurately identified using computed tomography (CT) brain scans, magnetic resonance imaging (MRI), positron emission tomography (PET), and other diagnostic procedures. Sickle vasculopathy eventually culminates in young adulthood as end-stage kidney failure (glomerulosclerosis), sickle chronic restrictive lung disease, intracranial hemorrhages and brain damage, retinopathy with blindness, disabling leg ulcers, and painful generalized osteonecrosis of many of the bones of the body. Specialized medical care is required for the diagnosis and management of these permanent incurable complications.

Treatment and Therapy

Most acute complications of SS disease can be treated successfully so that the patient can attend school, be involved in social activities, and have a pleasant childhood and adolescence. Intensive care units with sophisticated monitoring equipment that are dedicated to infants and young children can manage and maintain the vital function of patients during severe illness episodes.

The institution of appropriate immunization programs for children with sickle cell anemia has substantially decreased their mortality and morbidity throughout the world. The importance of preventing the usual childhood infectious diseases such as hepatitis, whooping cough (pertussis), red measles (rubeola), rubella (German measles), diphtheria, tetanus, mumps, poliomyelitis, and *Hemophilus influenzae* septicemia allows 90 percent of these children to reach adulthood. The use of prophylactic antibiotics such as penicillin during young childhood (four months to five years) decreases the incidence of invasive pneumococcal blood infections. However, a recent ominous increase has been seen in penicillin resistance to pneumococcal serotype-specific strains, making prophylactic antibiotic prevention less effective. Salmonella contamination of chicken is still a major source of septicemia and salmonella osteomyelitis (bone infection).

Over time, children with sickle cell disease and their families begin to recognize the things that may precipitate a painful sickle cell crisis. Severe episodes require hospitalization and analgesic treatment, often with narcotic agents in addition to intravenous fluids.

Perspective and Prospects

Sickle cell anemia is the prototypical molecular disease. The causative gene modifying the chemical structure of the hemoglobin β chain ($β^A$ to $β^S$)—replacing the amino acid glutamic acid with valine—originated in Africa. The disorder was transmitted to the United States, Arabia, Europe, and South and Central America as part of the slave trade. At that time, healthy persons carrying the sickle gene, who are said to have sickle cell trait, survived the rigors of a slave ship. As persons carrying the sickle cell trait migrated throughout the North and South American continents and Europe, genetic drift occurred, accounting for the 15 percent of patients with the various forms of sickle cell disease who are not phenotypically African in appearance.

Improvements in acute medical care during childhood and in the social and environmental situation for patients, as factors taken together, have made it possible for most children with sickle cell anemia and other forms of sickle cell disease to survive childhood. In the United States, Great Britain, and most European countries, umbilical cord blood diagnosis or peripheral blood sampling of newborns can diagnose the disorder at birth. This allows the children to be provided with responsive knowledgeable medical care and complete immunizations early in life.

The current focus of clinical investigations is prevention of the tissue destruction induced by the repeated endothelial damage caused when sickle cells obstruct blood vessels. Such prevention requires lifelong medical treatment. Drugs that can modify the rate of hemoglobin polymerization (precipitation) in the red blood cells include hydroxyurea, cytosine arabinoside, 5-azosididine, and other agents that increase the amount of fetal hemoglobin in red blood cells. By increasing the fetal hemoglobin, the rate of polymerization of hemoglobin S is modified so that there is less propensity for insoluble rods to be formed. The membranes of red blood cells become more flexible, allowing the cells to traverse the microvasculature and thereby decreasing the damage to blood vessels. Adhesion molecules (such as VCAM-1) act to provide the glue that binds the damaged sickle cell to the in-

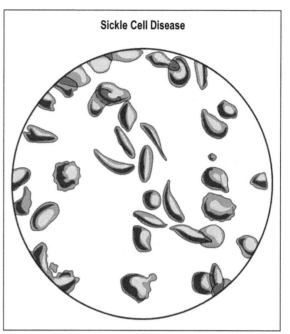

Sickle Cell Disease

The red blood cells are sickle-shaped rather than round, which causes blockage of capillaries.

ner lining of the blood vessel, inducing permanent endothelial damage. Intensive search is underway to identify blocking agents for these adhesion molecules that can prevent the blood vessel occlusion.

Bone marrow transplantation with normal bone marrow (normal red blood cell precursors) from a donor with identical human leukocyte antigens (HLAs) is the only cure now available for sickle cell anemia. Bone marrow transplantation is limited by the paucity of HLA-compatible sibling donors who do not have sickle cell anemia.

Gene therapy holds the promise of a cure but has not been successfully developed for use in patients with sickle cell anemia. The advantage of gene therapy is that no HLA-compatible donor is required.

—*Darleen Powars, M.D.*

See also African American health; Anemia; Blood and blood disorders; Bone marrow transplantation; Fatigue; Genetic diseases; Hematology; Hematology, pediatric; Pain management; Thalassemia.

For Further Information:

Ballas, S. K. "Sickle Cell Anaemia: Progress in Pathogenesis and Treatment." *Drugs* 62 (2002): 1143-1172. A clearly presented review of sickle cell anemia, with available treatment options described.

Edelstein, Stuart J. *The Sickled Cell: From Myths to Molecules.* Cambridge, Mass.: Harvard University Press, 1986. A historical description of ancient African cultural beliefs and how they correlated to the modern molecular understanding of sickle hemoglobinopathies.

Embury, Stephen H., Robert P. Hebbel, Narla Mohandas, and Martin H. Steinberg, eds. *Sickle Cell Disease: Basic Principles and Clinical Practice.* New York: Raven Press, 1994. Chapters 26, 30, 35,

38, and 40 offer an in-depth description of the molecular and bio-chemical nature of sickle hemoglobin and clinical correlations.

O'Malley, Paul D., ed. *New Developments in Sickle Cell Disease Research*. New York: Nova Science, 2006. Covers a range of topics, from psychobiological reactivity to acute chest syndrome.

Pauling, Linus, H. Itano, S. J. Singer, and I. C. Wells. "Sickle Cell Anemia: A Molecular Disease." *Science* 110 (1949): 543-548. The discovery of the electrophoretic mobility of sickle Hb S as compared to normal Hb A defines the first molecular disease to be identified.

Powars, Darleen R. "Management of Cerebral Vasculopathy in Children with Sickle Cell Anaemia." *British Journal of Haematology* 108 (2000): 666-678. Explains that brain infarction (stroke) is the most devastating complication of sickle cell anemia.

Serjeant, Graham R., and Beryl E. Serjeant. *Sickle Cell Disease*. 3d ed. New York: Oxford University Press, 2001. Offers clinical observations of sickle cell disease based on long-term studies in Jamaica.

SIDS. *See* SUDDEN INFANT DEATH SYNDROME (SIDS).

SIGNS AND SYMPTOMS
Procedure
Anatomy or system affected: All
Specialties and related fields: All
Definition: Characteristics of a disease state perceived either by the affected individual (symptom) or by someone other than the affected individual (sign).
Key terms:
asymptomatic disease: a disease that has no obvious symptoms
diagnosis: the act of identifying a specific disease using signs and symptoms as evidence
prognosis: the predicted outcome of a disease
symptomatic disease: a disease or disorder that displays overt symptoms

Introduction

It is common practice to use the words "sign" and "symptom" interchangeably. There is, however, a subtle difference between the two terms; it concerns who is making the observation. Symptoms are subjective qualities that indicate an abnormality or disease. In other words, they are perceived by the affected individual. Examples of symptoms that a patient may describe are an itchy sensation in the skin, headache, joint pain, or nausea.

Signs are objective. They can be noticed by persons other than the affected individual, such as physicians, nurses, and relatives. Examples of outward signs of disease include hyperactivity in a child, forgetfulness in an elderly person, fever, rash, a swollen ankle, or vomiting. Sometimes, signs may not be immediately apparent and further testing may be necessary in order to reveal them. For example, a physician or nurse may check a patient's blood pressure, blood may be drawn for analysis, or a colonoscopy may be ordered.

Health care professionals use a combination of the signs that they observe and the symptoms described by the patient in order to determine the presence of a particular disorder. This process is called diagnosis. Once a diagnosis has been made, an appropriate course of treatment is evaluated.

Types of Signs and Symptoms

Signs and symptoms come in many different guises, and the way in which they present themselves gives health care professionals further clues as to the nature of the disorder-not only which disease is present but also how severe it is.

Blood pressure, pulse rate, body temperature, and breathing rate are known as vital signs. They are used as standard markers when monitoring an individual's state of health.

A sign or symptom is described as chronic if it is present for an extended period of time. For example, a chronic cough may be indicative of asthma, or a response to an environmental allergen. If a sign or symptom lessens in intensity or disappears, then it is a remitting symptom; conversely, if it worsens or reappears after a period of abatement, then it is relapsing. Some conditions are characterized by these types of signs. Relapsing-remitting multiple sclerosis is an example. In the relapse stage of this disease, the body's immune system attacks the sheath of myelin that surrounds nerves in the central nervous system. When the immune response has calmed down, special cells in the central nervous system, called glia, repair the myelin; the remission period is entered.

The presenting symptom is the symptom that first prompts the affected individual to consult a health care professional. If a symptom is general, involving the whole body-such as fatigue, weight loss, or fever-then it is called a constitutional symptom.

A condition that manifests in a tangible way is said to be a symptomatic disease or disorder. An asymptomatic condition, however, can be present without the affected individual being aware of it. Sometimes, routine screening methods such as a mammogram or prostate examination expose the presence of asymptomatic conditions before they become symptomatic, thereby increasing the chance for successful treatment. An asymptomatic infection is an infection by viruses or bacteria that does not result in obvious signs or symptoms. Often, sexually transmitted infections are asymptomatic: Examples include infection by the *Chlamydia trachomatis* bacterium (chlamydia) or the human papillomavirus (HPV). Some infections are asymptomatic while the bacteria or virus is incubating, which is the period of time between exposure to the infectious agent and the onset of symptoms. For example, the incubation period of the seasonal influenza virus is one to four days. Asymptomatic infections can be problematic because it is possible for the affected individual to transmit them to other people unknowingly.

Diseases can have primary and secondary symptoms. Alzheimer's disease is characterized primarily by symptoms such as memory loss and difficulty with concentration. As a result of the burden caused by these primary symptoms, an affected individual may develop depression. In the case of Alzheimer's disease, depression is a secondary symptom.

Prognostic signs or symptoms are those that give clues

about the future course of the disease. The predicted outcome of the disease is called the prognosis. An example of a disease with an extremely poor prognosis is pancreatic cancer. Pancreatic cancer is rarely diagnosed in its early stages due to lack of symptoms; the chance of successful treatment becomes very low as the disease progresses. Less than 5 percent of pancreatic cancer patients survive for more than five years after diagnosis.

When an addictive substance is abruptly denied to an addicted body, withdrawal symptoms usually become apparent. In alcoholism, these symptoms range from headaches, nausea, and weakness to convulsions and delirium tremens (confusion and visual hallucination). Each addictive substance has a characteristic set of withdrawal symptoms.

Eponymous signs are named after the person who first described them. For example, Braxton Hicks' contractions (sometimes known as Hicks' sign), prelabor contractions occurring during pregnancy, were first described by John Braxton Hicks.

Perspective and Prospects

Many years ago, physicians could use only their limited powers of observation, along with patients' description of their symptoms, to make a diagnosis. The development of progressively sophisticated equipment and new methods for clinical testing has made the diagnostic procedure faster and more accurate. As a consequence, treatment is becoming increasingly effective.

A vast amount of medical information is now available to the layperson. Online discussion groups and "symptom checker" Web sites encourage the practice of self-diagnosis. In fact, the act of researching a disease using the Internet as a resource, and subsequently worrying that one is suffering from symptoms of that particular disease, is termed cyberchondria.

—Claire L. Standen, Ph.D.

See also Allied health; Alternative medicine; Biopsy; Blood pressure; Blood testing; Cancer; Cardiac rehabilitation; Death and dying; Diagnosis; Disease; Hospice; Imaging and radiology; Invasive tests; Laboratory tests; Noninvasive tests; Physical examination; Physical rehabiliation; Prognosis; Pulse rate; Screening; Syndrome.

For Further Information:

Kahan, Scott, Redona Miller, and Ellen Smith. *In a Page-Signs and Symptoms*. 2d ed. Philadelphia: Lippincott Williams & Wilkins, 2008.

Springhouse, ed. *Handbook of Signs and Symptoms*. 4th ed. Philadelphia: Lippincott Williams & Wilkins, 2009.

Tierney, Lawrence, and Mark Henderson. *The Patient History: Evidence-Based Approach*. New York: McGraw-Hill Medical, 2004.

Single photon emission computed tomography (SPECT)

Procedure

Also known as: Single photon emission tomography (SPET)

Anatomy or system affected: Blood, blood vessels, brain, circulatory system, head, heart

Specialties and related fields: Cardiology, nuclear medicine, psychiatry, pulmonary medicine, radiology

Definition: A nuclear imaging test used to provide three-dimensional information about the flow of blood through arteries and veins in order to diagnose a wide range of health conditions, including strokes, epilepsy, dementia, and tumors.

Key terms:

gamma rays: electromagnetic radiation emitted during radioactive decay with short wavelengths

ischemia: reduced blood flow

myocardial perfusion imaging (MPI): a type of cardiac stress test

neurotransmitter: a chemical that communicates nerve impulses from one nerve cell to another

photons: particles that travel at the speed of light

tracer: a substance that is injected into the body and releases energy which allows it to be followed along its path through the circulatory system and metabolism pathways

Indications and Procedures

Single photon emission computed tomography (SPECT) uses the radioisotopes xenon 133, technetium 99, and iodine 123 to acquire information about blood flow. A small amount of radioisotope is injected into a patient's vein to observe the flow of blood and metabolic pathways during the digestion of food. These radioisotopes are the radioactive forms of the naturally occurring elements of xenon, technetium, and iodine. These forms are referred to as radioactive because they emit gamma rays. These gamma rays can be measured directly by using a gamma ray detector containing a series of crystals that convert the gamma rays to photons of light.

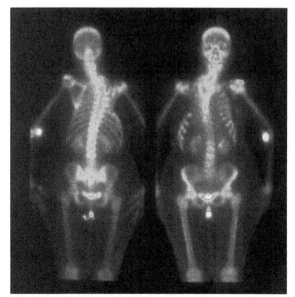

SPECT scan showing scoliosis, a curvature of the spine. (Oullette/ Theroux/Publiphoto/Photo Researchers, Inc.)

In the News:
Use of SPECT to Detect Pulmonary Embolism

Single photon emission computed tomography (SPECT) has been shown by researchers to be useful in the diagnosis of pulmonary embolism. According to the study titled "Detection of Pulmonary Embolism with Combined Ventilation-Perfusion SPECT and Low-Dose CT: Head-to-Head Comparison with Multidetector CT Angiography," SPECT plus low-dose CT had a sensitivity of 97 percent and specificity of 100 percent. This diagnostic effectiveness was much greater than that of the multidetector CT angiography alone, which had a sensitivity of 68 percent and specificity of 100 percent.

Pulmonary embolism is a blockage in an artery in the lung caused by a blood clot. Diagnosis can be problematic because a seemingly healthy individual can develop this condition quickly, often with no symptoms. Furthermore, the mortality rate is estimated to be a relatively high 30 percent.

The article published by researchers in Denmark in the December, 2009, issue of *The Journal of Nuclear Medicine* is one of several recent articles describing additional applications of SPECT to diagnose these types of blood flow abnormalities as well as coronary heart disease and even to diagnose brain damage and cancer. Researchers in Houston, Texas, have found that the combination of using SPECT along with the coronary artery calcium score (CACS) is more effective in diagnosing coronary heart disease than either method alone. These results were published in the November 10, 2009, issue of the *Journal of the American College of Cardiology*. ReGen Therapeutics has also reported that SPECT has shown the effectiveness of their drug zolpidem for treating brain damage.

—*Jeanne L. Kuhler, Ph.D.*

Photomultiplier tubes amplify the photons into electrical signals, which are then converted by a computer into detailed three-dimensional visual images on a screen.

SPECT is one of several nuclear imaging techniques used in medicine for diagnosis. Imaging is important as a noninvasive method of seeing inside the body, without requiring surgery. Other common techniques include X rays, magnetic resonance imaging (MRI) scans, computed tomography (CT) scans, and ultrasound. The other nuclear imaging techniques include cardiovascular imaging, bone scanning, and positron emission tomography (PET). All these techniques assist in the detection of inadequate blood flow to tissues, aneurysms (weak locations in the walls of blood vessels), various blood cell disorders, and tumors.

Of these techniques, SPECT is the most similar to PET, but SPECT is less expensive and more readily available. SPECT radioisotopes emit single gamma rays with longer decay times than in PET, and thus have the disadvantage of producing less detailed images than PET.

Tomography refers to the technique of using rotating X rays to record an image within the body. With today's computers, the terminology of computed tomography (CT) is used. The imaging process of SPECT combines CT with the use of radioisotopes. These radioisotopes are often referred to

as tracers because they allow physicians to follow the pathway traveled by the blood through the body. Tracers emit gamma rays that are collected by a computer, which then translates the data into two-dimensional cross sections that are added together to form a three-dimensional image. These radioactive tracers decay within minutes to hours and are eliminated in the urine, thus posing negligible harm to the body.

Uses and Complications

The sharp images that can be obtained using SPECT enable it to be a useful diagnostic tool for a variety of cardiovascular, cerebrovascular, and neurological disorders. SPECT is more sensitive than an electrocardiogram (ECG) for detecting ischemia. In order to diagnose ischemic heart disease, SPECT scanning enhances myocardial perfusion imaging (MPI) after a patient exerts stress in order to compare images from before and after stress to assess blood flow. SPECT has become an extensively used tool to diagnose coronary artery disease (CAD). Because it is such a useful tool for detecting reduced blood flow, SPECT has also been widely used to detect tumors. For example, as part of the diagnosis of patients suspected of having aneurysms or tumors at the base of the skull, the internal carotid artery temporary balloon occlusion (TBO) test is enhanced by the use of SPECT to evaluate the cerebral blood flow. SPECT is also used to detect lymphoma tumors in the chest and abdomen, neuroendocrine tumors, stress fractures and stress reactions in the spine (known as spondylolysis), and liver lesions.

The high resolution of SPECT allows it to be a very useful tool for obtaining images of the striatum, a specific area of the brain containing the neurotransmitter dopamine. This dopamine activity can be monitored to help diagnose schizophrenia and various mood and movement disorders, including epilepsy, Alzheimer's disease, dementia, and obsessive-compulsive disorder.

Perspective and Prospects

Although a SPECT scan exposes the body to less radiation than does a CT scan or a chest X ray, pregnant or nursing women should not receive a SPECT scan. A nuclear medicine technologist will inject a patient with a small amount of radioactive tracer. After enough time is allowed for the tracer to travel to the brain (usually ten to twenty minutes), a special camera called a gamma camera is used to acquire multiple images from multiple angles by rotating around the head. This gamma camera detects the gamma radiation emitted by the radioactive tracers. Thus, the patient needs to remain motionless during the scanning process so that clear images can be obtained. After the scanning process is finished, it is important for the patient to drink fluids to remove the radioactive tracers from the body.

—*Jeanne L. Kuhler, Ph.D.*

See also Angiography; Angioplasty; Computed tomography (CT) scanning; Echocardiography; Imaging and radiology; Magnetic resonance imaging (MRI); Mammography; Neuroimaging; Noninvasive tests; Nuclear medicine; Nuclear radiology; Positron emission tomography (PET) scanning; Radiation sickness; Radiation therapy; Radiopharmaceuticals; Ultrasonography.

For Further Information:

American Academy of Neurology, Therapeutics, and Technology Assessment Subcommittee. *Assessment: Brain SPECT*. Minneapolis: American Academy of Neurology, 1995.

Frankle, W. G., et al. "Neuroreceptor Imaging in Psychiatry: Theory and Applications." *International Review of Neurobiology* 67 (2005): 385-440.

Masdeu, J. C., et al. "Special Review: Brain Single Photon Emission Tomography." *Neurology* 44 (October, 1994): 1970-1977.

Van Heertum, R. "Single Photon Emission, CT, and Positron Emission Tomography in the Evaluation of Neurologic Disease." *Radiologic Clinics of North America* 39 (May, 2001).

SINUSITIS
Disease/Disorder

Anatomy or system affected: Nose, respiratory system

Specialties and related fields: Family medicine, internal medicine, otorhinolaryngology

Definition: Irritation and swelling of the sinuses.

Key terms:

deviated septum: a condition that causes a shift of the bones and cartilage from the middle of the nose to either side, making one side of the nasal passages much smaller than the other

nasal polyps: noncancerous growths inside the nose; usually associated with allergies or asthma, which can block the sinus drainage tract

orbit: the bones and other tissues that surround the eye, commonly known as the eye socket

Causes and Symptoms

The sinuses are airspaces in the skull that exist in the forehead just above the eyes, on either side of the nose below the eyes, and in the area just above the nose and in between the eyes. The sinuses are lined with mucus and tiny hairs, called cilia, which trap inhaled particles and bacteria and move them back out through the nose. This action serves as a natural defense system to eliminate these potential irritants that are inhaled during normal breathing. The tracts through which the sinuses drain are relatively small and easily blocked by swelling of the area. This blockage can impair drainage and cause the buildup of normal sinus secretions.

The term "sinusitis" refers to irritation or swelling of the sinuses and their membranes. Typical symptoms may include a feeling of congestion or pressure in the nose or face and runny nose with secretions that may vary in color from clear to yellowish green to bloody. The facial pressure is often worse when bending forward.

Most often, sinusitis is precipitated by the common cold. Another frequent cause is allergies, with typical symptoms of sneezing, runny nose, and itchy, watery eyes. An allergic patient who is sensitive to a particular airborne substance (pollen, ragweed, dust, animal dander) has a particularly vigorous response when these particles land in the nose and enter the sinuses. An increased production of mucus and the body's natural immune defenses combine to produce thick and copious nasal secretions that can fill the sinuses in an attempt to eliminate the offending agent.

Another factor that may predispose a patient to sinusitis is environmental exposure to smoke or air pollution, which are natural irritants to the sinuses. Problems that cause a blockage of the sinus drainage system by things such as nasal polyps, a deviated septum, or pregnancy (which leads to swelling of

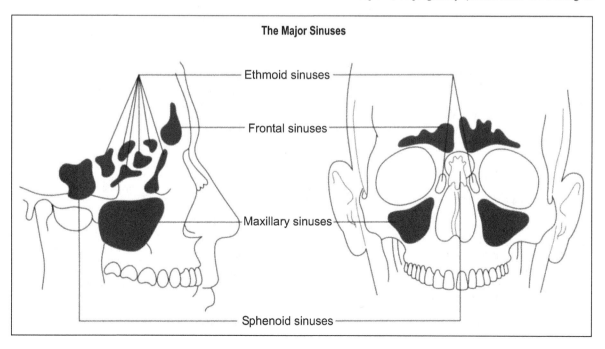

The Major Sinuses

Ethmoid sinuses

Frontal sinuses

Maxillary sinuses

Sphenoid sinuses

Information on Sinusitis

Causes: Common cold; allergies; environmental exposure to smoke or air pollution; blockage from nasal polyps, deviated septum, or pregnancy

Symptoms: Irritation or swelling of sinuses, congestion or pressure in nose or face, runny nose with secretions varying from clear to yellowish green to bloody, decreased sense of smell, productive cough, fever, tooth pain, bad breath

Duration: Acute

Treatments: Increased fluid intake, antihistamines, anti-inflammatory drugs, decongestants, humidified air, nasal irrigation, oral or nasal allergy medications, antibiotics if needed

---

the nasal membranes as a result of hormonal changes) can interfere with mucus drainage from the sinuses. Finally, other genetic diseases such as cystic fibrosis or disorders of the immune system can predispose patients to sinusitis.

Although most cases of sinusitis are caused by viruses or allergies, these can often lead to infection by bacteria if they do not resolve promptly. Bacterial sinusitis requires treatment with antibiotics to avoid the rare but serious complications of infection of the orbit or infection of the brain and its surrounding tissues.

The distinction between bacterial and other causes of sinusitis is most accurately based on the patient's symptoms and a physical examination. A patient is more likely to have bacterial sinusitis if two or three of the following symptoms are present for at least seven days: facial pressure, nasal congestion, discolored nasal mucus, decreased sense of smell, productive or "wet" cough, fever, tooth pain on the upper jaw, or bad breath.

Sinus X rays, done frequently in the past, are not considered a reliable diagnostic test for sinusitis. Though sinus computed tomography (CT) scans allow intricate visualization of sinus anatomy, they do not reliably distinguish bacterial sinusitis from other forms and are useful only in cases of long-standing, refractory symptoms for which sinus surgery is being considered.

Treatment and Therapy

The initial treatment of sinusitis involves extra fluids, anti-inflammatory drugs such as ibuprofen, antihistamines, short-term use of nasal decongestant sprays (no longer than three days), and oral decongestants such as pseudoephedrine. Humidified air (for example, steam from a hot shower) and nasal irrigation with water or saline can offer short-term symptom relief.

If allergies are the cause of sinusitis, then oral or nasal allergy medications are appropriate. Examples are nonprescription antihistamines such as chlorpheniramine or diphenhydramine; they can cause drowsiness in some patients. Loratadine and other related, newer generation antihistamines are also available over the counter. They offer once-daily dosing and are significantly less sedating. Other nasal sprays such as topical steroids are available by prescription and offer significant relief.

If symptoms persist longer than seven to fourteen days, then antibiotic therapy may be necessary and evaluation by a health care provider is warranted. Many different types of antibiotics are effective for sinusitis, and prescription practices vary. Initial treatment is typically for two weeks.

Perspective and Prospects

Prior to the antibiotic era, the treatment of sinusitis involved drainage of the sinuses by extracting a tooth, puncturing the roof of the mouth, or entering the nose and creating a drainage tract through which secretions could be removed and the sinuses could be irrigated with fluid for cleansing. Given the invasiveness of these procedures, they have become uncommon with the development of effective antibiotic therapy.

The development of tiny, high-resolution cameras known as endoscopes in the 1950s created a revolution in the understanding of sinus disease. Direct visualization of the nasal passages and sinus drainage tracts allowed a better understanding of the sinus anatomy and thus led to the use of this equipment to facilitate surgical treatment.

Occasionally, patients with recurrent symptoms require surgical removal of infected sinus tissue and enlargement of

---

In the News: Balloon Sinuplasty

In late 2005, the Acclarent Company received permission from the Food and Drug Administration (FDA) to market a device to clear blocked sinuses similar to that used to clear blocked arteries in the heart. A flexible catheter tube inserted into the nostril guides a balloon into the targeted sinus. The balloon is inflated, spreading the bones of the passageway sufficiently to permit accumulated mucus or pus to drain. A minimally invasive outpatient procedure, balloon sinuplasty is performed under local anesthesia and takes one to two hours. Patients report little or no pain and can often return to normal activity within twenty-four hours. The sinuplasty devices cost from $1,200 to $1,500 and are not reusable. Total costs for the procedure run $4,000 to $6,800; the procedure is covered by some private insurance plans.

The procedure cannot be used if nasal polyps need to be removed. Nevertheless, it provides a possible alternative for sinusitis sufferers who do not need, or prefer not to undergo, surgical procedures involving cutting away bone or other tissue to open the blocked sinus. Surgeons using the devices praised them. The American Rhinologic Society was more cautious in its October, 2006, position statement, asserting that the technology had limited indication at the time. In November, 2006, the California Blue Cross labeled the procedure investigational and not medically necessary, noting that since the FDA's clearance was based on the devices' comparability to already approved procedures, it did not require submission of safety or effectiveness data. The most extensive 2006 clinical trial, which claimed that the procedure was safe and effective, followed 109 patients over twenty-four weeks. Longer-term efficacy remains unknown.

—Milton Berman, Ph.D.

the natural drainage tracts to minimize sinus obstruction. A specialist in otorhinolaryngology can perform such surgery using an endoscope, without the need for general anesthesia. Patients do not typically require hospitalization, and complications are rare.

—*Gregory B. Seymann, M.D.*

See also Allergies; Antihistamines; Bacterial infections; Common cold; Decongestants; Ear infections and disorders; Hay fever; Headaches; Multiple chemical sensitivity syndrome; Nasal polyp removal; Nasopharyngeal disorders; Otorhinolaryngology; Polyps.

For Further Information:

Beers, Mark H., et al., eds. *The Merck Manual of Diagnosis and Therapy*. 18th ed. Whitehouse Station, N.J.: Merck Research Laboratories, 2006.

Brook, Itzhak, ed. *Sinusitis: From Microbiology to Management*. New York: Taylor & Francis, 2006.

Kennedy, David W., and Marilyn Olsen. *Living with Chronic Sinusitis: A Patient's Guide to Sinusitis, Nasal Allergies, Polyps, and Their Treatment Options*. Long Island, N.Y.: Hatherleigh Press, 2007.

McCaffrey, Thomas. "Functional Endoscopic Sinus Surgery: An Overview." *Mayo Clinic Proceedings* 68 (June, 1993): 571-577.

Mickelson, Samuel, and Michael Benninger. "The Nose and Paranasal Sinuses." In *Textbook of Primary Care Medicine*, edited by John Noble. 3d ed. St. Louis, Mo.: Mosby, 2001.

Younis, Ramzi T., ed. *Pediatric Sinusitis and Sinus Surgery*. New York: Taylor & Francis, 2006.

SJÖGREN'S SYNDROME

Disease/Disorder

Also known as: Dry eye/dry mouth or sicca syndrome
Anatomy or system affected: Eyes, immune system, mouth
Specialties and related fields: Dentistry, family medicine, rheumatology
Definition: An autoimmune disorder resulting in the loss of tears and saliva.

Causes and Symptoms

Sjögren's (pronounced SHOW-grins) syndrome is a chronic autoimmune disease in which the body's own immune cells attack and eliminate the glands that produce tears and saliva. This results in dryness of the eyes and mouth and is referred to as sicca syndrome. The causes of Sjögren's syndrome are not known, although evidence suggests that viral infection, heredity, and hormones may be involved. Sjögren's syndrome is one of the more prevalent autoimmune disorders, affecting as many as four million Americans. Nine of ten patients with Sjögren's syndrome are female.

Sjögren's syndrome can be difficult to diagnose because the symptoms are similar to those caused by other diseases. The symptoms can also mimic the side effects associated with a number of medications and may vary from individual to individual. Even when the symptoms are reported to a physician, dentist, or eye specialist, the proper diagnosis can be overlooked.

The classic symptoms are dry eyes (xerophthalmia) and dry mouth (xerostomia). Individuals with Sjögren's syndrome often have blurred vision, constant eye discomfort, re-

---

Information on Sjögren's Syndrome

Causes: Unknown; possibly viral infection, heredity, hormones
Symptoms: Dry eyes, dry mouth, blurred vision, eye discomfort, recurrent mouth infections, swollen salivary glands, hoarseness, difficulty swallowing and eating, extreme fatigue
Duration: Chronic
Treatments: Moisture replacement (eyedrops, saliva-stimulating drugs, salivary packets); immunosuppressive drugs or NSAIDs

---

current mouth infections, swollen parotid (salivary) glands, hoarseness, and difficulty in swallowing and eating. Dryness of other mucous membranes of the body, such as the intestines, lungs, and reproductive system, may also occur. Extreme fatigue can also seriously alter the quality of life.

Sjögren's syndrome is most commonly diagnosed in people in their mid-forties. In some individuals, primary Sjögren's syndrome affects only the tear ducts and salivary glands. In other patients, it is present in conjunction with other diseases such as rheumatoid arthritis, systemic lupus erythematosus, systemic sclerosis (scleroderma), or polymyositis/dermatomyositis (secondary Sjögren's syndrome).

Treatment and Therapy

Once Sjögren's syndrome is suspected, blood tests for autoantibodies against nuclear or cytoplasmic proteins may be performed. Schirmer's test, which measures tear production, and salivary scintigraphy, which determines salivary gland function, may also be performed. A lower lip biopsy, to determine the extent of inflammation, may also be needed.

Moisture replacement therapies are designed to ease the symptoms of dryness. The routine use of eyedrops aids in controlling dryness of the eyes, and saliva-stimulating drugs and salivary packets help with difficulties in chewing and swallowing food. For individuals with more severe complications, immunosuppressive or nonsteroidal anti-inflammatory drugs (NSAIDs) may be prescribed.

Perspective and Prospects

Sjögren's syndrome is named after the Swedish eye doctor Henrik Sjögren, who first identified the syndrome in 1933. There is no known cure for Sjögren's syndrome, nor is there a current treatment to restore gland secretion. The outlook for individuals with this condition is usually good because Sjögren's syndrome is generally not life-threatening.

—*Thomas L. Brown, Ph.D.*

See also Autoimmune disorders; Eyes; Glands; Otorhinolaryngology; Rheumatoid arthritis; Scleroderma; Systemic lupus erythematosus (SLE); Tears and tear ducts; Vision disorders.

For Further Information:

Parker, James N., and Philip M. Parker, eds. *The Official Patient's Sourcebook on Sjögren's Syndrome*. San Diego, Calif.: Icon Health, 2002.

Rose, Noel R., and Ian R. Mackay, eds. *The Autoimmune Diseases*.

4th ed. St. Louis, Mo.: Academic Press/Elsevier, 2006.

Wallace, Daniel J., et al., eds. *The New Sjogren's Syndrome Handbook*. 3d ed. New York: Oxford University Press, 2005.

SKELETAL DISORDERS AND DISEASES. *See* BONE DISORDERS.

SKELETON. *See* BONES AND THE SKELETON.

SKIN
Anatomy
Anatomy or system affected: Nerves, nervous system

Specialties and related fields: Dermatology, neurology, oncology, plastic surgery

Definition: The largest organ of the body, which is vital to the survival of an organism for its protection against dehydration and abrasion, regulation of body temperature, and sensory reception.

Key terms:
basal cell carcinoma: the most common type of skin cancer; it grows slowly and seldom spreads beneath the skin

collagen: a fibrous protein found in the connective tissue, including skin, bone, ligaments, and cartilage

contact dermatitis: a common skin allergy characterized by inflamed skin; it occurs when skin comes in contact with substances such as poison ivy or allergenic cosmetics

dermatologist: a physician who treats the skin, including its structures, functions, and diseases

dermis: the layer of skin beneath the epidermis, consisting of dense connective tissue and blood vessels

epidermis: the outermost part of the skin, composed of four or five different layers called strata

keratin: an extremely tough protein that is the chief constituent of the epidermis, hair, nails, and tooth enamel

melanin: the dark pigment of the skin or hair that accounts for variations in skin color

melanoma: a cancer arising from a pigmented mole; it tends to spread to internal organs if left unchecked

psoriasis: a chronic skin disease characterized by red, scaly patches overlaid with thick, silvery gray scales

Structure and Functions
The anatomy of the skin consists of two major parts: the outer epidermis and the underlying dermis. The epidermis is composed of a particular kind of tissue called stratified squamous epithelium. Epithelium consists of cells that are packed together very tightly, a feature that is most important to an organ that must cover and protect the rest of the body. It is called squamous, which means "flat" in Latin, because its cells are flat and fit together like tiles. The word "stratified" describes the dozens of layers of cells that are piled up to create the epidermis. These cells form four or sometimes five strata, with their own characteristics and roles to perform.

The stratum basale, or basal layer, lies on a thin piece of tissue called the basement membrane, which is next to the dermis. The basal layer cells divide continuously throughout life, supplying new cells called keratinocytes for all the layers above the basal layer. About one-fourth of the stratum basale cells are called melanocytes because they produce the pigment melanin. As the keratinocytes are pushed up, they acquire a spiny shape; for this reason, the layer above the basal layer is called the stratum spinosum. While in the spiny layer, the upward-moving cells begin to produce the protein fibers that will eventually become waterproof keratin. As the spiny cells are moved further upward, they begin to flatten out. The layer that they form at this point is called the stratum granulosum because the keratin being formed is visible here, under the microscope, as large clumps or granules. Langerhans cells, which are very important in immunity and protection from disease, are also found in the granular layer. Only in thick skin, such as that found on the palms of the hands and the soles of the feet, do some of the migrating cells form a transparent layer of dead cells full of a shiny substance called eleidin. The shininess of this fourth layer earned it the name stratum lucidum.

The outermost part of the epidermis, the stratum corneum, is what most people think of as "the skin"-dead, dry cells that are completely waterproof because they are packed with keratin. The twenty-five layers of corneum cells form an efficient barrier to water loss and to the entrance of microorganisms. The epidermis has no blood vessels. The living, reproducing basal-layer cells must be nourished by nutrients passed from blood vessels in the dermis. Nerve endings that pick up the sensations of touch and pain extend upward into the epidermis, while those that sense pressure, heat, and cold extend only into the dermis.

Directly beneath the epidermis's basement membrane is the dermis. The dermis extends in a wavy or vertical tonguelike fashion into the epidermis to anchor it. The top of the dermis, which is called the papillary layer, thus forms ridges that account for one's fingerprints and toe prints. There are small blood vessels and fibers scattered throughout the papillary layer. The larger, lower part of the dermis is called the reticular layer. This thicker dermal layer has many more elastic and collagen fibers than does the papillary layer, and it is the location of oil glands, sweat glands, fat cells, hair follicles, and large blood vessels.

Directly under the skin, which is often called the cutis, is the jellylike, fat-filled subcutaneous layer. This packaging material provides heat insulation and energy storage, and it serves to attach the skin to the muscles and organs below.

The anatomy of the skin makes it able to perform a variety of functions. All these roles have one major purpose: to enable the skin to maintain homeostasis-that is, to keep the body relatively stable inside, in spite of constantly changing conditions outside.

The intact skin acts as a barrier to invasion by the multitude of microorganisms that come into contact with its surface. The waterproof keratin in the epidermis prevents all substances that are able to dissolve in water from entering the body through the skin. The presence of the pigment melanin enables the skin to absorb harmful radiation from the sun safely, up to a point. Too much exposure to the sun causes

The Structure of the Skin

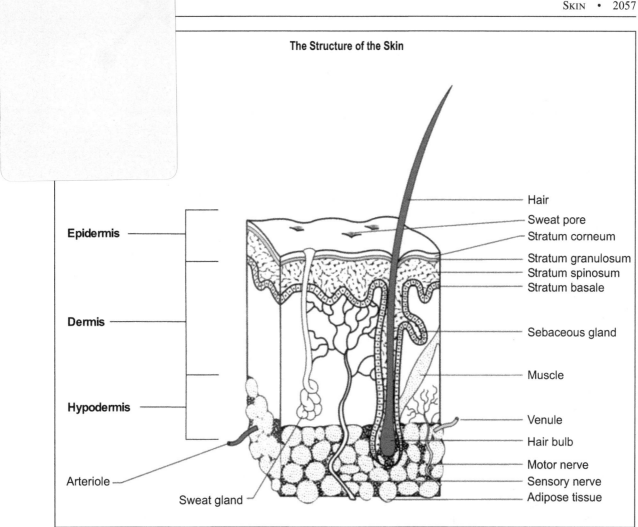

Epidermis

Dermis

Hypodermis

Arteriole

Sweat gland

Hair
Sweat pore
Stratum corneum
Stratum granulosum
Stratum spinosum
Stratum basale
Sebaceous gland
Muscle
Venule
Hair bulb
Motor nerve
Sensory nerve
Adipose tissue

sunburn, drying of the skin, a loss of elasticity, and wrinkling. More important, every sunburn increases the risk of skin cancer. Inheritance determines the amount of melanin possessed; although all races have the same number of melanocytes, people of different races differ greatly in the amount of melanin that their cells produce. The more melanin present, the darker the skin. The absence of a certain gene prevents melanin synthesis, causing those persons without the gene to be albinos. Skin color also varies because of the yellow pigment called carotene, which is found in the upper layers of the epidermis, and because of the red blood that is visible through the dermis of light-skinned people.

A very important function of skin is its role in temperature regulation. The body rids itself of excess heat by sweating. Excess heat passes from blood vessels into sweat glands, which conduct heat and perspiration to the surface. A large amount of heat can be lost as the sweat evaporates, thus maintaining normal body temperature. At other times, skin conserves heat by tightening blood vessels and reducing sweat secretion. Simultaneously, shivering, which is the involun-

tary contraction of skeletal muscles, releases internal heat to counteract excessive heat loss from the body. Only certain sweat glands-namely, those in the armpit and groin-produce the type of sweat that gives rise to an odor.

The waterproof quality of the skin prevents most substances from being absorbed through it into the body. Among the materials that can be absorbed are oxygen; vitamins A, D, E, and K; steroids such as cortisone cream; and, unfortunately, poisons such as insecticides.

The skin is able to produce a form of vitamin D that becomes active and useful to the body after passing through the kidneys. This synthesis requires a small amount of sunshine-far less than that necessary to cause a sunburn. If the skin does not produce enough vitamin D to enable the body to use calcium correctly, then vitamin D is needed in the diet.

Two very specialized accessory structures of the skin have their own particular functions. One of these skin derivatives is the pili, or hair. Except for the palms, soles, lips, and eyelids, the entire body contains hair. Each hair consists of a hair shaft that grows beyond the skin surface and a hair root lying inside a hair follicle. The follicle itself consists of epidermis that has grown downward into the dermis. Each hair follicle has an associated sebaceous gland that produces sebum, an oily substance, to lubricate the hair. Scalp hair protects the scalp from overexposure to the sun and from cold weather; eyelashes and tiny hairs inside the nose and ear canals help keep foreign material from entering.

The other important skin accessory is the nails. Each nail consists of a nail plate attached to a nail bed. Nails contain modified, highly keratinized cells from the stratum corneum. The basal cells that reproduce to make the nails grow lie under the cuticle at the base of the nail. Nails help to protect fingers and toes and enable humans to pick up tiny objects more efficiently.

Disorders and Diseases

The complex anatomy of the skin allows for the development of many possible defects and diseases. Three disorders that modern medical science attempts to understand and alleviate are psoriasis, cancer, and the many varieties of contact dermatitis.

Psoriasis, one of the most common of all skin conditions, is said to afflict about 3 percent of the American population. It commonly runs in families and affects both sexes equally. It may develop in childhood or old age but typically appears in the second or third decade of life. It most frequently occurs as scaly patches, or plaques, on the elbows, knees, and scalp but may appear on the back, belly, buttocks, and legs. Many people with psoriasis experience itching; surprisingly, some do not.

Human epidermis cells usually take about twenty-eight days to move from the stratum basale, where they are produced, to the top of the stratum corneum, where bathing removes them. This means that the cycle of normal epidermal cells in transit through the skin is accomplished in a month or more, allowing the cells time to mature. In psoriasis patients, this transit period is as short as four days. The reproducing basal cells divide five to ten times too rapidly, and the epidermis thickens enormously, but in patches. The skin cells of psoriasis patients are so abnormal that the patients' immune systems form antibodies that attack and destroy them, further damaging the ruptured, scaly surface. There is a notable tendency for psoriatic lesions or sores to form at sites of childhood injuries such as sunburns, scratches, scrapes, and areas where chickenpox was particularly widespread. These lesions often become pus-filled abscesses that contain enormous numbers of white blood cells. The epidermal cells no longer die at the stratum granulosum, and even the granules themselves are lost. The outermost corneum layer, which is usually dead, dry, and protective, is full of living but abnormally functioning cells. In the dermis below, large, dilated, thin-walled blood vessels appear, and the epidermis directly above them is disproportionately thin. Scratching or picking at the plaques causes bleeding.

The exact cause of psoriasis is not yet known. Genetic factors play a role in its development, since one-third of all patients have a family member who is also afflicted. In addition

to the physical discomfort and damage to self-esteem caused by this very obvious skin condition, it can lead to heat loss, fever, severe arthritis, heart failure, and even death.

The many forms of skin cancer can also cause great disfigurement and even death. Two frequently observed types are basal cell carcinoma and malignant melanoma. Basal cell cancers, which may begin in the hair follicle epithelium, are the most common skin cancers, accounting for almost 70 percent of all cases. Fortunately, they are also the most easily treated. They are most often found where sunlight strikes the hardest, on the neck, scalp, face, and shoulders. Basal cell cancers often start as small bumps but grow wider and more elevated, usually with a cavity in the center. Although their surface is shiny and filled with tiny blood vessels, their color may still be like that of normal skin. If left untreated, basal cell carcinomas may develop a crust or an ulcer that cannot heal. Although they seldom metastasize, shifting or spreading through the bloodstream to another part of the body, they often do great damage to the tissues and structures directly under them. Those that grow near ears and eyes can cause loss of function of those organs.

In almost all cases, the appearance of basal cell carcinomas is directly related to sun exposure. A few seem to be related to previous scars, burns, tattoos, or exposure to arsenic. It is important to be aware of the warning signs of basal cell carcinomas. Some can be felt as well as seen as reddish or dotted lumps; others look like open sores caused by scratches or insect bites that do not heal. Because these cancers, which often grow for two years before detection, have such varied appearances, they can be diagnosed accurately only by biopsy.

The most dangerous skin cancers are the malignant melanomas. They begin in the pigmented cells called melanocytes but usually and quite rapidly invade deeper tissue. Severe sunburns early in life seem to be their usual cause. Many start as small dark brown growths similar to moles, although they may become white, blue, or reddish and irregular in shape as they grow. Often they will bleed if rubbed. People who have acquired one hundred or more moles by young adulthood are considered genetically predisposed toward these dangerous melanomas; such people should use sunscreens every day all year long. It should be noted that half of all melanomas arise from apparently normal skin that has no moles. The malignant melanomas are much more dangerous than the basal cell carcinomas because they tend to release cancerous cells into the bloodstream that latch on to and grow into numerous internal organs.

Seldom life-threatening, contact dermatitis can still be very uncomfortable for a patient. Dermatitis is an inflammation of the skin that usually is a result of an allergic reaction and may include redness, swelling, blistering, crusting, and scaling among its symptoms. In all its many varieties, it probably forms the bulk of a dermatologist's practice. Contact dermatitis results from coming into contact with a causing substance, such as poison ivy, poison oak, or poison sumac. The sap from these plants contains urushiol, a substance to which 70 percent of all people are allergic.

Large numbers of persons are allergic to the metal nickel

and can develop inflammations from wearing nickel rings, watches, earrings, or other jewelry. Nickel zippers and clothing snaps, eyeglass frames and sewing needles, and even coins can cause a reaction.

The chemicals in permanent hair dyes cause terrible swelling and itching of the face and neck in some people. Oddly, the scalp under the dyed hair is often unaffected. When dermatitis seems to result from hair dyes, it is often because the affected person has simultaneously been using certain sunscreens, the pain reliever benzocaine, or one of many other common medicines.

The chemical potassium dichromate is found in many detergents. People who experience dermatitis caused by detergent use should avoid other chromate-containing products as well. These include inks, paints, bleaches, and spackling, to name only a few.

Other people contract dermatitis caused by a formaldehyde allergy. Permanent-press clothing and sheets are made wrinkle-proof by the use of a formaldehyde-based substance. Individuals with a formaldehyde allergy must also avoid many paper products, cosmetics, and disinfectants that contain formaldehyde derivatives.

Susceptibility to contact dermatitis from rubber products is widespread. Surprisingly, it often appears long after the exposure and is most common in manufacturing workers.

In modern society, with its heavy reliance on over-the-counter drugs, cleaning products of all kinds, deodorants and cosmetics, insecticides and weed-killers, and innumerable other chemical products, the potential causes of contact dermatitis have been and will continue to be multiplied.

Perspective and Prospects

Research in dermatology both borrows from and sheds light upon many other branches of medical science. Immunology, endocrinology, biochemistry, surgery, and oncology are just a few of many.

Diseases of the skin can reveal the presence of many otherwise unseen internal disease conditions. Shiny, thin, reddish-yellow patches on the shins may be a sign of diabetes. Prediabetics are also susceptible to repeated yeast and fungal infections of the skin and have poor wound-healing ability.

Too little thyroid hormone causes coarse hair; thickened, dry, cool skin; and rough plaques on the shins. Too much thyroid hormone causes thin hair, excessive sweating, and, surprisingly, identical rough plaques on the shins.

Abnormally dark skin can be a sign of drug side effects, the presence of heavy metals, poor adrenal gland output, or pituitary tumors. Skin may also darken from excess iron intake or, very noticeably, from a widespread malignant melanoma.

Various bowel diseases may also cause skin conditions. The small intestine defect involving a flattened, malfunctioning lining can produce severely itchy blisters on the limbs and the back. Ulcers in the large intestine often produce deep, dirty-looking skin ulcers.

The presence of cancer in the breast, bowel, or lungs may precipitate thousands of external wartlike growths or flat, waxy-surfaced growths. Similarly, the gradual appearance,

usually on the legs of the elderly, of fishlike skin may reveal the early presence of cancer of the lymph glands.

Alcoholism reveals itself in spider telangiectasia, webs of dilated capillaries on the skin surface. The presence of hepatitis, a serious viral infection of the liver, is indicated by the yellowing of the skin known as jaundice.

Two other links among dermatology, immunology, and oncology are the search for a vaccine against skin cancer and a new treatment called photopheresis. Since the late 1960s, there has been an ongoing attempt to develop a vaccine to prevent a recurrence of malignant melanoma. This is a particularly important pursuit because those who have survived one case of melanoma have a high risk of developing future ones.

Photopheresis patients take a drug called psoralen. Two hours later, their blood is drawn and exposed to ultraviolet light. The interaction between the psoralen and the light destroys abnormal white blood cells, after which the blood is returned to the body. Since 1987, photopheresis has been used to treat a cancer of the immune system that begins in the skin. Researchers hope eventually to use psoralen to treat arthritis and lupus, and to prevent the rejection of organ transplants.

For many years, drugs for internal conditions could be administered only orally or by injection. In both methods, the circulating amount may be too high to be safe immediately after it is given and too low to be effective as the hours go by. Dermatologists have greatly advanced medical science by developing transdermal patches. These patches enable a steady supply of a drug to enter the bloodstream by absorption through the skin. By the end of the twentieth century, patches had been developed to treat angina, high blood pressure, motion sickness, menopausal symptoms, and nicotine addiction.

One of the greatest traumas skin can suffer is a widespread burn. Although surgeons have had great success in transplanting many internal organs, they are unable to permanently transplant skin from another person. In 1981, they developed a marvelous technique to produce artificial skin. It uses animal skin protein seeded with a few skin cells taken from the patient. From this small patch, a large enough piece of skin can be grown to cover the wounds until the gradually healing skin replaces it.

From the earliest simple salves for skin rashes to the great discoveries of transdermal patches and artificial skin, dermatologists have done and continue to do their share in advancing medical science.

—*Grace D. Matzen*

See also Abscess drainage; Abscesses; Acne; Acupressure; Acupuncture; Age spots; Albinos; Allergies; Athlete's foot; Bedsores; Biopsy; Birthmarks; Bites and stings; Blisters; Boils; Bruises; Burns and scalds; Candidiasis; Canker sores; Cells; Chickenpox; Cold sores; Collagen; Corns and calluses; Cradle cap; Cryosurgery; Cyst removal; Cysts; Dermatitis; Dermatology; Dermatology, pediatric; Dermatopathology; Diaper rash; Eczema; Edema; Electrical shock; Electrocauterization; Face lift and blepharoplasty; Fifth disease; Frostbite; Fungal infections; Glands; Grafts and grafting; Hair; Hair loss and baldness; Hair transplantation; Hand-foot-and-mouth disease; Heat exhaustion and heatstroke; Hives; Host-defense mechanisms; Human papillomavirus (HPV); Hyperhidrosis; Impetigo; Insect-borne diseases; Itching; Jaundice; Kawasaki disease; Laceration repair; Laser use in surgery; Leishmaniasis; Leprosy; Lesions; Lice, mites, and ticks; Lower extremities; Measles; Melanoma; Moles; Morgellons disease; Nails; Necrotizing fasciitis; Numbness and tingling; Pigmentation; Pityriasis alba; Pityriasis rosea; Plastic surgery; Poisonous plants; Porphyria; Psoriasis; Radiation sickness; Rashes; Ringworm; Rocky Mountain spotted fever; Rosacea; Roseola; Rubella; Scabies; Scarlet fever; Scleroderma; Sense organs; Shingles; Skin cancer; Skin disorders; Skin lesion removal; Smallpox; Stevens-Johnson syndrome; Stretch marks; Styes; Sunburn; Sweating; Systemic lupus erythematosus (SLE); Tattoos and body piercing; Touch; Upper extremities; Vitiligo; Warts; Wrinkles.

For Further Information:

Goodman, Thomas, and Stephanie Young. *Smart Face*. Englewood Cliffs, N.J.: Prentice Hall, 1988. An easy-to-read explanation of skin structure, problems, and care, with special emphasis on delicate facial skin. Contains an extensive appendix of consumer product information.

Jacknin, Jeanette. *Smart Medicine for Your Skin*. New York: Putnam, 2001. An accessible and comprehensive guide to skin problems and solutions that include traditional therapies and alternative medicine choices.

Lamberg, Lynne. *Skin Disorders*. Philadelphia: Chelsea House, 2001. This brief volume is an introduction to the study of skin problems. Contains a very helpful glossary, a bibliography, and a list of organizations to contact for more information.

Lees, Mark. *Skin Care: Beyond the Basics*. 3d ed. Clifton Park, N.Y.: Thomson/Delmar Learning, 2007. A text for estheticians and students in the field that provides practical information on treating many kinds of skin problems and discusses topics such as rosacea, sensitive skin, hormones and menopause, and postlaser skin care.

Mackie, Rona M. *Clinical Dermatology*. 5th ed. New York: Oxford University Press, 2003. A text written for dermatology students but useful to the general public for more precise and detailed information than that contained in popular works. Illustrated in color.

Siegel, Mary-Ellen. *Safe in the Sun*. New York: Walker, 1995. Presents information from research of leading dermatologists and ophthalmologists showing the relationship between sun exposure and damage to skin and eyes. Easily understood by the general public. Contains an extensive glossary and many pages of helpful further sources of information.

Turkington, Carol, and Jeffrey S. Dover. *The Encyclopedia of Skin and Skin Disorders*. 3d ed. New York: Facts On File, 2007. More than one thousand entries on skin-related topics, including diseases, treatments, resources and organizations, skin cancer, acne treatment, FDA approvals of new treatments, and remedies for wrinkled skin.

Weedon, David. *Skin Pathology*. 3d ed. New York: Churchill Livingstone/Elsevier, 2010. Text with extensive photographs, covering tissue reaction patterns; the epidermis, dermis, and subcutis; the skin in systemic and miscellaneous diseases; infections and infestations; and tumors, among other topics.

SKIN CANCER
Disease/Disorder

Anatomy or system affected: Lymphatic system, skin

Specialties and related fields: Dermatology, environmental health, immunology, oncology

Definition: Malignancies of the skin (and sometimes spreading to the internal organs) caused by the ultraviolet radiation in sunlight.

Cancer is the common term used to describe the large class of

Information on Skin Cancer

Causes: Genetic factors, ultraviolet radiation from sun exposure

Symptoms: Lesion that increases in size and turns several colors (black, blue, white, brown); in later stages, itching, bleeding, and pain

Duration: Short-term to recurrent

Treatments: Surgical removal, chemotherapy, radiation therapy

diseases called neoplasms. Neoplasms, which occur only in multicellular organisms, develop and function in an autonomous way that does not abide by the biological mechanisms that govern the growth and metabolism of the individual cells and the reactions that take place in a living organism. When such neoplasms grow at a rate faster than the tissues from which they arise, while at the same time invading those tissues, they are called malignant and are commonly described as cancerous. Benign neoplasms, which do not invade surrounding tissues, generally are not as dangerous as malignant ones.

Sun radiation is life-sustaining, but the higher-energy part of the sunlight spectrum brings the danger of skin cancer. When living tissue is irradiated, its molecular structure is disrupted, thus initiating a chain of reactions, many of which are not the usual ones associated with the living organism. Therefore, a change in the chromosomal composition and the development of unwanted cells is likely to occur. Such changes take place because of the formation of free radicals in the deoxyribonucleic acid (DNA) molecules that constitute the genetic code. The result is skin cancer, the most common form of cancer in both men and women in the United States.

Types of skin cancer. Skin neoplasms may be benign or malignant, acquired or congenital, although the majority are benign and acquired. The common mole (the medical term for which is melanocytic nevus) is a neoplasm of benign melanocytes that is often present at birth and which is known as a birthmark. Such moles are generally harmless unless they are large in size, in which case they may have up to a 10 percent chance of becoming malignant. Other melanocytic nevi are strawberry hemangiomas and port-wine stains, which are of vascular origin.

The most common forms of skin cancer are the basal cell and squamous cell carcinomas, which arise from the corresponding part of the keratinocytes of the epidermis and are caused by the cumulative effects of ultraviolet radiation on the skin. They are generally localized, however, and rarely metastasize. These cancers are easily identified as persisting sores or crusting patches that grow mostly on sun-exposed parts of the body such as the hands, neck, arms, and nose. They can be treated with routine surgical procedures.

A malignant melanoma is formed from the pigment-forming melanocyte and almost certainly undergoes metastasis. It should therefore be removed surgically at the earliest possible stage. If the melanoma is detected at a later stage, chemotherapy and irradiation are the techniques usually applied. A malignant melanoma appears as a lesion that increases in size and turns several colors, such as black, blue, white, and brown. Symptoms such as itching, bleeding, and pain are not as common at first but are encountered at the later stages of development.

There are two additional skin malignancies that may be fatal: mycosis fungoides and Kaposi's sarcoma. Mycosis fungoides is a skin lymphoma that may be confined to one location for ten or more years before it metastasizes to internal organs, with death following. As a result, it is difficult to track this skin cancer, both clinically and histologically, and several biopsies (skin histological examinations) may be required to ascertain its presence. On the other hand, Kaposi's sarcoma occurs either as lesions (commonly among older Mediterranean men) or as skin abnormalities in HIV-infected people. The sarcoma is derived from skin blood vessels and appears as violet patches or lesions. As long as it is contained only in the skin, it is not fatal. Once the inner organs are affected, however, death is imminent, even though the lesions may be treated with irradiation and chemotherapy.

The effects of sunlight on skin. Extensive skin exposure to sunlight, such as at the beach, leads to the polymerization of skin chemicals (known as catecholamines) and the subsequent formation of different types of epidermal pigmentation (the melanins), which are responsible for tanning. Tanning occurs only if there is gradual exposure to sunlight; otherwise, a sunburn will arise. Photoprotection is believed to be one of the major biological functions of the melanin pigment. It appears that melanin formation can participate effectively in reducing the harmful effects of sunlight by an array of photoinduced chemical reactions, which result in the consumption of scavenging active oxygen species such as the superoxide anion and hydrogen peroxide. It has been determined that in biological systems, superoxide and hydrogen peroxide are formed in small quantities during normal processes. Both species are known to produce several biological effects, most of which are harmful to tissues. It should be pointed out, however, that although melanin may act as a free radical scavenger, it may also become energetically overloaded and may change to a toxic state. Evidence exists that melanin increases the radiative damage to cells, which leads to sunlight-induced skin cancer. In other words, melanin formation is good only when moderate exposure to sunlight occurs.

In the atmosphere 12 to 48 kilometers above the earth's surface lies a small layer of ozone. Although this layer does not contain much ozone-it is estimated to be about 3 millimeters thick under normal conditions of temperature and pressure-it has a profound effect on life. The ozone layer absorbs the harmful ultraviolet radiation from the sun, thus providing the mechanism for the heating of the stratosphere. A reduction in the ozone layer would lead to a large increase of ultraviolet rays intruding into the atmosphere, thus increasing the incidence of skin cancer. F. S. Rowland and M. J. Molina declared in 1974 that the presence of the volatile chlorofluorocarbons would eventually reduce the ozone layer. Some measurements done by scientists in 1979 showed a decrease in the

layer, which led to the action taken by several governments to decrease and replace the chlorofluorocarbons commonly used in aerosols. As the average life span steadily increases, the incidence of skin cancer will increase as well. The use of effective sunscreens and sunglasses with high ultraviolet blocking is recommended for people who are exposed to large amounts of sunlight.

—Soraya Ghayourmanesh, Ph.D.

See also Cancer; Carcinogens; Carcinoma; Chemotherapy; Dermatology; Dermatopathology; Kaposi's sarcoma; Lesions; Lymphadenopathy and lymphoma; Malignancy and metastasis; Melanoma; Moles; Radiation therapy; Skin; Skin disorders; Skin lesion removal; Sunburn; Warts.

For Further Information:
Dollinger, Malin, et al. *Everyone's Guide to Cancer Therapy.* 5th ed. Kansas City, Mo.: Andrews McMeel, 2008. An excellent source of medical information about cancer, written for the general public. Describes various cancer sites in the body. Includes a helpful glossary of medical terminology.

James, William D., Timothy G. Berger, and Dirk M. Elston. *Andrews' Diseases of the Skin: Clinical Dermatology.* 10th ed. Philadelphia: Saunders/Elsevier, 2006. Includes discussions of skin cancer.

McClay, Edward F., and Jodie Smith. *One Hundred Questions and Answers About Melanoma and Other Skin Cancers.* Boston: Jones and Bartlett, 2004. Uses a reader-friendly format to survey a range of topics related to skin cancer.

Siegel, Mary-Ellen. *Safe in the Sun.* New York: Walker, 1995. This comprehensive book describes the benefits of sunlight, the risks of exposure and how to protect the skin, and how damage that has already occurred can be treated.

Skin Cancer Foundation. http://www.skincancer.org. Promotes public education about skin cancer through campaigns against sun exposure and in support of early detection and research into new diagnostic techniques and therapies.

Weedon, David. *Skin Pathology.* 3d ed. New York: Churchill Livingstone/Elsevier, 2010. Text with extensive photographs, covering tissue reaction patterns; the epidermis, dermis, and subcutis; the skin in systemic and miscellaneous diseases; infections and infestations; and tumors, among other topics.

SKIN DISORDERS

Disease/Disorder

Anatomy or system affected: Skin

Specialties and related fields: Dermatology, family medicine, occupational health

Definition: Diseases and conditions that affect the skin, ranging from harmless to life-threatening.

Key terms:

benign: in reference to a neoplasm, having a nonmalignant character

dermatology: the study of the skin, its chemistry, physiology, histopathology, cutaneous lesions, and the relationships of these lesions to systemic disease

malignant: in reference to a neoplasm, having the property of uncontrollable growth and dissemination, recurrence after removal, or both

melanin: dark brown or black molecules of pigment that normally occur in the skin, hair, pigmented coat of the retina,

2062 • Skin disorders

and pupil of the eye and in selected cells of the brain

metastasis: the shifting of a disease, or its local manifestations, from one portion of the body to another; in cancer, the appearance of neoplasms in parts of the body remote from the primary tumor

Anatomy of the Skin

The skin is the largest organ of the body. It provides a barrier between the external world and the internal world: It protects against external contamination and helps to maintain the sterility of the internal body. The skin also assists in temperature regulation; humans can survive only within a narrow temperature range. The skin has nerve receptors that supply the brain with information, providing an interface with the world. There are specialized receptors for touch, temperature, vibration, and position in space (proprioception).

Appendages to the skin are fingernails, toenails, and hair. They are mainly of psychological importance. Nails protect the tips of fingers and toes in humans but are not needed for protection as claws are in lower animals. Hair is analogous to feathers. In birds, tiny muscles attached to the base of each feather cause them to be ruffled; this creates air pockets and allows birds to conserve heat and keep warm. The same muscles persist in humans, causing "goose flesh," but they do not serve any other function. The main importance of these appendages is cosmetic. For example, people spend billions of dollars on hair care products each year. The motivation for this activity is psychological.

The two main layers in skin are the epidermis and dermis. The epidermis is the upper or outermost layer, and cells are continually formed at its base. As new cells are formed, existing cells are pushed toward the surface of the skin. These cells gradually lose their watery central contents, causing them to dry out (desiccate) and become flattened. This process normally spans approximately a month. Thus, the surface of the body is largely composed of dead cells that have become flattened. These cells are normally lost on a continual basis and create dandruff when shed from the scalp. On other parts of the body, sloughed cells provide excellent conditions for bacterial growth, accounting for the unpleasant odors that accompany poor hygiene habits.

Two other important types of cells are found in the epidermis: melanocytes and Langerhans cells. Melanocytes contain melanin and provide all the variations of pigmentation found in the human species. They multiply when stimulated by the ultraviolet radiation in sunlight. This causes the skin to become darker, a protective mechanism against damage from ultraviolet radiation. Langerhans cells contain surface receptors for immunoglobulins. They play a central role in allergic reactions of the skin, such as contact dermatitis or delayed hypersensitivity reaction.

The dermis is an inner layer of skin located beneath the epidermis. Its main function is protection. Within the dermis are highly specialized cells containing microscopic filaments. These cells impart tensile strength to the skin in much the same way that fibers strengthen fiberglass or reinforcing steel mesh strengthens concrete. Because they are so dense,

Information on Skin Disorders

Causes: Infection, disease, allergies, environmental factors (e.g., ultraviolet radiation), hormonal changes, irritation, clogged sweat glands, eczema
Symptoms: May include inflammation, infection, flaking, pain, itching, redness, rashes, lesions, bleeding
Duration: Acute to chronic
Treatments: Topical ointments, antibiotics, corticosteroids, surgery, chemotherapy, radiation therapy

they also serve as a barrier to the entry of most pathogens and many chemicals. Eccrine sweat glands are found in the dermis throughout the entire body. These produce a salty secretion (essentially salt water) that assists in thermoregulation through evaporative cooling. They are also sensitive to emotional stress. Apocrine sweat glands are primarily in the armpits (axilla) and groin and produce a milky secretion. When these secretions are broken down by bacteria on the surface of the skin, a characteristic odor is produced. The bases of hair follicles are also found in the dermis. The small sebaceous, or oil-secreting, gland associated with most hair follicles has the function of softening and moisturizing the hair.

Hair is found on most surfaces of the body; exceptions are the palms of the hands, the soles of the feet, and the glans penis in men. The texture and length of the hair vary with location on the body, gender, genetic heritage, and age. Dramatic increases in the growth and distribution of hair occur at puberty. With increasing age, hair is typically lost from the scalp and other body parts. It also changes color, assuming a gray or white color because of the loss of melanin at the base of the hair follicle.

Complications and Disorders

When normal skin anatomy and physiology are upset, several common diseases or disorders result. When the barrier provided by the skin is broken, bacteria, viruses, fungi, and other pathogens can invade the body, leading to infections. Locally, these infections can cause inflammation (redness and pain) of the skin; if widespread, they can lead to systemic infections. When the cells and other substances found in the skin become irregular or are abnormal, skin disorders or conditions result.

Skin disorders and conditions. Pigmentation of the skin results from the presence of melanocytes, cells that manufacture and contain melanin. Most humans have pigmentation over their entire bodies; the degree of pigmentation varies with different racial and ethnic groups. Local areas of increased color have a range of names depending on the size of the pigmented area. A freckle is small and discrete. A nevus is a larger area of hyperpigmentation. These conditions are attributable to underlying variations in the distribution of melanocytes. They are genetic in origin and permanent; they are also accentuated by exposure to sunlight. Melasmas are irregular, flat, light brown areas on the neck, cheeks, or forehead. They are caused by hormonal changes associated with pregnancy or contraceptive pills and by exposure to sunlight. Melasmas fade with the reduction of excess hormones. There are also color changes in the labia of females during pregnancy; these changes are both harmless and permanent.

Generalized increases in skin coloration can occur with some metabolic diseases. Addison's disease involves an increase in melanocyte-stimulating hormone. This leads to an overall bronzing of the body, with accentuation in creases of the palms and soles. The condition subsides with treatment of the underlying cause of the disease. Similar pigment increases are associated with some forms of lung cancer, hemochromatosis, and chronic arsenic exposure. The latter two conditions are caused by the deposition of iron (hemochromatosis) and arsenic in the skin.

Generalized decreases in skin coloration can also occur. If melanocytes fail to migrate to the skin during embryologic development, hair follicles will lack color, resulting in a condition called piebaldism. Characteristically, this is a white patch in the hair of the forehead. Vitiligo is caused by an immunologically mediated loss of melanocytes. Individuals with phenylketonuria (PKU) experience a generalized depigmentation of hair and eye color, in addition to mental retardation, if the condition is not adequately and promptly treated. An individual totally lacking melanocytes is called an albino; because melanin is also responsible for eye color, albinos have red eyes. The loss of hair is called alopecia. It can occur because of aging, sustained pulling on the hair with some hairstyles, and genetics. Women do not usually experience much alopecia until after the menopause. Conversely, some men start to lose their hair during their twenties.

Skin diseases. Eczema or dermatitis is a general term that describes a skin disease involving vesicles that ooze fluid. These conditions are usually characterized by a rash; they are inflammatory reactions, commonly caused by contact with a chemical or plant material. They can be caused by an adverse reaction to a drug or by sunlight. Bacteria, yeasts, or other fungi on the skin can cause eczema. Most rashes itch or burn; they can be spread by scratching. Athlete's foot is a common example of an eczematous dermatitis.

Maculopapular diseases encompass several common skin conditions, such as red measles (rubeola), German measles (rubella), and scarlet fever. Viruses that land on the skin cause these diseases. They are characterized by relatively large, localized areas of changed skin color (macules) that are also raised (papules) but not fluid-filled. After their clinical course is run, they disappear without leaving a scar. The more dangerous toxic shock syndrome also belongs to this group of diseases; it is caused by toxin from the bacteria *Staphylococcus aureus*.

Thickening of the skin and the formation of red to purple areas having sharply defined borders characterize papulosquamous skin diseases. The most common example is psoriasis. Other examples are pityriasis and ichthyosis. The pathology responsible for psoriasis is an alteration in the normal development of skin cells. In individuals with psoriasis, new skin cells develop and migrate to the surface in only five days instead of the usual thirty. This fact alone explains the flaking (rapid cell turnover), redness (thinner skin and a rich blood supply for new skin), and pain and itching (less protection for sensory nerve endings) experienced. Pityriasis includes a group of different conditions caused by different viruses. Patches or large spots develop on the skin. They usually resolve within a few weeks. Aside from being locally photosensitive, they usually are not serious. Ichthyosis describes a group of genetic conditions characterized by extreme scaling of the skin.

Vesiculobullous diseases have fluid-filled blisters that can vary in size from relatively small (vesicles) to relatively large (bullae). Insect bites, herpes, and some bacterial infections lead to the formation of vesicles or bullae. Such conditions are attributable to an immune reaction that leads to the formation of blisters at the junction between epidermis and dermis. They can be accompanied by intense pruritus (itching); scratching often leads to scarring.

Pustular diseases of the skin include acne, folliculitis, and candidiasis. They are characterized by the inflammation of hair follicles caused by surface bacteria or yeasts. Adequate personal hygiene is the most effective method of prevention. These diseases are usually not serious, but prolonged or repeated attacks can result in scarring and disfigurement. The sebaceous glands, which secrete oil at the base of hair follicles, can increase in size. The subsequent increase in oil output worsens the condition.

Clogged sweat glands can lead to acne. While this is primarily a problem for teenagers, it can affect individuals of any age. Exposure to cutting oils and other hydrocarbons such as gasoline and paint thinners can cause a similar condition called chloracne, which is inflammation in the base of hair follicles found on exposed skin in areas such as the nape of the neck, forearms, and face. The inability to sense temperature and regulate body heat through sweating is called anhidrosis, a condition that can cause shock and potentially death.

Other diseases that can affect the skin. Five such diseases are worthy of mention: leprosy, scleroderma, lupus, atherosclerosis, and diabetes mellitus. Leprosy, or Hansen's disease, is caused by infection by *Mycobacterium leprae*, a relative of the bacteria that cause tuberculosis. In leprosy, the causative organism accumulates in the skin and peripheral nerves. This causes disfigurement and loss of sensation, the latter being similar to that experienced by an uncontrolled diabetic. Disfigurement is responsible for the stigma associated with leprosy since ancient times: loss of fingers and toes, as well as mutilation of the nose and ears. Leprosy is caused by long-term association with the organism and can be adequately treated with appropriate antibiotics.

Scleroderma (literally, "hard skin") is an uncommon disease characterized by fibrosis of the skin and involvement of visceral organs. The skin involvement can range from an isolated, hardened patch to a life-threatening, generalized condition described as an ever-tightening case of steel. The skin becomes stretched tightly over the underlying skeleton. Skin tone is lost with restriction of movement.

Systemic lupus erythematosus is a disease of unknown etiology that is characterized by inflammation in many different organ systems. The skin is usually involved, as nearly all individuals with lupus develop a characteristic butterfly-shaped rash on their faces. This red coloration covers the cheeks and nose. Persons with lupus are also sensitive to sunlight, and many develop alopecia. Most of those affected are female. The disease waxes and wanes; treatment depends on the particular organs involved.

Atherosclerosis and diabetes can block the arteries supplying the nerves of the skin, leading to a loss of sensory input. When the patient is unable to experience pain, cuts and other abrasions on the skin are not noticed. Untreated, these lesions can lead to gangrene, sometimes requiring amputation of a body part.

Skin cancer. The most commonly diagnosed form of cancer is that involving the skin. It is not the most fatal form, but millions of cases are discovered annually. The origin of most skin cancers can be traced to excessive exposure to radiation from the sun. They can occur on any surface of the body, although they are more common on areas that are usually exposed to the sun, such as the face, the backs of the hand, and the neck. Skin cancers can arise in the epidermis or dermis. The majority are noncancerous, or benign. Epidermal nodules are characterized by local thickening of the epidermis, often accompanied by scaling of the skin in the affected area. Nodules in the dermis may appear as lumps with no alteration of the epidermis above them.

There are three malignant forms of skin cancer. Basal cell carcinoma arises from cells deep in the epidermis. This form of tumor rarely spreads (metastasizes), but it can be extensive and destructive locally. Squamous cell carcinoma is less common but can be invasive (involving adjacent tissues) and can metastasize. Melanoma is relatively uncommon but can grow extremely rapidly; it has the potential to be fatal in a matter of months. It involves the uncontrolled growth of melanocytes. Melanomas have irregular borders and color or pigmentation. Any pigmented lesion or suspicious change in the skin should be evaluated by a medical professional in a timely manner.

Prevention is the preferred method of dealing with skin cancer. When outside, loose-fitting clothing can provide protection from the sun, and a hat can protect the head. When exposure is unavoidable, a product with a sun-blocking agent will reduce exposure. Limiting the time of exposure to the sun until the body has reacted by producing additional melanocytes (tanned) is recommended.

Prolonged exposure to the sun also accelerates changes in the skin associated with aging. Collagen fibers provide the characteristic firm feel to the skin of a young person. With aging the skin becomes less firm, losing some of its tone, and begins to sag. Inadequate moisture also contributes to the loss of skin tone. Excessive exposure to the sun hastens both of these processes.

—*L. Fleming Fallon, Jr., M.D., Ph.D., M.P.H.*

See also Abscess drainage; Abscesses; Acne; Age spots; Aging; Albinos; Allergies; Bedsores; Birthmarks; Bites and stings; Blisters; Boils; Bruises; Canker sores; Carcinoma; Chickenpox; Cold sores; Corns and calluses; Cradle cap; Cyst removal; Cysts; Dermatitis; Dermatology; Dermatology, pediatric; Dermatopathlogy; Diaper rash; Eczema; Fifth disease; Grafts and grafting; Hair; Hair loss and baldness; Hand-foot-and-mouth disease; Herpes; Hives; Human papillomavirus (HPV); Hyperhidrosis; Impetigo; Inflammation; Insect-borne diseases; Itching; Kawasaki disease; Leprosy; Lesions; Measles; Melanoma; Moles; Morgellons disease; Necrotizing fasciitis; Neurofibromatosis; Pigmentation; Pityriasis alba; Pityriasis rosea; Poisonous plants; Psoriasis; Rashes; Ringworm; Rocky Mountain spotted fever; Rosacea; Scabies; Scleroderma; Skin; Skin cancer; Skin lesion removal; Stevens-Johnson syndrome; Stretch marks; Styes; Sunburn; Sweating; Systemic lupus erythematosus (SLE); Tattoo removal; Tattoos and body piercing; Vitiligo; Warts; Wrinkles.

For Further Information:

Burns, Tony, et al., eds. *Rook's Textbook of Dermatology.* 7th ed. Malden, Mass.: Blackwell Science, 2004. This is a core text in dermatology that will appeal to professionals and members of the general public who want a concise introduction to the subject. The aim of the book is to integrate basic science with clinical practice.

Frankel, David H., ed. *Field Guide to Clinical Dermatology.* 2d ed. Philadelphia: Lippincott Williams & Wilkins, 2006. Frankel, a noted internist and dermatologist, has enlisted widely respected and talented colleagues to help in the production of this book. It is a uniquely organized and easily readable field guide complete with 220 pages of excellent color illustrations.

Freinkel, Ruth K., and David T. Woodley, eds. *Biology of the Skin.* New York: Parthenon, 2001. Covers the basic biology of the skin, how the skin functions, effects of the environment, the molecules that direct cutaneous function, genetic influences, and methods in cutaneous research.

Goldsmith, Lowell A., Gerald S. Lazarus, and Michael D. Tharp. *Adult and Pediatric Dermatology: A Color Guide to Diagnosis and Treatment.* Philadelphia: F. A. Davis, 1997. This book provides excellent pictures to accompany good descriptions of dermatologic diseases.

Grob, J. J., et al., eds. *Epidemiology, Causes, and Prevention of Skin Diseases.* Cambridge, Mass.: Blackwell Science, 1997. This well-written book presents data on large groups of people. The sections on skin cancer are especially noteworthy.

Kenet, Barney, and Patricia Lawler. *Saving Your Skin: Prevention, Early Detection, and Treatment of Melanoma and Other Skin Cancers.* 2d ed. Chicago: Four Walls Eight Windows, 1998. Skin cancer is the focus of this title, which reviews the early symptoms of melanoma, its causes, and its treatment. Very few skin care titles do more than offer a chapter on the problem.

Sams, W. Mitchell, Jr., and Peter J. Lynch, eds. *Principles and Practice of Dermatology.* 2d ed. London: Churchill Livingstone, 1996. This is a new edition of a dermatology reference guide and text emphasizing accurate diagnosis by succinct discussions in eighty-five presentations featuring color photographs.

Weedon, David. *Skin Pathology.* 3d ed. New York: Churchill Livingstone/Elsevier, 2010. Text with extensive photographs, covering tissue reaction patterns; the epidermis, dermis, and subcutis; the skin in systemic and miscellaneous diseases; infections and infestations; and tumors, among other topics.

SKIN GRAFTING. *See* GRAFTS AND GRAFTING.

SKIN LESION REMOVAL

Procedure

Anatomy or system affected: Arms, hands, nose, skin

Specialties and related fields: Dermatology, general surgery, oncology, plastic surgery

Definition: The removal of cancerous and precancerous skin lesions under local anesthesia with a curette or scalpel, an electric needle, or liquid nitrogen.

Indications and Procedures

Actinic (or solar) keratoses and skin cancers affect more than a half million Americans each year. Actinic keratoses, warty lesions that are considered to be premalignant, are often removed as a precaution. Among skin cancers, basal cell carcinoma is the least harmful. The lesion may appear on the skin surface as a small, flesh-colored or pale pink spot, usually with a raised edge that has a translucent, pearly appearance. It grows slowly and will rarely spread (metastasize) to other parts of the body. Squamous cell carcinoma is more dangerous. It appears on the surface as a small, firm, scaly tumor with an indistinct margin. Untreated squamous cell malignancies may metastasize. Malignant melanoma, called black cancer, is the most dangerous of the three types. Melanoma lesions may resemble a mole with an irregular shape and can be red, blue, black, brown, gray, or even white. Melanoma rapidly invades nearby tissue and can metastasize readily to other parts of the body.

The method of treatment will depend on the type of lesion and its location and size. Most are treated in the dermatologist's office under local anesthesia. More widespread lesions may be removed in the hospital under general anesthesia.

The site is cleaned with a germicidal swab, and a local anesthetic is injected under the skin. The lesion is scraped away with a curette, an instrument with a small, scoop-shaped cutting head. An electric cautery kills any remaining lesion cells and seals off small blood vessels.

The curette is used on basal cell carcinomas that are less than 1 or 2 centimeters in diameter. Larger lesions are removed with a scalpel, and stitches close the incision. Cancers on the eyelids, on the tip of the nose, or near facial nerves may be removed with radiation (using X rays or another source). If the area treated is large, cosmetic or reconstructive surgery is performed to restore the patient's physical appearance.

Uses and Complications

There is about a 95 percent cure rate for treated basal cell carcinomas. The cure rate for squamous cell carcinomas is only slightly less, especially if the lesion has been treated at an early stage. The cure rate for malignant melanomas is low unless they are diagnosed and treated early.

—Albert C. Jensen, M.S.

See also Biopsy; Cancer; Carcinoma; Cryosurgery; Dermatology; Dermatopathology; Electrocauterization; Grafts and grafting; Laser use in surgery; Lesions; Melanoma; Oncology; Pigmentation; Plastic surgery; Skin; Skin cancer; Skin disorders; Warts.

For Further Information:

Hall, John C., and Gordon S. Sauer. *Sauer's Manual of Skin Diseases.* 10th ed. Philadelphia: Lippincott Williams & Wilkins, 2010.

McKee, Phillip. *A Concise Atlas of Dermatopathology.* New York: Gower Medical, 1993.

Mehregan, Amir H., et al. *Pinkus' Guide to Dermatohistopathology.* 6th ed. Norwalk, Conn.: Appleton & Lange, 1995.

Turkington, Carol, and Jeffrey S. Dover. *The Encyclopedia of Skin and Skin Disorders.* 3d ed. New York: Facts On File, 2007.

Weedon, David. *Skin Pathology.* 3d ed. New York: Churchill Livingstone/Elsevier, 2010.

Sleep

Biology

Anatomy or system affected: Brain, cells, glands, nervous system, psychic-emotional system

Specialties and related fields: Biochemistry, endocrinology, family medicine, internal medicine, neurology, pharmacology, preventive medicine, psychiatry, psychology

Definition: A quiescent period of rest characterized by decreased motor activity and diminished voluntary thought.

Key terms:

electroencephalograph (EEG): a device that records the electrical activity of the brain through electrodes attached to the scalp

insomnia: long-term deprivation of adequate sleep

neurotransmitter: a chemical that is stored in a neuron (nerve cell) and crosses the synaptic cleft (gap between neurons) to cause a change in another neuron

rapid eye movement (REM) sleep: a type of sleep characterized by heightened brain activity, vigorous eye movements, and relaxed postural muscles

sleep stage: the type of sleep based primarily on the EEG record; additional recordings of eye movements and muscle tension are used to determine the presence of REM sleep

Structure and Functions

All multicellular animals cycle through daily fluctuations in biological activity known as circadian rhythms, with the alternation of sleep and wakefulness being the most obvious example. In humans, a polycyclic sleep/wake cycle-several periods of sleep and arousal during a twenty-four-hour period-becomes evident in the fetus during the latter stages of pregnancy. As children progress from infancy through childhood, they gradually settle into a mainly diurnal pattern, with one long period of sleep during the day. A complex interaction of several external and internal events determines the timing and duration of sleep.

The key exogenous factor that influences sleep is light. In the absence of the alternation of day and night, people will usually develop a sleep/wake cycle that is a little longer (from a few minutes to an hour) than a twenty-four-hour day. Two neurological structures detect light and synchronize the body's sleep/wake cycle with the presence or absence of light. The pineal gland is a photosensitive endocrine gland centrally located in the brain that secretes the hormone melatonin, which causes drowsiness. When darkness increases, the pineal gland steps up production of melatonin; levels of melatonin decline as light increases. Melatonin levels also affect the structure of the brain that plays the key role in regulating circadian rhythms, the suprachiasmatic nucleus of the hypothalamus (SCN). The SCN serves as the body's

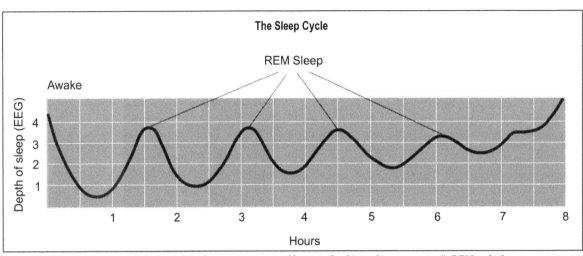

Over an eight-hour sleep period, depth of sleep fluctuates, punctuated by periods of "rapid eye movement" (REM), which appear necessary for restful sleep.

primary biological clock, containing cells that will pulse in rhythmic activity in the absence of light. The activity of these cells, however, is influenced by output from the pineal gland and also from the eye's retinal cells, providing two avenues by which light can affect the SCN. Light causes the SCN to alter levels of Tim, a protein which, when it interacts with two other proteins known as Per and Clock, will induce sleepiness at high levels. Levels of Tim, in turn, will increase activity in certain cells of the SCN. Thus, light serves as the *zeitgeber* (time-giver) for the sleep/wake cycle by changing the activity of the pineal gland and SCN, thereby altering levels of sleep-inducing chemicals.

Although damage to the pineal gland and SCN will significantly disrupt the quality and quantity of sleep, periods of sleep will still occur. That observation, in addition to the fact that animals will develop sleep/wake cycles in the absence of light changes, points to other, internal mechanisms that control sleep and arousal. One of these mechanisms is body temperature. Body temperature fluctuates from approximately 98 degrees Fahrenheit (36.7 degrees Celsius) to 99 degrees Fahrenheit (37.2 degrees Celsius) during the day. Rising body temperature is associated with arousal; declining body temperature is correlated with drowsiness. Vigorously rubbing the hands together can increase blood flow to the hands, dropping the blood supply to the brain, thereby decreasing the temperature of the brain and making it easier to fall asleep. While blood flow has an impact on the level of alertness, it is the flow of several neurotransmitters-chemicals that bridge the synaptic gap between one neuron (nerve cell) and another-that play the crucial role in regulating sleep and arousal.

Neurotransmitters generally have excitatory or inhibitory effects on arousal, but their impact on sleep is dependent on the neurological structures that they affect. Overall, more neurotransmitters appear to facilitate arousal rather than sleepiness. Acetylcholine and glutamate are the primary

neurotransmitters for learning, so it is not surprising that they mediate the brain's alertness to external stimuli. The pontomesencephalon portion of the reticular formation-the brain's major arousal system-releases these two neurotransmitters, which activate regions of the brain from top (the cortex) to bottom (the medulla). Acetylcholine is also released by excitatory basal forebrain cells that have direct connections with the thalamus, the brain's center for the integration and processing of sensory information. Close to the bottom of the brain in the pons is the locus coeruleus, which promotes wakefulness and helps to consolidate memories. Norepinephrine, the neurotransmitter that is involved in the display of active emotions such as fear or anger, is released from this structure and arouses many areas of the brain. Between the locus coeruleus and the basal forebrain is the hypothalamus, which influences many aspects of motivation and emotion, particularly through its regulation of the pituitary gland, the master gland of the endocrine system. Anterior cells of the hypothalamus release histamine, which, like acetylcholine, has widespread arousing effects on the brain. Taking antihistamine drugs to subdue the symptoms of allergies and colds will militate against those arousing effects. Lateral cells of the hypothalamus produce orexin, a neurotransmitter that is necessary for staying awake, especially as the day transpires.

Three neurotransmitters promote the induction and maintenance of sleep; two of them exert their effects via the basal forebrain. Gamma-aminobutyric acid (GABA), the brain's primary inhibitory neurotransmitter, is released by inhibitory cells in the basal forebrain and dampens arousal in the cortex and thalamus. Adenosine decreases activity in the acetylcholine-producing cells of the basal forebrain, thereby inhibiting arousal. Caffeine derives its stimulating effects by blocking adenosine receptors. Moderate levels of serotonin have a calming effect and can facilitate the induction of sleep. However, serotonin (and norepinephrine) can decrease the quantity of REM sleep. Other chemicals, such as prostaglandins, work in conjunction with these three neurotransmitters to promote the induction and maintenance of sleep.

The interplay of various levels of neurotransmitters and hormones effect changes in the electrical activity of the brain. Recordings of the electrical potentials of brain cells made with an electroencephalograph (EEG) have resulted in the identification of four succeeding distinct patterns of brain wave activity that occur in approximately ninety-minute cycles. Prior to falling asleep, a person manifests mostly alpha EEG readings-high amplitude (top-to-bottom distance), medium wavelength (peak-to-peak distance) brain wave activity-characteristic of an alert, relaxed state. When a person slips into the first stage of sleep, a theta EEG pattern-low amplitude, short wavelengths-predominates. As sleep progresses, brief periods of very short wavelengths (sleep spindles) and bursts of high amplitude waves (K-complexes) punctuate the theta EEG pattern, marking the appearance of stage 2 sleep. Eventually, high amplitude and long wavelength brain activity-a delta EEG record-becomes more prevalent and stage 3 sleep is evident. Finally, delta EEG waves predominate as the person settles into stage 4 sleep. The individual will then cycle back through the third and second stages before reaching stage 1 sleep again, completing the ninety-minute biorhythm. The second period of stage 1 sleep is usually accompanied by the first appearance of rapid eye movement (REM) sleep in humans (many species lack the eye movements), a phenomenon in which brain activity is high but many signs of physiological arousal, such as muscle tension, are low. The time spent in each stage varies, depending on how long the person has been sleeping: stages 3 and 4 predominate during the first half of a sleep period, while stages 1 and 2 predominate (stage 4 sleep is often absent) during the second half.

Differences in sleep stage characteristics and their associated phenomena have led some researchers to distinguish between two basic types of sleep: S-sleep (more neural synchrony, similar activity in diverse brain regions), which combines stages 3 and 4, and D-sleep (more neural desynchrony, diverse brain regions active at different times), which combines stages 1 and 2. S-sleep is characterized by many signs of a deeper physical rest: lower body temperature, generally lower autonomic arousal, difficult arousal. Moreover, sleep loss and physical injuries or deprivations tend to increase the percentage of S-sleep over D-sleep. In contrast, more signs of psychological restoration are associated with D-sleep: increased cortical blood flow and more vivid and prevalent dreams, especially during REM sleep. Additionally, deprivation of REM sleep tends to impair memory and increase irritability more so than deprivation of S-sleep. Because the distinctions between S-sleep and D-sleep are not always clear-cut-for example, S-sleep is essential for some types of memory formation-some researchers prefer to distinguish between REM sleep and non-REM (NREM) sleep.

Disorders and Diseases

Species vary in the amount of sleep that they require during a day, ranging from approximately two hours for a horse to twenty hours for a bat. Humans begin life averaging around sixteen hours of sleep a day as babies, progress to needing about half that much through most of adolescence and adulthood, and then typically get six to seven hours of sleep a day in later adulthood (partially due to age-related decreases in melatonin). No matter what the species or the age of the individual, problems with both the quantity and quality of sleep impair physical and psychological well-being.

Poor quantity of sleep, resulting in feeling tired during waking hours, is the primary characteristic of the most common class of sleep disorders known as insomnias. Insomnias may be characterized by difficulty initially falling asleep (onset), problems in staying asleep (maintenance), or inability to fall back asleep when waking up early (termination). Termination and maintenance insomnia become more likely as people leave early adulthood. Rising body temperature is a factor in both onset and termination insomnia; breathing problems often induce maintenance insomnia.

Trouble breathing, leading to a drop of oxygen in the blood and frequent awakenings, is the main symptom of sleep apnea. Apnea can be caused by many factors, including obstructions of airway passages (often the result of obesity), the use of drugs (such as alcohol and tranquilizers, which relax breathing muscles), or deterioration of areas in the brain that control breathing (the pre-Botzinger complex of the medulla). Left untreated by surgery or breathing aids, apnea can result in numerous health problems, such as loss of cells in multiple areas of the brain, memory deficiencies, heart problems, and diabetes.

Insomnias and apnea, as well as numerous other sleep disorders, can also lead to poor quality of sleep. In particular, depressed amount of REM sleep is a common problem associated with sleep dysfunctions. Neurological depressants, such as alcohol and tranquilizers, have commonly been used to treat insomnia. Unfortunately, such drugs can lead to iatrogenic (caused by medical treatment) insomnia in which a drug initially facilitates sleep but then tolerance develops, in which an increasing amount of the drug is needed to induce its primary effects, and insomnia recurs. Moreover, neurological depressants typically suppress REM sleep, further exacerbating the insomniac's condition.

In stress-induced insomnia, EEG records reveal that brain activity drifts in a twilight zone between sleep and wakefulness, with minimal REM sleep. People suffering from significant reactions to trauma, such as in post-traumatic stress disorder (PTSD), frequently reexperience their traumatic encounters in nightmares that are so vivid and horrifying that they are unable to stay asleep during REM periods. In contrast, it is the sleep partners of individuals with REM behavior disorder who have problems staying asleep, as the person with the dysfunction thrashes wildly about, perhaps acting out her or his dreams.

Overactive motor activity is also the primary symptom of two NREM disorders: restless leg syndrome, which is characterized by twitching and high muscle tension of the legs, and myoclonus, which involves body twitching, particularly of the arms and legs, while asleep. The extreme overactive muscle sleep disorder, however, is sleepwalking. Sleepwalking normally occurs in stage 4 sleep and is more common in children and adolescents. What sleepwalking is to motor activity, night terrors (extremely terrifying dreams) are to psychological activity. As with sleepwalking, night terrors are more common in children and adolescents and occur during stage 4 sleep. Sleeptalking is not restricted to any particular age-group or sleep stage.

Narcolepsy is a sleep dysfunction in which the main problem is evident during waking hours rather than during the sleep period. The four primary symptoms of narcolepsy are intense periods of sleepiness, cataplexy (muscle weakness), hypnogogic imagery (dreamlike hallucinations while slipping into sleep), and sleep paralysis (muscle immobility while moving into and out of sleep periods). Because most of the symptoms are associated with REM sleep, narcolepsy has been interpreted as a wakeful experience of REM-like sleep. Low levels of orexin have been implicated as a cause of this disorder.

Perspective and Prospects

In his book *The Promise of Sleep* (1999), William C. Dement, one of the foremost researchers of sleep, describes the breakthrough research in the early 1950s that gave birth to the modern era of sleep understanding. Dement, working with Nathaniel Kleitman and Eugene Aserinsky, conducted the first research to measure simultaneously the electrical activity of the eyes and brain while people were sleeping. The results of their work led to the identification of four distinct stages of sleep, the discovery of a ninety-minute sleep cycle, and the detection of REM sleep. REM sleep was later found to correspond with a discovery by Michel Jouvet called paradoxical sleep, so named because animals in this type of sleep manifest high brain activity but relaxed postural muscles. Dement and Kleitman also discovered that people awakened from REM sleep were usually dreaming. These discoveries of the 1950s opened up new avenues of research, from empirical studies of dreaming to the interrelationship between sleep and health, and led to the development of better methods to diagnosis and treat sleep disorders.

By the mid-twentieth century, benzodiazepines (tranquilizers, such as Halcion, Valium, and Xanax), which facilitate the action of GABA and adenosine, became the primary treatment for diverse kinds of sleep disorders. Such side effects such as REM suppression, increased likelihood of apnea, and drowsiness during waking hours, however, prompted researchers to search for alternatives to these highly addictive drugs. Safer alternatives for insomnia were developed in the late twentieth century as nonbenzodiazepine, GABA-facilitating sleep aids (such as Ambien, Lunesta, and Sonata) became more popular. Rozerem, a melatonin receptor stimulant, offered physicians a new approach to treating insomnia in the twenty-first century. While chemicals, such as dopaminergic agents (Sinemet) for restless leg disorder and stimulants (Ritalin) for narcolepsy, can be useful in treating various sleep disorders, for the person suffering from insomnia the best advice is often to avoid the chemicals-such as al-cohol, caffeine, and nicotine-that will interfere with the natural mechanisms designed to promote sleep.

—*Paul J. Chara, Jr., Ph.D.*

See also Apnea; Caffeine; Chronobiology; Hallucinations; Narcolepsy; Nightmares; Paralysis; Physiology; Sleep apnea; Sleep disorders; Sleepwalking; Stress.

For Further Information:

Dement, William C., and Christopher Vaughan. *The Promise of Sleep: A Pioneer in Sleep Medicine Explores the Vital Connection Between Health, Happiness, and a Good Night's Sleep*. New York: Delacorte Press, 1999. Renowned sleep expert Dement presents an authoritative, yet accessible overview of sleep research and sets forth principles for healthy sleeping. An extensive list of sleep centers in the United States of America is included.

Hirshkowitz, Max, Patricia B. Smith, and William C. Dement. *Sleep Disorders for Dummies*. Hoboken, N.J.: For Dummies, 2004. This easy-to-understand guide covers the causes, symptoms, and treatment options for numerous sleep disorders. Practical advice, humor, and numerous visual aids make this book a good reference for the person with little knowledge of sleep disorders.

Jacobs, Gregg D. *Say Goodnight to Insomnia*. London: Rodale, 2009. Jacobs outlines a drug-free program, developed at Harvard Medical School, for overcoming insomnia. Six basic strategies for conquering insomnia form the core of the program.

Kryger, Meir H., Thomas Roth, and William C. Dement, eds. *Principles and Practice of Sleep Medicine*. 4th ed. New York: Saunders/Elsevier, 2005. A comprehensive textbook (1,517 pages) that is the standard reference for the field of sleep medicine. Written with the scholarly audience in mind.

SLEEP APNEA

Disease/Disorder

Also known as: Obstructive sleep apnea

Anatomy or system affected: Respiratory system

Specialties and related fields: Otorhinolaryngology, pulmonary medicine

Definition: A sleep disorder characterized by intermittent cessation of airflow through the upper airway.

Key terms:

apnea: lack of airflow for more than ten seconds

hypopnea: a decrease in airflow greater than 50 percent

oxygenation: the process of getting oxygen into the bloodstream

Causes and Symptoms

Obstructive sleep apnea (OSA) is caused by upper airway obstruction. Soft tissue in the back of the mouth collapses during sleep and temporarily obstructs airflow into the lungs. People with sleep apnea experience many periods of apnea and hypopnea. During such periods, the oxygen level in the bloodstream can decline significantly. Since these episodes happen throughout the night, the sleep pattern is interrupted, and the person will feel sleepy during the day. Symptoms of OSA may include morning headaches, fatigue, difficulty with concentration, and daytime sleepiness (somnolence). The person might doze off while watching television, reading, or, more dangerously, driving. The person may not be aware of apnea or the resultant snoring. However, a sleeping partner will frequently notice these symptoms. It should be noted, however, that snoring alone, without apnea, is very common and does not indicate sleep apnea.

Risk factors for the development of OSA include obesity, a small jaw, a deviated septum of the nose, a big tongue, or enlarged tonsils. Smokers are also at higher risk of developing sleep apnea.

If OSA is left untreated, then medical complications may occur, such as increased risks of hypertension, heart failure, strokes, and pulmonary hypertension. In pulmonary hypertension, the lungs become stiff and fail to provide normal oxygenation. Therefore, it is extremely important to recognize and treat sleep apnea.

The clinical triad of snoring, apneic episodes, and daytime somnolence suggests OSA. A diagnosis can be made by an overnight oximeter or by a formal sleep study (polysomnography). An oximeter is a noninvasive device worn over a finger that measures the oxygen level in the bloodstream. It can be worn overnight at home and is useful for detecting any drop in oxygen level caused by apneic or hypopneic episodes. A formal sleep study requires an overnight observation in a sleep center where multiple monitors record brain waves, heart rate, breathing rate, abdominal muscle movement, and oxygen level. Based on these mea-

surements, an apnea-hypopnea index (AHI), the average number of apneic and hypopneic episodes in one hour, is reported. An AHI of 5 to 20 is considered mild sleep apnea. An AHI of 21 to 50 is moderate, and an AHI of greater than 50 is considered severe.

Treatment and Therapy

Obese individuals with OSA should lose weight, quit smoking, and avoid sedating medications and alcohol because they may impair breathing even further.

Initial OSA treatment consists of a nasal continuous positive airflow pressure (CPAP) machine. A triangular mask fits over the nose and is hooked up to a machine that pushes air under pressure into the upper airway to keep it open. A repeat sleep study using a CPAP machine can determine the level of pressure necessary to prevent apneic and hypopneic episodes. Such a device can be very effective in treating OSA. Side effects may include anxiety from using the mask, nasal congestion, nosebleeds, dry mouth, and irritation of the skin from the mask.

Some individuals require surgical treatment, especially those who cannot tolerate the use of a CPAP machine. The procedure called uvulopalatopharyngoplasty involves surgical removal of excess soft tissue including the tonsils in the

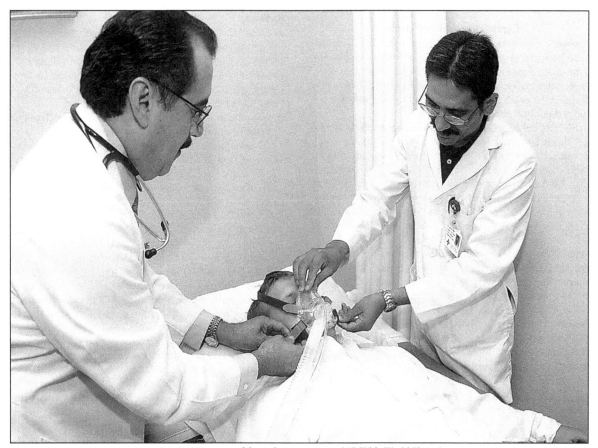

A patient is prepared for a sleep apnea test. (AP/Wide World Photos)

Information on Sleep Apnea

Causes: Upper airway obstruction; risk factors include obesity, small jaw, deviated septum, big tongue, enlarged tonsils, smoking

Symptoms: Periods of apnea and hypopnea during sleep, interrupting sleep pattern and resulting in snoring, daytime sleepiness, morning headaches, fatigue, difficulty with concentration; complications may include hypertension, heart failure, strokes, pulmonary hypertension

Duration: Chronic with acute episodes

Treatments: Lifestyle changes (weight loss, smoking cessation, avoidance of sedating medications and alcohol); continuous positive airflow pressure machine; in severe cases, surgery (removal of excess soft tissue, moving of tongue and jaw forward, tracheostomy)

back of the mouth. Laser-assisted uvulopalatoplasty, in which a laser is used to remove the soft tissue, can be performed in the office. Other surgeries can move the tongue and jaw forward in order to open up the airway in the back of the mouth. For very severe cases of sleep apnea, an opening can be made in the trachea (the windpipe in the upper neck) to bypass the obstruction in the mouth and nose.

Perspective and Prospects

Accounts of what may have been sleep apnea date back to 305 to 30 BCE and involve eleven members from seven generations of the Egyptian royal family. These individuals were obese and were reported by contemporary philosophers and historians to have a tendency toward falling asleep during social and political events.

Sleep apnea has sometimes made an appearance in literature. In the late sixteenth century, symptoms of OSA are suggested in characters created by William Shakespeare for this plays *Richard II* and *Henry IV*. In *Richard II*, the obese Sir John Falstaff snores and sleeps much of the day, interrupted by an apneic breathing pattern. In *Henry IV*, King Henry IV has trouble sleeping, with periods of not breathing in his sleep. Lewis Carroll described a character with sleep apnea in his book *Alice's Adventures in Wonderland* (1865). At the Mad Hatter's tea party, the Dormouse suffers from daytime sleepiness. The other characters try to help the Dormouse by putting him into a tight teapot, which would serve as a positive pressure to assist his breathing.

The famous composer Johannes Brahms (1833-1897) was thought to have developed sleep apnea in his later years when he gained weight. He was known to his friends to snore loudly at night. He also fell asleep during a performance by another famous composer, Franz Liszt.

—*Veronica N. Baptista, M.D.*

See also Apnea; Asphyxiation; Cyanosis; Hypoxia; Lungs; Obesity; Pulmonary diseases; Pulmonary medicine; Pulmonary medicine, pediatric; Respiration; Resuscitation; Sleep; Sleep disorders.

For Further Information:

Goldman, Lee, and Dennis Ausiello, eds. *Cecil Textbook of Medicine*. 23d ed. Philadelphia: Saunders/Elsevier, 2007.

Lavie, Peretz. *Restless Nights: Understanding Snoring and Sleep Apnea*. Translated by Anthony Berris. New Haven, Conn.: Yale University Press, 2003.

Mason, Robert J., et al., eds. *Murray and Nadel's Textbook of Respiratory Medicine*. 5th ed. Philadelphia: Saunders/Elsevier, 2010.

Randerath, Winfried J., Bernd M. Sanner, and Virend K. Somers, eds. *Sleep Apnea: Current Diagnosis and Treatment*. New York: S. Karger, 2006.

Rock, Peter, ed. *Obesity and Sleep Apnea*. Philadelphia: Saunders/Elsevier, 2005.

Terris, David J., and Richard L. Goode, eds. *Surgical Management of Sleep Apnea and Snoring*. Boca Raton, Fla.: Taylor & Francis, 2005.

SLEEP DISORDERS

Disease/Disorder

Anatomy or system affected: Brain, nervous system, psychic-emotional system

Specialties and related fields: Geriatrics and gerontology, neurology, psychiatry, psychology

Definition: Any abnormal pattern of sleep which threatens normal function, including conditions that cause too much as well as too little sleep, and which may be both organic and nonorganic in origin.

Key terms:

circadian rhythm: a physiological process that occurs in twenty-four-hour cycles; examples include the sleep-wake cycle and the maintenance of body temperature

hypersomnia: a group of disorders in which the patient complains of excessive daytime sleepiness or of an inability to stay awake during the day

insomnia: the complaint of poor-quality sleep, which can be caused by a difficulty in falling asleep or a difficulty in maintaining sleep; the most common sleep disorder

narcolepsy: a disorder in which sufferers experience an overwhelming need to sleep during the day; other characteristics include sudden muscle weakness, hallucinations, or sleep paralysis

parasomnias: disorders, occurring primarily in children, in which the patient exhibits abnormal behavior during sleep; examples are sleepwalking and night terrors

periodic leg movements: a disorder in which muscle spasms in the legs partially awaken the sleeper, preventing the proper staging of the sleep cycle

polysomnogram: a collection of physiological information regarding brain waves, breathing, muscle movements, and blood oxygen levels used to diagnose sleep disorders

rapid eye movement (REM) sleep: the period of sleep in which intense brain activity can be measured; the stage of sleep in which dreaming occurs

sleep apnea: a cessation of breathing during sleep, which interrupts the normal sleep cycle; the patient must partially awaken in order to resume breathing

Causes and Symptoms

Sleep is more than the absence of wakefulness. While a person sleeps, the brain continues to be quite active-indeed, this activity is essential for human survival. Brain activity can be measured in sleeping subjects and has been used to classify sleep into stages 1 through 4, where stage 1 is the lightest sleep and stage 4 is the deepest. A sleeper moves from stage 1, through stages 2 and 3, and to stage 4, and then back through stages 2 and 3 to stage 1. This cycle occurs every ninety to one hundred minutes throughout the night. During the latter part of the sleep period, stage 1 sleep is associated with brain activity that is as intense as that seen in waking subjects. During these periods of intense brain activity, rapid eye movements (REMs) are observed, and as a result these periods are referred to as REM sleep, and the other sleep stages are referred to as non-REM sleep. Although the precise function of sleep is still hotly debated in scientific circles, most people can verify from experience that adequate sleep has a major impact on their ability to function effectively and on their emotional stability. For those who suffer from a sleep disorder, life can become a daily struggle; sleep disorders often have severe physical, financial, and social consequences.

Patients who are having difficulty with sleeping usually complain of insomnia, feeling sleepy during the day, or abnormal behaviors during sleep. Sleep disorders have been divided into four broad categories by the Association of Sleep Disorders Centers: the insomnias, or disorders of initiating or maintaining sleep; the hypersomnias, or disorders of excessive sleep; disorders of the sleep-wake cycle; and the parasomnias, or disorders of partial arousal such as sleepwalking and night terrors. Of these, the most common complaint are the insomnias.

Insomnia is a subjective complaint of nonrefreshing sleep. Patients believe that their ability to function during the day is impeded by short or poor-quality sleep. Since most people experience transient insomnia at various times in their lives, chronic insomnia is defined as insomnia lasting longer than three months. Individuals with insomnia have a variety of sleep patterns: Some may require a long period to fall asleep, some wake up after a few hours and cannot fall asleep again, and some may not know that they have awakened briefly hundreds of times during the night. The sleep patterns of the insomniac can vary from night to night, which increases the anxiety of the patient. Electrical monitoring of brain activity shows that most insomniacs have only a slightly reduced total sleep time, with few changes in sleep stages. Physiologically, poor sleepers have been shown to maintain a higher body temperature during sleep than normal sleepers, which may reflect a higher level of arousal. Insomnia is not a disorder in itself; instead, it can be a symptom of a large number of underlying disorders. These can be physiological, psychological, or behavioral in nature, or they can be a normal part of the aging process.

Insomnia can be caused by medical problems that interfere with breathing, such as sleep apnea, in which patients have multiple episodes each night when they stop breathing. A single episode can last ten seconds to two minutes, and in some

Information on Sleep Disorders

Causes: May include sleep apnea, obesity, restless leg syndrome, stress, anxiety, caffeine use, aging process, jet lag, shift work, medications, psychiatric or medical problems
Symptoms: Varies widely; may include irregular snoring, daytime sleepiness, sudden muscle weakness, sleepwalking, night terrors
Duration: Acute to chronic
Treatments: Sleep clinic monitoring, drugs, technical aids, behavior modification

severe cases, up to 50 percent of sleep time can be spent without breathing. Sleep apnea is often seen in obese men and women because of obstruction of the air passage. Clinical signs include irregular snoring and daytime sleepiness. Insomnia can also be caused by neurological problems, muscular problems, or conditions that cause pain. Periodic leg movement can (but does not always) cause multiple awakenings during the night, as can a related disorder called restless leg syndrome, which is characterized by a creeping sensation in the legs. Psychiatric research has demonstrated that insomnia can be a symptom of clinical depression. Surveys have shown that insomniacs have a higher level of stress, tension, and anxiety than normal sleepers. In addition, insomnia can occur when behavioral patterns do not encourage sleep. The use of caffeine or engaging in arousing activities just prior to bedtime can contribute to poor sleep. The normal aging process usually causes a decrease in total sleep time and in stage 1 sleep and an increase in fragmented sleep, resulting in drowsiness and sometimes depression in the elderly.

In addition to all these causes, there are some individuals who complain of insomnia in which no abnormalities can be found. When comparing subjective reports from the patient to sleep recordings in the laboratory, there is a tendency for such insomniacs to report wakefulness even though the sleep recording indicates that the patient is sleeping normally. It appears that there are other sleep abnormalities that contribute to the quality of sleep which remain unknown.

The hypersomnias are defined by excessive daytime sleepiness (EDS) and include the group of patients who are unable to stay awake during the day. Several external circumstances can contribute to EDS, such as jet lag, shift work, medications, or some of the disorders underlying insomnia listed above. In addition, narcolepsy, a central nervous system disorder, is characterized by the overwhelming need to sleep several times a day. These sleep attacks often occur without warning. Narcoleptics can also experience cataplexy, or sudden muscle weakness when in emotionally charged situations that cause anger, laughter, or fear. They may also experience hallucinations when sleep begins or sleep paralysis upon waking that can last for several minutes. Narcolepsy affects 0.05 percent of the population and causes significant hardship to those afflicted. It can pose a danger if the person falls asleep while operating a car or when in a dangerous environment.

The daily cycle of wakefulness followed by a prolonged sleep period is controlled by circadian rhythms. People who travel across time zones or who work rotating shifts are often forced to sleep at a time when their circadian rhythm supports wakefulness and work when their circadian rhythm supports sleep. Other individuals have defects in the mechanisms that regulate circadian rhythms and may experience delayed or advanced sleep phase syndrome in which there is a shift of the normal twenty-four-hour cycle. If they follow their circadian rhythm, these patients will sleep for a normal amount of time; however, the social consequences of retiring at 7:00 P.M. or awakening at noon are prohibitive. Internal desynchronization between the sleep-wake cycle and the closely related circadian temperature cycle can also contribute to poor-quality sleep.

The parasomnias, or disorders of arousal, include sleepwalking and night terrors. Both of these disorders occur predominantly in childhood, although they can be experienced by adults. When brain activity is characterized by an electroencephalograph (EEG), there are elements of both wakefulness and REM sleep, often in the deepest stages (3 and 4). This finding dispels the myth that sleepwalkers are acting out dreams, since dreaming occurs during REM sleep. Sleepwalking activity can vary in length. The person usually has his or her eyes open, can respond verbally, and can move about normally. Sleepwalkers are usually aware of the environment at some level, although their judgment is impaired and they can sometimes injure themselves. Night terrors involve signs of panic such as shrieking, sweats, and frenzied movements and can be distinguished from nightmares, which involve little movement and more extensive memory. Both sleepwalking and night terrors are usually not recalled, and there is little connection between these syndromes and psychiatric disease. Both may be exacerbated by sleep deprivation, stress, fever, or medications.

Treatment and Therapy

One of the difficulties in diagnosing insomnia or one of the other sleep disorders is that there is much individual variability among normal sleepers in sleep needs and amount of sleep logged each night. Therefore, what may be adequate sleep for one person might cause another to report poor sleep. To determine the causes of poor sleep, a person is usually referred to a sleep clinic. There, a detailed history of the problem as well as a description of the patient's sleep habits, lifestyle, and psychological state is recorded. Often, a description of behavior during sleep from someone who shares the bedroom can provide additional important information. Next, a polysomnogram, in which the sleeping patient is monitored with electrodes, is performed so that information on brain waves, breathing, muscle movements, and blood oxygen levels can be obtained. Sometimes this test is administered in the sleep center, and sometimes it is done in the more natural sleep environment of the person's home using ambulatory monitoring devices. From this information, a diagnosis usually can be made and the appropriate therapy determined.

When insomnia is associated with an underlying psychiatric or medical problem, treatment usually begins with the primary problem rather than with the symptom of poor sleep. When the primary problem is solved, the sleep pattern usually returns to normal. Symptomatic treatment of the insomnia itself is provided only when the cause of the sleep disturbance cannot be treated. There are two major approaches: treatments that emphasize the use of drugs or technical aids and treatments that emphasize a change in behavior.

Although over-the-counter aids cannot improve sleep, large numbers of prescription drugs can affect sleep patterns and influence alertness during waking hours. Historically, barbiturates were administered for insomnia, but in 1970, benzodiazepines were introduced; they are now the most commonly prescribed drugs for sleeplessness. These drugs are usually taken about thirty minutes before bedtime, causing drowsiness and thus decreasing the amount of time it takes to fall asleep. Benzodiazepines alter the stages of sleep, decreasing the amount of stage 1 and REM sleep and increasing the amount of stage 2 sleep. The significance of these changes is not understood. When used alone, benzodiazepines are very safe and have few side effects; if they are combined with other drugs, however, there can be a toxic interaction. Although most people can tolerate these drugs and report no daytime grogginess, some impairment of function may exist upon waking. There is strong evidence to suggest that benzodiazepines be used for only a short period of time. With continued use (longer than thirty days), patients usually find that the drug becomes less effective unless the dosage is increased to an unsafe level. When the drug is discontinued, the original symptoms of insomnia usually recur and often a "rebound insomnia," which is even more severe than before the drug treatment began, may be present for a brief period. Because of these limitations, these "sleeping pills" are usually given when an acute but temporary situation exists. To treat insomnia that is caused by periodic leg movements, a muscle relaxant is sometimes used. For patients whose sleep apnea is not resolved by weight reduction, mechanical devices that hold the air passage open during sleep are usually employed. Orthodontic aids or tongue retainers may provide relief, and other patients wear masks that hold the air passage open, providing a continuous airflow during sleep.

Since insomnia is often caused by poor habits that condition the sleeper to remain awake, the problem can sometimes be solved by a simple commitment to avoid naps, reduce caffeine and alcohol intake, eat light meals in the evening, reduce noise in the sleep environment, and establish a regular bedtime. Many insomniacs are so preoccupied with the fear that they will not sleep well that they become tense as bedtime approaches. These fears may sometimes be put to rest by the knowledge that sleep needs vary greatly from individual to individual. In some cases, people may not physiologically require a "normal" amount of sleep but have been convinced that they have a sleep disorder by spouses who do. Another commonly held misperception that contributes to tension is the notion that, once sleep is lost, it can never be recovered. Studies have shown that sleep-deprived humans are able to

In the News:
Side Effects of Ambien and Other Sleep Aids

Ambien (zolpidem) and similar sleep-promoting hypnotic drugs were prescribed more than twenty-six million times in the United States in 2005, and they steadily continue to increase in use. Because so many people now use drugs such as Ambien, hundreds of people have reported unusual side effects with their use. The most publicized reports of Ambien side effects concern "sleepdriving" and "sleepeating," behaviors that are similar to sleepwalking, or somnambulism.

Sleepdriving under the influence of Ambien made headlines on May 4, 2006, when U.S. representative Patrick Kennedy of Rhode Island had a single-car accident at the U.S. Capitol in the early morning. The Capitol Hill Police cited Kennedy for failure to keep a proper lane, unreasonable speed, and failure to give full time and attention to the operation of a vehicle. Considerable attention was given by the media because no sobriety test was given to Kennedy. More than two months earlier, however, at the annual meeting of the American Academy of Forensic Sciences, Laura J. Liddicoat, supervisor of the toxicology section of the Wisconsin State Laboratory of Hygiene, stated, "A 'typical' Ambien driver [has]…a profound loss of balance, so pronounced that the standardized field sobriety tests, such as the walk-and-turn and one-leg-stand, are usually discontinued for fear that the subjects will fall or otherwise harm themselves." Liddicoat reported that Ambien was detected in the blood of 187 impaired drivers tested at her Wisconsin laboratory between 1999 and 2004. In March, 2007, the Food and Drug Administration (FDA) warned that all prescription sleeping pills may sometimes cause sleepdriving and ordered the makers of thirteen drugs to put warnings on their labels: Ambien, butisol sodium, Carbrital, Dalmane, Doral, Halcion, Lunesta, Placidyl, Prosom, Restoril, Rozerem, Seconal, and Sonata. The warning was also to include the threat of life-threatening allergic reaction and severe facial swelling.

When Michael H. Silber, codirector of the Mayo Clinic Sleep Disorder Center, was named president-elect of the American Academy of Sleep Medicine in 2006, he said that he had seen twenty cases of sleepeating in Ambien patients. Sleepeating occurs when a person under the influence of Ambien "awakens," goes to the kitchen, and prepares and eats food. Upon fully awakening, the person retains no memory of the event, but food is missing from the refrigerator. Some of these individuals have gained large amounts of weight—up to one hundred pounds—after taking Ambien. Patients with a history of nocturnal eating disorder, in which they awaken during the night and binge-eat, appear to convert to sleepeating after using Ambien.

—*Anita Baker-Blocker, M.P.H., Ph.D.*

return quickly to normal sleep patterns, and therefore a few nights of poor sleep is no cause for alarm.

For those whose anxiety about sleep persists, techniques that teach people to relax their muscles or meditation to decrease mental activity may reduce this anxiety and promote sleep. Patients who experience better sleep when away from their normal sleeping location may have "learned" to associate the bedroom environment with wakefulness. To overcome this problem, stimulus control is used to try to strengthen the bedroom as a cue for sleep. This method requires that patients use the bedroom only for sleeping and go to bed only when sleepy. Most important, if they do not fall asleep within ten minutes of lying down, they should get up, go into another room, and engage in a mundane activity, coming back to the bedroom only when sleepy. This may be done several times, but the main goal is to associate the bedroom with falling asleep quickly. Regardless of the length of sleep, patients should always get up at the same time and not nap during the day. This regimen may need to be continued for several weeks in order to overcome the previous habit and requires perseverance from the patient; however, the advantage of behavioral therapy lies in the absence of the side effects

caused by medication.

Excessive daytime sleepiness is usually diagnosed by a polysomnogram followed by a Multiple Sleep Latency Test. In this test, patients are allowed to fall asleep several times a day, and if sleep occurs within five minutes multiple times during the day, the diagnosis is positive. EDS is treated in different ways depending on its cause. If the cause is sleep apnea or periodic leg movements, the disorder is handled as described above. In other cases of sleep fragmentation, medication is used to prevent arousal during the night. The excessive daytime sleepiness found in narcoleptics is usually treated with drugs that act as central nervous system stimulants. Other symptoms of narcolepsy are usually treated with antidepressant drugs that suppress REM sleep. Of these, gamma hydroxybutyrate has been shown to be effective and to cause limited side effects. Short naps taken throughout the day seem to prevent many of the symptoms associated with sleep attacks.

Problems with the circadian rhythms of the sleep-wake cycle are usually not helped by medication. Instead, chronotherapy may be effective in resetting the biological clock. Over the course of two weeks, the patient's bedtime is gradually moved forward or backward around the clock until the desired bedtime is reached. Similar effects may be seen using strong light to shift the sleep period.

Perspective and Prospects

The field of sleep research is still in its infancy. For most of history, sleep was not studied at all because it was difficult to characterize the process without interrupting it. Early scientists such as Lucretius, however, made observations and suggested that the motions of sleeping animals might reflect their dreams. In the early nineteenth century, sleep was viewed simply as the absence of waking, and the treatment of lethargic patients with damage to the brain stem led doctors to postulate that this area of the brain had two centers-a waking center and a sleeping center. These two centers were thought to function and communicate with each other using chemical signals. As the field of neurobiology advanced, it became possible to measure the electrical properties of the brain using an electroencephalograph. By the 1930s, numerous studies had shown that the brain remains active during sleep and that the different stages of sleep have different patterns of electrical activity. REM sleep was first observed in 1953 and was linked to dreaming. Additional brain structures in the midbrain and pons were identified that controlled REM and non-REM sleep. An understanding of the neurotransmitters, or chemical substances involved in sleeping and waking, began in the 1960s when it was discovered that neurons in the pons contained serotonin and norepinephrine. Another neurotransmitter, acetylcholine, was found in neurons that were active during REM sleep.

It is only recently that the study of sleep disorders has been recognized as a legitimate pursuit. Most of the sleep disorders mentioned here were discovered in the 1960s and 1970s, and public opinion regarding those who complain of tiredness and fatigue is only gradually shifting from disdain to understanding that there might be a real physiological cause.

This greater acceptance might be due to a growing awareness of the toll of sleep deprivation. The 2000 Omnibus Sleep in America Poll completed by the National Sleep Foundation found that 43 percent of Americans reported that they are sleepy during the day and that the sleepiness was enough to interfere with daily activities. The National Sleep Foundation concluded that the consequences of sleep deprivation are more severe than most people realize and affect metabolism, endocrine functions, immune system function, memory, mood, and reaction time. The average adult sleeps about an hour less than the eight hours per night recommended by sleep experts. During the workweek, only 33 percent of adults get the necessary eight hours of sleep. Forty-three percent of the adults in the survey reported that they often stay up later than they should because of watching television or surfing the Web. Also, 58 percent of adults experienced the symptoms of insomnia, and 15 percent experienced restless leg syndrome. The factors most often identified for disrupting sleep were stress and pain. Fifty-one percent of Americans reported driving while drowsy, and one in five said they have actually fallen asleep at the wheel. Sleep deprivation has also negatively impacted work performance for 27 percent of adults. The list of work-related problems included being late for work, making errors, reductions in quality of work, lower productivity, diminished concentration, and suffering injuries.

Perhaps because of such statistics and a growing public recognition of the dangers of sleep problems, the number of sleep centers and laboratories that are studying sleep and its accompanying disorders has grown tremendously. These sleep centers have been instrumental in elucidating the primary disorders of sleep and in educating the general public concerning sleep management and the safety risks that result from abnormal sleep. Research laboratories are investigating the anatomical, chemical, and physiological mechanisms of sleep and sleep abnormalities. Some of the most interesting areas of current research include genetic studies that determine whether sleep disorders are inherited. There appears to be a significant genetic component to several sleep characteristics, including bedtime, sleep duration, insomnia, narcolepsy, snoring, and sleep apnea. It is expected that, as scientists come to understand more about the nature and

mechanisms of the brain and normal sleep, further understanding of the causes and treatments for sleep disorders will be forthcoming.

—Katherine B. Frederich, Ph.D.

See also Aging; Anxiety; Apnea; Caffeine; Chronobiology; Depression; Hallucinations; Memory loss; Narcolepsy; Nightmares; Paralysis; Phobias; Sleep; Sleep apnea; Sleepwalking; Stress.

For Further Information:

Caldwell, J. Paul. *Sleep: The Complete Guide to Sleep Disorders and a Better Night's Sleep.* Rev. ed. Toronto, Ont.: Firefly Books, 2003. A thorough examination of sleep disorders constitutes a good portion of this book, including such topics as what causes sleep apnea, sleep disorders in children and seniors, what drugs interfere and help with sleep, and treatment guidelines.

Carskadon, Mary A., ed. *Encyclopedia of Sleep and Dreaming.* New York: Macmillan, 1993. An extremely important and comprehensive resource that provides well-written articles on all facets of sleep and sleep disorders.

Dement, William C., and Christopher Vaughan. *The Promise of Sleep.* New York: Delacorte Press, 1999. Over this book's four sections, the authors cover the basics, such as "Daily Sleep Need," "Alternative Therapies," and "Sleeping Pills." Gives sleep, one of human beings' greatest basic needs, the attention it deserves.

Dotto, Lydia. *Losing Sleep: How Your Sleeping Habits Affect Your Life.* New York: William Morrow, 1990. Discusses the physical and social consequences of sleep disorders, with an emphasis on sleep loss. In an easy-to-read style, the author reports on the effects that a modern, frenetic lifestyle has on sleep and its ramifications for waking hours as well.

Hobson, J. Allan. *Sleep.* New York: Scientific American Library, 1995. This beautifully illustrated volume provides an overview of past and contemporary sleep research. The author draws upon neurology and psychology to provide an interdisciplinary approach to his topic.

Montplaisir, Jacques, and Roger Godbout, eds. *Sleep and Biological Rhythms.* New York: Oxford University Press, 1990. This collection of articles highlights the role that biological rhythms play in sleep, wakefulness, and psychological well-being. One chapter is devoted to explaining a possible mechanism for insomnia and another discusses drugs that are used in the treatments for restless leg syndrome and narcolepsy.

National Sleep Foundation. http://www.sleepfounda tion.org. Along with good information about the range of sleep disorders, the site also gives information on sleep tips, children and sleep, and sleep services, among other features.

Reite, Martin, John Ruddy, and Kim E. Nagel, eds. *Concise Guide to Evaluation and Management of Sleep Disorders.* 3d ed. Washington, D.C.: American Psychiatric Press, 2002. Gives an overview of the symptoms and treatments available for different types of sleep disorders.

Walsleben, Joyce A., and Rita Baron-Faust. *A Woman's Guide to Sleep: Guaranteed Solutions for a Good Night's Rest.* New York: Crown, 2001. Writing in an informal, easily comprehensible style, Walsleben, director of the Sleep Disorders Center at New York University School of Medicine, and freelancer Baron-Faust cover nearly every sleep disorder suffered by women.

SLEEPING SICKNESS
Disease/Disorder

Also known as: West African trypanosomiasis, Gambian sleeping sickness, East African trypanosomiasis

Anatomy or system affected: Brain, heart, lymphatic system, nervous system, psychic-emotional system

Specialties and related fields: Environmental health, epidemiology, internal medicine, microbiology, neurology, public health

Definition: A parasitic disease caused by protozoa and transmitted to humans by the bites of infected tsetse flies.

Key terms:

acute: having a sudden, severe onset

blood-brain barrier: an anatomical barrier created by the modification of brain capillaries that prevents certain chemicals in the blood from crossing the capillary walls into the brain tissues

chronic: having a slow onset with progressively more serious symptoms

edema: water retention

parasite: an organism that lives off or in another organism without benefit to the host organism

protozoa: a phylum or subkingdom of mostly unicellular, mobile organisms that includes disease-causing parasites

vector: an organism that transmits a pathogen to another organism

Causes and Symptoms

Sleeping sickness is a vector-transmitted parasitic disease caused by *Trypanosoma*. These protozoa are transmitted to humans by the tsetse fly, genus *Glossina*, which is found only in moist savannas and forests in parts of sub-Saharan Africa. Rarely, transmission can occur from a mother to her unborn child or through blood transfusion or organ transplantation. There are two types of sleeping sickness. West African trypanosomiasis is found in both Central and West Africa. Also called Gambian sleeping sickness, it is caused by *Trypanosoma brucei gambiense*. East African trypanosomiasis is caused by *T. brucei rhodesiense*. Another human form of trypanosomiasis, Chagas' disease, is found in the Western Hemisphere.

Symptoms of the East African type emerge in three stages. Untreated victims of this acute form of the illness may die within weeks or one year later. The first stage begins with the reaction to the tsetse fly's bite. A painful sore, called a chancre, appears about forty-eight hours after the bite and lasts from two to four weeks. It is accompanied by swollen lymph nodes. The second or early stage includes high fever, severe headache, joint pain, and fatigue; symptoms appear in waves, with symptom-free periods that can last up to two weeks. Rashes, swollen lymph nodes, enlargement of the liver and spleen, and edema may also occur. As the disease progresses, weight loss and debilitation increase. Heart involvement may appear early; some patients succumb to heart failure before the parasites invade the central nervous system. In the late stage, which appears within a few weeks to months of the infection, loss of appetite, personality changes, headache, listlessness, and insomnia are seen, along with tremors, slurred speech, and unsteady gait. Uncontrollable drowsiness occurs late in the course of the disease, progressing to coma and finally death, often from secondary infections.

West African sleeping sickness is a chronic illness, though

Information on Sleeping Sickness

Causes: Parasitic infection transmitted by tsetse flies

Symptoms: Painful sore at bite, swollen lymph nodes, high fever, severe headache, joint pain, fatigue, rashes, liver and spleen enlargement, edema, weight loss, debilitation, heart failure; in late stage, appetite loss, listlessness, personality changes, insomnia, tremors, slurred speech, unsteady gait, uncontrollable drowsiness, coma, and death

Duration: A few weeks to months; progressive and fatal if untreated

Treatments: Toxic drugs (suramin, melarsoprol) for both types; nontoxic drug (eflornithine) for West African type

---

just as deadly as the East African variety if left untreated. Instead of three distinct stages, there is usually a long symptom-free period. Often, no chancre appears, and the early stage may be so mild as to be overlooked, although swollen lymph nodes on the back of the neck, called Winterbottom's sign, may be visible. Symptoms gradually appear weeks or years later but are often so subtle that they continue to be ignored. Ironically, the lack of symptoms can be very dangerous for the patient because early treatment of sleeping sickness is critical in avoiding disability or death.

Treatment and Therapy

All but one of the drugs used to treat sleeping sickness are highly toxic. Mortality from drug toxicity can reach 5 to 10 percent. In addition, some of the drugs cannot cross the blood-brain barrier, so they are useless in late-stage illness. The one nontoxic drug, eflornithine, not only crosses the barrier but also is highly effective in treating both early-stage and late-stage West African infection. It is not used for East African illness, however, because it is not consistently effective for that type. In addition, it is expensive and difficult to administer correctly. Thus, for both types of early-stage infection, intravenous suramin (or suramine) is often used after giving a test dose to see how patients will tolerate the drug, with intravenous melarsoprol given for late-stage disease of both types. With treatment, most patients recover. However, irreversible brain damage or death is common when therapy is attempted at the later stage.

Perspective and Prospects

Sleeping sickness is endemic in about one-third of Africa's total land area and threatens more than sixty million people in thirty-six countries. The World Health Organization (WHO) estimates that between 300,000 and 500,000 people are infected annually, despite much smaller numbers of cases reported. In some areas of Angola, the Democratic Republic of Congo, and southern Sudan, sleeping sickness has become the first or second greatest cause of mortality, ahead of human immunodeficiency virus (HIV) or AIDS. Its worst effects are felt in remote, rural areas where health infrastructure is often nonexistent. War, poverty, and lack of education hamper efforts at controlling the disease by shrinking tsetse fly populations through insect abatement programs, treating livestock harboring the parasites, and testing and treating asymptomatic human carriers.

Suramin was discovered in 1921. Pentamidine, sometimes used in treating the early stage of West African sleeping sickness, was discovered in 1941. Melarsoprol, the last arsenic-based medicine still in use, was discovered in 1949. Eflornithine was registered for use in sleeping sickness in 1990 and is approved in the United States for topical use in removing facial hair. None is an ideal drug, and most are difficult to administer under less-than-ideal conditions. Early diagnosis is likewise not easy or inexpensive.

The tragedy is that sleeping sickness had almost disappeared by the early 1960s, but strict screening and control efforts were allowed to lapse, allowing the disease to reestablish itself and become endemic in many areas. In an effort to once again reverse the spread of the disease, WHO has created the Program for Surveillance and Control of African Trypanosomiasis (PSCAT), which unites national programs, nongovernmental organizations, private foundations, universities, regional centers, and donor countries in an effort to reach the common goal of permanent eradication.

—*Sue Tarjan*

See also Bites and stings; Insect-borne diseases; Parasitic diseases; Protozoan diseases; Tropical medicine.

For Further Information:

Dumas, Michel, Bernard Bouteille, and Alain Buguet, eds. *Progress in Human African Trypanosomiasis, Sleeping Sickness*. New York: Springer, 1999.

Hoppe, Kirk Arden. *Lords of the Fly: Sleeping Sickness Control in British East Africa, 1900-1960*. Westport, Conn.: Praeger, 2003.

Lyons, Maryinez. *The Colonial Disease: A Social History of Sleeping Sickness in Northern Zaire, 1900-1940*. New York: Cambridge University Press, 1992.

Ramen, Fred. *Sleeping Sickness and Other Parasitic Tropical Diseases*. New York: Rosen, 2002.

World Health Organization. *Control and Surveillance of African Trypanosomiasis: Report of a WHO Expert Committee*. Geneva: Author, 1998.

SLEEPWALKING

Disease/Disorder

Also known as: Somnambulism

Anatomy or system affected: Brain, musculoskeletal system, nervous system, psychic-emotional system

Specialties and related fields: Neurology, psychology

Definition: Repeated episodes of arising from bed during sleep and walking about, without being conscious of the episodes or remembering them.

Key terms:

electroencephalogram (EEG): a report of brain wave activity, achieved through attaching conductors to the scalp

parasomnia: normal waking behavior appearing within sleep (including sleepwalking) that is not caused by psychiatric illness

sleep stages: the division of sleep into rapid eye movement

(REM) sleep, in which dreaming occurs, and non-REM sleep divided into four progressive levels, the first two being drowsiness and light sleeping and the last two involving deep sleep

Causes and Symptoms

Sleepwalking occurs during stages 3 and 4 of non-REM sleep and most frequently between one to four hours after falling asleep. Electroencephalograms (EEGs) indicate that children usually make a sudden transition into lighter sleep at the end of the first period of deep sleep. Some children do not make the transition rapidly and engage in parasomnia, or a simultaneous functioning of deep sleep and waking known as sleepwalking. An episode lasts from a few minutes to about an hour.

An estimated 40 percent of children ranging from six to sixteen years have reported sleepwalking, with twelve being the age of prevalence. While sleepwalking before the age of four is rare, partial wakings can affect toddlers and infants. Although sleepwalking usually ends around the age of seventeen, it can continue on into the early twenties. It is slightly more common in boys. Although most children sleepwalk infrequently, some sleepwalk frequently and for a period of five years or longer.

Sleepwalkers may have blank, staring faces and remain unresponsive to the attempt of others to communicate with them. They can be awakened only through great effort. Although sometimes sleepwalking children possibly see and walk around objects during their episodes, their behavior may involve leaving the bed violently and running without regard for obstacles. Partial awareness of their environment may be evident in their ability to negotiate hallway turns or objects on the floor. Some children stumble on stairs, crash into glass windows or doors, or walk out of the house into traffic. Serious injuries have occurred. While memory of these episodes is often absent, there may be a dim recall of the need to escape.

During sleepwalking, aggression toward others or toward objects in the vicinity is rare. The activity may be accompanied by sleeptalking that is characterized by poor articulation. Sleepwalkers also have increased incidence of other sleep disorders associated with non-REM sleep, such as night terrors.

Hormones or other biological factors may affect the character of these nighttime arousals. Statistics show that as many as 50 percent of sleepwalking children have close relatives with a history of similar phenomena. Although sleepwalking in very young children is developmental, many older children exhibit both a biological and an emotional predisposition for frequent sleepwalking. Some children who struggle to avoid expressing their feelings develop sleep problems.

Treatment and Therapy

Ensuring adequate sleep and providing a normal schedule are the best ways to treat partial wakings in young children. Although these remedies can help, some parents may have to learn to live with their children's sleepwalking.

Information on Sleepwalking

Causes: Developmental disorder, hormones, hereditary factors

Symptoms: Blank, staring face; unresponsiveness; running without regard for obstacles; poor articulation

Duration: Acute to chronic

Treatments: Monitoring in sleep clinic, drugs, technical aids, behavior modification

---

Understanding what is happening will prevent the parents from intervening by attempting to awaken or question children or returning them to bed immediately. Instead, parents should talk quietly and calmly to sleepwalking children. If the children spontaneously awake after the episode, parents should avoid negative comments and treat the event matter-of-factly. In the case of agitated sleepwalking, restraint merely intensifies and increases the length of time of the episode. One should approach the child only to prevent injury, thus allowing the sleepwalking to run its course.

The child's environment should be made as safe as possible to prevent accidental injury. Floors and stairs should be cleared, and hallways should be lit. For young children, gates may be installed at their bedroom doors or at the stairs, and should they attempt to leave the house, chain locks above their reach should be affixed to the doors.

Richard Ferber, director of the Center for Pediatric Sleep Disorders in Boston and author of *Solve Your Child's Sleep Problems* (1985), believes that older children whose sleepwalking may involve both psychological and inherited factors will benefit from psychotherapy. They may find it very difficult to express their feelings, especially if they are involved in situations in which things are happening outside their control. In the event of changes, losses, or an absence of warmth or love within a family, Ferber believes that children are often quite angry about the circumstances but do not express it outwardly. Psychotherapy or counseling will encourage children to believe that their feelings are not dangerous and will help them express these feelings. Medication is prescribed reluctantly-only to prevent self-injury-and is decreased as the benefits from psychotherapy increase.

Perspective and Prospects

As late as the 1960s, sleepwalking was believed to be a neurotic or hysterical manifestation or an acting out of a dream. Contemporary studies have confirmed that sleepwalking is a sleep disorder that is not caused by psychiatric illness and is not a walking dream state.

Fortunately, sleepwalking can be outgrown by adulthood. Meanwhile, investigations into the nature of sleep, sleep and waking patterns, and biological rhythms continue to provide the best insight into this distressing family problem.

—*Mary Hurd*

See also Nightmares; Psychiatry, child and adolescent; Sleep; Sleep disorders.

For Further Information:

Ferber, Richard. *Solve Your Child's Sleep Problems*. Rev. ed. New York: Simon & Schuster, 2006. This concise volume is illustrated and includes an index.

McMillan, Julia A., et al., eds. *Oski's Pediatrics: Principles and Practice*. 4th ed. Philadelphia: Lippincott Williams & Wilkins, 2006. A text that offers clear descriptions of diseases and illustrations.

Parkes, J. David. *Sleep and Its Disorders*. London: W. B. Saunders, 1985. This volume is aimed at the medical professional and includes illustrations, bibliographical references, and an index.

Reite, Martin, John Ruddy, and Kim E. Nagel, eds. *Concise Guide to Evaluation and Management of Sleep Disorders*. 3d ed. Washington, D.C.: American Psychiatric Press, 2002. Gives an overview of the symptoms and treatments available for different types of sleep disorders.

Sutton, Amy L., ed. *Sleep Disorders Sourcebook: Basic Consumer Health Information About Sleep and Sleep Disorders*. 2d ed. Detroit, Mich.: Omnigraphics, 2005. Covers topics such as insomnia, sleepwalking, sleep apnea, restless leg syndrome, narcolepsy, and their treatment options.

SLIPPED DISK

Disease/Disorder

Also known as: Herniated disk, ruptured disk, prolapsed disk, intervertebral disk displacement

Anatomy or system affected: Arms, back, legs, musculoskeletal system, neck, nerves, nervous system, spine

Specialties and related fields: Exercise physiology, family medicine, occupational health, orthopedics, osteopathic medicine, physical therapy, preventive medicine, sports medicine

Definition: A condition in which the soft, gelatinous center part of an intervertebral disk pushes out through a weakened portion of the disk, often placing pressure on a spinal nerve.

Causes and Symptoms

The spinal column has small bones called vertebrae that connect the skull to the pelvis. It is divided into regions: cervical (neck), thoracic (chest), and lumbar (lower back). Separating

---

Information on Slipped Disk

Causes: Aging process (degeneration and loss of water in disks); trauma (improper lifting, excessive weight, vertical pressure on spine, twisting)

Symptoms: Varies with region affected and with degree of protrusion and nerve compression; may include low back pain (dull ache or sharp, burning sensation), neck pain, numbness, tingling, weakness, loss of bladder or bowel control, muscle spasms

Duration: Chronic

Treatments: Initially bed rest, then activity and physical therapy; medications (pain relievers, anti-inflammatory drugs, muscle relaxants, steroid injections); surgery (diskectomy, microdiskectomy, spinal fusion); chemonucleolysis

---

Slipped Disk

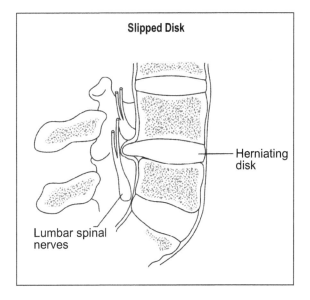

Herniating disk

Lumbar spinal nerves

the vertebrae are intervertebral disks that provide cushioning and shock absorption during movement. The spinal column also has a hollow center portion called the spinal canal, which contains the spinal cord and nerves.

A slipped disk occurs when the outer portion of the intervertebral disk, called the annulus fibrosus, becomes weakened and allows the center portion, called the nucleus pulposus, to push out or leak through. There are various reasons that such bulging may occur. The process of aging is associated with degeneration and loss of water content in the disk material, which causes it to weaken over time, becoming less elastic. Improper lifting, excessive weight or vertical pressure on the spine, twisting, or forceful trauma can also cause a disk to rupture. Slipped disks are most common in the lumbar region, occur less frequently in the cervical region, and occur rarely in the thoracic region.

Symptoms vary with the degree of disk protrusion and nerve compression. In the lumbar region, the main symptom is low back pain, which may be a dull ache or a sharp and burning sensation radiating to the buttocks, legs, and feet (sciatica). Other symptoms include weakness or tingling in one leg and loss of bladder or bowel control. In the cervical region, symptoms include neck pain, often radiating to the shoulder, arm, or hand, and numbness, tingling, or weakness in any of these areas. All cases may include muscle spasms, and pain may be worsened upon movement, coughing, or straining.

Treatment and Therapy

Conservative treatment with initial bed rest, over-the-counter pain relievers, and anti-inflammatory medications is standard for a slipped disk. Muscle relaxants may be prescribed for muscle spasms. After forty-eight hours, activity and physical therapy is recommended. Most patients recover with this regimen. In cases of acute pain, steroid injections in the back may be used to reduce inflammation. Various surgical approaches, involving diskectomy, microdiskectomy, and spinal fusion, exist for patients who do not improve with conservative treatment.

An often effective alternative to surgery is chemonucleoylsis, wherein the orthopedist injects an enzyme that dissolves the ruptured portion of the disk. In 2007, the Food and Drug Administration approved lumbar disc replacement as a treatment option for some types of low back pain. Some clinical researchers believe that as new materials and placement techniques are developed, spinal disc-replacement surgery may become a standard treatment for some types of low back pain.

—*Barbara C. Beattie*

See also Anti-inflammatory drugs; Back pain; Laminectomy and spinal fusion; Numbness and tingling; Orthopedic surgery; Orthopedics; Sciatica; Spinal cord disorders; Spine, vertebrae, and disks.

For Further Information:

Gunzburg, Robert, and Marek Szpalski, eds. *Lumbar Disc Herniation*. Philadelphia: Lippincott Williams & Wilkins, 2002.

Icon Health. *Herniated Disk: A Medical Dictionary, Bibliography, and Annotated Research Guide to Internet References*. San Diego, Calif.: Author, 2004.

"Information from Your Family Doctor: When You Have a Herniated Disk." *American Family Physician* 67, no. 10 (May 15, 2003): 2195-2197.

Porter, Robert S., et al., eds. *The Merck Manual Home Health Handbook*. Whitehouse Station, N.J.: Merck Research Laboratories, 2009.

SMALL INTESTINE

Anatomy

Also known as: Small bowel, small gut

Anatomy or system affected: Abdomen, endocrine system, gastrointestinal system, immune system, intestines, lymphatic system, nervous system

Specialties and related fields: Alternative medicine, biochemistry, endocrinology, gastroenterology, general surgery, histology, immunology, internal medicine, nutrition, oncology, osteopathic medicine, pathology, pediatrics, pharmacology

Definition: The section of the alimentary canal where the digestion of nutrients is completed and nutrients, vitamins, minerals, and fluids are absorbed. It is connected proximally to the stomach and distally to the large intestine and divided into the duodenum, jejunum, and ileum.

Key terms:

absorption: the passage of simple nutrients from the food compartment of the small intestine to the blood

chyme: food in a semifluid state that reaches the small intestine after partial digestion in the stomach

epithelium: tissue made up of tightly adherent cells, usually lining the surfaces of the body and organs

intestinal lumen: the inner cavity of the intestine; represents the food (chyme) compartment

Structure and Functions

In the average adult man, the small intestine is about 6 to 7 meters long, with a diameter of 2.5 to 3.0 centimeters. Its wall contains layers of smooth muscle and nervous tissue, which allow contraction movements and their control; its inner layer consists of absorptive mucosa, rich in blood and lymph vessels that drain into the portal vein. The mucosa is lined with absorptive epithelium.

Chyme from the stomach is mixed in the duodenum with bile and pancreatic enzymes, which neutralize its acidity and digest nutrients to simpler molecules. Proteins are degraded to smaller peptides, fats to fatty acids and glycerol, and carbohydrates to oligosaccharides. Enzymes linked to mucosal cells complete the breakdown, so nutrients can cross the epithelium and reach the bloodstream (absorption).

The mucosa is lined with millions of fingerlike projections (villi), 0.5 to 1.5 millimeters long, surrounded by moatlike invaginations (crypts), and each absorptive cell has microvilli protruding into the lumen. This yields an enormous absorptive area: about 250 meters^2 (the size of a tennis court). The mucosa includes absorptive, secretory, endocrine, and antimicrobial cells and is constantly renewed. Absorptive cells originate in the crypts and migrate up the villus, where they become mature and fully functional. Here they live for about three days, then are shed into the lumen. Nutrients enter the absorptive cells either via specialized cellular transport mechanisms (simple sugars and amino acids) or by simple diffusion (lipids), exit the cell through the basolateral membrane, and diffuse into the villus capillary vessels. Chyme is then moved down the intestinal lumen.

Three layers of smooth muscle allow segmentation contractions that mix the chyme and peristaltic movements that propel it distally. Between meals, periodic contractions called "migrating motor complex" propagate caudally along the small intestine and remove residual debris and bacteria. Intestinal movements are controlled locally by the enteric nervous system (a network of nerve fibers in the intestinal wall) and are modulated by the central nervous system. Hormones secreted by the small intestine regulate gastrointestinal secretion and motility and interact with the nervous system in modulating hunger and satiety.

Disorders and Diseases

Absorption-related disorders are linked to defects of mucosal enzymes or transporters and are usually genetic: In lactose intolerance (not to be confused with milk allergy), the enzyme lactase is lacking or insufficient; in glucose-galactose malabsorption, the mucosal transporter for glucose and galactose is defective. Unabsorbed sugars in the lumen cause gastrointestinal symptoms, which are reversed by avoiding the offending sugars.

Celiac disease is caused by an immunological response to gluten (a protein present in wheat, barley, and rye) and causes chronic intestinal inflammation with flattening of the villi. Mucosal surface and function are restored by a gluten-free diet.

Tropical sprue is a disorder of unknown cause (possibly an infection) in tropical areas, which causes abnormalities in the lining of the small intestine and anemia. It is treated with tetracycline.

In intestinal lymphangiectasia (idiopathic hypoproteinemia) the mucosal lymph vessels are enlarged and obstructed, so that fat and proteins cannot be absorbed. A low-fat, high-protein diet with supplements can help manage the resulting diarrhea. Short bowel syndrome occurs after surgical removal of a large portion of the small intestine. It causes diarrhea and malabsorption and often requires long-term total parenteral nutrition.

Whipple's disease (intestinal lipodystrophy) is a rare bacterial infection that damages the mucosa. It is successfully treated with antibiotics but can recur. Bacterial overgrowth syndrome is the result of slow peristalsis, which allows intestinal bacteria to grow excessively, causing diarrhea and malabsorption. It is treated with antibiotics.

Cancerous tumors in the small intestine are rare. Adenocarcinoma develops in the glandular cells of the mucosa. It requires surgical removal. Noncancerous (benign) tumors can affect different kinds of intestinal cells. Small noncancerous growths may be destroyed by endoscopic surgery.

Parasitic infestations include giardiasis (caused by a unicellular organism, mainly treated with metronidazole) and ascariasis (treated with mebendazole) and tapeworm infections (treatments vary widely), both caused by worms.

Perspective and Prospects

Intestinal ailments and remedies are documented in ancient civilizations. Medieval anatomists maintained the gut could influence the humoral balance of the body. In the seventeenth century, intestines were described as being "made up of tunics, and these from fibers, flesh, parenchyma, veins, arterie, mesenterics, mucous crust, and fat." It was not until the mid-twentieth century that the complexity and importance of the small intestine became apparent. The glucose-transport mechanism was discovered in the 1960s, and molecular mechanisms of absorption have been studied throughout the late century. Recent techniques now allow investigation of their regulation through transporter gene expression. Also, the discovery of a host of intestinal hormones has opened the exploration of the endocrine and neural pathways that regulate nutrient intake, particularly in connection with the problem of obesity control.

—*Donatella M. Casirola, Ph.D.*

See also Abdomen; Abdominal disorders; Appendicitis; Colitis; Colon; Colonoscopy and sigmoidoscopy; Colorectal cancer; Colorectal polyp removal; Colorectal surgery; Constipation; Crohn's disease; Diarrhea; Digestion; Diverticulitis and diverticulosis; Endoscopy; Gastroenterology; Gastroenterology, pediatric; Gastrointestinal disorders; Gastrointestinal system; Internal medicine; Intestinal disorders; Intestines; Irritable bowel syndrome (IBS); Laparoscopy; Nutrition; Obstruction; Peristalsis.

For Further Information:

Badman, Michael K., and Jeffrey S. Flier. "The Gut and Energy Balance: Visceral Allies in the Obesity Wars." *Science* 307 (March 25, 2005): 1909-1914. An article about intestinal hormones and nervous signaling, within a special section about the gut in a scientific magazine.

Levin, Roy J. "Digestion and Absorption of Carbohydrates: From Molecules and Membranes to Humans." *American Journal of*

Clinical Nutrition 59, 3d suppl. (March, 1994): 690S-698S. A scholarly article discussing intestinal sugar absorption in detail.

Sherwood, Lauralee. "The Digestive System." In *Human Physiology: From Cells to Systems.* 7th ed. Belmont, Calif.: Brooks/Cole Cengage Learning, 2010. A chapter in a textbook for undergraduate students, easily accessible to the nonspecialist.

SMALLPOX

Disease/Disorder

Also known as: Variola

Anatomy or system affected: Gastrointestinal system, muscles, skin

Specialties and related fields: Dermatology, environmental health, epidemiology, histology, immunology, pathology, preventive medicine, public health, virology

Definition: An acute, systemic, highly contagious disease caused by a viral infection; there are two forms, the more deadly and feared "classic" smallpox and a milder variety known as alastrim, which has a fatality rate of about 1 percent.

Key terms:

Centers for Disease Control and Prevention (CDC): a government facility, located in Atlanta, that coordinates investigations of disease occurrence in the United States; the CDC stockpiles smallpox vaccine for distribution if and when needed

incubation period: after initial infection, the period of time before any symptoms appear

quarantine: the sequestering of individuals who have been exposed to the infectious phase of a disease until any threat of contagion has passed; with smallpox, this period is seventeen days following last contact with a known case

vaccination: a process whereby live or attentuated virus is introduced into the skin tissue of healthy people in an effort to provide immunity

Causes and Symptoms

The variola virus that causes smallpox is spread through physical contact with infected victims, sometimes through droplets from nasal or oral secretions and sometimes through contact with scabs carried on bedding, towels, clothing, or other fabrics. After exposure to the variola virus, the incubation period ranges from seven to seventeen days. Early symptoms resemble influenza and include headache, muscle ache, and sometimes vomiting. When the characteristic rash appears, the infected person is already very ill. In unvaccinated persons not treated with antiviral medications, between 20 and 40 percent of persons infected with classic smallpox (variola major) would be expected to die. Death most often occurs between the fifth and seventh day of illness.

The initial deep-seated rash characteristic of smallpox develops into lesions, which then follow a progressive sequence of fluid-filled vesicles, then pustules, and finally scabs. Lesions often appear first on the face. In contrast to chickenpox, in which "crops" of lesions appear, all smallpox lesions are at the same phase in development. Smallpox cases become contagious when the first lesions appear and remain so until the

---

Information on Smallpox

Causes: Infection with variola virus

Symptoms: Rash (progressing from lesions to fluid-filled vesicles to pustules to scabs); flulike symptoms (headache, muscle ache, sometimes vomiting); complications may include blindness and sterility

Duration: About one week

Treatments: Prevention through vaccination, antiviral drugs

---

last scab separates from the skin. After the scabs are completely shed, the recovered smallpox victim is left with characteristic pitted scars over large portions of the body. Some victims are rendered permanently blind as a result of contracting smallpox; males may be left sterile. Survival is generally accompanied by lifetime immunity to further infections.

Treatment and Therapy

Smallpox may be prevented through vaccination. Live vaccinia virus is introduced into the skin tissue of healthy people in an effort to provide immunity against smallpox. The vaccinia virus is very similar to the variola virus that causes smallpox. Live vaccinia virus has been used for smallpox vaccinations since the time of Edward Jenner, the Englishman who pioneered vaccination in the late eighteenth century.

There is no treatment known to cure smallpox, although vaccination may be effective in lessening disease severity when administered within four days of exposure. In the 1970s, methisazone (N-methylisatin beta-thiosemicarbazone), trade name Marboran, was believed to afford some protection when administered early in the incubation period. Isolation of victims, burning of all contaminated discharges, concurrent disinfection of the isolation environment, and sterilization of bedclothes and fabrics, combined with quarantine and vaccination of all persons susceptible to smallpox, has been used to contain epidemics in the historical past.

One of the last outbreaks of smallpox in the United States occurred in New York in 1947. To prevent a nationwide outbreak that year, the New York City Board of Health vaccinated about six million people (80 percent of the city's population) within a four-week period.

The final smallpox outbreak in the United States occurred in the Rio Grande Valley of Texas in 1949. The last case reported in the Western Hemisphere was in Brazil in 1971. Prior to the official "last case" of smallpox observed in human populations in October, 1977, international travelers were responsible for introducing the disease into areas where people had not received vaccinations to prevent smallpox. A laboratory accident in England in 1978 caused several cases of smallpox. In 1980, the World Health Organization (WHO) officially declared that smallpox had been eradicated. Major world powers, including the United States and the Soviet Union, maintained stocks of viable smallpox virus for further study.

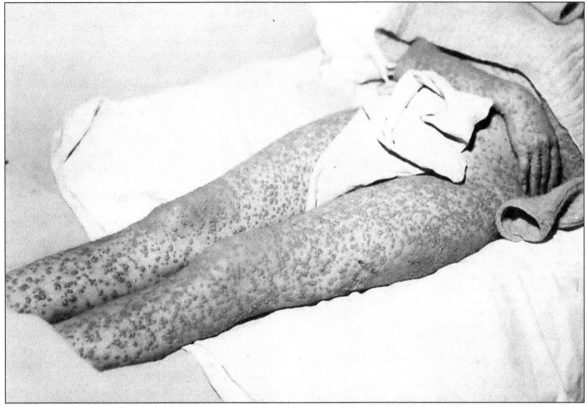

A man suffering from smallpox in the mid-twentieth century. (NMLM)

Perspective and Prospects

There are no natural carriers of smallpox virus; prior to its eradication, it was an endemic urban disease found only in humans, spread as healthy people came into contact with smallpox cases or with fabrics containing scabs shed by smallpox patients.

Following the terrorist attacks on the United States on September 11, 2001, a series of letters containing anthrax spores were sent through the U.S. mail. These letters caused inhalation anthrax, resulting in severe illnesses and several fatalities. Governments became concerned that terrorists would attempt to cause smallpox epidemics. Within the United States, a program was initiated in 2002 to vaccinate "first responder" health professionals in the event of a bioterrorist attack using smallpox. Few people volunteered for vaccination, but among the outwardly healthy people who were vaccinated, two died unexpectedly from cardiovascular disease. News reports of these deaths made people who were offered vaccination less willing to participate, although subsequent study seemed to indicate that these deaths were not directly attributable to receiving the vaccine.

Few Americans, even those now involved in research on the smallpox virus, have ever seen an active case. If a bioterrorist attack using the smallpox virus were to occur, then medical personnel might have some initial difficulty identifying the disease. The general public would need to be informed about the disease in a manner that would avoid widespread panic and ensure that those exposed were immediately vaccinated and quarantined.

By 2004, no medication had been approved to treat smallpox within the United States. Various antiviral agents had been investigated; the drug cidofovir (Vistide), at that time approved only to treat cytomegalovirus retinitis, was identified by several authorities as a potential agent to treat smallpox. Supportive measures that may be used include fever reducers, pain control medication, intravenous rehydration, and antibiotics to control secondary infections.

A single case of smallpox occurring anywhere in the world at any time in the future would constitute an immediate epidemiological emergency. Smallpox is a "Class 1" internationally quarantinable disease; any cases must be reported immediately to local, state, national, and international health authorities.

The resurgence of interest in smallpox at the start of the twenty-first century brought forth many new ideas about all aspects of the disease and its prevention. In 2003, several researchers noted that the increase in numbers of people infected by human immunodeficiency virus (HIV) corresponded with the decline in smallpox vaccinations worldwide. Laboratory research has since determined that prior infection with the vaccinia virus (through vaccination) may confer some immunity to HIV.

—*Anita Baker-Blocker, M.P.H., Ph.D.*

See also Biological and chemical weapons; Childhood infectious diseases; Epidemics and pandemics; Immunization and vaccination; Monkeypox; Rashes; Viral infections.

For Further Information:

Baciu, Alina, et al., eds. *The Smallpox Vaccination Program: Public Health in an Age of Terrorism*. Washington, D.C.: National Academies Press, 2005. A report from the Committee on Smallpox Vaccination Program Implementation from the Board on Health Promotion and Disease Prevention.

Benenson, Abram S., ed. *Control of Communicable Diseases in Man*. 16th ed. New York: American Public Health Association, 1995. This handbook, written after the last reported case of smallpox in the Western Hemisphere but before smallpox was declared eradicated, contains a complete description of methods of control, including preventive measures; the control of patients, contacts, and immediate environment; epidemic measures; and international measures.

Frieden, T., et al. "Cardiac Deaths After a Mass Smallpox Vaccination Campaign-New York City, 1947." *Morbidity and Mortality Weekly Report* 52, no. 39 (October 3, 2003): 933-936. Briefly reviews the history of the New York City 1947 epidemiological emergency and the Board of Health response. According to the New York City data, no unexpected increase in cardiovascular mortality occurred as a result of mass vaccination.

Glynn, Ian, and Jenifer Glynn. *The Life and Death of Smallpox*. New York: Cambridge University Press, 2004. Takes a historical view of the disease.

Heymann, David L., ed. *Control of Communicable Diseases Manual*. 19th ed. Washington, D.C.: American Public Health Association, 2008. An official report of the American Public Health Association. Includes an index.

SMELL

Biology

Anatomy or system affected: Nervous system, nose

Specialties and related fields: Neurology, otorhinolaryngology

Definition: One of the five special senses; chemicals interact with receptor sites in specialized structures of the nasal cavity, and the resulting nerve impulses are classified as certain kinds of odor.

Key terms:

anosmia: a loss of the ability to detect aromas; general anosmia describes a lost ability to detect or identify any odors, while specific anosmia describes a lost ability to detect or identify a specific class of odors

Bowman's glands: one of three sources of the olfactory mucus that moistens the membranes of the olfactory center, thereby allowing odoriferous molecules to adhere to the olfactory hairs; glands that are located between olfactory supporting cells

chemoreceptors: in olfaction, specific structures in the nasal cavity upon which odoriferous, gaseous molecules adhere; this attachment induces a neural response that the brain interprets as smell

olfaction: the sense of smell; a process in which nerve impulses caused by chemicals interacting with chemoreceptors in the nose arrive in the olfactory center of the brain and are classified as certain kinds of odor

olfactory adaptation: the relatively quick response to and subsequent fatigue of the sense of smell that allows the presence of odoriferous chemicals to be recognized quickly and then become less and less noticed until they are soon ignored

olfactory bulb: an extension of the brain located below the frontal lobes of the cerebrum and above the ethmoid bone (extending back from the nose); one of a pair of gray masses into which the olfactory nerves terminate, thus serving as the first synaptic sites in olfactory neural pathways

olfactory epithelium: the surface covering of the olfactory region of the nasal cavity from which tiny, hairlike projections monitor the external world; a mucus-coated layer made of olfactory cells, supporting cells, and basal cells

olfactory hairs: the small, cilia-like projections extending from olfactory knobs into the conchae of the nasal cavity; at these projection sites, odoriferous molecules may interact chemically with the hairs to cause a nervous impulse to be sent to the brain

olfactory knobs: unmyelinated, tiny, rounded nerve endings of the sensory cells found at the mucus-coated olfactory membrane; each knob has five to eight extensions, called olfactory hairs, that branch out into the nasal cavity and monitor the environment

olfactory receptor cells: bipolar nerve cells surrounded by supporting cells in the olfactory epithelium; each cell body has one dendrite that terminates as an olfactory knob with hairlike projections

olfactory tract: the canal running posteriorly from the nose into the primary olfactory area of the cerebral cortex of the brain; the tract that houses large, myelinated olfactory nerves

Structure and Functions

Smell, one of the five special senses, plays an important role in both conscious and subconscious thought. While the loss of smell (anosmia) is troublesome, in isolation it is not a life-threatening problem. Nevertheless, anosmia is frequently an indication of an underlying pathology in either the olfactory or related organs; some of these pathologies may be life-threatening.

Of the special senses-gustation (taste), sight, olfaction (smell), audition (hearing), and equilibrium (balance and direction)-smell is the most primitive. As such, the organs that compose the olfactory system in humans are essentially identical to those found in other animals, including lampreys, cats, or dogs. The olfactory region of the nose is a very discriminating organ. Humans are able to classify smells according to at least seven agreed upon, although vague, classifications of primary odors: camphorlike, musky, floral, minty, ethereal, pungent, and putrid. Other categories that have been suggested are woody, spicy, and burned.

Within each odor category, the olfactory nerves and the brain are able to identify specific aromas with precision. For example, within the category of pungent, smells of onion, garlic, or skunk spray are easily discerned as similar, yet different, odors. Within the floral category, the human mind can readily distinguish among rose, lavender, and gardenia. The human olfactory sense can even distinguish between "left-handed" or "right-handed" molecules. In other words, the olfactory system can identify mirror-image molecules, in which one molecule is the spatial reverse of the other. An example is the substance carvone: When a person sniffs one form of carvone, the smell is spearmint; a sniff of the other form of carvone smells of caraway seed.

While studies of the anatomy and physiology of olfaction have not been finalized, the most accepted model of olfaction depends on the concept of odoriferous molecules attaching to olfactory receptor sites; the size and shape of both the odor molecules and the receptor sites are essential elements in currently adopted theories and descriptions of the mechanics of olfaction. Molecules of an odor-emitting substance chemically interact at receptor sites within specialized structures of the nasal cavity. The olfactory dendrites that are in contact with the external environment are directly linked to the neural centers of the brain. The olfactory tract connects these nerves directly to the hypothalamus region of the brain, which is associated with basic instinctual responses including fight-or-flight cues, food intake, or sexual curiosity and drive. This direct link to the brain causes a rapid and powerful response in animals to odor stimuli.

Because there is no physical barrier to protect olfactory receptors from the outside world, these nerve endings have a certain vulnerability to harm or damage. Olfactory nerves constantly regenerate in about a twenty-eight-day cycle; they are the only nerves that are capable of readily regenerating themselves and returning to full function. Nevertheless, it is estimated that about 1 percent of all olfactory receptors in an individual die each year because of externally induced damage and general wear. Therefore, the sense of smell becomes less sensitive in older adults, which can minimize or repress the desire to eat and result in malnutrition.

The nasal cavity has two roles, one associated with respiration and the other with the sense of smell. The region that is dedicated to olfaction is small and evenly divided between the two septa of the nose. Within each nostril are folds called conchae. Humans have three conchae pairs-lower, middle, and upper. The specialized sensing structures for olfaction are found inside the middle and upper conchae. It is currently believed that olfactory receptors are regions of specialized molecular architecture located on cilia-like fibers called olfactory hairs. Olfactory hairs are extensions, or branches, of the olfactory sensing cells. The hairs, which are actually made of microfilaments, are dispersed over the surface of the

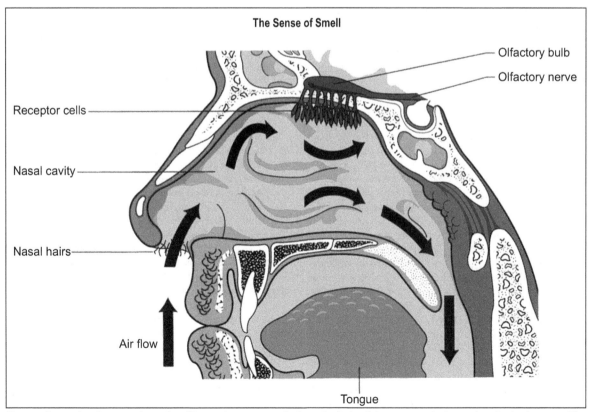

Humans detect odors by a complex series of interactions—some only theoretical—involving receptors in the nasal cavity that interact with odor molecules to send nerve impulses to the brain through the olfactory nerve.

olfactory sensing region of the nasal cavity.

While the size of the olfactory region of the nasal cavity is small (about the size of a dime), its surface area is comparatively large because of the many olfactory hairs coating the surface, or epithelium, of the olfactory cleft. It is estimated that humans have between 10 and 40 million olfactory receptors. The number of receptor hairs varies among species; dogs have about 1 million receptors on their olfactory cleft alone and are far more sensitive to specific odors than are humans. This feature explains why dogs can be trained for hunting game, finding missing persons, and locating drugs or explosives. A person can smell a pot of soup cooking and know it is soup, but a dog smelling the same pot of soup smells each ingredient of the soup, not the scent of the mixture. Nevertheless, among the senses, the sense of smell in humans is second only to vision in terms of number of receptors per unit of surface area.

The olfactory hairs are surrounded by a thick, brown-colored mucus and are partially covered and partially exposed. Thus, the mucosal lining on the epithelium of the olfactory region is a thin and poor protective barrier for the specialized structures that it coats. The mucus on the olfactory epithelium has three structures of origin: Bowman's glands, the goblet cells of the respiratory regions of the nose, and the supporting cells of the olfactory epithelium. Most of the mucus around the olfactory hairs is secreted from Bowman's glands, and only the Bowman's secretions contain the brown pigment that colors the mucus. It is known that, in other species, pigment is connected to olfactory ability; for example, albino pigs, which are lacking all pigments, are unable to smell toxic plants and often die from ingesting native plants that are poisonous to their species. The true significance of the brown pigment in humans, however, remains unclear.

The significance of the olfactory mucus itself is not in question. Odoriferous molecules must be trapped by the mucus so that they can travel to chemoreceptor sites on the olfactory hairs. The interaction between the odor molecules and the chemoreceptors of the olfactory hairs requires a mutual attraction, originating from small electrostatic forces. The shape, size, and polarity or nonpolarity of molecules causing odor are important factors in the creation of a smell stimulus.

From the olfactory hairs in the membrane structure, the odor molecules travel through the cribriform plate and into the olfactory tract, which leads directly to the hypothalamus in the brain. The olfactory hairs extend from the olfactory knobs, unexposed sensory cell endings completely covered by brown mucus. Five to eight hairs extend from each knob; electron micrographs show that the hairs are actually dendrites extending from the cell body into the external environment, while the axons of the cells carry nerve impulses toward the brain.

The sensory cells are found about midway in the olfactory epithelium. Other cells in the epithelium are the supporting cells and the basal cells. The supporting cells provide a scaffolding for the sensory cells and also contribute fluids to the mucus layer. Basal cells are able to assist in the replenishment of receptor cells.

The cribriform plate, often described as a wafer-thin structure, is an important separation point between unmyelinated sensory nerves, which are in touch with the environment, and the myelinated nerves that direct the tiny electrical impulses of smell to the brain. Myelinated olfactory nerves are large and function with great speed and efficiency in comparison to the unmyelinated sensory cells. Thus, the original nerve signal prompted by an odoriferous molecule is slow, but this time is more than recovered in the myelinated nerve fibers. Working together, the unmyelinated and myelinated nerve bundles detect, transmit, and deliver nerve impulses of smell in fractions of a second, aided by the relatively short path between the nasal cavity and the hypothalamus.

The hypothalamus is located under the thalamus in the brain. It is the center into which nerve impulses originating at the sensory organs of sound, taste, smell, and the somatic senses are delivered. The activity of this portion of the brain is closely linked to the activity of the pituitary gland. This association is important in the sense of smell and sexual maturation, which is triggered by hormones released by the hypothalamus. In addition to these attributes, the hypothalamus is essential to regulating the autonomic nervous system, body temperature, and food intake.

Disorders and Diseases

Loss of the ability to sense all smells is called anosmia. Hyposmia (a decrease of smell function), dysosmia (an altered sense of smell), and anosmia can manifest themselves in numerous ways.

Most people are well acquainted with the inability to smell during a heavy cold. This condition is a temporary one caused by the presence of excessive mucus. The presence of a cold virus causes the respiratory region of the nose to respond by producing excessive volumes of cleansing mucus from goblet cells. Unfortunately, there tends to be so much mucus that the olfactory region becomes flooded; instead of swimming in mucus, the olfactory hairs are drowning. A thick coating over the hairs prevents odoriferous molecules from reaching the chemoreceptors. The sense of smell is lost until partial recovery decreases the mucus levels and once again allows the olfactory hairs to be partially exposed to the exterior world. The ability to sense odors fully returns once recovery from the head cold is complete.

Because it is uncommon to lose the ability to smell all odors, true anosmia is a rare condition. Furthermore, anosmia is seldom a problem found in isolation. Often there are simultaneously occurring symptoms such as a loss of taste (gustatory) function, undeveloped ovaries and testes, or head injury. In diagnosing possible causes of anosmia or dysosmia, a physician must obtain a complete medical history and perform a thorough physical exam. Special attention is given to the nasal cavity, the head and neck area, and, perhaps surprisingly, to genital maturation and function. Smell function is measured by passing vials containing increasing concentrations of an odoriferous chemical under a patient's nose until a scent can be detected. It is also important to assess whether the patient can properly identify the smell; if not, further studies must be done.

Olfactory problems can originate in one of the three structures that are involved in olfaction: in the sensory receptors, which convert chemical signals arising from odor molecules into electrical impulses; in the sensory nerve cells, which transmit these electrical impulses to the brain; and in the brain, which interprets the incoming electrical signals.

Abnormalities in the nasal cavity that can modify or destroy olfaction may include nasal polyps, a tumor located in an olfactory bulb, or allergic rhinitis (irritated and swollen membranes of the nose). Other olfactory maladies may be of an indirect origin, such as nutritional abnormalities or the presence of a toxic trace metal. Endocrine imbalances can be particularly pertinent in olfaction function.

An example of an endocrine imbalance that can influence the olfactory sense is seen in the cooperative workings of the hypothalamus and the pituitary gland. The hypothalamus receives impulses from olfactory nerves. It also lies just above the major endocrine gland, the pituitary gland. The pituitary gland receives regulating chemicals from the hypothalamus that either stimulate or inhibit the anterior portion of the gland. The anterior region of the pituitary gland monitors the levels of steroid hormones circulating in the body. Steroid hormones are essential to complete sexual maturation in both males and females. A congenital defect that affects both the nose and sexual maturation is Demorsier's olfactogenital dysplasia. Individuals with this malady are anosmic as a result of underdeveloped olfactory lobes. Low levels of gonadotropic hormones are also found in afflicted persons, resulting in undeveloped ovaries or testes. A somewhat similar (but not congenital) problem can be seen in Kohn's syndrome. In this syndrome, the ovaries or testes are underdeveloped and the olfactory nerves are abnormally formed, halting the sense of smell.

Olfaction is believed to play a role in the timely onset of sexual maturation in puberty. It seems that both male and female pheromones, oily scents that subconsciously cause sexual excitement in a species, can assist in or accelerate the events of sexual maturation. Although researchers are still exploring the role of pheromones in the human species, it appears that smell is relevant to the onset of menstruation in pubescent girls. Scents also contribute to sexual arousal in males.

An altered sense of smell can occur with pregnancy because of the resulting changes in hormone levels. For some pregnant women, formerly pleasant aromas may become repugnant, sometimes contributing to the feeling of nausea that some pregnant women experience. In addition, the increased mucus production that occurs with pregnancy works to block full smell function.

Brain tumors or lesions can sometimes account for anosmia, hyposmia, or dysosmia. Head injury is another possible cause because nerves or the hypothalamus itself can be crushed or otherwise damaged. Tumors, lesions, and neural damage can be detected using positron emission tomography (PET) scanning or magnetic resonance imaging (MRI). Some neurological diseases may be considered when diagnosing these olfactory disorders since the sense of smell requires only organs found in the nervous system.

Treatment of olfactory malfunctions varies greatly depending on the origin of the problem. Surgery may be needed to remove tumors. Allergies may be treated by shots; corticosteroids may be used to prevent the inflammation of nasal mucous membranes. Drugs may be administered to either inhibit or activate nerve conduction. Treatment often results in the recovery of olfaction, but not in all cases.

Perspective and Prospects

The sense of smell has been recognized as one of the most primitive attributes of the human species, and it once held a high position in the hierarchy of skills required for species survival. Olfaction has long been a topic of intrigue in intellectual circles. The Greek philosopher Democritus of Abdera (384-322 BCE) proposed his theory of the atom in a time when modern science and scientific methods did not exist. Democritus incorporated his description of atoms into an explanation of olfaction. He presumed that the sense of smell in humans resulted from some kind of connection that formed when atoms of odor-emitting substances entered the nose. Different odor sensations, he proposed, would result from differences in the texture and shape of these atoms. The anatomy of the nose and brain was not considered in his philosophy. Democritus's idea of atoms was largely rejected in Greek circles of thought, however, and the concept of atoms combining to form molecules would not appear for hundreds of centuries. Modern understanding of the sense of smell is largely a more advanced, more informed, and more technical description of the very ideas imagined by this great Greek philosopher.

Another Greek contemplating the subject of smell was the physician Galen of Pergamum (129-c. 199 CE), who proposed an insightful description of the neuroanatomy of olfaction which also proved to be validated, with some alterations, centuries later. Whether he accepted the notion of atoms or not, Galen believed that particles actually tunneled into what are now called olfactory bulbs, thereby causing an odor to be detected. Galen also believed that these olfactory bulbs were extensions connected directly to the brain. Living in an era when microscopes and the scientific method did not exist, Galen could only describe what he saw with the unaided eye and reason intuitively. It is fascinating, therefore, to learn that his belief that the olfactory bulbs were extensions of the brain has been proven correct.

As the most primitive, and thus less evolved, of the five special senses, smell is associated with basic instincts, reactions or responses to external stimuli that aid an individual organism. Smell influences instincts of aggression when odors are released in fighting or battle through sweat and perhaps blood. These odors may inspire fight-or-flight responses in the brain and body. Social groups, such as a street gang, a group of soldiers, or a den of lions, can learn to recognize the scent (or the absence of scent) of its members in training or other group activities, helping to identify safe and unsafe groups in darkness or battle when other cues may be masked.

Thus, while it is a subtle form of recognition often registered in the subconscious, smell apparently plays a role in modern survival tactics as well.

Another basic instinct that utilizes the sense of smell is the so-called mothering instinct. For example, new mothers are better able to identify their newborns by scent than by sight only hours after delivery. This sense seems adaptively helpful to the exhausted mother-who may have been in labor for days and is likely to be suffering from general exhaustion and diminished energy-in locating and feeding her baby. In a primitive human culture, this ability would help mothers identify babies if a flight from danger or a search for food or water caused a temporary separation of the mother-child pair. In addition, a nursing baby is guided to the mother's nipple by the scent released from the sweat glands surrounding the nipples.

Mate selection is believed to be linked to scents and olfactory appeal. There is some evidence that even the most heavily perfumed person of modern society emits pheromones that are sexually alluring to some and repulsive to others. This allure or repulsion seems to occur in the subconscious mind, or the limbic region of the brain.

On a more conscious level, the sense of smell is sometimes useful as a warning of a health problem; thus odors can be helpful in either describing or diagnosing a disease. For example, some people with epilepsy, days or only minutes before the onset of an epileptic seizure, have olfactory hallucinations-they smell odors in the absence of any stimulating molecules. The odor is usually described as either a scent of decay, as at a fish market, or a chemical, such as ether or petroleum. The sweet smell of acetone on a person's breath can indicate a diabetic who is in danger of coma, or who is already in a coma and cannot ask for help. Vincent's angina can be suspected if a foul breath odor is present, while diphtheria causes a sweet scent.

Because of the unique regenerative capacity of the olfactory neurons, neurologists and other researchers are actively attempting to understand the mechanisms that allow these nerves to be so efficient and effective in nerve regeneration. Such research may have an impact upon the understanding and treatment of a variety of neurological disorders that are not directly affiliated with olfaction.

—Mary C. Fields, M.D.

See also Allergies; Anosmia; Antihistamines; Aromatherapy; Common cold; Decongestants; Nasal polyp removal; Nasopharyngeal disorders; Otorhinolaryngology; Polyps; Respiration; Rhinoplasty and submucous resection; Sense organs; Sinusitis; Taste.

For Further Information:

Engen, Trygg. *The Perception of Odors.* New York: Academic Press, 1982. Designed for the beginner, this text describes the anatomy, physiology, and psychology behind olfaction. Provides detailed explanations of the classification of odors, odor theories, and the tests that are used to assess olfactory function.

Finger, Thomas E., Wayne L. Silver, and Diego Restrepo, eds. *Neurobiology of Taste and Smell.* 2d ed. New York: Wiley-Liss, 2000. Introduces the study of taste and smell, focusing on the way chemical senses work, with coverage ranging from microorganisms to humans and from genetics to behavior.

Møller, Aage R. *Sensory Systems: Anatomy, Physiology, and Pathophysiology.* Boston: Academic Press, 2003. An excellent text that describes how human sensory systems function, with comparisons of the five senses and detailed descriptions of the functions of each of them. Also covers how sensory information is processed in the brain to provide the basis for communication and for the perception of one's surroundings.

Schmidt, Robert F., ed. *Fundamentals of Sensory Physiology.* Translated by Marguerite A. Biedermann-Thorson. Rev. 3d ed. Berlin: Springer, 1986. Chapter 9, "Physiology of Olfaction," addresses the organization of the olfactory system and its relevant connections in the brain.

Shier, David N., Jackie L. Butler, and Ricki Lewis. *Hole's Essentials of Human Anatomy and Physiology.* 10th ed. Boston: McGraw-Hill, 2009. Covers the sense of smell and related topics, such as the anatomy and organization of the brain and nervous system. Although this academic textbook is more advanced than an introductory biology book, its definitions and excellent diagrams and drawings assists readers at all levels.

Tortora, Gerard J., and Bryan Derrickson. *Principles of Anatomy and Physiology.* 12th ed. Hoboken, N.J.: John Wiley & Sons, 2009. This text offers a brief treatment of the topic of smell, but perusal of the book will allow the reader to place this special sense within the context of the whole human anatomy.

Wolfe, Jeremy M., et al. *Sensation and Perception.* 2d ed. Sunderland, Mass.: Sinauer, 2009. Addresses all five senses. Includes a detailed section on olfaction.

SMOKING

Disease/Disorder

Anatomy or system affected: Circulatory system, respiratory, throat, gastrointestinal, bladder

Specialties and related fields: Oncology, pulmonary medicine, vascular medicine, addiction medicine

Definition: The inhalation of tobacco in the form of cigarettes or cigars, which poses important health risks; those risks can be significantly decreased by smoking cessation, even in older age.

Causes and Effects

Cigarette smoking has long been known to have adverse effects. Smokers get more wrinkles than nonsmokers and brown/black discoloration of teeth so they tend to look older than their chronological age. They also are more likely to develop worsening of age-related problems such as gum disease, loss of teeth, and alteration in sense of smell and taste. Loss of teeth leads to difficulty chewing, which in turn leads to difficulties with digestion. Most people who lose teeth eventually develop loss of the bone that should support their teeth, making it increasingly difficult to fit dentures.

Smokers are ten times more likely to get lung cancer than nonsmokers. Lung cancer is now the number one cause of cancer death in women, as well as in men. In addition to lung cancer, smokers have a higher incidence of cancers of the head and neck, esophagus, colon, rectum, kidney, bladder, and cervix. Smokers are three to six times more likely to have a heart attack than are nonsmokers. In older people, the major risk factor for disease of the coronary arteries is hypertension, but smoking is still significant, especially when combined with other risk factors for heart disease, such as diabetes or high choles-

Information on Smoking

Causes: Addictive properties of drug

Symptoms: Increased incidence of lung cancer, pancreatic cancer, oral cancer, esophageal cancer, bladder cancer, emphysema, and chronic bronchitis; increased risk of gum disease; impaired sense of smell and taste; tooth loss; difficulty with digestion including acid reflux; decreased muscle strength, agility, coordination, gait, and balance; wrinkles

Duration: Often chronic

Treatments: Support groups, hypnosis, increased exercise; use of nicotine replacement systems (patches, gum), medications, electronic cigarettes

terol. Smoking and diabetes are also the two most important risk factors for diseases of the veins and arteries of the lower leg. Those who continue to smoke once these diseases develop are much more likely to require limb amputation than those who quit. Smokers may develop chronic obstructive pulmonary disease (COPD), which includes emphysema and chronic bronchitis, and are eighteen times more likely than nonsmokers to die of diseases of the lungs other than cancer. Older smokers also show a decrease in muscle strength, agility, coordination, gait, and balance. The changes in these areas make them seem older than their actual age.

Smoking has long been thought to be associated with peptic ulcer disease. In addition, smoking makes the symptoms of many diseases worsen or increases the risk of complications in patients with allergies, diabetes, hypertension, and vascular disease. Male smokers are at greater risk of experiencing sexual impotence. Female smokers tend to experience an earlier menopause, bone loss called osteoporosis and are therefore at increased risk for hip fracture than nonsmokers. Smokers are more likely to develop glaucoma than nonsmokers. (Studies completed in 1996 indicated an increased risk with smoking for macular degeneration, the leading cause of blindness in older adults. The evidence is mixed on smoking and Alzheimer's disease, but a 1998 study contradicted earlier work and found that the risk is greater in smokers than in nonsmokers.) Finally, smokers are at greater risk of death or injury caused by cigarette-related fires.

Cigarette smoking tends to speed up the processes in the liver for breaking down, using, and eliminating medications, both nonprescription and prescription. This means that medications may not perform as expected in the body. Smokers may need to take medications more frequently or in greater doses than nonsmokers, so it is important for health care providers to know that a person smokes. The drugs known to be affected by smoking include sedatives, narcotic and synthetic narcotic painkillers, certain antidepressants, anticoagulant medications, asthma medications, and certain blood pressure medications. These changes are of particular concern in the older population for a number of reasons. First, older people (whether smokers or nonsmokers) tend to need more medications than younger people. With each additional drug, the risk of serious drug interaction and other adverse effects in-

creases. Second, changes in body composition and function that alter the metabolism of drugs come with age, making medication use somewhat riskier in older persons, in terms of adverse effects and complications. The additional changes associated with smoking increase these risks significantly.

The dangers of passive smoking are well documented. More than fifty compounds in secondhand smoke are identified as carcinogens in humans. The effects seem to be more harmful in children than in adults, but adults who are affected are at increased risk for cancer, heart disease, noncancerous lung diseases, and allergies.

Treatment and Therapy

Numerous studies have shown that smoking cessation has health benefits in as little as one year, such as reducing the risk of heart attack and coronary artery disease. Within two years of smoking cessation, the risks of stroke and diseases of the blood vessels in the lower leg are reduced as well. Even though chronic lung disease is not reversible, those who quit smoking slow the decline in lung function considerably. Risks for cancers also decrease significantly with smoking cessation and are similar to the cancer risk for nonsmokers in ten to thirteen years. These findings indicate that it is worthwhile even for older people to give up smoking. An average forty-year-old gains approximately nine additional years of life by quitting smoking, and a sixty-year-old gains approximately three additional years.

Because smoking is an addiction, it may be difficult to quit, particularly after years of cigarette use. Most smokers have to stop several times before quitting permanently. Setting a quit date, attending support group meetings, taking it one day at a time, undergoing hypnosis, making a contract with a friend or a health care provider, substituting carrot sticks for cigarettes, increasing exercise (particularly swimming), and breathing deeply all seem to be helpful techniques. Nicotine replacement systems are available in the United States on a nonprescription

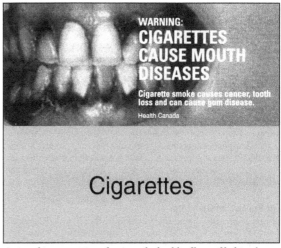

Antismoking campaigns focus on the health effects of habitual use, such as gum disease. (AP/Wide World Photos)

basis, but it is important for older people, particularly those with health problems or who are taking multiple medications, to consult a health care professional prior to using them. It is also important that anyone using these aids stop smoking completely. Continuing to smoke while using nicotine replacement could potentially cause toxicity, and it decreases the success of cessation attempts, since the behavior of smoking is still present. Two non-nicotine-containing medications are available by prescription for smoking cessation: bupropion SR (Wellbutrin, Zyban) and varenicline (Chantix). Both medications significantly increase the success rates at the end of treatment and one year later. The mechanism of action is by stimulating chemical messengers in the brain that are affected by nicotine.

Electronic cigarettes are used as a tool for smoking cessation. It is a battery-powered device that can deliver nicotine without the combustion or smoke. Use and awareness of e-cigarettes has dramatically increased over the past few years. Studies have suggested that physical and behavioral stimuli, such as holding a cigarette, can reduce the craving to smoke. Recent findings suggest that individuals who used e-cigarettes reduced the number of tobacco cigarettes they smoked. These findings suggest that the e-cigarettes may be an important tool for reducing the harm that tobacco cigarettes can cause. Unfortunately, the benefits and risks of electronic cigarette as of 2013 are still uncertain. More studies are needed for further investigation of their safety and efficacy.

Perspective and Prospects

Smoking is the main avoidable cause of death in the United States and many other developed nations. More than 10 percent of North Americans over the age of sixty-five smoke cigarettes This put them, and those with whom they live, at risk for significant health problems. These risks appear to increase both with age and with the number of years of smoking. After World War II, more women began smoking. Because the diseases related to smoking usually take years to develop, it was only in the last part of the twentieth century that rates of smoking-related disease among women began to approach those of men. Research indicates that smoking cessation appears to be beneficial, even in a person who has smoked for many years.

—Rebecca Lovell Scott, Ph.D., PA-C;
updated by Bianca Garcia, M.D.,
and Luzanna Plancarte, M.D.

See also Addiction; Amputation; Bronchitis; Caffeine; Cancer; Carcinogens; Chronic obstructive pulmonary disease (COPD); Dental diseases; Diabetes mellitus; Emphysema; Eyes; Fracture and dislocation; Gingivitis; Glaucoma; Heart attack; Lung cancer; Lungs; Macular degeneration; Nicotine; Osteoporosis; Pulmonary diseases; Pulmonary medicine; Respiration; Sexual dysfunction; Skin disorders; Strokes; Substance abuse; Teeth; Vision disorders; Wrinkles

For Further Information:

Britton, John. *ABC of Smoking Cessation.* Malden, MA: Blackwell, 2004. This guide provides practical information for smoking cessation and discusses the public health and individual health problems associated with smoking.

Hales, Dianne. *An Invitation to Health Brief.* Updated ed. Belmont, CA: Wadsworth/Cengage Learning, 2010. This updated, helpful resource covers many aspects of health, including mental health, physical fitness, stress management, and preventive medicine.

Jorenby, Douglas E., et al. "Efficacy of Varenicline, an α4β2 Nicotinic Acetylcholine Receptor Partial Agonist, versus Placebo or Sustained-Release Bupropion for Smoking Cessation." *Journal of the American Medical Association* 296, no. 1 (July 5, 2006): 56-63. This article compares two non-nicotine smoking-cessation products to a placebo in a smoking-cessation study with evaluation at the end of treatment and at fifty-two weeks. Varenicline was found to be significantly more effective than bupropion. Both agents were more effective than a placebo.

Marcus, Bess H., Jeffrey S. Hampl, and Edwin B. Fisher. *How to Quit Smoking without Gaining Weight.* New York: Simon & Schuster, 2004. This paperback book from the American Lung Association provides expert advice on quitting smoking without gaining substantial weight. It provides motivation and discusses physical activity and many strategies to help with cravings. Includes recipes and meal plans.

Parles, Karen, and J. H. Schiller. *One Hundred Questions and Answers about Lung Cancer.* 2nd ed. Sudbury, MA: Jones and Bartlett, 2010. A patient-oriented guide that covers a range of topics related to lung cancer, including risk factors and causes; methods of prevention, screening, and diagnosis; available treatments and how to choose among them; and ways of coping with common emotional and physical difficulties associated with the diagnosis and treatment.

Pirozynski, Michael. "One Hundred Years of Lung Cancer." *Respiratory Medicine* 100, no. 12 (December, 2006): 2073-2084. Lung cancer is the most common cause of cancer death in the world, and cigarette smoking remains the major risk factor. Discusses treatment and prognosis.

Sloan, Frank A., et al. *The Price of Smoking.* Cambridge, MA: MIT Press, 2006. This book contains a thorough analysis of the costs of smoking, which have often been ignored. These costs are carefully and comprehensively discussed by a group of economists.

SNAKEBITES
Disease/Disorder

Anatomy or system affected: Blood, circulatory system, nervous system

Specialties and related fields: Emergency medicine, hematology, serology

Definition: The penetration of skin or flesh by the fangs of a snake. Although a snakebite often involves a poisonous snake, not all bites include venom injection into the bloodstream.

Key terms:

antivenin: an antidote given to snakebite victims to combat the effects of venom that has been injected into the bloodstream

venom: the substance that is often injected into the affected part of the flesh during a snakebite

Causes and Symptoms

A snakebite is a wound that results from the flesh penetration created by the hollow teeth, or fangs, of a snake and sometimes the injection of venom into the bloodstream. Venom is usually encountered in snakes, although other animals and insects use it, often as part of their defense system. In Australia, for example, several creatures are classified as venomous,

Information on Snakebites

Causes: Penetration of skin or flesh by fangs of snake
Symptoms: Swelling or discoloration of skin, racing pulse, weakness, shortness of breath, nausea, vomiting, dilation of pupils, shock, convulsions, twitching, slurred speech
Duration: Acute
Treatments: Tight tourniquet to reduce lymphatic flow without cutting off blood supply, antivenin

such as twenty-two types of spiders, four types of ants, two types of beetles, two types of caterpillars, all platypus variations, two types of blue-ringed octopi, seven types of jellyfish, and eleven types of rays.

Venomous snakebites have a different effect based on the size of the victim, the location of the bite, the quantity of venom injected, and the time elapsed between the snakebite and the administration of antivenin therapy. Any part of the body is subject to this injury, but statistically legs, feet, and arms are by far the most commonly affected areas.

The symptoms of a snakebite include swelling or discoloration of the skin, a racing pulse, weakness, shortness of breath, nausea, and vomiting. Other symptoms include dilation of the pupils, shock, convulsions, twitching, and slurred speech. In extreme cases, severe pain and swelling and sometimes paralysis, unconsciousness, and even death may occur.

Snake venom contains an array of substances that are usually proteins in nature and that create tissue damage in several ways. The most important kinds of damage are nerve destruction, in which case the venom is called neurotoxic, and blood and tissue destruction, in which case the venom is hemotoxic. Neurotoxins have the tendency to paralyze the nervous system and lead to heart and respiratory failure. Hemotoxins destroy arteries, veins, and blood corpuscles and lead to internal hemorrhaging. Different snakes have various degrees of toxins. Cobra venom is usually neurotoxic, while rattlesnake venom is hemotoxic. The development of gangrene in the location of the snakebite is possible unless the victim is treated promptly.

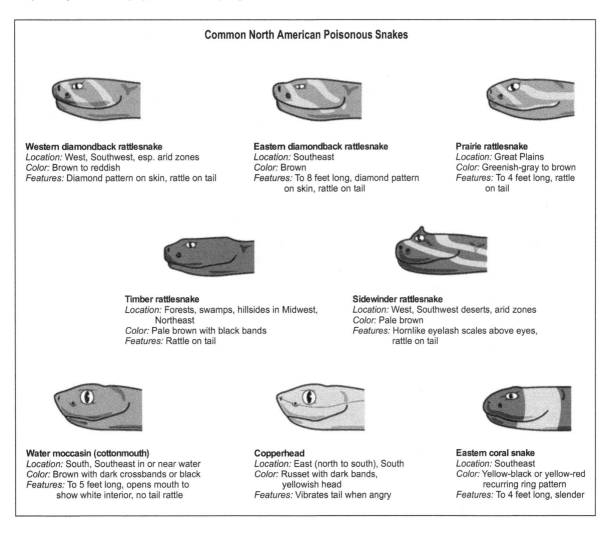

Common North American Poisonous Snakes

Western diamondback rattlesnake
Location: West, Southwest, esp. arid zones
Color: Brown to reddish
Features: Diamond pattern on skin, rattle on tail

Eastern diamondback rattlesnake
Location: Southeast
Color: Brown
Features: To 8 feet long, diamond pattern on skin, rattle on tail

Prairie rattlesnake
Location: Great Plains
Color: Greenish-gray to brown
Features: To 4 feet long, rattle on tail

Timber rattlesnake
Location: Forests, swamps, hillsides in Midwest, Northeast
Color: Pale brown with black bands
Features: Rattle on tail

Sidewinder rattlesnake
Location: West, Southwest deserts, arid zones
Color: Pale brown
Features: Hornlike eyelash scales above eyes, rattle on tail

Water moccasin (cottonmouth)
Location: South, Southeast in or near water
Color: Brown with dark crossbands or black
Features: To 5 feet long, opens mouth to show white interior, no tail rattle

Copperhead
Location: East (north to south), South
Color: Russet with dark bands, yellowish head
Features: Vibrates tail when angry

Eastern coral snake
Location: Southeast
Color: Yellow-black or yellow-red recurring ring pattern
Features: To 4 feet long, slender

Treatment and Therapy

The victim of a snakebite may exhibit mild to severe symptoms. Although the strength of venom of different snakes differs widely, snakebite treatment should be imposed as soon as possible in order to reduce the possibility of a fatality. This treatment should address two points: how to restrict the venom to the smallest body area possible and how to remove as much venom as possible. Thus, all contractions of the body and limb movement should be reduced immediately to a minimum to avoid spreading the venom. This is accomplished by immobilizing the affected area, preferably in a horizontal position and definitely lower than the heart. Any exertion and/or excitement by the bitten person increases the pulse rate and blood circulation, which leads to easier spreading of the venom. This is the same reason that stimulants should be avoided.

Statistically, more than three-quarters of snakebites occur on the lower leg or forearm. Current first aid recommendations do not include ice, any incision, the application of oxidizers such as potassium permanganate, or the administration of aspirin, ibuprofen, acetaminophen, or alcohol. Instead, the bitten part should be wiped, and a relatively tight tourniquet that reduces the lymphatic flow without cutting off the blood supply to the affected area should be applied. A nurse or other emergency medical service employee should check the pulse at the bitten area to ensure adequate blood flow. It is also recommended that the bandage be released every half hour for half a minute. It is also helpful to take the snake, whether alive or dead, to the hospital for proper identification.

If the swelling extends more than 5 inches within the first twelve hours after the bite, antivenin is given through intravenous transfusion in a hospital. Antivenin preparations are created through the immunization of animals such as horses, and their efficiency is dependent on the purification and concentration of the substance. Antivenins are usually specific, but some, such as that for tiger snake venom, appear to protect against the venom of more than one snake. If there is no swelling and increasing pain around the bite within thirty minutes, then the wound is one of the approximately one-third of bites by poisonous snakes in which venom is not injected. A notable exception is the bite of the coral snake, in which swelling takes place regardless of the venom infusion.

After the patient sees a doctor, several nutrients can be taken that appear to relieve pain and symptoms. They include vitamin C (approximately 10,000 milligrams every hour), which serves as a detoxifier and lessens infection; calcium gluconate (500 milligrams every four to six hours), which relieves pain; and pantothenic acid (500 milligrams every four hours for two days), which serves as an antistress vitamin.

Perspective and Prospects

Snakebites have been recorded in history for thousands of years, including such well-known examples as during Moses and the Israelites' flight from Egypt and Cleopatra's suicide with an asp. Traditionally, American Indians have had snakebite victims use echinacea, either by chewing the leaves and roots of the plant or drinking it in a tea form. They have also used its pulp placed on the affected area after making an incision and sucking the venom out until blood flows freely.

Approximately one-third of the three thousand snake species are poisonous, and only about three hundred can kill humans. The efficiency of emergency services and the wide availability of antivenins have reduced the death rates from snakebites dramatically. As a result, the number of people killed because of bee, wasp, and scorpion stings in the United States is higher than the deaths attributed to snakebites.

—*Soraya Ghayourmanesh, Ph.D.*

See also Bites and stings; Emergency medicine; Emergency medicine, pediatric; Nervous system; Neurology; Neurology, pediatric; Numbness and tingling; Poisoning; Seizures; Toxicology; Zoonoses.

For Further Information:

Altimari, William. *Venomous Snakes: A Safety Guide for Reptile Keepers*. St. Louis, Mo.: Society for the Study of Amphibians and Reptiles, 1998. This concise volume covers the handling of poisonous snakes, offering information on snakebites and venom. Includes bibliographical references and an index.

Campbell, Jonathan A., and William W. Lamar. *The Venomous Reptiles of the Western Hemisphere*. Ithaca, N.Y.: Cornell University Press, 2004. Provides valuable information about the medical aspects of snakebite.

Julivert, Maria Angels. *The Fascinating World of Snakes*. New York: Barron's Educational Series, 1993. Vivid, full-color illustrations provide much detail, especially of predatory activities. Includes a glossary and an index.

Mattison, Christopher. *The Encyclopedia of Snakes*. New York: Facts On File, 1995. This volume discusses aspects of the life cycle of snakes-their biology, history, and taxonomy. Chapter topics include origin and evolution, morphology and function, feeding, defense, and reproduction.

"Squamata." In *McGraw-Hill Concise Encyclopedia of Science and Technology*. 6th ed. New York: McGraw-Hill, 2009. A section in a reference for the nonspecialist that offers articles written by world-renowned scientists and engineers.

Thorpe, Roger S., Wolfgang Wüster, and Anita Malhotra, eds. *Venomous Snakes: Ecology, Evolution, and Snakebite*. New York: Oxford University Press, 2002. Offers a multidisciplinary approach to research into venomous snakes, focusing on the medical aspects of snake venoms and the effects of snakebites.

Tilton, Buck. *Backcountry First Aid and Extended Care*. 5th ed. Guilford, Conn.: Falcon, 2007. A small, portable guide to the myriad emergencies and medical problems encountered in the wilderness.

Tu, Anthony T., ed. *Reptile Venoms and Toxins*. New York: Marcel Dekker, 1991. In twenty-four contributed chapters, thirty-seven international specialists describe the latest developments in research on snake venom and summarize what is known to date on Gila monster and frog toxins.

SOILING

Disease/Disorder

Also known as: Encopresis

Anatomy or system affected: Anus, gastrointestinal system, intestines, psychic-emotional system

Specialties and related fields: Gastroenterology, pediatrics

Definition: The passage of fecal material into inappropriate places, usually underclothes.

Key terms:

functional megacolon: the rectal dilatation characteristic of fecal soiling

psychogenic megacolon: fecal soiling as part of a constellation of behavioral disorders

Causes and Symptoms

Some authors use the term "encopresis" to mean the passage of an entire bowel movement into the underwear and reserve the term "soiling" for the seepage of small amounts of semisolid feces. The term "encopresis" was derived by combining the Greek terms *enourein* (meaning "to pass urine") and *kopros* (meaning "feces") to form a term that is analogous to enuresis, which describes bed-wetting.

The term "functional megacolon" is used to describe the rectal dilatation characteristic of this disorder and distinguishes it from congenital aganglionic megacolon (Hirschsprung's disease). In this much less common and far more serious disorder, the failure of development of part of the autonomic nervous system in the intestines results in a failure of propagation of colonic contractions (peristalsis), which in turn results in distention of the colon. As a general statement, children with Hirschsprung's disease rarely, if ever, have fecal soiling.

The term "psychogenic megacolon" implies fecal soiling as part of a constellation of behavioral disorders. Although behavioral abnormalities occur in children with soiling, most recent studies indicate that they are no more common in soiling children than in normal children and that they tend to be a response to the soiling.

Soiling is caused by chronic constipation in school-aged children. About 1.5 percent of second-graders experience fecal soiling, which is six times more common in boys than in girls. Constipation and its associated complications are common symptoms in young children, accounting for 25 percent of visits to pediatric gastroenterologists. Constipation becomes less frequent with age and usually resolves as puberty approaches. The basis of constipation is slow motility of the colon, usually present in several family members, which allows excessive water absorption from the stool, causing hard stools that are difficult to expel.

Typically, the child will begin having frequent episodes of fecal soiling at ages five to seven. Parents are mystified by this symptom and bring the child to the physician because of the impending forced socialization of beginning school. Upon questioning, a history of infrequent, large-caliber bowel movements, sometimes too large to be accommodated by the plumbing, is often obtained. The size of these bowel movements is evidence of distention of the rectum as a result of long-standing constipation, which is the basis of this disorder.

The rectum normally functions as a sensory organ, responding to rectal distention by alerting the brain that a bowel movement is imminent and that appropriate arrangements should be made. Persistent rectal distention (megacolon) as a result of chronic constipation results in decreased sensitivity of the rectum to acute rectal distention. These children fre-

Information on Soiling

Causes: Behavioral disorders, chronic constipation, gastrointestinal disorders, disease
Symptoms: Loss of control of bowel movements
Duration: Acute to chronic
Treatments: Oral cathartic agents (citrate of magnesia, sodium phosphate, colonic lavage solutions), stool softeners, biofeedback training

quently admit that they do not sense an impending bowel movement before or during episodes of soiling, and studies with distention of balloons passed into the rectum bear out this lack of sensitivity to acute rectal distention. Much more air has to be pumped into a rectal balloon before a soiling child can sense it than for a normal child.

In soiling children, the rectum functions as a storage organ, and does so rather poorly. Storage of fecal material in the rectum bypasses the normal mechanisms of continence and leaves the external anal sphincter, a circular muscle holding the anus closed, as the sole mechanism of continence. The external anal sphincter is under voluntary control. To keep it closed, the child must keep all the muscles of the pelvic floor contracted. Any distraction or relaxation of the pelvic floor muscles to urinate can lead to leakage of semisolid stool.

Treatment and Therapy

Since soiling results from rectal distention (megacolon), effective therapy should empty the rectum (catharsis) and keep it empty (maintenance), allowing reversal of the rectal distention and return of normal rectal sensitivity. Several regimens are available, with most using a saline cathartic agent-that is, one that works by pulling water out of the circulation and into the colon, thus flushing out the contents of the colon. Hypertonic sodium phosphate enemas are frequently recommended but carry the risk of dehydration and electrolyte disturbances. In addition, these children are very sensitive to anorectal manipulation. For these reasons, using an oral cathartic is preferable. Such agents include citrate of magnesia, sodium phosphate, and colonic lavage solutions designed for cleaning the colon before an endoscopic examination.

Stool softeners are usually prescribed as maintenance therapy to keep the water content of the stool high. Preparations such as mineral oil, milk of magnesia, lactulose, and sorbitol are generally safe and effective. Stool softeners are safe for long-term use and, unlike stimulant laxatives such as senna and phenolphthalein, do not cause dependence.

The goal of therapy is resolution of the fecal soiling, since this is the only symptom that causes the child to suffer. Constipation is usually benign and self-limiting, and regularity of bowel movements should be seen not as a goal but rather as an indication that the rectal distention is reversing. Even with no treatment, soiling resolves spontaneously around the time of puberty as the underlying constipation resolves.

This therapy is usually very successful if applied consistently, and no child should have to suffer the humiliation of fecal soiling. Many studies indicate that an effort by the child and his or her family to keep track of the episodes of soiling, passage of bowel movements, and dosage of medicine is required for the best outcome. Even if the soiling is resolved, however, the tendency toward constipation remains until puberty, and if the problem falls on the family's list of priorities as it resolves, the chance of recurrence is high.

Perspective and Prospects

The demonstration of abnormalities of anorectal function has prompted the use of biofeedback training to resolve those abnormalities. Recent studies show equally good results with less invasive therapy with an initial catharsis followed by maintenance with stool softeners, casting doubt on the importance of these functional abnormalities and the advisability of expensive and invasive techniques.

—*Wallace A. Gleason, Jr., M.D.*

See also Anus; Bed-wetting; Colon; Constipation; Gastroenterology; Gastroenterology, pediatric; Gastrointestinal disorders; Gastrointestinal system; Hirschsprung's disease; Peristalsis; Psychiatry, child and adolescent; Rectum; Toilet training.

For Further Information:

Beach, R. C. "Management of Childhood Constipation." *The Lancet* 348, no. 9030 (September 21, 1996): 766-767. Childhood constipation and soiling can be a source of physical and mental anguish. Management of constipation in the early stages without anal manipulation could reduce the numbers requiring more extensive treatment.

Cooper, Candy J., Heidi Murkoff, and Teresa Martinez. "Bye-bye, Diapers." *Parenting* 14, no. 5 (June/July, 2000): 98-105. The authors highlight eight potty predicaments and how to solve them. Some suggestions for picking the perfect potty are offered as well.

Kuhn, Brett R., Bethany A. Marcus, and Sheryl L. Pitner. "Treatment Guidelines for Primary Nonretentive Encopresis and Stool Toileting Refusal." *American Family Physician* 59, no. 8 (April 15, 1999): 2171-2178. Six guidelines for managing children with primary nonretentive encopresis, or stool toileting refusal, are outlined. A case study demonstrates the efficacy and simplicity of these guidelines.

Loening-Baucke, Vera. "Clinical Approach to Fecal Soiling in Children." *Clinical Pediatrics* 39, no. 10 (October, 2000): 603. Fecal soiling is common in childhood and can be caused by stool toileting refusal, fecal incontinence due to organic disease, or encopresis due to functional constipation.

McClung, H. J., et al. "Is Combination Therapy for Encopresis Nutritionally Safe?" *Pediatrics* 91, no. 3 (March, 1993): 591-594. A study was conducted to determine whether, over a six-month period, the current combined therapeutic program of laxatives, lubricants, and fiber has any measurable deleterious effects on the nutritional status of pediatric primary care outpatients and whether a high fiber intake could be sustained in school-age and preschool-age children.

Wicks-Nelson, Rita, and Allen C. Israel. *Behavior Disorders of Childhood*. 6th ed. Upper Saddle River, N.J.: Pearson/Prentice Hall, 2008. An accessible text that details childhood behavior disorders, related clinical and research data, and updated coverage of treatment.

Woolf, Alan D., et al., eds. *The Children's Hospital Guide to Your Child's Health and Development*. Cambridge, Mass.: Perseus, 2002. An authoritative and comprehensive guide to children's health, providing a guide to every common illness or condition that affects children and a carefully designed emergency section.

SORE THROAT
Disease/Disorder

Anatomy or system affected: Nose, respiratory system, throat
Specialties and related fields: Family medicine, otorhinolaryngology, pediatrics
Definition: Discomfort and/or pain experienced in the throat, which sometimes indicates the presence of a more serious disorder.

Causes and Symptoms

Sore throat, termed pharyngitis by medical practitioners, is a common cause of patient discomfort and visits to the doctor's office. Though many people equate sore throat with strep throat, in reality there are many infectious and noninfectious causes of this symptom. Sore throat can even be a sign of disease in another part of the body. The sensation, which may be described by sufferers as scratchy, raw, tight, burning, or achy, may last from minutes to months, depending on the underlying cause, and may be accompanied by related complaints such as fever, runny nose, hoarseness, or difficulty swallowing.

Most sore throats are caused by infection in the upper respiratory tract, including the ears, nose, and sinuses as well as the throat and tonsils. Research has demonstrated that more than half of these infections are caused by common viruses. Epstein-Barr virus, which causes mononucleosis, accounts for less than 10 percent. Most of the remainder are caused by various bacteria. Of the bacterial causes, strep, more specifically group A beta-hemolytic *Streptococcus pyogenes*, is the most common pathogen (disease-causing organism). Additional bacterial causes include species of *Staphylococcus*, *Hemophilus*, *Mycoplasma*, non-group A streptococcus, and others. More rarely, fungi may account for a larger portion of throat infections in patients with weakened immune defenses.

Noninfectious causes of sore throat are quite varied. Although most are self-limited (resolving over time without treatment), some represent serious illness. These come into consideration especially if the duration of symptoms is longer than usual and if other aspects of the patient's health history suggest the likelihood of secondary causes.

Traumatic causes of throat discomfort include swallowing foreign objects, such as fish bones; thermal injury from a hot beverage; chemical injury from an ingestion, such as bleach; and external force from a blow to the neck. Environmental irritants, such as smoke and solvent fumes or allergies to dusts and pollens, cause symptoms in susceptible, exposed persons. Regurgitated stomach acid causes discomfort, which may be more pronounced when the patient is lying down. Enlargement of the thyroid gland or the salivary glands, cysts arising from embryonic structures such as the thyroglossal duct, or inflammation of lymph nodes can exert local pressure on the throat itself or on adjacent nerves, thereby eliciting symptoms. Cancer is the most ominous cause of sore throat symptoms, and it needs to be considered in patients with risk factors such as smoking and alcohol consumption.

Information on Sore Throat

Causes: Allergies, bacterial or viral infections, ingestion of foreign objects, thermal injury from hot beverage, chemical injury, external force from blow to neck, environmental irritants, lymph node inflammation

Symptoms: Scratchy, raw, tight, burning, or achy throat; may be accompanied by fever, runny nose, hoarseness, difficulty swallowing

Duration: Acute to several months

Treatments: Rest, increased fluid intake, analgesics, antibiotics if needed

---

Considering this expansive list of possibilities, which does not include every possible cause of sore throat, it is evident that the expedient diagnosis of sore throat is challenging. Though most sore throats resolve without treatment or complication, the practitioner must consider the possibility of rarer but potentially life-threatening diseases. The initial history and physical examination are sufficient in most cases to separate those patients who are likely to have an infectious cause from those who are unlikely to have one. Since most patients are initially concerned about the possibility of strep throat and the need for antibiotics, clinical algorithms, such as the Centor score, have been developed to assist this process. By tallying associated signs, symptoms, and patient characteristics, the practitioner may increase diagnostic accuracy. In some cases, additional testing, such as a rapid streptococcal antigen throat swab or a culture, is needed.

The search for noninfectious causes often begins when the patient returns with persisting symptoms. Since most throat infections resolve within a week or two, lingering discomfort suggests the need for further evaluation. In many cases, additional historical information from the patient and a follow-up physical examination will significantly narrow the list of possibilities. Clues such as weight loss, hoarseness, and a history of cigarette smoking and alcohol consumption increase the probability of cancer. Occupational information may uncover exposure to noxious dust or vapors. In difficult cases, diagnosis may require examination and biopsy of the throat during a procedure called laryngoscopy.

Treatment and Therapy

The treatments of noninfectious sore throat are as varied as the diagnoses themselves. The treatment of infectious sore throat depends on the underlying cause, ranging from rest, fluids, and analgesics (painkillers) for viruses to antibiotics for certain bacteria and fungi. Penicillin has been the mainstay of strep throat treatment since the mid-twentieth century. Before the discovery of penicillin, throat infection sometimes resulted in serious complications, such as rheumatic fever (which damages the heart valves) and glomerulonephritis (which damages the kidneys). Although group A *Streptococcus pyogenes* has remained remarkably sensitive to penicillin, reports have suggested that the treatment of strep throat is becoming more complex. The presence of other bacteria in

the throat, some of which have developed the ability to inactivate penicillin, may actually protect the strep bacteria from the antibiotic. Interestingly, some research suggests that antibiotic treatment very early in the course of disease may even increase the likelihood of subsequent recurrence. Infections by bacteria other than strep or by fungi are treated with other antibiotic and antifungal drugs.

Given this scenario, one may wonder why doctors do not treat everyone with antibiotics, rather than going to the trouble and expense of diagnosing strep throat. Antibiotic treatment is complicated by many factors, including cost, drug interactions, and the potential for fatal allergic reactions. Widespread use has led to the development of antibiotic-resistant strains of "super bacteria," which are very difficult if not impossible to treat.

—Louis B. Jacques, M.D.

See also Acid reflux disease; Antibiotics; Common cold; Epiglottitis; Influenza; Mouth and throat cancer; Multiple chemical sensitivity syndrome; Nasopharyngeal disorders; Otorhinolaryngology; Pharyngitis; Pharynx; Quinsy; Strep throat; Streptococcal infections; Tonsillectomy and adenoid removal; Tonsillitis; Tonsils; Voice and vocal cord disorders.

For Further Information:

Coutts, Cherylann. "A New Way to Treat Tonsil Trouble." *Parenting* 14, no. 10 (December, 2000/January, 2001): 33. If a child's physician determines that a tonsillectomy is required, a promising new procedure may be used. It uses radio-frequency energy to shrink tonsils, allowing for less pain and a much speedier recovery.

Evans, Julie A. "Thirteen Old-Fashioned Cold Remedies That Really Work!" *Prevention* 52, no. 11 (November, 2000): 106-113. Argues that good science is behind homemade elixirs for sniffles, sneezes, and other woes. Old-fashioned cold remedies, like honey and lemon for sore throats and chicken soup for a stuffy head, are discussed.

Ferrari, Mario. *PDxMD Ear, Nose, and Throat Disorders*. Philadelphia: PDxMD, 2003. A clinical yet accessible reference text that provides a comprehensive list of disorders, with a summary of the condition, background, diagnosis, treatment, outcomes, prevention, and resources.

Kemper, Kathi J. *The Holistic Pediatrician: A Pediatrician's Comprehensive Guide to Safe and Effective Therapies for the Twenty-five Most Common Ailments of Infants, Children, and Adolescents*. Rev. ed. New York: Quill, 2002. Integrates mainstream and alternative medicine to aid parents in dealing with the most common childhood health problems, such as fever, diaper rash, sore throats, ear infections, and allergies.

Kimball, Chad T. *Colds, Flu, and Other Common Ailments Sourcebook*. Detroit, Mich.: Omnigraphics, 2001. A comprehensive guide for general readers covering treatment issues and controversies surrounding common ailments and injuries. Includes discussions on ailments of the nose, throat, lungs, ears, eyes, and head; common injuries; alternative therapies; choosing a doctor; and buying drugs and finding health information online.

Litin, Scott C., ed. *Mayo Clinic Family Health Book*. 4th ed. New York: HarperResource, 2009. Perhaps the best general medical text for the layperson, this book covers the entire medical field. While the information is derived from a wide variety of highly technical sources, the articles are written to be easily understood by a general audience.

McIsaac, Warren J., Vivel Goel, Teresa To, and Donald E. Low. "The Validity of a Sore Throat Score in Family Practice." *Canadian Medical Association Journal* 163, no. 7 (October 3, 2000): 811.

This study assessed the validity of a previously published clinical score for the management of infections of the upper respiratory tract accompanied by sore throat.

Speech disorders
Disease/Disorder

Anatomy or system affected: Ears, muscles, musculoskeletal system, psychic-emotional system

Specialties and related fields: Audiology, psychiatry, psychology, speech pathology

Definition: Dysfunction in the brain-coordinated use of speech organs, such as problems with language, vocal quality, articulation, fluency, and dementia.

Key terms:

aphasia: a partial or total loss of the ability to articulate ideas; often results from brain damage

articulation: the act or process of speaking correctly, as a result of appropriate movement and coordination of the speech organs

connective tissue: tissues possessing a highly vascular structure that form support and connecting structures of the body (for example, cartilage, ligaments, and tendons)

dysfluency: another term for stuttering

dysfunction: the disordered or impaired function of a body system or organ

organic: pertaining to, arising from, or affecting a body organ

psychogenic: originating in the mind or in mental conditions and activities

stuttering: a disorder involving speaking with spasmodic hesitation, prolongation, and/or repetition of sounds

Causes and Symptoms

Learning to speak correctly is of great importance to all people. It involves the brain-coordinated use of the mouth, jaws, lips, and tongue, as well as of the vocal cords, lungs, and diaphragm. On average, children learn to talk during their second year by imitating the speech of those persons, mostly family members, with whom frequent and close contact is maintained. Hence, it is important that young children hear correct speech.

The development of speech is viewed as occurring in several distinct stages. First, babies make involuntary noises in response to physical stimuli. Then, they begin to enjoy making these noises at about two months of age. Next, about nine months after birth, they start to imitate the sounds and inflections of the speech of others around them. Beginning at twelve to eighteen months of age, children start to vocalize in a meaningful way, and in due time, they learn to speak.

In many cases, however, a child is quickly found to have some difficulties with the use of speech or with its development to levels viewed as appropriate within expected time spans. Such children suffer from speech disorders including stuttering, lisping, and lack of speech comprehension. They should receive appropriate professional help as soon as possible. Others are born with physical problems, such as cleft palate, which make appropriate speech impossible without medical intervention. Smaller numbers of people develop speech disorders later in life for various reasons, including accidents that damage the brain or the mechanical organs of speech, as well as the physical and mental ravages of advanced age.

Speech disorders fall into three main categories: problems associated with speech production, difficulties of articulation, and dysfunction in the ability to utilize language. These disorders have been known since antiquity and although they are frequently hereditary, the genetic cause is often unclear. In fact, there is often a psychogenic aspect to their origin as well.

Another broad means of categorizing speech disorders is by dividing them into causative organic and nonorganic groups. The term "organic speech disorder" is used to indicate birth defects or later injuries to the brain or the structures, muscles, and connective tissues that are required to produce speech. The disorders for which no such origin can be clearly identified with existing techniques fall into the nonorganic group. Usually, they are attributed solely to psychogenic factors. It is probable, however, that they have subtle organic causes that are beyond present methods of identification.

Speech disorders may be associated with articulation, voice, fluency, language, and dementia. The cures for all these types of speech disorders vary; they include the interactive participation of teachers in school systems and the attention of speech professionals such as audiologists, surgeons, psychiatrists, and physical therapists. Each case must be analyzed carefully and then treated individually. Even so, varied success is obtained from patient to patient, regardless of the disorder, the nature of the therapeutic procedures utilized, and the therapists who are involved.

Articulation disorders are attributable to the inappropriate sequential movement of the jaw, tongue, and related speech structures. Minor, nonpathological differences result in regional differences (accents) in the spoken language within a country. Pathological problems that cause speech that cannot be understood are most often organic in nature. Examples include cleft palate and neurologic dysfunction. Voice disorders include inappropriate pitch, sound quality (for example, hoarseness), lack of audibility, or inappropriate loudness. Fluency disorders are most often identified with stuttering, speech rate problems, and speech rhythm problems. The best-known language disorders are the aphasias, which are characterized by poor language comprehension and childhood language impairment (often resulting from developmental problems). Dementia can impair speech at any age, but it is most

---

Information on Speech Disorders

Causes: Dementia, brain injury, neurologic disorders, birth defects, cleft palate

Symptoms: Inappropriate pitch or sound quality (e.g., hoarseness), lack of audibility, inappropriate loudness, stuttering, speech rate and speech rhythm problems, aphasias

Duration: Temporary to chronic

Treatments: Surgical and dental treatment, behavior and speech modification

common in the elderly, for whom memory, language, and cognitive ability may be greatly impaired.

Treatment and Therapy

Many viewpoints exist concerning the treatment of speech disorders. All agree, however, that interaction between family, patient, teachers, and various clinicians is essential. Disorders of articulation are quite common and range from mild problems (for example, a lisp) to those which are so extreme that the speech of afflicted individuals becomes unintelligible. Many of the most severe of these speech disorders arise from the organic impairment of motor control in the speech musculature, which may be attributable to stroke, cleft palate, or even the loss of lips or other speech system components.

Frequently, efforts at remediating such problems must include surgical and dental treatment. After any necessary corrective surgery and/or dentistry, many treatment regimens focus on behavior modification. Affected individuals receive instruction regarding the physical basis of their problems and are then trained to overcome them as effectively as possible.

In many cases, the use of psychological and psychiatric counseling is considered to be of great value. Some experts suggest, however, that the main effect of such therapy is to enable afflicted individuals to live comfortably with the imperfections in articulation that remain after all treatments are tried.

Voice disorders occur when the phonatory mechanism is dysfunctional. They range from the consequences of laryngeal, oral, or respiratory disease to the misuse of the phonatory system, which may reflect psychological state. Such functional disorders, if left untreated for too long, may lead to organic damage. In the case of pitch abnormalities, causative factors may include psychological tension, an undersized larynx, misformed vocal cords, and hearing problems, either individually or in various combinations.

Disorders of voice quality likewise have many physical sources, including larynx and vocal cord abnormalities, and ones of psychogenic origin. The disorders associated with loudness range from overly loud voices caused by workplace noise or hearing loss to extremely soft ones that are generally psychogenic. Treatment of all such disorders begins with the disqualification of treatable organic problems. In the case of psychogenic disorders, psychiatric counseling can be extremely helpful. Psychological and medical treatments must be followed, however, by very thorough interaction with speech-language pathologists if optimum results are to be obtained.

Disorders of fluency most often involve stuttering, also called dysfluency, which features spasmodic hesitation and the prolongation or repetition of sounds. In addition, stuttering is often accompanied by tics and other uncontrolled body movements. The basis for the problem is unclear, and different experts point to learned behavior, psychogenic origins, or organic roots. There is no cure for dysfluency, but it (and the accompanying nonspeech problems) can be greatly diminished. Treatment usually involves both psychiatric counseling and behavior and/or speech modification by speech-lan-

guage pathologists as well as by other related speech professionals. Such therapy varies widely from individual to individual and with the age of the patient.

Language disorders are characterized by the diminished ability to use or to understand spoken language. In children, these disorders are often identified as language delay or development aphasias. They are most often thought to be attributable to mental retardation, hearing loss, or autism. When lost hearing is not the main problem, the treatments for such language problems often involve behavior modification techniques. In all cases in which hearing loss is an important component, its correction is the first effort; such efforts may work wonders. When hearing problems cannot be remediated entirely, however, the overall treatment will be much less successful because hearing the speech of others is so important to speech development.

True aphasia is very often viewed as speech impairment; it occurs in adults as a result of stroke, accidents that produce severe head trauma, or dementia. It is desirable to begin treatment of afflicted persons as soon as possible after aphasia is observed. Some rapid and spontaneous healing of lost language ability occurs, and this healing can be maximized by the efforts of speech-language pathologists. The continued treatment of aphasias is very important and usually follows careful evaluation of its causes. It is often possible to make progressive, long-term advances in healing aphasias. Complete recovery is rare, however, and the use of sign language or personal computers for interpersonal communication may be necessary.

Perspective and Prospects

For many years, it was thought that speech disorders were caused only by insoluble psychological problems in the very young or by severe head, facial, and brain trauma later in life. It is now clear that they have other causes, ranging from hearing loss to dementia. Furthermore, it is currently understood that speech problems of every type can attack anyone-young children, adolescents, and adults of all ages.

These problems often have disastrous psychological and economic effects on the afflicted person. Young children may be traumatized if speech disorders are not treated early; in severe cases, they may later be unable to enter the workforce in meaningful positions or to receive anything above the most rudimentary education. This is unfortunate because many such problems of childhood, adolescence, and even young adulthood can be almost completely solved by careful medical examination, followed quickly by appropriate corrective action.

There is also help available for older people who develop speech problems because of aging, dementia, or harmful workplace conditions. In all cases, once a sound treatment plan is developed, it is essential that the afflicted person follow it rigorously. Miracles should not be expected; rather, sustained interaction between the treatment team-especially the patient and a speech-language pathologist-must be undertaken. Furthermore, the psychological support of the patient's family and friends has been recognized as a crucial factor in many successful treatment plans.

In the case of the young child, the diagnosis of speech problems by schoolteachers can be another important means to treatment. Once a problem is observed, the child's family can be advised concerning special education available through the school system or local programs. Teachers should be cautioned, however, against attempts to treat the child in question unless they have adequate training. The job of unspecialized teachers should be diagnosis and the recommendation of an appropriate treatment group. When speech disorder therapy results in less-than-adequate treatment of extremely serious problems, the use of sign language, special typewriters, and computer-assisted communication, as well as psychotherapy, should be considered.

Overall, the treatment of speech problems has improved, and its sensible application can enable patients to enter into or return to the workforce at levels commensurate with their abilities, can prevent them from becoming maladjusted, and can enrich society as a whole. Dealing with such problems in the young is particularly important because it may help to prevent neuroses and psychoses from developing. It is hoped that ongoing research will continue to increase the avenues available for the prevention and cure of speech disorders, to identify additional methods for treating them, and to result in their eradication.

—Sanford S. Singer, Ph.D.

See also Alzheimer's disease; Aphasia and dysphasia; Audiology; Autism; Birth defects; Brain damage; Cerebral palsy; Cleft lip and palate; Cleft lip and palate repair; Deafness; Dementias; Developmental disorders; Dyslexia; Ear surgery; Ears; Electroencephalography (EEG); Jaw wiring; Laryngitis; Learning disabilities; Lisping; Paralysis; Strokes; Stuttering; Tics; Tonsillitis; Tourette's syndrome; Transient ischemic attacks (TIAs); Voice and vocal cord disorders.

For Further Information:

American Psychiatric Association. *Diagnostic and Statistical Manual of Mental Disorders: DSM-IV-TR*. 4th ed. Arlington, Va.: Author, 2000. This classic text contains diagnostic criteria and other useful facts about a variety of mental disorders, including those associated with speech dysfunction.

Beers, Mark H., et al., eds. *The Merck Manual of Diagnosis and Therapy*. 18th ed. Whitehouse Station, N.J.: Merck Research Laboratories, 2006. Contains useful data on the characteristics, etiology, diagnosis, and treatment of speech disorders and related processes. Although the text is designed for physicians, the material should be useful to general readers as well.

Cole, Patricia R. *Language Disorders in Preschool Children*. Englewood Cliffs, N.J.: Prentice Hall, 1982. This book by an expert speech-language pathologist explains the modalities associated with solving speech-language disorders. Solid and well referenced, it covers language development, disorders, diagnosis, and treatment. Much useful information concerning learning semantics and syntax.

Gelfand, Stanley A. *Essentials of Audiology*. 2d ed. New York: Thieme, 2009. Undergraduate text covering a wide range of relevant topics, including acoustics, anatomy and physiology, sound perception, auditory disorders and their related speech disorders, and the nature of hearing impairment.

Lubinski, Rosemary, and Carol M. Frattali, eds. *Professional Issues in Speech-Language Pathology and Audiology*. San Diego, Calif.: Thomson/Delmar Learning, 2007. For those interested in entering the field of audiology. Covers the practicalities of a career path, ethical-legal considerations, professional organizations, and ongoing issues in health care, among other topics.

Paul, Rhea. *Language Disorders from Infancy Through Adolescence: Assessment and Interventions*. 3d ed. St. Louis, Mo.: Mosby/Elsevier, 2007. An introductory text that covers pediatric language disorders across various ages, assessment and treatment of those disorders, public policy, and special pediatric populations.

Winitz, Harris, ed. *Human Communication and Its Disorders: A Review*. Vol. 4. Timonium, Md.: York Press, 1995. This authoritative text covers in detail the prominent disorders of human communications: their occurrence, symptoms, and treatment. Both organic and nonorganic aspects of these communication problems are carefully explored and referenced.

SPERM BANKS
Organizations

Anatomy or system affected: Genitals, psychic-emotional system, reproductive system, uterus

Specialties and related fields: Biotechnology, ethics, genetics, infertility, obstetrics, urology

Definition: The identification of suitable sperm donors and the evaluation, processing, storage and distribution of their semen for use in assisted reproductive technology.

Key terms:

insemination: the process of placing semen in the female reproductive tract; natural insemination occurs during sexual intercourse, while artificial (or donor) insemination is performed with medical instruments in a clinic

semen: the male reproductive fluid consisting of two parts, a liquid called seminal plasma and living reproductive cells called sperm

Indications and Procedures

Sperm banks exist primarily to help women with normal adult premenopausal reproductive function to become pregnant. A woman seeking pregnancy may need the services of a sperm bank if her male partner is infertile, if she is in a lesbian relationship, or if she chooses to be a single mother. When a man in a heterosexual relationship produces too few sperm for his female partner's pregnancy, sperm from a sperm bank can help the couple become pregnant through artificial (or donor) insemination. An additional purpose of sperm banking is to allow men who have cancer to preserve their sperm before undergoing chemotherapy or radiation, which might render them infertile or compromise the quality of their sperm.

A sperm bank makes available the sperm from a number of qualified donors. The primary task of a clinical sperm bank is to preserve sperm and identify suitable donors, based upon medical and biological criteria. The sperm bank does a medical physical examination of donor candidates and obtains an extensive medical and family history from them. Special attention is given to semen quality and to the risk of transmitting infectious or genetic diseases.

Semen quality has two major components. The first component is whether the semen has enough fertile sperm with

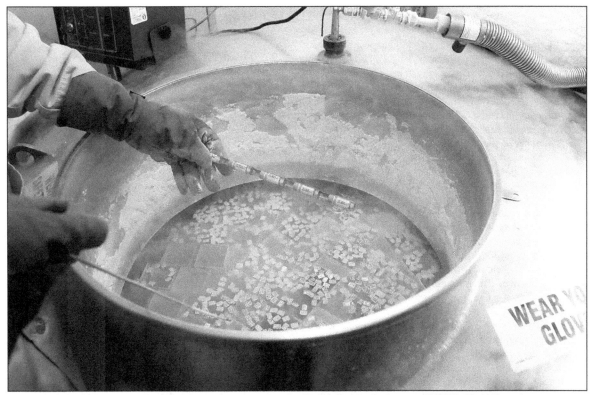

A cryogenic technician inserts a tube containing sperm into a tank of liquid nitrogen for storage. (AP/Wide World Photos)

appropriate motility and morphology to create a pregnancy. The second component is whether enough sperm in the semen survive freezing. Freezing in a special way (cryopreservation) to keep sperm alive is the only way a sperm bank can store its semen inventory. Another important reason for cryopreservation is related to infectious disease testing. For example, a donor is tested for acquired immunodeficiency syndrome (AIDS) at the time he produces the semen, but the test is repeated six months later to increase its certainty. The cryopreservation allows the semen to be stored during this "quarantine" period. Donors are tested for a variety of diseases that can be transmitted through semen: AIDS, gonorrhea, chlamydia, syphilis, trichomonas, and well-known sexually transmitted infections (STIs); and viral hepatitis, cytomegalovirus, and human T-lymphotropic virus (HTLV).

The genetics of a donor is very important. Genes are responsible for each person's positive attributes and negative ones (genetic diseases). There are no genetically perfect persons; there are no perfect donors. There are only a few hundred genetic tests for more than five thousand genetic conditions; therefore comprehensive testing for genetic disease is impractical. Sperm banks usually screen donors routinely for a few very common diseases with a genetic component, such as diabetes, gout, and high cholesterol. Additional tests may be done on donors of certain ethnic backgrounds for diseases linked to specific ethnicities: cystic fibrosis, Canavan disease, Gaucher disease, sickle cell disease, Tay-Sachs disease.

Each sperm bank will have its own list.

Fortunately, both parents determine a child's genetics. The genetic attributes of one often will compensate for the liabilities of the other. A person choosing a donor would be wise to seek the help of a certified genetics counselor. A genetics counselor will help match the genetics of the woman with the genetics of possible donors.

Considering all that is involved in identifying each suitable donor, a sperm bank requires donors to provide many "samples," not only of semen but also of blood. Additionally, there are annual physical exams, perhaps a psychological exam, and other tests. It is understandable that the bank compensates donors for their time and effort in participating; this is different from "buying sperm." Similarly, sperm banks receive a fee for their efforts in recruiting and evaluating donors plus their work in evaluating, processing, and providing semen to physicians and their patients.

Semen is normally available to a patient through a physician or other medical clinician trained in artificial insemination. Sometimes a patient will request self-inseminating at her home. This is possible with physician authorization, meaning that the physician retains responsibility for mistakes that might occur. The requested semen is delivered frozen by the sperm bank in a shipping container similar to a thermos. The semen is thawed immediately before insemination.

Uses and Complications

There are many personal decisions to be made regarding artificial insemination. Often there are psychological effects on the woman to be inseminated and her partner. Usually artificial insemination is done with semen from an anonymous donor, thus preventing any social contact between donor and recipient. The use of an anonymous donor usually conveys full parental rights and responsibilities on the partner of the recipient, relieving the donor of any responsibility. Sometimes the recipient or her partner want to use a donor known to them, a directed donor. Although this is possible, it raises legal and psychological issues that are not fully known. These issues about the kind of donor also have implications for the psychology of the offspring. There are many medical decisions to be made regarding artificial insemination. The procedure must be done at the time of ovulation, an event occurring between menstrual periods. The occurrence of ovulation can be determined in several ways, often by hormonal tests. The physician must decide whether to do one or more inseminations at ovulation. If the timing is off, the patient will not become pregnant. Another attempt can be made on the next monthly cycle.

Although many women will become pregnant with semen placed in the vagina at the entrance to the uterus, many physicians and other clinicians will increase the success of insemination by placing the semen into the woman's uterus. Intrauterine insemination (IUI) requires removing the semen from the seminal plasma, administering substances that cause the uterus to contract strongly, and discharging the sperm into the uterus through a catheter.

Other complications include the possibility of infection or genetic problems. Although the sperm has been properly tested, tests are not perfect. The patient must remember that even when all aspects of insemination are technically perfect, the complex biology of making a baby from a fertilized egg can go wrong.

Perspective and Prospects

Horse breeders may have successfully used artificial insemination as early as the fourteenth century. In 1776, John Hunter, an English surgeon, may have been the first person to successfully artificially inseminate a woman. Cryopreservation of bull semen was developed in England in the early 1950s. An American urologist, Raymond H. Bunge, was the first physician to successfully use cryopreserved human semen. Many sperm banks were established in the early 1980s so that semen could be quarantined to prevent the transmission of AIDS. Today, sperm banks are being used to guarantee male fertility for men with medical problems as well as to allow women to reproduce. Sperm banks have expanded to become embryo banks. Future technology will permit cryopreservation of human eggs. These banks will be contributing components of genetic medicine.

—Armand M. Karow, Ph.D.; updated by
Robin Kamienny Montvilo, R.N., Ph.D.

See also Assisted reproductive technologies; Childbirth; Cloning; Conception; Gynecology; Infertility, female; Infertility, male; Men's health; Obstetrics; Pregnancy and gestation; Reproductive system; Screening; Semen; Uterus.

For Further Information:

Bahadur, G., et al. "Factors Affecting Sperm Banking for Adolescent Cancer Patients." *Archives of Diseases in Children* 91, no. 8 (2006): 715-716.

Berger, Gary S., Mark Fuerst, and Marc Goldstein. *The Couple's Guide to Fertility*. 3d ed. New York: Broadway Books, 2001.

Critser, J. K. "Current Status of Semen Banking in the USA." *Human Reproduction* 13, supp. 2 (1998): 55-65.

Doherty, C. Maud, and Melanie M. Clark. *Fertility Handbook: A Guide to Getting Pregnant*. Omaha, Nebr.: Addicus Books, 2002.

Mohler, Marie, and Lacy Frazer. *A Donor Insemination Guide: Written by and for Lesbian Women*. New York: Alice Street Editions/Harrington Park Press, 2002.

Pence, Gregory E. *Re-creating Medicine: Ethical Issues at the Frontiers of Medicine*. Lanham, Md.: Rowman & Littlefield, 2007.

Schover, Leslie R., and Anthony J. Thomas. *Overcoming Male Infertility: Understanding Its Causes and Treatments*. New York: John Wiley & Sons, 2000.

Vercollone, Carol Frost, Heidi Moss, and Robert Moss. *Helping the Stork: The Choices and Challenges of Donor Insemination*. New York: John Wiley & Sons, 1997.

Zouves, Christo. *Expecting Miracles: On the Path of Hope from Infertility to Parenthood*. New York: Berkley, 2003.

SPHINCTERECTOMY

Procedure

Anatomy or system affected: Anus, bladder, eyes, intestines, muscles, musculoskeletal system

Specialties and related fields: General surgery, ophthalmology

Definition: The surgical removal of all or a portion of a sphincter, a ring of muscle that closes or constricts an opening or passage in the body when the muscles contract.

Indications and Procedures

In the human body, sphincters can be found in the internal and external region of the anus, in the area that joins the large and small intestine, between the urinary bladder and the urethra, at the lower end of the esophagus, and in the pupil of the eye. While located in a variety of areas of the body, each has in common the ability to allow or prevent the passage of something (solid, liquid, or light) through it when relaxed or constricted, respectively. A variety of conditions may lead to the need for surgical intervention to restore proper functioning of a sphincter or an associated organ.

Spinal cord injuries may lead to the need for bladder management intervention, especially in men. An option for those who do not prefer intermittent catheterization for bladder control is to slit the urethral sphincter to create a low-pressure bladder system that allows evacuation without need for muscular control of the sphincter.

Splits in the lining of the rectum called anal fissures can be caused by hard bowel movements. For chronic conditions that do not heal because of anal spasms, cutting the outermost portion of the anal sphincter may relieve the spasms and speed healing.

In patients afflicted with both cataracts and glaucoma, excision of a portion of the pupillary band of the iris can aid in removing the cataract while dealing with potential pressure buildup caused by glaucoma.

Uses and Complications

Although surgery to correct tears or defects in sphincters is more common than their removal, in cases of extreme damage or disease, useless sphincters must be surgically excised. For the removal of internal sphincters, the patient is opened surgically and the appropriate organs are moved to expose the sphincter in question; external sphincterectomies are performed without incisions in the body cavity. A scalpel is used to dissect the sphincter away from the surrounding tissue. Bleeding vessels are repaired, and the incisions are closed.

After removal, an individual will lack the control provided by the sphincter, such as control of defecation or urination, and alternative means of compensating for this loss will be presented to the patient. As in all surgeries, patients must be aware of any potential indications of infection such as fever, redness at the area of incision, and bleeding.

—*Karen E. Kalumuck, Ph.D.*

See also Anus; Cataract surgery; Cataracts; Colon; Esophagus; Eye infections and disorders; Eye surgery, Eyes; Gastroenterology; Gastroenterology, pediatric; Gastrointestinal disorders; Gastrointestinal system; Glaucoma; Intestinal disorders; Intestines; Muscle sprains, spasms, and disorders; Muscles; Peristalsis; Rectum; Small intestine; Urinary disorders; Urinary system; Urology; Urology, pediatric.

For Further Information:

Daniel, Edwin E., et al., eds. *Sphincters: Normal Function-Changes in Disease*. Boca Raton, Fla.: CRC Press, 1992.

Friedman, Scott L., Kenneth R. McQuaid, and James H. Grendell, eds. *Current Diagnosis and Treatment in Gastroenterology*. 2d ed. New York: Lang Medical Books/McGraw-Hill, 2003.

Griffith, H. Winter. *Complete Guide to Symptoms, Illness, and Surgery*. Revised and updated by Stephen Moore and Kenneth Yoder. 5th ed. New York: Perigee, 2006.

Holschneider, Alexander M., and Prem Puri, eds. *Hirschsprung's Disease and Allied Disorders*. 3d ed. New York: Springer, 2008.

Janowitz, Henry D. *Your Gut Feelings: A Complete Guide to Living Better with Intestinal Problems*. Rev. ed. New York: Oxford University Press, 1995.

SPIDER BITES. *See* BITES AND STINGS.

SPINA BIFIDA
Disease/Disorder

Also known as: Myelocele, meningomyelocele, lipomeningocele

Anatomy or system affected: Bones, brain, nervous system, spine

Specialties and related fields: Embryology, neonatology, perinatology, plastic surgery

Definition: A birth defect that results from a mistake early in the development of the spinal cord.

Key terms:

central nervous system: the brain and spinal cord

hydrocephalus: the abnormal accumulation of fluid within the developing brain

neural plate: a layer of tissue in the early embryo from which the brain and spinal cord will develop

neuropore: a small opening into the interior of the brain or spinal cord of the embryo

vertebra: an individual bone in the spine

Causes and Symptoms

The development of the fetal nervous system is the most complicated process during pregnancy. It starts a few weeks after conception and continues until well after birth. The earliest steps are the most crucial, because the basic plan of the nervous system must be established accurately if it is to work properly later.

The central nervous system begins with the formation of a thickened layer of tissue, called the neural plate, along the back of the embryo. The edges of this plate curl up to form ridges, and the whole plate rolls up into a slender tube running from the head to the rump. This cylinder is then covered over by tissues that will form the surface of the back. The front end of this tube will soon expand to become the brain, and the rest of the tube will form the spinal cord. In order for these processes to proceed properly, the tube must seal itself along its entire length. If there are any gaps where the tube does not close, it will leak and will not be able to expand and develop properly. Without such expansion, all the later stages of nervous system development will also be prevented from occurring properly.

If the neural tube fails to seal, a small opening called a neuropore will remain at some point along its length. Depending on where the opening is, a variety of abnormalities can result. When the posterior region of the neural tube fails to close, the result is spina bifida. This flaw in the neural tube in turn affects the assembly of the muscle, bone, and skin in this region. In spina bifida, which means "divided spine," the vertebrae of the backbone do not join together properly.

The severity of spina bifida depends on how much damage has been done to the lower spinal cord region. In its mildest form, the only evidence of a problem may be that two of the bones in the spine fail to form quite right. If several vertebrae are involved, the membranes that protect the surface of the spinal cord can bulge outward, forming a ball-like mass in this region. The problems that result depend on how much of the spinal membrane is involved in this bulge. In the most severe cases, the vertebrae fail to protect the spinal cord, so that

---

Information on Spina Bifida

Causes: Birth defect

Symptoms: Bulging spinal cord, hydrocephalus, paralysis in lower back and legs, bladder and bowel malfunction, loss of sensation, mental impairment

Duration: Chronic

Treatments: Surgery, catheterization, prostheses, physical therapy, sometimes fetal surgery

the nervous tissue itself is also involved and an opening to the outside remains at the base of the spinal cord. Additional problems with nervous system development may result, including improper fluid balances in the brain (hydrocephalus).

Because the brain and spinal column fail to develop properly in spina bifida, a variety of mental, behavioral, and physical symptoms can result. The nerve connections at the base of the spine are likely to be affected, resulting in paralysis in the lower back and legs, problems with bladder and bowel function, and loss of sensation. Because the development of the brain can also be affected, mental abilities may be impaired.

Treatment and Therapy

Effective measures have been developed to minimize the effects of spina bifida. Often, surgery is performed within twenty-four to forty-eight hours of birth to close any opening in the child's lower back and to reconstruct the spine and other tissues in this area. Problems with feet and legs may also be dealt with surgically. If the child has symptoms of hydrocephalus, the excess fluid will be drained. Bladder and bowel function will be regulated, such as by catheterization. Eventually, prosthetic devices may be fitted to assist the child's movement. Mental health and physical therapy experts will also be involved to assist in overcoming learning hurdles, monitoring physical development and training, and making emotional adjustments.

Perspective and Prospects

Spina bifida has been known since ancient times, but little could be done then to ease the mental and physical damage that it causes. By the 1960s, surgical procedures were being developed that could repair the damage to the spinal cord and other

parts of the lower back. Improvements in physical therapy methods, as well as improved prosthetic devices, also began to make physical activity a realistic prospect for these children.

Late in the twentieth century, new insights were gained into the causes of spina bifida. The mutated genes involved were identified, and it was learned why they do not work properly. Studies of neural tube defects in mice revealed how these defects occur and how best to prevent them.

It is now known that the diet of a pregnant woman can influence neural tube development. One of the most effective measures for preventing spina bifida has been shown to be the daily intake of folic acid. Recommended doses vary from 0.4 to 4.0 mg per day based on risk status, such as prior delivery of a baby with neural tube defects. Preconceptual counseling includes recommendations for prenatal vitamins (which contain significantly more folic acid than other multivitamins) to be taken even before pregnancy. In 2000, it was reported that a folic acid supplement program for pregnant women that took place over a six-year period in South Carolina cut in half the rate of neural tube defects, including spina bifida. Doctors now know that folic acid supplements starting at the point of conception can decrease the risk of spina bifida by as much as 75 percent.

For fetuses that develop spina bifida, fetal surgery, which occurs while the fetus is in the womb, has become an option for parents. Fetal surgery can improve brain malformations, making it unnecessary for many babies to need lifelong shunts-devices that allow drainage of fluid that has accumulated around the brain. Even with the demonstrated benefits of the surgery, however, there is no guarantee that the surgery can correct all neurological functions or that it will be successful for all babies. In fact, it has been shown that fetal sur-

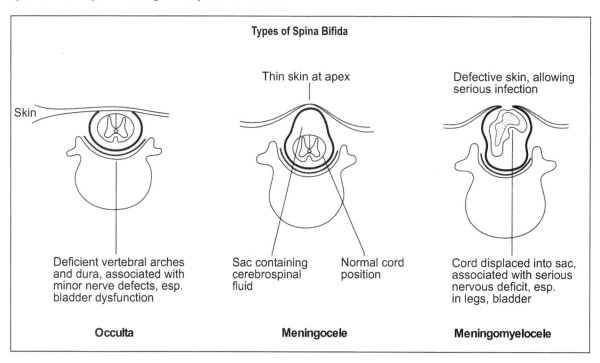

Types of Spina Bifida

Skin

Thin skin at apex

Defective skin, allowing serious infection

Deficient vertebral arches and dura, associated with minor nerve defects, esp. bladder dysfunction

Sac containing cerebrospinal fluid

Normal cord position

Cord displaced into sac, associated with serious nervous deficit, esp. in legs, bladder

Occulta

Meningocele

Meningomyelocele

gery increases the risk of a baby being born prematurely, which poses a whole new set of problems.

Support organizations for families can help them cope with the challenges of caring for children with spina bifida. Physical therapy, counseling, and various group activities are available. Thanks to improved treatment and support, it is now possible for children with this condition to lead long and healthy lives.

—Howard L. Hosick, Ph.D.

See also Amniocentesis; Birth defects; Brain damage; Chiari malformations; Congenital disorders; Embryology; Fetal surgery; Genetic diseases; Hydrocephalus; Mental retardation; Neonatology; Nervous system; Neurology; Neurology, pediatric; Neurosurgery; Perinatology; Plastic surgery; Spinal cord disorders; Spine, vertebrae, and disks; Stillbirth.

For Further Information:

Bloom, Beth-Ann, and Edward L. Seljeskog. *A Parent's Guide to Spina Bifida*. Minneapolis: University of Minnesota Press, 1988. Designed to assist the parents of children with spina bifida. The book includes chapters on the nature of the disorder and how it is treated, the medical problems associated with spina bifida, and how to help the afflicted child while he or she is growing up.

Kimball, Chad T. *Childhood Diseases and Disorders Sourcebook: Basic Consumer Health Information About Medical Problems Often Encountered in Pre-adolescent Children*. Detroit, Mich.: Omnigraphics, 2003. Offers basic facts about cancer, sickle cell disease, diabetes, and other chronic conditions in children and discusses frequently used diagnostic tests, surgeries, and medications. Long-term care for seriously ill children is also presented.

McLone, David. *An Introduction to Spina Bifida*. Reprint. Washington, D.C.: Spina Bifida Association of America, 1998. A concise report on spinal dysraphism and related disorders. Illustrations illuminate the text.

Martin, Richard J., Avroy A. Fanaroff, and Michele C. Walsh, eds. *Fanaroff and Martin's Neonatal-Perinatal Medicine: Diseases of the Fetus and Infant*. 2 vols. 8th ed. Philadelphia: Mosby/Elsevier, 2006. This classic reference work is one of the most comprehensive to date and features discussions on the diverse practice of neonatal-perinatal medicine, pregnancy disorders and their impact on the fetus, delivery room care, provisions for neonatal care, and the development and disorder of organ systems.

Moore, Keith L., and T. V. N. Persaud. *The Developing Human*. 8th ed. Philadelphia: Saunders/Elsevier, 2008. An outstanding textbook on human embryonic development, with specific information about the causes of congenital malformations and common defects occurring in each of the body's systems.

Nightingale, Elena O., and Melissa Goodman. *Before Birth: Prenatal Testing for Genetic Disease*. Cambridge, Mass.: Harvard University Press, 1990. Offering practical guidance to prospective parents, this volume addresses the question of whether or not to undergo testing, and if elected, how best to use the results.

Spina Bifida Association. http://www.sbaa.org. Promotes the prevention of spina bifida and strives to enhance the lives of all affected. Offers newsletter, physician referrals, and scholarship funds, among other services.

Spinal cord disorders
Disease/Disorder

Anatomy or system affected: Bones, musculoskeletal system, nerves, nervous system, spine

Specialties and related fields: Emergency medicine, neurol-

ogy, physical therapy

Definition: Conditions that adversely affect the spinal cord, which normally carries sensory information from the skin and muscles to the brain and returns with information to control movement.

Key terms:

congenital malformation: an abnormal condition that exists at birth

lesion: damage to cells, tissues, or organs that results in lost or impaired function; spinal cord lesion usually involves motor and/or sensory nerve fiber tracts

neuroglia: nonneuronal support cells of the central nervous system; oligodendrocytes are one type of neuroglia that myelinate nerve fibers

neuron: a nerve cell, the functional unit of the nervous system, containing dendrite and axon processes specialized for carrying information toward and away from the cell body, respectively

neurotrophic factor: a chemical signal that is required for the normal differentiation and function of neurons; this signal is often produced by neuroglia or by the cells with which neurons form synapses

plasticity: the ability of the nervous system to change its function over time by experience; includes changes in nerve fiber networks

teratogen: a chemical that causes abnormal embryonic development; often an environmental pollutant or something to which the mother is exposed during pregnancy, such as alcohol or other drugs

Causes and Symptoms

Most people take certain basic tasks for granted, such as walking up a flight of stairs, brushing their teeth, or using a personal computer. Motor neurons in the spinal cord control the hundreds of muscle fibers that are involved in each of these activities. At the same time, other neurons of the spinal cord serve as part of the sensory pathways that provide information regarding body position and motion that contributes to the coordination of these activities. In amyotrophic lateral sclerosis (ALS), also known as Lou Gehrig's disease, the motor neurons in the spinal cord die, leaving patients without control of their muscles. This example of a spinal disorder serves to emphasize the important role that the spinal cord plays as it serves as an interface (input-output system) between the brain and the body.

Similarly, most people have experienced pain in the hand, which is followed by an instantaneous, automatic movement of the hand away from the object causing that pain. Such reflexes represent the simplest of movements, yet they still require the integrative and relay action of neurons of the spinal cord to cause immediate hand withdrawal without requiring the individual to think about the act consciously. Only after the reflex has occurred does the spinal cord activity "inform" the brain that something happened. Therefore, in addition to sensory and motor interface functions for the brain, the spinal cord performs basic integration tasks as it controls reflexes, contributes to the coordination of movement between the left

Information on Spinal Cord Disorders

Causes: Injury, congenital or hereditary defects, disease, infection, tumors or cysts
Symptoms: Varies; may include impaired movement, pain, tingling or numbness, loss of sensation
Duration: Acute to chronic
Treatments: Depends on cause; may include surgery, antiviral drugs, antibiotics

and right sides of the body and prevents opposing muscle groups from trying to move a joint in opposite directions at the same time. As with any other vital organ of the body, spinal cord damage or defects have serious consequences for the health and well-being of humans.

In the medical research laboratory, paralysis results from complete or partial transection of the spinal cord. In the real world, a fracture or dislocation of vertebrae or damage done by a bullet can cause paralysis in the same fashion. Acute transection of the spinal cord can also result from an inflammatory condition or from any situation in which the spinal cord is compressed, such as by a tumor. The spinal cord is contained within the vertebral column, which is divided into the cervical, thoracic, lumbar, and sacral regions, each of which is associated with a specific set of functions. Transection typically results in the loss of sensory and motor functions below the level of the lesion.

Spinal cord injuries and defects are the result of three basic types of pathological conditions. The first of these conditions is traumatic physical injury to spinal cord tissue, such as the severing of the spinal cord during a car accident. The second condition is a congenital or inherited genetic problem with spinal cord development and function, as illustrated by spina bifida. The third is an acquired condition such as damage caused by a viral or bacterial infection. In each case, the severity of the pathological condition is dependent upon the location and extent of the resultant spinal cord lesion. In the clinical setting, physicians utilize information regarding all aspects of spinal cord function (such as sensory, motor, reflex, and coordination functions), as well as information from a variety of imaging techniques to diagnose pathological conditions and to select appropriate treatments.

Trauma. The neurons of the spinal cord carry out their functions by way of their long nerve processes (axons), which extend to form synapses with, and control, target cells (muscles and other neurons). Some of these nerve processes extend out of the spinal cord to the body, others extend either up to or down from higher-brain regions, and yet others extend from one side of the spinal cord to another. Trauma mainly damages the nerve process of cells and in this fashion disrupts their function in controlling target neurons and muscles. Often, after nerve processes have been damaged, the neuron itself will die because of loss of neurotrophic influences from their target cells. It has been estimated that every year between ten thousand and twelve thousand people in the United States are disabled by some degree of paralysis resulting from traumatic injury to the spinal cord. The spinal cord

can be also damaged by blocked blood flow to the cord, blood accumulation (hematoma) in or near the cord, or the presence of a ruptured or herniated disk, all of which can be caused by trauma.

Congenital defects. Spinal cord defects are not the result of trauma but rather are generally attributed to abnormal events during embryonic development. In particular, most major spinal cord defects arise around the third week of development. During this time, the flattened neural plate is beginning to fold upward as its lateral edges come together and fuse to form the top margin (dorsal aspect) of the neural tube. If this process is incomplete, then the spinal cord remains open and exposed along the embryo's back, accompanied by the failure of the vertebral bones to surround the spinal cord tissue completely. This condition is referred to as spina bifida. Often, rather than simply being exposed, some normal contents of the vertebral canal, including spinal cord tissue, protrude out of the back as a bulge. Spina bifida is most common in the lower lumbar and upper sacral regions of the spine, but more severe cases may involve the cervical and thoracic regions. Depending on the level and extent of the defect, the clinical symptoms of spinal abnormalities range from mild impairment to fatality. This type of neural tube defect often causes some degree of motor and sensory handicap. The cerebrospinal fluid is continuous from the ventricles of the brain to the central canal of the spinal cord. If the spinal defect impairs the normal flow of cerebrospinal fluid, other problems may occur, such as retardation resulting from hydrocephalus (fluid on the brain). Although there is still much to learn about the causes of spinal cord defects, in many cases scientific evidence points the finger at genetic problems (mutations) and the disruptive action of teratogens such as environmental pollutants and drugs.

Infections. Acquired spinal cord lesions are not the result of trauma or developmental problems but rather are related to such conditions as tumor development or viral and bacterial infections. In general, invasion of the spinal cord by viruses or bacteria can produce inflammation known as myelitis. Multiple sclerosis (MS) and ALS are the two most common nontraumatic disorders of the spinal cord. Many of the nerve fibers of the central nervous system are covered by a myelin sheath produced by neuroglia cells, known as oligodendrocytes. This sheath contributes to the speed and efficiency of the nerve cells as they carry electrical information. MS involves the destruction of this important myelin sheath, leading to the disruption of motor and sensory nerve pathway functions manifested by such symptoms as abnormal sensations, paralysis, and exaggerated reflexes. Although its cause is not clearly understood, researchers believe that viral infections are involved in some cases, while in others the individual's own immune system might be mistakenly destroying normal myelin tissue (an autoimmune disorder). ALS is a fatal condition that is restricted to the loss of motor neurons. As with MS, there is much speculation regarding the causes of ALS. Acquired immunodeficiency syndrome (AIDS) is a viral infection that can involve the disruption of spinal cord neuron function.

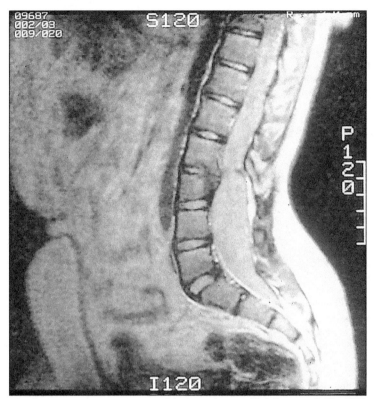

A nuclear magnetic resonance scan of the spine showing the defect spina bifida. (SIU School of Medicine)

alleviating serious problems. It is believed that better prenatal care may reduce the risk of spinal cord defects. For example, consumption of the vitamin folic acid in pregnancy greatly reduces the incidence of spina bifida. Numerous other causative factors have been implicated in spinal cord defects, including alcoholism, drug use, and even environmental pollution. In some cases, genetic screening may provide a method to reduce certain types of defects, while in other cases reduced exposure to risk elements is the most effective preventive action.

Treatments for acquired spinal cord injury involve antiviral and antibacterial drugs that combat infection and in so doing reduce inflammation and cell damage. It is clear that early detection and intervention is an important factor in being able to save as many neurons as possible and to limit the extent of the lesion. Neurotrophic factors are likely to be important therapeutic agents as doctors try to stimulate the maximum recovery of neuronal function. In cases in which the immune system itself may be damaging healthy neurons, as is suspected in some cases of MS, drugs are used to suppress immune function.

Other infections that can cause spinal cord lesions include tabes dorsalis, poliomyelitis, meningitis, and syringomyelia. Tabes dorsalis involves the degeneration of sensory neurons from the dorsal region of the spinal cord as a result of the invasion of the syphilis spirochete bacterium. The polio virus infects and kills spinal motor neurons in a disease called poliomyelitis; if the disease destroys the brain-stem neurons that control respiration and heart rate, then this condition is fatal. Meningitis is a bacterial inflammation of the layers of cells that cover the spinal cord (collectively referred to as meninges), producing high fever and sometimes inducing a comatose state that can lead to death.

Tumors and cysts. Growths within the spinal cord can also disrupt normal spinal cord function. Syringomyelia is such a condition, in which fluid-filled cysts develop among the neurons of the spinal cord. Cancerous tumors are often the result of uncontrolled growth of the neuroglia cells, which can damage neurons and nerve fiber pathways.

Treatment and Therapy

Spinal cord defects, either congenital or hereditary, pose serious challenges for the medical community. Surgical intervention is the only option in mild cases of spina bifida, but in severe cases there is no effective treatment. The advent of intrauterine surgery (prior to the birth of the baby) for the correction of minor cases of spina bifida is a major step toward

Perspective and Prospects

Medical researchers are taking numerous approaches to understand spinal cord development and function, in the hope of utilizing that information to develop new therapies to prevent or treat these clinical conditions. An interesting aspect of the problem is that, unlike most other organ systems, the adult nervous system appears to retain only a few selected stem cell populations after embryonic development. Stem cell populations are groups of cells that divide to produce cells for the growth and regeneration of tissues and organs.

It was believed that human babies were born with all the neurons in their central nervous system that they would ever have, meaning that no new neurons would be produced. Recent work in rodents and nonhuman primates, however, has unequivocally demonstrated that neural stem cells exist in the adult mammalian brain and give rise to millions of new neurons during an individual's life span. This process generates new neurons predominantly in two areas of the brain-in the olfactory bulb, which controls the sense of smell, and in the hippocampus, a memory center-but not to any appreciable extent in other brain areas. Scientists are beginning to identify stem cells in other brain regions, but there appear to be only a few, and those lack the ability to repair spinal cord injuries. Many laboratories are working on harnessing the potential of stem cells for cell replacement therapies, which hold significant promise for brain repair. As the individual ages, the nervous system becomes more efficient in processing information as neural networks are modified. This modification involves changes in nerve cell connections, a process referred to as plasticity, and new neuron generation (neurogenesis), but only in a few areas of the adult brain. Researchers hope to utilize information about the biological basis of normal plasticity to help repair damaged or impaired nervous systems.

Modern neuroscience research quickly vanquished the long-held belief that it is impossible to repair neurons damaged by trauma or disease. Experiments with animals and in tissue culture have demonstrated that damaged neurons can survive, regrow nerve processes, and once again carry electrical impulses. In fact, neurons from human spinal cords have been grown in tissue culture under conditions that stimulated them to regrow their axonal process. One of the most important aspects of understanding nervous system development is the fact that the cells communicate with one another not only with neurotransmitters but also with neurotrophic factors. Basic research and clinical trials are being done on neurotrophic factors with the expectation that they will become important parts of therapeutic treatments to stimulate the repair and regeneration of damaged neurons. These neurotrophic factors hold such promise because they are important in stimulating normal cell differentiation during embryonic development and for the subsequent survival of neurons after birth into adulthood. Therefore, clinical treatments are being designed to recreate the embryonic conditions that contributed to normal development. In addition, it is believed that one of the major factors in the lack of a regeneration response in damaged spinal cords is that the neuroglia cells, known as astrocytes, form scar tissue that is not conducive to nerve fiber regeneration. Therefore, medical researchers are looking at treatments that, in addition to prolonging the life of neurons, reduce the formation of scar tissue.

—*William L. Muhlach, Ph.D.;*
updated by W. Michael Zawada, Ph.D.

See also Amyotrophic lateral sclerosis; Anesthesia; Anesthesiology; Back pain; Bone cancer; Bone disorders; Bones and the skeleton; Brain damage; Cerebral palsy; Chiari malformations; Chiropractic; Congenital disorders; Disk removal; Fracture and dislocation; Head and neck disorders; Kinesiology; Kyphosis; Laminectomy and spinal fusion; Lumbar puncture; Meningitis; Motor neuron diseases; Multiple sclerosis; Muscle sprains, spasms, and disorders; Muscular dystrophy; Nervous system; Neuralgia, neuritis, and neuropathy; Neurology; Neurology, pediatric; Neurosurgery; Numbness and tingling; Osteoarthritis; Osteoporosis; Paget's disease; Paralysis; Paraplegia; Physical rehabilitation; Poliomyelitis; Quadriplegia; Radiculopathy; Sciatica; Scoliosis; Slipped disk; Spina bifida; Spine, vertebrae, and disks; Spondylitis; Sports medicine; Sympathectomy.

For Further Information:

Carey, Joseph, ed. *Brain Facts: A Primer on the Brain and Nervous System.* 5th ed. Washington, D.C.: Society for Neuroscience, 2006. A publication by the Society of Neuroscience directed at educating the general public about the value of neuroscience research.

Carlson, Bruce M. *Human Embryology and Developmental Biology.* 4th ed. Philadelphia: Mosby/Elsevier, 2009. This textbook presents human development in the context of modern scientific and medical research. Includes a consideration of basic normal spinal cord development, as well as a detailed look at developmental defects.

Kandel, Eric R., James H. Schwartz, and Thomas M. Jessell, eds. *Principles of Neural Science.* 5th ed. Norwalk, Conn.: Appleton and Lange, 2006. This massive, comprehensive book serves as the bible for the field of neuroscience. In spite of its tremendous breadth and depth, this book contains excellent basic explanations and illustrations, and thus serves as a valuable reference for people of all academic backgrounds.

Larsen, William J. *Human Embryology.* Edited by Lawrence S. Sherman, S. Steven Potter, and William J. Scott. 3d ed. New York: Churchill Livingstone, 2001. Basic coverage of human embryonic development, including both normal and abnormal spinal cord development.

Litin, Scott C., ed. *Mayo Clinic Family Health Book.* 4th ed. New York: HarperResource, 2009. Discusses both muscles and bones, underscoring the intimate relationship between disorders in the two systems. The text and illustrations are complete and easy to understand.

National Institute of Neurological Disorders and Stroke (NINDS). *Disorder Index.* http://www.ninds.nih .gov/disorders/disorder_index.htm. The site provides information about various spinal cord diseases and injury, current research, and support organizations.

Nicholls, John G., A. Robert Martin, and Bruce G. Wallace. *From Neuron to Brain.* 4th ed. Sunderland, Mass.: Sinauer, 2007. An excellent and detailed undergraduate neurobiology text that describes how nerve cells transmit signals, how signals are put together, and how higher functions emerge from this integration.

Palmer, Sara, Kay Harris Kriegsman, and Jeffrey B. Palmer. *Spinal Cord Injury: A Guide for Living.* Baltimore: Johns Hopkins University Press, 2000. Sets expectations for recovery from and life after a spinal cord injury. Covers initial hospitalization, rehabilitation therapy, readjusting to home, the effects of spinal cord injury on other family members, dating and sexuality, independent living choices, and current research.

Salter, Robert Bruce. *Textbook of Disorders and Injuries of the Musculoskeletal System.* 3d ed. Baltimore: Williams & Wilkins, 1999. Four sections of the book-"Basic Musculoskeletal Science and Its Applications," "Musculoskeletal Disorders: General and Specific," "Musculoskeletal Injuries," and "Research"-examine the diagnosis and treatment principles of disorders and trauma of the musculoskeletal system.

SPINAL FUSION. *See* LAMINECTOMY AND SPINAL FUSION.

SPINAL TAP. *See* LUMBAR PUNCTURE.

SPINE, VERTEBRAE, AND DISKS
Anatomy

Anatomy or system affected: Back, bones, musculoskeletal system, nerves, nervous system

Specialties and related fields: Alternative medicine, geriatrics and gerontology, neurology, orthopedics, physical therapy, preventive medicine, sports medicine

Definition: The supporting structures of the trunk, from the base of the skull to the end of the tailbone; the vertebrae form a small, central canal for the sensory and motor nerves that constitute the spinal cord.

Key terms:

disk: a soft, cushionlike structure that lies between bony vertebrae from the base of the skull to the sacrum of the pelvis; it has a soft liquid in the center (the nucleus pulposus) and is surrounded by a thickened ligament (the annulus fibrosis)

intervertebral foramina: openings between two adjacent vertebrae to permit the exit of nerve structures from the spinal cord

spinal cord: a cord in the trunk containing nerve cells that transmit impulses to and from the brain

spinous processes: bony projections from vertebrae (horizontally in the neck, tilting downward in the thoracic area, and horizontally in the lumbar area) that are connected to one another by the interspinous and supraspinous ligaments and that control extremes of trunk motion

transverse processes: projections from the sides of vertebrae, to which are attached muscles and ligaments, that assist in motor function by enhancing leverage and limiting extremes of motion

vertebra: a bony structure in the back with a central spinal canal surrounded by an arch; the back part of the arch (the lamina) and the front part of the arch (the pedicle) are joined together by muscles, ligaments, and cartilage for motion, stability, and posture

Structure and Functions

The spinal column undergoes developmental changes from infancy to the adult state and then degenerative changes with aging. The alignment of the spinal column at birth is in the shape of a C curve, the fetus having been curled up. This forward-tilted curve is retained except in the neck and lower back. As the infant raises its head and attempts to see things, head control and vision gradually require the head to tilt back, resulting in a posterior curve at the neck. As children progress to standing and walking, the lower spine also develops a posterior curve (a normal lumbar lordosis). As individuals increasingly use the predominant upper extremities, these muscles become stronger and increase the pull on that side of the spine, resulting in a lateral curve (a normal scoliosis).

Humans generally have thirty-three vertebrae, but abnormalities can occur in their numbers, shape, alignment, density, and maturation. There are seven vertebrae in the neck or cervical area, twelve in the chest or thoracic area, five in the lower back or lumbar area, five usually joined together in the pelvic region to form the sacrum, and three or four rudimentary vertebrae partially fused to form the coccyx. The typical vertebra develops embryologically from two bone growth centers. The front of one bone growth center becomes the body and part of the arch, while the other bone growth center evolves into the spinous processes, the transverse processes, the articular processes, and the back portion of the arch.

The thirty-three vertebrae of the spine have various defined parts and characteristics. The oval or round vertebral body has a spongy center surrounded by a dense bone. Above and below it are layers of cartilage. Lack of the mineral calcium reduces the density of the bone, resulting in osteoporo-sis. This condition may occur in postmenopausal women, causing pain, fractures, and kyphosis (a thoracic humpback). The pedicle portions of this anterior arch have an upper and lower notch called the intervertebral foramina, through which the spinal nerves exit from the spinal canal. At the junction of pedicle and lamina are projections upward and downward that form the articular processes, or joints. The alignment and direction of these joints vary with the spinal region and serve to control spinal motion. The transverse processes assist in the movement of muscles and at the chest level act as links between the ribs. There are generally twelve

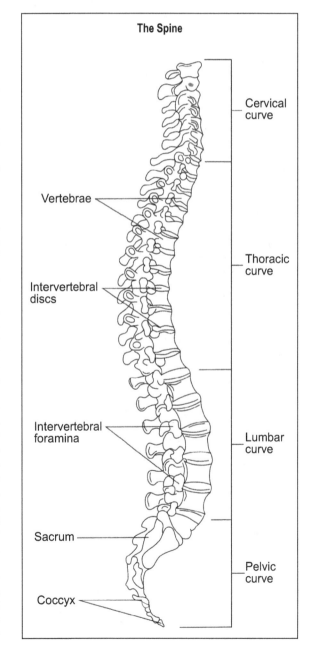

The Spine

Vertebrae

Intervertebral discs

Intervertebral foramina

Sacrum

Coccyx

Cervical curve

Thoracic curve

Lumbar curve

Pelvic curve

thoracic vertebrae and twelve ribs. On occasion, an extra cervical rib may be present; this extra rib narrows the exit space at the neck and can pinch the cervical nerves and blood vessels.

The upper two cervical processes are different from all other vertebrae. The first cervical vertebra supports the head and is called the atlas. Instead of a body, it has an enlarged anterior arch and a groove on which the head rests. Its transverse processes are long, but its spinous process is a little knob. The second cervical vertebra is also unique, with an upward projection called the dens that is like a pole fitting into the ring of the first cervical vertebral arch. It represents the body of the first cervical vertebra. This pole and ring permit the head to rotate.

The cervical transverse processes or lateral projections have holes, the transverse foramina, through which the vertebral arteries send blood to the brain. As one progresses downward, the vertebrae become larger and bear more weight. The thoracic vertebrae have their joint surfaces in the frontal plane, and the transverse processes are solid. The ribs share half of the joint surfaces with the adjoining vertebrae, except for the first, tenth, eleventh, and twelfth vertebrae; these vertebrae join only their corresponding ribs. As one continues down the spine, the spinous processes become more slender and project downward, almost touching one another. The lower thoracic vertebrae are closer to the lumbar vertebrae in appearance.

The lumbar vertebrae are more massive, carry more stress, and support the weight of the body. The transverse processes in this region are thinner but longer, increasing the leverage action for muscles. The joint surfaces tilt upward, backward, and toward the center, opening the joint space when one bends forward. This action permits side bending, increasing the side pressures on the disks. The five sacral vertebrae are fused, with small ridges representing the sites of fusion. Small openings allow the upper four sacral nerves to exit the spine. The sacrum contributes the back portion of the pelvis. The coccyx, or tailbone, is composed of three or four rudimentary vertebrae, with the first distinct and separate from the other two or three, which are fused. The back of the spine is layered with muscles going to the upper extremities, with long vertical muscles underneath, intermediate-length muscles under these, and the deepest muscle groups closest to the spine and only two or three vertebrae in length.

Vertebrae are separated by washers called disks. The central portion of a disk is a gel-like substance, the nucleus pulposus, which offers hydraulic cushioning and allows some movement. This substance is enclosed in a ligamentous covering called the annulus fibrosis. Disks contribute approximately one-fourth of body length, can add about eight degrees in motion per vertebra, and can alter their shape to accommodate the solid vertebrae when the body is bent. The nucleus pulposus is 70 to 80 percent water, and about 14 kilograms (30 pounds) of pressure must be exerted constantly by ligaments to maintain the shape of the disk. Dehydration, aging, compressive forces, and simply a day of normal activity can temporarily reduce the amount of the watery nucleus

pulposus, increase the bulging of the disks, and shorten one's stature.

The spinal cord connects the peripheral structures of the body to the brain and the nerve cells in the spinal cord itself. Until about the third month of life, the spinal cord occupies the entire length of the spinal canal. The vertebrae grow faster than the spinal cord, however, and later in life it occupies two-thirds of the length of the spinal canal (approximately 42 to 45 centimeters) and ends at about the second lumbar vertebra. The coverings on the cord continue as the filum terminale, which is attached to the sacral vertebrae.

There are three coverings of the spinal cord within the spinal canal. The outermost, toughest, and fibrous covering, called the dura, is separated from the bony surfaces by fat and blood vessels. The spinal cord is covered by a thin layer called the pia that enters into the spinal cord and separates various portions of the cord. Surrounding the pia is a protective fluid, the spinal fluid, which is held in place by the arachnoid layer; this fluid can be aspirated for analysis, as in a lumbar puncture, or spinal tap. The nerves exiting from the spinal cord are also segmental. There are only seven cervical vertebrae but eight cervical nerves. The eighth cervical nerve exits below the seventh cervical vertebra, and thereafter all roots from the vertebrae leave below the corresponding vertebra. These segmental nerves then join, divide, send messages to the brain and other organs, and control bodily functions and motion.

Ligaments run vertically in front of the vertebral bodies (the anterior longitudinal ligament) and in back of the vertebral bodies and within the spinal canal (the posterior longitudinal ligament). These ligaments support the vertebrae and disks and limit excessive motion forward and backward. The posterior longitudinal ligament ceases at about the fourth lumbar vertebra, and thus farther down the spine the fibrous rings about the disks are weaker, permitting herniations. Such leakages from the disks may press on nerve roots exiting at these levels and cause pain. These ruptures of the disks occur mostly when lifting with the trunk bent forward and sideways. There are additional ligaments between the spinous processes at the tips (the supraspinous ligament) and along the length of the spinous processes (the interspinous ligament). The portion of the arch between the spinous processes and the transverse processes is the lamina. Between the laminae are the ligamentum flavum. The interspinous ligament, ligamentum flavum, and nucleus pulposus have no pain fibers. The laminae and disks may be removed when disk surgery is performed, and pieces of bone from the hip may be used to fuse and reduce motion at this level.

Motion between each vertebra is about eight degrees. Motion is enhanced by the facets, vertical bony projections with joint surfaces. They are structured like the other joints of the body, and thus are subject to irritation and arthritic changes. Flexion of the trunk opens the spaces in the lumbar joints and allows side bending and rotation in the same direction. Extension of the trunk compresses and limits motion in these facets.

The blood supply to the spinal cord and the surrounding tissues diminishes progressively downward. Excessive activ-

Some Types of Spinal Disorder

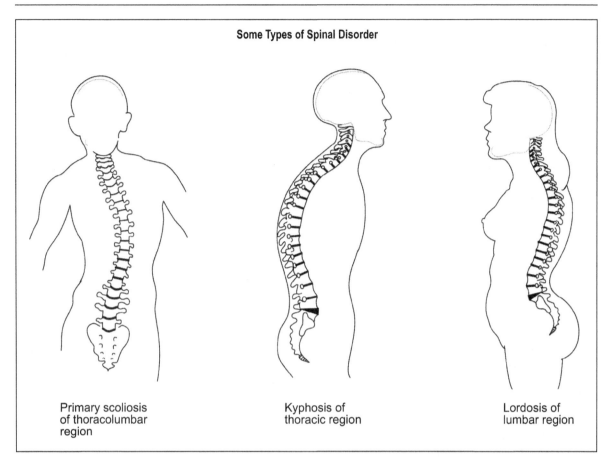

Primary scoliosis
of thoracolumbar
region

Kyphosis of
thoracic region

Lordosis of
lumbar region

ity can lead to insufficient circulating blood to these nerves and give rise to symptoms in the lower extremity called intermittent claudication. The front portion of the spinal cord contains motor nerve cells, leading to the trunk and the muscles of the extremities, that can be inhibited or activated by impulses. The lateral areas of the spinal region contain messenger tracts and the autonomic nervous system. The back portion of the spinal cord has sensory structures that carry messages of pain, temperature, position, and touch to the brain. The different levels within the spinal cord connect to different segmental structures of the body. The fifth cervical nerve down to the first thoracic nerve connect to the upper extremities, and the second lumbar to second sacral roots connect to the lower extremities. Compression of these nerve roots at the spine may cause symptoms in areas distant from the spine.

Disorders and Diseases

The anatomy of the trunk regulates the erect, or standing, posture. It is influenced by the structure of the vertebrae and extremities and even by the tilt of the head. It is also influenced by cultural factors, emotion, habits, and occupation. Good posture involves standing straight with the head up, the shoulders back and up, the stomach in, and the hips and knees straight. This position also is most efficient in energy expenditure, since it requires the least amount of muscle activity in order to balance the weights in the front and back of the trunk, as well as the weights on the left and right sides of the body. Looking at the front of the body, the central gravitational, or weight-bearing, line falls in line with the nose and between the pelvis, knees, and ankles. From the back, the gravitational line follows the center of the head, the spinous processes, the gluteal fold between the buttocks, and between the knees and ankles. The weight stresses should be balanced between the right side and the left side of the body and between the front and the back. The head should be maintained so that the eyes and the labyrinth in the inner ear are level. Any deviations cause imbalance in the trunk, resulting in muscle strain, ligament sprains, pain, and possibly deformities. Abnormalities in posture and gait may be attributable to muscle imbalance, deformities at birth, problems in development, disease, or surgical procedures.

There are several birth defects that affect the spine. Occasionally, during embryonic development, the two bone growth regions that form a vertebra do not fuse together, causing an opening in the arch in the back called spina bifida. Spondylolysis occurs when the articular process remains unattached. Ligaments, muscles, and tendons are unable to attach to these areas securely, and the result is weakness in the vertebra and a reduction in stability. Occasionally, this weakness permits the upper vertebra to slide forward, a condition called spondylolisthesis. The misalignment and narrowing of the spinal canal can compress the nerve structures within it, a condition known as spinal stenosis. The lower cervical and lower lumbar regions, which need more nerve tissue to supply the extremities, are especially vulnerable to pressure symptoms.

Inequality in leg lengths or pain in the lower extremities, upper extremities, abdomen, chest, or neck can lead to compensatory reactions in the trunk. These may then cause misalignment in the spine with side deviations (scoliosis), backward deviations (kyphosis, or humpback, in the thoracic area), and forward deviations (lordosis in the low back). Other contributing factors are overuse, muscle spasm or weakness, birth defects, developmental abnormalities, diseases, aging, and trauma. Some misalignments occur after surgery on the chest, back, or abdomen. Idiopathic scoliosis (scoliosis of unknown cause) may occur in adolescent girls; when it is severe, lung and heart functions can be impaired. Temporarily increased lordosis can occur in pregnancy, to compensate for the extra weight in the abdomen. Lordosis may be permanent because of structural changes in the spine, pendulous abdomen and/or breasts, or poor muscle balance. Therefore, back problems may be caused by poor posture, behavior, occupation, and structural, neurologic, or muscular factors. Pain located only in the back is generally attributable to poor posture, trauma, or inflammation. If pain extends below the knees, the cause may be nerve pressure at the fifth lumbar or first sacral nerve roots. Bladder and rectal sphincter disturbances may indicate sacral nerve or cord involvement and may require immediate surgical care.

The body's center of gravity is in the front portion of the second lumbar vertebra. Thus, the compressive force of body weight is increased when one lifts an object with the arms in front of the trunk. The greater the distance of the object from the center of the body, the greater the need for the back muscles to contract. Lifting a 45-kilogram (100-pound) object may require a 545-kilogram (1,200-pound) muscle pull and compressive force. The posterior longitudinal support for the disks that is provided by ligaments narrows in the sides at the level of the fourth and fifth lumbar vertebrae. Herniations through the fibrous disk ring at these levels are more likely, and a ruptured disk can pinch the nerves exiting at these levels.

Stresses that bear on the spine are categorized as compressive, shearing, elongating, or rotational. Compressive forces may involve the muscles, disks (possible ruptures), vertebrae (fractures), and the facet joints. Shearing stress may lead to forward slippage of the fourth or fifth vertebra from the segment below. This is most common in individuals with incomplete bony union of vertebrae. Rotatory stress may affect the joints, the facets of the spine, the short spine muscles, or the ligaments. On rare occasions, an elongating stretch or traction may strain muscles and sprain or tear ligaments.

Perspective and Prospects

Examinations of the spine usually include the history of the problem: whether it is sudden or gradual and whether it is influenced by certain activities or climates. The physician checks the patient's posture for abnormal curvatures and determines whether they are fixed or functional. Functional curves disappear when the patient is lying down. The gait should be evaluated for symmetry, balance, and deviations. The physician will measure leg lengths for inequalities, the circumference of the chest for rib flare, and the circumferences of extremities for swelling or shrinkage. Next, the trunk's range of motion will be evaluated, followed by palpation to discover tender spots and muscle spasms.

With spinal problems, a full examination of the entire body is indicated since pain can be referred to the back from other organs. Changes in function, sensation, and motor strength can indicate spinal cord or nerve involvement. Simple X rays of the spine will indicate alignment of the vertebrae, bone density, fracture lines, extraneous bone growth, cartilage thickness, and unusual soft tissue densities caused by hemorrhage or calcification. For problems other than bone and cartilage tissue involvement, a computed tomography (CT) scan or magnetic resonance imaging (MRI) may be needed; these techniques provide images of the area to be examined that are at different levels or depths.

—Eugene J. Rogers, M.D.

See also Anesthesia; Anesthesiology; Back pain; Bone cancer; Bone disorders; Bones and the skeleton; Braces, orthopedic; Cerebral palsy; Chiari malformations; Chiropractic; Disk removal; Fracture and dislocation; Head and neck disorders; Kinesiology; Kyphosis; Laminectomy and spinal fusion; Lumbar puncture; Meningitis; Motor neuron diseases; Multiple sclerosis; Muscle sprains, spasms, and disorders; Muscular dystrophy; Nervous system; Neuralgia, neuritis, and neuropathy; Neurology; Neurology, pediatric; Neurosurgery; Numbness and tingling; Orthopedic surgery; Orthopedics; Orthopedics, pediatric; Osteoarthritis; Osteoporosis; Paget's disease; Paralysis; Paraplegia; Physical rehabilitation; Poliomyelitis; Quadriplegia; Radiculopathy; Sciatica; Scoliosis; Slipped disk; Spina bifida; Spinal cord disorders; Spondylitis; Sports medicine; Stenosis; Sympathectomy; Whiplash.

For Further Information:

Fine, Judylaine. *Conquering Back Pain: A Comprehensive Guide.* Rev. ed. Englewood Cliffs, N.J.: Prentice Hall, 1987. This softcover book summarizes the anatomy of the back, discussing its various structures, types of pain, and areas where pain may be distributed. Also enumerates the treatments, both conservative and surgical, of back pain.

Jenkins, David B. *Hollinshead's Functional Anatomy of the Limbs and Back.* 9th ed. Philadelphia: Saunders/Elsevier, 2009. An easy-to-understand and well-illustrated book designed for physical therapy students. It can be useful for those individuals wishing more information about the muscles of the back and extremities, their nerve and blood supplies, and the function of these structures.

Palastanga, Nigel, Derek Field, and Roger Soames. *Anatomy and Human Movement: Structure and Function.* 5th ed. New York: Butterworth Heinemann/Elsevier, 2007. This large volume contains excellent illustrations, definitions, and indexes and is written to simplify the more complex aspects of anatomy using understandable terms.

Scott, Judith. *Good-bye to Bad Backs: Stretching and Strengthening Exercises for Alignment and Freedom from Lower Back Pain.* 3d ed. New York: Princeton Book, 2002. Provides visualizing techniques, gentle exercises, and specific workouts for alleviating back pain. Medical line drawings illustrate and teach about muscles and their relationship to posture and lower back pain.

Tortora, Gerard J., and Bryan Derrickson. *Principles of Anatomy and Physiology*. 12th ed. Hoboken, N.J.: John Wiley & Sons, 2009. This introductory college textbook offers an excellent survey of human anatomy and physiology. Several chapters are devoted to the musculoskeletal system. In addition to normal structure and function, each chapter includes sections on abnormalities (including both injuries and diseases) and their treatment.

SPINOCEREBELLAR ATAXIA
Disease/Disorder

Also known as: Olivopontocerebellar atrophy, Maria's ataxia, Cerebellar degeneration

Anatomy or system affected: Arms, brain, eyes, feet, hands, head, legs, muscles, musculoskeletal system, nerves, nervous system

Specialties and related fields: Genetics, occupational health, ophthalmology, optometry, physical therapy, speech pathology

Definition: A group of inherited diseases that cause degeneration in the brain and spinal cord, resulting in progressive loss of coordination.

Key terms:

ataxia: poor coordination and unsteadiness that result from damage to the brain

dysarthria: speech disorder as a result of nerve damage

macular degeneration: damage to the photoreceptors in the retina that causes loss of vision in the center of the visual field

Causes and Symptoms

Located at the base of the brain, the cerebellum receives neural input from the overlying cerebral hemispheres, spinal cord, and sensory receptors, and integrates these inputs in order to precisely coordinate movement. Damage to the cerebellum causes dizziness, nausea, poor balance, and coordination problems.

Spinocerebellar ataxia (SCA) is a group of hereditary diseases of the nervous system characterized by the progressive onset of ataxia or inability to coordinate muscle movements. The symptoms of SCA are a consequence of gradual, progressive damage to the cerebellum.

Over 30 different types of SCA have been described, and they are named SCA1, SCA2, and so on. Mutations in distinct genes cause the different types of SCAs, and their inheritance patterns also vary.

The specific symptoms of each type of SCA vary as do the age when symptoms first appear, but virtually all of them cause ataxia and tremors. For example, people with SCA1 begin with an abnormal gait and gradually progress into ataxia of all four limbs and speech problems (dysarthria). Within 15-20 years, the disease confines most patients to a wheelchair. SCA2 has similar symptoms except that the fast, jerky movements the eyes make when changing their focus from

---

Information on Spinocerebellar Ataxia

Causes: Inherited mutations in various genes that cause the death of brain cells

Symptoms: Symptoms vary but they have in common progressive loss of coordination and tremors

Duration: Onset of symptoms varies; disease lasts a lifetime

Treatments: Physical and occupational therapy, speech pathology, supportive devices to help with movement

---

one object to another (saccades) significantly slow. In addition to ataxia, SCA7 causes macular degeneration and blindness, and SCA10 and 17 cause seizures.

Treatment and Therapy

Diagnosis of SCA requires brain imaging, which can detect atrophy of the cerebellum, the symptoms of the patient, and, since these diseases are inherited, their family history. However, because the symptoms of these diseases show so many similarities, molecular genetic tests remain the only way to definitively determine which type of SCA ails a patient.

No cure exists for SCA, and treatments consist of addressing symptoms. Balance and mobility problems may require a cane, walker, or wheelchair. Physical therapy has been shown to improve mobility for patients, and occupational therapy can also assist patients with independent living. Speech pathology can also help with speech problems. Sleep disorders afflict some SCA patients, and prescribed sleep aids may provide relief.

Experimental treatments with stem cell transplantations have shown promise in laboratory animals, and a small clinical trial in China with umbilical cord stem cells showed definite promise, but such treatments remain in the experimental stages.

—*Michael A. Buratovich, Ph.D.*

See also Genetic counseling; Neurology; Occupational health; Quadriplegia; Terminally ill: extended care

For Further Information:

Hong, Sunghoi, ed. *Ataxia: Causes, Symptoms and Treatment.* Hauppauge, NY: Nova Science Publishers, 2012.

McArthur, Sara. *Ataxia: How I Had to Cope with an Untreatable, Incurable Neurodegenerative Cerebellum Disease.* Frederick, MD: PublishAmerica, 2010.

Schuman, Tammy L. Scooter Sagas: *Coping With Ataxia.* Bloomington, IN: iUniverse, 2013.

SPLENECTOMY
Procedure

Anatomy or system affected: Abdomen, lymphatic system, spleen

Specialties and related fields: Emergency medicine, general surgery

Definition: The surgical removal of the spleen.

Indications and Procedures

Splenectomy is often performed after trauma to the upper left abdominal cavity that results in injury to the spleen. When the spleen is damaged in such cases, life-threatening intra-abdominal hemorrhage may occur. Surgical repair of the damaged spleen is sometimes difficult, but the lack of a spleen has relatively few ill effects, as other organs such as the liver and tissues of the lymphatic system compensate for its absence. Therefore, splenectomy is usually the indicated treatment for damage to the spleen.

Patients undergoing splenectomy are first anesthetized by an anesthesiologist. Surgical assistants then prepare the patient by scrubbing the upper abdomen to rid the skin of pathogens. The surgeon than makes an incision in the upper left abdomen or along the midline of the abdomen. He or she will then expose the spleen and tie off blood vessels to the spleen with sutures. The surgeon then cuts the attachments that anchor the spleen in the abdomen and removes the organ. This procedure takes approximately one hour to complete, provided that there are no complications. Most patients are allowed to leave the hospital after about one week or less. Although surgical infections are rare, they may require the patient to remain hospitalized for a few more days.

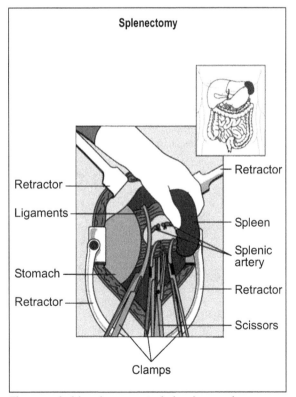

Splenectomy

Retractor
Retractor
Ligaments
Spleen
Splenic artery
Stomach
Retractor
Retractor
Scissors
Clamps

The removal of the spleen is required when the organ has sustained damage from injury or disease; the inset shows the location of the spleen.

Uses and Complications

Splenectomy is also performed to treat patients with certain types of anemia and hypersplenism. Since the normal function of the spleen is to destroy aged or nonfunctional red blood cells and platelets, overactivity of the spleen in hypersplenism results in excessive destruction of these blood cells and leads to anemia and blood-clotting disorders.

Even though splenectomy has few long-term adverse effects, some adult patients have a slightly increased risk of contracting infections. Splenectomy in children, however, results in greater susceptibility, particularly to pneumococcal pneumonia. Physicians often recommend that children who have undergone splenectomy be immunized against this bacterial pneumonia, and many of these patients even receive long-term prophylactic antibiotic therapy to prevent the disease.

—Matthew Berria, Ph.D.,
and Douglas Reinhart, M.D.

See also Abdomen; Abdominal disorders; Anemia; Bleeding; Hematology; Hematology, pediatric; Immune system; Immunology; Internal medicine; Lymphatic system; Metabolism; Pneumonia; Wounds.

For Further Information:

Griffith, H. Winter. *Complete Guide to Symptoms, Illness, and Surgery.* Revised and updated by Stephen Moore and Kenneth Yoder. 5th ed. New York: Perigee, 2006.

Hiatt, J. R., E. H. Phillips, L. Morgenstern, eds. *Surgical Diseases of the Spleen.* New York: Springer, 1997.

Kasper, Dennis L., et al., eds. *Harrison's Principles of Internal Medicine.* 16th ed. New York: McGraw-Hill, 2005.

Schwartz, Seymour I., James T. Adams, and Arthur W. Bauman. *Splenectomy for Hematologic Disorders.* Chicago: Year Book Medical, 1971.

Wilkins, Bridget, and Dennis H. Wright. *Illustrated Pathology of the Spleen.* New York: Cambridge University Press, 2000.

Zollinger, Robert M., Jr., and Robert M. Zollinger, Sr. *Zollinger's Atlas of Surgical Operations.* 8th ed. New York: McGraw-Hill, 2003.

SPLIT-BRAIN

Disease/Disorder

Anatomy or system affected: Brain

Specialties and related fields: Neurology, neuroscience, psychiatry, psychology

Definition: A condition that results from cutting the corpus callosum, which is the major connection between the two cerebral hemispheres of the brain.

Key terms:

cerebral hemispheres: refers to the two halves of the cerebrum that includes the cerebral cortex, containing both white and gray matter of the brain

commissure: a connection or link between two structures such as the two cerebral hemispheres

contralateral: referring to the opposite side

epilepsy: a neurological condition that results in seizure activity

epileptic focus: the point in the brain where a seizure originates

glia: the most numerous cells within the brain; in contrast to neurons, they do not conduct impulses but provide various supportive functions such as cleaning up waste products

laterality: refers to unique functions that occur within only one cerebral hemisphere

myelin: glia cells that wrap themselves around nerve axons

Causes and Symptoms

Split-brain is a condition that develops when the two cerebral hemispheres in the brain cannot easily and efficiently communicate with each other. In early usage, it was referred to as the bisected brain. The corpus callosum (CC) is the largest of several connections between the two hemispheres. The CC is made up of mostly nerve axons (approximately 350 million in the human brain), which are covered with glia cells that form a myelin sheath. The density of the myelinated axons is such that it alters the color of the CC giving it a whitish appearance-hence, the name "white matter" as opposed to "gray matter" found in the brain. The central purpose of the CC is to allow for the transference of massive amounts of information to flow across the two hemispheres. When this connection is severed, the brain receives information but becomes limited in how it can process it.

Immediately after the CC is surgically cut, a patient will typically experience trouble coordinating their behavior. Investigators have described the split-brain condition as though two people are in control of a single body. For example, a split-brain person who removes an item from a closet with one hand could find that the opposite hand attempts to put it back. Fortunately, the internal competition that results from two independent hemispheres dissipates after a few weeks. The brain, through the process of neuroplasticity, begins to alter itself in ways that allow the two hemispheres to cooperate better. One way it does this is by allowing additional commissures (e.g., anterior commissure) to transfer information that had been previously sent across by the CC. It is also believed that the left hemisphere suppresses the right hemisphere's ability to interfere with coordination by taking control.

Although severing the CC is an intrusive surgical procedure, it usually does not lead to a permanent debilitating outcome. Most patients lead a normal life postsurgery. For physicians and neuroscientists, one unexpected windfall from the procedure was that it created an opportunity to learn more about the independent nature and functionality of the two hemispheres. Although it was previously known that each hemisphere controlled the sensory and motor information on the contralateral side of the body, the split-brain condition revealed the laterality for different language functions, memory processes, and different types of attentional processes. Experimental testing performed by Michael Gazzaniga and his colleagues found that visual information could be presented in such a way that only one hemisphere could learn it. If a word such as "spoon" was presented to the right hemisphere, the split-brain person showed signs of knowing the word yet could not verbalize it. The inability to say "spoon" was due to the lack of language centers in the left hemisphere for the vast majority of people. However, when the person is

asked to point to the object from a group of objects, he has no difficulty identifying the spoon. This apparent lack of "knowing" how to verbalize the object is due to the fact that information was placed into the nonspeaking hemisphere, which could not transfer the information into the left hemisphere via the CC.

Treatment and Therapy

The split-brain procedure is most often performed on patients who suffer from epilepsy. Epilepsy occurs in one to two percent of the population. In the majority of cases, epileptic seizures can be controlled using antiseizure medication such as tegretol. When medicines do not adequately control seizure activity, surgical procedures are considered to remove the epileptic focus with the goal of eliminating the seizures. In rare instances, a patient might have multiple focus points within the same hemisphere whereby surgically removing all of them would be too dangerous. An alternative surgical procedure is a corpus callostomy. This is a procedure that severs the CC, resulting in the split-brain condition. Surgeons will consider cutting about two-thirds of the CC and then evaluating the results as a means to avoid some of the split-brain symptoms. This procedure does not prevent seizures from occurring; instead, it isolates the seizures in one hemisphere by preventing the malevolent electrical signals to propagate through the CC to the opposite hemisphere, thus minimizing its disrupting influence on the brain. A corpus callostomy is a last resort treatment to stop the hemispheres from sharing seizure activity, but it can come at a cost.

Different degrees of split-brain conditions can occur as a result of abnormal neural development. A rare genetic disorder, callosal agenesis, occurs when the CC forms improperly or not at all. This condition can lead to developmental delays and difficulties in language as well as spatial reasoning. Whether the split-brain condition arises from corpus callostomy or from callosal agenesis, cognitive rehabilitation can be prescribed as a means to improve overall cognitive functioning.

Perspective and Prospects

While William P. van Wagenen and R. Yorke Herren, in 1940, were the first to create the split-brain condition by surgically cutting the CC as a means to control epileptic seizures, it was Michael Gazzaniga, Joseph Bogen, and Roger Sperry who adapted more modern techniques, which were initially performed on animals, to human patients in the early 1960s. Today, while corpus callostomy surgeries are still being performed to help patients suffering from epileptic seizures, most neuroscientists have turned to functional brain imaging technologies such as fMRI and PET as a means to investigate the unique processing capabilities of the two cerebral hemispheres.

—*Bryan C. Auday, Ph.D., and Daruenie Andujar*

See also Epilepsy; Neurology; Neuroscience

For Further Information:
Epilepsy Foundation of America. http://www.epilepsyfoundation.org.

Gazzaniga, Michael. "Forty-Five Years of Split-Brain Research and Still Going Strong." *Nature Reviews Neuroscience* (August, 2005): 653-659.

Gazzaniga, Michael. "The Split Brain Revisited." *Scientific American: The Hidden Mind; Special Editions* (May, 2002): 27-31.

Reuter-Lorenz, Patricia Ann, and Michael S. Gazzaniga. *The Cognitive Neuroscience of Mind: A Tribute to Michael S. Gazzaniga.* Cambridge, MA: MIT Press, 2010.

Springer, Sally, and Georg Deutsch. *Left Brain Right Brain Perspectives from Cognitive Neuroscience.* New York: W.H. Freeman and Company, 2003.

Stirling, John D. *Cortical Functions.* London: Routledge, 2000.

SPONDYLITIS

Disease/Disorder

Also known as: Ankylosing spondylitis

Anatomy or system affected: Joints, spine

Specialties and related fields: Cardiology, ophthalmology, orthopedics

Definition: A form of arthritis that affects the spine.

Causes and Symptoms

Spondylitis, also known as ankylosing spondylitis, is a form of arthritis that is chronic and affects the spine. It is a specific disease within a family of diseases called spondyloarthropathies. Examples include psoriatic arthritis, Reiter's syndrome, and arthritis associated with inflammatory bowel disease (IBD). Spondylitis has unique features differentiating it from the other spondyloarthropathies and its own prognosis. The cause of spondylitis is unknown, but the condition may be genetic. Most people with this condition or other spondyloarthropathies are born with a particular gene, HLA-B27. However, having the gene does not mean that a person will develop spondylitis.

Symptoms include mild to severe back and buttock pain that is often worse in the early morning hours. This pain usually decreases with activity. The condition may begin in the teens or twenties and appears gradually over time. Continued inflammation of the ligaments and joints of the spine can cause the spine to fuse together, leading to deformity and disability. The inflammation of ankylosing spondylitis can affect other parts of the body, most commonly other joints and the eyes, but sometimes the lungs and heart valves. Other complications include arthritis of the hip joints and the joints between the ribs and sternum, bone spurs and inflammation in the feet, inflammation of the eyes, scarring of the lungs, inflammation of the prostate, and inflammation of the aorta and aortic valve. Severe disease may lead to poor posture and deformities.

It is reported that men are more likely than women to develop spondylitis; however, females may develop milder cases that sometimes go undiagnosed. Most symptoms of spondylitis appear in early adulthood, prior to age forty, although young males may have symptoms in early adolescence, or even in childhood.

The hallmark signs and symptoms are stiffness and pain in the lower back, buttocks, and hips upon waking in the morning or after a period of inactivity; back pain relieved by movement and exercise; difficulty bending the spine; pain in the hips and difficulty walking; pain in the heels and soles of the feet; bent posture; straightening of the normal curvature of the spine; fever; loss of appetite and weight loss; fatigue and decreased energy; eye swelling, redness, and pain; sensitivity to light; difficulty with chest expansion for deep breathing; heart failure; and heart block.

No definitive test can diagnose ankylosing spondylitis. Most doctors expect to see X-ray evidence of inflammation of the joint between the sacrum and the ilium, as well as any one of the following: inflammatory back pain, reduced mobility of the spine, and reduced ability to expand the chest. Blood tests results that can suggest spondylitis include an elevated erythrocyte sedimentation rate and anemia. The aspiration of synovial fluid from the joint will confirm inflammation.

Treatment and Therapy

Treatment includes exercise and physical therapy to help reduce stiffness and to maintain good posture and mobility. Medications for pain and inflammation, such as nonsteroidal anti-inflammatory drugs (NSAIDs), are prescribed. Treatment of iritis involves regular eye examinations. Assistive devices, such as a cane or walker, are used to help reduce joint stress and inflammation. Surgery is rarely performed. Patients should choose chairs that help them avoid slumped or stooped postures. Other treatments include hip replacement surgery, treatment for iritis with steroid and dilating drops, and a pacemaker for severe heart block.

—*Jane C. Norman, Ph.D., R.N., C.N.E.*

See also Arthritis; Back pain; Joints; Paralysis; Rheumatoid arthritis; Rheumatology; Spine, vertebrae, and disks.

For Further Information:

Klippel, John H., Paul A. Dieppe, Fred F. Ferri. *Primary Care Rheumatology.* Philadelphia: W. B. Saunders, 2002.

Koopman, William J., and Larry W. Moreland, eds. *Arthritis and Allied Conditions: A Textbook of Rheumatology.* 15th ed. Philadelphia: Lippincott Williams & Wilkins, 2005.

Royen, Barend J. van, and Ben A. C. Dijkmans, eds. *Ankylosing Spondylitis: Diagnosis and Management.* New York: Taylor & Francis, 2006.

Information on Spondylitis

Causes: Unknown; possibly genetic

Symptoms: Pain in lower back, buttocks, and hips in morning or after inactivity; difficulty bending spine; bent posture; difficulty walking; pain in heels and soles; fever; appetite loss and weight loss; fatigue and decreased energy; eye swelling, redness, and pain; sensitivity to light; difficulty with chest expansion for deep breathing; heart failure; heart block

Duration: Chronic

Treatments: Exercise and physical therapy; medications (pain relievers, NSAIDs); assistive devices (canes, walkers)

Van der Linden, S., and D. van der Heijde. "Ankylosing Spondylitis: Clinical Features." *Rheumatic Disease Clinics of North America* 24, no. 4 (1998): 663-676.

Weisman, Michael H., Désirée van der Heijde, and John D. Reveille, eds. *Ankylosing Spondylitis and the Spondyloarthropathies*. St. Louis, Mo.: Mosby/Elsevier, 2006.

SPORTS MEDICINE

Specialty

Anatomy or system affected: Bones, circulatory system, feet, hands, head, heart, joints, knees, legs, ligaments, muscles, musculoskeletal system, nervous system, spine, tendons

Specialties and related fields: Cardiology, emergency medicine, exercise physiology, family medicine, internal medicine, nutrition, orthopedics, pharmacology, physical therapy, preventive medicine, psychology, rheumatology

Definition: A medical subspecialty concerned with the care and prevention of athletic injuries, primarily those related to the musculoskeletal system.

Key terms:

joint: a specialized structure in the body where bones come together and motion occurs

ligament: a tough, rubber-band-like structure that connects one bone to another and prevents the abnormal motion of these bones in relationship to each other

musculoskeletal: a term used to describe the relationship between bones and muscles within the framework of the body and the way in which they provide stability and locomotion

musculotendinous unit: a structure that consists of a muscle that provides motion of a bone and its attachment to the bone, the tendon, which is a tough, inelastic fibrous structure

orthopedic surgery: the field of surgery that deals with the musculoskeletal system

Science and Profession

Sports medicine is a field that has become popular as the number of people who exercise has increased. More than 50 percent of people in the United States exercise on a daily basis. People all over the country are participating in sports, from recreational sports to professional competitive sports. There has been a growing trend of participation in exercise as more and more studies have proved that exercise is beneficial to health; however, exercise places people at risk for injuries that a sedentary person would not have. This fact has led to the emergence of sports medicine, with its specially trained health care professionals. These professionals include physical therapists, athletic trainers, nutritionists, exercise physiologists, cardiologists, sports psychologists, family practitioners, internists, and orthopedic surgeons. They all contribute by bringing special knowledge and understanding to the care of athletes and athletic injuries. Such knowledge can relate to nutrition, strength training, cardiovascular conditioning, psychosocial issues, musculoskeletal care, or one or more of many other areas related to the health of athletes. Therefore, sports medicine is a very broad and diverse field that requires a team approach.

Athletic injuries occur with regularity, but very few injuries are unique to sports. Yet treating an injured athlete does not necessarily require the same process as that used to treat an injured sedentary person. The athlete tends to have greater expectations than does the average sedentary person. These expectations usually increase proportionately with the competitive level of the athlete. For example, the athlete with an ankle sprain will spend ten to twelve hours per day performing treatment and rehabilitation supervised by a physical therapist or athletic trainer. The sedentary person, however, might go to physical therapy three times per week. Although the philosophy of the treatment is the same, the number of treatments and the desired outcomes are completely different. Athletes also require an extensive amount of information regarding their injuries, treatment, and rehabilitation. Athletes are not afraid to ask questions regarding their injuries because they want to know when they will be able to return to competition. The average patient, however, is quite uncomfortable asking the physician about an injury or illness.

Sports medicine is a challenging and rewarding profession. It is enjoyable working with patients who have a high level of compliance and motivation. The reward of watching an athlete recover from an injury and compete is exceptional. The sports medicine physician must realize, however, that he or she will also be called upon by the athlete and the athlete's coach and parents to communicate the severity of the injury and its significance-a process which can be quite difficult at times, especially when what the physician has to say is not what anyone wants to hear. Nevertheless, it is the role of the physician to act in the best interest of the athlete. In order for the physician to be prepared to handle this, he or she must fully understand the demands of each and every sport. Attendance at games is usually not enough to achieve this level of knowledge and experience. Observing practice sessions and workouts is often quite useful. With the exception of high-impact collision sports such as hockey and football, most injuries occur during practice and workout sessions. Furthermore, such observation gives the physician an opportunity to be involved in education and injury prevention. Many athletic injuries are witnessed by an athletic trainer or physician who may be called upon to administer first aid in the field or, in some instances, provide treatment for injuries.

By attending practices or competitions, the physician may also have the opportunity to observe the actual mechanism of injury, which can be quite useful in evaluating the type and severity of the injury. Many physicians call the first twenty minutes after an injury has occurred, prior to the onset of swelling and spasm, the "golden period." It is at this time that an accurate and meaningful physical examination can be performed on the injured athlete. The recreational athlete, however, usually will arrive at the physician's office one to two days after the injury, when swelling and spasm are maximal. At this time, examining the injured body part is quite difficult and may not be meaningful. This may result in delays in diagnosis and definitive treatment. For the sedentary person and the occasional athlete, such delays will probably not be significant. The highly competitive athlete, however, would be quite dissatisfied if an injury delayed his or her return to competition. So, although most athletic injuries differ very little from other cases of musculoskeletal trauma, the finer points of managing them are unique.

Most athletic injuries affect one of three structures in the body: bones, ligaments, or musculotendinous units. These injuries may be acute or chronic in onset. Most acute injuries occur as a result of trauma, with presentation being rather soon after the incident. Chronic injuries, which are often insidious in onset, usually result from a change in the athlete or the athletic environment. Chronic injuries tend to be difficult to recognize and treat effectively. The best approach to chronic injuries is prevention. Most acute injuries can be classified as sprains, strains, or fractures, and most chronic injuries can be classified as strains or stress fractures.

Sprains are injuries to ligaments; strains are injuries to the musculotendinous unit. Sprains occur when there is excessive abnormal motion at a joint. This results in overstretching of the ligaments and produces local pain, swelling, limitation of motion, and a sense of instability. Such overstretching can result in partial tears (mild) or complete tears (severe) of the ligament. Strains are usually the result of an abrupt increase in the tension of the musculotendinous unit (for example, they may occur when one lifts weights that are too heavy). This increase may result in partial or complete tears of the muscle, the tendon, or the bone to which the tendon is at-tached. The most important principle is to realize that strains are not the result of overstretching but occur well within the normal limits of motion. Strains are also graded from mild to severe. Often, there is an obvious deformity at the site of injury because the muscle rolls up into a ball. Fractures are simply breaks in the bones of the body. Stress fractures occur when excessive demands are placed on the bone. Eventually, the bone fails to accommodate these demands, and microscopic breaks result.

Diagnostic and Treatment Techniques

The initial management of acute injuries is the same in athletics as it is in other musculoskeletal trauma. Treatment should be directed at prevention of bleeding and edema. These conditions usually lead to pain and decreased function of the injured body part, which requires the application of ice, compression, elevation, and rest. There are other methods of treatment used in the professional setting that are also useful in preventing or reducing bleeding and edema. These include electric stimulation, contrast baths, ultrasound, and compression stockings. After the initial phase of bleeding and edema, therapy should be directed at restoring range of motion, strength, and, finally, functional tasks that will ultimately result in the athlete's return to competition. Chronic injuries, however, usually require elimination of the precipitating factors as well as increased rest while the injured body part is allowed to heal. This may require a special taping procedure, a brace, a change in footwear, the alteration of practice

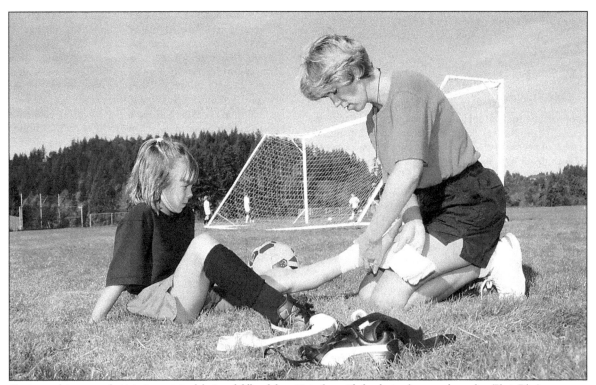

Doctors seek to ensure that injuries sustained during childhood do not interfere with developing bones and muscles. (PhotoDisc)

sessions, or simply refraining from that activity for a short period of time.

Chronic injuries and overuse injuries are usually caused by change. Change can occur in the athlete, the environment, or the activity. Identifying these changes can be helpful in injury prevention, since the majority of injuries in athletics are chronic. Also, the treatment requires elimination of the offending change and restoration of the proper condition. Strains to the musculotendinous unit can also occur chronically. They tend to result from muscle fatigue, too much training too fast, or poor training conditions. Many of these injuries are called "tendinitis," which means inflammation of the tendon. The most prominent aspect of such an injury is pain. The pain is almost always located in the region of the injured structure. Management is directed at avoidance of painful activity, elimination of the offending factor, and symptomatic relief of pain with ice, ultrasound, injections, electric stimulation, and medicines. Rehabilitation is aimed at restoring strength and flexibility as well as avoiding the initial cause.

Most sprains can be treated with routine physical therapy and rehabilitation, but many severe sprains will require surgery. Average time lost from athletics ranges from seven days (for example, for a mild ankle sprain) to one year (for example, for a severe knee sprain with reconstruction of ligaments). With strains, complete tears of the tendon usually require surgery, while injury to the muscle itself does not. Treatment is similar to that for sprains; rehabilitation should be directed at regaining strength and flexibility. The diagnosis of a fracture can be made only with the aid of an X-ray picture. Treatment of fractures requires immobilization either in a cast, special splint, or brace. Some fractures will require the placement of plates or screws by an orthopedic surgeon. Rehabilitation of fractures involves restoration of motion, strength, flexibility, and proprioception. Proprioception is simply the unconscious awareness of where a body part is in space (for example, a person can tie his or her shoes with eyes closed because the brain knows where the hands are in space). The treatment of stress fractures is different from treatments of other fractures in that immobilization is almost never necessary. Adaptation of activity and relative rest are usually all that is required. Return to competition averages three to six weeks but may be longer.

Sports medicine personnel also provide education and guidance to coaches, athletes, and parents. They make themselves available to provide the best and most efficient care possible. It is the responsibility of the sports medicine physician to coordinate this care. This all begins with the preseason screening history and physical exam.

Prior to the commencement of each athletic season, athletes are usually required to provide a medical history and undergo a physical examination. The requirements of such examinations vary from state to state, college to college, and professional league to professional league. The purpose of these examinations is to identify athletes who may have potential problems in the sport in which they have chosen to compete.

For example, Johnnie is a thirteen-year-old high school freshman trying out for the football team. The doctor listens to his heart and lungs and hears a small heart murmur. The physician recommends that Johnnie see a cardiologist prior to beginning football practice. A further workup by the cardiologist reveals that Johnnie has a condition in which the arteries that supply his heart are abnormal. The cardiologist recommends that Johnnie not participate in athletic activity that requires stress on the heart. Although this scenario is uncommon, it is a perfect example of the benefits of preseason history and physical exams. Johnnie could have died as a result of his condition if it had gone unnoticed.

The preseason screening also identifies athletes who are at risk for developing strains and sprains because their flexibility is lower than normal. Identifying these athletes allows the athletic trainer to work with them on a stretching program intended to reduce the number and severity of such injuries. It is during the preseason that the athletes are at greatest risk for injury, since the workouts are long and numerous and most athletes are not yet in shape. Injuries may occur at any time during practice or a game. Most injuries occur during practice, however, and especially at the end of the session, because athletes are tired and their concentration level is low.

Dean is a twenty-year-old junior college soccer player who is kicked in the side during a slide tackling drill. He is taken out of practice by the coach and then sent to the training room to see the athletic trainer. The athletic trainer astutely examines Dean's urine and finds blood in it. Also, he finds that Dean's blood pressure is somewhat low and that his heart rate is mildly elevated. Because of this, the trainer is concerned about injury to Dean's kidney or spleen. He promptly phones the team physician, who advises that they meet him in the emergency room at the hospital. After being evaluated by the team doctor, Dean is brought to the operating room by a surgeon, who removes Dean's extensively damaged spleen. Dean recovers quickly and returns to exercise within six weeks but is not allowed to play soccer until the following season. Without the aid of the trainer and prompt attention by the team physician, Dean might not have had such favorable results.

Mary is a fifteen-year-old high school all-state cross country runner. She is now entering her junior year and is expected to compete on the national level. Mary is also an excellent student with a grade-point average of 3.6. She has always been an overachiever. Six weeks into the fall season, Mary's times begin to fall off slightly. When asked about her performance, she states that she has been experiencing pain in both her shins, particularly the one on the right, for two weeks. Her coach, because of her concern, asks Mary to see her family doctor, since Mary's school does not have an athletic trainer or team physician. Mary's doctor, who is not trained in sports medicine, simply tells Mary that she has shin splints and that she should rest. Mary does not accept this, because everyone is counting on her to win for her school. She continues to run against his advice. In the next race, Mary finishes dead last. The pain has become quite unbearable. Mary is finally referred to a sports medicine physician, who discovers several relevant facts. Mary has not been eating well and has in fact been forcing herself to vomit for a number of days prior to each race. Also, Mary has not experienced her first menses, and her secondary sexual characteristics are somewhat immature. X rays of Mary's right leg reveal a stress fracture that is quite severe. Mary is referred to several people, including an orthopedic surgeon who places her in a cast, a nutritionist and a psychologist who evaluate and treat her eating disorder, and a gynecologist who proceeds with a workup for her late development. After several months of treatments from all three doctors, Mary begins retraining on a bicycle under the direction of an athletic trainer and a physical therapist. She moves on to compete in the spring season of track and field and becomes a national champion. Without the aid of the sports medicine team, Mary might have continued to have difficulty and might not have been evaluated properly until it was too late. This is a quite common scenario among adolescent athletes. The pressures placed upon them by friends, coaches, and parents can become detrimental to their emotional and physical well-being.

Henry is a fifty-five-year-old businessman who spends five days a week playing tennis at the local health club to stay in shape. After buying a new racket, he begins to experience pain in his right elbow. He is seen by an orthopedic surgeon in town who specializes in sports medicine. After speaking with Henry and examining his elbow, the doctor recommends anti-inflammatory medication, a special forearm strap, and use of the old racket. Henry's condition, which is called tennis elbow, or lateral epicondylitis, is quite common. After several weeks of the initial treatment, Henry does not feel any better. His doctor, therefore, injects him with a medicine to ease the pain and calm the inflammation. Henry is instructed to rest his arm for a week prior to starting tennis again. Henry follows the doctor's instructions carefully. He begins to play tennis again and feels fine for about a month, after which he begins to experience the same discomfort. This time, the doctor recommends surgery for Henry's elbow. Three months after the surgery, Henry is free of pain.

These examples have demonstrated how sports medicine can be beneficial to athletes. Each scenario differs in type of athlete, location, diagnosis, and treatment.

Perspective and Prospects

Sports medicine is assuming a significant role in the medical profession today. Sports medicine was first recognized in the days of the early Olympics. It was not until the final decades of the twentieth century, however, that it emerged into a field of its own. Sports medicine training programs have been developing at an exponential rate. Interest in sports medicine can be pursued in various ways. Most sports medicine physicians undergo a one-year fellowship after either a five-year orthopedic residency training program or a three-year family medicine residency training program. Athletic trainers must pass a national examination for certification. Most have master's degrees, and all have some form of bachelor's degree. Their expertise is in the prevention, treatment, and rehabilitation of athletic injuries. These are the primary caregivers of the sports medicine world. Certified athletic trainers are

being hired at all major universities, many high schools, and many health clubs across the country. Various types of sports medicine centers are continually being developed. These centers offer a wide range of services to both professional and amateur athletes. As more and more people begin to exercise, the need for sports medicine professionals will increase.

Athletes' needs and goals are different from those of most other people. Although the injuries that they experience are not unique to sports, the rapidity with which they recover is of utmost importance. This identifies them as a distinct group of people with special demands for medical care. It is because of this and because of the growing number of people who exercise on a daily basis that sports medicine has evolved into a viable medical field. Sports medicine will continue to grow and will play an important role in preventing many of the injuries that afflict people in the United States.

—*Paul Freudigman, Jr., M.D.;*
updated by Bradley R. A. Wilson, Ph.D.

See also Acupressure; Anorexia nervosa; Arthroplasty; Arthroscopy; Athlete's foot; Biofeedback; Bones and the skeleton; Braces, orthopedic; Bruises; Cardiology; Concussion; Critical care; Eating disorders; Emergency medicine; Ergogenic aids; Exercise physiology; First aid; Fracture and dislocation; Fracture repair; Glycolysis; Head and neck disorders; Heat exhaustion and heatstroke; Hydrotherapy; Joints; Kinesiology; Muscle sprains, spasms, and disorders; Ligaments; Muscles; Nutrition; Orthopedic surgery; Orthopedics; Orthopedics, pediatric; Oxygen therapy; Over-the-counter medications; Overtraining syndrome; Physical examination; Physical rehabilitation; Physiology; Preventive medicine; Psychiatry; Psychiatry, child and adolescent; Rotator cuff surgery; Spine, vertebrae, and disks; Steroid abuse; Steroids; Tendinitis; Tendon disorders; Tendon repair; Whiplash.

For Further Information:

Blumenstein, Boris, Michael Bar-Eli, and Gershon Tenenbaum, eds. *Brain and Body in Sport and Exercise: Biofeedback Applications in Performance Enhancement.* New York: John Wiley & Sons, 2002. Notes that technical advances in biofeedback have made it a vital method of training athletes in order to increase individual awareness and control over the body and reduce habitual physiological tensions. Brings together current research and applications and shows how different biofeedback approaches can be used in various sports.

Delforge, Gary. *Musculoskeletal Trauma: Implications for Sport Injury Management.* Champaign, Ill.: Human Kinetics, 2002. Covers the therapeutic management of sport-related soft tissue injuries, fractures, and proprioceptive/sensorimotor impairments. Reviews the major categories of intervention and presents fifty illustrations to accompany the text.

Landry, Gregory L., and David T. Bernhardt. *Essentials of Primary Care Sports Medicine.* Champaign, Ill.: Human Kinetics, 2003. This book explains general health issues for athletes.

McArdle, William, Frank I. Katch, and Victor L. Katch. *Exercise Physiology: Energy, Nutrition, and Human Performance.* 7th ed. Boston: Lippincott Williams & Wilkins, 2010. A wide-ranging text on exercise and the human body, covering topics such as nutrition, energy transfer, exercise training, systems of energy delivery and utilization, enhancement of energy capacity, the effect of environmental stress, and the effect of exercise on successful aging and disease prevention.

Scuderi, Giles R., and Peter D. McCann, eds. *Sports Medicine: A Comprehensive Approach.* 2d ed. Philadelphia: Mosby/Elsevier,

2005. This text covers all types of athletic injuries and offers useful illustrations. Includes a bibliography and an index.

Small, Eric, et al. *Kids and Sports: Everything You and Your Child Need to Know About Sports, Physical Activity, and Good Health.* New York: Newmarket Press, 2002. Reminds parents that children are physiologically and psychologically different from adults and thus experience sports and their injuries in different ways. Covers which sports are suitable for which age, how to prevent and treat injuries, how to plan sports programs for children with chronic conditions such as asthma or diabetes, and the importance of good nutrition and exercise.

SPRAINS. *See* MUSCLE SPRAINS, SPASMS, AND DISORDERS.

SQUAMOUS CELL CARCINOMA. *See* SKIN CANCER.

STAPHYLOCOCCAL INFECTIONS
Disease/Disorder

Also known as: Staph infections

Anatomy or system affected: Blood, circulatory system, gastrointestinal system, musculoskeletal system, nervous system, respiratory system, urinary system

Specialties and related fields: Bacteriology, cardiology, dermatology, epidemiology, general surgery, internal medicine, microbiology, orthopedics, urology

Definition: Infections caused by bacteria from the genus *Staphylococcus*.

Causes and Symptoms

Under the microscope, staphylococci bacteria are observed to grow in irregular, grapelike clusters from which they derive their name. Individually, the organisms are spherical and appear purple (positive) when stained with Gram technique. Staphylococci are found predominantly living on the skin and mucous membranes of mammals and birds and usually exist in a benign symbiotic relationship with their hosts. When the barrier imposed by either the skin or mucous membranes is breached, however, staphylococci may then cause disease, assisted by a variety of enzymes and toxins that they are able to manufacture. Many strains of staphylococci, such as *Staphylococcus aureus*, produce coagulase, which catalyzes the formation of a clot from fibrinogen proteins in the blood. Hyaluronidases, lipases, and other proteolytic enzymes carve out a cavity within the clot, which is covered by a coagulase-generated fibrin coat, and an abscess is formed. Abscess formation is one of the hallmarks of staphylococcal infection and can be found in virtually any organ in the body as a result of local invasion or spread to the site via the bloodstream.

Staphylococcal strains are able to produce a variety of proteins called exotoxins that have significant roles in determining the type of illness that results. Superantigens, such as toxic shock syndrome toxin-1 (TSST-1), target the circulatory system and can markedly lower blood pressure. TSST-1 producing strains have caused disease not only by growing in vaginal tampons but also while simultaneously causing

postsurgical wound infections. Food poisoning results after ingesting food that is contaminated with staphylococcal strains that produce enterotoxins. The toxins are produced in the food after contamination from the colonized noses or infected skin of food handlers through sneezing or direct contact. The enterotoxins are relatively heat-stable and do not result in any unusual taste, odor, or appearance of the food. Abdominal cramps, nausea, vomiting, and diarrhea occur one to six hours after ingestion of the contaminated food containing the toxin. This is not a true infection, as it is the preformed toxin that produces the illness. Exfoliative toxin is produced by the strains causing scalded skin syndrome. The illness is manifested by fever and reddened skin that subsequently peels off.

Staphylococci are able to form a variety of cytotoxins that damage the membranes of bodily tissues. These toxins are able to destroy red and white blood cells as well as organ cells. Leukocytolytic activity from staphylococci was first reported in 1932 and the Panton-Valentine leukocidin (PVL) was named in honor of these scientists. PVL is produced by strains of *S. aureus* causing skin and soft tissue infection and pneumonia in the community (outside the hospital).

S. aureus is the preeminent pathogen causing infection in hospitalized patients. It is the most common cause of surgical wound infections. It is joined by another species, *S. epidermidis*, which can produce slime enabling the bacteria to adhere to the surfaces of medical devices such as vascular catheters, central nervous system shunts, artificial heart valves, and prosthetic joints. Together, these two species account for a large number of hospital-acquired infections.

Infection of skeletal muscle and contiguous tissues is called pyomyositis or necrotizing fasciitis. This type of infection has been common in developing countries with tropical climates, but since the 1970s it has been seen more frequently in modern countries with temperate climates. The pathogenesis of pyomyositis is not completely understood. Some cases follow trauma, and there are a number of risk factors, such as intravenous drug abuse, human immunodeficiency virus (HIV) infection, and skin diseases. Other cases occur in healthy individuals without any apparent risk factor. Recently, virulent strains of community-acquired methicillin-resistant *S. aureus* (MRSA) have caused pyomyositis in the United States.

S. saprophyticus is an important cause of urinary tract infections in young women. The infection may be manifested

---

Information on Staphylococcal Infections

Causes: Bacterial infection with staphylococci; often from food poisoning, contamination of catheter or shunt

Symptoms: Depends on type; may include vomiting, fever, rashes, pus-producing lesions

Duration: Acute

Treatments: Depends on type; may include alleviation of symptoms, drainage or cleansing of site, antibiotics (vancomycin, methicillin, oxacillin)

2118 • STEM CELLS

In the News: Methicillin-Resistant Staphylococci

Staphylococcal infections, especially methicillin-resistant *Staphylococcus aureus* (MRSA), occur most frequently in patients with weakened immune systems. Hospital, nursing home, and dialysis patients may develop surgical wound infections, bloodstream infections, pneumonia, prosthetic joint or heart valve infections, and other types of staphylococcal infections as a result of acquiring hospital-associated MRSA (HA-MRSA) as a consequence of medical treatment. These bacteria may come from the patients themselves, other patients, or health care workers. Whatever the source, these infections are potentially preventable. Efforts are under way to reduce staphylococcal infections in health care facilities. Patients scheduled to undergo elective surgery, such as joint replacement, are being screened for staphylococcal colonization by nasal culture, and those that are positive are being treated with nasal mupirocin or even oral antibiotics to eradicate the staphylococci prior to surgery. Patients harboring staphylococci who are admitted to hospitals are being isolated to prevent transmission to both health care workers and other patients. Many states have passed legislation requiring health care institutions to report their records publicly, including infection rates, and this awareness is accelerating these preventive measures.

MRSA is no longer limited to patients in health care facilities. Community-associated MRSA (CA-MRSA) also has come into prominence. CA-MRSA most commonly manifests as a skin or soft tissue infection such as a boil or abscess. Close skin-to-skin contact, cuts or abrasions, and contaminated items may lead to infection. Skin lesions have allowed CA-MRSA to cause infections in wrestlers, fencers, rugby players, and football players. Similarly, skin abrasions in hot tub users in Alaska have resulted in CA-MRSA outbreaks. Prisoners, gay men, and military recruits are among other groups who have been associated with outbreaks. Children, some without any identified predisposing risk, have also become infected with CA-MRSA. Typing of CA-MRSA strains using a technique called pulsed-field gel electrophoresis has identified a specific strain of CA-MRSA called USA 300 as being responsible for nearly all infections in the United States.

Both HA-MRSA and CA-MRSA are treatable with antibiotics, but those that are effective in each type are quite different. HA-MRSA infections are treated with vancomycin, daptomycin, or linezolid. These antimicrobial agents are very expensive and usually require intravenous administration. CA-MRSA infections are treated with cheaper oral agents such as trimethoprim-sulfamethoxazole, tetracylines, fluoroquinolones, or clindamycin. Neither HA-MRSA nor CA-MRSA infections can be treated successfully with beta-lactam antibiotics, which are the antibiotics of first choice for other *S. aureus* infections. Recognition of the persons at risk and the differences in effective antibiotic therapies are critical because lack of appropriate initial treatment may result in spread of the infection into the bloodstream, with more severe illness.

—*H. Bradford Hawley, M.D.*

---

by cloudy or blood-tinged urine and dysuria. It is associated with sexual intercourse or swimming. Various adhesions and the enzyme urease contribute to its ability to produce infection of the urinary tract.

Treatment and Therapy

Specific treatment of a staphylococcal infection hinges on administering an effective antibiotic. MRSA is a type of *S. aureus* that is resistant to antibiotics called beta-lactams, which include methicillin and other related, commonly used antibiotics. Vancomycin, an antibiotic developed in the 1950s, has remained effective for nearly all strains, but it must be given intravenously and has some serious potential side effects. Some newer antibiotics, daptomycin and linezolid, are effective against MRSA and have been used successfully to treat infections.

Antibiotics are not the only measure necessary to cure these infections. Surgical or percutaneous catheter drainage of abscesses, surgical debridement of dead tissue, and the removal of medical devices or protheses are often necessary. Other medical supportive modalities, such as fluid replacement, vasopressors, or mechanical ventilation, may be required.

Perspective and Prospects

The Centers for Disease Control and Prevention (CDC) is collaborating with other medical organizations to develop and promote strategies to reduce the transmission of staphylococci, primarily MRSA, in both health care and community settings. The CDC has also launched a campaign to prevent antimicrobial resistance by educating both the public and health care providers about unnecessary and inappropriate antibiotic usage. Legislative efforts have been directed at eliminating the use of antibiotics in animal feed to assist in preventing resistance.

Newer antimicrobial agents continue to be developed, but the stream has slowed. Molecular-based treatments directed toward toxins and other virulence factors are being actively pursued.

—*H. Bradford Hawley, M.D.*

See also Abscess drainage; Abscesses; Antibiotics; Bacterial infections; Blisters; Boils; Drug resistance; Iatrogenic disorders; Infection; Methicillin-resistant *Staphylococcus aureus* (MRSA) infections; Necrotizing fasciitis; Opportunistic infections; Osteomyelitis; Pneumonia; Septicemia; Skin; Skin disorders; Styes; Toxic shock syndrome; Urinary disorders.

For Further Information:

Crossley, Kent B., and Gordon L. Archer, eds. *The Staphylococci in Human Disease*. New York: Churchill Livingston, 1997.
Kasper, Dennis L., et al., eds. *Harrison's Principles of Internal Medicine*. 16th ed. New York: McGraw-Hill, 2005.
Koneman, Elmer W. *The Other End of the Microscope: The Bacteria Tell Their Own Story*. Washington, D.C.: ASM Press, 2002.

STEM CELLS
Biology
Anatomy or system affected: All
Specialties and related fields: Biochemistry, biotechnology, cardiology, cytology, embryology, endocrinology, ethics,

genetics, hematology, immunology, neurology, oncology, pulmonary medicine, vascular medicine

Definition: Unspecialized cells derived from embryos, fetuses, or adults that retain the capacity to develop into specialized cells and regenerate themselves; scientists manipulate and study stem cells in the hope of using them to cure diseases.

Key terms:

cell: the fundamental unit of a living organism

differentiation: the process by which unspecialized cells develop into cells with highly specific form and functions

mitosis: the process of cell division

multipotent: referring to stem cells derived from adults that may develop into one or more specific types of tissue

pluripotent: referring to stem cells that have the capacity to develop into most of the specialized tissues of the body, but not an entire individual

tissue: specialized cells organized to form a specific function; tissue is further organized into organs

totipotent: referring to stem cells that have the capacity to develop into all the specialized cell types of the body

Structure and Functions

Stem cells are unspecialized cells that can develop into all the specialized cell types that organize themselves into the tissues, organs, and organ systems making up an entire individual. An egg fertilized by a sperm is a totipotent stem cell, in that this single cell has the capacity to divide repeatedly and ultimately to contribute cells to each specialized body component. For example, from the single cell that is a fertilized human egg, cells must ultimately specialize to become the beating cells of the heart, pancreatic cells that produce insulin, skin cells that cover the body, and bone cells that support the body, among scores of other types of cells.

After fertilization, an egg divides repeatedly to form an embryo. The three- to five-day-old embryo is a hollow ball of cells called a blastocyst. Inside the blastocyst, a group of about thirty cells called the inner cell mass constitutes the stem cells of the embryo. Embryonic stem cells are referred to as pluripotent because they have the capacity to develop into most, but not all, of the specialized cell types that will form the structures needed for the embryo to develop into an adult. Embryonic stem cells do not form the placenta, the structure that provides the essential connection between mother and embryo during gestation.

Adults also harbor several types of stem cells, although a very small number in each tissue. The major function of adult stem cells is to provide new cells to replenish aging or damaged ones. Many adult stem cells are believed to be sequestered in a specific area of tissue and remain nondividing until activated by tissue disease or injury. Others are required to provide new cells with greater frequency. For example, skin

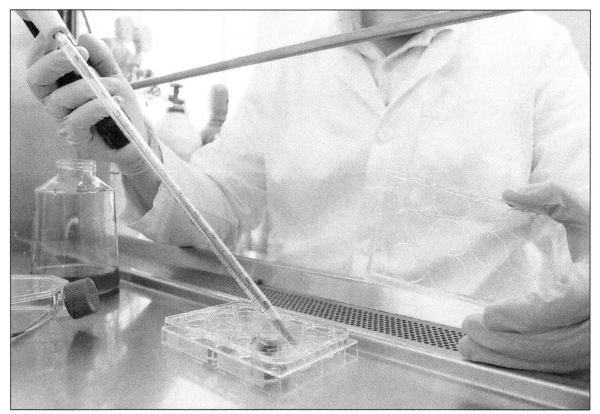

A technician cultures stem cells. (© Andrei Tchernov/iStockphoto.com)

stem cells are constantly differentiating into mature skin cells to replace the large numbers of cells naturally lost each day.

Pluripotent hematopoietic (blood) stem cells reside in the bone marrow and are also very active. They regenerate themselves through mitosis but also divide into the numerous specialized cells found in the blood, including the red blood cells that carry oxygen, the various types of white blood cells involved in body defenses, and the platelets critical to clot formation.

Unlike specialized cells such as heart cells, brain cells, and muscle cells, which do not normally replicate themselves, stem cells may replicate many times, even when isolated from the body and propagated in the laboratory. Because of their capacity to regenerate themselves and their ability to differentiate into specific tissue types, scientists are isolating and studying stem cells in the hopes of understanding diseases such as cancer. They are exploring the prospect of using stem cells as therapeutic agents in treating a host of diseases and disorders, including Parkinson's disease, diabetes mellitus, and some forms of heart disease.

Embryonic stem cells are studied in the laboratory by isolating the inner cell mass from a three- to five-day-old embryo. The embryos are typically donated for research, with informed consent, by individuals who have extra, unneeded embryos created by in vitro fertilization for the treatment of infertility. The cells are added to a culture dish containing a nutrient medium and coated with mouse cells that provide a sticky surface to which the stem cells adhere. New methods now allow stem cells to grow in the absence of contaminating mouse cells. The stem cells replicate repeatedly and fill the dish, then are divided and added to fresh culture dishes. After six months of repeated growth and repeated division and transfer to fresh culture dishes, the original thirty stem cells may yield millions of embryonic stem cells. The cells are analyzed at six months of growth, and if they have not differentiated, remain pluripotent, and appear genetically normal, then they are referred to as an embryonic stem-cell line.

Adult stem cells have proved to be much more difficult to grow in culture, and doing so has been a major focus of work by scientists. Unlike embryonic stem cells, adult stem cells are generally limited to differentiating into the cell type of their tissue of origin. Some evidence suggests, however, that certain types of adult stem cells may be manipulated in the laboratory to differentiate into a broader range of tissue types.

Medical Applications

There are three major areas of stem cell research, each with potential medical applications. One branch of research seeks to discover and understand the many steps in the complex process of cellular differentiation. Other researchers are exploring the potential uses of stem cells in pharmaceutical development. A third major line of research focuses on the use of stem cells in the treatment of a host of diseases.

Embryonic stem cells are used to study the processes by which undifferentiated stem cells differentiate into specialized cell types. Through this work, scientists will gain a greater understanding of normal cell development. Understanding the mechanisms of normal cell development will provide insights into situations of abnormal growth and development. Scientists already know that turning specific genes on and off at critical times in the differentiation process is what leads to one cell becoming a muscle cell, another a lung cell, and still another a red blood cell, but the signals that influence these genes are only partially understood. Many serious medical conditions, such as cancer and certain birth defects, are the result of abnormal cellular differentiation and division. A better understanding of these processes in normal situations could lead to major insights in the development of such disorders and perhaps point the way to preventive measures or new therapeutic tools.

Established cell lines are often used by pharmaceutical companies when testing potential products. For example, cancer cell lines are used to test antitumor drugs. If human stem cell lines were available, then many drugs could be tested for both beneficial and toxic effects in stem cell cultures in one of two general fashions. In one case, drugs could be tested for their effects, either positive or negative, on the normal differentiation of stem cells into specialized cells. In a second scenario, pluripotent stem cells could be used to create new lines of a variety of differentiated cell types that are currently not

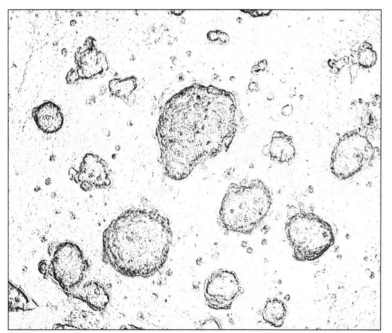

Embryonic stem cells under a microscope. (© Andrei Tchernov/iStockphoto.com)

available, and drugs specific for that cell type could be tested on these cell cultures. In either case, screening drugs with cell lines derived from human stem cells would have the advantage of testing directly on human cells. Such testing would decrease the number of nonhuman animals used in drug testing and could decrease the number of human clinical trials needed to prove the efficacy and safety of a drug, thus speeding it through the governmental approval process and making it available to the public. To screen drugs effectively, however, the cells must be identical from culture to culture and for each drug being tested. To achieve this, scientists must understand the cellular signals and biochemical pathways that control cellular differentiation into the desired cell type so that the process can be controlled precisely in repeated experiments. Scientists do not currently understand differentiation well enough to initiate drug testing in stem cells, but many are working toward that goal.

Perhaps the most exciting area of stem cell research is the possibility of using pluripotent stem cells to treat disease. Organ and tissue transplantation are commonly used to treat a number of medical conditions. Heart and kidney transplants are a few examples. These treatments are available only when organs fail and often put the patient at serious risk of death. The donor material often must come from donation of the organs after the death of another individual. There are serious shortages of transplantable organs, and many patients die before suitable donor organs become available. Even if a transplant can be performed, the body will attack the transplanted organ because it is perceived as foreign, thus risking the destruction and rejection of the organ. Even with powerful drugs to suppress this response, some organs are still rejected, with dire consequences to the recipient.

Pluripotent stem cells, if directed to differentiate into specific cell types, have the potential to provide a renewable source of cells and tissue. For example, it may be possible to generate healthy heart cells from stem cells in the laboratory, then transplant these cells into a damaged heart. The hope is that the transplanted cells would proliferate and grow into healthy, functioning tissue that would rejuvenate the damaged heart and circumvent the need for heart transplantation. Other conditions that could be treated with stem cell therapy are diabetes, Alzheimer's disease, Parkinson's disease, stroke, burns, and spinal cord injury. Although a great deal of research is ongoing in this area of regenerative medicine, not all stem cell therapies are experimental. For example, transplantation of blood-forming hematopoietic stem cells found in bone marrow has been in use since the 1960s. More pure preparations of adult hematopoetic stem cells are currently approved for the treatment of leukemia, lymphoma, and several inherited blood disorders.

Perspective and Prospects

In the 1960s, researchers first discovered that bone marrow contains at least two types of stem cells. One type, termed hematopoietic stem cells, was found to form all of the different types of blood cells. The second line, termed stromal cells, generates fat, cartilage, and connective tissue. Also in the 1960s, scientists studying adult rat brains discovered areas that contained undifferentiated cells that divided and differentiated into nerve cells. At that time, scientists did not believe that brain cells could regenerate themselves and discounted the results of this study. In the 1990s, enough evidence had accumulated for scientists to agree that adult brains, including those of humans, contain stem cells that are able to differentiate into the three major types of cells found in the mature brain. The two main neurogenic areas of the adult mammalian brain are now known to be the olfactory bulb, which controls the sense of smell, and the hippocampus, a memory center.

Much of what scientists know about stem cells and their differentiation has come from studies in mice. The first stem cells were isolated from mouse embryos in 1981. Scientists treated these cell lines with various growth factors to stimulate the development of a particular cell type. For example, cells treated with vitamin A derivative differentiated into nerve cells. All types of blood cells and cardiac cells have been generated in similar fashions, and in 2000 scientists from StemCells, Inc., produced mature liver cells from the hematopoietic stem cells of mice. That same year, neuroscientists at Johns Hopkins University announced that they had successfully reversed paralysis in rats and mice by injecting them with embryonic stem cells. The cells migrated to a region of the spinal cord that contains motor nerve cells. Half of the rats regained movement in their hind feet. This success was heralded as a first step toward curing human neurological disorders with stem cells.

While mice are excellent models for research on human biology, they are not human. Ideally, research would be conducted on human cells. Human pluripotent stem cells were isolated for the first time by scientists Michael Shamblott and James Thomson, working independently, in 1998. In 2000, scientists were successful in isolating stem cells from human cadavers and directing their development from bone marrow stem cells into nerve cells. In the late 1990s and early twenty-first century, a body of research accumulated to indicate that adult stem cells exist in more body tissues than originally believed. This finding has led scientists to explore the possibility of using adult stem cells, rather than embryonic stem cells, as sources of transplant material. Use of adult stem cells would have the advantage of the transplant material being from the recipient, so it would not be rejected by the body as with a foreign transplant.

Some adult stem cells have been shown, under the right conditions, to differentiate into a variety of cells that are not the tissue from which they were derived. In April, 2003, it was reported that fourteen patients with severe heart disease improved after being injected with stem cells harvested from their own bone marrow. Other studies suggest that stem cells derived from umbilical cord blood could be stored and provide a source of stem cells for therapeutic use at a later time.

In 2007, American and Japanese scientists created adult human stem cells from differentiated skin cells. The process used to achieve this involved taking adult skin cells and infecting them with several genes known to be highly active in embryonic stem cells but less active in differentiated cells. The cells, called induced pluripotent stem cells (iPS), are therefore reprogrammed into an embryonic state. In 2009, another group produced iPS from adult fat cells. This case is particularly exciting because there is no shortage of fat cells available for reprogramming. Essentially, each human is carrying a supply of potential stem cells. However, severe problems are associated with the efficiency of the reprogramming process, and there are also concerns that some of the genes used to create iPS could cause cancer. Intense research is being performed, and in the future, iPS technology could be used as a therapeutic tool.

Because of the small amounts, scarcity, and lower developmental potential of adult stem cells, scientists believe that they must experiment with cells derived from fetuses and embryos if stem cell research is to progress and fulfill the promise of therapy for a host of dread diseases. Because embryos must be destroyed in order to isolate stem cells, the use of embryonic stem cells is controversial, particularly within the United States. In 2001, President George W. Bush banned the use of federal funds for embryonic stem-cell research except for the sixty-four stem-cell lines in existence at the time. In 2006, Bush vetoed a bill that reversed his previous decision and allowed use of federal funds for embryonic stem-cell research. As of 2006, fewer than one-third of the original sixty-four embryonic stem-cell lines were being studied because most either acquired deleterious mutations or propagated poorly and were discontinued.

Great Britain instituted no such restrictions on stem cell research, however, and in September, 2002, plans were unveiled for the United Kingdom Stem Cell Bank, to be located in Hertfordshire. It was to be the world's first center for storing and supplying tissue from human embryos and aborted fetuses to be used to repair diseased and damaged tissues. Subsequently, in 2005, the National Stem Cell Bank (NSCB) was established in the United States at WiCell Research Institute in Madison, Wisconsin, to acquire, characterize, and distribute the twenty-one of the original sixty-four human embryonic stem-cell lines that have been approved for federal government funding.

In 2004, the unfavorable attitude toward embryonic stem-cell research started to change, and voters in California passed Proposition 71, the California Stem Cell Research and Cures Initiative, which authorizes the sale of bonds to allocate $3 billion over ten years to stem cell research, with priority given to studies examining human embryonic stem cells. The initiative allowed formation of the California Institute for Regenerative Medicine (CIRM), a stem cell agency that oversees the direction of research and distributes funding.

In 2009, President Barack Obama overturned the ban on the use of federal funding for embryonic stem-cell research. Also, with a huge increase in funding to scientists, the United States can now be competitive in the fast-moving, exciting field of embryonic stem-cell research. This should open doors to the future use of embryonic stem cells or iPS to cure human diseases.

—*Karen E. Kalumuck, Ph.D.;*
updated by W. Michael Zawada, Ph.D.

See also Abortion; Animal rights vs. research; Assisted reproductive technologies; Cancer; Cells; Clinical trials; Cloning; Diabetes mellitus; Embryology; Ethics; Fetal tissue transplantation; Genetic engineering; In vitro fertilization; Paralysis; Spinal cord disorders; Transplantation.

For Further Information:

Campbell, Neil A., and Jane B. Reece. *Biology.* 8th ed. San Francisco: Pearson/Benjamin Cummings, 2009. The clearly written text and informative illustrations make this introductory college textbook accessible to interested nonspecialists. The background information on cells and genetics and the introduction to stem cells will provide the reader with an excellent foundation for grasping some of the complexities of stem cell research.

Committee on Guidelines for Human Embryonic Stem Cell Research. National Research Council. *Guidelines for Human Embryonic Stem Cell Research.* Washington, D.C.: National Academies Press, 2005. This book provides updated information on research, regulations, and ethics of embryonic stem cell use. Of interest to scientists, physicians, ethicists, or anyone wanting to delve into this field.

Cookson, Clive, et al. "The Future of Stem Cells." *Scientific American* (July, 2005). This special report from *Scientific American* and *Financial Times* synthesizes the research, ethics, politics, and commercialization of stem cells in view of potential regenerative therapies.

Holland, Suzanne, K. Lebacqz, and L. Zoloth, eds. *The Human Embryonic Stem Cell Debate: Science, Ethics, and Public Policy.* Cambridge, Mass.: MIT Press, 2001. The twenty essays in this book are written by scholars of biology, medicine, theology, and bioethics, among other disciplines, and provide foundational information about the science of stem cell research. Ethical and philosophical issues intimately tied with this research, including the nature of human life, the meaning of existence, and issues surrounding the use of embryonic and fetal tissues in research, are addressed.

Lanza, Robert, et al., eds. *Essentials of Stem Cell Biology.* 2d ed. San Diego, Calif.: Academic Press, 2009. This abridged version of the best-selling *Handbook of Stem Cells* is a detailed textbook for any student of this field and an excellent reference book on the subject.

National Institutes of Health (NIH). *Stem Cell Information.* http://stemcells.nih.gov. This site provides information on therapeutic potential of stem cells, a description of the U.S. policy on stem cell research, the NIH stem cell registry, and a link to the National Stem Cell Bank.

National Research Council. Institute of Medicine. *Stem Cells and the Future of Regenerative Medicine.* Washington, D.C.: National Academy Press, 2002. Using terms accessible to the interested nonspecialist, this book summarizes the current state of knowledge about embryonic stem cells and examines the moral and ethical issues that arise from their use and the role of the government in the regulation of this research. An excellent introduction to the field for students, educators, and the concerned public.

STENOSIS
Disease/Disorder

Also known as: Stricture, arctation, coarctation

Anatomy or system affected: Blood vessels, circulatory system, gastrointestinal system, heart, spine

Specialties and related fields: Cardiology, exercise physiology, gastroenterology, nephrology, neurology, oncology, orthopedics

---

Information on Stenosis

Causes: Buildup of plaque; swelling of tissue, cells, or organ; deformity
Symptoms: Varies by area affected
Duration: Temporary or permanent
Treatment: Various medications, invasive interventions, surgery

---

Definition: An abnormal narrowing or constriction of a canal or passageway in the body that is caused by the buildup of cholesterol, fats, or other substances (called plaque); the swelling or overgrowth of cells, tissue, or an organ; or a deformity.

Causes and Symptoms

Stenosis can occur in many areas of the body, such as an artery, heart valve, or vertebral (spine) canal. It may stem from many causes, depending on the area affected. In an artery, stenosis occurs with the buildup of cholesterol, fats, or other substances (called plaque). A stenotic heart valve can be a congenital (birth) defect or result from an infection (endocarditis), rheumatic fever, or aging. The septum (dividing wall in the heart) can enlarge and lead to an abnormally small ventricle (heart chamber). Spinal stenosis is caused by a deteriorating or herniated disk, arthritis, tissue enlargement inside the spinal canal, deformities of the spinal column (Paget's disease), or an injury.

Symptoms of this disorder relative to an artery, heart valve, or ventricle include high blood pressure, pain or tightness in the chest (angina pectoris), shortness of breath, dizziness or fainting with exertion, fatigue, palpitations (rapid heartbeat), or a heart murmur. In more severe cases, it can develop into a heart attack or stroke. The symptoms of spinal stenosis include back, neck, leg, or buttocks pain or numbness that worsens with standing or exercising.

Treatment and Therapy

Medication is commonly used to treat or relieve the symptoms caused by a stenosis. Blood thinners (aspirin, Coumadin) allow easy passage of blood through a stenosed area to lower the risk of high pressure. Cholesterol-lowering medications slow the buildup of plaque in the artery. Antibiotics help repair damaged heart valves, with a long course and high dosage used if the cause is infectious endocarditis. Finally, anti-inflammatory medications or steroid injections are the first line of treatment for spinal stenosis.

A number of interventions can be used to correct this disorder. Balloon angioplasty flattens plaque buildup, while valvuloplasty widens the valve opening. Stent placement (wire mesh tube) often follows an angioplasty to hold the artery open. An alternative is atherectomy, in which a laser or rotary shaver breaks up the plaque. If a patient has multiple severely stenosed arteries, then coronary artery bypass surgery may be recommended. Finally, artificial heart valve replacement surgery or corrective surgery for spinal stenosis may be warranted.

—Christine G. Holzmueller

See also Angiography; Angioplasty; Arteriosclerosis; Bypass surgery; Cholesterol; Circulation; Claudication; Endocarditis; Heart; Heart attack; Heart disease; Hypercholesterolemia; Hypertension; Plaque, arterial; Spine, vertebrae, and disks; Stents; Strokes; Vascular medicine; Vascular system; Venous insufficiency.

For Further Information:

American Heart Association. http://www.american heart.org.
Dorland's Illustrated Medical Dictionary. 30th ed. Philadelphia: Saunders, 2003.
North American Spine Society. http://www.spine.org.

STENTS
Procedure

Anatomy or system affected: Abdomen, blood vessels, circulatory system, heart
Specialties and related fields: Cardiology, radiology, vascular medicine
Definition: Wire mesh tubes permanently implanted to prop open arteries or veins.

Indications and Procedures

A stent is a stainless steel or Nitinol mesh tube implanted into a blood vessel to keep it propped open. The need for such a device arose in the 1980s. Doctors were performing a new procedure, called angioplasty, to clear narrowed arteries. The procedure involved inserting a small catheter into a blood vessel in the groin and threading it up to an area where a vessel was being narrowed by a fatty material called plaque. A small balloon on the end of the catheter was then inflated to push against the plaque, thus reducing the degree of narrowing of the vessel. This procedure was very successful, saving many patients the risks and complications of traditional surgeries. However, 35 to 45 percent of patients would experience renarrowing of the artery within four to six months because the plaque would spring back after the catheter was removed.

The idea of leaving a wire mesh tube to act as scaffolding to keep the plaque from springing back resulted in the first use of a stent device in 1986. The federal Food and Drug Administration (FDA) finally approved the use of stents in human patients in 1993. Since that time, many kinds of stents have become available. The first stents were made by soldering wires together around a pencil. Today, stents are made of steel etched by lasers that are controlled by computers.

Most stents are mounted on the balloon of an angioplasty catheter. Once the balloon reaches the narrowed area of the artery, it is inflated and the stent expands with it. The balloon is deflated and removed, leaving the deployed stent permanently in place to keep the vessel propped open.

Uses and Complications

Most stents are placed in the coronary arteries, the arteries that take blood to the heart. However, stents can be placed in any number of other blood vessels, including the peripheral arteries and veins (which serve the arms and legs), the carotid arteries (which serve the brain), or vessels in the abdomen.

Ironically, the complications that befall stents are similar to the problems they were designed to solve. Once a stent is placed, a mysterious scar may form on the stent, causing it to narrow. About 20 percent of stents will develop this problem. This scar is similar to, but not exactly the same as, the plaque in the artery. Studies are being done to reduce this problem. Coating the stent with materials that might retard the scar and radiating the stent to inhibit scar formation are being tried, and these measures appear promising. Clots may also form in the stent. For this reason, blood thinners and antiplatelet agents are commonly used to lessen the chances of clot formation on the stent.

—Steven R. Talbot, R.V.T.;
updated by Bradley R. A. Wilson, Ph.D.

See also Angioplasty; Arteriosclerosis; Blood vessels; Bypass surgery; Cardiology; Circulation; Claudication; Heart disease; Vascular medicine; Vascular system.

For Further Information:

American Heart Association. *What Is a Stent?* Dallas, Tex.: Author, 2005.

Heuser, Richard R., and Giancarlo Biamino, eds. *Peripheral Vascular Stenting*. 2d ed. New York: Taylor & Francis, 2005.

Serruys, Patrick W., and Benno Rensing, eds. *Handbook of Coronary Stents*. 4th ed. Malden, Mass.: Blackwell Science, 2002.

White, Christopher J., et al. *Quick Guide to Peripheral Vascular Stenting*. Royal Oak, Mich.: Physicians' Press, 2001.

STERILIZATION

Procedure

Anatomy or system affected: Abdomen, genitals, reproductive system, uterus

Specialties and related fields: Family medicine, general surgery, gynecology, urology

Definition: The surgical prevention of pregnancy, as performed on males through the cutting of the vas deferens (vasectomy) or on females through the blockage or cutting of the Fallopian tubes, the removal of the ovaries, or the removal of the uterus (hysterectomy).

Key terms:

contraception: the prevention of pregnancy

corpus luteum: a yellow cell mass produced from a graafian follicle after the release of an egg

endometriosis: a disease of the female reproductive system that occurs when cells of the uterine lining (endometrium) grow outside the uterus and cause severe pain

Fallopian tubes: the two tubes that connect the ovaries to the uterus and through which an egg travels during ovulation

graafian follicle: any of the ovarian follicles that produce eggs

hormone: a substance made by a body organ and carried through the blood to a second (or target) organ in order to optimize the operation of that target organ

hysterectomy: a surgery that removes part or all of the uterus

laparoscopy: a surgical procedure in which a small incision is made near the navel and the organs of the abdominal cavity, including the uterus and Fallopian tubes, are viewed with a lighted tube called a laparoscope

ovariectomy: the removal of the ovaries

peritoneal cavity: the abdominal cavity that contains the visceral organs

Indications and Procedures

Sterilization, of either a woman or a man, is a permanent method of surgical contraception that is used to render a couple incapable of conceiving children. Female sterilization involves the blockage or removal of the Fallopian tubes, the ovaries, or the uterus. Male sterilization involves the interruption of the vas deferens, the pathway of sperm from the testicles. The vas deferens may be reconnected, while many of the sterilization procedures performed on women are considered irreversible. Although the most frequently utilized types of female sterilization possess the potential for reversal at a later date, attempted reversals are often unsuccessful. Therefore, a woman choosing this type of contraception should be quite sure that she does not want another child. By the beginning of the twenty-first century, sterilization was the most prevalent form of contraception worldwide, with an estimated one hundred million women choosing the procedure. In the United States, approximately 700,000 women are sterilized each year. One reason that female sterilization is a popular form of contraception with women is because it represents a onetime effort that is usually both simple and the cause of only mild side effects. Another advantage of sterilization over the use of birth control pills is its high success rate: Less than a tenth as many sterilized women will become pregnant (as a result of improperly performed or incomplete procedures) as will women who rely on birth control pills for their contraception. The use of condoms, diaphragms, and all the other barrier pregnancy prevention devices are even less effective than birth control pills.

Before considering the various aspects of sterilization, it is useful to describe the female reproductive system and its biological operation. This organ system consists of two ovaries connected to paired Fallopian tubes that open up into the uterus. The entire system passes through a monthly menstrual cycle that is controlled by the female hormones progesterone and the estrogens. During each menstrual cycle, an ovary produces one egg (sometimes more) in a graafian follicle. The egg then enters one of the Fallopian tubes, which carries it to the uterus. If an egg is fertilized, it then implants in the endometrial tissue that lines the interior of the uterus and subsequently develops into an embryo.

Egg formation and uterus preparation for implantation are controlled by the female hormones. Once an egg implants, the uterus is kept in a state that optimizes pregnancy with the production of progesterone and related hormones, first by the corpus luteum (originally the graafian follicle that yielded the egg) and then by the placenta that forms from commingled uterine and fetal tissue. In the absence of fertilization, the menstrual cycle continues, most of the endometrium breaks down into the monthly menstrual flow, and the process begins over again.

Menstruation stops between forty-five and fifty-five years of age in most women, causing them to undergo a process called the menopause. After hundreds of repeated menstrual cycles since puberty, the graafian follicles stop producing eggs. Cessation of the menstrual cycle means that female hormone production stops almost entirely. Therefore, the menopause is accompanied by gradual atrophy of the sex organs and possible related symptoms, including hot flashes, depression, and irritability. When ovariectomy or hysterectomy is performed to achieve sterilization, these symptoms of the menopause may be induced prematurely.

For pregnancy to occur, then, a woman must have at least one functional ovary that produces eggs, an intact and operational Fallopian tube to transport the egg, and a functional uterus. The surgical methods that are used for sterilization must, therefore, make one of these reproductive organs nonfunctional. Most often, sterilization cuts and then blocks or removes the Fallopian tubes. Such interruption of the Fallopian tubes is the preferred form of female sterilization surgery for three reasons. First, these operations are relatively minor surgical procedures and are unlikely to be very risky. In addition, premature menopausal symptoms are not produced because the menstrual cycle continues. Finally, when carried out appropriately, interruption of the Fallopian tubes can sometimes be reversed if the patient changes her mind as a result of altered marital arrangements, lifestyle, or financial circumstances.

In many cases, a 1-centimeter to 1.5-centimeter section in the middle of each Fallopian tube is removed surgically or burned away via electrocoagulation. Alternatively, plastic or metal clips are used to close off each tube, or similar tube closure is effected by making a loop in each Fallopian tube and closing it off with a tight plastic ring or band.

Very frequently, the method that is used to damage the Fallopian tubes is a form of surgery called a laparoscopic procedure. The patient is given a general anesthetic, a very small incision is made close to the navel, and a flexible lighted tube-a laparoscope-is inserted into the incision. The laparoscope is equipped with fiber optics and enables an examining physician to see into the abdominal (peritoneal) cavity. Visibility of the Fallopian tubes and the other abdominal organs with laparoscopic examination is enhanced by pumping harmless carbon dioxide gas or nitrous oxide gas into the abdomen, to distend it. This process is called pneumoperitoneum.

After laparoscopic examination identifies the operation site in the peritoneal cavity, the surgical tools for cauterization, cutting, banding, and other aspects of interrupting the Fallopian tubes are passed through the laparoscope, and the chosen surgical interruption procedure is carried out. An entire laparoscopic procedure often takes less than thirty minutes, which is one of the reasons for its great popularity. In addition, women who choose to undergo such surgery can usually go home in a few hours and are fully recovered after only one to two days of postoperative bed rest, followed by a week or so of curtailed physical and sexual activity.

Despite the popularity of the laparoscopic procedure for sterilization, some physicians prefer to carry out sterilization by use of a larger surgical incision through which the tubes are altered directly. Despite the larger size of the incision, the physicians who use this method believe that it is safer and more sure of success and that it has a greater potential for reversibility.

Other methods for sterilization through Fallopian tube surgery are culdoscopy and chemical means. Culdoscopy, in which an optical instrument and surgical tools reach the Fallopian tubes through the uterus, has a somewhat lower success rate than do the laparoscopic procedure and the direct method. Chemical methods for tubal closure have also been attempted and are not viewed as viable because of a low success rate and frequent, serious postoperative complications.

The other avenues available for sterilization are ovariectomy (removal of the ovaries) and hysterectomy (removal of the uterus). Both of these types of sterilization surgery are much more serious and risky. In addition, ovariectomy and hysterectomy are totally irreversible. Ovariectomy, a more complicated procedure than the one inactivating the Fallopian tubes, is usually utilized only when both ovaries are diseased. This procedure produces an early menopause because most of a woman's female hormones are made by the ovaries' graafian follicles.

Hysterectomy is the most uncommon form of female sterilization because it requires even more extensive surgery and can have fatal complications. While the operation is sometimes carried out when a woman has completed her desired family, most hysterectomies are curative. They are performed in cases of very severe and widespread endometriosis and in the presence of other serious gynecological problems.

An alternative available to couples is sterilization of the male partner. This type of surgery, a vasectomy, is quite simple, brief, and relatively painless and only rarely results in physical or psychological complications. In addition, after vasectomy only one-tenth of a percent of involved couples experience undesired pregnancies. Vasectomy has no effect on sexual desire or male hormone production. It is also relatively easy to reverse such surgery, if so desired later in life. Consequently, the method has become quite popular. In the United States, for example, it was estimated in the early twenty-first century that approximately 500,000 men undergo this sterilization surgery each year.

Vasectomy involves the surgical interruption of the tube-the vas deferens-through which sperm leave the testicle. Vasectomy is carried out after identifying the position of each tube and injecting it with a local anesthetic. A 1-inch-long incision is made in the scrotum, each tube is cut near its middle, a small piece of the tube is removed to keep the cut ends apart, and all the ends are closed with sutures, by cauterization, or with metal or plastic clips.

Vasectomy has a short recovery period and does not stop ejaculation during postoperative intercourse. It is important to note, however, that azoospermia (a lack of sperm in the ejaculate) is achieved only after six to fifteen postoperative ejaculations. Therefore, to ensure sterility, it is critical that the condition of azoospermia has been achieved before the patient carries out intercourse without using condoms or other protective measures. After two consecutive sperm counts indicate azoospermia, unprotected intercourse is deemed safe.

Uses and Complications

The most popular method of female sterilization is to block or damage both Fallopian tubes so that eggs cannot pass through them to the uterus. In some cases, the tubes are removed completely. While removal ensures successful sterilization, it is irreversible and considered too drastic by women who might someday wish to reverse the operation. Several popular alternatives to removal are the methods that interrupt the tubes, retaining the potential for reversal at a later date. Women undergoing this type of surgery are warned, however, that such reversal may be impossible.

When the Fallopian tubes are damaged but not entirely closed off, they may reconnect and cause an ectopic pregnancy, in which a fertilized egg implants in one of the tubes and begins to grow into a fetus. Ectopic pregnancy can be fatal to the pregnant woman, and when identified, it is corrected by surgical removal of the fetus. Although the cause of this problem is not clear, there is some thought that alteration of the interior wall of the tube or slowed passage of an egg through the tube may be the causative agent. Fortunately, ectopic pregnancy is relatively uncommon.

Whether the laparoscopic method or the direct approach is utilized, the best time to carry out female sterilization is at the end of a menstrual cycle; at this time, early pregnancies cannot be compromised. It is advised that the patient discontinue intercourse and the use of birth control pills for at least a month prior to the surgery. The cessation of intercourse eliminates the chance of unexpected pregnancy at the time of surgery, while stopping the use of birth control pills decreases the possibility of blood-clotting problems.

The complications of all types of Fallopian tube surgery can include internal bleeding, blood-clotting problems, injury to the intestines and the other abdominal organs, and abnormal postoperative menstrual cycles. It is estimated, however, that these complications occur in less than 1 percent of patients. A more frequent problem is the difficulty of restoring fertility by reconnecting the Fallopian tubes (with only a 20 to 40 percent success rate).

Hysterectomy is never a highly recommended female sterilization operation. Rather, it is used mostly in those cases where other uterine health problems are sufficiently severe to make the process sensible. These problems may include recurrent and heavy vaginal bleeding, severe endometriosis, and chronic pelvic inflammatory disease (PID). This extensive surgery results in a high rate of complications and a significant number of deaths.

A woman may seek sterilization when she is having an abortion or soon after giving birth to an undesired child. Such a decision, perhaps made hastily at a time of intense emotional stress, is not advisable. It is essential that a sterilization operation be performed only after careful reflection. Divorce or the death of a spouse and subsequent remarriage may cause a sterilized woman regret should she desire more children.

Severe psychological problems for both the patient and her family may accompany female sterilization. Therefore, it is highly recommended that these women, their families, and both partners in married couples consult a gynecologist and a psychological counselor before proceeding with female sterilization surgery.

In contrast to the complications associated with female sterilization, with vasectomy a day of bed rest and a week of avoidance of all strenuous physical activity usually produce complete recovery. Health complications occur in less than 5 percent of vasectomy patients. In addition, these problems are usually minor and almost never lead to fatalities. Skin discoloration, swelling, and oozing of clear fluid from the scrotum incision are common symptoms immediately following the surgery, but they spontaneously disappear as the healing process continues. Less frequently, inflammation and a condition called sperm granuloma can occur when sperm leak out of the cut portion of the vas deferens closest to the testicle. A granuloma produces severe inflammation, pain, and swelling. When this condition does not subside spontaneously, the granuloma must be removed surgically.

Perspective and Prospects

While surgical sterilization was first described in the nineteenth century, it was not widely available for contraception until the 1920's, nor did it become popular immediately. Though voluntary sterilization began slowly in the 1950s, its use accelerated until it became a popular form of fertility control in the industrial and developing nations of the 1970s.

A source of discontent with the sterilization techniques that are available is their total or poor reversibility when fertility reinitiation is desired later in life. This discontent has occurred because, with passing time, an unexpectedly large segment of sterilized men and women have come to regret their decisions regarding sterilization. All hysterectomies and Fallopian tube removals are forever irreversible, and a low reversibility rate is seen even in the two most popular-and potentially reversible-sterilization methodologies: Fallopian tube interruption and vasectomy.

Consequently, the development of sterilization surgery has been directed toward devising methods that will enable much larger incidences of reversibility, where desired. One direction has been to expand the understanding of Fallopian tube and vas deferens anatomy and functionality. Particularly useful results obtained include the realization that destruction of the nerves that control the operation of these organs can make the recovery of fertility incomplete or impossible even when excellent corrective surgery reverses the original interruption of continuity. This discovery has led to the development of more sophisticated interruption surgery that is less likely to damage the vas deferens or Fallopian tube nerve integrity. Some improvement of the reversibility of these operations has been obtained in this manner, but the overall results are still far from satisfactory.

Consequently, many other surgical techniques have been attempted, including the placement of removable plugs in the Fallopian tubes or of tiny, faucetlike valves in the vas deferens that allow or stop the ejaculation of sperm. Other useful methods to ensure reversible sterilization may include hormones, vaccines against eggs and sperm, and chemical treatments. It is hoped that improved antifertility methodologies will be developed that combine more reversible surgical sterilization, vaccines, chemicals, and various contraceptives.

—*Sanford S. Singer, Ph.D.*

See also Conception; Contraception; Gynecology; Hysterectomy; Laparoscopy; Menopause; Men's health; Menstruation; Ovaries; Pregnancy and gestation; Reproductive system; Tubal ligation; Uterus; Vas deferens; Vasectomy; Women's health.

For Further Information:
Ammer, Christine. *The New A to Z of Women's Health: A Concise Encyclopedia.* 6th ed. New York: Checkmark Books, 2009. A respected classic that covers the full spectrum of women's health issues, including reproduction and methods of contraception.

Connell, Elizabeth B. *The Contraception Sourcebook.* Chicago: Contemporary Books, 2002. A straightforward guide that provides comprehensive coverage of each contraceptive method, including a clear and understandable analysis of its advantages and disadvantages as well as a lively discussion of its origins.

Denniston, George C. *Vasectomy.* Victoria, B.C.: Trafford, 2002. Provides a range of information for men who are considering a vasectomy.

Mastroianni, Luigi, Jr., Peter J. Donaldson, and Thomas T. Kane. *Developing New Contraceptives: Obstacles and Opportunities.* Washington, D.C.: National Academy Press, 1990. This book on contraceptive measures other than sterilization by surgery also contains considerable useful information on sterilization practices and legalities. Provides useful insights and allows the reader to consider other effective, long-term methods of contraception, excluding surgery.

Parker, James N., and Philip M. Parker, eds. *The Official Patient's Sourcebook on Vasectomy.* San Diego, Calif.: Icon Health, 2002. Draws from public, academic, government, and peer-reviewed research to provide a wide-ranging handbook for patients considering a vasectomy.

Sherwood, Lauralee. *Human Physiology: From Cells to Systems.* 7th ed. Pacific Grove, Calif.: Brooks/Cole/Cengage Learning, 2010. This college text provides details about the menstrual cycle, hormones, and the endometrium. Many useful definitions, diagrams, and glossary terms are included.

Wigfall-Williams, Wanda. *Hysterectomy: Learning the Facts, Coping with the Feelings, and Facing the Future.* New York: Michael Kesend, 1986. Discusses sterilization as a motive for hysterectomy, in addition to severe endometriosis. Offers guidelines for the choice of a physician or surgical procedure and explores possible aftereffects, such as depression and changes in sexual function.

STEROID ABUSE
Disease/Disorder

Anatomy or system affected: Circulatory system, endocrine system, heart, muscles, psychic-emotional system, reproductive system

Specialties and related fields: Exercise physiology, psychiatry, psychology, sports medicine

Definition: The use of illegal anabolic steroids to increase athletic performance, with negative side effects on physical and psychological health.

Causes and Symptoms

Steroids provide many valuable medical benefits for various conditions ranging from asthma, infections, and delayed

---

Information on Steroid Abuse

Causes: Psychological and emotional factors, competitive sports

Symptoms: Relatively rapid gain in muscle tone, increased aggressiveness, violent temper, increased acne, premature balding, abnormal breast development

Duration: Temporary to long-term

Treatments: Cessation of drug use, counseling

---

puberty to spastic colon. Unfortunately, steroid abuse has become an increasingly prevalent issue. Steroid abuse has gained attention in the past few years mainly due to its relation to professional sports. Numerous well-known athletes have admitted to using steroids in order to increase their athletic edge. A lack of social acceptability around steroid use has resulted from the more than seventy side effects associated with steroid use, including such immediate problems as rage, depression, and highly aggressive behavior. Reports have included findings of teenagers committing acts as brutal as murder, without any prior history of criminal or aggressive behavior, while under the influence of steroids. While such acts are rare, the connection between steroids and out-of-control rage is well known. In addition, steroid abuse has been linked with such long-term problems as heart attacks, strokes, and changes in the reproductive system. It is likely that increasing attention will be focused on these kinds of long-term effects, both in research and in terms of problem reporting. Increases in the access to anabolic steroids are also partly responsible for an increase in the visibility of and attention to such problems.

Social research also has demonstrated important findings related to steroid use in college students and in athletes. One study, for example, demonstrated that college students consistently rated anabolic steroid-using athletes more negatively than drug-free athletes. In fact, students tended to evaluate anabolic steroid-using athletes just as negatively as they would an athlete who was using cocaine. In another study, researchers demonstrated that steroid use is not only physically reinforcing but also psychologically reinforcing. Specifically, in interviews with thirty-five male self-reported anabolic steroid users, lower levels of anxiety related to the perception of one's physique and higher levels of satisfaction with one's upper body were demonstrated, relative to the control subjects. There was a psychological gain associated with the steroid use that was directly related to the shorter-term physical benefits of their use.

Perspective and Prospects

Recent estimates suggest that about 1.4 percent of college athletes are using anabolic steroids. A 2001 report by the National Collegiate Athletic Association (NCAA) demonstrated that this was a decrease from the 4.9 percent of student athletes who reported using steroids in 1985. Nationwide, according to the NCAA, collegiate football players were reported to have the highest rate of use, at 3.0 percent. The survey suggested, however, that this lowered rate may reflect underreporting. Factors such as the illegality of drug use or a lack of social acceptability in acknowledging such personal behavior may be responsible. Such assertions of underreporting also are based on other reports that 2.6 percent of male high school students and 0.4 percent of female high school students have used anabolic steroids. Furthermore, among athletes not in college, reported rates are much higher. The highest reported usage rates were found in weight lifters, power lifters, track-and-field athletes, football players, and sprinters. Major League Baseball banned steroids in 2002 and instituted a testing program after several top players admitted to steroid use. Future work in this area will likely explore these psychological factors and focus on how to intervene effectively. Additionally, it is likely that social interventions will be explored. Athletics remain competitive and financially lucrative, so special attention will need to be paid to the social context in which steroid abuse occurs. There is little research or studies on the treatment of steroid abuse. Most knowledge on treatment comes from the experience of a small number of physicians who have treated steroid withdrawal themselves. The most effective treatment is prevention.

—*Roman J. Miller, Ph.D. and Nancy A. Piotrowski, Ph.D.; updated by Samar Aslam, M.D.*

See also Addiction; Ergogenic aids; Ethics; Exercise physiology; Hormones; Hypertrophy; Muscles; Psychiatry, child and adolescent; Puberty and adolescence; Sports medicine; Steroids

For Further Information:

http://www.drugabuse.gov/publications/drugfacts/anabolic-steroids
Craig, Charles R., and Robert E. Stitzel, eds. *Modern Pharmacology with Clinical Applications.* 6th ed. Philadelphia: Lippincott, 2004.
Kronenberg, Henry M., et al., eds. *Williams Textbook of Endocrinology.* 11th ed. Philadelphia: Saunders/Elsevier, 2008.
Taylor, William N. *Anabolic Steroids and the Athlete.* 2nd ed. Jefferson, NC: McFarland, 2002.
Yesalis, Charles E., ed. *Anabolic Steroids in Sport and Exercise.* 2nd ed. Champaign, IL: Human Kinetics, 2000.
Yesalis, Charles E., and Michael S. Bahrke. "Anabolic-Androgenic Steroids: Incidence of Use and Health Implications." *President's Council on Physical Fitness and Sports Research Digest* 5, no. 5 (2005): 1-8.

STEROIDS

Biology

Anatomy or system affected: Endocrine system, glands

Specialties and related fields: Biochemistry, endocrinology, pediatrics, pharmacology, sports medicine

Definition: Organic compounds, both natural and synthetic, that enhance specific activities of the body and that can be used as therapeutic agents in the treatment of many clinical disorders.

Key terms:

anabolic steroids: a class of steroids that stimulate body reactions to build up more complex molecules and structures from simpler molecules; most are synthetic derivatives of testosterone

cholesterol: a fatlike steroid alcohol that is found in animal fats, oils, and tissues; most of the body's supply is manufactured in the liver, while some is absorbed from the diet

corticosteroids: the group of steroid hormones produced by the adrenal cortex, which includes the classes of mineralocorticoids, glucocorticoids, and sex steroids

glucocorticoids: steroid hormones that regulate the metabolism of glucose and other organic molecules

mineralocorticoids: steroid hormones that regulate the body levels of sodium and potassium

sex steroids: steroid hormones such as androgens and estrogens that influence the activity of sexual organs and activity

steroid nucleus: the molecular arrangement of four carbon rings that makes up the backbone of all steroids

sterol: a steroid that has long side chains of carbon compounds attached to it and contains at least one hydroxyl group; cholesterol is one type of sterol

Structure and Functions

Steroids are a group of organic compounds that are distinguished by a unique molecular arrangement of seventeen carbon atoms situated in four adjacent rings. This set of four rings is referred to as the steroid nucleus and is common to all steroid compounds. Three of these rings are hexagonal six-carbon rings arranged in a bent-line fashion to form what is called a phenanthrene group. The fourth group or ring contains only five carbon atoms. Steroids vary with the nature of the attached groups, the position of a given attached group, or some alteration to the configuration of the steroid nucleus. Small chemical differences in the structure of steroids can reflect very great differences in specific biological effects. Steroids are included in the lipid category of biological molecules because they are nonpolar and insoluble in water.

Any steroid that contains a hydroxyl group (-OH) is called a sterol. This term comes from a Greek word meaning "solid"; sterols were so named because they were among the earliest compounds that were found to be solid at room temperature. Once chemical structures were determined, then other compounds with similar structures were given the name steroid, which means "sterol-like." The suffix "-oid" comes from the Greek and means "similar to."

Chemists have isolated hundreds of different steroids from plants and animals; additionally, thousands have been made by chemically modifying natural steroids or by synthesizing the entire molecule. The parent compound for steroids is acetic acid. Assisted by a variety of enzymes, acetic acid is altered and transformed into several other compounds before cholesterol is formed. Cholesterol serves as the parent, or precursor compound, for bile acids and for the steroids that are biologically important to the body.

Cholesterol is the most common steroid in the human body, as it is a structural component of cellular membranes. The prefix "chole-" comes from the Greek word for liver bile, which is a digestive fluid manufactured by the liver and secreted into the intestines. The name is appropriate since the bile contains a considerable amount of cholesterol. Bile is stored in the gallbladder and becomes concentrated there. Cholesterol is not very soluble, and if it accumulates in great enough quantities, it will form small crystals in the bile. These crystals may join together to form larger particles that can block the narrow duct that leads from the gallbladder to the intestines. These aggregations of particles are called gallstones and are composed of almost pure cholesterol. The blockage can result in a buildup of pressure and cause much pain. Often, a surgical operation is required to remove the obstruction.

Cholesterol is also an important molecule because it is the precursor or parent molecule for the steroid hormones produced by the gonads and the adrenal cortex. The gonads, a collective term referring to the testes and ovaries, secrete the sex steroids. These sex steroids include estradiol and progesterone from the ovaries and testosterone from the testes. The adrenal cortex secretes the corticosteroids, which include cortisol and aldosterone as well as other steroid compounds. Most of the steroid hormones are specialized in their function and do not produce general effects on metabolism. The sex hormones influence reproduction by acting on sexual organs to stimulate their development and function, by influencing sexual behavior, and by stimulating the development of secondary sex characteristics. Some of the steroids secreted by the adrenal cortex have more general effects on the metabolism of carbohydrates and proteins in many tissues.

Steroid hormones combine with specific receptors that are located in the cytoplasm of the responsive tissues. Since these hormones are lipid-soluble, they pass readily through cell membranes, which are largely composed of lipids. Inside the cytoplasm, a steroid-specific protein receptor will bind to the hormone. Upon binding, the hormone-receptor complex becomes activated or transformed and is then translocated to the nucleus. In the nucleus, the activated steroid receptor complex binds to the chromatin, or genetic material, causing an activation of a certain set of genes. Gene activation results in the production of messenger molecules that induce the production of specific proteins that are either used by the cell or secreted elsewhere.

The steroid hormones of the adrenal cortex fall into three categories, each having separate actions and sites of actions. Aldosterone is the principal mineralocorticoid and plays an important role in regulating body levels of sodium and potassium. Cortisol, the major glucocorticoid, regulates carbohydrate metabolism. Adrenal androgens are also produced, but they have only weak activity and play a minor physiological role under most conditions. All adrenal steroids are derived from cholesterol.

Mineralocorticoids are the adrenal steroids that regulate levels of potassium and sodium in the body. Aldosterone, the most potent mineralocorticoid, is secreted by the adrenal cortex at the rate of about 0.1 milligram per day. Mineralocorticoids affect the distal tubules of the kidney by stimulating the excretion of potassium and the reabsorption of sodium. The net effect of these actions is to increase the volume of body fluids.

Glucocorticoids are the adrenal steroids that regulate glucose metabolism. In humans, cortisol is responsible for most of the glucocorticoid activity. It is secreted by the adrenal cortex at the rate of about 20 milligrams per day and metabolically affects tissues throughout the body. Cortisol is regulated by the central nervous system and by permissive or stimulatory messenger molecules of the body. Generally, glucocorticoids stimulate the production of glucose and enhance the use of fat and protein as energy sources.

Androgens are steroid hormones that are secreted primarily by the testes but also by the adrenal glands and ovaries. Testosterone is the principal androgen that is secreted by the testes; it regulates the development and function of male sex accessory organs. Increased testosterone secretion during puberty is required for the growth of the seminal vesicles and prostate. Removal of androgens by castration results in these organs undergoing atrophy.

Androgens stimulate growth of the larynx and cause lowering of the voice. They increase hemoglobin synthesis, which is higher in males than females, and affect bone growth by causing the conversion of cartilage to bone. Androgens also promote protein synthesis or anabolic activity in skeletal muscle, bone, and kidneys. As a class of compounds, androgens are reasonably safe drugs, since they have a limited and relatively predictable set of side effects. In human males, testosterone is synthesized by the testes at the rate of about 8 milligrams per day.

Estrogens and progesterones are primarily produced in the ovaries of nonpregnant adult women. In pregnancy, the placenta is the major site of estrogen and progesterone production. Smaller amounts of estrogen synthesis involve the liver, kidney, skeletal muscle, and testes. Estrogens cause the growth of the female reproductive organs and are responsible for the expression of female secondary sex characteristics, such as breast enlargement, female body contours, skin texture, and distribution of body hair. Estrogens are thought to protect against atherosclerosis and heart attacks since occurrence of these health problems in mature women is much lower than in males of similar ages.

Uses and Complications

When cortisone was initially discovered, it was labeled a "wonder drug" and was thought to possess widespread effectiveness in many areas of medicine. Although these expectations have not been realized, a variety of steroids are found to be effective in medical practice and treatment. Steroids are commonly prescribed to serve as replacements for those persons whose bodies are unable to produce specific steroid hormones in adequate quantities. Steroids are effective as anti-inflammatory agents, reducing inflammatory reactions in a variety of body tissues. They are also prescribed for patients who have undergone an organ transplantation or have highly sensitive allergies because they inhibit the responsiveness of the immune system.

The primary therapeutic use of androgens is for testicular deficiency in which the induction and maintenance of male secondary sex characteristics are desired. In these cases, supplemental doses of androgens are given to stimulate and enhance the development of sexual and accessory sex characteristics. Androgens are effective also in the therapy of some anemias when persons have reduced levels of red blood cells. Androgens are used to treat osteoporosis, which is a decrease in bone or skeletal mass. Androgens are given to women in the treatment of breast cancer and are effective about 20 percent of the time. They are used to treat the abnormal growth of endometrial tissue in the peritoneal cavity of women, a disease called endometriosis, and are effective in that role.

Steroids also have anabolic activities that are manifested by stimulating increases in protein production, by enhancing the uptake of amino acids into cells, and by inhibiting the glucocorticoids from breaking down proteins. They influence embryonic development, especially the differentiation of the central nervous system and the male reproductive tract. The excitatory function of androgens occurs at puberty, during which the reproductive organs are activated to produce sex cells. Androgens also maintain the body's sexual characteristics in the adult. Thus, in cases of androgen deficiency there is a regression of male sexual behavior, libido, and reproductive function; this regression is reversible with treatment.

It should be noted that anabolic steroids are frequently abused because of these kinds of effects. Athletes and body builders in search of accelerated muscle building or physical definition are two groups in which such abuse has been seen. A complication has been that the stimulatory effects of the anabolic steroids make the drug administrations reinforcing and therefore loaded with addiction potential. As such, frequent users of anabolic steroids should be aware of conditions such as dependence, as well as withdrawal and other problematic side effects of heavy steroid use. Such effects may include increased periods of sleep disturbance, paranoia, anger and agitation, mood swings or instability of mood, violence or other impulsive behavior, and concentration and memory disturbance. Physical problems may include severe acne, jaundice, excess water retention, decreased sperm count, high cholesterol, liver problems, and difficulty with blood sugar control.

Addison's disease is caused by a failure of the adrenal gland to secrete adequate amounts of both glucocorticoids and mineralocorticoids. The symptoms of this disease are imbalances of body levels of sodium and potassium, dehydration, reduced blood pressure, rapid weight loss, and generalized weakness. A person with Addison's disease will die if not treated with corticosteroids because of the severe electrolyte imbalance and dehydration.

Cushing's syndrome results when the adrenal gland secretes corticosteroids in excessive quantities. Symptoms include high blood pressure, alterations in protein and carbohydrate metabolism, high blood sugar concentrations, and muscular weakness. This syndrome is often caused by a tumor in the adrenal gland that promotes the secretion of corticosteroids. Surgical intervention is often used to remove the portion of the gland that is malfunctioning. Symptoms similar to those seen in Cushing's syndrome are found in people with inflammatory diseases who receive lengthy treatments with corticosteroids in order to reduce the inflammation.

Adrenogenital syndrome results from an excessive level of sex steroids, usually caused by hyperactivity of the adrenal gland. Androgen is the major sex steroid involved in this clinical condition, which causes a premature puberty and enlarged genital sex organs when it occurs in young children. Other characteristics are increased amounts of body and facial hair as well as deepening of the voice.

The greatest use of estrogens as therapeutic agents is in oral contraception, or "the pill." This method is convenient, reversible, and relatively inexpensive; its use is worldwide and includes 25 percent of American women of childbearing age. Most oral contraceptives are active combinations of estrogen and progesterone. Users take a daily pill containing both steroids for twenty or twenty-one days of the menstrual cycle and then a placebo for seven or eight days. Withdrawal bleeding occurs two to three days after discontinuing the pill. The mechanism for the effectiveness of these steroids involves inhibiting the release of hormones that would normally stimulate ovulation. Hormone therapy was the primary treatment for menopausal symptoms. However, the Women's Health Initiative Study showed that while hormone therapy had some benefits, it also increased the risk for blood clots, breast cancer, heart attacks, and strokes.

Antiandrogens are substances that prevent or depress the action of androgens, or testosterone, on the body. They are of value in the management of patients whose bodies are producing abnormally high levels of androgens, who are undergoing a premature puberty, or who are affected with acne, hirsutism (excessive hairiness, especially in women), and certain tumors or neoplasms. Potentially, these drugs can be utilized to cause sterility in males.

Natural body androgens stimulate the growth of the prostate gland in males and enhance the proliferation of many prostate cancers. Treatment of abnormal growths, malignant cancers, or benign tumors in the male prostate gland has frequently used either natural or synthetic steroids. Estradiol, a form of the female sex steroid estrogen, is used to control the advancement of prostate carcinoma in some males and can induce remission in 50 to 80 percent of the cases of prostate tumors. Estrogens exert their effect by interfering with androgen production or by inhibiting the function of androgen-responsive tissues. Thus in some cases estrogens inhibit abnormal cellular growth. A manufactured synthetic drug, cyproterone acetate, is also used in the treatment of benign prostatic enlargement in men. Cyproterone acetate is very effective in treating prostate cancers and tumors, and it does not have the feminizing side effects of the estrogens; however, it does cause inhibition of sperm production and loss of sexual drive.

Perspective and Prospects

The use of steroids as therapeutic agents began in the early 1930s. At that time, Philip Showalter Hench, who was working in the Mayo Clinic, noticed that the symptoms of arthritic women were alleviated when they became pregnant. He suggested that increased secretions from the adrenal cortex might be the responsible agents. Later, clinical trials were conducted to test the role of corticosteroids in treating acute arthritis. With the use of adequate dosages, the clinical response was impressive. The 1950 Nobel Prize in Physiology or Medicine was awarded to Hench and his coworkers for their finding that cortisone was effective in treating arthritis.

Pharmaceutical firms have manufactured numerous steroid derivatives, all of which have different effectiveness levels as glucocorticoids, mineralocorticoids, or sex steroids. Organic chemists synthesize analogues of adrenal steroids in order to create compounds that produce heightened biological effects with a minimum or lack of side effects. As a consequence, hundreds of different steroids are available. Most of these are characterized according to their biological effectiveness, such as their ability to reduce inflammation or to inhibit the immune system. When determining a course of treatment, a physician chooses a particular steroid that enhances the effects that are desired and has minimal effects in related areas. Some pharmaceutical derivatives of adrenal steroids are very poorly absorbed by the skin. These derivatives are especially useful to apply to the skin when a maximal local effect is desired without a generalized effect on other body regions.

Steroids, however, can also have negative, and sometimes dangerous, effects on the body, whether they are ingested (cholesterol) or injected (anabolic steroids). Evidence indicates that high blood cholesterol levels are associated with an increased risk of atherosclerosis, a clinical condition in which localized plaques (or atheromas) build up in the walls of arteries, reducing blood flow. Atheromas serve as locations for blood clot formation, which can further block the blood supply to a vital organ such as the heart, brain, or lung. High blood cholesterol may result from a diet rich in cholesterol and saturated fat, or it may result from an inherited condition in which affected individuals have extremely high cholesterol concentrations, regardless of their diet. These persons usually suffer heart attacks during their childhood.

Cholesterol is found in foods that are based on animal products. Cholesterol-rich foods include most meats, eggs, and dairy products such as cheese, cream, and butter. Humans readily absorb cholesterol from dietary sources. Most Western diets contain 400 to 600 milligrams of cholesterol per day, of which about 75 percent is readily absorbed into the bloodstream from the dietary tract. Cholesterol is carried to the arteries by proteins in the blood plasma called low-density lipoproteins (LDLs). A given cell may engulf the LDLs and use the cholesterol for different purposes. The LDLs in a given location may stimulate other cells to secrete growth factors that either begin or contribute to the development of an atheroma. Thus the risk of atherosclerosis is greatly increased. Most people can significantly lower their blood cholesterol levels through controlled exercise and diet. Since saturated fat raises blood cholesterol levels, foods such as fatty meat, egg yolk, and liver should be eaten sparingly so that fat contributes less than 30 percent to the total calories of a diet.

The use and abuse of anabolic steroids to increase muscle mass and strength are widespread in both amateur and professional sports. Although those promoting steroid use claim increases in muscle mass, strength, and endurance, controlled clinical trials show minimal, if any, enhancement of muscle mass and strength. Testosterone may also enhance training efforts by promoting aggressive behavior. Use of these compounds poses ethical questions and increases the risk of serious toxicity because of the extremely high doses that are administered, often as much as one hundred times the usual therapeutic dosages.

—Roman J. Miller, Ph.D.;
Nancy A. Piotrowski, Ph.D.; updated by
Sharon W. Stark, R.N., A.P.R.N., D.N.Sc.

See also Addison's disease; Adrenal glands; Cholesterol; Contraception; Cushing's syndrome; Endocrine disorders; Endocrine glands; Endocrinology; Endocrinology, pediatric; Ergogenic aids; Glands; Growth; Gynecology; Hormone therapy; Hormones; Hypercholesterolemia; Metabolism; Muscles; Ovaries; Pain management; Pharmacology; Prostate cancer; Prostate gland; Puberty and adolescence; Reproductive system; Sports medicine; Steroid abuse.

For Further Information:

Craig, Charles R., and Robert E. Stitzel, eds. *Modern Pharmacology with Clinical Applications*. 6th ed. Philadelphia: Lippincott, 2004. This college-level pharmacology text contains easy-to-comprehend sections on steroids, including their chemistry, synthesis, physiological activity, and pharmacological activity.

Guyton, Arthur C., and John E. Hall. *Human Physiology and Mechanisms of Disease*. 6th ed. Philadelphia: W. B. Saunders, 1997. Guyton is a nationally recognized authority on medical physiology, having written and edited numerous college-level and medical school textbooks on the subject. His writing style is flowing and understandable to the nonmedical specialist and student.

Henry, Helen L., and Anthony W. Norman, eds. *Encyclopedia of Hormones*. 3 vols. San Diego, Calif.: Academic Press, 2003. A comprehensive overview of the role of hormones, the major physiological systems in which they operate, and the biological consequences of an excess or deficiency of a particular hormone.

Kronenberg, Henry M., et al., eds. *Williams Textbook of Endocrinology*. 11th ed. Philadelphia: Saunders/Elsevier, 2008. Comprehensive information regarding endocrine diseases, pathophysiology, diagnoses, treatment, and prognoses.

Montgomery, Rex, et al. *Biochemistry: A Case-Oriented Approach*. 6th ed. St. Louis, Mo.: Mosby Year Book, 1996. Surveys the field of biochemistry, examining steroids and steroid hormones in that context. A major section describes the essential role of cholesterol in the body, as well as in the synthesis of other steroids.

Tortora, Gerard J., and Bryan Derrickson. *Principles of Anatomy and Physiology*. 12th ed. Hoboken, N.J.: John Wiley & Sons, 2009. This popular college-level undergraduate anatomy and physiology text contains well-written sections on major biological molecules such as steroids, as well as longer sections on steroid hormones and their specific effects.

Zelman, Mark, et al. *Human Diseases: A Systemic Approach*. 7th ed. Upper Saddle River, N.J.: Pearson, 2010. This well-written and interesting book uses a case-oriented approach to explore the essential concepts of physiology and health. Numerous examples of pathologies relating to steroids or steroid hormones are illustrated.

STEVENS-JOHNSON SYNDROME
Disease/Disorder

Also known as: Toxic epidermal necrolysis

Anatomy or system affected: Abdomen, back, breasts, eyes, feet, gastrointestinal system, genitals, hands, head, immune system, knees, legs, lungs, neck, nose, reproductive system, respiratory system, urinary system

Specialties and related fields: Critical care, dermatology, emergency medicine, family medicine, gastroenterology, immunology, internal medicine, ophthalmology, pediatrics, pulmonary medicine, urology

Definition: A severe immune response-mediated hypersensitivity reaction to particular drugs or infections that causes a rash, sloughing of the skin, and the disruption of mucous membranes.

Key terms:

dermis: the middle layer of the skin, which lies below the epidermis and above the subcutaneous layer

epidermis: the outermost layer of the skin

erythema multiforme: a skin disorder that produces multiple skin lesions and results from an allergic reaction or infection

Fas ligand: a membrane protein that is a member of the tumor necrosis factor family of signaling proteins; it binds to a Fas receptor and induces programmed cell death

Causes and Symptoms

Stevens-Johnson syndrome begins with a nonspecific upper respiratory tract infection or after the consumption of a particular drug. The early symptoms last for one to fourteen days and consist of fever, sore throat, headache, cough, body aches, and sometimes vomiting and diarrhea. Subsequently, a flat, red rash (erythema multiforme) breaks out over the face and trunk that later spreads to the rest of the body. Painful blisters form in the center of the rash, and the skin around the blisters is quite loose and rubs off easily. Patients have a headache, fever, weakness (malaise), and a cough that produces thick, pus-filled material.

Blisters can form on the mucous membranes that line the mouth (preventing the patient from eating or drinking), throat, genitals, eyes, and anus. If the urinary tract is involved, then the patient will not be able to urinate. Eye involvement causes the eyes to swell and fill with pus so that they seal shut. Blisters on the surface of the eyes (corneas) can scar them. Lesions in the respiratory tract restrict breathing, and tissue sloughing can cause respiratory collapse. Sores in the digestive tract can cause diarrhea and narrowing of the esophagus. The open, skinless sores are also susceptible to infections.

Stevens-Johnson syndrome is classified according to the percentage of the skin affected. If 10 percent or less of the body surface area detaches, then the patient has Stevens-Johnson syndrome. If 10 to 30 percent of the skin detaches, then the patient has overlapping Stevens-Johnson syndrome/toxic epidermal necrolysis (TEN). If more than 30 percent of the skin is detached, then the patient has TEN.

Information on Stevens-Johnson Syndrome

Causes: Hypersensitivity to infections and drugs

Symptoms: Fever, headache, cough, rash, blistering

Duration: Lasts minimum of two to three weeks; convalescence can be very long

Treatments: Discontinuation of offending drug, intravenous fluids and salts, symptom management, treatment of secondary infections

---

Drug reactions cause most cases of Stevens-Johnson syndrome. The drugs that may trigger it include antibiotics, such as penicillin, ciprofloxacin, and sulfa drugs; anticonvulsant drugs, such as phenytoin, carbamazepine, and barbiturates; nonsteroidal anti-inflammatory drugs (NSAIDs); the antigout drug allopurinol; the narcolepsy treatment modafinil (Provigil); anti-human immunodeficiency virus (HIV) drugs; diuretics; and topical ocular medications. Viral, bacterial, fungal, and protozoan infections can also cause the disease, as can various types of cancers. Between one-quarter and one-half of all cases of Stevens-Johnson syndrome are idiopathic, which means that there is no discernable cause. There is also a genetic basis for this disorder.

Diagnosis requires a skin biopsy, which shows extensive cell death, detachment of the upper layer of the skin (epidermis) from the middle layer of the skin (dermis), and infiltration of the skin with particular white blood cells called lymphocytes.

The large amount of skin loss in TEN is similar to a severe burn and is life threatening. Water and salts leak through the denuded areas and can produce organ failure. Infection at the damaged areas is also a major cause of death in TEN patients.

Treatment and Therapy

The most important therapeutic step is to discontinue all drugs suspected of triggering the disease. Management of symptoms is also essential. Mouthwashes can treat oral lesions and allow fluid intake, which, when coupled with the intravenous replacement of fluid and salts, can prevent dehydration and electrolyte imbalance. Skin lesions are treated as burns. Topical anesthetics can reduce pain, and denuded skin areas are covered with saline compresses. Any secondary infection that develops must be rapidly identified and treated.

There is no universally accepted drug treatment for Stevens-Johnson syndrome. Oral corticosteroids appear to help during the first few days, but not after that. In advanced cases of TEN, corticosteroids increase the incidence of complications. Intravenous delivery of antibodies (immunoglobulins) against the Fas ligand that mediates cell death has helped small groups of TEN patients, but this treatment has not been systematically evaluated. Also, drugs that down-regulate the immune system have been used, but too little data exist to evaluate their efficacy properly.

Perspective and Prospects

Stevens-Johnson syndrome was first described in 1922 by Albert Mason Stevens and Frank Chambliss Johnson. They encountered two young boys who showed inflammation of the mucous lining of the cheeks, pus-filled eyes, and the generalized skin blisters that are now commonly associated with the disease. Stevens and Johnson originally thought that the boys suffered from a type of unknown infectious disease. Bernard Thomas named the condition in 1950. The condition gained public attention in 2010 when it contributed to the death of former professional basketball player Manute Bol.

No treatment for Stevens-Johnson syndrome provides consistent benefits to patients in systematic studies. Nevertheless, several treatments have shown promise in small studies. For example, intravenous immunoglobulin treatments, skin grafts, the antitransplant rejection drug cyclosporine, and a blood filtration procedure called plasmapheresis have successfully treated small groups of patients with few complications and little mortality. However, until larger, double-blind, placebo-based studies establish the efficacy of these treatments, they will remain experimental.

—*Michael A. Buratovich, Ph.D.*

See also Allergies; Antibiotics; Blisters; Eye infections and disorders; Eyes; Human immunodeficiency virus (HIV); Immune system; Lesions; Necrosis; Pus; Rashes; Skin; Skin disorders; Ulcers.

For Further Information:

Boyer, Woodrow Allen. *Understanding Stevens-Johnson Syndrome and Toxic Epidermal Necrolysis.* Raleigh, N.C.: Lulu Press, 2008.

Koh, Mark-Jean-Aan, and Kwang-Yong Tay. "An Update on Stevens-Johnson Syndrome and Toxic Epidermal Necrolysis in Children." *Current Opinion in Pediatrics* 21, no. 4 (August, 2009): 505-510.

Parrillo, Steven J. "Stevens-Johnson Syndrome and Toxic Epidermal Necrolysis." *Current Allergy and Asthma Reports* 7, no. 4 (July, 2007): 243-247.

Warn, Dana, and Nancy Matharu. *Stevens-Johnson Syndrome: A Booklet for Children and Their Families.* Vancouver, B.C.: Provincial Health Services Authority, 2006.

STILLBIRTH
Disease/Disorder

Also known as: Intrauterine fetal demise, fetal death, fetal wastage, miscarriage
Anatomy or system affected: Reproductive system, uterus
Specialties and related fields: Obstetrics
Definition: Birth of a fetus or infant who has died prior to delivery.

Causes and Symptoms

There are many causes of stillbirth, but in many cases, the precise cause of a fetal death is not known. The causes of stillbirth can be grouped into general categories such as fetal asphyxia; hematologic, chromosomal, or developmental problems with the fetus; and maternal illness. Fetal asphyxia occurs when the blood supply to the fetus is reduced or cut off, such as in cases of umbilical cord entanglement or placenta abruptio (abnormal detachment of the placenta from the uterus caused by such factors as maternal high blood pressure or preeclampsia, trauma, or certain drugs). Hematologic causes of stillbirth include isoimmunization (in which

Information on Stillbirth

Causes: Often unknown but may include lack of oxygen to fetus (umbilical cord entanglement, placenta abruptio); hematologic factors (isoimmunization, thrombophilias); chromosomal or developmental problems with fetus; maternal illnesses (diabetes, infections)
Symptoms: Absence of fetal movement or heartbeat, sometimes bleeding and contractions in mother
Duration: Acute
Treatments: Grief counseling, induction of labor, minimization of trauma to mother during labor, control of any maternal illnesses, investigation into cause (fetal autopsy, karyotyping)

maternal antibodies attack fetal blood cells) or thrombophilias (abnormalities in blood clotting). Maternal illnesses such as diabetes, infections (such as listeria), cholestasis, and antiphospholipid syndrome are also associated with increased risk of stillbirth.

The primary symptom of fetal demise is the absence of fetal movement. The death can be confirmed on ultrasonography or fetoscopy, which reveals the absence of a fetal heartbeat. Stillbirth may be associated with other symptoms, depending on its cause. For instance, if it results from placenta abruptio, then the woman may experience bleeding and contractions.

Treatment and Therapy

Once a stillbirth has been confirmed, treatment is directed at helping the woman and her family cope with the loss. Grief counseling is an important component of therapy. If the patient is already in labor, then minimizing obstetric trauma to the mother is of prime concern. If the patient is not in labor, then plans regarding the induction of labor are made, since prolonged retention of the dead fetus and placenta may result in disseminated intravascular coagulation (DIC), a dangerous blood condition. The patient also receives treatment aimed at controlling any maternal illnesses, such as diabetes or preeclampsia. If no obvious conditions contributed to the stillbirth, then the patient may be offered an investigation into causes of the demise. This investigation may involve tests on maternal blood for abnormalities of blood clotting, infections, abruption, diabetes, and liver abnormalities. With appropriate consent, witnessed sampling, and chain of custody handling, a urine specimen may be evaluated for the maternal ingestion of toxic substances. The stillborn fetus may be sent for autopsy and karyotyping.

No effective means exist for preventing stillbirth, although with advances in medical care, by 2003 the stillbirth rate in the United States had fallen to about 7.5 per 1,000 births, about half of what it was in the mid-1940s. If a pregnant woman has conditions putting her at increased risk of fetal demise or a history of stillbirth, then increased surveillance using ultrasonography and fetal heart tone monitoring may be indicated.

—*Anne Lynn S. Chang, M.D.*

See also Asphyxiation; Birth defects; Childbirth; Childbirth complications; Death and dying; Depression; Disseminated intravascular coagulation (DIC); Grief and guilt; Miscarriage; Obstetrics; Placenta; Postpartum depression; Preeclampsia and eclampsia; Pregnancy and gestation; Premature birth; Teratogens; Toxemia; Umbilical cord; Uterus.

For Further Information:

Creasy, Robert K., and Robert Resnik, eds. *Maternal-Fetal Medicine: Principles and Practice*. 5th ed. Philadelphia: W. B. Saunders, 2004.

Cunningham, F. Gary, et al., eds. *Williams Obstetrics*. 23d ed. New York: McGraw-Hill, 2010.

Gabbe, Steven G., Jennifer R. Niebyl, and Joe Leigh Simpson, eds. *Obstetrics: Normal and Problem Pregnancies*. 5th ed. Philadelphia: Churchill Livingstone/Elsevier, 2007.

Kohner, Nancy, and Alix Henley. *When a Baby Dies: The Experience of Late Miscarriage, Stillbirth, and Neonatal Death*. Rev. ed. New York: Routledge, 2001.

STINGS. *See* BITES AND STINGS.

STOMACH, INTESTINAL, AND PANCREATIC CANCERS

Disease/Disorder

Anatomy or system affected: Abdomen, gastrointestinal system, intestines, pancreas, stomach

Specialties and related fields: Gastroenterology, immunology, oncology

Definition: Malignant tumors of the small intestine, stomach, or pancreas, the latter two types being difficult to detect and treat.

Key terms:

carcinogen: anything that initiates cancer

endoscope: a long, flexible fiber-optic tube used to examine the gastrointestinal tract; the tube's accessories can also remove tissue or stones

gastric: pertaining to the stomach

jaundice: a yellowing of the skin and eyes from an excess of bile pigment caused by a blocked duct or injured liver

metastasis: the dispersal of cancer cells from a tumor to other parts of the body, where they begin secondary tumors

pancreas: a secretory organ behind the stomach and connected to the duodenum; it produces enzymes to digest food and insulin to metabolize sugar

small intestine: the region of gut between the stomach and the colon that comprises the duodenum, jejunum, and ileum; also called the small bowel

tumor: a mass of new cells growing independent of surrounding tissues; either benign (noncancerous) or malignant (cancerous)

Causes and Symptoms

The section of the gut from the esophageal sphincter in the upper stomach to the ileocecal valve at the end of the small intestine digests food taken into the body and absorbs its nutrients. This vital function also exposes the gut and its organs, the liver and pancreas, to ingested toxins that can initiate

---

> ### Information on
> ### Stomach, Intestinal, and Pancreatic Cancers
>
> **Causes:** Gastric carcinogens (high-nitrate diet, alcohol consumption, radiation exposure, cigarette smoking); chronic gastritis; genetic predisposition; chronic stomach infection; gallstones; chronic pancreatitis; cirrhosis; exposure to chemicals
> **Symptoms:** May include abdominal pain, appetite loss, weight loss, diarrhea, black blood in stool, general weakness, vomiting blood, swollen abdomen, noticeable mass in stomach, iron-deficiency anemia
> **Duration:** Chronic, possibly recurrent
> **Treatments:** Surgery, chemotherapy, radiation therapy

cancer and to materials that damage the gut lining, also potentially leading to cancer. Because diet greatly influences the chances for contracting these cancers, it is understandable that stomach cancer is the world's most common type. Surprisingly, however, cancers of the small bowel are rare. Pancreatic cancer is the most lethal of these cancers and one of the most difficult to detect before irreversible damage has been done: Few patients live long after diagnosis. These facts and the large number of suspected carcinogens make the stomach and pancreatic cancers a pressing challenge for physicians and public health.

Broad similarities characterize the types of cancers throughout the upper gastrointestinal (GI) tract. The majority, adenocarcinomas, grow in and mimic gland tissue, but possible as well are cancers of the lymph tissue (lymphoma), hormone-secreting cells (carcinoid tumors), and the muscle wall of the bowel (sarcoma). Early symptoms tend to be vague and do not necessarily point specifically to cancer: abdominal pain, loss of appetite, weight loss, and perhaps diarrhea or vomiting.

While diet is a major factor in stomach cancer, its role in pancreatic and intestinal cancers is not as clear. A diet consisting mainly of pickled, smoked, or salted food with few fruits and vegetables, especially those containing vitamins A and C, is thought to be risky. In fact, countries with the highest rates of gastric cancer, such as Japan, are those that have long relied on such chemical preservation techniques rather than on refrigeration. It is probably no coincidence that the stomach cancer rate in the United States declined sharply after refrigeration became widespread in the 1930s; moreover, Japanese immigrants to the United States have sharply fewer gastric cancers than do their relatives in the homeland.

The presence of nitrites in the diet, alcohol consumption, radiation exposure, chronic gastritis (inflammation of the stomach lining), and cigarette smoking have also been suspected as gastric carcinogens. Hereditary susceptibility may sometimes play a role, although it is also possible that family members, living under the same conditions, are simply exposed to the same carcinogens and that no genetic susceptibility is involved. Finally, chronic stomach infection with the bacterium *Helicobacter pylori* has been linked to gastric cancer development.

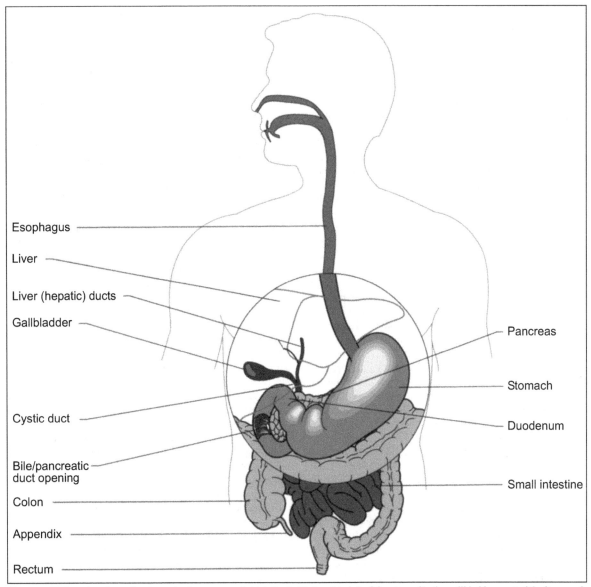

Esophagus

Liver

Liver (hepatic) ducts

Gallbladder

Cystic duct

Bile/pancreatic duct opening

Colon

Appendix

Rectum

Pancreas

Stomach

Duodenum

Small intestine

The magnified section shows the stomach, the pancreas (which lies behind and to left of the stomach), the gallbladder, part of the liver, and the midsection of the large colon.

Risk factors for the pancreas and small intestine are much less clear. Chronic pancreatitis, gallstones, and cirrhosis (scarring) of the liver pose some danger of initiating pancreatic cancer, and smokers and diabetics are twice as likely to develop it than are others. Chemists and others who work with organic solvents and petrochemicals also run a slightly higher risk. Intestinal cancer becomes more likely after the immune system has been damaged or late in the course of chronic intestinal diseases, such as Crohn's disease and sprue.

Risky foods, diseases, or occupations do not inevitably lead to cancers. Tumor growth requires at least three factors:

some agent that initiates a change in a cell's genetic structure so that a new type of cell is created, called a mutation; an agent that enhances the cell's response to the initiator, encouraging it to reproduce; and the failure of the immune system to destroy the abnormal cells. Most small bowel and gastric cancers probably result from long-term overstimulation of the glands or mucosa. This overstimulation occurs when the body fights chemical irritants that have been ingested with food, drink, or air; the body's defense mechanisms lead to inflammation in the damaged area. Chronic inflammation and continually stimulated cell division to repair damage eventually is likely to produce a mutated cell. If adapted to the harsh environment that produced it, the cell can multiply unchecked, overwhelm the immune system, and invade normal tissue; eventually, it may metastasize. A potentially lethal cancer can grow for months or years before its victim notices any definite changes in particular body functions or general health.

Eventually, however, danger signs begin. After initially complaining of abdominal pain, loss of appetite, and difficulty keeping food down, stomach cancer patients may have black, digested blood in the stool, weight loss, general weakness, bouts of vomiting blood, a swollen abdomen, a noticeable mass in the stomach, and iron-deficiency anemia. When the disease is well advanced, metastases become increasingly common, invading the lymph nodes, bile ducts, and liver and eventually spreading to the lungs, bones, and brain. The cancer becomes symptomatic relatively quickly. On average, patients go to their doctors about six months after noticing symptoms.

Pancreatic cancer is much less likely to cause early symptoms, and by the time patients seek medical help, the cancer is usually too far advanced to cure. Physicians suspect pancreatic adenocarcinoma when a patient complains of food aversion, progressive weight loss, and abdominal and back pain, especially when accompanied by vomiting, diarrhea, and jaundice. A rare form of pancreatic cancer (less than 5 percent of cancers in the pancreas) develops from the insulin-producing cells of the organ and makes abnormally high amounts of insulin; in this case, the symptoms are attributable to low blood sugar (hypoglycemia) and include weakness, loss of energy, dizziness, chills, muscle spasms, double vision, and, in extreme cases, coma.

Adenocarcinomas, lymphomas, carcinoid tumors, and sarcomas may form in the small bowel, and most of these grow slowly. Intestinal adenocarcinomas show up primarily in the jejunum or duodenum of elderly patients. Often, they first become apparent when they clog the bowel or bleed. Usually appearing in the stomach, lower jejunum, or ileum, lymphomas are suspected when the patient has fever, night sweats, weight loss, and abdominal pain. Intestinal carcinoid tumors may actively secrete hormones. If they metastasize, release of the hormones sometimes causes a bizarre group of symptoms that are collectively known as carcinoid syndrome: diarrhea, flushing, itching, low blood pressure, and heart disease. Intestinal sarcomas can occur anywhere in the small bowel and reveal themselves by bleeding.

Treatment and Therapy

Since other diseases also cause the weight loss, abdominal pain, and nausea common to these cancers-for example, pancreatitis, malabsorption, inflammatory bowel disease, and gastritis-the diagnosis of cancer requires specific evidence from chemical tests, imaging, endoscopic procedures, or surgery. Suspecting stomach cancer, the physician may send the patient for an upper GI barium study. For this procedure, the patient drinks a mixture containing barium sulfate; the radio-opaque barium coats the stomach and under X-ray photography can be seen to outline a tumor if one is present. Tests to

check for anemia and blood in the stool may also be ordered. If imaging and tests support a diagnosis of cancer, a gastroenterologist, inserting an endoscope through the patient's mouth, will obtain biopsies of the tumor so that a pathologist can determine if the tumor is malignant. Since biopsies remove such small samples and can miss a cancerous portion of a tumor (especially a lymphoma or sarcoma), surgical biopsy may be necessary to settle the diagnosis beyond doubt.

Similarly, initial tests for pancreatic and intestinal cancer rely on imaging and chemical assays. A barium X-ray study of the small bowel, a computed tomography (CT) scan, or ultrasonography may locate the tumor. Again, endoscopic or surgical biopsy alone can verify the diagnosis of malignancy. Tumors in the small bowel usually lie beyond the reach of endoscopy, so when a barium study reveals a tumor, surgical biopsy is most often necessary to obtain tissue samples; at the same time, the tumor is usually removed to relieve or prevent obstruction of the bowel.

If a tumor has not spread and is well defined, cutting it out provides the best chance of a cure for cancers throughout the stomach, pancreas, and small bowel. Such surgeries are often technically difficult, however, because the patients are typically malnourished and weak and have difficulty enduring the rigors of surgery. When a stomach tumor is single and small, surgeons remove it and a small margin of tissue around its edges. Larger or multiple tumors force the removal of larger portions of the stomach and adjacent lymph nodes. For pancreatic cancer, if more than a single area of the pancreas is involved, the surgeon may remove the entire organ and, depending on the size and location of the tumor, parts of the duodenum and stomach as well. Cancers of the intestines are cut away along with a section of bowel, whose ends are then reconnected by suturing. Chemotherapy and radiation on their own have not proved reliable for shrinking stomach, pancreatic, and intestinal cancers (except lymphomas) and are usually used in conjunction with surgery, especially when a primary tumor has metastasized.

Sometimes endoscopic maneuvers can stop bleeding or relieve pain by clearing out obstructions or, in the case of an obstructed bile duct, by inserting a small perforated tube called a stent to ensure that bile and pancreatic juices flow freely. Pain management, whether with manipulative procedures or with drugs, becomes the primary focus of treatment when surgical cure for a cancer is unlikely. Surgeons do not attempt curative operations if the cancer has metastasized. At this point, surgery, if possible at all, is for relieving pain, preventing blockage, or minimizing blood loss.

Perspective and Prospects

The frequency of these cancers and their distribution in the world vary considerably. Intestinal cancers make up less than 1 percent of all cancers and less than 5 percent of gastrointestinal cancers; pancreatic cancer accounts for only about 3 percent of all cancers. Yet the incidence of both cancers has been rising. In the United States, for example, pancreatic cancer increased about 25 percent from the 1950s to the 1990s. By

2002, it was the fourth leading cause of cancer death, and more than 30,000 Americans were diagnosed with the disease annually. At the same time, stomach cancer decreased dramatically, dropping from the United States' most common cancer in the 1930s to about 2 percent of all cancers in the 1990s. Yet in Japan, Iceland, and parts of Central and South America and of Eastern Europe, the stomach cancer rate is very high, accounting for most of the nearly 700,000 new cases yearly. In some countries, such as Japan, it is higher than all other cancer types combined. Until the 1990s, men contracted and died from stomach, pancreatic, and intestinal cancers more often than women; thereafter, however, women and men began to die from pancreatic cancer in nearly equal numbers. In the United States, African Americans get these cancers more often than Caucasians. Probably because of their diet, poor people develop them more often than middle-class or upper-class people. The peak age group is fifty to fifty-nine years for stomach cancer and seventy to seventy-nine years for pancreatic and intestinal cancer.

The chances for successfully treating or drastically curtailing small bowel cancer are reasonably good; 20 percent of patients with adenocarcinomas in the small intestine survive for at least five years following diagnosis, and patients with carcinoid tumors have lived ten and even fifteen years after surgery. Treatment of small bowel or stomach lymphomas can result in a cure or prolonged survival in a significant percentage of cases. The prospects for pancreatic and stomach adenocarcinomas, however, are another story entirely. Overall, in the United States about 10 percent of gastric cancer patients are alive five years later. Pancreatic cancer is even deadlier, with 90 percent of patients dying in the first year after diagnosis, regardless of treatment. Of those with cancer of the pancreatic duct, only about 4 percent survive three years. Those with cancer in the insulin-producing cells fare better-a 30 percent survival rate-but this is a very rare type of cancer.

Japan has higher survival rates of stomach cancer than does the United States; 50 percent of Japanese patients survive at least five years. The reason is simple. Because gastric cancer is common in Japan, doctors routinely screen patients for it by endoscopy or photofluorography (a type of X ray). Many more cancers are caught early, while they are still surgically treatable. Endoscopic and chemical screenings for pancreatic cancer are also possible, but since the disease is so much less common, doctors do not perform the tests unless they already have good reason to suspect cancer. Avoidance of carcinogens, especially alcohol, remains the most promising way to escape gut cancers.

—*Roger Smith, Ph.D.*

See also Alcoholism; Bladder cancer; Cancer; Carcinoma; Chemotherapy; Colorectal cancer; Gallbladder cancer; Gastrectomy; Gastroenterology; Gastroenterology, pediatric; Gastrointestinal disorders; Gastrointestinal system; Gastrostomy; Ileostomy and colostomy; Intestinal disorders; Intestines; Jaundice; Kidney cancer; Liver cancer; Malignancy and metastasis; National Cancer Institute (NCI); Oncology; Pancreas; Pancreatitis; Radiation therapy; Small intestine; Tumor removal; Tumors.

For Further Information:

American Cancer Society (ACS). http://www.cancer .org. Web site is divided into sections for patients, family, and friends; survivors; health information seekers; ACS supporters; and professionals. Information on all cancers is wide ranging.

Daly, John M., Thomas P. J. Hennessy, and John V. Reynolds, eds. *Management of Upper Gastrointestinal Cancer.* New York: W. B. Saunders, 1999. This book addresses such topics as surgical management of gastric cancer, gastric lymphoma, esophageal cancer, and the various treatments associated with these and other ailments.

Eyre, Harmon J., Dianne Partie Lange, and Lois B. Morris. *Informed Decisions: The Complete Book of Cancer Diagnosis, Treatment, and Recovery.* 2d ed. Atlanta: American Cancer Society, 2002. This text from the American Cancer Society is intended for the layperson. It is exemplary in its discussion of cancer.

Kapadia, Cyrus R., James M. Crawford, and Caroline Taylor. *An Atlas of Gastroenterology: A Guide to Diagnosis and Differential Diagnosis.* Boca Raton, Fla.: Parthenon, 2003. Provides a fully illustrated, nonspecialist understanding of myriad gastrointestinal diseases, including gastrointestinal cancers. Includes bibliographic references and an index.

Levine, Joel S., ed. *Decision Making in Gastroenterology.* 2d ed. Philadelphia: B. C. Decker, 1992. This text for physicians contains detailed information about the symptoms and development of cancers. Accompanying charts explain the sequence of examination, testing, and treatment, and dedicated laypersons can glean much of value from them.

O'Reilly, Eileen, and Joanne Frankel Kelvin. *One Hundred Questions and Answers About Pancreatic Cancer.* 2d ed. Sudbury, Mass.: Jones and Bartlett, 2010. Gives both a doctor's and patients' points of view and covers treatment options, post-treatment quality of life, and sources of support.

Parker, James N., and Philip M. Parker, eds. *The Official Patient's Sourcebook on Gastric Cancer.* San Diego, Calif.: Icon Health, 2002. Guides patients in using the Web to educate themselves about the disease and draws from public, academic, government, and peer-reviewed research to provide information on virtually all topics related to gastric cancer, from the essentials to the most advanced areas of research.

Rustgi, Anil K., and James M. Crawford, eds. *Gastrointestinal Cancers.* New York: W. B. Saunders, 2003. This book discusses cancer of the digestive organs, as well as the growth and development of the gastrointestinal system. Includes a bibliography and an index.

Sachar, David B., Jerome D. Waye, and Blair S. Lewis, eds. *Pocket Guide to Gastroenterology.* Rev. ed. Baltimore: Williams & Wilkins, 1991. Contains outlines of the medical subspecialty's basics. An invaluable reference for symptoms, tests, and treatments.

Steen, R. Grant. *A Conspiracy of Cells: The Basic Science of Cancer.* New York: Plenum Press, 1993. Thorough, lucid explanations of all physiological aspects of cancer make this book instructive for readers willing to slog through the subject's complexity and terminology.

STOMACH REMOVAL. *See* GASTRECTOMY.

STONE REMOVAL
Procedure
Anatomy or system affected: Abdomen, bladder, gallbladder, kidneys, urinary system
Specialties and related fields: Gastroenterology, general surgery, nephrology, urology

Definition: An operation that extracts solidified substances (stones) from an organ; typically, these stones block the organ's ability to release fluid.

Key terms:

calculus: an abnormal crystalline formation of a mineral salt; also called a stone

cholecystectomy: the removal of a diseased gallbladder or one that contains many gallstones

cholelithiasis: the formation of gallstones in the gallbladder or the ducts that connect the gallbladder to the liver or small intestine

ureterolithotomy: the surgical removal of a stone in the ureter

ureters: the two muscular tubes that connect the kidneys to the urinary bladder and that serve as conduits for urine

urolithiasis: the formation of stones in the urinary tract

Indications and Procedures

Urinary tract stones can occur in the kidneys, ureters, or urinary bladder. These stones, or calculi, are caused by substances that precipitated in the urine. The most common substance that solidifies in the urine is calcium oxalate. Stones referred to as infective, however, are present in about 20 percent of patients with urinary tract stones. These stones typically occur in patients with chronic urinary tract infections. Bacteria in the urinary tract produce ammonia, which combines with calcium or magnesium. Infective stones have the potential to block large areas of the urinary tract.

Patients with urinary tract calculi may experience a variety of symptoms depending on where the stones are located. If a stone is in the ureter, then a sharp pain that extends from the middle of the back to the groin is felt; this pain is called renal colic. Bladder stones are usually not as painful, but they may obstruct the flow of urine from the urinary bladder.

The patient's physician will have the urine examined for the presence of blood (hematuria) and crystals. X rays and/or ultrasound will show the location of the stone. Blood tests may or may not be ordered depending on whether a metabolic disorder is suspected. Hypercalcemia and hyperparathyroidism can be detected by a blood test; both indicate a problem of excess calcium.

If the urinary tract stone is relatively small, the renal colic is treated with bed rest and an analgesic, along with adequate fluid intake to promote passing of the stone. Larger stones, infective stones, or severe obstruction of urinary flow requires surgery to remove the stone. The patient is usually under general anesthesia and has a small surgical scope (a cystoscope for the bladder or a ureterorenoscope for the ureter) passed up the urethra. These scopes give the surgeon the ability to visualize and crush the stones with attachments on the instruments.

The gallbladder, which stores and concentrates bile, also has the potential for stone formation. Gallstones are usually composed of cholesterol and may be found in the ducts that connect the gallbladder to the small intestine or liver. If a stone has obstructed one of these ducts, the resulting symptoms can include intense pain known as biliary colic. This pain is usually felt in the upper right side of the abdomen or between the shoulder blades.

Ultrasound scanning of the upper abdomen can almost always detect the presence of gallstones. If the gallstones do not cause symptoms, they may be left alone, or drugs such as chenodiol and ursodeoxycholic acid may be tried to dissolve them. When symptoms are severe, removal of the gallbladder (cholecystectomy) is indicated. This surgery involves an incision under the ribcage on the right side. A laparoscope may be used or a larger incision made for an open procedure. In either case, the liver is gently lifted to expose the gallbladder, and the blood vessels and cystic duct are tied off so that blood and bile do not leak from the excised organ. The wound is then closed, and the patient may return home within a week.

Uses and Complications

Complications from removing urinary tract stones include infections, scarring, bleeding, and anesthesia risks. These complications are rare when the operation is performed by a competent surgical team. An uncommon but significant adverse result from obstruction relief is an excessive amount of urine loss, sometimes greater than 10 liters per day, which places the patient at risk for dehydration. Reducing fluid intake helps the kidney return to normal function slowly. Occasionally, this complication does not resolve. If the obstruction is not removed, however, the patient is at risk for developing chronic urinary tract infections and even renal failure.

The major risk in performing cholecystectomy is damage to the bile duct that leads to the small intestine. If scarring or inflammation occurs in this duct, it may lead to obstruction of the flow of bile from the liver. This in turn may lead to obstructive jaundice, in which pigments normally released into the intestines accumulate in the liver and blood. The patient may have a yellowish tinge to the skin and eyes until the obstruction is corrected.

If there are no complications during the cholecystectomy, then the outcome of the surgery is usually good. Approximately 90 percent of the patients have no further symptoms and recover completely in about three weeks.

Perspective and Prospects

Advances in medical technology have aided physicians in the removal of stones. Kidney and urethral stones now can be broken up using a technique called lithotripsy. An ultrasonic lithotripsy probe can break the stones using externally applied sound waves that penetrate the skin and other soft tissues. For some patients, a noninvasive technique takes advantage of sound waves transmitted through the abdominal cavity and directed at the stones. This procedure is known as extracorporeal shock-wave lithotripsy. The latter technique is also used to treat some patients with gallstones.

—Matthew Berria, Ph.D.,
and Douglas Reinhart, M.D.

See also Bile; Cholecystectomy; Cholecystitis; Cystoscopy; Gallbladder; Gallbladder diseases; Hematuria; Kidney disorders; Kidneys; Laparoscopy; Lithotripsy; Nephrology; Stones; Ultrasonography; Urinary disorders; Urinary system; Urology.

For Further Information:

Alexander, Ivy L., ed. *Urinary Tract and Kidney Diseases and*

Disorders Sourcebook: Basic Consumer Health Information About the Urinary System. 2d ed. Detroit, Mich.: Omnigraphics, 2005. Covers diagnosis and treatment of a range of disorders, including kidney and bladder stones.

Blumgart, L. H., and Y. Fong, eds. *Surgery of the Liver and Biliary Tract.* 3d ed. 2 vols. New York: W. B. Saunders, 2000. This authoritative text offers a comprehensive, detailed description of the subject.

Leikin, Jerrold B., and Martin S. Lipsky, eds. *American Medical Association Complete Medical Encyclopedia.* New York: Random House Reference, 2003. A concise presentation of numerous medical terms and illnesses. A good general reference.

Parker, James N., and Philip M. Parker, eds. *The 2002 Official Patient's Sourcebook on Kidney Stones.* San Diego, Calif.: Icon

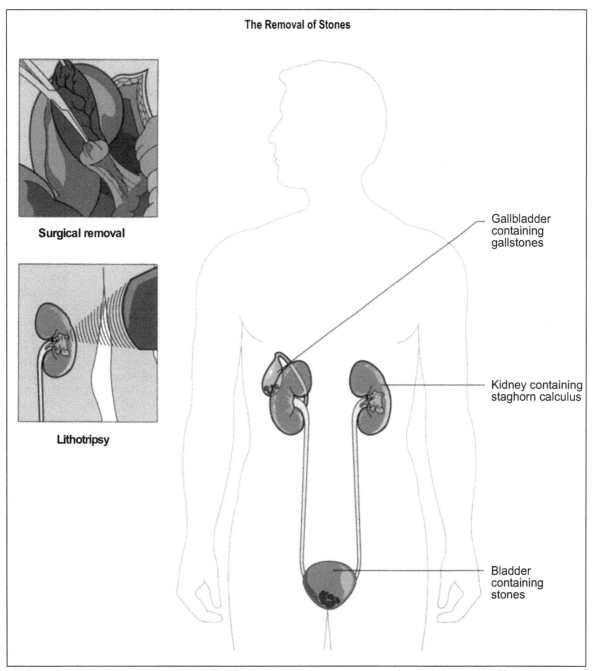

The Removal of Stones

Surgical removal

Lithotripsy

Gallbladder containing gallstones

Kidney containing staghorn calculus

Bladder containing stones

The formation of large calcium deposits in the gallbladder and parts of the urinary system such as the kidneys and bladder can cause pain and obstruction of the ureters or bile ducts. In the case of gallstones, treatment may involve the removal of the entire organ, while kidney or bladder stones can be destroyed using lithotripsy, in which shock waves are used to break up the stones.

Health, 2002. Draws from public, academic, government, and peer-reviewed research to provide a wide-ranging reference about the causes, treatments, and risk factors of kidney stones.

Tierney, Lawrence M., Stephen J. McPhee, and Maxine A. Papadakis, eds. *Current Medical Diagnosis and Treatment 2007.* New York: McGraw-Hill Medical, 2006. This book is revised annually. Contains several chapters that address stones. An excellent and concise text, but written for professionals.

Walsh, Patrick C., et al., eds. *Campbell-Walsh Urology.* 4 vols. 9th ed. Philadelphia: Saunders/Elsevier, 2007. A classic urology text.

STONES

Disease/Disorder

Also known as: Calculi

Anatomy or system affected: Abdomen, bladder, gallbladder, kidneys, urinary system

Specialties and related fields: Gastroenterology, internal medicine, nephrology, urology

Definition: Hard deposits of material in the body associated with urine and bile.

Information on Stones

Causes: Metabolic disorders, chronic urinary infection, high levels of cholesterol, prostate enlargement, narrowed urethra, abnormal pouching of bladder, neurologic dysfunction leading to poor bladder emptying

Symptoms: Sharp and sudden pain in lower abdomen that worsens with movement, intermittent blockage of urine stream, weak urine stream, increased frequency of urination, urgency, recurrent urinary tract infections, blood in urine

Duration: Acute

Treatments: Extracorporeal shock-wave lithotripsy, surgery (laser and conventional), endoscopy

---

Causes and Symptoms

Stones may form in the kidneys, ureters, bladder, and gallbladder. Kidney and ureter stones are typically calcium-based, while bladder stones are most frequently composed of uric acid (a by-product of protein metabolism) or struvite (a result of chronic urinary infection). Gallstones contain very little calcium; they are primarily composed of cholesterol.

The symptoms that accompany urinary stone disease are dependent on the location of the stone, the size of the stone, how long the stone has been present, whether infection is associated with the stone, and the degree of obstruction to urinary flow caused by the stone. Urine, which is produced by the kidneys, located beneath the ribs of the back, is collected into a structure just outside the kidney known as the renal pelvis. From the renal pelvis, urine passes into a thin narrow tube called the ureter and travels a relatively long distance to the urinary bladder. It is easy to envision how a stone traveling along such a narrow, long tube can get stuck and dam the further flow of urine.

Stones caught in the renal pelvis, prior to entry into the ureter, generally cause an intermittent, sharp pain in the back or side. Stones that pass into the ureter can cause pain in the back as well as points distant from the urinary system (the groin, the lower abdomen, and the testicles and penis in men); this phenomenon is known as referred pain. Occasionally, stones in the lowest portion of the ureters will cause pain only with urination or produce the desire to urinate frequently but only in small amounts. Often, blood not visible to the naked eye can be found in the urine with a simple chemical dipstick or by looking at the urine under a microscope, both easily accomplished in most doctors' offices.

Several radiological tests can be performed to pinpoint the location of a stone lodged in the urinary tract. An intravenous pyelogram (IVP) is a series of X rays performed following the administration of a dye into the patient's vein. This dye is concentrated in the urine and can be visualized as it travels through the urinary tract. High-frequency sound waves, or ultrasound, can determine if obstruction is present in the kidneys but will frequently miss stones lodged in the ureters. A computed tomography (CT) scan is similar to an IVP but uses advanced computer technology to visualize better all contents of the body. While the CT scan is the most sensitive test for the detection of urinary stones, certain situations may necessitate the use of different tests. Frequently, people with poor renal function cannot receive the X-ray dye because of its potential harmful effects on the kidneys. A CT scan without contrast or ultrasound will frequently be performed in this situation.

Bladder stones are found much less frequently than stones in the kidney and ureter. Perhaps the most famous person to have suffered from bladder stones is Benjamin Franklin, who reportedly stood on his head to urinate. Throughout the world, bladder stones are almost exclusively a disease of the older, male population. They are most frequently found in association with enlargement of the prostate that obstructs the bladder's ability to empty and allows these stones to crystallize in the urine. Other causes of bladder stone formation should be excluded, such as a narrowed urethra, an abnormal pouching of the bladder, a chronic urinary infection, or a neurologic dysfunction leading to poor bladder emptying.

Symptoms of a bladder stone are pain in the lower abdomen that worsens with movement, intermittent blockage of the urinary stream, a weak urine stream, increased frequency of urination often associated with a strong and urgent need to void, recurrent urinary tract infections, or blood in the urine. Definitive diagnosis of a stone can be made with a simple X ray of the abdomen alone; however, the physician will often need to perform additional tests, including a direct look into the bladder.

Diseases affecting the gallbladder and bile ducts occur commonly in the elderly. By the age of seventy, stones in the gallbladder and bile duct represent the most frequently occurring disorder affecting this organ system. In the late 1990s, it was estimated that 33 percent of the U.S. population over seventy would be diagnosed with gallstones at some point in their lives.

The symptoms associated with stones in the gallbladder or bile duct are numerous and depend on the location and size of the stone and whether there is an associated infection. Frequently, patients complain of pain in the right upper part of the abdomen. This pain often occurs after the consumption of a fatty meal, which causes the gallbladder to contract and release its bile. Fever, sweats, and chills may accompany the pain if there is infection present. Jaundice, a yellowish discoloring of the skin, may occur if the common bile duct or hepatic duct becomes obstructed with a gallstone. As with stones in the urinary tract, it is the blockage of flow of bile from the gallbladder that leads to the symptoms. Elderly patients who appear jaundiced may not always be suffering from gallstones, especially if there is no associated pain. Other diseases of the liver and biliary system, such as cirrhosis of the liver or hepatitis, will also cause jaundice and are frequently found in the elderly.

The biliary system stores bile formed in the liver and delivers it to the intestines following a meal, aiding in the digestion of fat and the absorption of certain vitamins. The gallbladder is a blind-ending pouch that comes off of the bile duct as it courses from the liver to the small intestine. After consumption of a fatty meal, its muscle-lined wall contracts to release bile into the intestine. Stones can form in the gallbladder and can cause pain or infection when lodged in the bile duct or common hepatic (liver) duct. If a stone causes blockage and infection, the patient can become very sick and require emergency medical care.

Unlike kidney stones, gallstones are frequently not visible upon plain X-ray examination of the abdomen. Despite their hard nature, gallstones contain very little calcium. They are primarily composed of cholesterol, which, unlike calcium, is not dense enough to be visible on an X ray. Ultrasound examination of the liver and gallbladder is almost always the first test ordered by a physician who is suspicious that a patient may have a gallstone. To determine if obstruction of the bile duct is present, a physician can also use nuclear medicine studies, which use a radioactive material concentrated by the gallbladder, similar to the concentration of X-ray dye used in the diagnosis of kidney stones. On occasion, the diagnosis of a gallstone lodged in the bile duct requires the placement of a telescope into the patient's stomach and intestine and direct visualization of the common bile duct's entry into the intestine.

Treatment and Therapy

Treatment of any stone depends on the location of the stone, its size, the time it has been in place, and any complicating issues such as infection. The methods for treatment are broad, and the specific means by which a stone should be removed are often debated among the experts in this field. Some stones-especially if they are small, cause no pain, and are not significantly obstructing-are given a chance to pass on their own, a treatment termed watchful waiting. The most frequent noninvasive means to treat a small stone located in the urinary tract above the pelvic bone is extracorporeal shock-wave lithotripsy (ESWL). This procedure involves the use of high-energy sound waves created by a machine outside the body and focused through the skin onto the stone. These

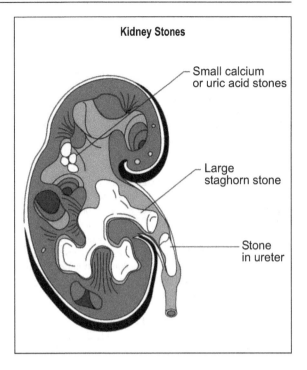

Kidney Stones

Small calcium or uric acid stones

Large staghorn stone

Stone in ureter

sound waves break the stone into fine sand, which passes in the urine without symptoms. This is frequently the best method to deal with stones in elderly patients who have other medical problems that can make surgical means of removing a stone risky. Endoscopic removal of a stone involves the use of small telescopes passed into the urinary tract either through the urethra or through the back directly into the kidney. Different means of fragmenting the stone into smaller pieces for direct removal are then employed through the telescopes. This method is highly successful and often used for larger stones. Like ESWL, this low-invasive, endoscopic means of removing the stone places minimal stress on the elderly patient with other medical problems.

The development of these minimally invasive procedures for stone removal has led to a significant decrease in the need for open surgery. Nevertheless, there are special situations when an open surgical procedure may be the first reasonable option for the elderly patient with a urinary stone. These situations include abnormal urinary tract anatomy, concurrent urinary tract pathology other than the stone, or the failure of less invasive means to remove the stone.

Treatment of bladder stones is very successful and appropriate for the elderly. As with stones of the kidney and ureter, endoscopic removal of a bladder stone using small telescopes frequently can be performed. Most bladder stones, however, are removed with open surgery. Paramount to the successful treatment of a bladder stone is the treatment of the underlying cause for its formation, which frequently dictates the method of removal. Whether endoscopic or open surgery is chosen, both are generally well tolerated by elderly patients even if significant other medical problems exist.

Treatment of symptomatic gallstones almost always involves surgery using lighted telescopes passed either directly into the abdomen (laparoscopes) or through the stomach and intestine (endoscopes), or open surgery. Unlike the removal of kidney and bladder stones, which most often merely involves the removal of the actual stone and not the kidney, ureter, or bladder, treatment of gallstones usually also involves the removal of the gallbladder itself. The loss of this unpaired organ often does not lead to significant digestive problems, though in the elderly loose, foul-smelling bowel movements may result from the altered digestion of fats.

The choice of surgical approach again depends on whether an infection is associated with the stone, how severe the symptoms are, whether any liver dysfunction is associated with the stone, and the overall health of the patient. Gallstones not causing symptoms are generally not removed. Patients with diabetes mellitus and other complicating medical conditions are dealt with in a more cautious manner and frequently undergo surgery to remove the gallstone and gallbladder even if symptoms do not exist.

Perspective and Prospects

While there is no evidence of increased incidence of urinary stones with increasing age, stones of the biliary tract (cholelithiasis) do increase with age, affecting approximately 33 percent of the U.S. population over seventy years old.

Kidney stones or stones in the urinary tract affect 5 to 10 percent of the general population of the United States. The likelihood of a person to form a stone for the first time in their life decreases with advancing age. In people who have a prior history of urinary stone formation, however, the incidence, recurrence, and severity of urinary stone disease is similar between the geriatric and younger populations. The composition of urinary stones in the older population is no different from that of those found in younger patients; however, the underlying urinary abnormality leading to the stone formation is different. More frequently, urinary stones in the elderly are caused by high uric acid levels and low citrate levels in the urine. Similar difficulties in the disposal of protein metabolites can lead to gouty arthritis.

—John F. Ward, M.D.,
and Prodromos G. Borboroglu, M.D.

See also Bile; Cholecystectomy; Cholecystitis; Endoscopy; Gallbladder; Gallbladder diseases; Gout; Jaundice; Kidney disorders; Kidneys; Laparoscopy; Lithotripsy; Nephritis; Nephrology; Nutrition; Stone removal; Urethritis; Urinary disorders; Urinary system; Urology.

For Further Information:

Gillenwater, Jay Y., et al., eds. *Adult and Pediatric Urology.* 4th ed. Philadelphia: Lippincott Williams & Wilkins, 2002. A three-volume clinical set that covers a range of urologic diseases and disorders in adults and children.

Moran, M. E. "Uric Acid Stone Disease." *Frontiers in Bioscience* 8 (September, 2003): 1339-1355. Details the rise of uric stone formation throughout the world, examining its history, diagnosis, treatments, and risk factors.

Saunders, Carol S. "Urolithiasis: New Tools for Diagnosis and Treatment." *Patient Care* 33, no. 15 (September 30, 1999): 28-44.

Noncontrast helical CT has replaced IV pyelography as first-line imaging for suspected acute renal colic, and treatment decisions have been simplified with new guidelines. This and other advances in prevention are discussed.

Walsh, Patrick C., et al., eds. *Campbell-Walsh Urology.* 4 vols. 9th ed. Philadelphia: Saunders/Elsevier, 2007. This edition of a classic urology text maintains its encyclopedic approach while following a new organ systems orientation. Halftone illustrations and contributions by multiple authors. Includes a CD-ROM.

STRABISMUS

Disease/Disorder
Also known as: Crossed eyes
Anatomy or system affected: Eyes, muscles
Specialties and related fields: Ophthalmology
Definition: The improper alignment or crossing of the eyes.

Causes and Symptoms

Strabismus affects approximately 5 percent of the population. It may be caused by a problem with the nerve supply to the muscles that move the eye or by poor vision or obstruction of vision in one or both eyes.

The most common type of strabismus is an esotropia (inward deviation) of the eye, which accounts for 75 percent of the cases of crossed eyes. There is also exotropia (outward deviation), hypertropia (upward deviation), and hypotropia (downward deviation) of the eye. When a child with strabismus has a penlight shone in the eye, the light reflected back does not fall on the pupil in the same place. This is referred to as the corneal light reflex test. When the eyes are aligned, the corneal light reflex will be placed symmetrically on the pupil. It is important to identify strabismus and to have it evaluated to prevent amblyopia (dimness of vision) or blindness in the eye that is deviated. It is also important because without input from both eyes, it is difficult to perceive depth.

A condition called pseudostrabismus gives the appearance of having crossed eyes. It occurs because there is a flat bridge of the nose or extra skin near the nose. In this situation, the corneal light reflex will be symmetrical in the pupil.

Information on Strabismus

Causes: Improper alignment of eyes
Symptoms: Appearance of having crossed eyes
Duration: Temporary to long-term
Treatments: Surgery, glasses and bifocals

Treatment and Therapy

Treatment of strabismus is aimed at avoiding amblyopia and realigning the eyes to restore depth perception. This realignment frequently requires surgery. Some cases can be treated with glasses and bifocals. An ophthalmologist should be consulted for the treatment of strabismus.

—Sheila J. Mosee, M.D.

See also Blindness; Botox; Eye infections and disorders; Eyes; Optometry; Optometry, pediatric; Sense organs; Vision; Vision disorders.

For Further Information:

Buettner, Helmut, ed. *Mayo Clinic on Vision and Eye Health: Practical Answers on Glaucoma, Cataracts, Macular Degeneration, and Other Conditions*. Rochester, Minn.: Mayo Foundation for Medical Education and Research, 2002.

Eden, John. *The Physician's Guide to Cataracts, Glaucoma, and Other Eye Problems*. Yonkers, N.Y.: Consumer Reports Books, 1992.

Flynn, John T. *Strabismus: A Neurodevelopmental Approach*. New York: Springer, 1991.

Riordan-Eva, Paul, and John P. Whitcher. *Vaughan and Asbury's General Ophthalmology*. 17th ed. New York: Lange Medical Books/McGraw-Hill, 2007.

Sutton, Amy L., ed. *Eye Care Sourcebook: Basic Consumer Health Information About Eye Care and Eye Disorders*. 3d ed. Detroit, Mich.: Omnigraphics, 2008.

Van Noorden, Gunter K., and Emilio C. Campos. *Binocular Vision and Ocular Motility: Theory and Management of Strabismus*. 6th ed. St. Louis, Mo.: Mosby, 2002.

STREPTOCOCCAL INFECTIONS

Disease/Disorder

Also known as: Strep infections

Anatomy or system affected: Arms, back, chest, circulatory system, ears, feet, genitals, hands, heart, joints, legs, muscles, neck, skin, throat

Specialties and related fields: Bacteriology, critical care, dermatology, emergency medicine, family medicine, general surgery, microbiology, obstetrics, pediatrics

Definition: Infections caused by bacteria belonging to the genus *Streptococcus*, such as strep throat, scarlet fever, impetigo, cellulitis, rheumatic fever, and necrotizing fasciitis.

Causes and Symptoms

Among the many bacteria that belong to the genus *Streptococcus*, two groups are distinguished for their pathogenicity, the group A streptococci and the group B streptococci. Group A streptococci, common pathogens found in the throat and skin, cause a variety of symptoms in the body, ranging from skin lesions and sore throat to severe, life-threatening infections. The most common infection caused by the group A streptococci is a sore throat commonly known as strep throat. If untreated, the disease may spread to involve other organs, causing otitis media, sinusitis, or tonsillitis. Some children may exhibit later sequelae such as rheumatic fever, and organs such as the heart and joints may be involved. Scarlet fever is another manifestation, with a rash that starts on the face and moves downward. Group A streptococci can also affect the skin and cause impetigo (yellow-crusted, pus-filled lesions), cellulitis, and even infection with the dreaded "flesh-eating bacteria," necrotizing fasciitis. These bacteria have also been implicated in toxic shock syndrome, previously thought to be caused only by *Staphylococcus* bacteria.

Group B streptococci, on the other hand, cause mostly severe disease and mainly affect newborns and pregnant women. These bacteria, found in the genital and intestinal tracts of 20 to 35 percent of healthy adults, can infect a newborn during the birth process. They are the most common cause of neonatal meningitis and sepsis and are a cause of neonatal death. Group B streptococci also affect pregnant

---

Information on Streptococcal Infections

Causes: Bacterial infection with streptococci

Symptoms: Depends on type; may include sore throat, otitis media, sinusitis, tonsillitis, impetigo, cellulitis, necrotizing fasciitis, toxic shock syndrome

Duration: Acute

Treatments: Depends on type; may include antibiotics (penicillin, cephalosporins), prevention through good hygiene and wound cleansing, emergency care if severe

---

women and can cause amnionitis, urinary tract infections, and stillbirth. They have also been implicated in causing disease in the elderly and in adults with chronic medical conditions.

Treatment and Therapy

Strep throat is diagnosed readily in the clinic by a rapid strep test and can be treated easily with common antibiotics, such as penicillin or cephalosporins. Prevention is the key to avoiding complications of the disease. Maintenance of hygiene (such as washing hands after sneezing or coughing), visiting a doctor to rule out streptococcal disease in case of severe sore throat, and taking any antibiotics prescribed should keep complications at bay. Keeping all wounds clean should prevent the occurrence of skin infections. Streptococcal toxic shock syndrome is an emergency siuation and requires hospitalized care.

Pregnant women should be screened for group B streptococci, and antibiotics are administered during labor to women who are carriers of these bacteria. This practice is quite effective in preventing neonatal meningitis and sepsis. Babies affected by the disease can be treated effectively with antibiotics and management of symptoms.

—*Rashmi Ramasubbaiah, M.D.,*
and Venkat Raghavan Tirumala, M.D., M.H.A.

See also Antibiotics; Bacterial infections; Ear infections and disorders; Impetigo; Infection; Necrotizing fasciitis; Peritonitis; Pharyngitis; Pneumonia; Quinsy; Rheumatic fever; Scarlet fever; Sinusitis; Sore throat; Strep throat; Tonsillitis; Toxic shock syndrome.

For Further Information:

Frazier, Margeret Schell, and Jeanette Wist Drzymkowski. *Essentials of Human Diseases and Conditions*. 4th ed. St. Louis, Mo.: Saunders/Elsevier, 2009.

Kasper, Dennis L., et al., eds. *Harrison's Principles of Internal Medicine*. 16th ed. New York: McGraw-Hill, 2005.

Tapley, Donald F., et al., eds. *The Columbia University College of Physicians and Surgeons Complete Home Medical Guide*. Rev. 3d ed. New York: Crown, 1995.

STRESS

Disease/Disorder

Anatomy or system affected: All

Specialties and related fields: Dermatology, environmental health, epidemiology, family medicine, immunology, internal medicine, oncology, psychiatry, psychology

Definition: A psychophysiological response to perceived pressures in the environment, including danger; prolonged stress contributes to hormonal imbalances, immune system collapse, susceptibility to disease, cancer, and death.

Key terms:

alarmone: a type of intracellular hormone which alerts the cell to various chemical imbalances in the cellular environment

anxiety: a type of stressful condition in which heightened neural activity accentuates an individual's anticipation of a stress-producing event

cellular transformation: carcinogenesis; the biochemical conversion of a cell from a normal state to a cancerous one of uncontrollable proliferation

chaos: a disorderly shift from predictable, linear behavior to nonlinear randomness, a situation which often occurs in stress and homeostatic breakdown

fight-or-flight response: a stressful biochemical reaction in animals, usually involving the adrenal hormone epinephrine, that prepares the animal for confrontation with predators or competitors

homeostasis: the maintenance of constant, linear conditions within a system, such as the maintenance of human body temperature, pH, and hormonal levels at stable states

hormone: a gene regulatory molecule which is produced in one body tissue region and which targets or controls cells in another region

nonlinear system: a process which is unstable and unpredictable in nature; such a process often results from a disturbance to a linear, predictable system

tend-and-befriend response: a neuroendocrine-linked stress response observed in females characterized by a tendency to respond to stressful situations by protecting self and young through nurturing behaviors and forming alliances with a larger social group

type A behavior: a psychological behavior classification for individuals who exhibit stressful, time-conscious lifestyles

type B behavior: a psychological behavior classification for individuals who exhibit unstressed, relaxed lifestyles

---

Information on Stress

Causes: Nervous system and hormonal reactions to internal and external stimuli

Symptoms: Hormonal imbalances; immune system collapse; increased susceptibility to disease, cancer, ulcers, high blood pressure, and heart disease

Duration: Temporary to chronic

Treatments: Lifestyle modification, relaxation, time management, peer counseling and support, strengthening family bonds, improving self-esteem, exercise

---

Causes and Symptoms

Stress is a psychophysiological response, within an individual animal, to a perceived danger. Stress involves a complex interplay of nervous and hormonal reactions to internal and external stimuli. All living organisms respond to stimuli, usually by means of gene-regulating chemical messengers called hormones.

Chemistry of stress. Hormones are produced in certain cells within the individual and then target tissues elsewhere in the body; these hormones control by controlling the gene regulation within their target cells. Hormones will activate certain genes within target tissue cells while inactivating other genes. If a hormone activates the control region of a gene so that the gene is "on," then it can be "read" by an enzyme (RNA polymerase), thereby leading to RNA and protein production. The produced protein may affect cellular chemical processes or may affect the expression (the on/off status) of other genes. In the latter case, the protein would be a type of intracellular hormone called an alarmone.

If a hormone inactivates the control region of a gene so that the gene is "off," then RNA polymerase will be unable to read the DNA nucleotide sequence of the gene. Therefore, no RNA and no protein will be produced. In this fashion, a hormone may activate certain genes while inactivating others. Consequently, a hormone controls what happens within the cell.

Such control is critical within complex multicellular organisms such as animals. Different cells specialize to become different tissues and organs (such as eyes, ears, hair, intestines, the heart, and so on) under the specific influence of hormones. Additionally, changes in the development of an organism over time involve changes in gene expression caused by hormones. Critical developmental changes in an individual must occur at precise times when a hormone is produced and acts correctly upon the proper array of genes in target cell tissues. When a hormone does not act correctly or issues incorrect instructions to genes, the homeostatic stability of the organism becomes disrupted. Incorrect proteins are produced in the wrong cells at the wrong times, thereby disturbing development and possibly threatening the organism's survival.

In higher animals, including humans, the body is regulated by hormones and by complex nervous systems that evolved from hormones. Most hormones are produced and secreted from the glands of the endocrine system, including the pituitary, thyroid, and adrenal glands as well as numerous organs, tissues, and cells throughout the body. The nervous system is an array of several trillion nerves concentrated in the brain and spinal cord and extending peripherally to virtually every cellular region of the body. The two systems are tightly interconnected. Both the endocrine and nervous systems at some point involve the secretion of hormones. Nerve tissue secretes hormones called neurotransmitters between electrically conducting cells called neurons.

Physiological responses to stress. Stress is therefore a biochemical response to danger that occurs within animals. The nervous system detects danger from internal or external stimuli, usually external stimuli such as predators, competitors, or life-threatening events. Increased electrical conductivity along millions of nerve cells targets various tissues to prepare the body for maximum physical activity. Among the tissues affected will be the skeletal muscles, the heart muscle, the hormone-secreting glands of the endocrine system, the immune system, the stomach, and blood vessels. Under nerve-activated stress, skeletal muscles will be poised for contraction. The heart will beat faster, thereby distributing more blood and nutrients to body cells, in the process accelerating the breathing rate to distribute more oxygen. Blood vessels will constrict. The stomach and other intestinal organs will decrease their activity, including a decreased production of mucus that protects against acid.

Heightened nerve activity also will trigger the production of various hormones from the immune system, specifically hormones that influence bodily metabolism such as thyroxine and epinephrine (adrenaline). These hormones target body tissue cells to prepare the body for increased output in the face of danger. Massive production of epinephrine will trigger maximum physical readiness and extraordinary muscular output, a phenomenon often referred to as the fight-or-flight response.

These physiological changes within an animal facing danger are important survival adaptations that evolved very early in the history of animal life on earth. Stress is a fact of life for animals because they must eat to survive. Competition for available food resources and avoidance of predators must be faced by all animals, including humans. While predation by larger animals is of little worry to current-day modern humans, the struggle for available resources remains. Furthermore, human technology has created stresses of an entirely different character.

The fight-or-flight stress response and other evolutionary stress adaptations endure within the individual for only seconds or minutes. Such natural stresses are to an individual's advantage, ensuring survival. The stresses that humans face are based on these behavioral adaptations. Much human stress is artificial, however, and lasts not for minutes but for hours, days, weeks, months, and years. Such stresses involve the same nervous and endocrine system responses, but they are usually brought about by perceived danger, not true danger.

Human societies impose norms and rules for the behavior of the individuals who compose the society. People must adhere to the societal norms or face punishment. In fast-paced technological societies, increasing bureaucratization and organization place less emphasis on the individual and more emphasis on process and productivity. People must face deadlines, be on time, produce quotas, generate company profit, and meet the demands of family, colleagues, and administration simultaneously. The result is a continuous fight-or-flight response in which individuals fear losing their jobs and thus the means of supporting themselves and their families.

The physiological manifestations of prolonged stress are devastating. Continued hyperactivity of nerve impulses and overproduction of hormones at incorrect developmental stages lead to the abnormal functioning of internal organs. The stomach undersecretes mucus, thereby leading to ulcers. The heart muscle contracts too rapidly, leading to higher pulse and respiration rates. The blood vessels constrict for lengthy periods of time, thereby causing the heart to pump harder and leading to high blood pressure and heart disease. Hormone overproduction leads to incorrect cell instructions and gene activation/inactivation, causing abnormal tissue functioning and cellular transformation leading to cancer. The immune system weakens under abnormal signaling by hormones, thereby decreasing the body's ability to defend itself from disease.

Newer research on stress response in women has uncovered a mechanism of stress response that is of interest given this upswelling of constant stress. Work by Shelley E. Taylor has documented an alternative to "fight or flight" known as "tend and befriend." Potentially linked to oxytocin, such tend-and-befriend behavior may help to facilitate relaxation and interpersonal bonding in response to stress. The potential stress response promises longer-lasting benefits, adaptively connecting humans to their social groups.

Stress and disease. A wide variety of human illnesses and disorders have been associated with stress. Heart disease, cancer, stroke, mental illness, allergies, accidents, asthma, chronic fatigue, depression, suicide, and deviant behavior are among the many illnesses and disorders that are considered by scientists to be stress-related illnesses. These stress-related diseases and disorders are responsible for the majority of deaths, hospitalizations, and visits to physicians by people in highly technological societies such as the United States, Japan, and Western Europe. In the United States alone, several billion dollars are spent each year for medications to treat stress-related illnesses that otherwise could be prevented by antistress methodologies.

Before the advent of industrialization in Europe and North America, the leading killers of humans were bacterial and viral diseases, which continue to be the principal killers of humans in the pretechnological and emerging technological countries of the Middle East, Asia, Africa, Latin America, and Oceania. European and North American industrialization has been accompanied by prodigious advances in medical science and the eradication or control of many microorganismal diseases. The psychological demands of fast-paced living and the dehumanized expectations of technological societies, however, have produced a plethora of stress-generated diseases and disorders, some of which had been masked by microorganismal diseases.

There still is some debate concerning the causal relationship between stress and illness, despite overwhelming scientific evidence demonstrating bodily responses to stressful situations. Abnormal nerve hyperactivity and prolonged, abnormal secretions of gene regulatory hormones from various endocrine glands disrupt the balanced homeostasis of many different body systems. Immune system reduction often occurs during stress, thereby making a stressed individual more susceptible to contracting infectious bacterial and viral diseases.

A clear linkage exists between the occurrence of stress in people and their subsequent susceptibility to infectious disease. Furthermore, there is a tendency for strokes, heart attacks, cancer, and sudden death to occur in individuals who recently have experienced major traumatic events in their lives. Too little attention has been given to the effects of everyday living upon the physical well-being of people. Environmental stimuli, nervous and endocrine systems, and physiological rhythms within the body are intricately connected.

Most bodily processes follow a self-regulatory, homeostatic pattern that is rhythmic, linear, stable, and predictable. For example, the beta cells of the islets of Langerhans in the pancreas secrete the hormone insulin in response to elevated blood glucose levels, whereas the alpha cells in these same islets secrete the hormone glucagon in response to low blood glucose levels. Likewise, the body chemically maintains a constant blood temperature (37 degrees Celsius), pH (7.35 to 7.45), calcium levels, and so on. The heart muscle requires an electrical stimulus approximately once per second to trigger a wave of muscular contractions throughout the myocardium via the sinoatrial and atrioventricular nodes.

Linear, balanced physiological rhythms are sensitive to subtle chemical changes in the cellular and organismal environment. An orderly, homeostatic process in the body can collapse into disorderly, nonlinear, and unpredictable chaos because of the slightest disturbance. Stress is a disturbance that imbalances the nervous and endocrine systems, which subsequently imbalance cells and organ systems throughout the human body. Physiological systems become unstable, and disease or cancer may ensue.

Treatment and Therapy

Psychologists, psychiatrists, physicians, and other medical professionals are becoming more aware of the physiological effects of stress. Through this awareness, professionals have sought to examine whether there are any characteristic styles of stress response. In response, psychologists have identified two principal behavioral types when it comes to stress among humans: type A behavior pattern and type B behavior pattern. Type A individuals are highly anxious, task-oriented, time-conscious, constantly in a rush to accomplish their jobs and other objectives, and somewhat prone to hostility. Research indicates that type A individuals may have a higher incidence of heart disease. Increasingly, the hostility component of type A behavior is seen as a very important contributing factor. On the other hand, type B individuals are more relaxed and experience less stress. Nevertheless, it should be emphasized that behavior is a continuum: Different people may exhibit varying degrees of type A and B behavior patterns. Given this discovery, it is not uncommon for professionals to recommend to their stressed clients to monitor their participation in type A behavior and to try behaving more in kind with type B behavior patterns.

Another important focus for health care has become the prevention, management, and treatment of stress itself. Health education programs emphasize the importance of physical fitness and stress reduction in everyday living. Stress-reducing methodologies for the individual include time management, peer counseling and support, spending longer amounts of time relaxing, strengthening family bonds, improving self-esteem, exercise, and learning to reframe how daily life events are interpreted, such as may be done through cognitive behavior therapy. These approaches greatly enhance an individual's quality of life and help the individual to cope positively with stressful events. All these stress reduction techniques emphasize an individual's personality and the more efficient use of an individual's free time. Relaxation, social interaction, and physical activity help the body to return to normal physiological rhythms following the numerous stressful events that every person faces daily. Individuals in American and Western societies are coming to realize that a slower, more relaxed living pace is essential for reducing stress and the millions of cases of stress-related disease that occur each year.

Perspective and Prospects

Because stress is a major contributor to illness and disease in American and Western societies, a major objective of health care professionals in these countries is the identification of stress initiators and the reduction of stress in the general population. Stress cannot be eliminated entirely in any individual. Humans always will experience stress as a result of their continuous interactions with one another and with the environment. Stress is an important survival adaptation for animal life on earth. Nevertheless, stressful events in an individual's life serve as negative environmental stimuli that hyperactivate the human nervous and endocrine systems to create a fight-or-flight response. When this fight-or-flight response is maintained for abnormally long periods of times, prolonged elevations in nervous and hormonal activity modify body tissues and the developmental gene expression within cells to produce abnormal growths (such as cancers) and abnormal system functioning (such as diabetes mellitus). Breakdown of the human immune system under stress makes the body less capable of fighting spontaneous tumors, cancers, and infectious disease. The net result from physiological stress is illness, disease, rapid aging, and death.

Stress reduction should be a prime focus of medical research and education. The simplicity of educating the public with respect to stress can yield incredible savings in terms of lives saved, quality of lives improved, length of human life spans increased, and money saved. Some researchers propose that stress reduction not only can yield enormous health benefits but also can produce greater industrial productivity, happier people, and considerably less crime. It is expected that additional research into oxytocin, the tend-and-befriend response, and yet undiscovered mechanisms of stress response will contribute meaningfully to decreased stress and increased mental and physical well-being.

—David Wason Hollar, Jr., Ph.D.;
updated by Nancy A. Piotrowski, Ph.D.

See also Addiction; Alcoholism; Alternative medicine; Antianxiety drugs; Antidepressants; Anxiety; Appetite loss; Bipolar disorders; Caffeine; Cancer; Canker sores; Death and dying; Depression; Domestic violence; Eating disorders; Factitious disorders; Grief and guilt; Hallucinations; Hormones; Hypochondriasis; Midlife crisis; Neurosis; Obsessive-compulsive disorder; Panic attacks; Phobias; Postpartum depression; Post-traumatic stress disorder; Psychiatric disorders; Psychiatry; Psychiatry, child and adolescent; Psychiatry, geriatric; Psychoanalysis; Psychosis; Psychosomatic disorders; Schizophrenia; Sexual dysfunction; Sibling rivalry; Sleep; Sleep disorders; Stress reduction; Suicide.

For Further Information:

Bremner, Douglas J. *Does Stress Damage the Brain? Understanding Trauma-Related Disorders from a Neurological Perspective.* New York: W. W. Norton, 2002. Questions whether what one sees, hears, feels, and in other ways experiences, especially during times of stress, can result in permanent changes to the brain and argues that extreme stress may result in lasting damage to the brain, especially a part of the brain involved in memory.

Day, Stacey B., ed. *Cancer, Stress, and Death.* 2d ed. New York: Plenum Press, 1986. This informative work is a collection of scientific survey papers that demonstrate the relationship between stress and disease. The papers are clearly written for both scientific and general audiences.

Goodman, H. Maurice. *Basic Medical Endocrinology.* 4th ed. Boston: Academic Press/Elsevier, 2009. Focuses on research advances in the understanding of hormones involved in regulating most aspects of bodily functions. Includes in-depth coverage of individual glands and regulatory principles.

Henry, Helen L., and Anthony W. Norman, eds. *Encyclopedia of Hormones.* 3 vols. San Diego, Calif.: Academic Press, 2003. A comprehensive overview of the role of hormones, the major physiological systems in which they operate, and the biological consequences of an excess or deficiency of a particular hormone.

Kronenberg, Henry M., et al., eds. *Williams Textbook of Endocrinology.* 11th ed. Philadelphia: Saunders/Elsevier, 2008. Text that covers the spectrum of information related to the endocrine system, including hormones and their relation to stress.

Monroe, Judy. *Coping with Ulcers, Heartburn, and Stress-Related Stomach Disorders.* New York: Rosen, 2000. Designed for students in grades seven and up, this book discusses different types of ulcers, irritable bowel syndrome, food intolerances and allergies of all types, and heartburn and acid reflux.

Newton, Tim, with Jocelyn Handy and Stephen Fineman. *Managing Stress: Emotion and Power at Work.* Newbury Park, Calif.: Sage, 1996. This book addresses job stress and offers stress management techniques for coping with it. Includes a bibliography and an index.

Orth-Gomér, Kristina, Margaret A. Chesney, and Nanette K. Wenger, eds. *Women, Stress, and Heart Disease.* Mahwah, N.J.: Lawrence Erlbaum, 1998. This is a comprehensive and ground-breaking book on women's heart health.

Taylor, Shelley E. *The Tending Instinct: How Nurturing Is Essential to Who We Are and How We Live.* New York: Times Books, 2002. Presents a discussion of stress response in women and explores a strategy of tend and befriend instead of fight or flight.

STRESS REDUCTION

Treatment

Anatomy or system affected: All

Specialties and related fields: Alternative medicine, environmental health, immunology, occupational health, preventive medicine, psychiatry, psychology

Definition: A set of procedures with the goal of decreasing bodily and mental tension by increasing rest and coping skills.

Key terms:

palliative treatments: therapies that reduce symptoms without completely eradicating a disorder

psychotherapy: treatment using the mind to remedy problems related to disordered behavior or thinking, emotional problems, or disease

stress: physical, environmental, or psychological strain experienced by an individual that requires adjustment

Indications and Procedures

Stress can exacerbate difficulties in daily functioning, slow recovery from mental or physical problems, and impede immunological functioning. Stress reduction techniques represent a cluster of procedures that share the goal of reducing bodily and emotional tension: drug and physical therapies, exercise, biofeedback training, meditation, hypnosis, psychotherapy, relaxation training, and stress inoculation therapy.

The drugs used in stress reduction are designed to provide overall bodily relaxation, to induce rest, or to decrease the anxious thinking that exacerbates stressful experiences. Sedatives, tranquilizers, benzodiazepines, antihistamines, beta-blockers, and barbiturates are examples of such drugs. Similarly, physical therapies and exercise are recommended for these purposes. Baths (hydrotherapy), massages, and moderate exercise can also be part of a stress reduction program.

Psychotherapy is a common treatment for stress implemented by psychiatrists, psychologists, social workers, psychiatric nurses, and counselors. Not only does it help individuals to sort out their problems mentally but it is also an effective stress management strategy. When individuals analyze their lifestyles and life events, stress-inducing behaviors and life patterns can be explored and targeted for modification.

Biofeedback training, meditation, hypnosis, and relaxation training all focus on inducing relaxation or altered consciousness by shifting a person's attention. Biofeedback uses monitoring devices attached to the body to provide visual or aural feedback to the trainee. Such devices include the electromyograph (EMG), which measures muscle tension, and the psychogalvanometer, which measures galvanic skin response (GSR). An EMG involves placing sensors on various muscle groups to record muscular electrical potentials. GSR also relies on sensors, but these sensors record bodily responses caused by sweat gland activity and emotional arousal. The feedback from such devices allows a trainee to learn to control certain bodily processes (for example, muscle tension, brain waves, heart rate, temperature, and blood pressure). Biofeedback training is used to treat headaches, temporomandibular joint (TMJ) syndrome, high blood pressure, and tics, and it can also facilitate neuromuscular responses in stroke patients.

Meditation is a focused thinking exercise involving a quiet setting and the repetition of a word or phrase called a mantra. By blocking distracting thoughts and refocusing attention, meditation reduces anxious thinking. It is useful for mild anxiety, minor concentration difficulties, and daily relaxation.

Hypnosis involves the use of suggestion, concentrated attention, and/or drugs to induce a sleeplike state, or trance. Hypnosis can be induced by a hypnotist or via self-hypnosis. Hypnotic states are characterized by increased suggestibility, ability to recall forgotten events, decreased pain sensitivity, and increased vasomotor control. The ability to be hypnotized varies from person to person based on susceptibility to suggestion and psychological needs. Hypnosis is used as a brief therapy targeting such problems as insomnia, pain, panic, and sexual dysfunction. In addition, hypnosis is sometimes used when drugs are contraindicated for anesthetic use, particularly for dental procedures.

Relaxation training involves three primary methods: autogenic training, which involves such techniques as head, heart, and abdominal exercises; progressive relaxation, which involves becoming aware of tension in the various muscle groups by relaxing one group at a time in a specific order; and breathing exercises. Relaxation training is best learned when a therapist trains an individual in person and then the exercises are practiced independently. Relaxation can be practiced several times daily, as well as in response to stressful events. High blood pressure, ulcers, insomnia, asthma, drug and alcohol problems, spastic colitis, tachycardia (rapid heartbeat), pain management, and moderate-to-severe anxiety disorders are treated with relaxation training.

Stress inoculation therapy is a specific type of psychotherapy involving techniques that alter patterns of thinking and acting. It comprises three steps: education about stress and fear reactions, rehearsal of coping behaviors, and application of coping behaviors in stress-provoking situations. It is useful for treating anxiety disorders related to stress.

Uses and Complications

Individuals should not apply stress reduction procedures without proper consultation; medical conditions that might be causing symptoms should be assessed or ruled out first. Biofeedback training for headaches, for example, would be unwarranted until other, more serious causes of headaches had been eliminated from consideration. Similarly, exercise, drug, and physical therapies could actually worsen conditions such as high blood pressure, alcohol and drug problems, and chronic pain if applied incorrectly. For example, where stress or pain is chronic, drug therapies might encourage the development of drug dependence.

Instead, skilled providers should administer these procedures. Training via self-help materials alone or by an unskilled provider may provide no benefit or create difficulties. Poor training could result in frustration, hypervigilance, heightened anxiety, depression, or pain caused by overattention to symptoms or conflicts. In fact, some individuals are prone to these effects even with good training. Therefore, ongoing assessment is necessary. Finally, interpretation of any memories provoked by hypnosis should be done with caution because of the suggestibility that is characteristic of hypnotic states.

Perspective and Prospects

Stress reduction techniques evolved from ancient meditation practices and simpler methods of pain management predating the development of modern anesthetics. The palliative and preventive effects of these techniques have given these procedures a sure hold in future medical practice, while benefits such as decreased absenteeism and increased feelings of wellness in employees have secured these strategies in the workplace. The expanded use of stress reduction procedures in prenatal care and with the elderly is likely.

—*Nancy A. Piotrowski, Ph.D.*

See also Acupressure; Acupuncture; Alternative medicine; Antianxiety drugs; Antidepressants; Anxiety; Aromatherapy; Biofeedback; Caffeine; Cardiac rehabilitation; Chiropractic; Electrocardiography (ECG or EKG); Environmental health; Headaches; Hypertension; Hypnosis; Meditation; Occupational health; Palliative medicine; Stress; Temporomandibular joint (TMJ) syndrome; Tics; Yoga.

For Further Information:

Davis, Martha, Elizabeth Robbins Eshelman, and Matthew McKay. *The Relaxation and Stress Reduction Workbook*. 5th ed. Oakland, Calif.: New Harbinger, 2000. Provides guidance for different stress management techniques.

Humphrey, James H. *Stress Among Older Adults: Understanding and Coping*. Springfield, Ill.: Charles C Thomas, 1992. A rich overview of general and geriatric stress management issues and techniques.

Manning, George, Kent Curtis, and Steve McMillen. *Stress: Living and Working in a Changing World*. Duluth, Minn.: Whole Person Associates, 1999. Road rage and workplace violence are but two of the more obvious symptoms of increasingly stressful times. Manning and his partners have put together this comprehensive manual to show individuals how to manage stress and help managers, counselors, and teachers develop programs that reduce stress.

Newton, Tim, with Jocelyn Handy and Stephen Fineman. *Managing Stress: Emotion and Power at Work*. Newbury Park, Calif.: Sage, 1996. This book addresses job stress and offers stress management techniques for coping with it. Includes a bibliography and an index.

Pelletier, Kenneth. *The Best Alternative Medicine*. New York: Fireside, 2002. Explains mind/body medicine, herbal and homeopathic remedies, spiritual healing, and traditional Chinese systems, and discusses their effectiveness, the ailments each is most appropriate for, and how they can help prevent illness.

Schafer, Walt, and Sharrie A. Herbold. *Stress Management for Wellness*. 4th ed. Belmont, Calif.: Thomson/Wadsworth, 2000. Describes how stress affects the body and how it may contribute to illness and death. Includes tests for identifying high personal stress levels and discusses stress reduction measures.

Seaward, Brian Luke. *Managing Stress: Principles and Strategies for Health and Well-Being*. 6th ed. Sudbury, Mass.: Jones and Bartlett, 2009. Blends techniques from stress management with health psychology to offer a holistic approach to a healthy, relaxed lifestyle.

STROKES

Disease/Disorder

Also known as: Cerebrovascular accidents (CVAs)

Anatomy or system affected: Blood vessels, brain, circulatory system, head, heart, nervous system, psychic-emotional system

Specialties and related fields: Emergency medicine, neurology, speech pathology, vascular medicine

Definition: Stroke, or a cerebrovascular accident (CVA), is the severe reduction or cessation of blood flow to the brain, resulting in a variety of serious and often permanent impairments depending on the area of the brain affected. A transient ischemic attack (TIA) is a temporary, brief loss of blood to the brain, accompanied by temporary impairment of vision, numbness, or other symptoms; it may herald a stroke.

Key terms:

amaurosis fugax: temporary blindness in one eye

angiography: radiological modality to visualize the arteries in the body; involves the placement of a catheter in an artery and the injection of dye

embolus: a small piece of atherosclerotic plaque, thrombus, or other debris that breaks off and lodges in a blood vessel

endarterectomy: a surgical technique in which an atherosclerotic plaque is excised

infarct: tissue death resulting from lack of blood flow

ischemia: lack of blood in a particular tissue

revascularization: procedures to reestablish the circulation to a diseased portion of the body

thrombosis: the aggregation of platelets and other blood cells to form a clot

transient ischemic attacks (TIAs): commonly known as ministrokes; associated neurological deficits last less than twenty-four hours and usually only minutes

Causes and Symptoms

Strokes produce damage to portions of the brain as a result of decreased blood supply. Strokes are commonly known as cerebrovascular accidents (CVAs). Symptoms of strokes will vary depending on the part of the brain that is affected. Resulting speech disorders may include aphasia (loss of the ability to speak) or dysarthria (difficulty in speaking). A sudden weakness or numbness of one side of the body is known as hemiparesis or hemiplegia. The eyes can also be involved. A dimness or transient loss of vision, particularly in one eye, is called amaurosis fugax. Occasionally, it can involve the same portion of the visual field in both eyes. Other symptoms of stroke may include dizziness, unsteadiness, sudden falls, headaches, confusion, or stupor. Coma is less commonly involved in a stroke.

Predisposing factors to strokes include hypertension (high blood pressure), diabetes, high cholesterol, smoking, atherosclerotic disease in other portions of the body (such as the heart or legs), and a previous or family history of strokes or transient ischemic attacks. Gender and age are also associated with the incidence of strokes.

In cerebrovascular disease, atherosclerosis affects the arteries that circulate blood to the brain. The brain receives blood from two major sets of arteries. The carotid arteries, in the front of the neck, supply the anterior (front) portions of the brain. The vertebral arteries travel through the transverse processes of the spine and join the basilar artery to provide blood to the posterior (back) portion of the brain. Both circu-

---

Information on Strokes

Causes: Hypertension, diabetes, cerebral aneurysm, high cholesterol levels, smoking, atherosclerosis, personal or family history of strokes or TIAs

Symptoms: Vision impairment, numbness, aphasia, slurred speech, relaxed facial muscles, general muscle weakness, dizziness, unsteadiness, sudden falls, headaches, confusion, stupor

Duration: Acute

Treatments: Surgical revascularization (endarterectomy), balloon angioplasty, drugs, physical therapy

---

latory systems are joined within the brain in a structure known as the circle of Willis, a composite of arteries that join to form an anatomical circle. The various arteries supply the necessary blood flow to different areas of the brain. Only 25 to 50 percent of people have a complete circle of Willis; this anatomical variance may be a factor in the severity of the stroke.

In atherosclerotic disease, fat, cholesterol, and calcium deposits are laid down along the walls of the arteries, primarily at sites where arteries divide and natural turbulence tends to occur. These components build up to form plaques, which may cause stenosis (narrowing) and occlusion (closure) of the arterial lumen. Accumulation of platelets and other blood cells can form a thrombus (blood clot) along with plaque buildup, which also may obstruct the arteries. Pieces of plaque or thrombotic material may break off and cause emboli to lodge acutely in the main vessels or their more distant branches.

The most common components of cerebrovascular disease are transient ischemic attacks (TIAs), also referred to as ministrokes. By definition, TIAs last less than twenty-four hours; usually, they last only a few minutes or hours. Most TIAs are produced by emboli. An embolus occurs when a piece of plaque from the lining of a major artery breaks off and temporarily blocks the blood flow to a particular area of the brain. If the symptoms last for more than twenty-four hours, a cerebrovascular accident, cerebral infarct, or stroke has occurred. A reversible ischemic neurological deficit (RIND) is similar to a stroke in that it is an event that lasts for more than twenty-four hours but resolves in about seventy-two hours.

The majority of strokes (88 percent) are the result of impaired blood flow (ischemia) to the brain. Atherosclerosis in the cerebrovascular system will cause similar symptoms of ischemia in other portions of the body. There is increasing narrowing, or stenosis, of blood vessels. Eventually, they will close off completely and become occluded. The development of new, small vessels that bypass a diseased artery is called collateralization. This process requires weeks or months to occur. Collateralization seems to be especially prominent in the cerebrovascular system, since the brain is an organ that requires constant blood flow at all times. Eventual occlusion or thrombosis of a major vessel causes the majority of CVAs, producing significant ischemia in a portion of the brain.

In certain cases, the blockage is acute, having resulted from an embolus or thrombus that blocks an artery. If collateralization has not developed, the damage to an affected structure is more severe. A thrombus or embolus can also arise from the heart. This is most common in individuals who have had a recent heart attack, who have disease that involves the mitral valve, or who have atrial fibrillation, a variety of irregular heartbeat. Another cause of stroke is cerebral hemorrhage, or bleeding into the brain, which is also occasionally referred to as apoplexy. Hypertension is the most common cause of intracranial bleeding and accounts for 10 to 15 percent of cases. Other causes of strokes are cerebral aneurysms (5 to 7 percent), tumors that have developed blood supplies (3 to 5 percent), and genetic bleeding tendencies (1 to 2 percent).

A cerebral aneurysm occurs when the wall of an artery becomes weak and enlarges like a balloon. These aneurysms often rupture. With a ruptured cerebral aneurysm and subsequent hemorrhage, by-products of red blood cell degeneration may produce a condition called vasospasm, wherein the arteries will constrict. This often leads to ischemia. One or more thrombi are often formed in an aneurysm. If they break loose, they can become emboli, float until they become lodged in a small blood vessel, block the flow of blood, and cause ischemia. This can ultimately lead to a stroke.

Stroke refers to the disease process that is mainly produced by atherosclerotic changes in the arteries to the brain. Contributing or significant risk factors in the development of atherosclerosis include hypertension (high blood pressure), hyperlipidemia (high levels of cholesterol in the blood), smoking, diabetes mellitus, and a family history of similar incidents. Evidence of atherosclerotic disease in other portions of the body, such as the heart or legs, increases the risk of stroke. Atherosclerosis is a generalized disease process that affects arterial beds throughout the body.

Symptoms of TIAs in structures near the front of the brain, the area supplied by the carotid arteries, include hemiparesis, a numbness or loss of function in half of the body. Hemiplegia, a weakness of an arm or leg (or both), can be attributable to disease in the carotid artery on the side of the body opposite to the affected body part. Another relatively common problem usually caused by disease in the left carotid artery is aphasia, a speech disorder. Disease in either carotid artery can cause amaurosis fugax, or blindness in one eye. Victims often describe this condition as a shade being drawn over the eye.

Other, more generalized symptoms are the result of problems in the vertebral arteries or the blood vessels at the base of the brain, which supply the back portions of the brain. Associated symptoms include dizziness, a loss of orientation often produced by decreased blood flow to the brain. Dizziness is frequently caused by abrupt positional changes, in which blood pressure will suddenly fall with rapid standing or sitting, or by cardiac arrhythmias (irregular heartbeats), which prevent adequate amounts of blood flow from being delivered during certain cardiac cycles.

Vertigo is different from dizziness. Individuals suffering

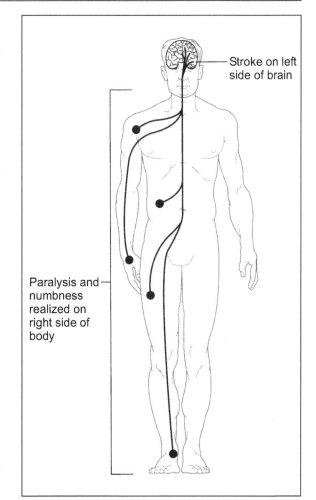

A major stroke to one hemisphere of the brain generally results in impairment of motor functions on the opposite side of the body. In addition, because the two brain hemispheres control different mental and autonomic functions, impairments will vary; for example, left-brain stroke is usually associated with some degree of speech impairment, because the speech centers are located in the left brain.

from vertigo experience a spinning sensation that may be accompanied by nausea. A common cause for vertigo is a condition known as subclavian steal, in which atherosclerotic disease affects the arteries of the arms just prior to the point where the vertebral arteries branch off. As an arm is used, or with abrupt changes in head position, blood will flow out of the vertebral arteries in a reverse manner (the so-called steal) to aid circulation in the arm (via the subclavian arteries) and vertigo will ensue. In addition, imbalance and other visual disturbances may be associated with problems in the vertebral arteries. These symptoms may also result from cerebrovascular disease in which inadequate blood supply to multiple areas of the brain can produce diverse symptoms.

In the majority of strokes, symptoms last twenty-four to seventy-two hours. Approximately 25 percent of patients will develop permanent deficits that will affect them for the rest of their lives. Approximately 20 percent of individuals who have strokes will experience no symptoms (be asymptomatic) and not know that they have had a stroke. They are unlikely to even develop TIAs. Such unheralded events result from occlusion or thrombosis of the blood vessels in the brain. This causes ischemia that leads to infarction or cell death in a particular section of the brain.

Asymptomatic cerebrovascular disease, however, can often be detected by the presence of a bruit, a French word meaning "noise." Stenosis in arteries can be compared to rapids in a river. Blood will flow very quickly through the narrow area and create turbulence, producing a bruit that can be heard with a stethoscope. Patients with narrowing in the carotid arteries ranging from 20 to 80 percent may possess a bruit. The absence of a bruit does not mean that the carotid arteries are disease-free. Once the stenosis reaches critical proportions, the flow is diminished and turbulence may be negligible, indicating a severe stenosis or an occluded artery. Often, doctors will recommend elective surgery to patients with coronary artery stenosis between 60 and 80 percent in an effort to reestablish blood flow and prevent eventual occlusion and possible stroke. About 75 percent of strokes are caused by ischemia that results from the above process. Crescendo TIAs, in which multiple TIAs occur in a brief period of time, and evolving strokes require immediate medical treatment. Appropriate diagnosis and treatment may prevent a stroke or decrease its severity.

Although disease caused by an aneurysm is a separate entity, it may be associated with atherosclerotic disease in certain cases. Most aneurysms within the brain produce no symptoms. As aneurysms increase in size, the probability of rupture increases; therefore, elective surgery may be recommended. Occasionally, diagnoses of cerebral aneurysms are made during investigations of other cerebral events, such as headaches. Acute onset of severe headaches or stiff neck should mandate immediate medical attention, since rupture of a cerebral aneurysm often manifests itself in this manner.

Treatment and Therapy

Strokes and TIAs often occur quickly and without warning. The best treatment for them is preventive behavior to avoid the atherosclerotic disease leading to such events. When a stroke or TIA is suspected, however, a complete history and physical examination is usually the first component of diagnosis. Eliciting symptoms and noting significant risk factors and findings upon physical examination will help a physician determine the primary area of the brain affected, schedule the appropriate tests for further diagnosis, and choose the best course of therapy.

Because of the high incidence of death and disability associated with strokes, a variety of diagnostic tests have been developed since the 1950s. One of the oldest noninvasive methods is the directional Doppler test. A Doppler device employs a probe with one or two piezoelectric crystals. An ultrasonic signal using a frequency of 2 to 5 megahertz (MHz) is sent into the body. Movement of red blood cells causes a shift in the frequency of the signal that is transmitted back. The amount of shift is proportional to the speed of blood flow. This device can also be used to determine the direction of blood flow. By listening with a continuous-wave Doppler over a branch of the ophthalmic artery at the corner of the eye and performing certain compression maneuvers on the arteries that supply the face, information regarding possible collateral pathways can be obtained concerning internal carotid artery blockages of greater than 75 percent.

The vascular surgeon William Gee developed another device, called an ocular pneumoplethysmograph (OPG). The OPG utilizes cups placed in the eye to measure the ocular pressure. A vacuum is applied to the eyes, effectively blocking the ophthalmic arteries, which are the first major branches of the internal carotid artery. As the vacuum is released, the blood flow is reestablished and the appearance of arterial pulsations is noted on a strip chart. These pulsations denote systolic blood pressure in the ophthalmic arteries. A pressure difference of 5 millimeters of mercury (mm Hg) between the two eyes or an index of less than 0.66 (comparing the systolic blood pressure in the ophthalmic artery with that in the brachial artery) is consistent with carotid artery blockage of more than 50 to 75 percent.

Both of these methods are indirect tests, in which significant internal carotid artery disease is implied if the test is positive. Deficiencies in the test procedures include quantification of the percentage of carotid artery disease or differentiation of significant stenosis from occlusions. They also may be wrong if the vertebral or basal arteries contribute significant collateral blood flow. The OPG is still used in certain situations as a quick screening tool, but the directional Doppler has lost favor as an accurate diagnostic test.

Duplex ultrasound machines, first employed in the early 1980s, utilize B-mode (brightness-mode) ultrasound to visualize the vessels and type of plaque. In comparison, Doppler ultrasound can audibly evaluate the blood flow in the vessels. Using real-time spectrum analyzers, the Doppler signals are then analyzed in terms of velocity (speed of the blood flow) and waveform characteristics. The greater the velocity, the greater the amount of stenosis. Absence of blood flow will denote occlusions.

Much research has been done in evaluating plaque morphology and its association with the incidence of TIAs, but results have been controversial using the standard gray-scale duplex devices. The use of color duplex ultrasound, in which the Doppler signals are color-coded in terms of flow direction and speed to denote the various flow patterns in normal and diseased vessels, has enhanced the diagnostic accuracies of the examinations. The use of color Doppler in many ultrasound machines is allowing more rapid detection of arterial lesions in blood vessels both inside and outside the skull.

Transcranial Doppler uses a MHz pulsed Doppler probe through various normal anatomic windows (holes) in the skull. Measurements can be made through the side of the head (transtemporal), from the back of the head (transoccipital), and through the eye (transocular). The purpose of the examination is to assess the blood circulation in the circle of Willis. The transcranial Doppler gives information concerning various collateral pathways established when significant disease is present in blood vessels outside the skull. It is also useful when there is stenosis of arteries inside the skull. It is extremely accurate in detecting and monitoring early vasospasm in individuals with bleeding inside the skull. Additional research with this device is ongoing in other areas, such as in the detection of cerebral aneurysms and arteriovenous malformations in which there is an abnormal connection between the arteries and the veins.

Computed tomography (CT) scanning is a radiological technique that provides a three-dimensional picture of the brain and its structures. Occasionally, a contrast medium is also used in this examination. CT scanning is especially useful in the diagnosis of cerebral aneurysms and areas of infarct. Magnetic resonance imaging (MRI) is a nonradiological technique that also provides exceptional three-dimensional images of the soft tissue structures of the brain. MRI can detect cerebral infarcts at an earlier stage than can CT scanning.

Arteriography or angiography is an invasive procedure that is performed in a hospital setting. A catheter is placed in one of the arteries, and dye containing iodine is injected. Multiple X rays are then taken to visualize the circulation. Arteriograms are considered to be standard in diagnosis. The delineation of the blockages and collateral pathways is then used primarily to plan surgical procedures.

Aspirin is often prescribed to alleviate symptoms of TIAs and to help protect patients from strokes or heart attacks. Although it is a powerful drug in decreasing the incidence of embolus formation, a national study has demonstrated that patients with a history of TIAs and carotid artery stenosis of greater than 60 percent should undergo surgical revascularization to protect against major strokes. The chances of having a stroke after suffering a TIA are approximately 40 percent greater.

Endarterectomy is a surgical technique in which the inner wall and part of the middle wall of the carotid artery are excised, effectively scraping out atherosclerotic plaques. Although used in other arterial segments, endarterectomy is the most common surgical procedure used to revascularize the carotid arteries. Occasionally, procedures are performed to bypass diseased segments of the cerebral vessels. Long-term research has shown that they have limited effectiveness. Consequently, many have been abandoned.

Other techniques for intervention have been developed. Percutaneous balloon angioplasty involves placing a balloon catheter in the diseased segment during an angiogram. When the balloon catheter is inflated, it opens up the area of stenosis or small segment of occlusion. This method has been employed in the coronary arteries as well as in the vessels leaving the aorta, the iliac arteries, and arteries in the lower extremities. It is not used often in the treatment of atherosclerotic plaques in the cerebral circulation because of the possibility of emboli traveling to the more distant blood vessels of the brain or eye. Some success in the use of balloon angioplasty has been reported in the treatment of vasospasm.

New drugs that dissolve clots may be used alone or in combination with balloon angioplasty or surgery. Although effective in the treatment of coronary artery and peripheral vascular disease, their use in the cerebral circulation has been restricted because of the risk of embolus formation or bleeding complications.

Perspective and Prospects

Stroke is the third-leading cause of death in the United States, with approximately 158,000 deaths annually. There are 700,000 strokes annually, and about one-fourth of all nursing home patients are permanently impaired from strokes. These statistics have a great impact on the amount of money spent annually on care for victims of strokes.

Since the 1960s, the death rate from strokes in the United States has decreased significantly, by about 60 percent. Control of blood pressure and diet, the development of new drugs and diagnostic techniques, and the advent of cardiovascular surgery in the early 1950s have contributed to these results. Unfortunately, strokes are still prevalent given the extent of atherosclerotic disease in the American population, which is largely attributed to a high-fat diet. Autopsies of U.S. soldiers killed in the Korean and Vietnam Wars demonstrated evidence that atherosclerosis begins at a very early age, often by age eighteen. Atherosclerosis is more prevalent in males. Females have more protection until the onset of the menopause. Within five years of the menopause, however, the stroke and death rates of men and women tend to equalize.

High-salt diets, which contribute to hypertension, also contribute to the development and progression of atherosclerosis, as well as hemorrhagic strokes. Ethnic African and Asian populations appear to be at greater risk in this respect. Since the 1960s, however, extensive education of the American public concerning diet and the control of blood pressure has had a favorable impact. More recently, the increase in individuals who have stopped smoking and who have undertaken regular exercise has helped to lower stroke rates further.

Since the 1950s, a number of both noninvasive and invasive procedures have been developed to diagnose atherosclerotic disease. Cardiovascular surgical techniques were developed in the 1950s. The first bypass surgery (arterial autograft) probably occurred during the Korean War. The development of ultrasound devices in the 1950s initiated the research into using these noninvasive devices to diagnose cerebrovascular disease. The duplex devices introduced commercially in the late 1970s and early 1980s have spurred the development of new diagnostic devices for detecting atherosclerotic disease. These devices allow for visualization of plaque morphology (composition of the plaque, such as thrombus, calcium, hemorrhage, and other particulate matters) and blood flow characteristics for a better understanding of the disease process. Future developments in the field of ultrasound include holographic imaging for the three-dimensional visualization of plaques. These noninvasive technologies will also allow physicians to monitor the effects of new drugs and techniques in the treatment of atherosclerosis. Advances in digital subtraction and computer enhancement of angiographic techniques, along with new contrast media, have made arteriograms safer and more accurate.

Color duplex devices are utilizing low-frequency probes to visualize and produce color scans of blood vessels that lie inside the skull. By analyzing the blood flow direction and velocity in the circle of Willis and within the blood vessels of the skull, physicians will come to a better understanding of the formation of collateral pathways and will learn how to detect other pathological conditions that lead to cerebrovascular disease. Magnetic resonance imaging (MRI) is also being utilized to measure actual flow in individual arterial segments of the body.

Carotid endarterectomies, which lost favor for a period of time, have become the preferred therapeutic treatment for individuals with episodes of TIAs and severe atherosclerotic plaques in the carotid arteries. Additional studies will further delineate which other patient populations may benefit from this surgery. Aspirin still remains a potent drug in the treatment of TIAs in patients with lesser degrees of disease and in postsurgery patients. Recognition and prompt treatment of symptomatic cerebrovascular symptoms remain the key to better survival rates.

—*Silvia M. Berry, M.Sc., R.V.T.;*
L. Fleming Fallon, Jr., M.D., Ph.D., M.P.H.;
updated by Bradley R. A. Wilson, Ph.D.

See also Angiography; Angioplasty; Aphasia and dysphasia; Arteriosclerosis; Blood vessels; Brain; Brain disorders; Bypass surgery; Carotid arteries; Cholesterol; Circulation; Congenital heart disease; Edema; Embolism; Endarterectomy; Heart attack; Heart disease; Heart failure; Hyperlipidemia; Hypertension; Ischemia; Numbness and tingling; Paralysis; Physical rehabilitation; Plaque, arterial; Speech disorders; Thrombolytic therapy and TPA; Thrombosis and thrombus; Vascular medicine; Vascular system.

For Further Information:
American Medical Association. *American Medical Association Family Medical Guide.* 4th rev. ed. Hoboken, N.J.: John Wiley & Sons, 2004. Provides updated, understandable medical information about various diseases including stroke.
American Stroke Association. http://www.stroke association.org. Gives information on warning signs, stroke care, and stroke programs. Offers newsletters and scientific and professional research links, among other features.
Marler, John R. *Stroke for Dummies.* Indianapolis, Ind.: John Wiley & Sons, 2005. Offers general information about strokes for nonscientists.
Rao, Paul R., Mark N. Ozer, and John E. Toerge, eds. *Managing Stroke: A Guide to Living Well After Stroke.* Washington, D.C.: ABI Professional, 2000. The staff of the National Rehabilitation Hospital in Washington, D.C., has created an instructional guide for those who have suffered a stroke.
Senelick, Richard C., and Karla Dougherty. *Living with Stroke: A Guide for Families.* 3d ed. Albany, N.Y.: Delmar, 2001. Provides a range of information for stroke patients and their families, including data on strokes, current theories on neural plasticity, and the process of rehabilitation, especially the emotional component of recovery.
Wiebers, David O., Valery L. Feigin, and Robert D. Brown, Jr. *Handbook of Stroke.* Philadelphia: Lippincott Williams & Wilkins, 2006. Based on extensive experience at the Mayo Clinic, this book provides a concise and easy-to-read guide for the evaluation and management of stroke. It is filled with algorithms that put pertinent information at the reader's fingertips.

STURGE-WEBER SYNDROME
Disease/Disorder

Also known as: Sturge-Weber-Dimitri syndrome, encephelotrigeminal angiomatosis

Anatomy or system affected: Blood, blood vessels, brain, circulatory system, eyes, head, nerves, nervous system, skin

Specialties and related fields: Dermatology, neurology, ophthalmology, pediatrics, plastic surgery, psychology, vascular medicine

Definition: A disorder associated with partial facial disfigurement which involves vascular accumulations that affect the central nervous system.

Causes and Symptoms

Although the precise causation of Sturge-Weber syndrome has not been established, medical researchers have found a relationship to excess circulatory vessels remaining from embryonic development. Professionals estimate that approximately 15 percent of newborns with port-wine stains have this syndrome. Patients usually exhibit a facial port-wine stain along the trigeminal nerve on one side. The size of the birthmark and the area covered depend on which, and how many, of the three branches of this nerve-found in the brow, cheek, and jaw-are affected by excessive capillaries delivering blood to the skin. Sometimes, the birthmark appears on other parts of the body or the entire head. Infrequently, patients with this syndrome do not have a port-wine stain.

Neurological activity is often disrupted and slowed in these patients because of the massing of circulatory vessels on the brain adjacent to the port-wine stain. As a result, patients sometimes experience calcium buildup in brain tissues and epileptic seizures on the side without the birthmark. Approximately half of patients suffer developmental problems, including mental retardation. Because circulation to the eyes is altered, fluid drainage is sometimes disrupted and pressure intensifies, resulting in swelling, glaucoma, and possible blindness. Partial paralysis occasionally accompanies this syndrome.

Treatment and Therapy

Many patients with Sturge-Weber syndrome suffer only facial birthmarks and mild neurological symptoms that do not affect their life span. Lasers can erase port-wine stains, and cosmetics are a less expensive but temporary solution.

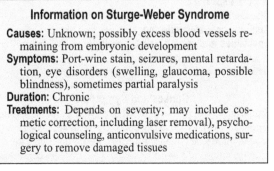

Information on Sturge-Weber Syndrome

Causes: Unknown; possibly excess blood vessels remaining from embryonic development
Symptoms: Port-wine stain, seizures, mental retardation, eye disorders (swelling, glaucoma, possible blindness), sometimes partial paralysis
Duration: Chronic
Treatments: Depends on severity; may include cosmetic correction, including laser removal), psychological counseling, anticonvulsive medications, surgery to remove damaged tissues

Psychological counseling can help patients cope with societal reaction to their birthmarks, including bullying and rejection.

Patients whose brains are significantly affected have higher risks. Medications can treat convulsions. In extreme cases, surgery may be required to remove damaged tissues. Medical professionals X-ray patients to assess brain calcification and to locate any tumors. The eyes are examined regularly to detect problems and are treated with medication or surgery as applicable. Physical therapy can strengthen weakened muscles in cases of partial paralysis.

Perspective and Prospects

William Allen Sturge hypothesized in 1879 that a six-year-old patient suffering from seizures had a brain lesion on the same side as her port-wine stain. His peers rejected his theory. By 1901, Siegfried Kalischer verified Sturge's hypothesis through pathological studies. In 1922, Frederick Parkes Weber used radiography to document calcification inside the craniums of patients with port-wine stains. The next year, Vincente Dimitri added his insights; he is sometimes incorporated into the name of this syndrome. E. Steve Roach described three types of Sturge-Weber syndrome in 1992. His categories are based on trait occurrence and extent.

Established in 1987, the Sturge-Weber Foundation has created a registry of individuals with this syndrome. In the early twenty-first century, researchers continued their investigations of possible genetic factors in this syndrome.

—*Elizabeth D. Schafer, Ph.D.*

See also Birthmarks; Blood vessels; Brain damage; Circulation; Congenital disorders; Dermatology; Dermatology, pediatric; Eyes; Glaucoma; Nervous system; Neuralgia, neuritis, and neuropathy; Neurology; Neurology, pediatric; Paralysis; Plastic surgery; Seizures; Skin; Skin disorders; Vascular medicine; Vascular system.

For Further Information:

Ball, Karen Fisher, ed. *Sturge-Weber Syndrome: The Resource Guide for a Reason, a Season, and a Lifetime.* Mt. Freedom, N.J.: Sturge-Weber Foundation, 2003.

Bodensteiner, John B., and E. Steve Roach, eds. *Sturge-Weber Syndrome.* Mt. Freedom, N.J.: Sturge-Weber Foundation, 1999.

Guttman, Cheryl. "Location of Port-Wine Stains May Signal Syndromal Associations." *Dermatology Times* 19, no. 7 (July, 1998): 25.

Sturge-Weber Foundation. http://www.sturge-weber .org.

STUTTERING

Disease/Disorder

Anatomy or system affected: Nervous system
Specialties and related fields: Family medicine, neurology, pediatrics, speech pathology
Definition: Breaks in the smooth flow of speech.

Causes and Symptoms

Stuttering is usually recognized as a child develops enough language skill to speak in complete sentences, beginning around three years of age. Typically, the child repeats the beginning sounds of a word, or whole words, before continuing

---

> ### Information on Stuttering
>
> **Causes:** Developmental and physical defects, emotional stress, anxiety
> **Symptoms:** Repeating beginning sounds of word or whole words; concomitant eye blinking, finger snapping, or foot tapping
> **Duration:** Often short-term, may be chronic
> **Treatments:** Speech therapy, reading aloud, singing

---

with the sentence, as in, "I l-l-l-like to p-p-p-pet my ca-ca-cat." True stuttering must be differentiated from developmental dysfluency and dysfluency caused by unusually severe environmental or social pressures. Developmental dysfluency is normal, occurring in the three- or four-year-old child whose brain works faster than his or her mouth. This child may repeat parts of words, words, or parts of phrases, especially when excited. When a child feels significantly anxious, language may become dysfluent, or broken up and difficult to understand. This is not true stuttering, and treatment should be aimed at alleviating the anxiety or stress.

True stuttering is less common than the two dysfluencies just described, and it occurs more often in boys. Frequently, the true stutterer is consistently dysfluent on the same sounds or words. There is consistency in repetitions, prolongations, pauses, grammatical forms, and rate of emission of dysfluency. Often, the child will overcome a verbal hurdle by using certain actions such as eye blinking, finger snapping, or foot tapping.

Treatment and Therapy

Treatment of true stuttering by a competent speech pathologist is imperative, and the prognosis, although variable, can be good. Parents and teachers should be alerted to alleviate any emotional stress that is unusual or severe. Absolutely essential is the ability of all adults to deal with the stuttering child without calling attention to the speech patterns or mannerisms. Practicing reading aloud, especially poetry, and singing-all in the privacy of the company of a caring adult-may help.

Perspective and Prospects

The great ancient Greek orator Demosthenes was dysfluent and allegedly practiced talking with pebbles in his mouth until he could speak clearly. Stuttering does not preclude a person becoming successful in any endeavor. Modern speech therapy and understanding adults can be of great benefit to a child who stutters.

—*Robert W. Block, M.D.*

See also Antianxiety drugs; Anxiety; Lisping; Phobias; Psychiatry, child and adolescent; Speech disorders.

For Further Information:

Cole, Patricia R. *Language Disorders in Preschool Children.* Englewood Cliffs, N.J.: Prentice Hall, 1982.

Hamaguchi, Patricia McAleer. *Childhood Speech, Language, and Listening Problems: What Every Parent Should Know.* 2d ed.

New York: Wiley, 2001.

Martin, Katherine L. *Does My Child Have a Speech Problem?* Chicago: Chicago Review Press, 1997.

Pinker, Steven. *The Language Instinct: How the Mind Creates Language*. New York: HarperCollins, 2007.

Plante, Elena, and Pelagie M. Beeson. *Communication and Communication Disorders: A Clinical Introduction*. 3d ed. Boston: Pearson/Allyn & Bacon, 2008.

Stuttering Foundation. http://www.stuttersfa.org.

STYES

Disease/Disorder

Also known as: External hordeolum

Anatomy or system affected: Eyes, skin

Specialties and related fields: Bacteriology, dermatology, family medicine

Definition: Inflammations of hair follicles or glands of the eyelids that become infected by bacteria, usually *Staphylococcus aureus*.

Causes and Symptoms

The most common symptoms that accompany styes are swelling, redness, and pain to an area of the eyelid. A pimple often appears in the area of the swelling. There may also be excessive watering of the infected eye and an increased sensitivity to light. A chalazion can sometimes be mistaken for a stye because it too is marked by swelling. A chalazion is a lump on the edge of the eyelid that is caused not by bacteria but rather by a blocked mucous gland under the eye. Unlike a stye, a chalazion is a painless swelling.

While styes have no specific causes, they often develop when staphylococci bacteria are transferred from nose to eye by excessive rubbing. Stress has also been named as an influence on the frequency of recurring styes. Styes are not harmful to vision and can occur at any age.

Treatment and Therapy

Some styes heal on their own within a few days. Healing may be encouraged by applying localized warm compresses (with a clean cloth) to the infected area for ten minutes, four to eight times throughout the day. The warmth of the compress assists in speeding the white blood cells to the infected area, which in turn accelerates the crowning of the stye and subsequent drainage of the abscess through the opening at the margin or underside of the eyelid. Once drainage of the pus begins, the swelling and pain associated with most styes begin to subside. Though the temptation may be great, styes should never be ruptured or "popped," as is often done with a pimple. This may spread the infection to other follicles of the eyelid, or it may spread the infection to the tissue of the eye, causing eyelid cellulitis.

Antibiotic creams and ointments are sometimes prescribed in cases of persistent and recurrent styes. Rarely do styes require lancing by a doctor. However, a health care provider should be consulted if the swelling on the eyelid continues to enlarge or if it does not cease on its own within a two-week period.

Information on Styes

Causes: Bacterial infection with staphylococci; may be triggered by rubbing or stress

Symptoms: Swelling, redness, and pain in eyelid; excessive eye watering; increased sensitivity to light

Duration: Usually a few days; sometimes recurrent

Treatments: Warm compresses, antibiotic creams or ointments if infection persists

---

To prevent stye recurrence, it is important to keep the eyelid and lashes clean. Careful attention should be placed on cleaning excessive oil from the edges of the lids. Hands should be washed regularly, especially if they have touched the nose. Separate washcloths and towels should be used among members of a shared household. Styes pose no danger to the eye, and therefore the prognosis is usually quite positive.

—Nicholas Lanzieri

See also Abscess drainage; Abscesses; Bacterial infections; Boils; Dermatology; Dermatology, pediatric; Eye infections and disorders; Eyes; Ophthalmology; Skin; Skin disorders; Staphylococcal infections.

For Further Information:

Anshel, Jeffrey. *Smart Medicine for Your Eyes: A Guide to Safe and Effective Relief of Common Eye Disorders*. Garden City Park, N.Y.: Avery, 1999.

Porter, Robert S., et al., eds. *The Merck Manual Home Health Handbook*. Whitehouse Station, N.J.: Merck Research Laboratories, 2009.

Riordan-Eva, Paul, and John P. Whitcher. *Vaughan and Asbury's General Ophthalmology*. 17th ed. New York: Lange Medical Books/McGraw-Hill, 2007.

SUBDURAL HEMATOMA

Disease/Disorder

Anatomy or system affected: Blood, brain

Specialties and related fields: Hematology, neurology, ophthalmology, speech pathology

Definition: Collection of blood (clotted and partially clotted) in the subdural space.

Key terms:

dura mater: tissue layer between the brain and the skull

hypoxia: lack of oxygen

subdural space: space between the brain tissue and the dura mater

tonic-clonic seizure (grand mal seizure): two-phase seizure common in epilepsy attacks that consists of a tonic phase, in which the body becomes rigid, and a clonic phase, which involves uncontrolled jerky movements

Causes and Symptoms

Subdural hematomas are caused by either a major head injury (acute subdural hematomas) or by a relatively minor head injury (chronic subdural hematomas). Acute subdural hematomas usually occur after a major head injury in which the rotational or linear forces cause veins in the subdural space to break. These types of subdural hematomas are the most common form of sports-related brain injury, especially in professional boxers because of the multiple head blows that they receive. Chronic subdural hematomas, on the other hand, typically develop days to weeks after relatively minor head injuries. This type of hematoma mainly afflicts the elderly, who are more likely to have brain shrinkage, which causes the subdural veins to stretch in order to cover the greater distance created between the brain and the dura mater. These stretched veins are more vulnerable to breakage, even from a minor head injury. Some cases of subdural hematomas occur without apparent head injury, which may be due to the fact that many minor head injuries go unnoticed. Blood-thinning drugs such as Coumadin, alcohol abuse, seizures, repeated falls, shunts draining excess cerebrospinal fluid (CSF) from the brain, and very young or very old age increase the risk of developing a subdural hematoma.

A subdural hematoma can compress the brain, frequently leading to brain injury. Symptoms in adults and older children include a persistent headache, drowsiness, loss of consciousness, paralysis on the opposite side of the body, seizures, memory problems, confusion, nausea, numbness, visual abnormalities, slurred or confused speech and language, and weakness. An elderly person with memory loss or drowsiness may be mistakenly thought to have dementia when he or she actually has a subdural hematoma. In professional boxers, symptoms include neurological abnormalities, deteriorating dementia, and death.

In infants, subdural hematomas occur as part of shaken baby syndrome. Symptoms of a subdural hematoma in infants include swollen fontanelles ("soft spots" in a baby's skull), focal seizures, generalized tonic-clonic seizures, increased sleepiness, irritability, and vomiting. In all cases, acute subdural hematomas carry a high risk of death and are considered medical emergencies. The cause of shaken baby syndrome remains controversial. Initially, shaking was thought to induce shear forces that cause breakage of the bridging veins in the subdural space, resulting in the subdural hematomas, retinal hematomas, and encephalopathy characteristic of shaken baby syndrome. However, more recent research suggests that these symptoms are more likely caused by vein damage due to impact and hypoxia. Subdural hematomas may also be caused by the birth process.

Treatment and Therapy

Computed tomography (CT) scanning and magnetic resonance imaging (MRI) can detect most subdural hematomas. MRI is more sensitive and may be able to detect hematomas that may not show up on CT scans.

Treatment is based on the type and size of hematoma and the amount of pressure that has accumulated in the brain. Small subdural hematomas may resolve when head injuries heal. For small subdural hematomas that do not resolve, a hole may be drilled in the skull and the blood mass drained from the subdural space via a catheter. This procedure can be performed at the patient's bedside. Large hematomas, how-

---

Information on Subdural Hematoma

Causes: Usually major or minor head injuries; some cases arise without apparent head injury

Symptoms: In adults and older children, persistent headache, drowsiness, loss of consciousness, paralysis, seizures, memory problems, confusion, nausea, numbness, visual abnormalities, slurred or confused speech and language, weakness; in infants, focal seizures, generalized tonic-clonic seizures, increased sleepiness, irritability, vomiting

Duration: May occur immediately or develop in days to weeks

Treatments: For smaller hematomas, hole drilled in skull for drainage; for larger hematomas, craniotomy

---

ever, may require a surgical procedure known as a craniotomy, in which the skull is surgically opened and the blood mass removed. Surgical removal of acute subdural hematomas is associated with a significant risk of death. On the other hand, treatment of chronic subdural hematomas has a relatively good prognosis.

Perspective and Prospects

In 1946, pediatrician John Caffey described the relationship between long bone injuries and subdural hematomas. Since then, subdural hematomas have been reported in the elderly, professional athletes such as boxers and hockey players, and in abused children.

There is considerable uncertainty about the long-term effects of subdural hematomas. Although it is not known if suffering a subdural hematoma puts someone at greater risk of experiencing subdural hematomas in the future, boxing commissions in several states have banned boxers with a history of subdural hematomas from competing. Boxers diagnosed with subdural hematomas risk being banned from boxing, a fact that prevents some professional boxers from seeking a diagnosis. A well-known case involves a thirty-one-year-old boxer, Joe Mesi, who was suspended by the Nevada Athletic Commission after he developed subdural hematomas as a result of head injuries sustained in a March, 2004, fight. Mesi lost an appeal to lift his medical suspension in 2005. Another athlete, a professional hockey player, suffered a subdural hematoma after receiving a hit to the head during a game. However, his wounds healed and his doctors allowed him to return to professional hockey, believing that there would be no negative consequences. Until more is known about the long-term effects of subdural hematomas, there will continue to be controversy over whether athletes with a history of hematomas should be allowed to compete.

—*Ing-Wei Khor, Ph.D.*

See also Accidents; Bleeding; Blood and blood disorders; Brain; Brain damage; Circulation; Emergency medicine; First aid; Hematology; Hematology, pediatric; Hematomas; Hemorrhage; Intraventricular hemorrhage; Sports medicine; Vascular medicine.

For Further Information:

Heller, J. L. "Subdural Hematoma." http://www.nlm .nih.gov/ medlineplus/ency/article/000713.htm. This MedLine Plus page (a service of the National Library of Medicine and the National Institutes of Health) provides an overview of the topic that is appropriate for a lay audience. Brief descriptions of symptoms, tests, treatment, and prognosis are included.

Miele, V. J., et al. *Subdural Hematomas in Boxing: The Spectrum of Consequences*. Medscape Today. http://www.medscape.com/ viewarticle/553965_3. The causes and effects of subdural hematomas in professional boxers are presented, along with a discussion of the conflict between the need for diagnosis and treatment and the risk of being barred from boxing.

Squier, W. "Shaken Baby Syndrome: The Quest for Evidence." *Developmental Medicine & Child Neurology* 50, no. 1 (January, 2008): 10-14. Discusses the causes of shaken baby syndrome.

Squier, W., and J. Mack. "The Neuropathology of Infant Subdural Hemorrhage." *Forensic Science International* 187, nos. 1-3 (May 30, 2009): 6-23. Describes the neurological symptoms of subdural hematomas in infants.

SUBSTANCE ABUSE

Disease/Disorder

Also known as: Substance-related disorders

Anatomy or system affected: All

Specialties and related fields: All

Definition: A pattern of social, psychological, and/or biological problems caused by the way in which a person uses drugs such as alcohol, nicotine, and prescription or illegal drugs.

Key terms:

abuse: a pattern of substance use observed in a twelve-month period resulting in occupational, safety-related, legal, and/ or social problems as a consequence of the substance use

addiction: a condition in which an individual is compelled to use a drug, such as alcohol, despite the fact that it is causing significant problems

co-occurring disorders: a situation in which a person has more than one diagnosable problem

dependence: a pattern of substance use problems in a twelve-month period that demonstrates physiological or psychological reliance on a specific substance that results in conditions such as tolerance, withdrawal, inability to regulate one's use, and desire to control or reduce one's use

psychotropic drugs: substances that affect the mind through their influence on the central nervous system

substance of abuse: a drug that affects the mind and body in a reinforcing manner, causing a person to want to repeat use of the drug for its positive effects

tolerance: using a drug and getting less and less effect from the same amount of the drug, or needing more of the drug to get the same effect

withdrawal: symptoms that result when a person ceases or abstains from using a drug; vary from substance to substance and may range from mild irritability to hallucinations, seizures and death

Causes and Symptoms

There are many substances of abuse, including ubiquitous drugs such as caffeine, alcohol and nicotine, and the misuse of the latter two cause the greatest harm psychologically, medically, and economically. Substances of abuse also include illegal and regulated drugs such as marijuana, cocaine, amphetamines, heroin, and hallucinogens. Often overlooked, however, are medicinal drugs, such as one might get via a prescription from a doctor, and even common household substances ingested as inhalants, including glue and paint.

According to the Diagnostic and Statistical Manual of Mental Disorders, Fifth Edition (DSM-V), the diagnostic handbook for mental health professionals, in order to be diagnosed with a substance abuse problem a person must have significant difficulty in fulfilling social and work-related obligations. These persons have frequent encounters with the law due to their drug problem and put themselves in danger physically either through the use of the substance itself or by driving under the influence, for example, over a twelve-month period. Substance dependence differs by definition in that those who have a substance abuse problem may require more of the drug to achieve the same effect, develop withdrawal symptoms when they do not have the drug, have difficulty quitting, and/or use the drug despite the negative social, legal, psychological, or physical effects.

Problems with substance use may result from many different causes. For conditions such as substance dependence, there can sometimes be a biological component related to genetics. Individuals who have a family history of these problems may carry a genetic risk. It is not a guarantee that they will have a problem, but they can have increased risk of developing one. In the same way, even if a person does not have a family history of a problem, it does not mean that they are risk-free. Using substances repetitively, particularly in large doses or very frequently, can also cause problems such as dependence. Patterns of use and frequent use can develop because an individual regularly has access to the drugs through family and/or friends. Also, people may learn how to use the drugs in ways that are not adaptive through these same individuals. Peers who use are a risk factor for their teenage friends.

Family history of other problems or characteristics can also contribute to having a greater risk for substance use problems. For instance, a family history of other mental health problems, such as depression, can be a risk factor for developing a substance use problem. Even social characteristics, such as a high amount of family stress, can be a risk factor because individuals may use substances to cope with stress and other life difficulties. Additionally, some individuals may never learn of the risks and consequences associated with substance use because of lack of education or prior exposure to the problems, and so they may use unwittingly and develop problems.

Treatment and Therapy

Treatments for substance-related disorders vary by the substance involved and the specific type of problem. For instance, if one is experiencing withdrawal from alcohol as compared to another drug such as heroin, different medications are given for treatment. This is the case because the

```
┌─────────────────────────────────────────────┐
│         Information on Substance Abuse        │
│                                               │
│  Causes: Exposure to addictive substances,    │
│    repetitive use, genetic risks, other       │
│    biological risk factors such as other      │
│    diseases and disorders, social risk        │
│    factors such as peer and family use,       │
│    stress, poverty                            │
│  Symptoms: For abuse, impaired occupational   │
│    functioning, using in unsafe situations,   │
│    legal problems, social problems; for       │
│    dependence, sometimes tolerance,           │
│    withdrawal, loss of control of use,        │
│    desire to control use, excessive time      │
│    spent related to use, reduction of other   │
│    activities, use despite psychological or   │
│    physical problems caused or made worse     │
│  Duration: Repeated pattern of problems       │
│    established within any twelve-month        │
│    period and time-limited, intermittently    │
│    repeating, or continuing lifelong          │
│  Treatments: Medications, psychotropic drugs, │
│    cognitive and behavioral treatments,       │
│    motivational treatments, family-based      │
│    treatment, harm reduction treatments,      │
│    self-help treatments, group-based          │
│    support, integrated treatments with        │
│    co-occurring disorders                     │
└─────────────────────────────────────────────┘
```

different drugs affect different neurotransmitters in the brain. Also, depending on the severity of the problems or presence of other problems, more than one drug treatment may be used. If a person withdrawing from alcohol was also showing signs of depression, that individual might be given an additional psychotropic drug to address the depression. In fact, many patients have co-occurring problems, so integrating treatment of the varied problems is important.

It is also important to note that while some treatments focus on reducing symptoms such as withdrawal or sleep problems that are biological in nature, others focus on the more social and behavioral aspects of the problem. Treatments may also vary in their goal. Some treatments may focus on having an individual achieve abstinence from the problem drug(s), while other treatments may focus on reducing the amount or frequency of drug use, or even reducing other harm from the substance use. Approaches focusing on reducing frequency and amount of use are often focused on moderation as a goal. Approaches focusing on reducing harm are usually known as harm reduction treatments and may focus on reducing associated problems. An example of harm reduction is having individuals who use drugs avoid doing dangerous things such as driving after they have used (thereby reducing risks related to driving while under the influence) or having individuals who inject drugs not share needles (thereby reducing risks related to blood-borne problems such as hepatitis or human immunodeficiency virus, or HIV).

Nonpharmacological treatments include therapies that focus on changing specific behaviors or thoughts related to the problem use. They may also include treatments focusing on helping address the motivation of the individual to change. More specifically, not all people with substance use problems are ready to change immediately. Therefore, sometimes the first treatment needed may be to work on the motivation to change. In fact, sometimes individuals work on their problem on their own, using self-help materials before seeking out treatment professionals. Additionally, it is not uncommon for individuals to seek help for substance use problems through support groups, such as twelve-step groups (e.g., Alcoholics Anonymous).

Perspective and Prospects

Problems related to substances of abuse have been affecting human behavior for all of human existence. Exposure to substances initially tried as foods or medicines that may have had psychotropic effects, such as fermented berries or mushrooms and plants, are probably some of the first experiences leading to both positive and negative consequences related to substance use. In fact, addictive substances have been an integral part of human society, used in religious and medicinal ceremonies from our beginnings as hunter-gatherers to Ancient Greece and beyond. As such, it is a long-standing problem that is likely to stay with human society and require management as time goes on.

While the formal diagnosis known as substance abuse is likely to change in terms of how it is recognized, the problems related to the condition as currently defined will remain a target of intervention and concern. For example, the parameters defining legal consequences may adjust with new laws as legislation evolves and even new substances of abuse are identified. In 2012, Washington and Colorado became the first states in the United States to legalize the recreational use of marijuana, and as a result, several other states are now showing increased pressure from voters and advocates alike to follow suit. The long-term legal and social effects of these measures are yet to be determined. Similarly, the type and scope of social and safety problems may increase as substances are used in new contexts and with new behaviors. Problems related to role functioning, legal issues, use in unsafe situations, and use resulting in consequences that disturb social relationships remain significant problems and will need continued attention by treatment providers and prevention specialists to address the problem of substance use whether it stands as a condition on its own or as part of a larger spectrum of substance dependence problems and formally diagnosable conditions.

The future is likely to bring continued fine-tuning of diagnoses to isolate and identify genetic and physiological aspects of these problems so as to refine prevention and treatment of drug problems involving more biological causes. The balance of the work to refine prevention and treatment will focus on the behavioral and social causes of these conditions which, on their own, may cause problems and also may interact with biological risk factors. Continued understanding of how substance-related conditions interact with other mental health problems, physical conditions, and even cultural differences are also efforts that will improve treatment and prevention.

—*Nancy A. Piotrowski, Ph.D;*
updated by Luzanna Plancarte, M.D.,
and Bianca Garcia, M.D.

See also Addiction; Alcoholism; Antidepressants; Caffeine; Club drugs; Geriatrics and gerontology; Herbal medicine; Homeopathy;

Metabolism; Narcotics; Nicotine; Over-the-counter medications; Pain; Pain management; Pharmacology; Pharmacy; Polypharmacy; Prescription drug abuse; Psychiatry; Psychiatry, child and adolescent; Psychiatry, geriatric; Self-medication; Smoking; Toxicology

For Further Information:

Bellinir, Karen, ed. *Tobacco Information for Teens: Health Tips about the Hazards of Using Cigarettes, Smokeless Tobacco, and Other Nicotine Products.* Detroit: Omnigraphics, 2007. This resource focuses on one of the most abused drugs in society, nicotine, and provides basic descriptions of key health problems related to its use in varied forms.

DiClemente, Carlo C. *Addiction and Change: How Addictions Develop and How People Change.* New York: Guilford Press, 2006. Provides an easy-to-understand description of problems with addictions, along with useful concepts for thinking about how these problems develop for many people, as well as practical strategies for thinking about how to change.

Julien, Robert M. *A Primer of Drug Action.* 11th ed. New York: Worth, 2007. This is a more technical work that presents a more academic description of what different drugs are, how drugs are processed by the body, their safety issues, and their other effects on the body and brain.

McNeece, C. Aaron, and Diana M. DiNitto. *Chemical Dependency: A Systems Approach.* 3rd ed. New York: Pearson, 2005. This textbook provides an integrated way of thinking about substance use problems and their treatment, starting with definitions, epidemiology, etiology, and the biological aspects and other consequences of these problems, while also addressing more advanced topics related to treatment of different types of individuals, such as adolescents, adults, elders, and whole families.

Rosen, Winifred, and Andrew T. Weil. *From Chocolate to Morphine: Everything You Need to Know about Mind-Altering Drugs.* Rev. ed. Boston: Houghton Mifflin, 2004. Source for varying ages provides insight into the broad range of substances that affect the mind.

Trends & Statistics: National Institute on Drug Abuse (2013). Retrieved October 14, 2013. http://www.drugabuse.gov/related-topics/trends-statistics. This website offers current statistical information on various substance abuse trends in America, ranging from prescription drugs to teenage substance abuse.

Sudden infant death syndrome (SIDS)
Disease/Disorder

Anatomy or system affected: All

Specialties and related fields: Neonatology, pediatrics, psychiatry, psychology

Definition: The abrupt and inexplicable death of any infant or young child, and the most common cause of infant death between the ages of two weeks and one year; postmortem examination fails to demonstrate a definitive cause of death.

Key terms:

apnea: absence of breathing

bradycardia: slowness of the heartbeat

hyperthermia: environmentally influenced elevated body temperature

hypothermia: environmentally influenced lower-than-normal body temperature

hypoxemia: subnormal oxygenation of arterial blood

neonatal: the period of time succeeding birth and continuing through the first twenty-eight days of life

prone: lying face-downward

supine: lying face-upward

tachycardia: rapid beating of the heart

thermolabile: unstable when heated

Causes and Symptoms

The distribution of sudden infant death syndrome (SIDS) is worldwide. Incidence rates vary from 0.12 to 3.0 for every thousand live births. In the United States, rates range from 1.6 to 2.3 for every thousand live births, with considerable ethnic variation: 0.5 among Asians, 1.3 among whites, 1.7 among Latinos, 2.9 among African Americans (5.0 for those of low socioeconomic status), and 5.9 among American Indians.

Cultural practices may make the incidence rate vary. In England, a Birmingham study found that 22 percent of Asian babies were put to sleep on their backs, compared with 3 percent of white babies. Sleeping prone is significantly more common in infants dying of SIDS than in controls. In the same study, 98 percent of Asian babies slept in the same room as their parents for the first year, 34 percent in the same bed. Only 65 percent of white infants slept in the same room as their parents. Perhaps the risk of sudden infant death increases in proportion to the amount of time an infant spends asleep out of parental earshot. In Zimbabwe, SIDS practically does not exist. According to English pediatrician Duncan Keeley, who served in that country for two years, black Zimbabwean infants almost invariably sleep with their mothers, at least until they are six months old and often until they are a year old.

The cause of sudden infant death syndrome is unknown, but a variety of genetic, environmental, and social factors have been associated with an increased risk of SIDS. Besides sleeping in the prone position, other associations include cold weather, overheating, the hours of the day from midnight to 9:00 A.M., and poor socioeconomic conditions, including overcrowding. The young, unmarried mother, especially if she has had no prenatal care, is more likely to have an infant with SIDS; so is the mother who smokes (either before or after the birth), is anemic, or ingests narcotics. Prematurity, especially with a history of apnea or damage to the immature lungs from elevated levels of inspired oxygen while on a respirator, also increases the risk.

Males are at a higher risk for SIDS than are females; so are the brothers and sisters of infants with SIDS. Likewise, a previously aborted episode of SIDS (that is, a "near miss") increases risk. On average, Apgar scores (a measure of infant health immediately after birth) are lower in infants with SIDS than they are in surviving peers. In a family that has lost an infant to SIDS, the risk for the next or subsequent child is about five times the usual risk. Most risk factors, however, are associated with only a twofold or threefold elevation of incidence. Therefore, predicting which infants will die unexpectedly is extremely difficult. Recent immunization is not a risk factor. Breast-feeding is not associated with a decreased risk, as was originally thought. Although the peak incidence of SIDS is around three months of age and coincides with normally low levels of circulating immunoglobulins, the syndrome is not

Information on
Sudden Infant Death Syndrome (SIDS)

Causes: Unknown; may involve interrelated genetic, environmental, and social factors (sleep disorders, sleep position, cold weather, overheating, poor socioeconomic conditions, premature birth)

Symptoms: Varies and often has no warning signs or symptoms; may include sleep apnea, slow heart rate, low body temperature

Duration: Acute, with little warning

Treatments: Parent education, placing infants to sleep on their backs

associated with any known pathogen.

Pathologists report a wide variety of findings in their postmortem reports-especially changes in the brain and other parts of the body that suggest chronic or intermittent hypoxemia. Yet pathologists also fail to find an increase in the number of cells in tissue of the carotid bodies, a chemoreceptor that responds to decreases in blood oxygen tension; such a finding weighs against the presence of chronic hypoxia.

Like many other aspects of this disease, the mechanism or mechanisms of death in SIDS are unknown. Does the infant stop breathing, or does some cardiac irregularity occur? An immature cardiorespiratory control mechanism involving the nervous system is the most common hypothesis.

D. P. Davies and Madeleine Gantley of the University of Wales College of Medicine believe that an important mechanism underlying SIDS is failure of respiratory control at a vulnerable stage of development-more a physiological syndrome than a disease in the accepted sense. These doctors hypothesize that the disturbance to this delicate equilibrium might upset the regulation of breathing, sometimes leading to death. Epidemiological risk factors, such as an upper respiratory infection (which is not uncommon), are somehow linked with destabilizing influences to breathing. By avoiding or modulating these factors, the risk of death can be reduced.

Although the pathogenesis of SIDS remains unclear, Anne-Louise Ponsonby and her colleagues at the University of Tasmania in Australia propose that SIDS be considered as a biphasic event, with the first set of factors operating to predispose the infant and the second set of factors acting as loading factors that operate at a critical stage of the infant's development. The Australian doctors believe that a warm environment could lead to sudden infant death through direct hyperthermia; a thermolabile, sudden fall in blood pressure leading to a diminished oxygen supply to the brain; impaired respiratory control; altered sleep state; or depressed arousal. An asphyxial mode of death would also be more likely, particularly in heavily dressed infants found prone (face down).

Concern for the confusion of SIDS with child abuse should not be ignored, nor should the efforts of the National Sudden Infant Death Syndrome Foundation to provide information about psychosocial support groups and counseling for families of SIDS victims.

Treatment and Therapy

Since the causes and mechanisms of death from SIDS may continue to be unknown, strategies that might reduce the incidence of this syndrome seem imperative. Cold weather and the hours of midnight to 9:00 A.M. bring increased risks for SIDS. A closer look explains that other risk factors are involved. Overheating as a response to cold weather and leaving the infant alone at night (particularly in Western countries) may be more important. Babies sleeping alone might lose external sensory stimulation that may help stabilize breathing patterns. Davies and Gantley, citing experimental work with mothers and infants co-sleeping in sleep laboratories, have shown how patterns of breathing may interact. They say that the alertness of the babies' caregivers to early symptoms of illness might also be important.

French doctors studied the seasonal variation of death from SIDS in their country for a two-year period in the early 1980s. They concluded that for babies born in the spring, the third month of age was not necessarily associated with the highest SIDS risk. Babies born during other seasons, however, exhibited a normal pattern of increasing risk between the first and third months. Age was an especially critical factor among babies who reached three months of age during the winter months. If they reach this age in July or August, they are less susceptible to SIDS.

This finding, then, leads to a consideration of the risk of overheating. Explanations for the association between cold weather and SIDS include hypothermia, increased viral illness, and indirect hyperthermia. New Zealand doctors looked at the role of thermal balance in SIDS by investigating the death scene. They found that infants who died of SIDS were significantly more likely to be overdressed for the room temperature at the death scene and in the prone position, when compared to control infants. They also suggest that parents may have responded to infections in their babies by increasing the amount of clothing and bedding or by otherwise warming the infant.

The government of New Zealand initiated a program of education for parents recommending that the prone sleeping position be avoided, that mothers not smoke, and that breastfeeding be encouraged. (Most experts believe that breastfeeding itself does not reduce risks for SIDS. Rather, closer and more frequent contact with mothers is the operative factor.)

A similar education program for parents in Avon, England, was initiated, but it omitted advice on breast-feeding and included suggestions to avoid overheating after a retrospective case-control study that suggested a nearly ninefold relative risk for SIDS from infants sleeping prone. New Zealand and Avon both reported fewer deaths from SIDS after their parental education programs were introduced. The Department of Health extended Avon's campaign nationally.

In an editorial note in 1986, the National Center for Health Statistics acknowledged that "the rapid decline of infant mortality rates in the 1970s has been attributed largely to the advent of medical technology in the area of premature and other clinically ill newborns." Yet, "in the 1980s, this decline has slowed considerably-partly because of a lack of progress in primary prevention of conditions which lead to infant death." Undoubtedly, the United States would benefit from a massive, national program of education for parents. For example, cigarette packages carry a warning of the harmful effects of smoking on the fetus; perhaps they should also include a warning about the dangers to infants of maternal smoking. Another possibility for intervention exists in the area of infections: Pertussis (whooping cough) could be prevented by the immunization of infants under six months of age. In the long term, all nations should work toward improving the socioeconomic status and health care of the poor.

Finally, improved medical technology will be less important over the long haul than will efforts to educate parents in infant care practices. The ability of parents and other members of the household to monitor infants and respond appropriately to both true and false alarms is crucial, as is appropriate training in infant CPR (cardiopulmonary resuscitation) and the proper use of monitory equipment. Even if all SIDS is eliminated in at-risk children, there will continue to be cases among children not known to have been at risk.

Perspective and Prospects

The term "sudden infant death syndrome" was popularized by Abraham Berman's book on SIDS in 1969, which grew out of a conference on that subject. Since then, recognition of the syndrome has led to the creation of organizations dealing with it. The Sudden Infant Death Foundation merged, on January 1, 1991, with the National Center for the Prevention of SIDS to form one organization, the Sudden Infant Death Alliance.

In dealing with SIDS, one factor looms most important: Education of parents makes all the difference. In 1991, for example, England's Scarborough district reported a 50 percent fall in the SIDS death rate after parents were advised not to overwarm their small infants. That same year, four other districts in England reported a similar reduction after parents were advised not to let their infants sleep in a prone position. The Foundation for the Study of Infant Deaths and the Department of Health recommend both procedures: a supine sleeping position and prevention of overwarming.

These successes raise two issues: the overall decline in rates of SIDS worldwide in industrial countries and parental guilt. For a number of years, the incidence of SIDS was generally falling. This decline slowed considerably in the 1980s. How much, then, did the parental education programs actually lower the incidence rate in these English districts? No one can say with certainty, but one thing is clear: If doctors make recommendations regarding sleeping positions and warming, they run the risk of inducing guilt in parents who have not followed their recommendations-or, alternatively, who have followed the recommendations but have still lost an infant to SIDS. Parents who have lost a child to SIDS are grief-stricken. They are not prepared for such a tragedy, and their grief is compounded by guilt, because no definitive

cause for SIDS has been identified and, as a result, parental behavior seems to be implicated. Investigations conducted by police, social workers, or others who become involved only add to this guilt. Parents may be confronted by questions of whether they positioned their infant correctly or overdressed the child. Regardless of these behaviors, however, the factors causing the death may not have been under the parents' control.

SIDS will continue to occur until the exact etiologies of the syndrome, its mechanisms, and its correct treatment-based on fact, not simply risks alone-are identified. Until that time, it is expected that incidence rates will continue to go down, based on what is now known of the risk factors and recommendations against prone sleeping positions and overwarming.

—*Wayne R. McKinny, M.D.*

See also Apnea; Death and dying; Grief and guilt; Hyperthermia and hypothermia; Neonatology; Premature birth; Respiration.

For Further Information:
Beers, Mark H., et al., eds. *The Merck Manual of Diagnosis and Therapy.* 18th ed. Whitehouse Station, N.J.: Merck Research Laboratories, 2006. Published since 1899, this classic medical book covers SIDS thoroughly and is easy to read.
Behrman, Richard E., Robert M. Kliegman, and Hal B. Jenson, eds. *Nelson Textbook of Pediatrics.* 18th ed. Philadelphia: Saunders/Elsevier, 2007. This standard pediatric textbook has been around for years and deservedly so. Its excellent chapter on sudden infant death syndrome is a thorough review of the disease.
Byard, R. W., and H. F. Krous. "Sudden Infant Death Syndrome: Overview and Update." *Pediatric and Developmental Pathology* 6, no. 2 (March/April, 2003): 112-127. Details the research advances in the understanding of SIDS since 1990 and discusses historical background, epidemiology, pathology, and pathogenesis.
Samuels, M. "Viruses and Sudden Infant Death." *Pediatric Respiratory Reviews* 4, no. 3 (September, 2003): 178-183. Examines the role of viral respiratory tract inflammation in SIDS, as well as a preceding history of symptoms of minor illness.
SIDS Network. http://sids-network.org. Provides news about current research, frequently asked questions about SIDS, and fact sheets on such topics as sleep, smoking, and apnea.
Southall, D. P., and M. P. Samuels. "Reducing Risks in the Sudden Infant Death Syndrome." *British Medical Journal* 304 (February 1, 1992): 265-266. These acknowledged experts in SIDS have written a thoughtful, thorough review on reducing the risks of SIDS. They strongly suggest that current interventions and socioeconomic factors need monitoring.

SUFFOCATION. *See* ASPHYXIATION.

SUICIDE
Disease/Disorder
Anatomy or system affected: Psychic-emotional system, all bodily systems
Specialties and related fields: Geriatrics and gerontology, psychiatry, psychology
Definition: The deliberate taking of one's own life, usually the result of a mental disorder although sometimes deliberated in the face of life-threatening physical illness, significant interpersonal stress, or when under the influence of one or more substances of abuse.

Key terms:

"no suicide" contract: an agreement, verbally or in writing, that a suicidal person will not act on his or her urges to commit suicide and instead will take other more adaptive action

psychosomatic: referring to physical symptoms interacting with psychological problems

rational suicide: suicide to avoid suffering when there is no underlying cognitive or psychiatric disorder

ritual suicide: a formal, ceremonial, and proscribed form of suicide performed for social reasons in Japanese history

serotonin: an abundant neurotransmitter in the brain that affects many emotional states

suicide cluster: the occurrence of several suicides immediately following a much-publicized suicide

suicide gesture: a superficial suicidal action in which the intention is not to die but to solicit help

Causes and Symptoms

Suicide is the deliberate taking of one's own life. Most often, suicidal individuals are trying to avoid emotional or physical pain that they believe they cannot bear; sometimes, they are very angry and take their lives to lash out at others. Suicide is seen as a solution to an otherwise insoluble problem. Each year, there are about 500,000 self-inflicted injuries and 30,000 completed suicides, with 200,000 family survivors in the United States. In 2006, there were 33,000 suicides, and estimates suggest there were between twelve and twenty-five times as many attempted suicides the same year. Women attempt suicide more often than men, but men complete suicide more often than women because men tend to use more lethal means, such as a gun. It should also be noted that adolescents and the elderly are two high-risk groups.

When an individual contemplates suicide to avoid the physical pain of a terminal illness and does not have a mental disorder, that form of suicidal thought is often called "rational" suicide. This does not imply that this form of suicide is appropriate, moral, or legal but merely that the suicidal thoughts do not arise from a mental disorder (nonrational). Social views on rational suicide vary by culture. For example, many Dutch people consider rational suicide to be acceptable, whereas most Americans do not.

Most suicidal people encountered by physicians, psychologists, social workers, and other mental health professionals experience suicidal thoughts as a result of a mental disorder. The suicidal thoughts and impulses are seen as symptoms of the underlying disorder and require treatment just as any other symptom. The treatment may involve protecting the person against his or her suicidal actions, even to the point of involuntary commitment to a mental hospital.

The rationale behind society's willingness temporarily to deny suicidal individuals' usual civil rights by involuntary commitment is that they are considered to be not "acting in their right mind" by virtue of their mental illness. Thus, they deserve the protection of society until their illness is treated. In fact, suicidal thoughts usually do abate when suicidal patients are treated. The vast majority of these individuals are

Information on Suicide

Causes: Psychological and emotional factors, depression, mental disorders, substance abuse

Symptoms: Depressed and/or anxious mood, hopelessness, loss of normal pleasure in life activities, diminished problem-solving skills, borderline personality disorder, unstable relationships

Duration: Temporary or recurrent

Treatments: Psychotherapy, counseling, drug therapy

appreciative afterward; they are glad that they were prevented from killing themselves, as they no longer wish to do so.

The most common mental illness that causes suicidal thoughts is depression. In fact, suicidal thoughts are considered to be a symptom of clinical depression. Other mental disorders associated with suicidal ideation include anxiety disorders such as panic disorder, psychotic disorders such as schizophrenia, substance use disorders such as alcohol dependence, and certain personality disorders such as borderline personality disorder.

Although suicide may occur at any time of the year, there is a seasonal variation in its peak incidence. Suicides are most common in both men and women in May; women have a second peak around October and November. This seasonal variation may be attributable to seasonal differences in the incidence of depression.

Suicide appears to have multiple factors involved in its etiology. There are biological, psychological, social, and contextual factors that interact in a complex way to contribute to the causes of suicide in any given individual. The biological factors include genetic contributions to the development of mental disorders such as clinical depression. This may be attributable in part to problems in the neurotransmitter systems in the brain, such as those that control levels of serotonin and dopamine.

Alcohol and other substances of abuse may also cause suicidal ideation. Suicidal thoughts may occur while the individual is using, intoxicated, or in withdrawal. Paradoxically, suicidal thoughts may also arise while the patient is taking antidepressant medications. Fortunately, this side effect is uncommon, and most antidepressant medications do not have such effects. The fact that suicidal thoughts may occur even when on medication, however, underscores the need for individuals taking medications to stay in regular contact with the prescribing physician and to never discontinue their medication without medical consultation. If family members observe a depressed individual taking medication become more depressed, hostile or angry, or suddenly happy or relieved, or if the individual has no apparent response to the medication, then it would be wise to consult with the prescribing physician. This is especially true for family members of children or elders on antidepressant medication.

Psychological factors contributing to suicide include a depressed and/or anxious mood, hopelessness, and a loss of normal pleasure in life activities. Chronically depressed people often have diminished problem-solving skills during periods of depression and can see no way out of their difficulties; suicide is seen as the only solution. There are also personality characteristics that contribute to suicide. In women, borderline personality disorder is often associated with suicide attempts. This disorder is characterized by widely fluctuating moods, rages, feelings of emptiness or boredom, and unstable relationships.

The social factors involved in suicide include cultural acceptance or rejection of suicide. Historically, Japanese people have accepted ritual suicide within their culture and somewhat sanction suicide as a response to a severe loss of face or social esteem. This does not mean that they embrace it, but rather that the history contributes to cultural norms where this is thought of as an option for dealing with shame. Similarly, the Dutch government has legalized rational suicide as an option for dying. In contrast, most Americans have a more negative view of the suicide act. Other social factors that increase the likelihood of suicide include social instability, divorce, unemployment, immigration, and exposure to violence as a child. In the United States, European Americans commit suicide more often than African Americans. Native Americans have a high incidence of suicide. In general, good social support reduces the risk of suicide.

Some patients engage in suicidal gestures; that is, they say they want to kill themselves and take actions such as swallowing some pills or superficially cutting their wrists, but there is no real intention to die. They act this way as a cry for help. For some, this may be the only way to receive attention for what troubles them. Unfortunately, the suicide gesture may go awry and unintended death may occur. Anyone who speaks of suicide or engages in what may appear to be a gesture should be taken seriously.

Most people who are suicidal have ambivalent feelings: Part of them wants to die, part does not. This is one of the reasons that the majority of suicidal people tell others of their intention in advance of their attempts. Most have visited their personal physician in the months prior to the suicide. Adolescents sometimes hint at their wish to die by giving away their prized possessions just prior to an attempt.

Contextual factors, or the circumstances in which people find themselves, can also contribute to individuals attempting suicide. Access to means of self-harm, such as weapons or drugs, can increase the likelihood of a suicide attempt. Similarly, physical isolation from others can also increase the odds, as there is no one to readily intervene. Even painful emotional or physical states, such as exhaustion or those that might be brought on by substance use, can set the stage for impulsive behavior to increase the likelihood of suicide attempts. In contrast, simply talking to someone about suicidal thoughts will not cause someone to commit suicide and instead may be a way to get help from a professional.

Anyone experiencing suicidal thoughts should be thoroughly evaluated by a professional trained in the assessment of suicidal patients. If the risk of suicide is considered to be high enough, the patient will have to be protected. This may require hospitalization, either voluntary or involuntary. It may mean removing suicidal means from that person's environment, such as removing guns from the home. Having someone stay with the patient at all times may be required. These steps should be individualized, taking into account the patient's situation.

Treatment of the underlying cause of the suicidal ideation is very important. Depression and anxiety can be treated with medications and/or psychotherapy. There are treatment programs for alcoholism and drug abuse. Usually, successful treatment of the underlying mental disorder results in the suicidal thoughts going away.

While they await the resolution of the suicidal ideation, patients need to be offered support and hope. Sometimes, a "no suicide" contract is helpful. This is simply a commitment on the part of the patient not to act on any suicidal thoughts and to contact the health professional if the urges become worse. While this contract may be written down, it is usually verbal.

Suicide prevention includes the early detection and management of the mental disorders associated with suicide. Because social isolation increases the risk of suicide, patients should be encouraged to develop and actively maintain strong social supports such as family, friends, and other social groups (church, clubs, and sports teams).

It may also be helpful to provide counseling to teenagers after an acquaintance has committed suicide, as this may prevent social contagion and suicide clusters. A suicide cluster is when several individuals (often teenagers) commit suicide after learning of the suicide of an acquaintance or a person who is attractive to them, such as a music or film star. Suicide clusters have increased among the young.

Family members of a suicide victim often go through a grieving process which is more severe than that which occurs after death from other causes. The stigma of suicide and mental illness is strong, and surviving family members often have greater feelings of both guilt and abandonment. Family survivors also have increased psychosomatic complaints, behavioral and emotional problems, and risk of suicide themselves. Referral to a suicide survivor group may be helpful.

Treatment and Therapy

An understanding of the causes, detection, and treatment of suicide has led to the development of a number of suicide hotlines and suicide prevention centers. There is evidence that, after these support groups are introduced into a community, the suicide rate for young women decreases. It is not yet known if they have any effect on other groups, such as young men or the elderly.

Most people who contemplate suicide do not seek professional treatment even if they tell people around them of their suicidal ideas. Thus, it is important for physicians, clergy, teachers, parents, and mental health workers to remain alert to the possibility of suicidal thoughts in those in their care. Someone who is depressed or very anxious should be asked about suicidal thoughts. Such a question will not plant the idea in his or her head, and the person may feel relieved after being asked. Once someone with suicidal ideation is identified, evaluation and treatment should proceed quickly. The following sample composite cases illustrate the application of the concepts described in the overview.

Mary is a seventeen-year-old senior in high school. She is from a broken home and was severely abused by her father prior to her parents' divorce ten years ago. Her teachers think that she is a bright underachiever who has a rather dramatic personality. Her friends see her as moody and easily angered. Her relationships with boyfriends are intense and always end with deep feelings of hurt and abandonment. Her mother is best described as cold, aloof, and preoccupied with herself.

Mary is brought to the school counselor by one of her friends when Mary threatens to kill herself and superficially scratches her wrists with a safety pin. The counselor learns that Mary has just broken up with her boyfriend, a young man at a local junior college. She is devastated. When she tried to tell her mother about it, her mother seemed uninterested and said that Mary always makes too much of such little things. It was the next morning that she scratched herself in front of her friend.

While more information is needed, this case illustrates a suicide gesture. In this case, Mary does not want to die but instead wants someone to realize how distressed she is. She feels rejected by her boyfriend and then by her mother. One can suspect a gesture rather than a serious suicide attempt by the superficial, nonlethal means (scratching with a safety pin) and by the likelihood of discovery (done in front of a friend).

Here is a second case. Tom is a forty-eight-year-old accountant. He is separated from his wife and three children and lives alone in an apartment. He has no real friends, only drinking buddies. Like his father and two uncles, Tom is an alcoholic. Each day after work, he stops at his favorite bar and drinks between eight and twelve beers.

He is brought to the emergency room of the local hospital by the police, who found him sitting on the steps of a church sobbing. He threatened to kill himself if his wife did not take him back. The emergency room doctor noted the strong odor of alcohol on his breath and ordered a blood alcohol test, which showed that he was legally intoxicated. Tom insisted that he would kill himself by running in front of a moving bus if he could not be with his family. The emergency room doctor had Tom's belt, pocketknife, and other potentially dangerous items taken from him and arranged for a staff member to sit with him until he was sober. Six hours later, his blood alcohol had returned to near zero. Tom no longer felt despondent and had no more suicidal thoughts. He was embarrassed by his statements a few hours before. An alcoholism counselor was called, and outpatient treatment for his alcoholism was arranged.

This case illustrates suicidal ideation caused by alcohol intoxication. As often happens, the suicidal ideation resolves when the patient becomes sober. The primary treatment is for the underlying addictive disorder.

Here is a third case. Sally is a fifty-three-year-old married mother of two. She is a part-time hairdresser and normally a very active, happy person. For the past three weeks, however, she has gradually lost all interest in her job, her children, her home, and her hobbies. She feels irritable and sad most of the time. Although she is tired, she does not sleep well at night, waking up very early each morning, unable to return to sleep. She is worried by the fact that she is having intrusive thoughts of killing herself. Sally imagines she could end all this dreariness by overdosing on sleeping pills and never waking up. She is a strict Catholic and knows it is against her religion to commit suicide. She calls her parish priest.

After a brief conversation, her priest meets her at the office of a psychiatrist who acts as a consultant for the diocese. The psychiatrist diagnoses major depression as the cause of Sally's suicidal ideation. She has a good social support network, so the psychiatrist decides to treat her as an outpatient and has her agree to a "no suicide" contract. Sally is also started on antidepressant medication, which gradually lifts her depression over a period of two to three weeks. Simultaneously, her suicidal thoughts leave her.

This case illustrates suicidal thoughts caused by depression. If Sally had been more depressed or her suicidal urges stronger, she would probably have needed hospitalization. If she had required hospitalization and had refused to go voluntarily, the psychiatrist could have had her committed according to the laws of the state where he practiced. Most states require a signed statement by two physicians or one physician and a licensed clinical psychologist. They must attest that the patient is a danger to himself or herself and that no less restrictive form of treatment would suffice.

Finally, here is a fourth case. Harry is a sixty-seven-year-old resident of a hospital, where he has been for the past two years. He has a serious neurological disorder called amyotrophic lateral sclerosis (also called Lou Gehrig's disease). It has caused progressive weakness such that he cannot even breathe on his own. Harry is permanently connected to a respirator attached to a tracheotomy tube in his throat. He has few visitors and mostly stares off and thinks.

Harry tells his nurse that he is "sick of it all" and wants his doctors to disconnect him from the respirator and let him die. His neurologist requests a psychiatric evaluation. The psychiatrist confirms the patient's wish to die. There is no evidence of dementia or other cognitive disorder, nor is the patient showing any evidence of a mental illness. Subsequently, a meeting is called of the hospital ethics committee to make recommendations. Membership on the committee includes physicians, nurses, an ethicist, a local minister, and the hospital attorney.

This case illustrates a difficult example of rational suicide request. The patient has a desire to die and is not suffering from any mental disorder. In this case, he is requesting not to take his own life actively but to be allowed to die passively by removal of the respirator. Some people do not consider this to be suicide at all. They make a distinction between passively allowing a natural process of dying to occur and actively taking one's own life. If this patient requested a lethal overdose of potassium to be injected into his intravenous tubes, such action would be considered suicide and ethically different. In either event, these matters are more ethical, social, and legal than psychiatric.

Perspective and Prospects

Throughout history, there have been numerous examples of suicide. In Western culture, early views on the subject were mainly from a moral perspective and suicide was viewed as a sin. Mental illness in general was poorly understood and often thought of as weakness of character, possession by evil spirits, or willful bad behavior. Thus, mental illness was stigmatized. Even though society now has a better medical understanding of mental illness, there is still a stigma attached to mental illness and to suicide. This stigma contributes to underdiagnosis and undertreatment of suicidal individuals, as many sufferers are reluctant to come forth with their symptoms.

Suicide remains an important public health problem. In 2006, it was the eleventh most common cause of death in the United States (although it was third for adolescents and second for young adults). Each year, there are about thirty thousand known suicides in the United States. The actual incidence may be higher because an unknown number of accidental deaths or untreated illnesses may actually be undiagnosed suicides. For every suicide death, between eight and twenty-five other individuals attempt suicide.

Unfortunately, most cases of suicidal ideation never come to the attention of health professionals. Therefore, when someone talks of suicide, a high index of suspicion should be maintained. Those people who express suicidal thoughts should be taken seriously and thoroughly evaluated. Increased levels of awareness of suicide may help to improve detection and treatment of this potentially preventable cause of death. Research in this area continues to focus on prevention and early identification and treatment for individuals who are distressed.

—Peter M. Hartmann, M.D.;
updated by Nancy A. Piotrowski, Ph.D.

See also Addiction; Alcoholism; Antidepressants; Anxiety; Death and dying; Dementias; Depression; Euthanasia; Grief and guilt; Hypochondriasis; Midlife crisis; Neurosis; Panic attacks; Phobias; Postpartum depression; Post-traumatic stress disorder; Psychiatric disorders; Psychiatry; Psychiatry, child and adolescent; Psychiatry, geriatric; Psychoanalysis; Psychosomatic disorders; Puberty and adolescence; Schizophrenia; Stress; Terminally ill: Extended care.

For Further Information:

DePaulo, J. Raymond, Jr., and Leslie Alan Horvitz. *Understanding Depression: What We Know and What You Can Do About It.* New York: Wiley, 2003. A leading expert on depression examines the disease's nature, causes, effects, and treatments.
Hafen, Brent Q., and Kathryn J. Frandsen. *Youth Suicide: Depression and Loneliness.* 2d ed. Evergreen, Colo.: Cordillera Press, 1986. An excellent review of all aspects of teenage suicide, with practical suggestions for helping the suicidal young person.
Jamison, Kay Redfield. *Night Falls Fast: Understanding Suicide.* New York: Alfred A. Knopf, 2000. Jamison, a distinguished psychologist and academic, brings a rare combination of personal and academic experience to bear in this monumental work on suicide.
Kolf, June Cerza. *Standing in the Shadow: Help and Encouragement for Suicide Survivors.* New York: Baker Books, 2002. The author, a veteran of hospice work, addresses the impact of suicide on family members and friends, and explores such emotions as forgiveness and depression, as well as the search for answers.
Koplewicz, Harold S. *More than Moody: Recognizing and Treating Adolescent Depression.* New York: Penguin, 2003. A leading clinician and researcher helps parents distinguish between normal teenage angst and depression, examining the warning signs, risk factors, and key behaviors, as well as treatment options.
Lester, David. *Making Sense of Suicide: An In-Depth Look at Why People Kill Themselves.* Philadelphia: Charles Press, 1997. This book may be helpful for beginning counselors and family members or friends interested in learning more about suicidal behavior.
Peck, M. Scott. *Denial of the Soul: Spiritual and Medical Perspectives on Euthanasia and Mortality.* New York: Random House, 1998. This book discusses controversial issues related to euthanasia and suicide.
Roesch, Roberta. *The Encyclopedia of Depression.* 2d ed. New York: Facts On File, 2001. This volume was written for both laypersons and professionals. Covers all aspects of depression, including bereavement, grief, and mourning. The appendixes include references, self-help groups, national associations, and institutes.
Suicide Awareness Voices of Education. http://www .save.org. Offers resources for suicide prevention, suicide survivors, and for families coping with a suicide loss.

SUPPLEMENTS

Treatment

Anatomy or system affected: All

Specialties and related fields: Alternative medicine, family medicine, internal medicine, nutrition

Definition: Chemical compounds, concentrated into pills, powders, and capsules, that are taken to prevent or treat diseases.

The Role of Supplements

Adequate nutrition is the foundation of good health. Everyone needs the four basic nutrients: water, carbohydrates, proteins, and fats. It is important to choose the proper foods to deliver these nutrients and, as necessary, to complement the diet with supplements.

Health-conscious adults have heard the message repeatedly that they can get the vitamins they need from the foods they eat, but surveys have shown that people in many countries fail to eat adequate amounts of fruit, vegetables, whole grains, and low-fat dairy foods. Should public health officials or registered dieticians recommend that people take supplements to compensate for poor eating habits? The answer to this question can be found in a discussion of vitamin supplements.

The 1990s brought to light much new information about human nutrition, its effects on the body, and the role that it plays in disease. The fuel for the body's engine comes directly from the food that one eats, which contains many vital nutrients. Nutrients come in the form of vitamins, minerals, enzymes, water, amino acids, carbohydrates, and lipids (fats). These nutrients provide people with the basic materials that human bodies need to sustain life.

One of the latest types of dietary supplements are nutraceuticals. These supplements are obtained from naturally derived chemicals in plants, called photonutrients, that make the plants biologically active. They are not nutrients in the classic sense. They are what determine a plant's color,

---

In the News:
Dietary Supplement Crackdowns by the FDA

In the past, the dietary supplement industry has been loosely regulated. Even though the Food and Drug Administration (FDA) required all the ingredients to be label-listed, there were no rules that limited the manufacturers' recommendations regarding serving sizes or the actual content amount of the nutrients. Moreover, no proof was required to guarantee product safety. However, as a result of the increasing problem of cross-contamination and misleading labeling of dietary supplements, coupled with adverse health outcomes, in March, 2003, the FDA proposed new labeling and manufacturing standards. A final rule was announced in June, 2007, indicating that the current Good Manufacturing Practices (cGMPS) would apply to the dietary supplement business. These standards were already in effect for the pharmaceutical and veterinary industries. The new rulings will establish industry-wide standards to guarantee consistent manufacturing standards in order to assure the public that the dietary supplement industry is safe and provides pure products with known strengths and compositions.

The FDA had been averaging about 550 supplement-related adverse event reports yearly since 1993; however, that figure doubled in 2002. For instance, dietary supplements had to be recalled by one manufacturer because of excessive lead contamination. Another manufacturer of niacin supplements mistakenly marketed a product that contained ten times the safe limit of niacin, which was not reflected on the label. The product was recalled after health reports of nausea, vomiting, and liver damage were received. Dietary supplements containing ephedra, used for weight loss, increased energy, and athletic performance enhancement, have been linked to several deaths, resulting in the banning of ephedra-enhanced products. A sports supplement abuse case involved the use of vitamins by a world-class athlete who failed a drug doping test; the results were later reversed when the product was tested and found to be cross-contaminated by an anabolic steroid compound that was also manufactured at the same laboratory where the vitamins were packaged.

Under the cGMPS ruling, manufacturers are required to document the identity, composition, purity, quality, and strength of the ingredients in dietary supplements. If the product is found to deviate from what the manufacturer has claimed to be the ingredients, the FDA considers the product adulterated. The minimum standards require physical plants to be constructed to ensure proper manufacturing operations, facility maintenance and cleaning, the establishment of quality control procedures, final product testing before going to market, and better methods for handling and resolving consumer complaints. These rulings do not limit consumer's access to dietary supplements but rather ensure a safer product.

—*Bonita L. Marks, Ph.D.*

---

ability to resist disease, and flavor.

Nutritionists have discovered that fruits and vegetables, grains, and legumes contain other healthful nutrients called phytochemicals. Researchers have identified thousands of phytochemicals and have the ability to remove these chemical compounds and concentrate them into pills, powders, and capsules. Phytochemicals are believed to be powerful ammunition in the war against cancer and other cellular mutations. In simple terms, cancer is a mutation of body cells through a multistep process. Phytochemicals are hypothesized to fight that disease by stopping one or more of the steps that lead to cancer. For example, a cancer process can be kindled when a carcinogenic molecule invades a cell, possibly from foods eaten or from air breathed. Sulforaphane, a phytochemical commonly found in broccoli, is then hypothesized to activate an enzyme process that removes the carcinogen from the cell before harm is done.

Researchers and pharmaceutical companies sell concentrated forms of various phytochemicals found in such vegetables as broccoli, brussels sprouts, cauliflower, and cabbage.

Because no single supplement can possibly compete with nature, some nutritionists recommend a shopping basket full of fruits and vegetables, as opposed to using expensive bottled supplements. Tomatoes, for example, are believed to contain an estimated ten thousand different phytochemicals.

Natural food supplements can be high in certain nutrients. Examples are aloe vera, bee pollen, fish oils, flaxseed, primrose oil, ginseng, ginkgo biloba, garlic, and oat bran. In general, natural food supplements are composed of by-products of foods that can provide a multitude of health benefits. One caution, however, is that supplements of this type may not have the same kind of quality control or oversight as medications prescribed by a doctor and bought from a pharmacy. As such, the effects of supplements may vary from pill to pill and bottle to bottle.

The Promise of Antioxidants

No discussion of supplements would be complete without mention of antioxidants. They are a group of vitamins, minerals, and enzymes that help to protect the body from the formation of free radicals. Free radicals are groups of atoms that can cause damage to cells and thus impair the immune system. This damage is also thought to be the basis for the aging process. Free radicals are believed to be formed through exposure to radiation and toxic chemicals such as cigarette smoke, as well as overexposure to the sun's rays.

Some common antioxidants are vitamin A and its precursor, beta carotene; vitamin C; and vitamin E. Zinc and the trace mineral selenium are thought to play an important role in neutralizing free radicals. Each vitamin or mineral has a recommended daily allowance (RDA).

Some in the field of nutrition have recommended higher supplementation doses of antioxidants and specific use of four antioxidant supplements-vitamins C and E, selenium, and mixed carotenes-to protect the immune system even further. Recommendations such as this are numerous and related to different kinds of supplement use, and they must be weighed carefully against data obtained from controlled clinical trials. While many of the substances touted as beneficial to health may have some benefits, supplements can be harmful in the wrong person; at the wrong dose; if taken in combination with the wrong medications or diet; or if taken in the presence of certain health conditions. For example, it is possible to overdose on vitamins such as A, B, and E, or on iron supplements. Some supplements, like St. John's wort, may

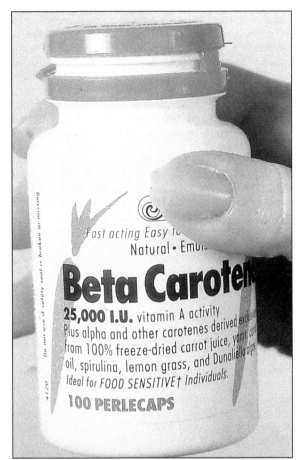

Dietary supplements such as these beta carotene pills have become increasingly popular in the United States, despite a lack of government regulation regarding safety and claims. (SIU School of Medicine)

create a side effect of light sensitivity, and discontinuing drugs such as valerian root can lead to heart problems. Also, it is easy to succumb to the temptation to seek "health in a bottle" instead of engaging in proven preventive practices. For these reasons, careful consideration and consultation with one's doctor should occur before embarking on any regimen of supplements.

Perspective and Prospects

Use of supplements is based both on modern research and development and on discoveries by mainstream scientists about the benefits of various substances. Substances such as garlic and aloe vera are examples of home remedies that have shown some promise for different kinds of ailments. Natural supplements have been used for centuries in many parts of the world as alternative medicines.

Considered and careful examination of supplement regimens in controlled clinical trials will serve as the ultimate test on the utility of these substances for health purposes. Simultaneously, consumers must remain aware that personal use of these supplements may, at times, be somewhat experimental.

Quality control concerns and interactions between supplements and prescribed medications are an important consideration. Additionally, knowledge of the supplements found in pills or popular beverages and how they may interact with street drugs of different types is also important in order to avoid unnecessary harm. This is especially true for children and elders.

—Lisa Levin Sobczak, R.N.C.;
updated by Nancy A. Piotrowski, Ph.D.

See also Aging; Alternative medicine; Antioxidants; Digestion; Ergogenic aids; Food biochemistry; Herbal medicine; Macronutrients; Malnutrition; Nutrition; Osteoporosis; Over-the-counter medications; Phytochemicals; Self-medication; Vitamins and minerals.

For Further Information:
Balch, James F., and Phyllis A. Balch. *Prescription for Nutritional Healing: A Practical A to Z Reference to Drug-Free Remedies Using Vitamins, Minerals, Herbs, and Food Supplements*. 4th rev. ed. Garden City Park, N.Y.: Avery, 2008.

Hendler, Sheldon Saul. *The Doctors' Vitamin and Mineral Encyclopedia*. New York: Simon & Schuster, 1990.

Murray, Michael. *The Pill Book Guide to Natural Medicines: Vitamins, Minerals, Nutritional Supplements, Herbs, and Other Natural Products*. New York: Bantam, 2002.

The PDR Family Guide to Nutritional Supplements: An Authoritative A-to-Z Resource on the One Hundred Most Popular Nutritional Therapies and Nutraceuticals. New York: Ballantine Books, 2001.

Weil, Andrew. *Eight Weeks to Optimum Health: A Proven Program for Taking Full Advantage of Your Body's Natural Healing Power*. Rev. ed. New York: Ballantine Books, 2007.

SURGERY, GENERAL
Specialty
Anatomy or system affected: All
Specialties and related fields: Anesthesiology, radiology
Definition: A field of medicine that involves a wide range of surgical procedures, from the simple removal of warts and bunions in the doctor's office to complex organ transplantation requiring a large staff in the operating room.
Key terms:
aseptic techniques: procedures that allow surgeons to operate in a germ-free environment
excision: the surgical removal of an organ or tissue

Science and Profession

In all probability, surgery has been practiced as long as humans have had cutting tools. Ample reports of battlefield amputations exist almost from the beginning of reported time. Historians tell of rough field surgery, the hacking off of wounded limbs and the sealing of the wounds by searing the lacerated flesh. There are even suggestions that ancient civilizations, such as that of the Egyptians, practiced trepanning, cutting into the skull to operate on the brain.

Until the latter half of the nineteenth century, surgery was a brutal, dirty, and dangerous practice. About this time, the relationship between microorganisms and diseases was first enunciated, a relationship which explained why so many surgery patients sickened and died. It was also at this time that anesthetics were developed, which for the first time allowed the surgeon to deaden the patient's pain.

Surgery today is one of the most respected medical specialties, requiring full training in the disciplines of medicine, as well as years of extensive work in surgical procedures. After becoming physicians, candidates for surgery spend years working under established surgeons learning the techniques that they will use in practice. They are subjected to intensive examination and receive certification only when their peers are convinced that they can perform their duties capably.

The tools and techniques of surgery that the surgical candidate must master present multiple challenges. In their training phase, surgeons learn to become skilled in the manipulation of all the basic instruments used in surgery, such as the various designs of scalpels, scissors, retractors, forceps, and sutures. The training surgeon learns a wide variety of stitching techniques and the materials used in suturing. Most challenging perhaps is mastery of the many new techniques and instruments that modern surgeons use.

After training and certification, some surgeons elect to practice general surgery. As the term implies, this field covers such diverse areas of the body as the stomach, gallbladder, liver, intestines, appendix, breasts, thyroid gland, salivary glands, main arteries and veins, lumps under the skin, hernias, and hemorrhoids. Other surgeons choose to specialize in disciplines that require still more training, such as heart surgery, bone (or orthopedic) surgery, and eye (or ophthalmic) surgery, to name some of the more prevalent specialties.

Modern surgery is a far-ranging practice involving all body structures and systems. It is also a practice that sees constant advancements and improvements in operating techniques, in instrumentation and tools, and in high-tech equipment. Microsurgery, in which the surgeon uses a microscope to view the operating field and manipulates tiny instruments to repair or excise tissue, was virtually unheard of at the middle of the twentieth century. It is now common practice in virtually every surgical facility in the United States. At one time, a severed limb could never be reconnected, largely because it was impossible to repair severed nerves. Now, because of microsurgery, arms, legs, hands, digits, and other severed body parts can be stitched back on to the body, often with much of their mobility restored.

Much minor surgery takes place in the physician's office or clinic. These procedures are generally simple, involving the excision of skin growths such as warts or cancers, hemorrhoids, and other surface conditions. Emergency surgery in the office, clinic, or emergency room may be necessary to open an airway for a patient whose breathing is impaired or to remove obstructions.

Major surgery usually requires a hospital stay, and its main characteristics are anesthesia and aseptic technique. Anesthesia may be local, regional, or general. For local anesthesia, anesthetic is injected into the site of the operation. The patient is usually fully awake during the surgery but feels no pain in the affected area. In regional anesthesia, a whole part of the body is anesthetized, such as a leg or an arm. As with local an-

esthesia, the patient is awake during the procedure but may be sedated for comfort. In general anesthesia, the patient is put to sleep and immobilized, usually by injections, and inhaled anesthetics are administered throughout the course of the operation.

To create an aseptic, germ-free environment, the operating room and everything in it are subjected to rigorous sterilization. Surgeons and all operating room staff scrub with antiseptic soaps. They don complete uniforms of sterilized cloth or paper: caps, masks, gowns, gloves, and foot coverings. Avoiding transmission of disease in the operating room can be said to be as important as the operation itself. It is vital that the patient be made safe from infection by the staff and from pathogenic organisms in the ambient atmosphere of the hospital.

It is equally important that staff be protected from infection by the patient. Operating room personnel are particularly vulnerable to blood-borne infections, such as hepatitis B and human immunodeficiency virus (HIV). Surgery can be a bloody procedure. In some operations, copious blood spurts are common, and the likelihood of staff being spattered is high, as is the possibility of disease transmission. It is possible that there will be a cut or tear in the staff's protective clothing and that the patient's blood or other body fluids can make contact with an abrasion on the body or even land on mucous membranes of the mouth, nose, and throat, where they can infect the caregiver. This has happened so often that the U.S. government has issued rigorous guidelines to high-risk health care personnel-particularly operating room staff-detailing specific procedures to follow to avoid disease transmission.

Diagnostic and Treatment Techniques

The surgeon is rarely the first physician whom the patient sees. Usually, a primary care physician makes a diagnosis and may confer with or send the patient to a specialist for confirmation of the diagnosis. When surgery is recommended, the surgeon confers with the primary care physician and/or the consulting specialist and is fully apprised of the patient's condition. He or she reviews the patient's history and inspects all relevant documents and diagnostic reports, such as X rays, computed tomography (CT) scans, and other information that he or she needs to plan and perform the procedure.

For the most part, surgeons deal with their patients only in the immediate context of the operation. They meet before the operation, and surgeons look in on patients afterward to check their progress and recovery. In some cases, follow-up visits to the surgeon are required.

In the operating room, the surgeon assembles the staff needed for the particular procedure. There will be an anesthesiologist, perhaps other specialized surgeons, and various general and specialized operating room nurses. The surgeon or the staff will also order everything needed for the procedure. There is an enormous range of specialized equipment that surgeons can use in their procedures. Cardiac surgeons use heart-lung machines, which take over the task of circulating the patient's blood and allow the surgeon to open and en-

A Typical Operating Room

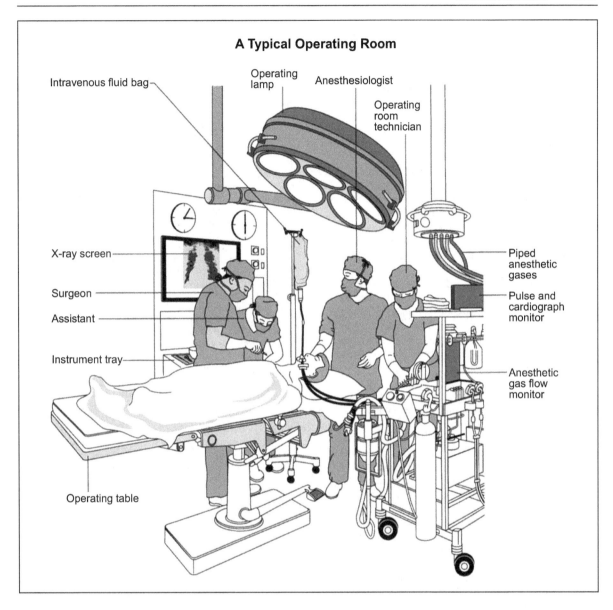

Intravenous fluid bag

Operating lamp

Anesthesiologist

Operating room technician

X-ray screen

Surgeon

Assistant

Instrument tray

Operating table

Piped anesthetic gases

Pulse and cardiograph monitor

Anesthetic gas flow monitor

ter the heart itself. The neurosurgeon may operate through specialized microscopic instruments.

A catalog of specialized endoscopes is now available to surgeons, many of which allow them to operate through a tiny hole in the patient's skin, rather than having to make massive cuts with a scalpel. Pulmonary surgeons use a bronchoscope to look down into the patient's bronchial tubes, where they can perform such surgical operations as removing obstructions and excising cancerous tissue. Gastrointestinal surgeons use a gastroscope both to investigate conditions in the stomach and to take small tissue samples for biopsy. Colon and rectal surgeons use a colonoscope to remove polyps from the colon and rectum, a major step in the prevention and treatment of colon cancer. Major surgery, however, still involves cutting the patient open to repair what has gone wrong inside

the body. Fortunately, this procedure is now safer and more specialized than it has ever been before.

Management of disease in the United States has reached the point where there are surgical specialties to cover virtually all parts of the body individually. Some surgeons specialize in individual organs, such as the heart, lungs, brain, eyes, and ears. Some surgeons specialize in body systems such as bones or circulation. Furthermore, many surgeons hone their skills in certain specialized surgical techniques and become so adept that they are recognized as experts in highly complex and critical procedures, such as repairing detached retinas, performing heart transplants, correcting slipped disks, or sealing brain aneurysms.

Surgeons are major inventors and designers. Much of the instrumentation and many of the surgical tools that are used in the operating room were invented by surgeons. They often direct the fabrication of specialized tools and instruments to help them in their work. Most of the metal and plastic prostheses implanted to replace damaged internal structures were designed by surgeons. Orthopedic surgeons design prosthetic hips, knees, and other implants. Ophthalmic surgeons design corneal implants. The specialized surgeon knows his or her area of the body better than anyone else does and can visualize what sort of equipment or device is needed to improve the patient's condition.

Surgeons are also at the forefront of major technical innovations that reach across the entire surgical field. They are adept at recognizing potential applications for new technology and adapting it to surgery. For example, fiber-optic science has been applied in surgical endoscopes. Cryosurgery, a technique of freezing tissue, is used in a wide range of procedures, from the removal of hemorrhoids to the reattachment of retinas.

Laser technology is employed in hundreds of surgical procedures. The laser is used for making incisions, for repairing tissue, and for excising diseased tissue, among other applications. One of the major areas that can benefit from the unique advantages of laser use is eye surgery. Ophthalmic surgeons use lasers to relieve diabetic retinopathy, glaucoma, macular degeneration, cataracts, and certain tumors, as well as to reattach torn retinas.

One of the critical qualities of the competent surgeon is judgment. No matter how thoroughly a surgeon may prepare for a procedure, there may be some surprises on the operating table. The surgeon learns the patient's history and status and also reviews all the appropriate diagnostic documents, X rays, and other visualizations, but unforeseen complications may arise during the operation. The surgeon must have the experience and competence to deal with the unexpected.

Perspective and Prospects

Up to the mid-nineteenth century, surgical procedures were probably responsible for as many deaths as cures. Today, surgery extends the lives of millions: heart disease victims, cancer patients, and victims of infection and accidents. Surgery helps improve the quality of life for patients with arthritis and rheumatism, gastrointestinal problems, lung disorders, and circulation problems.

Furthermore, surgery is entering new areas of medicine. For example, operations can now be performed in the uterus to correct anomalies in unborn fetuses. Many more such procedures are predicted for the future.

New areas of surgical expertise are opening constantly; new techniques, instrumentation, and equipment are making many old procedures obsolete. Practicing surgeons face a constant challenge in keeping abreast of what is happening all over the world and deciding what avenues to explore for the benefit of their patients.

—*C. Richard Falcon*

See also Abscess drainage; Adrenalectomy; Amputation; Anesthesia; Anesthesiology; Aneurysmectomy; Appendectomy; Biopsy; Bladder removal; Bone marrow transplantation; Breast biopsy; Breast surgery; Bunions; Bypass surgery; Cardiac surgery; Cataract surgery; Catheterization; Cervical procedures; Cesarean section; Cholecystectomy; Cleft lip and palate repair; Colorectal polyp removal; Colorectal surgery; Corneal transplantation; Craniotomy; Cryosurgery; Cyst removal; Disk removal; Ear surgery; Electrocauterization; Endarterectomy; Endometrial biopsy; Eye surgery; Face lift and blepharoplasty; Facial transplantation; Fistula repair; Ganglion removal; Gender reassignment surgery; Gastrectomy; Grafts and grafting; Hair transplantation; Hammertoe correction; Heart transplantation; Heart valve replacement; Heel spur removal; Hemorrhoid banding and removal; Hernia repair; Hypospadias repair and urethroplasty; Hysterectomy; Kidney transplantation; Kneecap removal; Laceration repair; Laminectomy and spinal fusion; Laparoscopy; Laryngectomy; Laser use in surgery; Liposuction; Liver transplantation; Lung surgery; Mastectomy and lumpectomy; Myomectomy; Nail removal; Nasal polyp removal; Nephrectomy; Neurosurgery; Ophthalmology; Oral and maxillofacial surgery; Orthopedic surgery; Parathyroidectomy; Penile implant surgery; Periodontal surgery; Phlebitis; Plastic surgery; Prostate gland removal; Refractive eye surgery; Rhinoplasty and submucous resection; Shunts; Skin lesion removal; Sphincterectomy; Splenectomy; Sterilization; Stone removal; Surgery, pediatric; Surgical procedures; Surgical technologists; Sympathectomy; Tattoo removal; Tendon repair; Testicular surgery; Thoracic surgery; Thyroidectomy; Tonsillectomy and adenoid removal; Tracheostomy; Transfusion; Transplantation; Tumor removal; Ulcer surgery; Vagotomy; Varicose vein removal; Vasectomy.

For Further Information:

Brunicardi, F. Charles, et al., eds. *Schwartz's Principles of Surgery.* 9th ed. New York: McGraw-Hill, 2010. A standard textbook on the topic. Intended for practicing surgeons, but valuable to general readers for its details.

Griffith, H. Winter. *Complete Guide to Symptoms, Illness, and Surgery.* Revised and updated by Stephen Moore and Kenneth Yoder. 5th ed. New York: Perigee, 2006. Covers more than five hundred diseases and disorders and includes information about causes and risk factors, preventive techniques, diagnostic tests, and surgical treatment.

Litin, Scott C., ed. *Mayo Clinic Family Health Book.* 4th ed. New York: HarperResource, 2009. This book covers the surgical aspects of medicine admirably, with clear and concise descriptions of surgical procedures.

Mulholland, Michael W., et al., eds. *Greenfield's Surgery: Scientific Principles and Practice.* 4th ed. Philadelphia: Lippincott Williams & Wilkins, 2006. Covers scientific reviews of wound biology, inflammatory mediators, immunology, and the management of trauma and transplantation in the first part and an overview of surgical practice according to anatomic region and specialty in the second part.

Zollinger, Robert M., Jr., and Robert M. Zollinger, Sr. *Zollinger's Atlas of Surgical Operations.* 8th ed. New York: McGraw-Hill, 2003. A comprehensive examination of surgery. Covers basic surgical anatomy and vascular, gynecologic, gastrointestinal, and miscellaneous abdominal procedures.

Surgery, pediatric

Specialty

Anatomy or system affected: All

Specialties and related fields: Anesthesiology, general surgery, neonatology, pediatrics

Definition: The surgical correction of medical conditions of infants and children.

Key term:

congenital defect: an anatomic defect present at birth; it is not necessarily hereditary

Science and Profession

A pediatric surgeon is a general surgeon who has received additional training in operating on infants and children. The full course of training includes four years of medical school, followed by five years of general surgery residency and two years of pediatric surgery residency. Pediatric surgeons generally practice in large referral hospitals or children's hospitals. The relatively small number of American training programs in this specialty are all located at major teaching hospitals.

Children are not simply small adults. They experience some different surgical disorders than adults, especially congenital defects. Their ability to withstand the stress of surgery is less than that of an older person. Also, many of their surgical problems require years of follow-up care by a surgeon who understands child growth and development.

In the first half of the twentieth century, when pediatric surgery was developing as a specialty, the pediatric surgeon was trained to operate on all parts of the child's body. As the specialty matured, however, the pediatric surgeon came to perform only general surgical procedures on infants and children. This trend was made possible by the development of pediatric subspecialties in the other surgical fields, such as neurosurgery and cardiac surgery. In addition, pediatric surgeons work closely with pediatricians. As a team, they share in evaluating the patient and in providing preoperative and postoperative care.

To a degree, pediatric surgeons differ from general surgeons in their point of view. Infants and children change constantly as they grow, and common surgical diagnoses also change with the age of the patient. Additionally, the ability of a child's body to cope with disease and with surgery alters with age. It is therefore necessary for the pediatric surgeon to understand child growth and development.

Although a disorder may be surgically corrected in infancy, the child may continue to have postoperative difficulty for many years. An example is the removal of a large amount of intestines, which must sometimes be done with premature infants. It takes considerable patience and expertise to follow this sort of patient for years, adjusting the child's diet and treatment to achieve as nearly normal growth as possible. The pediatric surgeon is specially trained to provide this care.

The organs and tissues of an infant or child are much smaller than those of an adult. The pediatric surgeon must develop expert skills to perform surgery on these small structures. Also, the pediatric surgeon is trained to work rapidly when performing surgery. It is important to complete procedures quickly to minimize stress on the pediatric patient.

Congenital defects are, fortunately, relatively uncommon. The pediatric surgeon treats relatively more of these conditions than a general surgeon would and therefore has greater experience in caring for them. Examples of congenital defects treated by pediatric surgeons include defects of the abdominal wall and diaphragm and the obstruction or absence of a part of the intestinal tract.

Because the patient is a child, the pediatric surgeon must also deal with the patient's family. This specialist is trained to build a supportive relationship with parents and to teach them about their child's disorder so that they can be informed participants in decisions regarding the patient's care. Especially with chronic diseases, the parents must be kept aware of their child's progress and changing needs so that they can participate fully in the child's recovery.

Diagnostic and Treatment Techniques

The pediatric surgeon's day is split between the operating room and the clinic. This specialist spends relatively more time in the clinic than does a general surgeon. Surgical correction is only one step in pediatric surgery: Careful evaluation and planning must precede any procedure. Afterward, extended follow-up care is often necessary, sometimes for years. This type of care requires patience and an interest in long-range planning on the surgeon's part.

The pediatric surgeon relies heavily on history taking and physical examination of the patient. This information, plus knowledge of the incidence of specific disorders at different ages, leads the surgeon to the most likely diagnosis. Specific laboratory and radiographic tests are ordered to aid in the diagnostic process.

The pediatric surgeon works very closely with the anesthesiologist, the physician responsible for keeping the patient anesthetized and his or her vital functions stable during surgery. The needs of a child are different from those of an adult during surgery. Many hospitals with pediatric surgeons are also staffed with pediatric anesthesiologists.

Like other surgeons, the pediatric surgeon also performs minor surgery on children, often in the clinic. Examples of minor procedures are the suturing of lacerations, the drainage of small abscesses, and the excision of small benign growths under the skin.

Perspective and Prospects

Pediatric surgery began in the United States as an offshoot of general surgery in the first half of the twentieth century. For decades, the specialty met resistance from general surgeons. The American Academy of Pediatrics was first to recognize the value of pediatric surgeons and, following a meeting by the academy in 1948, established a surgical section. C. Everett Koop, the surgeon general under President Ronald Reagan, was a vigorous advocate of pediatric surgical education and a developer of new surgical techniques for children from 1946 through the 1990s. He was an important proponent in the eventual recognition of pediatric surgery as a surgical specialty. It was not until 1973, however, that the Board of Pediatric Surgery certified the first specialists in the field.

In 1995, there were twenty-eight training programs for pediatric surgeons in the United States. Because of the limited number of graduates of these programs, pediatric surgeons will continue to be in great demand.

—*Thomas C. Jefferson, M.D.*

See also Abscess drainage; Adrenalectomy; Amputation; Anesthesia; Anesthesiology; Aneurysmectomy; Appendectomy; Biopsy;

Bone marrow transplantation; Cardiac surgery; Cardiology, pediatric; Catheterization; Cleft lip and palate repair; Craniotomy; Cryosurgery; Ear surgery; Electrocauterization; Endocrinology, pediatric; Eye surgery; Fistula repair; Gastroenterology, pediatric; Genetic diseases; Genetics and inheritance; Grafts and grafting; Heart transplantation; Heart valve replacement; Hernia repair; Hypospadias repair and urethroplasty; Kidney transplantation; Laceration repair; Laparoscopy; Laser use in surgery; Lung surgery; Nasal polyp removal; Nephrectomy; Nephrology, pediatric; Neurology, pediatric; Neurosurgery; Ophthalmology; Oral and maxillofacial surgery; Orthopedic surgery; Orthopedics, pediatric; Parathyroidectomy; Pediatrics; Plastic surgery; Pulmonary medicine, pediatric; Shunts; Splenectomy; Surgery, general; Surgical procedures; Surgical technologists; Sympathectomy; Tattoo removal; Tendon repair; Thoracic surgery; Thyroidectomy; Tonsillectomy and adenoid removal; Tracheostomy; Transfusion; Transplantation; Urology, pediatric.

For Further Information:

Cockburn, Forrester, et al. *Children's Medicine and Surgery.* New York: Oxford University Press, 1996. This volume discusses the basics of pediatrics and features illustrations and an index.

Glick, Philip L., et al. *Pediatric Surgery Secrets.* New York: Hanley & Belfus, 2001. An accessible question-and-answer format addresses general and critical care, thoracic surgery, cardiovascular surgery, gastroenterology, hepatobiliary and spleen surgery, head and neck surgery, genitourinary surgery, trauma, tumors and oncology, and special topics.

Koop, C. Everett. "Pediatric Surgery: The Long Road to Recognition." *Pediatrics* 92 (October, 1993): 618-621. The history of pediatric surgery is discussed. Some believe that pediatric surgery would never have gotten off the ground without the development of pediatric anesthesiology.

O'Neill, James A., Jr., et al., eds. *Principles of Pediatric Surgery.* 2d ed. St. Louis, Mo.: Mosby, 2004. This is a new edition of a classic textbook of pediatric surgery. It is the most comprehensive text available on the subject, a must for all practicing and aspiring pediatric surgeons. Perhaps a bit too comprehensive for nonpediatric surgeons looking for a simple reference book to keep on their shelf.

SURGICAL PROCEDURES

Procedures

Anatomy or system affected: All

Specialties and related fields: Anesthesiology, general surgery, nursing, plastic surgery

Definition: The treatment of diseases or disorders by physical intervention, which usually involves cutting into the skin and other tissues.

Key terms:

anesthesia: the use of drugs to inhibit pain and other sensations

hemostasis: the control of bleeding

incision: a cut made with a scalpel

suture: a thread used to unite parts of the body

Indications and Procedures

Surgery has progressed as rapidly as other areas of medicine. Early surgeries consisted of gross excision (the cutting out of abnormal or diseased tissue). Today, surgery has been transformed by scientific advances so that surgeons commonly use microscopes, lasers, and endoscopes that allow the surgeon to make small incisions in order to gain access to the surgical site. Modern operations are much more precise and emphasize repair or replacement rather than excision.

When a patient requires surgery, several preoperative procedures are performed to increase the chances of a successful outcome. First, the patient is asked to abstain from eating for at least eight hours prior to surgery. This action reduces the chances of the individual vomiting during surgery and aspirating the gastric contents into the trachea (windpipe). After arriving at the hospital or clinic, the patient removes his or her clothes and puts on a gown, allowing the medical staff easy access to the patient for catheter insertion, intravenous line insertion, monitor placement, and preparation of the surgical site. Next, an intravenous (IV) line is placed in a vein of the hand or arm and connected to a bottle or bag of solution, which is suspended above the level of the patient's arm. The intravenous line gives the physician rapid vascular access for sampling blood and injecting drugs. Just before the actual surgery, the patient is usually given a sedative by an anesthesiologist, and electrocardiogram (ECG or EKG) leads and a blood pressure cuff are applied to the patient to monitor heart rate, heart rhythm, and blood pressure. The anesthesiologist will then anesthetize the patient further while the surgical team begins to prepare the site for the operation. Preoperative antibiotics may be given if there is a significant risk of infection.

The surgery may require either general anesthesia, in which the patient is unconscious, or local anesthesia, in which a specific region of the body is anesthetized. For general anesthesia, the patient will be injected with an intravenous anesthetic and quickly intubated, a procedure in which a tube is inserted into the trachea and attached to a ventilator. This arrangement gives the anesthesiologist the ability to administer gaseous drugs such as nitrous oxide and halothane as well as to control the patient's breathing. Surgical assistants prepare the operative site by cleansing the skin with a disinfectant. A sterile drape is used to cover all areas of the body except the surgical site. Surgeons and assistants must mask themselves and prepare for surgery by thoroughly washing their hands and arms. They then carefully put on a sterile gown and gloves. At this point, they must not come into contact with anything nonsterile.

The surgeon uses a scalpel to make an incision through the skin and any underlying structures in order to gain access to the area of the body needing attention. When blood vessels are cut, bleeding must be controlled by cauterizing, clamping, tying off with sutures, or applying direct pressure to the vessel; this process is known as hemostasis.

After the surgery, the incision sites are closed with sutures, and the anesthetic is reversed. The patient is then taken to a recovery room to be monitored closely. Routine care of the patient recovering from anesthesia includes repeated evaluation of body temperature, pulse, blood pressure, and respiration. Postoperative pain medication (such as meperidine, morphine, or fentanyl) is given as needed.

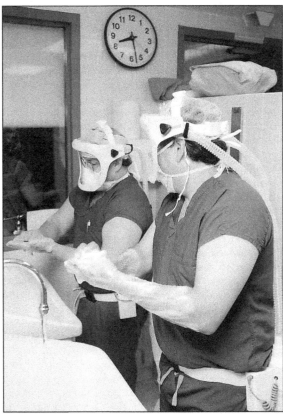

Surgeons scrub their hands and arms before performing an operation. Such procedures are essential to the maintenance of an antiseptic environment. (Digital Stock)

Uses and Complications

Complications from surgery can result from surgical errors, infections, and abnormal patient reactions to the procedure or medications (idiosyncratic reactions). Occasionally, surgery involves damage to healthy tissues, including nerves and blood vessels. Significant intraoperative blood loss may also occur, requiring transfusion. An incision into any part of the body provides an opportunity for bacteria to enter and infect the surgical wound; prophylactic antibiotics help reduce the chance of surgical infection. Rarely, a patient may have an unexpected response to the procedure or drugs, which could result in permanent disability or death. These very infrequent reactions may include a blood clot causing a stroke or heart attack, an abnormal heart rhythm, or severe allergic reactions to medication.

Perspective and Prospects

Modern surgery includes the use of surgical implants, microsurgery, laser surgery, endoscopic surgery, and transplant surgery. Surgery implants are used to replace a part of the body with an artificial implant. These implants include joints, heart valves, eye lenses, and sections of blood vessels or of the skull. During microsurgery, the surgeon uses specially designed instruments and a microscope to perform an operation on minute structures such as blood vessels, nerves, and parts of the eyes or ears. Microsurgery is also being used to reattach severed fingers and toes. Laser surgery utilizes a high-energy, narrow beam that can cut through tissues like a scalpel but that also cauterizes blood vessels during the incision. Lasers can be used on the retina, skin blemishes, and even tumors. Recovery from endoscopic surgery, in which a fiber-optic tube is inserted into the body to view the surgical site, is generally faster than from conventional operations because a smaller incision is made and less tissue damage results. Endoscopes are used to remove stones from the urinary tract and gallbladder and to remove or repair damaged cartilage in joints. With the availability of drugs that suppress tissue rejection, damaged organs can now be surgically replaced by donated organs. The most common examples are the heart, lungs, liver, kidneys, and bone marrow.

—Matthew Berria, Ph.D.,
and Douglas Reinhart, M.D.

See also Anesthesia; Anesthesiology; Biopsy; Bypass surgery; Catheterization; Cervical procedures; Colon and rectal surgery; Craniotomy; Cryosurgery; Cyst removal; Electrocauterization; Eye surgery; Fistula repair; Ganglion removal; Grafts and grafting; Hernia repair; Laparoscopy; Laser use in surgery; Lung surgery; Neurosurgery; Orthopedic surgery; Periodontal surgery; Plastic surgery; Shunts; Surgery, general; Surgery, pediatric; Surgical technologists; Thoracic surgery; Tracheostomy; Transfusion; Transplantation; Tumor removal.

For Further Information:

Brunicardi, F. Charles, et al., eds. *Schwartz's Principles of Surgery.* 9th ed. New York: McGraw-Hill, 2010. A standard textbook on the topic. Intended for practicing surgeons, but valuable to general readers for its details.

Leikin, Jerrold B., and Martin S. Lipsky, eds. *American Medical Association Complete Medical Encyclopedia.* New York: Random House Reference, 2003. A concise presentation of numerous medical terms and illnesses. A good general reference.

Mulholland, Michael W., et al., eds. *Greenfield's Surgery: Scientific Principles and Practice.* 4th ed. Philadelphia: Lippincott Williams & Wilkins, 2006. Covers the scope and practice of surgery and includes reviews of wound biology, immunology, the management of trauma and transplantation, surgical practice according to anatomic region and specialty, and musculoskeletal, neurologic, genitourinary, and reconstructive surgery.

Zollinger, Robert M., Jr., and Robert M. Zollinger, Sr. *Zollinger's Atlas of Surgical Operations.* 8th ed. New York: McGraw-Hill, 2003. A comprehensive examination of surgery. Covers basic surgical anatomy and vascular, gynecologic, gastrointestinal, and miscellaneous abdominal procedures.

SURGICAL TECHNOLOGISTS
Specialty

Anatomy or system affected: All

Specialties and related fields: Anesthesiology, emergency medicine, general surgery, nursing

Definition: Surgical team members whose primary functions are to prepare surgical instruments and hand them to the surgeon as needed and to prevent infection by maintaining a sterile field in the operating room.

Key terms:

analgesia: the absence of pain

anesthesia: the absence of sensation; anesthesia may be achieved systemically (general anesthesia) or in a specific region of the body (regional or local anesthesia)

aseptic techniques: the standard procedures that help prevent wound contamination during the performance of surgical procedures; contamination may be followed by infection or death

circulator: the worker in the operating room whose responsibility is to keep records and to open sterile supplies for the team members wearing gowns and gloves

inpatient procedure: a surgical procedure performed on a patient who comes from a room in the hospital and who will return to a room in the hospital

operating room: a room in which surgical procedures are performed

outpatient procedure: a surgical procedure performed on a patient who comes from outside the hospital and who will most likely leave the hospital after a short stay in the recovery room

prep: a short form of the word "prepare"; to prep means to wash and shave the surgical area and to clean the skin surface immediately before a surgical procedure

recovery room: the room where a patient returns to full consciousness after a surgical procedure; in an outpatient facility, patients can change clothes in the recovery room, which may serve double duty as the preoperative waiting room

scrub: to wash one's hands and forearms in preparation for donning gown and gloves, which protect the patient from the surgical technologist and protect the surgical technologist from the patient

sterile field: an area where only sterile supplies may be placed and that only those wearing sterile gowns and gloves may touch; includes the surgical wound, the surgical drapes, and the extra tables

surgical team: the people working together in the operating room during a surgical procedure, including the surgeon, first assistant, surgical technologist, anesthesiologist and/or anesthetist, and circulator

Science and Profession

Surgical technologists work as part of the surgical team in an operating room, so they must be familiar with many aspects of patient care. The surgical team typically includes at least one of each of the following: a surgeon, a first assistant, a surgical technologist, an anesthesiologist and/or anesthetist, and a circulator. As a member of the surgical team, a surgical technologist anticipates the needs of the surgeon, prepares the instruments to be used for surgery, hands instruments to the surgeon, promotes efficiency, and at the same time helps prevent infection by maintaining the sterile field. A surgical technologist may also be referred to as a scrub nurse, a surgical assistant, a private scrub, or simply a scrub.

Surgical technologists work in many types of operating rooms, so their training must be fairly extensive. Courses may be taken at community colleges in one-year or two-year programs. Some of the two-year programs are accredited by the Association of Surgical Technologists. In 2001, the Commission on Accreditation of Allied Health Education Programs (CAAHEP) recognized 350 accredited programs. The courses taken include medical terminology, anatomy, and physiology. Classes specifically focused on surgical technology may include surgical conscience and ethics, the organization of an operating room, principles of microbiology, sterilization and disinfection, aseptic techniques, preoperative preparation and care of the patient, anesthesia, medications used during surgery, proper positioning of a surgical patient, preparation of the surgical site, methods of closing the surgical wound, surgical routines, the supplies found in the operating room, and the legal aspects of surgery.

A surgical technologist may work in one or all of many surgical services, so coursework must provide information about general surgery; obstetrical and gynecological surgery; plastic and reconstructive surgery; ear, nose, and throat procedures; surgery on the mouth and face; orthopedic surgery; neurosurgery; open-heart surgery; lung surgery; pediatric surgery; and surgery on blood vessels not located in the chest.

Students are required to gain experience in an operating room, which is usually done under supervision at a local teaching hospital. At such a hospital, a student gains experience in appropriate operating room procedures and learns the universal precautions against the transmission of infectious diseases.

Although the surgical technologist may work in any of the available medical services, some hospitals require their surgical technologists to specialize-that is, to rotate through different services so that they will gain familiarity with many operative procedures. At other facilities, the surgical technologist will work primarily in one area. For example, if the facility is a plastic surgeon's clinic, only these types of procedures will be performed.

A surgical technologist who has gained some experience may gain a specific area of interest within a broader field and decide to become a specialist. Common areas in which to specialize include eye surgery, neurosurgery, orthopedics, and plastic surgery. If this is the case, the technologist might be invited to work for a certain doctor or may find a number of (perhaps unaffiliated) doctors with whom to work. Working as a private scrub offers a different way to practice in the field. The surgical technologist works directly for the surgeon, instead of working for the hospital or surgical facility, and can usually expect to charge and earn more. There is also the possibility of greater camaraderie with the physician and more trust of the surgical technologist by the physician. Concentrating in a specific area may offer greater remuneration to the surgical technologist, greater rapport with a familiar surgeon, and a more regular schedule, with no requirement for working on the weekends.

Duties and Procedures

Surgical technologists typically work in many areas, both inside and outside the operating room. Within the operating room, they may be either scrubbed or not scrubbed. After washing his or her hands, the surgical technologist dons a gown and gloves, which provides a sterile surface to reduce the possibility of transmission of infection, either from the patient to the surgical technologist or from the surgical technologist to the patient. When scrubbed, surgical technologists perform many duties. They assist surgeons during surgical procedures by handing them instruments, following routine procedures. They promote efficiency by keeping the instrument tables neat and organized. They must anticipate the needs of surgeons, so it is necessary that they know the steps of a procedure and monitor its progress. A surgical technologist places instruments in the surgeon's hands so that the surgeon does not have to look away from the wound in search of an instrument. Surgical technologists also help prevent injuries to the patient.

When necessary, the scrubbed surgical technologist may be asked to act as a first assistant for a procedure. In this capacity, it may be necessary for the surgical technologist to hold tissue out of the way (retract it), so that the surgeon can reach deeper tissues. Surgical technologists may also be required to sponge blood out of the wound or to rinse the surgical site to promote visibility of the tissues. They may also cut sutures. Surgical technologists help count sponges, needles, and instruments when such counts are required; items must be counted so that none are left behind in the patient. These items are counted before, during, and after the surgical procedure, in a specified and orderly manner. It is also the responsibility of the scrubbed surgical technologist to keep track of surgical specimens, pieces of tissue removed from the patient that will be sent to the laboratory for analysis. Many specimens may be taken from a particular procedure, so the surgical technologist must hand them off the sterile field to the circulator and make sure that the circulator labels the specimens properly. Specimens must also be handled and treated properly. Some are sent to the laboratory in preserving solutions, some are sent in salt water, and some are sent dry. It is important to keep track of specimens, to identify them, and to put them in the proper container for transportation to the laboratory.

When the surgical technologist is working in the operating room and is not scrubbed, a registered nurse must be immediately available in case there is an emergency. A registered nurse must also be present if medications are needed on the sterile field. A surgical technologist who is not scrubbed may function as a circulator. The circulator opens sterile supplies onto the operative field. Supplies are wrapped in many different ways, and the circulator must be able to pass the contents of a sterile package to the scrubbed surgical technologist without dropping them. Expiration dates must be checked on all supplies opened. Once the patient for a particular procedure is brought into the operating room, the circulator will help position the patient on the surgical table. The surgical technologist knows the position necessary for the particular procedure. Safe positioning methods prevent injury to patients. Once the patient is on the surgical table, the circulator washes the area with specified soaps and solutions and, if

necessary, will shave the area around the surgical wound so that the area can be cleaned for the incision. The circulator ties the gowns of the scrubbed surgical technologist as well as the surgeon and other scrubbed assistants. If the anesthesiologist or anesthetist asks for help, the circulator provides that help, which may include holding, informing, or reassuring the patient.

It is the function of the circulator to connect tubings and electrical wires from instruments that may be needed on the sterile field, including power cords for cautery units, special lights, and drills, as well as fluid lines and suction cords. The circulator may need to focus or aim the surgical lights. With the scrubbed surgical technologist, the circulator performs the count of the items that need to be counted, including the sutures, sponges, and instruments. The circulator keeps the official legal record of the procedure, the operative report. On this document, the circulator records the particulars of the procedure, including the counts, what was done, and the medications that were given. It is the responsibility of the circulator to receive surgical specimens from the surgical technologist, and to record properly where they came from, before they are sent to the laboratory. It might be necessary for the circulator to wipe the brow of any of the scrubbed personnel, so that sweat will not fall onto the sterile field; however, this is a rare event. The circulator handles all the nonsterile equipment present in the operating room during the surgical procedure. This could involve moving or connecting equipment. In addition, the circulator helps to move the patient from the operating room to the recovery room after the procedure is over.

When not scrubbed for a procedure or functioning as a circulator, a surgical technologist may be asked to perform other duties in the surgery department. Surgical technologists need to be familiar with the protocols for receiving patients in the department. They may be asked to take patients to and from the surgical area or within the surgery department. Surgical technologists may help to order supplies for a department and, when they arrive, may help transport the supplies to the appropriate storage cupboard. Supplies need to be ordered from the central supply department or directly from manufacturers. In the operating room, not only must supplies be restocked but the expiration dates on sterile items must be inspected as well, to ensure that no outdated supplies are present in the operating room and given inadvertently to the patient. Surgical technologists may assist in cleaning instruments and supplies after a surgical procedure and preparing them for sterilization and subsequent reuse. They must be familiar with ways to sterilize instruments and supplies and must know which methods to use for which items. If equipment is working improperly, it is the responsibility of the surgical technologist to make sure that the equipment is repaired or replaced.

Working in an operating room is a very demanding occupation. It requires first of all personal integrity. As with any professional, the surgical technologist must be willing to admit mistakes. Often mistakes can be corrected if they are detected early. For example, the surgical technologist might have to say, "I forgot to sterilize the instruments, so we'll have to wait another fifteen minutes," rather than rush ahead to meet a particular deadline. In addition, a surgical technologist has to be able to handle stress-from providing fast and accurate care to a very sick patient, to having a patient die on the operating room table, to working with individuals with whom one does not get along on a personal level, to changing schedules for emergency procedures, to not being able to take a break to go to the restroom, to standing in one position for a whole day or a whole procedure.

No discussion of surgical technology would be complete without some mention of its legal aspects. As of the early twenty-first century in the United States, no state had licensed or defined the practice of surgical technology, although several states, including Texas, Oregon, and Georgia, were working on licensing initiatives. Therefore, the surgical technologist has only the common rights of a citizen on the street. Although no special license is required for surgical technologists, most hospitals prefer, and others require, certification. Surgical technologists can become certified surgical technologists by completing an approved program of at least one year and passing an examination given by the Association of Surgical Technologists (AST). One thing is certain: The surgical technologist is not allowed to practice medicine or nursing.

Since surgical technologists are not physicians, they may not diagnose or treat disease, inject medicine into the human body, or pronounce death. These actions are limited to physicians, and in some states, a physician may not delegate certain actions (such as suturing, cutting or penetrating the human body, and clamping) to a surgical technologist. Similarly, since the surgical technologists are not nurses, they may not administer medications, which is a practice relegated to the field of nursing. At one time, only registered nurses were permitted to act as circulators. Many hospitals now allow surgical technologists to circulate, with a registered nurse standing by for emergencies. When circulating, however, a surgical technologist must remember that only nurses may select and measure medications, a right that cannot be delegated to someone without a license.

Surgical technologists must obey the laws in the performance of their duties. They can be prosecuted for breaking a law or for failing to perform a proper job. Surgical technologists must pay attention to laws involving the respecting of property rights, both of patients and of hospitals. In addition to not exceeding the scope of practice, there is another area of concern for surgical technologists: negligence. Any act of carelessness is called negligence, which is legally defined as "the failure to exercise the care that a reasonably prudent person would exercise under similar circumstances." Although negligence itself is not a crime, surgical technologists must remember that carelessness could endanger the safety of the patient.

The most common areas of negligence (and subsequent malpractice lawsuits) that affect surgical technologists involve the following: proper positioning of side rails and patient supports, abandonment of the patient, surgical consent, patient identification, loss of items inside the patient, specimen collections, burns, and explosions. Carelessness involv-

ing side rails could result in an anesthetized patient falling on the floor. Abandonment refers to the careless act of leaving an incompetent patient alone. The patient must sign a consent, in which he or she agrees to the surgical procedure; this detailed legal document must be present before the procedure is begun, and the procedure may not wander from the permission given. Sponges, instruments, and needles are counted many times before, during, and after the surgical procedure, which helps to reduce the possibility of leaving anything inside the patient. Burns could be caused by the improper grounding of electrical devices used in the operating room, by the application of the wrong soap to the wrong area, or by the use of recently sterilized instruments, which may be too hot to be placed directly in contact with the patient. Explosions are less likely now than they used to be, because explosive medications are no longer used for general anesthesia. Nevertheless, the presence of oxygen in tanks and tubing increases the possibility of explosion and fire. In summary, there are many things about which the surgical technologist must be careful in order to avoid legal complications and injuries to patients.

Perspective and Prospects

Historically, surgical technology began during World War II, when medical and nursing personnel in the armed forces trained men and women to assist in surgery in order to increase the availability of surgical procedures for the wounded. At that time, workers in this area were called operating room technicians. The name has gradually evolved to reflect the many areas where surgical procedures now take place-not only in hospitals but also in outpatient clinics, delivery rooms, and doctors' offices. In the beginning, surgical technologists had to work directly under the supervision of a registered nurse, who was legally required to be present in the operating room at all times.

The Association of Surgical Technologists began as a wing within the Association of Operating Room Nurses, but it later broke away to become the Association of Operating Room Technicians before later changing its name to the current one. Its headquarters are located in Littleton, Colorado. The AST provides many services for its members. It is a private organization that provides a certificate to those surgical technologists who pass a national examination. Certification, however, has little legal significance. States may not delegate their power to provide licenses to a private organization. The certified surgical technologist has demonstrated a level of skills and knowledge; however, one does not have to be certified in order to work as a surgical technologist. The AST also provides continuing education credits, insurance programs, and a magazine, as well as other services.

As the baby boom generation ages, the numbers of surgical procedures are expected to increase. Technological advances, such as fiber optics and laser technology, also allow new surgical procedures to be performed. For these reasons, the U.S. Bureau of Labor projects that employment opportunities for surgical technicians will grow by approximately 35 to 40 percent through the year 2010.

Working as a surgical technologist can be very demanding,

but satisfaction, as in any profession, comes from working with a team in a complex situation in order to achieve a goal. There is satisfaction in a job well done, in being able to work well in stressful situations. There is great satisfaction in seeing the human body in all its complexity and in helping restore it to health. There is satisfaction in knowing in advance what the surgeon is going to use and having it ready at the moment it is needed. It is the excellent surgical technologist who can give the surgeon what is needed and not merely what is asked for.

—*William F. Taylor*

See also Allied health; Anesthesia; Anesthesiology; Education, medical; Malpractice; Nursing; Surgery, general; Surgery, pediatric; Surgical procedures.

For Further Information:

Caruthers, Bob, et al., eds. *Surgical Technology for the Surgical Technologist: A Positive Care Approach*. Florence, Ky.: Cengage Learning, 2009. Includes bibliographical references and an index.

Fuller, Joanna Kotcher. *Surgical Technology: Principles and Practice*. 4th ed. St. Louis, Mo.: Saunders/Elsevier, 2005. An accessible work that functions as a textbook for surgical technologists. Fuller has assembled a wealth of practical clinical information about caring for patients in surgery.

Miller, Benjamin F., Claire Brackman Keane, and Marie T. O'Toole. *Miller-Keane Encyclopedia and Dictionary of Medicine, Nursing, and Allied Health*. Rev. 7th ed. Philadelphia: Saunders/Elsevier, 2005. A comprehensive work which contains much information about the full spectrum of allied health.

Phillips, Nancymarie Fortunato. *Berry and Kohn's Operating Room Technique*. 11th ed. St. Louis, Mo.: Mosby/Elsevier, 2007. Another accessible textbook. This one contains much practical information about what goes on in the operating room.

Rothrock, Jane C., ed. *Alexander's Care of the Patient in Surgery*. 13th ed. St. Louis, Mo.: Mosby/Elsevier, 2007. The bible of surgical techniques and practices. A detailed reference work of the most common surgical procedures.

SWEATING

Biology

Also known as: Perspiration

Anatomy or system affected: Glands, skin

Specialties and related fields: Dermatology, exercise physiology

Definition: The excretion of fluid from the sweat glands in order to cool the body.

Structure and Functions

Sweat glands are exocrine glands, which secrete products that are passed outside the body. There are two major types. Eccrine sweat glands excrete sweat that contains water and several salts. They are located in the skin throughout the body but are found in greater concentrations in the palms of the hands, soles of the feet, and forehead. Apocrine sweat glands excrete sweat that contains water and fatty substances. They are primarily found in the armpits and genital area. When bacteria break down the fatty materials, distinctive sweat odors develop.

The primary function of sweating in humans is to regulate body temperature. When the body temperature rises, the blood flow to the skin increases by opening more capillaries in the skin. Since blood can hold heat and circulates through-

out the body, the blood can transport heat from the inner core of the body, where the temperatures are higher and the heat is more insulated, to the surface, where the heat is less insulated. In the skin, the warm blood will transfer the heat to the surface, where sweat glands release sweat. When the sweat evaporates, changing its physical state from a liquid to a gas, significant amounts of heat are removed from the body.

Disorders and Diseases

Sweating is a normal process that is important for the temperature regulation (thermoregulation) of the body, but complications can arise. The most critical result of excess sweating is dehydration. The biggest risk for dehydration occurs when people exercise in hot, humid environments. Therefore, it is important to drink plenty of water. Additionally, when sweating a lot for a period of days, additional salts may be beneficial. Most sports drinks supply adequate salts. In extreme conditions, the excess loss of water in sweat can lead to heatstroke and death. When the body loses too much water, the sweating mechanism shuts down. Without the advantage of sweat evaporation to cool the body, the temperature will continue to rise until death ensues. Anyone who has symptoms of heat stress-such as a body temperature over 105 degrees Fahrenheit, cessation of sweating, or altered mental state-should get immediate medical attention. The intravenous administration of fluids by medical personnel will rehydrate the body quickly.

A less concerning disorder of sweating is hyperhidrosis. People with this condition sweat frequently and in excess of what is required to regulate body temperature. About 1 percent of people have this condition; it is often linked to obesity. There are numerous treatments but no cure. Typical treatments include surgery, medications, biofeedback, relaxation, hypnosis, and weight loss.

—*Bradley R. A. Wilson, Ph.D.*

See also Dehydration; Dermatology; Exercise physiology; Fever; Glands; Heat exhaustion and heatstroke; Host-defense mechanisms; Hyperhidrosis; Physiology; Signs and symptoms; Skin; Sympathectomy.

For Further Information:

Brooks, George A., Thomas D. Fahey, and Kenneth M. Baldwin. *Exercise Physiology: Human Bioenergetics and Its Applications*. 4th ed. Boston: McGraw-Hill, 2007.

McArdle, William, Frank I. Katch, and Victor L. Katch. *Exercise Physiology: Energy, Nutrition, and Human Performance*. 7th ed. Boston: Lippincott Williams & Wilkins, 2010.

Powers, Scott K., and Edward T. Howley. *Exercise Physiology: Theory and Application to Fitness and Performance*. 7th ed. New York: McGraw-Hill, 2009.

SYMPATHECTOMY

Procedure

Anatomy or system affected: Back, neck, nerves, nervous system, spine

Specialties and related fields: General surgery, neurology

Definition: The surgical interruption of part of the sympathetic nerve pathway.

Indications and Procedures

The autonomic nervous system controls the involuntary internal environment of humans, and the sympathetic nerves increase energy expenditures by accelerating the heart rate, increasing the metabolic rate, and constricting and dilating blood vessels, among other actions. Occasionally, the proper regulation of vasoconstriction or vasodilation goes awry, and the sympathetic nervous system causes prolonged and inappropriate constriction of the blood vessels to a specific area. In Raynaud's phenomenon, there is intermittent constricting of blood vessels when the fingers, toes, ears, or nose is exposed to cold. The affected areas change color from white to blue to red, and the condition can be associated with numbness, tingling, burning, and pain. Symptoms of long-term blood vessel constriction associated with decreased blood flow include cold and clammy skin, areas of gangrene, and painful fibrous growths and infections. In other cases, excessive sweating and facial blushing may be candidates for correction with sympathectomy.

After the specific nerves are located, the patient is prepared for surgery and opened in the location of the nerves, typically the neck or back area. Organs are moved or adjusted as needed. The offending region of nerve is clipped from the remainder and removed. The organs are replaced or repaired, and the incisions are closed. Normal vascular dilation will return rapidly and with it warmth to the area and healing of the infections, fibrous tissue, and areas of gangrene.

In the treatment of excessive sweating, often sympathectomy can be performed as an outpatient procedure under local anesthesia. A small incision is made under the armpit and air is introduced into the chest cavity. The surgeon inserts a fiber-optic tube, or endoscope, which projects an image onto a screen. Lasers are used to destroy the ganglia involved in the excessive sweating.

Uses and Complications

To determine if sympathectomy is an appropriate treatment, the nerve in question is injected with a steroid and anesthetic to block the nerve function temporarily. If the condition in question is relieved, then the patient will likely benefit from sympathectomy. After surgery is completed, Doppler ultrasonography, which uses sound waves to measure blood flow, can be used to determine whether the procedure has succeeded in increasing circulation.

Potential complications include those common to all major surgeries. Depending on the type of sympathectomy performed, side effects may involve a decrease in blood pressure when standing, which can lead to fainting spells. About 30 percent of cases of sympathectomy for treatment of excessive sweating result in an increase in sweating of the chest, but the procedure is 90 percent effective in alleviating excessive sweating of the face, hands, and feet.

—*Karen E. Kalumuck, Ph.D.*

See also Circulation; Nervous system; Neuralgia, neuritis, and neuropathy; Neuroimaging; Neurology; Neurosurgery; Sweating; Vascular medicine; Vascular system.

For Further Information:

Ernst, Calvin B., and James C. Stanley, eds. *Current Therapy in Vascular Surgery.* 4th ed. St. Louis, Mo.: Mosby, 2001.

Ganong, William F. *Review of Medical Physiology.* 23d ed. New York: Lange Medical Books/McGraw-Hill Medical, 2009.

Griffith, H. Winter. *Complete Guide to Symptoms, Illness, and Surgery.* Revised and updated by Stephen Moore and Kenneth Yoder. 5th ed. New York: Perigee, 2006.

Rutherford, Robert B., ed. *Vascular Surgery.* 6th ed. Philadelphia: Saunders/Elsevier, 2005.

SYNDROME

Disease/Disorder

Also known as: Condition, disease, disorder

Anatomy or system affected: All

Specialties and related fields: All

Definition: A group or pattern of recognizable symptoms or conditions that occur together and indicate a specific disease, psychological disorder, or other abnormal condition.

Key terms:

disorder: abnormal physical or mental condition

symptom: indication of a disorder

Causes and Symptoms

A syndrome is a collection of symptoms that characterize a disorder. For example, metabolic syndrome is the name given to a group of symptoms that warn of potential heart disease, stroke, or diabetes. The symptoms of metabolic syndrome are obesity, high blood pressure, low levels of insulin, and high cholesterol.

Syndromes can be grouped into roughly fourteen categories: environmental (caused by the environment); congenital (existing at birth); gastrointestinal (affecting the stomach and intestines); cardiovascular (involving the heart and blood vessels); iatrogenic (induced by a treatment or procedure); neoplastic (caused by a malignant or benign tumor); endocrine (affecting glands, including sex glands); pulmonary (involving the lung); infectious (caused by a virus, bacterium, or fungus); renal (involving the kidneys); reticuloendothelial (affecting cells, including blood cells); neurological (affecting the nervous system); psychopathological (affecting the mind and behavior); and medically unexplained (cause uncertain).

The causes of syndromes vary. Some come from a single, clear source. For example, toxic shock syndrome is caused by the bacterium *Staphylococcus aureus.* The bacterium enters the body through wounds from injuries or surgery incisions. It also breeds in superabsorbent tampons and contraceptive sponges. Symptoms of this syndrome include fever, headache, vomiting, diarrhea, and muscle aches.

Chinese restaurant syndrome is caused by monosodium glutamate (MSG), a chemical compound widely used to enhance the flavor of foods. MSG can induce headache, dizziness, giddiness, a feeling of facial pressure, tingling sensations over parts of the body, and chest pain.

Some syndromes result from any one of an array of causes. Fanconi syndrome, for instance, activates the release of certain substances from the kidney into the urine instead of the bloodstream. It can be caused by genetic defects, inherited diseases, exposure to heavy metals, a kidney transplant, or any number of medicines or diseases that damage the kidneys.

Other syndromes, such as carpal tunnel syndrome, arise from a combination of causes. This syndrome stems from increased pressure on certain nerves and tendons in the carpal tunnel in the wrist. Most people prone to carpal tunnel syndrome are born with a comparatively small carpal tunnel. This condition is complicated by injury to the wrist, an overactive pituitary gland, an underactive thyroid, rheumatoid arthritis, or repeated use of vibrating hand tools.

The causes of some syndromes remain uncertain. For example, Reye's syndrome is a rapidly appearing, deadly disorder that affects all body organs, most seriously the brain and liver. It attacks adults but is primarily a children's disease. Symptoms include personality changes, seizures, and loss of consciousness. There is no cure. The cause is unknown, but there seems to be a link to the use of aspirin taken for a previous viral disease.

Restless legs syndrome is the nighttime twitching of the legs that often leads to insomnia. The cause is unknown, but there seems to be some connection to a family history of the disorder. Also associated with this syndrome are anemia, diabetes, kidney failure, and certain prescription and nonprescription medicines.

Just as the causes vary, so too do the number and severity of symptoms, depending on the syndrome. Barrett's esophagus, for example, is a condition in which the esophagus (the tube that carries food to the stomach) develops new cells similar to those found in the intestines. Symptoms are nonexistent, and the cause is unknown. It can, however, lead to a deadly type of esophageal cancer.

The symptoms of premenstrual syndrome (PMS) vary widely in number and severity from woman to woman. Some women experience few symptoms; others need several days of bed rest. Symptoms include irritability, headache, backache, weight gain, swelling or tenderness of the breasts, depression, fatigue, and loss of sex drive.

Some fifty different symptoms, or characteristics, are associated with Down syndrome. Characteristics include mental retardation; short stature; slow physical growth; weak muscles; short, stocky arms and legs; a wide space between the big toe and second toe; small, low-set ears; a narrow roof of the mouth; crooked teeth and other dental problems; heart defects; an underactive thyroid; and hearing problems. So many symptoms require a lifetime of care.

Asperger's syndrome produces no symptoms that require medical attention, but people with this disorder display abnormal behaviors and have limited social skills that can bring on unwanted consequences, such as being shunned by others. Some people with this disorder seem "normal" most of the time. Others just seem odd or different from other people, quieter and disinterested. Still others exhibit somewhat bizarre, or at least socially unacceptable, behaviors, such as inflexible routines, a narrow but intense focus of interests, an inability to empathize with other people, and difficulty understanding some types of humor, especially teasing and sarcasm. Yet they are often above average in intelligence and do no more harm than so-called normal people. The odd behaviors lead people to think that Asperger's syndrome is a mental disorder. In fact, it is a type of autism, a developmental disorder that affects how the brain processes information. The cause is unknown.

Treatment and Therapy

Treatment of a syndrome depends on the underlying causes and the severity and number of symptoms. Because syndromes run the full range of medical problems, treatments run the full range as well. Drugs, surgery, physical therapy, diet and lifestyle changes, alternative medicine, and psychotherapy are all used to treat syndromes.

Perspective and Prospects

Both Western and Eastern medical practitioners have long recognized that a set of symptoms can describe an abnormal condition. Syndromes are researched, diagnosed, and treated no differently than individual diseases are.

—*Wendell Anderson*

See also Acquired immunodeficiency syndrome (AIDS); Acute respiratory distress syndrome (ARDS); Asperger's syndrome; Blue baby syndrome; Carpal tunnel syndrome; Chronic fatigue syndrome; Cornelia de Lange syndrome; Cushing's syndrome; Diagnosis; DiGeorge syndrome; Disease; Down syndrome; Fetal alcohol syndrome; Fragile X syndrome; Guillain-Barré syndrome; Gulf War syndrome; Hemolytic uremic syndrome; Irritable bowel syndrome (IBS); Klinefelter syndrome; Klippel-Trenaunay syndrome; Kluver-Bucy syndrome; Marfan syndrome; Metabolic syndrome; Multiple chemical sensitivity syndrome; Münchausen syndrome by proxy; Overtraining syndrome; Polycystic ovary syndrome; Prader-Willi syndrome; Premenstrual syndrome (PMS); Reiter's syndrome; Respiratory distress syndrome; Restless legs syndrome; Reye's syndrome; Rubinstein-Taybi syndrome; Severe acute respiratory syndrome (SARS); Severe combined immunodeficiency syndrome (SCID); Signs and symptoms; Sjögren's syndrome; Stevens-Johnson syndrome; Sturge-Weber syndrome; Sudden infant death syndrome (SIDS); Temporomandibular joint (TMJ) syndrome; Tourette's syndrome; Toxic shock syndrome; Turner syndrome; Wiskott-Aldrich syndrome.

For Further Information:

Kirmayer, Laurence, et al. "Explaining Medically Unexplained Symptoms." *Canadian Journal of Psychiatry* 49, no. 10 (October, 2004): 663-672.

McConnaughy, Rozalynd. "Asperger Syndrome: Living Outside the Bell Curve." *Journal of the Medical Library Association* 93, no. 1 (January, 2005): 139-140.

Pease, Roger, Jr., ed. *Merriam-Webster's Medical Desk Dictionary*. Rev. ed. Springfield, Mass.: Merriam-Webster, 2002.

Rice, Shirley. "Reye's Syndrome Isn't Just Child's Play." *Nursing* 33, no. 9 (September, 2003): 32hn1-32hn4.

Wallis, Claudia. "The Down Syndrome Dilemma." *Time* 166, no. 20 (November 14, 2005).

SYNESTHESIA
Disease/Disorder

Anatomy or system affected: Brain, nervous system, psychic-emotional system

Specialties and related fields: Genetics, neurology, psychiatry, psychology

Definition: A phenomenon wherein one sensory stimulus-a word or a musical note, for example-automatically induces a second, unstimulated sensory perception, typically a color.

Key terms:

functional magnetic resonance imaging (fMRI): a radiologic technique that shows regional oxygen uptake, indicating brain activity

grapheme: a written character or element-letter, word, or number

photism: in synesthesia, a vivid light or color sensation induced by a different sensory stimulus

positron emission tomography (PET): a technique that creates three-dimensional computer images from particles emitted after radioactively tagged substances are incorporated into body tissues; particle concentrations identify areas of increased energy metabolism

synesthete: a person who experiences synesthesia by virtue of having a second sensation evoked by a single stimulus

Causes and Symptoms

The term "synesthesia" derives from the Greek *syn-* (union/together) and *aisthesis* (sensation/perception). Regarded as an intriguing but perhaps bogus curiosity, synesthesia was once disparaged as a subjective experience unworthy of scientific interest. Since the 1980s, however, neuroimaging techniques have established the synesthetic experience as a genuine sensorineural phenomenon and a legitimate subject for scientific research. Described as rare by some and as common by others, synesthesia gives rise to widely divergent estimates of its prevalence: from 1 in 20,000 people to 1 in 23.

Various combinations of synesthetic experiences have been documented, but color is the most common concurrent perception. Of the many different types, none has been more intensively studied than grapheme-color synesthesia; specific characters written in black print induce the experience of a specific color. The induced color experiences, termed "photisms," are vivid and consistent; a specific grapheme always induces the same color in the same synesthete. A spoken word or musical note can act as the stimulus, and days of the week or months of the year also trigger colors-for some, Friday will always be chartreuse. Rarer synesthetic experiences involve touch or taste. Mirror-touch synesthesia activates a tactile sensation in the synesthete's body when someone within sight is touched. In tactile-emotion synesthesia, textures induce distinct emotions. Some synesthetes experience a specific taste on hearing a word or piece of music.

Synesthesia has a strong genetic component, although the mode of inheritance is unclear. Familial aggregation in synesthesia was first noted by Sir Francis Galton in 1880.

Information on Synesthesia

Causes: Unknown; probably increased connectivity and cross-wiring in contiguous brain regions

Symptoms: Subjective manifestations involve two or more concurrent sensory perceptions when only one has been stimulated

Duration: Generally lifelong

Treatments: Primarily occurs in neurologically and psychologically normal people, does not warrant medical treatment

One study found a greater than 40 percent prevalence of synesthesia among first-degree relatives of synesthetes. A report of monozygotic (identical) male twins discordant for grapheme-color synesthesia casts doubt on what was initially believed to be X-linked dominant inheritance; documented male-to-male transmission also argues against it. Genetic linkage studies suggest a complex pattern of inheritance, perhaps with multiple gene loci. Different types commonly coexist in the same family, and heterogeneity is characteristic. Within one type, the same word or letter evokes different colors in different individuals, and the subjective experience differs as well.

Diagnosis and Detection

Recognition begins with a self-report. Various psychological tests can distinguish between synesthetes and nonsynesthetes; neuroimaging is generally limited to research. Some diagnostic criteria have been generally accepted: synesthetic sensory experience is involuntary, automatic, and durable-synesthetes typically report their sensory associations as consistent over years.

Considerable evidence supports the neural basis of synesthesia. Neurologic injury can evoke synesthetic associations, and drugs such as mescaline can induce them. Brain imaging, however, identifies synesthesia as a neural phenomenon. The pattern of cerebral blood flow during a synesthetic experience, first recorded in the 1980s, was described as abnormal. Subsequent studies have used positron emission tomography (PET) and functional magnetic resonance imaging (fMRI) to show differences in brain structure and activity between synesthetes and nonsynesthetes.

Grapheme-color synesthesia has been the main focus of fMRI studies. According to posited models, increased connectivity between contiguous brain areas in the cerebral cortex facilitates cross-activation. The fusiform gyrus, involved both in color and grapheme processing, has shown increased activation in addition to increased cortical thickness, volume, and surface area. Increased white matter volume and connectivity has been observed in brains of some synesthetes compared with those of nonsynesthetic counterparts.

Can developmental mechanisms explain synesthesia? Some investigators suggest that incoming sensory information in infants is normally jumbled together, and pruning of comingled neural and synaptic connections comes with development. According to this hypothesis, sensorineural connections in synesthetic adults somehow escaped the pruning process, perhaps via mutation.

Perspective and Prospects

Synesthesia has a long and distinguished history. Around 1710, an English ophthalmologist reported a blind patient who experienced color visions that were induced by sound. Jonathan Swift's title character in *Gulliver's Travels* (1726) encountered a group of blind apprentices taught by their blind master to mix colors by touch and smell. Swift's source was believed to be the Royal Society scientists of his day, notably Robert Boyle. Francis Galton established synesthesia as a scientific entity in 1880.

The idea that the various senses are fused could be found in literature much before it resonated in neurology. Mary Shelley described the creature in *Frankenstein* (1818) as having a difficult time separating his various sensations because he simultaneously saw, felt, heard, and smelled. Later in the nineteenth century, psychologist William James expressed his view that incoming information from different senses is fused in a child before it is later untangled.

The renaissance of scientific research into synesthesia is prompted by the recognition that synesthesia can be a window into the nature of perception. Among the remaining questions is its true prevalence, which is of more than theoretical interest. Some evidence suggests that synesthetic crossmodal mechanisms are universal, even if below the level of consciousness in most adults. Human sensory experiences and their interconnections will undoubtedly continue to intrigue scientists and artists alike well into the future.

—*Judith Weinblatt, M.A., M.S.*

See also Hearing; Nervous system; Neurology; Neurology, pediatric; Sense organs; Smell; Taste; Touch; Vision.

For Further Information:

American Synesthesia Association. http://synesthesia .info. Raises awareness of synesthesia and sponsors periodic conferences that provide a forum and information source for researchers and synesthetes.

Beeli, Gian, et al. "Synaesthesia: When Coloured Sounds Taste Sweet." *Nature* 434 (March 3, 2005): 38.

Mass, Wendy. *A Mango-Shaped Space*. Boston: Little, Brown, 2003.

Ramachandran, Vilayanur, and Edward Hubbard. "Hearing Colors, Tasting Shapes." *Scientific American* 288, no. 5 (May, 2003): 42-49.

Van Campen, Cretien. *The Hidden Sense: Synesthesia in Art and Science*. Cambridge, Mass.: MIT Press, 2007.

SYPHILIS

Disease/Disorder

Also known as: "Bad blood," bejel (endemic syphilis)

Anatomy or system affected: Anus, bones, brain, eyes, genitals, heart, joints, kidneys, nervous system, reproductive system

Specialties and related fields: Bacteriology, embryology, epidemiology, gynecology, internal medicine, microbiology, neonatology, neurology, pediatrics, public health, rheumatology

Definition: A sexually transmitted disease caused by the spirochete bacterium *Treponema palladum* that can progress from a genital lesion to a systemic disorder involving multiple organs.

Causes and Symptoms

Syphilis is a sexually transmitted disease (STD) resulting from infection by *Treponema palladum*. The history of the disease is unclear. Evidence exists that its origin may have been linked with a disease, yaws, found in the Western Hemisphere at the time of explorer Christopher Columbus (1451-1506). Yaws is a relatively mild disease generally transmitted through contaminated objects or open skin lesions, but not generally through sexual transmission; it results from infection by a subspecies of *Treponema* called *T. palladum ssp. pertenue*. The theory suggests that this may have been the form of the disease brought back to Europe on one of Columbus's ships. Mutation and sexual transmission in the population of Europe may have produced the more serious form of the disease.

The disease is characterized by several distinct stages. Initial exposure to the organism during sexual intercourse results in formation of a painless skin lesion called a chancre at the site of infection (primary syphilis), developing anywhere from a week to months after infection. Spirochete bacteria may be isolated from the lesion, as well as being found live inside white blood cells (macrophages and neutrophils) that infiltrate the area. The white cells may be a mechanism for systemic spread of the organism. The lesion generally heals spontaneously, leaving the impression that the disease has been eliminated.

During the weeks after formation of the chancre, the spirochetes multiply to large numbers and become disseminated throughout the body. A second stage (secondary syphilis) often appears within two months following regression of the chancre. Symptoms are often described as flulike, with malaise, headache, fever, and joint aches. A skin rash often appears, covering most of the body. Sores may develop in the mouth and throat and on many of the mucous membranes in the body. The organism is highly transmissible during this period. The rash and other symptoms generally fade over a period of weeks.

Approximately 10 percent of untreated cases develop a third, or tertiary, stage of syphilis. The organism can infiltrate any organ or system in the body, resulting in soft tumors (gummas) in the eyes, lungs, bone, brain, or other organs. Symptoms are characteristic of the organ infected. For example, infection of the brain or other areas of the central nervous system are described as neurosyphilis or syphilitic dementia, characterized by memory loss, personality changes, and neurodegeneration. Even if tertiary syphilis is treated, prognosis for the patient at this stage is often poor.

Treponema has the ability to cross the placenta, and the infection of a pregnant woman may result in congenital syphilis, or infection of her unborn child. Infection may kill the fetus or cause it to be born with obvious deformities such as blindness or physical abnormalities. The infant may also be

Information on Syphilis

Causes: Bacterial infection transmitted through sexual contact or congenitally

Symptoms: In sexually transmitted form, painless skin lesion (chancre), malaise, headache, fever, joint aches, rash, sores in mouth and throat, and soft tumors in eyes, lungs, bone, or brain if untreated; in congenital form, stillbirth, blindness, physical abnormalities

Duration: Progressive, fatal if untreated

Treatments: Antibiotics (penicillin; also erythromycin, tetracyclines, chloramphenicol)

asymptomatic. An undiagnosed infection will likely progress, with symptoms appearing within weeks after birth. It is common for a rash to appear, with evidence of tertiary stage neurosyphilis or cardiovascular syphilis.

A diagnosis of syphilis can be made through microscopic examination of lesion exudates, noting the presence of spirochetes. However, *Treponema* is notoriously unstable, and the test must be made shortly after obtaining the specimen. More commonly, diagnosis is based upon serological testing for serum antibodies against the organism or tissue lipids released from infected or damaged cells.

Treatment and Therapy

Penicillin is the preferred method of treatment for both primary and secondary syphilis. If the disease has progressed to the tertiary stage, then antibiotic treatment will still eliminate the organism, but it will not reverse organ damage that may have occurred. Treatment for related organ involvement is symptomatic.

Alternative antibiotics include erythromycin, tetracyclines, and chloramphenicol, if necessary. However, only penicillin is effective during the tertiary stage or for use in pregnant women.

Perspective and Prospects

Despite the long-time existence of effective therapy, penicillin or alternative antibiotics, and the absence of any reservoir for *T. palladum* other than humans, syphilis remains the third most common sexually transmitted bacterial disease in the West. Only gonorrhea and chlamydia are more common.

As a result of effective therapy and the generally obvious symptoms of the disease, tertiary syphilis has largely disappeared. However, sexual practices continue to sustain spread of the disease, with approximately fifty thousand cases reported each year in the United States. Three factors are primary contributors to the resurgence of the disease: prostitution, the increase in riskier sexual practices among homosexual men, and general apathy toward a disease that is relatively easy to treat in its early stages. An increase in congenital syphilis also reflects the presence of the disease in women of childbearing years. In the absence of condom use, both unwanted pregnancy and the spread of STDs such as syphilis may result.

No vaccine currently exists for syphilis. The inability to culture the organism in the laboratory has made research related to *Treponema* difficult, and the organism does not infect animals other than humans to act as a method of vaccine production. However, genetic engineering has resulted in the cloning of several bacterial gene products related to surface proteins and virulence factors, allowing the possibility for a vaccine in the future. For now, the best means of controlling syphilis remains the prevention of its spread through education and safer-sex practices, as well as early treatment of those infected.

—*Richard Adler, Ph.D.*

See also Antibiotics; Bacterial infections; Birth defects; Chlamydia; Genital disorders, female; Genital disorders, male; Gonorrhea; Lesions; Neonatology; Pregnancy and gestation; Rashes; Sexually transmitted diseases (STDs).

For Further Information:

Centers for Disease Control and Prevention. *The National Plan to Eliminate Syphilis from the United States*. Atlanta: U.S. Department of Health and Human Services, 2006.

Mandell, Gerald L., John E. Bennett, and Raphael Dolin, eds. *Mandell, Douglas, and Bennett's Principles and Practice of Infectious Diseases*. 7th ed. New York: Churchill Livingstone/Elsevier, 2010.

Murray, Patrick R., Ken S. Rosenthal, and Michael A. Pfaller. *Medical Microbiology*. 6th ed. Philadelphia: Mosby/Elsevier, 2009.

Parker, James N., and Philip M. Parker, eds. *The Official Patient's Sourcebook on Syphilis*. San Diego, Calif.: Icon Health, 2002.

Quetel, Claude. *The History of Syphilis*. Baltimore: Johns Hopkins University Press, 1990.

Sutton, Amy L., ed. *Sexually Transmitted Diseases Sourcebook*. 3d ed. Detroit, Mich.: Omnigraphics, 2006.

SYSTEMIC LUPUS ERYTHEMATOSUS (SLE)

Disease/Disorder

Also known as: Lupus

Anatomy or system affected: All

Specialties and related fields: Cardiology, dermatology, endocrinology, family medicine, gastroenterology, histology, immunology, internal medicine, nephrology, nutrition, orthopedics, pharmacology, physical therapy, psychiatry, psychology, pulmonary medicine, rheumatology, vascular medicine

Definition: A chronic, inflammatory autoimmune disease in which the immune system attacks the body's own structures. SLE can affect any organ or body system, especially the skin, joints, blood vessels, and kidneys. It is distinguished from two other forms of lupus: drug-induced lupus, which is caused by certain prescription medications, and discoid lupus, which primarily affects the skin.

Key terms:

antibodies: proteins manufactured by the body to attack and neutralize foreign substances, such as bacteria

antinuclear antibody (ANA): an unusual antibody that is directed against structures within the nucleus of cells

autoantibodies: antibodies that attack the body's own cells and tissues

autoimmune: a term describing a disease in which the body

produces antibodies against its own cells

connective tissue: the substance holding the body and organs together

cytotoxic: having a damaging effect on cells

discoid rash: raised red patches

erythematosus: characterized by redness of the skin

hyperlipidemia: an excess of lipids (for example, cholesterol and triglycerides) in the blood

malar rash: a redness or rash on the face covering the cheeks and the bridge of the nose; also called butterfly rash

photosensitivity: a sensitivity to light or sunlight

Raynaud's phenomenon: discoloration and pain in the fingertips induced by cold

serositis: inflammation of the lining of the lung or heart

Causes and Symptoms

The cause of lupus is unknown, but scientists believe that both genetic and environmental factors are involved. Although there is a genetic predisposition to lupus, and researchers have identified an associated gene in some cases, only 10 percent of lupus patients have a familial connection and only 5 percent of children born to individuals with lupus will develop the disease. People of African, American Indian, Asian, and Hispanic origin seem to develop the disease more frequently than do non-Hispanic Caucasians. Lupus affects both men and women, but the incidence is ten to fifteen times higher in women and between 85 and 90 percent of patients are women. The majority of lupus diagnoses occur in young women in their late teens to thirties. It is possible that hormonal factors play a role in this disparity, because it is known that symptoms in women increase before menstrual cycles and during pregnancy. Environmental triggers include infections, exposure to ultraviolet light, and extreme stress, as well as antibiotic usage (particularly penicillin and those in the sulfa group). Certain other drugs, particularly hydralazine, procainamide, and isoniazid, can also cause lupus, but this type of drug-induced lupus usually disappears after the offending drug is discontinued.

Symptoms may begin suddenly with fever or may develop gradually over the course of months or years. The clinical course is usually marked by remissions, periods when symptoms are minimal or absent, and relapses (called flare-ups), when the patient experiences an aggravation of symptoms and general malaise.

SLE can affect all organ systems of the body. The production of autoantibodies is the underlying physiologic problem in lupus. These autoantibodies can appear in a great number and variety, differing from patient to patient, thus causing their varying symptoms. General symptoms include fatigue, fever, anemia, weight loss, Raynaud's phenomenon, and headaches. Joint inflammation and pain (arthritis) occurs in about 90 percent of patients and is often the earliest manifestation of the disease. It usually occurs intermittently and generally does not cause permanent joint damage or deformity. Skin manifestations are present in most patients and include malar (butterfly) and/or discoid skin rashes; redness on the hands, fingertips, and nails; mucous membrane ulcers in the

---

Information on Systemic Lupus Erythematosus (SLE)

Causes: Unclear; possibly related to paramyxoviral infection

Symptoms: Red or purple facial lesions, joint pain and swelling, fatigue, low-grade fever

Duration: Chronic

Treatments: None; alleviation of symptoms

---

mouth and nose; and photosensitivity. Inflammation of the sac around the lungs (pleurisy) or heart (pericarditis) is a frequent occurrence, resulting in pain upon deep breathing or chest pain. On rare occasions, there may be severe complications, such as bleeding into the lungs, which is life-threatening, or cardiac failure. Neurologic complications may also occur, including headaches, thinking impairment, personality changes, seizures, strokes, depression, dementia and psychosis. Kidney involvement may be either minor or progressive, leading to severe nephritis that can be fatal. Ocular changes sometimes occur, causing conjunctivitis or blurred vision. In rare cases, retinitis, inflammation of the blood vessels at the back of the eye, can occur, leading to blindness if not treated quickly.

SLE is difficult to diagnose, due to its variety of symptoms and similarity to many other diseases. The constellation of symptoms appears and progresses differently for each patient and initially may seem vague and unrelated. Usually, patients will first see their family doctors. Upon diagnosis or the discovery of particular body system involvement, the family doctor may refer the patient on to one or more specialists. There is no single test for lupus. A physician will perform several laboratory tests as part of the differential diagnostic process, including various blood and urine tests and biopsies of the skin and kidney. For a positive diagnosis of SLE, a patient must have at least four of the eleven criteria established by the American College of Rheumatology: malar rash, discoid rash, photosensitivity, oral ulcers, arthritis, serositis, renal disorder, neurologic disorder, hematologic disorder, immunologic disorder, and the presence of antinuclear antibodies (ANA).

Treatment and Therapy

There is no cure for lupus. Treatment is aimed at minimizing symptoms, reducing inflammation, and maintaining normal bodily functions. The treatment approach will vary according to the specific symptoms and organ involvement of the individual patient.

Preventive therapy involves lifestyle strategies aimed at reducing the risk of flare-up episodes. Patients are advised to follow a healthy diet, get adequate rest, and participate in moderate weight-bearing exercise in order to combat fatigue and muscle weakness. Counseling, support groups, and patient education help reduce stress and protect emotional well-being. Other recommendations include smoking cessation, limited alcohol intake, and adequate intake of vitamin D and calcium. Avoidance of excessive sun exposure through the use of protective clothing and sunscreens can reduce the occurrence of skin rashes and possibly systemic disease flares. Patients can learn to recognize the warning signs of an impending flare-up, such as increased fatigue, headaches, dizziness, stomach upset, fever, or the appearance of a rash. Regular laboratory tests can also detect an imminent flare-up. Early treatment of flare-ups can make them easier to control, can prevent tissue damage, and may reduce the length of time that the patient is given high doses of drugs.

Medications are an integral part of the treatment of lupus, and fall into four main categories: nonsteroidal anti-inflammatory drugs (NSAIDs), corticosteroids, antimalarial drugs, and cytotoxic and immunosuppressive agents.

NSAIDs are used to control symptoms and reduce muscle and joint pain and inflammation. Commonly used NSAIDs include acetylsalicylic acid (aspirin), ibuprofen, naproxen, indomethacin, sulindac, nabumetone, tolmetin, and ketoprofen. Since these drugs can cause stomach upset, patients are usually advised to take them with meals or to take antacids or prostaglandins as well. Some NSAIDs have a prostaglandin added to the capsule. Patients taking NSAIDs must be monitored because of the potential adverse effects to the liver, kidney, and central nervous system.

Corticosteriods are synthetic hormones that have excellent anti-inflammatory and immunoregulatory effects and reduce symptoms promptly. They are used to treat a spectrum of lupus manifestations, especially in cases when organs are threatened. Prednisone is the most commonly used, followed by hydrocortisone, methylprednisolone, and others. Topical formulations are used for skin rashes, and oral doses are given for systemic involvement. Dosages are monitored carefully and tapered after initial inflammation reduction is achieved in order to reduce possible side effects. Corticosteroids may also be administered by injection into the skin or joint. For severe cases, intravenous administration of large doses of methylprednisolone (called pulse steroids) for three days is given. Unfortunately, high doses of corticosteroids over long periods of time can produce unpleasant side effects, such as weight gain, rounded face, acne, emotional lability, hypertension, hyperlipidemia, increased risk of infection, diabetes, and osteoporosis.

Antimalarial drugs are frequently used in the management of skin rashes, joint inflammation, and serositis, though it may take months before their beneficial effects become apparent. They also help protect against the damaging effects of ultraviolet light. The most common agents are hydroxychloroquine (Plaquenil), chloroquine (Aralen), and quinicrine (Atabrine). These medications can be taken in combination with NSAIDs and other drugs to increase their effectiveness. They are particularly helpful when used with corticosteroids in order to decrease the amount of steroid needed. Damage to the retina is a potential side effect and is dose-related. Patients must be evaluated by an ophthalmologist twice a year.

Cytotoxic and immunosuppressive agents are potent drugs utilized in cases requiring aggressive therapy to protect major organs. They are used in conjunction with, or in place of, corticosteroids in order to spare the patient the side effects of the corticosteroids. Cytotoxics are not approved by the Food and Drug Administration (FDA) for use in the treatment of SLE; however, they are considered part of standard practice. These drugs target autoantibodies, thus suppressing the overactive immune response of lupus patients. Cyclophosphamide (Cytoxin) and azathioprine (Imuran) are both used in the treatment of lupus nephritis and are also effective in combating blood cell deficiencies, pulmonary bleeding, vasculitis, and central nervous system disease. Imuran is less potent but causes fewer side effects than does Cytoxin. Methotrexate, mycophenolate mofetil (CellCept), cyclosporine, chlorambucil, and nitrogen mustard are other cytotoxic agents that have been used in the management of lupus. Intravenous immunoglobulin injections are given to some patients to increase the production of blood platelets. Side effects of cytotoxic drugs include nausea, hair loss, increased risk of certain cancers, increased risk of infection, sterility, and bone marrow suppression.

Pregnancy in a lupus patient requires special care. Even though more than 50 percent of lupus pregnancies follow a normal course, all lupus pregnancies are considered high risk. Doctors recommend planning pregnancy during times of remission. Recent studies contradict the traditional belief that pregnancy increases the chance of flare-ups and also suggest that most flare-ups during pregnancy are mild, consisting only of rashes, fatigue, and arthritis. Frequent doctor visits are a necessity in order to detect and treat any problems early. The obstetrician will regularly check the baby's growth and heartbeat in order to detect any abnormalities that might signal problems. Some lupus medications, such as prednisone, are safe to take during pregnancy because they do not cross the placenta. Others, such as cyclophosphamide, need to be used with caution or discontinued during the pregnancy.

About 20 percent of women with lupus experience preeclampsia during their pregnancy. This is a serious condition in which there is a sudden increase in blood pressure and/or protein in the urine requiring immediate treatment of the patient and delivery of the baby.

About one-third of women with lupus have antiphospholipid antibodies. These antibodies cause blood clots, which puts the patient at risk for developing them in the placenta, interfering with the nourishment of the baby. Since these blood clots usually form in the placenta in the second trimester, often the baby has developed enough to be delivered prematurely. The mother can be treated with heparin, which reduces the chance of clots and miscarriage.

About 50 percent of lupus pregnancies result in birth before full term. The majority of babies born between thirty and thirty-six weeks will grow normally with no problems. Those born before thirty-six weeks are considered premature. Approximately 3 percent of women with lupus will have a baby with a syndrome called neonatal lupus. This syndrome consists of a transient rash and blood count abnormalities and disappears by three to six months of age. Sometimes, a permanent abnormality in the heartbeat also occurs, but it is treatable and the baby is able to grow normally.

Perspective and Prospects

The identification of lupus as a distinct medical entity dates back to the twelfth century, when the term "lupus" (Latin for "wolf") was used to describe ulcerative facial lesions, because they looked similar to either a wolf's bite or a wolf's facial markings. Other descriptions of the various dermatologic manifestations of lupus were noted by physicians over the next several centuries; the first medical textbook illustration occurred in 1856. The Viennese physician Moriz Kaposi, in 1872, was the first physician to recognize and describe the systemic manifestations of lupus, as well as the fact that there seemed to be two distinct forms of lupus, discoid and systemic. This was soon expanded upon by Canadian physician Sir William Osler, who detailed the major organ manifestations. In the late nineteenth century, the usefulness of quinine and salicylates in the treatment of lupus was reported. In the mid-twentieth century, the discovery of the immunologic aspects of lupus were discovered, when the presence of antinuclear antibodies were identified. Around this same time, the first animal models were used for the study of lupus, and the genetic component of lupus was also recognized. A major advance was the discovery of the effectiveness of cortisone in the treatment of systemic lupus. Corticosteroids remain the primary treatment modality, complemented by antimalarials (for skin and joint involvement) and cytotoxic agents (for severe kidney manifestations and other life-threatening complications).

The prognosis for lupus patients has improved dramatically as a result of earlier diagnosis and better treatment. The long-term prognosis for a given patient is still variable, however, and is often related to the severity and the controllability of the initial inflammation. Also, the morbidity patterns of lupus patients have changed because of the increased usage of corticosteroids and cytotoxic drugs. Infections, accelerated atherosclerosis, and osteoporosis have become significant risk factors. Overall, however, the outlook for survival and quality of life has greatly improved. As of 2005, more than 90 percent of lupus patients lived more than ten years postdiagnosis. Those with organ-threatening disease had a lower rate, with only 60 percent surviving fifteen to twenty years.

A proliferation of research into the treatment of lupus that began in the 1950s continues and brings much promise for additional insight into the pathogenesis of lupus as well as new treatment modalities and agents. Some focus areas of current research include investigations into patterns of gene activity, the role of the protein interferon-alpha in the progression of lupus, environmental factors, immune ablation, stem cell transplantation, and the targeting of destructive white blood cells. An intensified effort by the federal government, private industry, and nonprofit organizations, such as the Alliance for Lupus Research and the Lupus Foundation of America, fuels the hope that better treatments, prevention, and ultimately a cure for lupus will be found.

—*Barbara C. Beattie*

See also Arthritis; Autoimmune disorders; Fatigue; Joints; Kidney disorders; Light therapy; Rashes; Skin disorders; Stress; Tuberculosis; Vision disorders.

For Further Information:

Hanger, Nancy C. *Lupus-The First Year: An Essential Guide for the Newly Diagnosed*. New York: Marlowe, 2003. A "patient-expert" guides the reader step-by-step through the first year after diagnosis.

Kasitanon, Nuntana, Laurence S. Magder, and Michelle Petri. "Predictors of Survival in Systemic Lupus Erythematosus." *Medicine* 85, no. 3 (May, 2006): 147-156. This large study correlates various factors, such as demographics, clinical manifestations, and disease activity, to overall survival rates.

Lahita, Robert G., and Robert H. Phillips. *Lupus Q & A: Everything You Need to Know*. Rev. ed. New York: Avery, 2004. Written jointly by an expert on lupus and a psychologist, this book provides straightforward information about all aspects of lupus in an easy-to-read, question-and-answer format.

Lupus Foundation of America. http://www.lupus.org. An organization dedicated to improving the diagnosis and treatment of lupus, supporting individuals and families affected by the disease, increasing awareness of lupus among health professionals and the public, and finding a cure.

Meadows, Michelle. "Battling Lupus." *FDA Consumer* 39, no. 4 (July/August, 2005): 28-34. A complete overview of lupus written for the patient. Includes symptoms, diagnosis, treatment, and future prospects.

Phillips, Robert H. *Coping With Lupus: A Practical Guide to Alleviating the Challenges of Systemic Lupus Erythematosus*. 3d ed. New York: Avery, 2001. Written by an eminent psychologist, this book provides valuable assistance to patients and families on coping with the medical and psychological problems caused by lupus.

Seppa, N. "Self-Help: Stem Cells Rescue Lupus Patients." *Science News* 169, no. 5 (February 4, 2006): 67-68. A description of a promising new therapy procedure for patients with severe forms of lupus.

Wallace, Daniel J. *The Lupus Book: A Guide for Patients and Their Families*. 3d ed. New York: Oxford University Press, 2005. A complete compendium of information from a leading authority, this book provides thorough coverage of the pathogenesis and management of lupus as well as a discussion of standard, alternative, and promising new therapies. Includes references and sources of additional information.

Zonali, M. "Taming Lupus." *Scientific American* 292, no. 3 (March, 2005): 70-77. Authoritative coverage on the complexities of managing the various manifestations and complications of lupus.

SYSTEMIC SCLEROSIS

Disease/Disorder

Also known as: Systemic scleroderma

Anatomy or system affected: All

Specialties and related fields: All

Definition: A systemic disease characterized by extensive scarring in the skin, connective tissue, and internal organs.

Key terms:

autoimmune response: an inappropriate immune response against the patient's own cells

cytokines: small proteins released by immune cells that elicit specific effects from other cells

fibroblast: an immature cell that manufactures connective tissues

fibrosis: an increase in the fibrous scar tissue deposited between cells

Causes and Symptoms

During the process of wound healing, specific cells known as fibroblasts deposit a protein called collagen to heal the breach in our tissues. Large areas of collagen deposition compose what we commonly call a scar. Our bodies carefully regulate collagen deposition to prevent scarring in unneeded places. People with systemic sclerosis (SSc) experience unregulated deposition of collagen.

In SSc patients, the immune system malfunctions and attacks the body's own tissues and organs. This continuous damage and inflammation leads to continuous collagen deposition and scarring, which stiffens, hardens, and thickens those tissues and organs affected by the inflammation.

Typically, the SSc-specific autoimmune response begins with damage to blood vessels, which summons immune cells to the injury site. The immune cells secrete small signaling proteins called cytokines, in particular platelet-derived growth factor (PDGF), transforming growth factor-β1 (TGF-β1), and interleukin-6 (IL-6). These cytokines signal to antibody-producing B-lymphocytes to produce antibodies against blood vessels, and also signal to fibroblasts to differentiate into myofibroblasts. In response to the tissue destruction caused by the immune response, myofibroblasts deposit collagen and other molecules in an attempt to mitigate the damage. This repeated cycle of damage and collagen deposition leads to the formation of large, stiff scars that harden the tissue or organ and compromise its function.

What causes the initial damage to blood vessels remains unknown, but several factors seem to act as triggers. Exposure to silica, organic solvents (e.g., toluene, hexane, vinyl chloride, xylene, etc.), epoxy resins, pesticides, certain drugs (e.g., bleomycin cocaine, carbidopa, and others), appetite suppressants, silicone or paraffin implants, or vibrational injuries seem to act as triggers that initiate the cascade of events that lead to SSc. Genetic factors also clearly play a vital role in the propensity someone has to develop SSc. Finally, particular viral infections (e.g., cytomegalovirus) that infect and damage blood vessels might act as triggers.

Internationally, SSc afflicts 2.3-10 people per one million, and affects women three to six times more often than men. SSc is rare in Japan and China and more common in African-American and American Indian women than in white women.

The first signs of SSc tend to be Raynaud's phenomenon or a whitening of the hands in response cold exposure, and itching (pruritus). Damage to blood vessels causes puffy, swollen hands. Afterwards, the skin begins to thicken and harden, usually beginning with the hands and face. Lack of blood flow to the hands can produce ulcers at the tips of the fingers. Also, calcium deposits form under the skin (calcinosis). Calcium deposits and thickening of the skin can restrict movement around joints, especially the smaller joints of the hand. Patients can also experience arthritis and muscle weakness.

Lung damage causes shortness of breath upon exertion and later also at rest. Elevation in blood pressures in the pulmonary arteries (pulmonary hypertension) follows. Scarring of the gastrointestinal tract usually begins with narrowing of the esophagus (peptic stricture), which causes difficulty swallowing (dysphagia), and increased scarring reduces gastrointestinal motility. Severe gastroesophageal reflux disease (GERD) follows, which predisposes the patient to esophageal cancer. Reduction in intestinal motility compromises nutrient absorption, leading to malnutrition.

In the kidney, SSc produces scleroderma renal cysts. Kidney involvement substantially raises blood pressure (malignant hypertension) and blood levels of ammonium (azotemia), and causes the leakage of blood (hematuria) and protein (proteinuria) into urine.

Heart involvement scars the heart, leading to life-threatening heart failure. Vascular damage can also induce strokes.

Those who suffer from limited cutaneous SSc usually experience symptoms restricted to the skin. However, those who have diffuse cutaneous SSc show rapid scarring (fibrosis) of the skin, and internal organs, in particular the lungs, heart, gastrointestinal tract, and kidneys.

Treatment and Therapy

Serological tests of blood from SSc patients typically reveal particular auto-antibodies or antibodies that bind to patient's own tissues; antinuclear antibodies are characteristic of SSc. Imaging studies can document the fibrotic changes in the lungs, heart, and gastrointestinal tract, as can histological examinations of biopsied tissues.

Treatment focuses on decreasing fibrosis and preserving organ function. To stifle fibrosis, antiscarring drugs such as D-penicillamine, interferon-α, interferon-γ, methotrexate, chlorambucil, cyclosporine, thalidomide, tacrolimus, corticosteroids, cyclophosphamide, and statins have provided some patients relief, albeit not consistently. For patients with gastrointestinal involvement, proton pump inhibitors and H2 receptor blockers can control the symptoms of GERD. To treat inflammation of muscles, high dose corticosteroids can halt the advance of fibrosis. In patients with lung involvement, calcium-channel blockers, prostaglandins such as prostacyclin, and cyclophosphamide have provided relief for some, though not all, patients. For

---

Information on Systemic Sclerosis

Causes: An immune response against blood vessels leads to massive inflammation and scarring of the skin and internal organs

Symptoms: Itching, Raynaud's phenomenon, difficulty swallowing, nausea, vomiting, weight loss, abdominal cramps, diarrhea, fecal incontinence, shortness of breath, chest pain, fatigue, high blood pressure, joint pain and swelling, muscle pain and weakness, blood and protein in urine

Duration: Usually arises between the ages of 30 to 50 and remains for a lifetime

Treatments: Skin moisturizers, avoiding cold, calcium-channel blockers, blood vessel dilating drugs, antihypertensive agents, proton pump inhibitors, immunomodulatory agents, and bone marrow transplants

those with kidney involvement, angiotensin-converting enzyme (ACE) inhibitors or angiotensin II receptor blockers are essential to control hypertension. For Raynaud's phenomenon, avoiding exposure to cold temperature and warm clothing can prevent the onset of symptoms.

Pulsed dye laser treatments can effectively clear fibrotic areas, but multiple treatments are required and recurrence remains a problem.

Procedures and Prospects

Early paintings and written descriptions possibly recount cases of SSc, but the first codified description of SSc comes from Carlo Curzio in 1752. Curzio treated a 17-year-old woman at the Royal Hospital in Naples who suffered from a diffuse hardness of her skin. The Milanese physician Giovambattista Fantonetti in 1836 was the first to use the term "scleroderma," which comes from a combination of the Greek words "skleros" or hard and "dermos" or skin. Fantonetti described a 30-year-old patient named Antonia Alessandri whose skin was as dark, tense, and firm as leather. Fortunately, Ms. Alessandri miraculously recovered three months later, which casts doubt on Fantonetti's diagnosis, but medical professionals continued to use the term he coined.

Perhaps the most exciting development in SSc is the use of bone marrow stem cell transplantations to treat SSc patients. Patients treated with hematopoietic stem cell transplantations (HSCTs) survive better, have significantly improved skin flexibility, and some improvements in lung function. Refining this procedure should make it more mainstream rather than experimental.

—*Michael A. Buratovich, Ph.D.*

See also Antihypertensives; Cardiology; Dermatology; Dermopathology; Histology; Hypertension; Immunology; Immunopathology; Nephrology; Pulmonology; Raynaud's syndrome; Wounds

For Further Information:

Clearview, Darrell. *Your Scleroderma Symptoms, Treatments and Self-Help Guide.* Seattle, WA: Amazon Digital Services, 2011.
Jacob, Elliot, ed. *Medifocus Guidebook on: Scleroderma.* Silver Spring, MD: Medifocus, Inc., 2013.
Ruscitto, Louis. *Scleroderma-Understand Connective Tissue Disease.* Seattle, WA: Amazon Digital Services, 2012.

SYSTEMS AND ORGANS
Anatomy
Anatomy or system affected: All
Specialties and related fields: All
Definition: Groups of tissues and organs dedicated to particular functions, all of which must work together to perform efficiently.

Key terms:
atrium: the chamber of the heart where veins terminate; the atrium receives blood returning to the heart and delivers it to the ventricle
bronchi: the airways conducting air from the mouth to the depths of the lungs
carbon dioxide: the gas produced by the body from the use of oxygen; carbon dioxide and the hydrogen ions it can create may become toxic if not excreted by the body
foodstuffs: the basic components of food that the body can use-carbohydrates (which break down to sugars, primarily to glucose), proteins (which break down to amino acids), and fat
hormone: a chemical released by a tissue to signal another tissue to modify its function
ions: small chemical substances that have a positive or negative charge; the most important ions with a positive charge are sodium, potassium, hydrogen, and calcium, while the most important negative ion is chloride
ventricles: the large chambers of the heart that pump blood into the arteries; the left ventricle pumps blood into the aorta, and the right ventricle pumps blood into the lung's arteries

Structure and Functions

There are essentially nine systems in the human body: the nervous, cardiovascular, respiratory, gastrointestinal, renal, endocrine, reproductive, thermoregulatory, and skeletomuscular systems. All these systems are essential to sustain life, and many work together to perform their functions efficiently. All the other systems need the nervous system to operate or to coordinate their functions. The first six of these systems will be discussed in this article.

The nervous system is composed of the central nervous system (the brain) and the peripheral nervous system (the spinal cord and nerves extending to every part of the body). The brain receives information from the body by way of the sensory nerves. It then evaluates all the information and sends out the appropriate signals to respond. For example, the ears send information to the brain that there are noises coming from behind; the brain tells the head to turn in the direction of the sounds. The eyes send the signals that the noises are coming from, for example, a gorilla. The brain must decide to run, fight, or stand and try to reason with the gorilla. Meanwhile, the brain tells the heart to beat faster and harder. It also tells the stomach and intestines to stop digestion and reduce its blood flow because blood may be needed by the muscles for running. This is called the "fight or flight" response to stress, which the nervous system controls.

Sensory information can come from any of the five senses-sight, smell, hearing, touch, or taste-but it can also come from other sensors. Sensory nerves send the brain information on pain, temperature, blood pressure, and what is going on in the stomach and intestines (hunger or a full feeling). The brain receives millions of signals each second from every part of the body and must constantly decide how to respond. Humans can choose not to respond instinctively as animals do. For example, humans often eat when they are not hungry.

Different areas of the brain are dedicated to specific functions. The upper portion of the spinal cord and lower portion of the brain (the brain stem) are dedicated to controlling involuntary functions such as breathing, the maintenance of blood pressure and heart rate, and the responses to hot and cold. The middle portion of the brain coordinates movement. The middle brain also coordinates information from upper portions of the brain and generates emotions. The uppermost and outermost portions of the brain (the cerebrum) process the information from the senses and generate responses, such as telling the body to move. The cerebrum also performs such intellectual functions as reasoning.

The cardiovascular system is composed of the heart and blood vessels. Its job is to pump blood containing oxygen and foodstuffs (sugars, proteins, and fat) to every part of the body. Blood is composed of red and white blood cells suspended in plasma, a pale yellow fluid which flows through the cardiovascular system. Red blood cells are the carriers of oxygen, the main source of energy for the body. White blood cells help fight disease and are delivered to parts of the body that are hurt or diseased. The plasma contains platelets that help blood to clot when necessary. Blood also transports wastes produced by the body from tissues to organs that can dispose of them. For example, carbon dioxide is produced by the tissues when oxygen is used for energy. Blood carries carbon dioxide back to the lungs to be removed from the body in exhaled air.

Blood is pumped by the heart in a circuit in the cardiovascular system (also called the circulatory system). The heart has four chambers, two atria and two ventricles. Blood enters the heart through the left atrium, a small pocket of muscles that help pump blood into the left ventricle. The ventricle is a larger chamber with a thick wall of muscle that can pump very hard; it pushes blood into the arteries. The left ventricle pumps blood into the main artery of the body, the aorta. The aorta branches many times into smaller arteries, which in turn branch into capillaries. Every part of the body has millions of tiny capillaries just big enough for a blood cell to pass through them; in fact, blood cells must fold to get through some capillaries. In capillaries, oxygen and foodstuffs leave the blood, and then carbon dioxide and other waste products enter the blood to be taken away. Blood flows from the capillaries into small veins, which join to make larger and larger veins. The largest veins, the venae cavae, empty into the heart, in the right atrium. The blood is pumped from the right atrium to the right ventricle. Blood is then pumped by the right ventricle through the lung and back into the left atrium to start its journey again.

The lungs are the major organ of the respiratory system. The function of the respiratory system is to bring fresh air into the lungs, getting it very close to the blood, and to expel used air. Air enters the respiratory system through the nose and mouth, which connect to the main windpipe, the trachea. The trachea branches into smaller airways called bronchi. Bronchi in turn branch into smaller airways, bronchioles. The ends of bronchioles form many rounded sacs (alveoli) that resemble a bunch of grapes. These sacs of air have very thin walls that are shared with the walls of the lung's capillaries. This close arrangement of air and blood provides a minimal distance for oxygen to travel into the blood and for carbon dioxide to leave the blood.

Air is moved into the lungs when the muscles of respiration contract and expand the lungs. The diaphragm is a large sheet of muscle which separates the chest from the abdomen. When the diaphragm contracts, it pulls the lungs down. At the same time, muscles on the chest wall contract, pulling the lungs up and out. This expansion of the lungs causes air to be sucked into and fill the air sacs. During exhalation, the respiratory muscles are relaxed, the lung collapses somewhat, and air rushes out, carrying carbon dioxide with it.

Blood, specifically red blood cells, is specialized to carry large amounts of oxygen and carbon dioxide. Red blood cells contain hemoglobin, a special substance that attaches to these gases. When the amounts of oxygen and carbon dioxide in the plasma increase, they tend to leak back into the air sacs or tissues, respectively. These gases are effectively removed from the fluid by hemoglobin, allowing more gases to enter the blood without leaking back out. Hemoglobin also coordinates the release of these gases-oxygen to the tissues and carbon dioxide to the lungs-at the correct time.

The gastrointestinal system is a multiorgan system that breaks down food to be absorbed into the blood. Initially, food is broken down by chewing and by mixing with saliva. Then it is swallowed into the esophagus, a tube which travels through the chest to empty into the stomach. The stomach adds acid and other chemicals to the food, which breaks it down even more. The food, now called chyme, passes into the upper small intestine (the duodenum). The pancreas adds enzymes; a chemical called bicarbonate, which neutralizes the acid added by the stomach; and the hormones insulin and glucagon. Insulin is the major hormone secreted by the pancreas. It is absorbed into the blood by the intestine and signals the body to get ready to receive the products of digestion, primarily sugar (glucose). Bile is also added to the contents of the upper duodenum by the liver. Bile helps to break down fat to be absorbed into the blood. As the intestinal contents move along the small intestine, from the jejunum to the ileum, water and mucus are added to help move it along, and carbohydrates are absorbed in their smallest form, glucose. Enzymes attached to the wall of the intestine break up proteins to be absorbed as their component parts, amino acids. Water in chyme is constantly being reabsorbed. Finally the colon, or large intestine, absorbs most of the remaining water. The remaining solids are excreted through the rectum.

Food is moved through the gastrointestinal system by a special type of muscle called smooth muscle. The walls of the gastrointestinal tract are composed of muscle arranged in circular fashion around the tube and along its length. Initially, a circular group of muscles contracts, narrowing a short segment of intestine. This process is called segmentation. The contraction spreads down the muscles arranged lengthwise, squeezing the contents down the length of intestine. Movement of chyme is aided by relaxation of the muscles ahead of the contraction. This motion is called peristalsis. Peristalsis is coordinated by the nervous system, but the intestines have their own set of nerves. These intestinal nerves can control the motion of the intestine without help from the central nervous system.

The kidneys are the primary organs of the renal system. It is the function of the kidneys to regulate both the amount and the composition of the fluid in the body, in spite of wide variations in the human environment and in an organism's intake of food and water. Since blood circulates everywhere in the body, the kidneys can change the composition and amount of plasma, and the other fluids of the body then equalize with it. Therefore, the kidneys can regulate all body fluids. The body has sensors for both the amount of fluid in the blood and the concentration of the important elements in the blood, such as sodium, hydrogen, and potassium.

The kidneys regulate plasma volume and composition by filtering the plasma and returning only the appropriate amounts of fluid and substances back to the blood. Arteries entering the kidneys rapidly branch into capillaries. Approximately 20 percent of all plasma flowing into the kidneys leaves the capillaries and is collected in the capsules that surround them. This fluid is funneled into specialized tubes.

Substances are taken out and put into the fluid in the tubes in order to regulate fluid volume and composition. In the beginning of the tube (the proximal tubule), most of the salt, water, glucose, and amino acids are taken back into the blood. The next sections (the loop of Henle, distal tubule, and collecting ducts) help to regulate the final amount of water excreted in urine. The collecting ducts join to form the ureter, which carries the remaining fluid, urine, to the bladder, where it is stored. From the bladder, the urine is expelled through the urethra.

The endocrine system is another multiorgan system that helps to control and modify the function of almost all other systems. Endocrine glands produce chemicals and release them into the blood to direct the functions of cells and tissues elsewhere in the body. There are three classes of hormones: amines, peptides and proteins, and steroids. Adrenaline is an example of the amine group, insulin is a protein hormone, and estrogen is a steroid hormone. Each of these is produced by a different gland.

The adrenal glands, small glands located near the kidneys, make several hormones. The outer portion, the cortex, produces three types of steroid hormones referred to as corticosteroids: glucocorticoids, mineralocorticoids, and small amounts of androgenic hormones. The major glucocorticoid, cortisol, regulates the production and use of glucose, fats, and amino acids by many cells and tissues. It also plays a helper role for other hormonal actions, such as making them more potent during stress, and it helps prevent inflammation and swelling. The major mineralocorticoid, aldosterone, can modify the kidneys' excretion of sodium, potassium, and hydrogen. A person unable to produce mineralocorticoids will die in a few days without treatment but can be saved by aldosterone therapy. Therefore, these steroids are said to be lifesaving. The androgenic steroids can cause the development of adult male sexual characteristics, the same effect as the male sex hormone, testosterone.

The interior portion, or medulla, of the adrenal glands makes catecholamines, such as adrenaline (epinephrine). Adrenaline helps the cardiovascular system during exercise and stress. It is the hormone that stimulates much of the "fight or flight" response, making the heart beat faster and harder. Adrenaline also helps to increase blood flow to muscles, in case flight is the action of choice.

The pituitary gland, also known as the hypophysis, is located at the base of the brain and produces many hormones with a variety of actions. The pituitary is divided into two areas: the anterior lobe (also known as the adenohypophysis) and the posterior lobe (also known as the neurohypophysis). The anterior pituitary produces growth hormone, a protein that has a major influence on all metabolic activity. It causes the body to store carbohydrates, to make proteins for growth, and to use fat for energy. The other anterior pituitary hormones cause other glands to increase their production of hormones. The glands stimulated by distinct pituitary hormones are the thyroid, adrenal cortex, ovaries, testicles, and mammary glands. The posterior pituitary produces the peptide hormones antidiuretic hormone (also known as vasopressin) and oxytocin. Antidiuretic hormone (ADH) decreases the amount of water that the kidneys can excrete, which keeps the body from dehydrating. ADH can also cause the blood pressure to rise, which helps if fluid is lost as a result of bleeding. Oxytocin causes the uterus to contract during the birthing process, and it also stimulates the production of milk in new mothers. The pituitary has direct regulating control over many glands and tissues, and it regulates nearly all tissues and organs indirectly by way of its stimulating hormones. This gland is regulated in a similar fashion by the hypothalamus, a small part of the brain just above the pituitary.

The thyroid gland is located in the neck around the voice box, or larynx. The parathyroid glands are located next to the thyroid gland. Thyroid hormones (peptides) cause almost all tissues in the body to increase the use of foodstuffs for the production of proteins, aiding in growth. In addition, the thyroid gland produces calcitonin. Calcitonin and the parathyroid hormones regulate the amount of calcium in the blood. Parathyroid hormone acts by freeing calcium from bone when more calcium is needed in the blood, while calcitonin causes the opposite action. Therefore, when the level of one of these hormones goes up, the other must go down.

The sex organs are also endocrine glands. The ovaries make estrogen and progesterone, while the testes produce testosterone. These steroid hormones cause the body to develop primary and secondary sexual characteristics. When a woman is pregnant, the placenta (the part of a woman's uterus that nourishes the fetus) produces hormones that prepare her body for childbirth and breast-feeding.

Disorders and Diseases

The body has control mechanisms to ensure that its systems function properly. Many systems use what is called negative feedback to fine-tune their functioning. An example of negative feedback is the control of blood pressure. Sensors in the arteries allow the brain to monitor the body's blood pressure level. When pressure is too high, the brain tells the cardiovascular system to decrease pressure by slowing the heart and

2190 • Systems and Organs

opening the blood vessels and tells the kidneys to excrete fluid. Thus, when blood pressure is high, the feedback that the brain provides is negative, because it causes a response that is opposite to the unwanted change from the normal state.

The endocrine system uses negative feedback to regulate many hormones. The simplest endocrine feedback system involves insulin and glucose. When blood glucose increases, insulin secretion increases, which in turn decreases blood glucose. A decrease in blood glucose tells the pancreas to slow down the secretion of insulin. The failure of this system results in diabetes mellitus, a disease in which the ability to regulate blood sugar is lost. When this control is lost, other systems are damaged as a result, such as the renal and cardiovascular systems.

There are also much more complex feedback control systems. The regulation of the adrenal hormone cortisol serves as an example of such a system. Cortisol secretion is controlled by secretion of the pituitary hormone adrenocorticotropic hormone (ACTH), also called corticotropin. The secretion of ACTH is controlled by a hypothalamic hormone called corticotropin-releasing factor (CRF). Stress causes CRF to be released, which causes the release of ACTH and in turn stimulates the secretion of cortisol. In general, when the level of any of these hormones becomes too high, the release of one of the others can be shut down. High levels of cortisol turn off CRF and ACTH secretion. High levels of ACTH can turn off the secretion of the hormone that triggers its secretion, CRF. It is also thought that CRF can provide feedback to its organ of origin, the hypothalamus, and halt its own secretion. Thus, if one of the control systems fails to function, a backup system guards against total malfunction.

The systems and organs of the body are dedicated to specific functions, but each needs the others to function properly. In addition, each system requires the coordination from the central nervous system to perform efficiently. The lungs bring vital oxygen to the cardiovascular system, and all systems need the nutrients brought to them by the cardiovascular system. Some organs of the endocrine system, such as the adrenal glands, are essential to life. The kidneys keep the blood clean and maintain the body's fluid volume. The reproductive system is essential to maintaining the existence of a species. All these systems must perform their functions for the body to work well. If one system malfunctions, frequently other systems become involved and may malfunction as well.

An example of one system malfunction that causes the failure of many others is renal failure. Kidney failure can be caused by a malfunction of the cardiovascular system such as clogging of the capillaries, which prohibits the kidneys from doing their job. As a result, hydrogen and potassium ions will accumulate. The effects of high levels of hydrogen and potassium ions on the cardiovascular system are a weakened heart and lower blood pressure. The nervous system can sense the increase in hydrogen ions and will tell the respiratory system to breathe faster and deeper to rid the body of carbon dioxide and its hydrogen ions. The increase in breathing helps to lower the hydrogen ion levels in the blood but cannot com-

pletely compensate for the kidney malfunction; in fact, the increase in work by the respiratory muscles can produce more hydrogen ions. When levels of hydrogen become too high, the brain begins to malfunction. The patient may experience dizziness, have seizures, or lose consciousness. If these symptoms are not reversed, the malfunction of each system will aid in the deterioration of other systems. The brain will be irreversibly damaged, and the heart will stop.

There are several ways to treat renal failure to avoid multiple-organ sickness. Treatment of infections with antibiotics before they become severe can help to avoid early and mild kidney failure. In severe, long-term kidney failure, kidney transplantation may become necessary. The damaged kidney (or kidneys) is removed and replaced with an organ from a deceased donor or from a living donor (a person can live a normal life with only one functioning kidney). Kidneys, even from deceased donors, are rare, and many people in need of a transplant must wait for years to receive one that will not be rejected by the body's immune system. For such patients, dialysis is necessary for survival. Dialysis is the use of a machine to perform some of the functions of the kidneys. Patients with total kidney failure must be hooked up to an artificial kidney machine for several hours several times per week. Even with this treatment, they will still be very sick because the machine cannot perform all functions of the kidneys.

Perspective and Prospects

In the Middle Ages, it was believed that "spirits" were the essence of life or "vitality"; thus, the treatment for many ailments was bloodletting, the application of leeches to remove the "evil spirit" causing the sickness. It was not until the seventeenth century that William Harvey discovered that blood circulated from arteries to veins in both the lungs and the rest of the body. Oxygen was discovered at the end of the eighteenth century by Joseph Priestley. Knowledge of chemistry, biochemistry, and physiology grew in the nineteenth century, but most of the information about systems and organs contained in this article was revealed in the twentieth century.

Many discoveries have been in the area of how the body's systems and organs interact with and influence one another. New anatomical techniques of investigation have revealed the minute structures of many organs and tissues. As a result, the presence of previously unknown nervous and other tissue parts has been recognized; their functions are under investigation. Chemical techniques have revealed many new hormone and hormonelike substances through which one tissue or organ can influence another. Research into the molecular structure of some of these biochemical signals is helping to explain how they work.

In addition, the events that occur inside a cell or group of cells have been described in greater detail. How a group of cells produces unified organ function and how this function is altered is currently under investigation. Studies into how a cell can change its function in conjunction with surrounding cells have added to the knowledge of how systems and organs can fine-tune their functions. This research involves information regarding how the genes inside cells carry messages and how these messages in turn are expressed in unified physiological functions.

—J. Timothy O'Neill, Ph.D.

See also Adrenal glands; Anatomy; Brain; Circulation; Colon; Ears; Endocrine glands; Endocrine system; Eyes; Gallbladder; Gastrointestinal system; Glands; Heart; Immune system; Kidneys; Liver; Lungs; Lymphatic system; Nervous system; Pancreas; Pituitary gland; Reproductive system; Sense organs; Skin; Small intestine; Thyroid gland; Urinary system; Vascular system.

For Further Information:

Asimov, Isaac. *The Human Body: Its Structure and Operation*. Rev. ed. New York: Penguin Books, 1992. Asimov offers an easy-to-understand overview of all the body's organ functions.

Guyton, Arthur C., and John E. Hall. *Human Physiology and Mechanisms of Disease*. 6th ed. Philadelphia: W. B. Saunders, 1997. This physiology text deals with the function of the body in considerable detail. Excellent advanced reading for the physiology student.

Kittredge, Mary. *The Human Body: An Overview*. Reprint. Philadelphia: Chelsea House, 2003. This text explains the general workings of the human body. Provides background to the historical development of medical knowledge and addresses many of the pathologies that can arise in the body.

Page, Martyn, ed. *Human Body: An Illustrated Guide to Every Part of the Human Body and How It Works*. New York: DK, 2009. The first part of the book covers basic human anatomy with full color illustrations, explaining how each individual body system functions. The second part covers diseases and disorders.

Parsons, Jayne, ed. *Encyclopedia of the Human Body*. New York: DK, 2004. A beautifully illustrated and accessible guide to the human body designed for children and teens, covering anatomical concepts, disease mechanisms, and the history of medicine and its pioneers.

Thibodeau, Gary A., and Kevin T. Patton. *The Human Body in Health and Disease*. 4th ed. St. Louis, Mo.: Mosby/Elsevier, 2005. Examines the mechanisms of the human body by examining each system in detail.

TAPEWORMS
Disease/Disorder

Anatomy or system affected: Gastrointestinal system, intestines

Specialties and related fields: Gastroenterology, public health

Definition: Flatworms of the phylum Platyhelminthes and class Cestoda that are parasitic in the digestive tract of humans and other animals.

Causes and Symptoms

Humans are the definitive hosts for several tapeworm species. Infection is usually caused by ingestion of undercooked muscle tissue with encysted larvae. The larvae attach to the upper part of the small intestine and mature into adults. Adult tapeworms are hermaphrodites, having both male and female reproductive organs, and a single tapeworm can produce millions of eggs during its normal life span of up to twenty-five years. The eggs pass out through the feces and are ingested by intermediate hosts. Larvae emerge from the eggs, invade the muscle tissue of the intermediate host, and form cystlike structures called cysticerci. When an intermediate host's muscle tissue containing cysticerci is eaten by humans, the life cycle continues. Most tapeworm infestations are asymptomatic or cause only minor gastric distress.

The beef tapeworm, *Taenia saginata*, infects humans when undercooked beef containing cysticerci is eaten; it is the most common human tapeworm worldwide. *T. solium*, the pork tapeworm, although less common, is more serious. When humans ingest the cysticerci, an infection much like the one caused by the beef tapeworm usually occurs. However, when humans ingest *T. solium* eggs, larvae emerge that can burrow into human muscle and connective tissue and form cysticerci. They can cause major problems, especially when the cysticerci form in the brain or eyes. Seizures, severe headaches, and loss of consciousness can result from neurocysticercosis, while ocular cysticercosis can lead to many visual problems.

Diphyllobothrium latum is a tapeworm with two intermediate hosts. Eggs hatch into larvae that are ingested by copepods, which are themselves eaten by fish that may in turn be eaten by larger fish. The larvae become encysted in the fish muscle. Humans are infected when they ingest the undercooked fish. In this infection, vitamin B_{12} deficiency and associated megaloblastic anemia can occur as the worm competes with the host for vitamin B_{12}.

The dwarf tapeworm, *Hymenolepsis nana*, normally uses mice as the definitive host and grain beetles as the intermediate host. Unlike all other tapeworms, however, it can go through its entire life cycle in a single host. Humans, especially children, ingest *H. nana* eggs from contaminated soil. The eggs mature into larvae, which then mature into adults that attach to the intestinal wall.

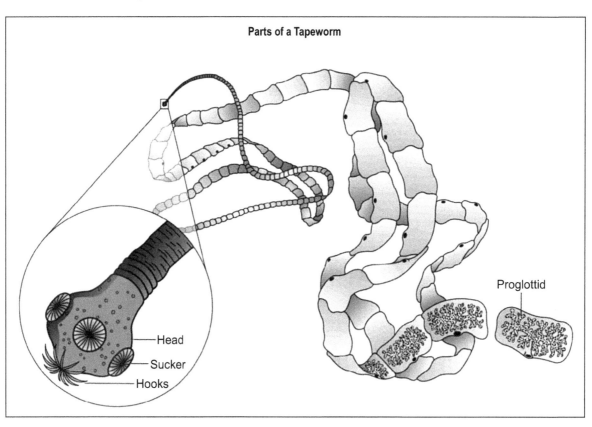

Parts of a Tapeworm

Head

Sucker

Hooks

Proglottid

Information on Tapeworms

Causes: Parasitic infection transmitted through ingestion

Symptoms: Depends on type; ranges from asymptomatic or minor gastric distress to seizures, severe headaches, loss of consciousness, visual problems, vitamin B_{12} deficiency, megaloblastic anemia

Duration: Chronic

Treatments: Praziquantel, niclosamide, albendazole

Treatment and Therapy

T. saginata, *T. solium*, and *D. latum* are usually treated by a single 5 to 10 milligram per kilogram dose of praziquantel. Alternatively, niclosamide and albendazole can be used. The preferred treatment for *H. nana* is a single 25 milligram per kilogram dose of praziquantel. Good personal hygiene, proper waste handling, and effective sewage treatment can break the cycle of infection. In addition, meat and fish from areas where these tapeworms are endemic should be cooked thoroughly.

—*Richard W. Cheney, Jr., Ph.D.*

See also Food poisoning; Insect-borne diseases; Intestinal disorders; Intestines; Parasitic diseases; Worms; Zoonoses.

For Further Information:

Icon Health. *Tapeworms: A Medical Dictionary, Bibliography, and Annotated Research Guide to Internet References*. San Diego, Calif.: Author, 2004.

Kearn, G. C. *Parasitism and the Platyhelminths*. New York: Springer, 1997.

Roberts, Larry S., and John Janovy, Jr., eds. *Gerald D. Schmidt and Larry S. Roberts' Foundations of Parasitology*. 7th ed. Boston: McGraw-Hill Higher Education, 2005.

TARDIVE DYSKINESIA

Disease/Disorder

Anatomy or system affected: Nervous system disorder, extrapyramidal disorder

Specialties and related fields: Psychiatry, neurology, pharmacology

Definition: A medication-induced movement disorder characterized by involuntary movements.

Key terms:

antipsychotics: a group of medications used to treat the symptoms of psychosis

DSM-5: the Diagnostic Statistical Manual, version 5, which includes behavioral diagnostic criteria for determining psychiatric illnesses

neuroleptics: another term for classes of drugs used to treat psychosis

neurotransmitters: chemicals manufactured by the brain for the purpose of facilitating or inhibiting neural signals

Background Information

The term tardive dyskinesia was coined in 1964 by Faurbye to refer to a movement disorder that occurred sometime after exposure to certain drugs. Today tardive dyskinesia is classified by the American Psychiatric Association's DSM-5 as a medication-induced movement disorder. It is characterized by involuntary movements that are associated with the long-term use of neuroleptic drugs (also known as antipsychotic drugs or major tranquilizers), and is a reasonably common side effect. It is also seen as a side effect of the antinausea drug metaclopramide. Studies indicate that tardive dyskinesia is seen in up to 30 percent of individuals on long-term neuroleptics. Tardive dyskinesia is categorized as a rare disease (by the National Organization for Rare Disorders) indicating that there are under 200,000 people suffering from this disorder in the United States.

Causes and Risk Factors

The causes of tardive dyskinesia are unclear. While some believe that neuroleptics stimulate the production of dopamine receptors in the part of the brain controlling movement, others hypothesize that it is more likely tied in to serotonin receptors. Some recent evidence suggests that rather than being tied to one of the major neurotransmitter per se, tardive dyskinesia may be related to a problem with an inhibitory neurotransmitter. If this is the case, the culprit is felt to be gamma-aminobutyric acid (GABA).

There are multiple risk factors for tardive dyskinesia. Obviously occurring in people who are using neuroleptics, certain factors seem to make this side effect of the medications more likely to occur. It is more commonly seen in people who have used more than one neuroleptic drug as well as in individuals who have had a substance use disorder (drug, alcohol, or cigarettes) during their lifetime. It is also seen more commonly in people of advanced age, with evidence indicating that it is much more common in people over the age of 50. Tardive dyskinesia is found more commonly in females, especially if they are postmenopausal. It has also been found more commonly in individuals who are developmentally disabled. Currently, it is unclear whether these factors actually increase the likelihood of developing this disorder as a side effect of the drugs, or whether they merely increase the likelihood of being prescribed neuroleptic drugs long term.

Symptoms

Individuals with tardive dyskinesia display sudden, often continuous, uncontrollable movements of groups of voluntary muscles. Individuals with tardive dyskinesia may develop their symptoms very abruptly or gradually over time. Patients who are on drugs known to cause tardive dyskinesia should be advised to keep a record of any symptoms that they develop, being sure to describe the symptom, note the date and time that it occurred, the body part affected, and the severity of the symptom. The involuntary movements occur most often in the area of the face (especially the mouth, jaw, and eyelids). Such movements have also been found to occur in the neck, any or all limbs, and the torso.

Screening and Diagnosis

When an individual is placed on   neuroleptics they are

typically evaluated using a tool known as the Abnormal Involuntary Movement Scale (AIMS) to obtain baseline level functioning and then followed up with this tool on a yearly basis. This screening may allow early identification of tardive dyskinesia. Alternatively, an individual who becomes aware of symptoms like those noted above should clearly be seen by a physician immediately. In order to make a differential diagnosis the physician would need to rule out a number of other disorders with similar symptoms. To make this diagnosis of exclusion (eliminating other possible etiologies) one would typically do blood work, EEGs (electroencephalograms), CT scans (computed axial tomography), or MRIs (magnetic resonance imaging). If most other causes are eliminated, and if the patient has been on one of the drugs known to cause medication induced movement disorders, then the diagnosis will likely be tardive dyskinesia. Typically by the time this diagnosis is made the patient has been seen by a psychiatrist and a neurologist. Once this diagnosis has been made, the patient will continue to be evaluated using the AIMS in order to determine the severity of the disorder.

Treatment and Therapy

Since the onset of tardive dyskinesia is clearly medication related, the first order of treatment is to identify and discontinue the offending medication. This process can be very complex, and should only be done under the direct supervision of a physician. Symptoms may often persist after the medication is discontinued. Hopefully, other medications can be described to deal with the underlying disorder. Newer neuroleptics (antipsychotics) are less likely to produce tardive dyskinesia, but it may still occur. When alternative drug use is not a possibility or does not treat the underlying disorder, the offending medication may still have to be taken. If that is the case or if the symptoms do not subside long after the medication is discontinued, then there is a drug available for the treatment of the symptoms of tardive dyskinesia. Tetrabenazine is widely used in Canada for this purpose, but is available only for use as an Orphan drug in the United States to treat tardive dyskinesia. Currently this is an off-label use for tetrabenazine, which is approved in this country only for the treatment of Huntington's chorea.

Perspective and Prospects

As indicated above, symptoms may disappear soon after the offending drug is discontinued. Yet in other cases, symptoms may persist for years. At present, research is being done to definitively determine the underlying mechanism of the disorder, develop drugs that do not create these side effects, and find ways to alleviate the symptoms should they occur.

—*Robin Kamienny Montvilo, Ph.D.*

See also Pharmacology; Psychosis; Schizophrenia

For Further Information:

Loonen, A.J.M., and S. A. Ivanova. "New Insights into the Mechanism of Drug-induced Dyskinesia." *CNS Spectrums* 18, no. 1 (2013): 15-20.
NAMI: Tardive Dyskinesia. http://www.nami.org/Content/Content Groups/./Tardive_Dyskinesia.htm.
Parker, J.N., and P. M. Parker. *The Official Patient's Sourcebook on Tardive Dyskinesia: A Revised and Updated Directory for The Internet Age.* San Diego, CA: ICON Health Publications, 2002.
Tardive Dyskinesia: https://www.bcm.edu/departments/neurology/parkinsons/?pmid=14198.
Tarsy, D., C. Lungu, and R. J. Baldessarini. "Epidemiology of Tardive Dyskinesia before and during the Era of Modern Anti-Psychotic Drugs." *Handbook of Clinical Neurology* 100 (2011): 601-616.

TASTE

Biology

Anatomy or system affected: Gastrointestinal system, mouth, nervous system, nose

Specialties and related fields: Gastroenterology, neurology, nutrition, otorhinolaryngology

Definition: One of the five special senses; chemicals interact with receptor sites in specialized structures of the tongue, and the resulting nerve impulses are classified as certain kinds of taste.

Key terms:

chemoreceptors: specific structures upon which tastant molecules (chemicals that cause a taste sensation on the tongue) adhere; it is presumed that taste receptors have some structural uniqueness because sweet, salty, sour, and bitter can be distinguished there

facial nerve: the seventh cranial nerve pair, which relays signals from the face and the front region of the tongue up to the pons of the brain stem; conducts impulses related to taste, salivation, and facial expression

filiform papillae: the small, rounded projections that form the tough, yet velvetlike, texture of the tongue surface; lacking any chemoreceptors, these papillae do not function in taste

foliate papillae: the folded papillae found on the soft edges of the rear of the tongue and just ahead of the V shape formed by the vallate papillae; although found in the regions that detect bitter or sour tastes, foliate papillae are not specific receptors for bitter or sour tastes

fungiform papillae: the papillae scattered about the tongue surface, in no specific array, that are responsive to tastant molecules; these do not exhibit specificity for a particular type of taste

glossopharyngeal nerve: the ninth cranial nerve, which relays signals pertaining to or controlling salivation; sends neurological information to and from the posterior region of the tongue to the medulla oblongata of the brain stem

gustation: the ability to taste, which is independent of smell (olfaction) or textural and temperature enhancements; ageusia, or apogeusia, is the loss of taste sensation

gustatory stimulation threshold: the minimal quantity of tastant molecules that must be present in a water or saliva solution for a neural response at the taste cell to be initiated and the correct taste perceived; below this threshold, taste is either absent or identified incorrectly

taste bud: a special sensing structure for taste found on taste-responsive papillae; taste buds are made of three cell types-gustatory or taste cells, supporting cells, and basal cells

taste cell: the cellular compartment of a taste bud that contains chemoreceptors; taste hairs, one type of chemoreceptor, are found at the taste pore, or entry point, of a taste cell

vagus nerve: the tenth cranial nerve, which carries taste messages from the limited number of taste buds located in obscure sites such as the palate, epiglottis, uvula, and other structures at the entrance of the esophagus; also sends important information from the thoracic and abdominal viscera to the brain

vallate papillae: the seven to ten papillae mounds, arranged in a V shape, which can be seen when the tongue is fully extended; these taste sensors lack taste specificity

Structure and Functions

For many people, the thought of biting into a lemon causes a puckering or a tingling sensation in the mouth. A real taste sensation is evoked even though the actual taste stimulus, a lemon, is absent. This kind of response indicates the power of the sense of taste. Taste is also called the "gustatory sense," a term derived from the Latin word *gustatus,* meaning "taste." This sense evolved to aid animals in the selection of safe, nontoxic foods. Although loss of the ability to experience taste (ageusia) is not a life-threatening condition, it may indicate the presence of other maladies, some of which are life threatening. A diminished or absent ability to taste may account for loss of appetite or weight loss in some ill persons; for these persons, sufficient and proper nutrition can become a critical issue.

There are five special senses of the human body: gustation, olfaction (smell), vision, hearing, and equilibrium. The organs associated with the special senses take in information from the environment in the form of chemical, light, sound, or mechanical energy and convert that energy into nerve impulses. Nerve impulses are tiny electrical signals that are carried by the peripheral and central nervous systems to the brain, where the information is integrated in order to assess how dangerous or secure an individual may be in any given environment. Taste is a primitive sense, meaning that it need not be taught; it evokes instinctual responses or reactions.

Although taste is not as essential to survival as the sense of vision, it is an important sense for a variety of organisms. Taste preferences can be observed in humans, elephants, monkeys, fish, and even some microorganisms. Yet not all organisms respond equally to the same tastant; one example is sugar. Cats lack taste receptors for sugar; therefore, if a cat eats a sweet food, it does so for other flavors. Just as a cat does not taste sweetness, however, a human might not notice a tastant that a cat recognizes. A tastant is any food or chemical (such as soap) that causes a taste sensation.

Taste is a nerve impulse that is interpreted by the brain. (In organisms lacking a brain, taste is interpreted by some other structure that serves as the center of integration and coordination.) For humans, and for many of the larger land animals, taste sensations begin upon the intake of food or other sub-

stances into the mouth. This signal is prompted by the interaction of tastant molecules or ions and chemoreceptors located in specialized regions within taste buds.

Composed mostly of muscle fiber, the tongue not only serves as a receptor site for taste stimuli but also is responsible for the refined and coordinated movements that produce speech—an important form of communication in the human species. Different sections of the tongue are in contact with specific nerves that allow coordinated and specialized movements of the tongue. The palatine section of the tongue is easily seen when the tongue is fully extended from the mouth; it constitutes the front two-thirds of the tongue. The back one-third is the pharyngeal section; the palatine and pharyngeal sections are visibly, but subtly, separated by a transverse groove.

The surface of the palatine section of the tongue is coated with small, closely spaced projections called "papillae." These structures give the tongue the dual properties of being rough and textured while remaining velvety smooth. Papillae are arranged, from the tongue's tip to the back, in more or less parallel rows that run along the medial groove of the tongue. The medial groove divides the tongue lengthwise into equal halves that are independently coordinated by nerves and muscle working together.

Most papillae covering the tongue are of the filiform type. Unlike the other three papillae forms, filiform papillae do not contain taste buds and thus are not responsive to tastants. Instead, filiform papillae aid in the tearing and grating of food

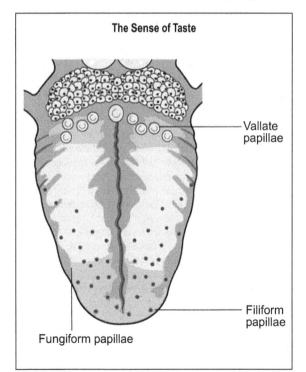

The Sense of Taste

Vallate papillae

Filiform papillae

Fungiform papillae

Special receptors on the tongue send nerve impulses to the brain that are registered as various tastes, such as bitter, sweet, salty, and sour.

particles. Although filiform papillae are not barbed, they do have a rasping mechanical action that aids in cleansing the body through licking (as observed in cats) and moving food particles about in the mouth.

All other papillae—the fungiform, the foliate, and the vallate—are actively involved in tasting, even though they are not present in great abundance or distributed uniformly over the tongue surface. Fungiform papillae, whose projections are shaped like a mushroom cap, are widely scattered on the tip and lateral sides of the tongue. Foliate papillae mimic the texture and appearance of smooth, folded leaves; they are located on both sides of the tongue, flanking the vallate papillae. The vallate papillae make a semicircular pattern (or a V shape) at the back of the tongue. Located on the palatine region just before the pharyngeal segment of the mouth, vallate papillae resemble rounded, soft cushions. Humans have between seven and twelve of these projections, making the vallate papillae the least abundant form of papillae.

Four tastes have commonly been recognized by humans: sweet, salty, sour, and bitter. These tastes are strongly registered in specific zones of the tongue. Much to the frustration of scientists, however, the recognition of taste is not specific to any particular type of taste-responsive papillae (fungiform, foliate, or vallate). Sweet receptors are plentiful at the tip of the tongue, while salty receptors are grouped together on either side just beyond the tip. Sour sensations are detected more strongly along the middle sides of the tongue, and bitter sensations are detected at the rear.

Since the vallate papillae are located in the region where only bitterness is tasted and the fungiform papillae are located in the regions sensitive to sweetness, one might assume that a match between papillae structure and taste type exists. Scientific studies, however, prove this to be a false correlation. A simple relationship between kind of taste and type of papillae does not exist, nor is there a complete explanation of the anatomy and physiology of the gustatory sense.

Taste-responsive papillae seem to respond to all tastants that enter their taste buds, whether they are classified as sweet, salty, sour, or bitter. The distinguishing factor seems to be a variation in the intensity of the neural message that a tastant induces. The variable levels of nervous impulses caused by a tastant constitute what is called a "taste profile." Taste profiles are mixed neural codes that a taste bud receives from certain tastants.

A tastant molecule causes a nervous impulse to be sent to the brain for interpretation. It has been learned that all three taste-sensitive papillae are fired, to a greater or lesser extent, by all tastant molecules. A neural response is triggered when tastant molecules arrive at specialized sites on the taste buds. Then there is a certain ratio, or firing pattern, that is interpreted as sweet, salty, sour, or bitter. Oddly, this kind of mixed signal can be misread in the brain. For example, if a sweet solution of table sugar and water (tasted and properly identified as sweet) is greatly diluted with very pure water, the sugar solution may be erroneously classified in the brain as salty. The taste sensation is simply able to recognize when something has interacted with a taste chemoreceptor; a weak stimulus

may cause a misinterpretation to occur.

For decades, researchers have been on the trail of an elusive fifth taste. While salty, bitter, sour, and sweet were all well-defined tastes, scientists have long suspected the presence of a fifth taste, called "umami." Umami is known more familiarly as the flavor enhancer monosodium glutamate (MSG). In the late 1990s, scientists at the University of Miami School of Medicine found compelling evidence of umami. Molecular biologists there demonstrated that a modified form of a brain glutamate, mGluR4, is a taste receptor for umami. Because its receptor was identified, many researchers now recognize umami as the fifth taste. Umami is difficult to describe, but foods such as Parmesan cheese, steak, seafood, mushrooms, and tomato juice have an umami component to them, though it is generally mixed in with other tastes as well.

Taste buds are relatively large, bulbous-shaped structures located on the tips of fungiform papillae and in the grooves of the foliate and vallate papillae. It is within the taste bud structure that sweet, salty, sour, or bitter begin the journey of becoming distinguished taste sensations. A taste bud is not a wholly sensing bundle; it can be divided into at least three distinct parts—taste (or sensing) cells, support cells, and basal cells.

The number of taste buds in humans ranges from two thousand to nine thousand. About half of these are located in the grooved edges of the vallate papillae, making this a very sensitive taste area of the tongue. Taste buds are abundant in infants and children, but a continuous decline is observed from adolescence throughout adulthood. This explains why adults often like to add rich sauces, gravies, and seasonings to foods; adults need to enhance food so that a greater range of taste sensations is triggered in each mouthful. Children tend to shun sauces and spices because they may experience almost overwhelming taste sensations when they consume adult-prepared foods. In the elderly, low numbers of taste cells can contribute to poor eating habits or food selection, putting them at risk during the most vulnerable stage in adult life. It is often recommended that foods be made readily available and prepared in colorful and aromatically pleasing ways to entice the elderly to eat properly.

Tastant particles must dissolve in saliva in order to cause a taste response that can be identified properly. The minimum amount of tastant that must be present for it to be identified correctly is called the "gustatory stimulation threshold." The requirement that a tastant be soluble in saliva is particularly true of sweet molecules (sugars and carbohydrates) or sour and some salty ions (salts and acids can release charged groups of atoms called "ions" when dissolved in saliva). Bitter substances seem to adhere to lipid sites on the papillae and thus could be thought of as fat-soluble molecules. Sweet, salty, and sour chemicals are generally hydrophilic (water loving), while bitter chemicals tend to be hydrophobic (water hating).

Whether hydrophilic or hydrophobic, tastant molecules or ions must get through the entry point on at least some taste cells located on taste buds. At the entry point of a taste cell, a tiny pore has small taste hair projections that are believed to be the true sensors of taste. The basic premise, according to current theory, is that the ions or molecules of the tastant substance enter the pore and then physically or chemically interact with specialized regions of the taste hairs. This interaction causes an action potential (a nerve impulse) to occur as the permeability of the nerve fibers innervating the taste cell is altered. An action potential will cause a wave of permeability changes all the way up the nerve fibers and into the brain. The medulla oblongata is the first site of the brain to receive the action potentials that will be registered as taste.

The exposure of taste cells to the environment renders them at risk to potential damage. Fortunately, new taste cells are regenerated every seven to ten days; regeneration occurs within the basal cells of the taste buds. It is important to note, however, that this is a regeneration of the taste cells, not of the nerves that innervate them. Olfactory nerves are the only nerve cells in the human body that can regenerate.

Disorders and Diseases

In the medical sciences, gustatory problems are generally not a cause but an effect. A diminished sense of taste (hypogeusia), an alteration of taste (dysgeusia), or the complete absence of the sense of taste (ageusia or apogeusia) is generally a symptom of an underlying pathology. It is rare for true ageusia to be an isolated symptom of a malady; it is even rarer for true ageusia to exist as an isolated physical malady. Yet ageusia does, in fact, exist in human populations. Among some descendants of the Ashkenazi Jews, for example, a double recessive genetic code mandates that taste papillae will not develop, resulting in congenital ageusia.

In discussing when or how noncongenital ageusia, hypogeusia, or dysgeusia can become a problem, it is important to review the critical components of a taste message. Three discrete structures are involved: taste cells, which contain taste hairs at their pores; nerve fibers, which connect the chemoreceptors (taste hairs) to the brain; and the brain itself. Alterations in the ability to taste can originate in any or all three of these discrete steps along the path.

Some pathologies that can cause a miscommunication at the receptor sites include actual physical or chemical damage to the taste buds, such as a burn that covers the tongue's surface or the ingestion of lye; accidental or therapeutic exposure to radiation; lingual (tongue) or palatal (palate) carcinomas; tumors or lesions of the tongue surface; or a leukemic infiltrate of the tongue surface.

The ability to taste may be altered or lost if damage occurs to certain cranial nerves. Specifically, damage to any of these cranial nerves may be responsible for taste disorders: the facial nerve (the seventh cranial nerve), which carries sweet and salty messages from the front of the tongue; the glossopharyngeal nerve (the ninth cranial nerve), which carries bitter and sour signals; and the large vagus nerve (the tenth cranial nerve), which carries taste sensations from the throat and epiglottis. Damage to these nerves may occur if they are crushed, severed, or pinched or if tumors, lesions, or neural disease interferes with normal function.

Finally, a head injury or malady can account for ageusia, hypogeusia, or dysgeusia. Regions of particular concern include damage to the medulla oblongata, the thalamus, or the gustatory cortex, which is located in the parietal lobe of the brain. Lesions, tumors, or head injuries resulting from sudden or severe impact can give rise to true taste pathology. In these cases, the brain can either no longer identify tastes properly or no longer receive or interpret taste impulses.

Indirect impairment of taste may occur as a result of an imbalance in body chemistry. Such imbalances may result from exposure to or ingestion of trace metal poisons or other toxins, insufficient dietary intake to allow for cellular repair or development, incomplete intake of essential vitamins or minerals, or metabolic imbalances, such as hypothyroidism (an underactive thyroid gland). In addition, taste-modifying pathologies, whose origins are not directly associated at the chemoreceptor sites, can involve allergic or drug reactions.

Other taste disorders that can be clinically assessed include cacogeusia, the alteration of once-pleasant tastes to ones that are repulsive (for example, the perception that all foods taste rotten); phantogeusia, the presence of a taste sensation in the absence of any tastant; heterogeusia, a distortion of tastes for all foods (for example, sweets may taste salty, salts may taste bitter, and so on); and parageusia, an unusual taste distortion of one taste type that does not cause a repulsive taste response (for example, bitter foods may taste salty).

In diagnosing a taste disorder, the physician must first obtain a full medical history from the patient and perform a physical examination. Because of the anatomy involved in taste function, special attention will be given to the head and neck area. General laboratory analysis of kidney, liver, and endocrine function must be performed, as well as a complete blood study. Also, tests may be administered to determine the possible role of allergies in a given pathology.

The issue of taste disorder is often complicated by the common use of terms that have specific meaning in a clinical setting. Three of these troublesome terms are "taste," "flavor," and "palatability." "Taste" means, quite literally, the chemoreceptor response of taste cells embedded in taste buds (located on the papillae), which is caused by tastant molecules. The interaction between the tastant and the chemoreceptors produces a nerve signal that travels from the taste receptor site to the brain. In stringent use of the term "taste," other factors, such as aroma, texture, or color, should not be considered in the assessment of this sense.

"Flavor" generally means the response of the olfactory and gustatory systems, working in unison, to assess the pleasure or displeasure prompted by a tastant. Smell is fundamentally integrated with taste to the point that people generally salivate more when exposed to an appealing odor, especially if the aroma is associated with a particularly pleasing food, such as freshly baked bread. A common exercise used to demonstrate the close connection between the olfactory and gustatory systems is a blind study in which the subjects close their eyes, pinch their noses shut, and sample uniformly sized cubes of solid foods kept at room temperature. Under such circumstances, most humans cannot distinguish among raw potato, raw onion, white cheese, and peeled fresh apple. Taste-testers may be shocked to discover that raw onions seem much the same as raw apples without visual or aromatic cues. This exercise speaks strongly to the significance of how humans integrate all of their senses in gathering data from the environment.

A loss or a decrease in the ability to smell greatly alters one's sense of flavor, even though there is no true loss of the ability to experience taste. A common example of this interrelationship between ability to smell foods or beverages and the connected ability to enjoy flavor has been experienced firsthand by anyone who has ever suffered from a severe head cold. When the nasal passages are coated with thick mucus, as generally occurs during a viral cold, eating is no longer pleasurable; foods are generally described as tasting flat or bland. The cold virus does not in any way interrupt the mechanics of the taste cells, nor does it disrupt the neurons associated with the taste cells. What is disrupted during a cold is the ability to smell and, therefore, enjoy the flavor of foods and beverages. Thus, a head cold alters the ability to experience fully all the sensory aspects of the foods or beverages that create a complete food sensation.

"Palatability" describes the association of taste with texture, temperature, and feeling. If a slice of bread is expected to be warm, soft, and sweet but what is ingested is cold, hard, and salty, then palatability is greatly diminished. If a person is truly hungry, however, then the lack of palatability, or even flavor, may be overruled by the greater need for nourishment. In the absence of the ability to see or to smell food (as in blindness or anosmia, respectively), texture and temperature take on heightened importance in the consumption of foods and beverages.

Taste disorders can be quantitatively assessed through various stimuli tests to measure the extent and type of taste disorder present. In addition, magnetic resonance imaging (MRI) and computed tomography (CT) scanning can be used to identify problems that may originate in the central nervous system. Positron emission tomography (PET) scanning can also be used to determine if brain lesions are responsible for a taste disorder. Treatments are as highly varied as the pathologies that cause taste disorders. Those disorders that arise from tumors may be treated by the surgical removal of the tumor. For certain metabolic imbalances, supplements rich in zinc ions may be administered. Some cases require simply restoring the patient to a healthy and balanced diet, while some rare disorders are untreatable.

Perspective and Prospects

Tasting is an inborn sense; it requires no training or skills. So-called acquired tastes are attained by adults mainly as a result of the declining population of taste cells, a natural aspect of the aging process. Because adults cannot sense food as fully as children, they may seek out heightened taste sensations, consuming salty foods such as caviar, drinking strong beverages such as whiskey, or enjoying spicy foods such as curry or hot peppers. Given their divergent taste responsiveness, it is reasonable to expect children to have natural aversions to certain foods, as compared to adults. A child is simply more aware of the mixed flavors of a given food, some of which may be bitter or sour relative to the way in which an adult senses the same food.

Like their primitive ancestors, modern humans let the tip of the tongue sample a new food before actually ingesting it. It is believed, therefore, that sweet receptors evolved to occupy the tip of the tongue to help humans seek out and consume safe foods in nature. Sweet foods, such as carbohydrate-rich vegetables, fruits, and (to some extent) proteins, are generally safe and nourishing. Therefore, humans tend to seek sweet flavors, especially in the infant stages, over salty, sour, or bitter ones. This instinctual drive may account for the powerful attraction many people have for sweet desserts and candies.

Bitterness is detected in the mouth nearer the esophagus. This location seems to prevent humans from naturally seeking bitter foods. Furthermore, it allows for the rejection of a bitter food before it enters the esophagus, where the food would be well on its way to digestion and absorption. This adaptation to the environment aids in human survival. Many naturally bitter substances are poisons or potential toxins. Included in the list of bitter taste sources are caffeine-containing tea leaves and coffee beans, cocaine, nicotine, almond bitters, and lye (sodium hydroxide). At the turn of the twenty-first century, scientists identified a new family of genes that encode proteins that function as bitter taste receptors. The discovery opens the way for the identification of additional receptors that detect bitter and sweet tastes and also gives researchers new probes with which to trace the wiring of the taste perception pathways into the brain itself.

In 2002, scientists reported the discovery of a new taste receptor that recognizes most of the twenty naturally occurring amino acids. They theorize that this receptor was evolutionary important because it helps humans select foods rich in these essential nutrients.

Researchers also continue to investigate the influence of genetics on food preferences, diminishment of tasting ability with age, regeneration of taste and smell receptors, relationship between the sweet taste receptors and glucose regulation, and better means of diagnosis and treatment for taste disorders.

Taste is a special sense that facilitates the ability of an organism to survive in or interact with an environment. More than this, however, taste provides the body with great sensory pleasure. Serving as both a tool to survive and as a pleasure-seeking sensor, taste is a unique and enriching sense.

—*Mary C. Fields, M.D.*

See also Aging; Appetite loss; Digestion; Food biochemistry; Food poisoning; Malnutrition; Nervous system; Nutrition; Otorhinolaryngology; Poisoning; Sense organs; Smell; Toxicology.

For Further Information:

A.D.A.M. Medical Encyclopedia. "Taste - Impaired." *MedlinePlus*, March 5, 2011.

Atkins, Peter. *Atkins" Molecules*. 2d ed. New York: Cambridge University Press, 2003.

Mã„ller, Aage R. *Sensory Systems: Anatomy, Physiology, and Pathophysiology.* 2d ed. Richardson, Tex: Author, 2012.

National Institute on Deafness and Other Communication Disorders. "Taking the Bitter out of Bittersweet." *U.S. Department of Health and Human Services, National Institutes of Health,* July 5, 2011.

National Institute on Deafness and Other Communication Disorders. "Taste Disorders." *U.S. Department of Health and Human Services, National Institutes of Health,* June 7, 2011.

National Institute on Aging. "Smell and Taste: Spice of Life." *U.S. Department of Health and Human Services, National Institutes of Health,* June 26, 2013.

Schmidt, Robert F., ed. "Physiology of Taste." *Fundamentals of Sensory Physiology.* Translated by Marguerite A. Biedermann-Thorson. Rev. 3d ed. Berlin: Springer, 1986.

Shier, David N., Jackie L. Butler, and Ricki Lewis. *Hole's Essentials of Human Anatomy and Physiology.* 11th ed. Boston: McGraw-Hill, 2011.

"Smell and Taste." *American Academy of Otolaryngology " Head and Neck Surgery,* 2013.

Tortora, Gerard J., and Bryan Derrickson. *Principles of Anatomy and Physiology.* 13th ed. Hoboken, N.J.: John Wiley & Sons, 2012.

Wolfe, Jeremy M., et al. *Sensation and Perception.* 2d ed. Sunderland, Mass.: Sinauer, 2009.

Tattoo Removal
Procedure
Anatomy or system affected: Skin
Specialties and related fields: Dermatology, general surgery
Definition: The use of lasers to break up tattoo ink under the skin.

Indications and Procedures
Application of a tattoo is relatively easy, although the process is painful. A design is drawn on the skin. Needles are used to push the ink down into the skin. When the skin heals from the multiple punctures, the design remains permanently in place. Attempts have been made to remove tattoos since the first one was applied. Scrubbing with sandpaper or table salt has been tried to scour the surface of the skin and remove the tattoo. The results have usually been disfigurement or scarring.

Currently, laser therapy is the most effective way of removing unwanted tattoos. The Food and Drug Administration (FDA) has approved several types of lasers for tattoo removal. The standard device now used is some form of Q-switched laser, which produces a pulsed beam with much higher power at the peak of the pulse than a continuous wave laser. When applied to a tattoo, the ink embedded in the skin absorbs the pulse of energy. The laser energy causes the tattoo ink to break up into fragments that can be removed by cells of the body's immune system. The treatment feels like a rubber band snapping against the skin, and local anesthetics may be necessary when attempting to remove large tattoos. Immediately after the laser treatment, the treated area turns white and might swell slightly; over the next few days, blisters and scabs may form. Within seven to ten days, the skin will look normal. Several such treatments are required, spaced a number of weeks apart.

Other, significantly less popular methods of tattoo removal include dermabrasion, where the outer layers of skin that hold the ink are abraded (scraped or rubbed away) with a spinning abrasive pad, and surgical excision, in which small tattoos can be removed by cutting them out and closing the skin with stitches

Uses and Complications
The number of treatments required to remove a tattoo depends on several factors: the color of ink, the amount of ink, the depth of the tattoo, and the location of the tattoo. Professional tattoos may require more treatments to remove than those applied by amateurs, because professionals tend to use more ink and to apply the ink deeper into the skin. Ideally, treatments are spaced several weeks apart to allow the body's immune system to remove the maximum amount of ink between sessions; this time is also necessary to allow the skin to recover fully before the next treatment.

It is more problematic to remove tattoos from areas of the body with thin skin, such as the face, genitals, and ankles. In the case of tattoo removal, laser treatments are designed to remove the unwanted buildup of abnormal pigment (ink) in the skin; however, people with dark skin have high amounts of natural pigment (melanin) in their skin. Sometimes, lasers cannot distinguish between tattoo ink pigment and normal skin pigment. As a result, both types of pigment are destroyed, leaving pale patches on the skin; these patches can fade with time. Conversely, an increase in pigmentation can be seen after treatment, causing dark patches on the skin; these patches can also fade with time. It is recommended that patients stay out of the sun before and after treatment for tattoo removal. Tattoo removal can lead to scarring, but with the modern laser methods, this is becoming rarer. The most striking side effect of laser tattoo removal is the cost, typically much higher than the cost of the original tattoo. Nonetheless, according to the American Society for Dermatologic Surgery, its members performed some 100,000 tattoo removals in 2011, up from 86,000 in 2010.

—*L. Fleming Fallon, Jr., M.D., Ph.D., M.P.H.*

See also Blisters; Dermatology; Healing; Laser use in surgery; Pigmentation; Skin; Skin disorders; Tattoos and body piercing.

For Further Information:
Ahluwalia, Gurpreet S., ed. *Cosmetic Applications of Laser and Light-Based Systems.* Norwich, N.Y.: William Andrew, 2009.

Camphausen, Rufus C. *Return of the Tribal: A Celebration of Body Adornment: Piercing, Tattooing, Scarification, Body Painting.* Rochester, Vt.: Park Street Press, 1997.

Graves, Bonnie B. *Tattooing and Body Piercing.* Mankato, Minn.: LifeMatters, 2000.

Hewitt, Kim. *Mutilating the Body: Identity in Blood and Ink.* Bowling Green, Ohio: Bowling Green State University Popular Press, 1997.

"Inked and Regretful: Removing Tattoos." *U.S. Food and Drug Administration,* January 30, 2013.

Kirby, William, Emily Holmes, Alpesh Desai, and Tejas Desai. "Best Clinical Practices in Laser Tattoo Removal." *Dermatologist* (June 2012): 23–28.

Miller, Jean-Chris. *The Body Art Book: A Complete, Illustrated Guide to Tattoos, Piercings, and Other Body Modifications.* Rev. ed. New York: Berkley, 2004.

Wilkinson, Beth. *Coping with the Dangers of Tattooing, Body Piercing, and Branding.* New York: Rosen, 1998.

"Unwanted Tattoos." *American Society for Dermatologic Surgery,* 2013.

TATTOOS AND BODY PIERCING

Procedure

Anatomy or system affected: Muscles, skin

Specialties and related fields: Dermatology, plastic surgery, public health

Definition: Piercing of the skin to implant devices or make designs.

Key terms:

dermis: the deepest skin layer

epidermis: the outer skin layer

mortification: self-induced physical pain

proof of ordeal: a painful surgical procedure that leaves a scar, design, or skin mutilation

tattooing: piercing of the skin with pigments or dyes

Indications and Procedures

Tattooing is accomplished by a variety of techniques, usually by persons who are specialists. In traditional cultures, a shaman or other religious practitioner would create a tattoo by piercing the skin with a sharpened object (such as a bone splinter or a piece of metal) or with a bundle of porcupine quills or ponderosa pine needles, or by passing a colored string on a needle through the skin. The colors were from mineral salts, charcoal, certain plant juices, and even the feces of dogs that had been fed charcoal.

Coloring inks were available from the end of the nineteenth century and are now supplied in liquid forms. They can be applied in either the so-called European fashion, in which the coloring ink is applied over a small surface and an electric vibrating needle impregnates the epidermis and the dermis, or the American procedure, in which the needle contains the desired pigment.

The skin is prepared in a variety of ways, usually by smearing a thin layer of petroleum jelly over the site to minimize the seepage of blood and tissue fluids that would otherwise obscure the artist's view. When the tattoo is completed, the area is washed and then covered with an antiseptic ointment. Tattoos assume various geometric or curvilinear designs and can be executed over all of a person's body or simply within a restricted area. Extensive tattooing may take several years to complete.

The most obvious forms of body piercing, by both males and females, are performed in the ears, nose, nasal septum, tongue, navel, lips, scalp, eyelids, or cheeks. In some cultures, the lips or ears may be grossly distorted by inserting over time increasingly large objects, such as pieces of horn, bone, wood, and even metal. In some cases, the particular style of body piercing may indicate a person's marital status, group membership, or religious affiliation, or it may simply be cosmetic mutilation. Body piercing has become increasingly common in Western culture since the later twentieth century. The breasts, particularly the nipples, are another common site for the insertion of either closed or threaded rings on both men and women. Less commonly, body piercing may also be performed on the male or female genitals. An example of male genital piercing is the Prince Albert, in which a ring or curved barbell enters the urethra and exits through the underside or, in some cases, the top of the glans penis. Women may have clitoral or labial piercings.

Uses and Complications

Tattoos and body piercing of the human body have been practiced by all cultures throughout the world to serve different functions: for religious purposes, as an indication of certain status changes or the accomplishment of culturally significant tasks, as a proof of ordeal, for medical reasons, as body art, as identification marks, to signify membership in either sacred or profane organizations, or to attain visions through mortification of the flesh. Depending on the culture or specific group, men, women, and children may undergo these frequently painful rituals. Various cultures believe that the soul's transition to a life hereafter is facilitated by having certain tattoos and body piercings. Often, the degree of pain experienced during the rituals of tattooing and body piercing, and from the subsequent wounds, not only is a proof of ordeal but also may serve as a physical and spiritual atonement for a person's moral transgressions. Certain groups, such as the Newar of Bhaktapur in Nepal, believe that they may gain a higher incarnation when they sell their tattoos in heaven.

In the United States during the early twentieth century, it became popular for women to be tattooed for eyeliner, cheek blush, and even colored lips. Although tattooing and body piercing were once associated with motorcycle gang members, prisoners, and military personnel, these procedures have become more popular with the general public. Tattooing and self-mutilation by body piercing are gaining popularity as forms of personal expression, particularly with women, who make up approximately 70 percent of the new business.

A concern, however, is the increasing frequency of adolescents engaging in tattooing and body piercing. Today, body piercing in Western cultures is often viewed by teenagers and young adults as a rite of passage, sometimes symbolically in defiance of the established social order. When self-practiced, tattooing and body piercing can lead to infection and even septicemia, particularly when people use instruments and inks that are not sterile.

Perspective and Prospects

Some anthropologists believe that the first documented examples of tattooing were practiced in Egypt approximately four thousand years ago. These conclusions are supported by tattooed female mummies and by clay figurines that have puncture "tattoos." Although there is not agreement among scholars, some believe that the practice of tattooing may have diffused from Egypt to other parts of the world.

Perhaps the most artistic and dramatic full-body tattooing was done by the Japanese as early as the fifth century BCE and the Maori of New Zealand; even today, many young male Maori follow this traditional custom. The Maori were noted for facial tattoos, called *moko*, that served to frighten and intimidate their enemies. The word "tattoo," however, comes from the Tahitian word *ta-tau*; it was encountered by eighteenth- and nineteenth-century European explorers in Polynesia, who introduced tattoos to Europe and America.

—*John Alan Ross, Ph.D.*

See also Acquired immunodeficiency syndrome (AIDS); Dermatology; Dermatology, pediatric; Hepatitis; Plastic surgery; Puberty and adolescence; Skin; Skin disorders; Tattoo removal.

For Further Information:
Brown, Kelli McCormack, Paula Perlmutter, and Robert J. McDermott. "Youth and Tattoos: What School Health Personnel Should Know." *Journal of School Health* 70, no. 9 (November, 2000): 355–360.
DeMello, Margo. *Bodies of Inscription: A Cultural History of the Modern Tattoo Community.* Durham, N.C.: Duke University Press, 2000.
Gard, Carolyn. "Think Before You Ink: The Risks of Body Piercing and Tattooing." *Current Health* 25, no. 6 (February, 1999): 24–25.
Gay, Kathlyn, and Christine Whittington. *Body Marks: Tattooing, Piercing, and Scarification.* Brookfield, Conn.: Millbrook Press, 2002.
Gilbert, Steve. *The Tattoo History: A Source Book.* New York: Juno Books, 2000.
"Support for Body Piercing Checks." *Nursing Standard* 14, no. 30 (April 12–18, 2000): 8.
"Tattoos and Body Piercings." *American Academy of Dermatology*, 2013.
"Tattoos: Understanding Risks and Precautions." *Mayo Clinic*, March 20, 2012.

TAY-SACHS DISEASE
Disease/Disorder
Anatomy or system affected: Nervous system
Specialties and related fields: Genetics, neonatology, neurology, pediatrics
Definition: An inherited disorder in which products of fat metabolism (gangliosides) accumulate in and destroy the brain and spinal cord.

Causes and Symptoms
Tay-Sachs disease is a genetic disorder of lipid (fat) metabolism resulting from a missing enzyme. This enzyme normally breaks down special nerve lipids known as gangliosides, which are present in the brain and spinal cord. These substances accumulate and destroy the cells, often killing the child by age three or four years.

Several features at birth may raise the possibility of early detection, particularly cherry-red spots on the retina of the eye. Most newborns with Tay-Sachs disease, however, appear normal at birth. Between the ages of three months and six months, the progressive neurologic damage becomes apparent: deafness, blindness, muscle paralysis, and developmental disorders. By eighteen months, the infant is usually already in a vegetative state, requiring complete care. The child may survive until three or four years of age, dying from complications associated with comatose and bedridden patients, usually infections.

Information on Tay-Sachs Disease
Causes: Genetic disorder
Symptoms: Initially, cherry-red spots on retina; in later stages, deafness, blindness, muscle paralysis, mental retardation, vegetative state
Duration: Three or four years, until death
Treatments: Supportive therapy only

Treatment and Therapy
Tay-Sachs disease has no cure, and only supportive measures can be used. Feeding tubes for nutrition and fluids, suctioning of throat secretions, meticulous skin care for bed sores, and oxygen to assist breathing are among the types of support needed. Full-time skilled nursing care at home or at a facility is often necessary.

Perspectives and Prospects
While Tay-Sachs disease is the most common lipid (or lysosomal) storage disease, it is rare in the general population—about one in 250 people carry the genetic mutation that causes Tay-Sachs. It is much more common, however, in people of Ashkenazi (Eastern European) Jewish ancestry, as well as those of French Canadian and Cajun ancestry. Among these populations, approximately one person in twenty-seven is a carrier of the genetic defect. If two such carriers have children, they have a 25 percent chance of having a child with Tay-Sachs disease. Prenatal testing using amniocentesis or chorionic villus sampling can detect affected fetuses. More important is genetic counseling and screening of couples with a family history. A blood test can identify carriers.

Ongoing research is attempting to correct the disease in the developing fetus through the insertion of the missing gene.

—*Connie Rizzo, M.D., Ph.D.*

See also Amniocentesis; Chorionic villus sampling; Coma; Embryology; Enzymes; Gaucher's disease; Gene therapy; Genetic counseling; Genetic diseases; Genetics and inheritance; Lipids; Metabolic disorders; Metabolism; Neonatology; Niemann-Pick disease; Pediatrics; Screening.

For Further Information:
Bartoshesky, Louis E. "Tay-Sachs Disease." *KidsHealth.org.* Nemours Foundation, May 2011.
Behrman, Richard E., Robert M. Kliegman, and Hal B. Jenson, eds. *Nelson Textbook of Pediatrics.* 19th ed. Philadelphia: Saunders/Elsevier, 2011.
Bellenir, Karen, ed. *Genetic Disorders Sourcebook: Basic Consumer Information About Hereditary Diseases and Disorders.* 3d ed. Detroit, Mich.: Omnigraphics, 2004.
Gormley, Myra Vanderpool. *Family Diseases: Are You at Risk?* Baltimore: Genealogical Publishing, 2002.
Harper, Peter S. *Practical Genetic Counselling.* 7th ed. New York: Oxford University Press, 2010.
Hollenstein, Jenna, and Kari-Kassir. "Tay-Sachs Disease." *Health Library*, Nov. 26, 2012.
McCance, Kathryn L., and Sue M. Huether. *Pathophysiology: The Biologic Basis for Disease in Adults and Children.* 6th ed. St. Louis, Mo.: Mosby/Elsevier, 2010.
Milunsky, Aubrey, ed. *Genetic Disorders of the Fetus: Diagnosis, Prevention, and Treatment.* 6th ed. Hoboken, N.J.: Wiley-

Blackwell, 2009.

"NINDS Tay-Sachs Disease Information Page." *National Institute of Neurological Disorders and Stroke*, Oct. 6, 2011.

Parker, James N., and Philip M. Parker, eds. *The Official Parent's Sourcebook on Tay-Sachs Disease*. San Diego, Calif.: Icon Health, 2002.

"Tay-Sachs Disease." *MedlinePlus*, May 9, 2013.

"Tay-Sachs Disease." *National Tay-Sachs and Allied Diseases Association*, 2012.

Tears and tear ducts

Anatomy

Also known as: Lacrimal ducts, nasolacrimal ducts, tear film

Anatomy or system affected: Eyes, head, nose

Specialties and related fields: Ophthalmology, optometry

Definition: Fluid produced by the eye and the channel that carries it from the eye to the nasal cavity.

Key terms:

canaliculus: a small canal linking the upper and lower puncta to the lacrimal sac

cornea: the transparent front portion of the eye

fluorescein: a brightly colored dye used for diagnostic purposes

instill: to slowly put a liquid into the eye, drop by drop

lacrimal: pertaining to the secretion and conduction of tears

lysosyme: an enzyme found in body secretions that destroys bacteria by breaking down their walls

ophthalmologist: a medical doctor who specializes in the treatment of disorders of the eye

Structure and Functions

The lacrimal gland is located beneath the upper eyelid, on the outer edge of each eye, and its key function is to produce tears. Tears flow constantly across the conjunctiva, which is the front surface of the eye, in order to keep it clean and lubricated. Blinking spreads tears across the eye. This constant flushing of the eye surface also supplies oxygen and nutrients to the cornea. Tears provide an important barrier to infection as they contain the antibacterial enzyme lysosyme, which destroys microorganisms on the eye surface. As new tears are produced, old tears drain from the eye at its inner edge, called the "canthus," by being drawn into two small holes, the upper and lower puncta, through capillary action. Tears flow through the canaliculus, entering the lacrimal sac, then to the tear duct (called the "nasolacrimal duct"), and at last into the nasal cavity. This is the reason that a surplus of tears results in a runny nose.

Tears, or tear film, are made up of three distinct layers: an outer oily layer to prevent drying, which is produced by the meibomion glands; a watery middle layer, which contains the oxygen and nutrients; and an inner mucous layer, produced by the conjunctival goblet cells, reducing the surface tension of the tears and allowing them to be spread evenly on the surface of the eye.

The body naturally produces tears in order to maintain and protect the eye, but in humans, tears are also produced in response to emotion in the form of crying. During a normal twenty-four-hour day, 0.75 to 1.1 grams of tears are secreted; however, this rate declines with age. Also, approximately 10 to 15 percent of tear secretion is lost to evaporation, dependent on the environment.

Disorders and Diseases

The most common disorder associated with tears is excessive tearing. This can occur for many reasons and may require evaluation by an ophthalmologist. An excessive amount of tears can be caused by infection, environmental irritants, glaucoma, certain medications, allergic reaction, eyestrain, dry eyes, foreign material in the eye, scratch on the surface of the eye, or other eyelid or eyelash disorders.

Dry eye, also described as "scratchy eye," can occur when too few tears are being produced, or they are draining from the eye too rapidly or evaporating too quickly. Symptoms of dry eye may also include photosensitivity, blurred vision, redness, and an itching or burning sensation. Often the treatment is to instill drops of artificial tears or lubricating gel, to apply compresses, and to avoid potential irritants such as excessively dry or warm rooms to prevent evaporation. If the cause of dry eye is that tears are draining too quickly, then a surgeon may modify the tear duct to slow or limit tear drainage.

Another common disorder associated with tear ducts is obstruction. If there is an obstruction of the tear duct (nasolacrimal duct), then tears are not able to drain easily into the nasal cavity. Blockage of the tear duct can occur in early childhood as a congenital blockage or later in life as a result of chronic infection or irritation, injury, or tumor. In order to test the tear duct for obstruction, a drop of fluorescein dye will be instilled into the lower lid and then the patient will be observed at regular intervals to determine if the dye has traveled through to the nasal cavity. Treatment varies depending on the underlying cause.

A congenital blockage occurs in 6 to 20 percent of infants when a membrane remains between the tear duct and nasal cavity. This results in the inability for the eye to drain, and the eye appears excessively watery or filled with mucus. Often the membrane will rupture spontaneously before one year of age, thus resolving the obstruction, but sometimes a probe will need to be inserted by an ophthalmologist.

Tear duct obstruction may cause an acute infection of the lacrimal sac, located at the upper, wider end of the nasolacrimal duct. This form of infection is called "dacrocystitis," and patients normally have an overflowing of tears (epiphora) and a swollen painful mass over the area of the lacrimal sac. Dacrocystitis may be treated with warm compresses and gentle massage but may require systemic antibiotics and drainage of the mass.

Perspective and Prospects

Research is being conducted to determine if tears not only provide nutrients and moisture to the eye but also have diagnostic uses. Tears are created from blood that has been filtered; therefore, tears can provide medical clues as to things happening in the blood. Studies are being done to determine if biological changes in the eye and eye health can be measured through small variations in the level of inflammatory proteins found in tears. Also, in 2000, a group of contact lens researchers in Australia found that tears contain protein markers that may be used to detect certain types of cancer. Research is continuing in this area in the hope that tears may provide useful information in future diagnoses.

—*April D. Ingram*

See also Eye infections and disorders; Eyes; Glands; Host-defense mechanisms; Ophthalmology; Sense organs; Sjögren's syndrome; Vision; Vision disorders.

For Further Information:
A.D.A.M. Medical Encyclopedia. "Dry Eye Syndrome." *MedlinePlus*, November 20, 2012.

"Blocked Tear Duct." *Mayo Foundation for Medical Education and Research*, February 13, 2013.

Cohen, Adam, Michael Mercandetti, and Brian Brazzo, eds. *The Lacrimal System: Diagnosis, Management, and Surgery.* New York: Springer, 2006.

Howson, Alexandra, and Christopher Cheyer. "Lacrimal Duct Stenosis." *Health Library*, June 4, 2012.

Kohnle, Diana, and Michael Woods. "Dacryocystitis." *Health Library*, November 26, 2012.

Sullivan, David, Darlene Dartt, and Michele Meneray, eds. *Lacrimal Gland, Tear Film, and Dry Eye Syndromes 2: Basic Science and Clinical Relevance.* New York: Plenum Press, 1998.

"Tear System." *American Society of Ophthalmic Plastic and Reconstructive Surgery*, 2012.

Van Haeringen, N. J. "Aging and the Lacrimal System." *British Journal of Ophthalmology* 81 (1997): 824–26.

TEETH
Anatomy

Anatomy or system affected: Bones, brain, gastrointestinal system, gums, heart, musculoskeletal system, nervous system

Specialties and related fields: Dentistry, orthodontics

Definition: Structures that aid animals in processing food prior to swallowing, bringing food into the mouth and grinding; they may also be used for defense, the killing of prey, and displays of either hostility or pleasure.

Key terms:

cementum: the outer covering of the root of a tooth

crown: the portion of the tooth, normally covered with enamel, that is exposed in the oral cavity above the gingiva (gums)

cusp: the conical projection of the chewing surface of the tooth

cuspid: the longest anterior tooth; also called the canine tooth or the eyetooth

dentin: the substance that composes the major portion of the tooth internally

enamel: the tissue that covers the crown of the tooth; the hardest tissue in the body

gingiva: the gum tissue surrounding the neck of the tooth

incisor: one of the front teeth, used primarily to cut or shear food with a scissoring motion

molars: the back teeth used to grind food into smaller portions prior to swallowing

periodontium: those tissues supporting the tooth in the jaws, including the gingiva, the jawbone, and the periodontal ligament that attaches the root of the tooth into the jaw

premolars: the teeth between the cuspids and the molars, used in crushing and grinding food; also called bicuspids

pulp: the internal, living tissue of the tooth, consisting of nerves, blood vessels, and dental cells

root: the portion of the tooth that is below the crown and is embedded in a bony socket of the jaw

Structure and Functions

Teeth are functional portions of the mouths of animals that assist them in processing food prior to swallowing. This process is called chewing, or mastication. Teeth are also primary offensive and defensive weapons for most animals. Many animals have no hands to grasp or capture food, and their teeth become the principal means of grabbing and killing prey. In humans, teeth not only process food but also have a sociological significance in displaying anger, friendliness, and desirability.

A tooth is composed of three basic parts: the crown, the dental pulp, and the root. The crown of the tooth is that portion exposed above the gingiva, commonly called the gums. The outer surface of the crown is covered by a hard, crystalline substance called enamel. Enamel is an almost completely inorganic material, calcium hydroxyapatite, and it is the hardest tissue in the human body. Underneath the enamel, the bulk of the crown is made up of a substance known as dentin. It, too, is quite hard, but it has more organic material, ground substance and nerve fibers, within it. The dentin is honeycombed by small tubules radiating from the dental pulp chamber at the center of the tooth. These tubules carry nerve

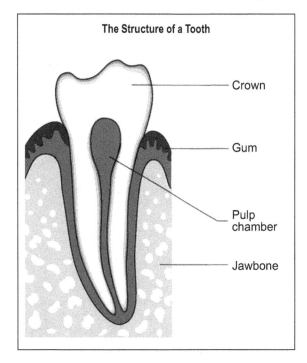

The Structure of a Tooth

Crown

Gum

Pulp chamber

Jawbone

fibers from the central nerve within the pulp to the junction of the enamel and dentin.

In the center of the crown is the pulp chamber. The pulp contains nerves and blood vessels that give sensations to and nourish the tooth. These nerves and blood vessels enter at the tip of the root, the apex, and arise from nerve trunks and blood vessels that run through the jawbone.

The root is the portion of the tooth joining the crown to the jawbone. The outer surface of the root is covered by a thin layer of bonelike substance called cementum, and it runs from the junction of the enamel of the crown to the apex of the root. Under the cementum, dentin composes the bulk of the root, continuing from the crown to the apex. The root is attached from the cementum to the bony socket in the jaw by the periodontal ligament. This ligament is composed of elastic connective tissue fibers that act not only as part of the attachment apparatus for the tooth but also as a shock absorber from chewing forces. The pulp chamber narrows into a thin, constricted channel from the pulp chamber to the apex; this is known as the root canal. In some animals, such as rodents, the root canal of incisors remains relatively large throughout life and is called "evergrowing." In most animals, including humans, the root canal constricts to prevent further growth while still providing sufficient blood flow for proper tooth nourishment. These teeth are termed "rooted" (although all teeth are actually rooted). The tooth is surrounded by the tissues of the attachment apparatus called the periodontium, consisting of the gingiva, the periodontal ligament, and the alveolar bone of the jaws.

In humans, there are normally thirty-two adult teeth and twenty deciduous (or baby) teeth. Deciduous teeth start calcifying in the embryo at about five to six weeks of development. Teeth start to form from two types of cells at an interface in the tooth bud, which becomes the dentoenamel junction. The enamel is formed by a cell called an ameloblast, and the dentin is formed by a cell known as an odontoblast. The enamel grows outward and the dentin inward from the interface. The pulp is formed from nerves and blood vessels in the developing jawbone. While the crown is growing, the root starts to form, lengthening as the tooth develops. After the crown is formed, the ameloblast cells rest on the outer surface of the enamel, while the odontoblasts line the internal cavity of the pulp chamber.

When the tooth erupts through the gum tissue, the ameloblasts are compressed and destroyed. Enamel is one of the two tissues in the human body that cannot repair itself (the other being the cornea of the eye). The odontoblasts can be activated inside the pulp chamber to form a secondary or reparative dentin. This formation of insulating dentin is in response to aging, advancing tooth decay, or trauma to the tooth or in reaction to the placement of restorative materials into a tooth.

The deciduous teeth begin to erupt through the gums in infancy and continue to do so until the full complement of primary dentition has erupted. Most of the adult teeth develop below the baby teeth, and as they push on the roots of the primary teeth, these roots are resorbed from the pressure of erupting permanent crowns. The primary teeth are shed throughout childhood and into adolescence. Other animals have both primary and permanent teeth. Sharks continually develop full sets of teeth, sometimes as many as seven or eight at a time; as their teeth loosen or break off, new teeth replace them. Humans, however, possess only one set of permanent teeth, and they are not naturally replaced if they are lost through trauma or disease.

Mammals differ from all other animals in having teeth set in sockets (thecodont) and in having several different kinds of teeth (heterodont), compared to the homodont teeth of animals such as sharks and reptiles.

The shape and size of teeth are closely related to their functions. The four front incisor teeth, both upper and lower, are used to shear and cut food. The movement of the mobile lower jaw, the mandible, against the static upper jaw, the maxilla, causes these teeth to work as scissors on food. Horses crop grasses with their large incisors. Cusps are conical projections of the cuspids and posterior teeth. They act as crushing and grinding segments of the posterior teeth, reducing the food into smaller portions that may be swallowed and digested efficiently. The four cuspids, or canines, are conical and pointed. Their primary function is to grasp and tear food. The fangs of a tiger are cuspids, as are those of lions. The eight premolars have two conical cusps and are called bicuspid teeth. They too are used for tearing, but working against the opposing teeth, they also function as a mill, crushing and grinding the food.

The twelve molars are multicusped teeth that grind food into smaller portions; mixed with saliva, the food is then readied for swallowing. The grooves of the occlusal (chewing) surfaces act as sluiceways to channel the food in the oral cavity. The tongue folds the food back onto the surfaces of the grinding teeth until it is chewed sufficiently.

The third molars are commonly called wisdom teeth. These teeth are the last to develop and are more prone to irregular calcification and morphology. In the course of human evolution, the jaws have shortened, and the third molars often do not have enough room in the jaw to erupt in a normal, perpendicular mode. The result is an irregular angle of eruption. When the third molars lock and push against the second molars and are unable to erupt normally, the condition is called impaction. Thus, in many cases, the wisdom teeth must be removed.

Teeth and their supporting tissues are susceptible to disease. The primary disease of the tooth is dental caries, or tooth decay. Caries (cavities) begin with the decalcification of the enamel crystals by acids. These acids are products of bacteria caught in a sticky film that forms on the teeth called plaque. These bacteria use refined hydrocarbons, principally sugars, for their food. If the plaque is not removed from the surface of the teeth, the acids are kept close to the enamel. Over a period of time, the decalcification of the enamel reaches the internal dentin, and the acid begins to decay the less calcified enamel at a more rapid rate. The acids also can touch the nerve fibers within the dental tubules, causing sensitivity and pain. If this process is not stopped, the decay can penetrate into the pulp and cause infection.

When the pulp becomes infected, it invariably dies. The dead tissues gradually seep through the apex, and bacteria feed on the necrotic material. Inflammatory cells from the blood vessels in the bone try to fight the infection, which can cause swelling, pain, and pus. The result is a periapical abscess.

The periodontium is also susceptible to disease, and again, the bacterial plaque is the chief cause. Surrounding the neck of the tooth is a cuff of gum tissue. The bacteria in the plaque release their waste products into the cuff and irritate the lining. Inflammatory white cells, known as lymphocytes or chronic inflammatory cells, are brought from the blood vessels in the gum tissue to the point of irritation in order to attack the bacteria and their by-products. This disease is called gingivitis, which can be reversed by removing the dental plaque.

If the plaque is allowed to remain on the surface of the tooth, it may calcify into a hard, rough, and porous substance called dental calculus or, more commonly, tartar. This material attracts and entraps more bacteria, and it is abrasive to the soft lining of the gingiva. The gums become further inflamed, bringing more lymphocytes into the area. These cells try to attack the bacteria and dissolve the dead and dying cells of the diseased gingiva.

Over a period of time, the inflammatory cells move deeper into the periodontium, dissolving and detaching the elastic fibers of the periodontal ligament and eroding the crest of the bony socket. This inflammation of the periodontium is called periodontitis. With the destruction of the fibers attaching the gingiva and bone to the root, the cuff of gum tissue deepens into a pocket around the neck of the tooth. The depth of the pocket facilitates the further entrapment of bacteria and makes it more difficult to clean.

If the condition is not corrected, eventually there is enough destruction of the periodontium that the tooth becomes loose. Often, the chronic inflammatory cells at the bottom of a deep pocket are joined by acute inflammatory cells, producing painful swelling and pus. This condition is known as a periodontal abscess. Most extractions of adult teeth are the result of periodontitis.

Disorders and Diseases

The principal scientific professions requiring knowledge of teeth and their surrounding structures are those of dentistry and dental hygiene. Dentists need to have thorough knowledge of the anatomy and physiology of the teeth and their surrounding structures in the mouth. They must be able to detect and treat diseases of the mouth and all its tissues. Dental caries, infected pulp, diseases of the periodontium, and tooth loss are treated by dentists. Dental hygienists aid dentists by treating and identifying diseases of the mouth. Their principal duty is to remove harmful deposits on the teeth, but hygienists also identify diseases of the teeth and periodontium. Using their anatomical and physiological knowledge of the teeth and surrounding structures, hygienists teach patients preventative techniques that can help prevent or halt the spread of dental disease.

Since the teeth and oral tissues are only a part of the body, knowledge of general human anatomy, physiology, and pathology is a must for dentists. Oral symptomatology discovered by dentists is often the first sign of a serious systemic disease. For example, a certain fruity odor on the breath is a sign of ketosis, which is a symptom of diabetes. Kaposi's sarcoma, a rare type of skin cancer, is often manifested as lesions of the oral tissues; the presence of such lesions may be a strong indication that the patient has acquired immunodeficiency syndrome (AIDS).

The successful treatment of diseases of the teeth and periodontium must be based on a thorough understanding of the anatomy and physiology of these tissues. To restore a decayed tooth, the dentist must know how deep to cut into the tooth, the probable location of the pulp, the irritating factors of the restorative material, the possible traumatic chewing forces on the new restoration, and the compatibility between the restoration and the tissues of the periodontium.

The treatment of tooth loss is literally as old as the pharaohs. An X ray of the skull of an Egyptian mummy displayed an attempt to construct a dental bridge using gold wire to secure a tooth between two natural teeth. At present, there are several ways to restore lost teeth. Cemented fixed bridges constructed of metal and porcelain are often the treatment of choice when there are sound teeth to support them. In the case of a partial or total loss of the teeth, removable dentures constructed of plastic or porcelain teeth fixed in an acrylic plastic base are used.

Introduction of newer materials and techniques for the restoration of teeth is a constant challenge for the dental scientist. While the theory of implanting restorations into the jaw to replace teeth is not new, some of the materials are. The recent use of titanium implants into the jaw reinforces the dentist's need to know the anatomy and physiology of the surrounding tissues. It is known that the bone of the jaw attaches to the surface of titanium, a process called osseointegration. Great care must be used, however, in placing correct chewing forces on the supporting bone, and nonirritating restorations must be placed near the periodontal tissues for the implants to be successful.

Special acrylic plastics called composites are sometimes used in restoring lost tooth structure by chemically bonding to the enamel and dentin. Thin films of these materials are placed in the grooves of the newly erupted posterior teeth. This treatment has been shown to prevent decay in the chewing surfaces of the teeth. Laser technology is being explored by scientists to see if the enamel surface might be fused to withstand decay.

While the bone lost as a result of periodontal disease cannot be regenerated, new techniques of grafting the patient's own bone, freeze-dried sterile bone, and other materials show some promise in strengthening the weakened tooth.

A number of recent studies clearly demonstrate a close connection between oral health and disease of other body systems. Patients with serious gum disease or tooth decay are at increased risk of cardiac arrhythmias, stroke, and kidney disease. Several studies reveal that older patients are especially susceptible. The American Geriatric Society, for example, published a study showing that patients over the age of eighty with three or more active root caries were twice as susceptible to cardiac arrhythmias when compared to individuals with disease-free teeth and gums.

Increased risk of heart attack and stroke may come from acute and or chronic inflammation caused by bacterial infection originating from bacterial pockets in gums and rotting teeth. Such inflammation leads to platelet activation and elevated levels of clotting factors in the blood, which increases the risk of cryptogenic stroke and cardioembolism.

Periodontal disease has been linked to another heart health problem called subacute bacterial endocarditis, a severe bacterial infection of the lining of the heart that can cause heart irregularities and heart attacks. This disease is also caused by bacterial infections that originate and reside in periodontal pockets known as gingival crevices. These bacteria eventually spread via the blood to all parts of the body and lodge in the tissues that line the heart, causing subacute bacterial endocarditis. Links between heart disease, stroke, and gum diseases are elevated in individuals who have lost teeth because the bacteria colonize the residual periodontal pockets, from which they leach into the bloodstream. Both periodontal disease and the secondary but important inflammations of the heart, brain, and other body systems that result are treatable and preventable conditions for many patients. Periodic cleaning and prompt attention to dental caries, along with complete removal of old amalgam fillings and other metals, have proven very helpful.

Perspective and Prospects

Recorded history and archaeological findings show that humans have tried to treat the teeth and their related diseases probably since the Stone Age. There has been speculation among archaeologists that the practice of trepanning, the surgical opening of the skull, could have been in response to severe toothaches as well as other pain in the head. Mutilation of the teeth by the Incas and Mayans was common in noble families; skulls have been discovered in burial sites of both nations showing the insertion of jade disks in slots filed into the front teeth.

In ancient Greece, Hippocrates wrote of treating a severe tumor of the jaw of a young man. After lancing the lesion, he wrote that the condition was morbid and that the young man would surely die. The Greeks also supposed that tooth decay was caused by small worms that bored into the tooth and ate it from within.

In medieval Japan, dentists were trained to extract teeth with their thumb and forefingers. They practiced on tapered wooden pegs pounded into a board. A soft wood was used at first for easier removal, then successively harder boards and pegs were introduced until the dentist could then remove a tooth from the jaw.

Most of the dentistry in the past was surgical removal of painful teeth. From the Middle Ages to the mid-nineteenth century, barbers performed extractions. Without the benefit of anesthetic, this practice was quite painful. Horace Welles found in 1894 that a patient could be put to sleep with ethyl ether, allowing painless tooth extraction. With the introduction of local anesthetics in the 1920s and later of intravenous drugs, pain during the extraction of a tooth has been virtually eliminated.

In modern practice, the study of the teeth has found new applications. For example, dental forensics contributes to the identification of abusers and criminals who bite their victims. The dental arch and the relationship of the teeth within it are unique, and bite marks are like fingerprints: No two are alike. The forensic scientist can take impressions of the bite marks on the victim's body with an accurate impression material. Plaster casts are formed in the impressions and compared to a cast of the suspect's dental arch. The evidence may either confirm or rule out the suspect's participation in the crime. In addition, dental forensics is used to identify the remains of people who are burned beyond recognition or whose bodies are badly decomposed. The teeth and their dental restorations are often the only way that a deceased person may be identified, especially in a major disaster such as an airplane crash.

The restoration and replacement of diseased teeth is an ongoing challenge, but with the new materials and technology available, humans should have healthier teeth in the future.

—*William D. Stark, D.D.S.;*
updated by Dwight G. Smith, Ph.D.

See also Braces, orthodontic; Cavities; Crowns and bridges; Dental diseases; Dentistry; Dentistry, pediatric; Dentures; Endodontic disease; Fluoride treatments; Forensic pathology; Fracture repair; Gastrointestinal system; Gingivitis; Gum disease; Jaw wiring; Nutrition; Orthodontics; Periodontal surgery; Periodontitis; Plaque, dental; Root canal treatment; Teething; Tooth extraction; Toothache; Veterinary medicine; Wisdom teeth.

For Further Information:

Cook, Allan R., ed. *Oral Health Sourcebook: Basic Information About Diseases and Conditions Affecting Oral Health*. Detroit, Mich.: Omnigraphics, 1998. This handy reference source, which covers all aspects of dental health, includes helpful statistics on dental disease.

Ferracane, Jack L. "Using Posterior Composites Appropriately." *Journal of the American Dental Association* 123 (July, 1992): 53-58. A discussion of the mechanical properties of acrylic composites, including resistance to wear and the use of bonded seals with this restorative material.

Foster, Malcolm S. *Protecting Our Children's Teeth: A Guide to Quality Dental Care from Infancy Through Age Twelve*. New York: Insight Books, 1992. This book, meant for parents, is clear and easy to understand. A good starting point.

Langlais, Robert P., and Craig S. Miller. *Color Atlas of Common Oral Diseases*. 4th ed. Philadelphia: Lippincott Williams & Wilkins, 2009. Provides six hundred color photographs of the most commonly seen oral problems accompanied by descriptive text for each condition.

Parker, James N., and Philip M. Parker, eds. *The Official Patient Sourcebook on Tooth Decay*. San Diego, Calif.: Icon Health, 2002. Self-described as a reference manual for self-directed patient research, this book describes in clear detail relationships among types of tooth decay and relationships between dental problems and overall health. Includes lists of Web links for many topics treated within.

Standring, Susan, et al., eds. *Gray's Anatomy*. 40th ed. New York: Churchill Livingstone/Elsevier, 2008. The definitive book on human anatomy. With 780 illustrations in the text, the interrelationship of nerves, blood vessels, bones, and other anatomical structures of the human body is displayed in a practical manner as a fascinating biological machine.

Zablotsky, Mark H. "The Periodontal Approach to Implant Dentistry." *Journal of the California Dental Association* 19, no. 12 (1991): 39. An excellent article outlining the important relationships between dental implants and the restorations attached to them and the periodontal tissues.

TEETHING

Biology

Also known as: Deciduous dentition, tooth eruption

Anatomy or system affected: Mouth, gums, teeth

Specialties and related fields: Dentistry, orthodontics, pediatrics

Definition: The eruption of the primary, or deciduous, teeth in infancy.

Key terms:

central incisors: the two center top and two center bottom teeth

cuspids: the teeth on either side of the lateral incisors; also known as the canines or eyeteeth

deciduous teeth: a child's first set of teeth, which will be replaced by the child's permanent teeth; also known as the primary or baby teeth

lateral incisors: the teeth on either side of the central incisors

molars: the grinding teeth located at the back of the mouth

Structure and Functions

A child's teeth begin to develop about the second month of pregnancy. The first tooth does not usually appear above the gum line, however, until the sixth or seventh month after birth. The tooth is pushed upward through the gum by growth at the base of the tooth. At the same time, the root sheath grows downward toward the jaw. Studies indicate that dental development does not seem to be affected by nutrition, illness, or climate. In addition, there seems to be little difference between girls and boys in their dental development.

Dental development follows a typical pattern. The teeth generally emerge in pairs. Usually, the lower central incisors are the first teeth to erupt, between five and seven months after birth, followed by the upper central incisors at six to eight months. The upper lateral incisors make their appearances between nine and eleven months, followed by the lower lateral incisors at ten to twelve months. The first molars, two upper and two lower, usually emerge between twelve and sixteen months. The cuspids follow next, at about sixteen to twenty months. The final deciduous teeth to emerge are the second molars, at twenty to thirty months. Most children will have twenty teeth, ten on the top and ten on the bottom, by their third birthday. By the time that they are six, most children begin to lose their primary teeth as the permanent teeth emerge.

While this is the typical pattern, there is much individual variation in both the time frame and the order of tooth eruption. Some children do not get the first tooth until their first birthday. On the other hand, children are sometimes born with teeth or have their first teeth erupt in the first month after birth. Those teeth present at birth are called "natal teeth," and those that emerge soon after birth are called "neonatal." Natal and neonatal teeth have been associated with other oral abnormalities, including cleft palate and cleft lip, although many children with these teeth have no abnormalities. Natal and neonatal teeth can present problems for babies, who may cut their tongues on the teeth, and for nursing mothers, who may experience lacerated nipples.

Although not permanent, a child's primary teeth are important. The primary teeth are necessary for the child to chew solid food. In addition, they are important as space holders and guides for the permanent teeth.

Disorders and Diseases

Some children have a more difficult time teething than do others. Common symptoms of teething in an infant include wakefulness, excessive drooling, fussiness, refusal to nurse, and chewing on fingers or hard objects. An infant's gums may also be swollen and tender. These symptoms have also been observed in animals as their teeth erupt.

Some debate exists over other commonly held beliefs concerning symptoms associated with teething. Historically, fever, diarrhea, and ear pulling have been attributed to teething; however, there is no scientific evidence to suggest that teething causes any of these symptoms. In a 1992 article, "Teething," in the *Journal of Pediatric Health Care*, Patricia T. Castiglia suggests that parents often attribute behaviors such as wakefulness to teething because it alleviates parental worry. She further argues that wakefulness at six to nine months is caused by separation anxiety, not teething.

Those researchers who have attempted to associate teething with disease have found it difficult to do so. The teething period is also the period when babies are no longer fully protected by the mother's antibodies but have not yet built up antibodies of their own, thus rendering them susceptible to disease. Consequently, while diseases may coincide with the teething period, it is difficult to associate teething with disease. The risk of infection during the teething period can be reduced by regularly cleaning the objects with which the child comes in contact.

Nevertheless, most pediatricians agree that babies experience some discomfort from teething. Many believe that allowing the child to chew on a cold rubber teething ring or damp washcloth will relieve the pain. While some experts suggest offering frozen teething rings and/or frozen bagels or bread, others argue that neither should be given. They contend that the frozen teething ring can damage the baby's gums, while bits of the frozen bagel can break off, potentially choking the baby. Likewise, there is little agreement about whether acetaminophen or teething gels should be used.

Most experts discourage using breast-feeding, a bottle, or a sweetened pacifier to help a teething baby fall asleep. The milk or sugar pools around the new teeth, potentially causing decay. Indeed, many pediatricians suggest that a baby's gums and new teeth should be wiped with a clean, damp gauze pad several times a day to remove traces of milk or juice from the mouth. Nonfluoridated toothpastes can be used to brush an infant's or toddler's emerging teeth; fluoridated toothpastes may be used once the child can spit on his or her own.

Perspective and Prospects

Teething has been a concern for doctors and parents for many years. Theorists as early as Hippocrates attributed fever, convulsions, and diarrhea to teething. During the eighteenth and nineteenth centuries, many writers considered teething to be the leading cause of death among infants.

During the last quarter of the twentieth century, however, the use of teething as a diagnosis for diarrhea, fever, and other childhood illnesses diminished among pediatricians, although studies indicated that some pediatricians continued to connect teething with diarrhea.

—*Diane Andrews Henningfeld, Ph.D.*

See also Cleft lip and palate; Cleft lip and palate repair; Dental diseases; Dentistry; Dentistry, pediatric; Neonatology; Pain; Pain management; Pediatrics; Teeth.

For Further Information:

A.D.A.M. Medical Encyclopedia. "Teething." *MedlinePlus*, November 12, 2012.

American Association of Pediatrics. "Teething and Dental Hygiene." *HealthyChildren.org*, May 11, 2013.

Gorfinkle, Kenneth. *Soothing Your Child's Pain: From Teething and Tummy Aches to Acute Illnesses and Injuries—How to Understand the Causes and Ease the Hurt.* Lincolnwood, Ill.: Contemporary Books, 1998.

Josephson, Laura. *A Homeopathic Handbook of Natural Remedies: Safe and Effective Treatment of Common Ailments and Injuries.* New York: Villard Books, 2002.

Kellicker, Patricia Griffin, and Michael Woods. "Discharge Instructions for Teething." *Health Library*, March 18, 2013.

Kemper, Kathi J. *The Holistic Pediatrician: A Pediatrician's Comprehensive Guide to Safe and Effective Therapies for the Twenty-five Most Common Ailments of Infants, Children, and Adolescents.* Rev. ed. New York: Quill, 2002.

Kump, Theresa. "The Facts About Baby Teeth: From Teething Pain to First Cleanings, Here's What You Do." *Parents* 70, no. 6 (June, 1995): 65–66.

Nemours Foundation. "Teething Tots." *KidsHealth.org*, November, 2011.

Rogoznica, June. "Teething Time." *Parents* 74, no. 3 (March, 1999): 139–40.

Shelov, Steven P., et al. *Caring for Your Baby and Young Child: Birth to Age Five.* 5th ed. New York: Bantam Books, 2009.

Woolf, Alan D., et al., eds. *The Children's Hospital Guide to Your Child's Health and Development.* Cambridge, Mass.: Perseus, 2002.

TELEMEDICINE. *See* INTERNET MEDICINE.

TEMPORAL ARTERITIS
Disease/Disorder
Also known as: Giant cell arteritis
Anatomy or system affected: Blood vessels, circulatory system, immune system

Specialties and related fields: Geriatrics, rheumatology
Definition: Inflammation of the medium and large blood vessels that bring blood to the temporal area of the head; may also occur in vessels in other parts of the body.

Causes and Symptoms

Arteries are blood vessels that carry oxygenated blood away from the heart to supply oxygen and nutrients to cells. A blockage of an artery can cause damage to the body and may even lead to death. The temporal artery is located in front of the ear and is a major supplier of blood to the head.

In some adults, the medium- and large-sized arteries in the head can become swollen and can decrease or block the flow of blood. The cause of the swelling is unknown, but it is thought to be an autoimmune disorder, where the body mistakenly attacks its own healthy cells, and may be triggered by a virus. Temporal arteritis is almost always found in adults who are older than 50 and is more common in women who are white. A person is more likely to get temporal arteritis if someone else in the family has had the condition.

The first symptom of temporal arteritis is usually a severe headache in the temple, which does not get better after taking pain medication. A person with temporal arteritis typically has pain in their jaw or other parts of their face and has some change in their vision. Almost half of the people who are diagnosed with temporal arteritis also have polymyalgia rheumatica, a condition where they are stiff in the morning and have aches in the neck, shoulder, chest, or hip.

People with this condition might also have a fever, feel tired, lose their appetite, or lose weight. While these symptoms are considered "classic," 40 percent of people will experience different symptoms.

Treatment and Therapy

Temporal arteritis is diagnosed by a temporal artery biopsy, but most medical providers will begin treatment for this disorder if the person has symptoms because it is so important to start treatment quickly to prevent blindness. In addition to the biopsy, blood work may be done to look for an increased number of white blood cells (WBC) and an elevated erythrocyte sedimentation rate (ESR), which are both indicators of inflammation in the body.

The treatment is high doses of steroids that are taken for a long period of time, sometimes as long as two years. The initial treatment is so strong that it needs to be given intravenously (IV) but the dose will begin to be tapered, or decreased, once the person's symptoms go away and their white blood cell level decreases. Taking steroids for long periods of time puts a person at a higher risk for developing osteoporosis.

Prognosis

Permanent blindness can happen if this disorder is not treated quickly. Long-term use of steroid medications help to make the bothersome symptoms go away, but half of the people with this disorder will have a flare-up within a year, even while taking steroids. Many people have to take steroids at a lower dose for several years to keep the symptoms from happening again.

—*Allison Dussault, RN*

See also Aging; Autoimmune disorders; Biopsy; Blood testing; Blood vessels; Corticosteroids; Fever; Head and Neck disorders; Headaches; Inflammation; Pain; Vascular system; Vision disorders

For Further Information:

Firestein, Gary S., Ralph C. Budd, Sherine E. Gabriel, Iain B. Mcinnes, and James R. O'Dell. *Kelley's Textbook of Rheumatology.* 9th ed. Philadelphia: Saunders Elsevier, 2012.

Goldman, Lee, and Andrew I.Schafer. *Goldman's Cecil Medicine.* 24th ed. Philadelphia: Saunders Elsevier, 2012.

Halter, Jeffrey B., Joseph G. Ouslander, Mary E. Tinetti, Stephanie Studenski, Kevin P. High, and Sanjay Asthana. *Hazzard's Geriatric Medicine and Gerontology.* 6th ed. New York: McGraw-Hill, 2009.

TEMPOROMANDIBULAR JOINT (TMJ) SYNDROME

Disease/Disorder

Anatomy or system affected: Bones, head, joints, mouth, muscles, teeth

Specialties and related fields: Dentistry, family medicine, psychology

Definition: A disorder that produces pain and stiffness in the joint between the lower jawbone (mandible) and the temporal bone of the skull.

Causes and Symptoms

The exact cause of temporomandibular joint (TMJ) syndrome, or myofacial pain-dysfunction syndrome, is not known. Possible causes include arthritis, bad bite (malocclusion), grinding or clenching of the teeth (bruxism), muscle tension, and psychological stress. X-rays and laboratory tests carried out on people with this disorder usually reveal no abnormalities. Another potential cause of pain and stiffness in the temporomandibular joints at either side of the jaw is rheumatoid arthritis. With rheumatoid arthritis, however, the symptoms are most severe the first thing in the morning, which is not typically the case with TMJ syndrome.

TMJ syndrome affects the temporomandibular joints, producing mild to severe spasms and pain in the jaw muscles that sometimes make it difficult to open the jaw fully. Other symptoms can include blurred vision, clicking or popping of

---

Information on Temporomandibular Joint (TMJ) Syndrome

Causes: Unclear; possibly arthritis, malocclusion, grinding or clenching of teeth, muscle tension, psychological stress

Symptoms: Joint pain and stiffness, mild to severe spasms, blurred vision, sinus problems

Duration: Chronic

Treatments: Heat therapy, injections or sprays of local anesthetics, analgesics, jaw exercises, dental procedures, surgery

---

the jaw, and pain that extends into the head, neck, ears, and even as far as the shoulders.

Treatment and Therapy

If spasmodic pain exists in the jaw muscles, a physician should be consulted. Treatment to provide relief varies according to the underlying cause but typically includes local heat therapy, injections or sprays of local anesthetics, and simple analgesics, such as aspirin, ibuprofen, or acetaminophen. Prescribed jaw exercises and relaxation techniques are also often helpful. Some cases may require dental procedures to improve jaw alignment or retainers to prevent clenching and grinding of the teeth. In the most severe cases, surgery may be necessary to correct the problem.

Perspective and Prospects

TMJ syndrome is fairly common; most people who have spasmodic pain in the jaw muscles have this condition. It is estimated that between 5 and 12 percent of the world's population suffers from some form of TMJ syndrome, ranging from mild to very severe. The majority of cases, however, go untreated.

—*Alvin K. Benson, Ph.D.*

See also Arthritis; Dental diseases; Head and neck disorders; Joints; Muscle sprains, spasms, and disorders; Muscles; Orthopedic surgery; Orthopedics; Orthopedics, pediatric; Pain management; Rheumatoid arthritis; Stress; Stress reduction.

For Further Information:

Bumann, Axel, and Ulrich Lotzmann. *TMJ Disorders and Orofacial Pain: The Role of Dentistry in a Multidisciplinary Diagnostic Approach.* Translated by Richard Jacobi. New York: Thieme, 2002.

Gremillion, Henry A., ed. *Temporomandibular Disorders and Orofacial Pain.* Philadelphia: Saunders/Elsevier, 2007.

Hollenstein, Jenna. "Temporomandibular Disorder." *Health Library,* September 30, 2012.

"Less Is Often Best in Treating TMJ Disorders." *National Institute of Dental and Craniofacial Research,* March 25, 2011.

Mitchell, David A. *An Introduction to Oral and Maxillofacial Surgery.* New York: Oxford University Press, 2006.

Okeson, Jeffrey P. *Management of Temporomandibular Disorders and Occlusion.* 7th ed. Philadelphia: Mosby/Elsevier, 2012.

Sarnat, Bernard G., and Daniel M. Laskin, eds. *The Temporomandibular Joint: A Biological Basis for Clinical Practice.* Philadelphia: W. B. Saunders, 1992.

TENDINITIS

Disease/Disorder

Also known as: Epicondylitis, tendinosis, tendon overuse syndrome, tendonitis

Anatomy or system affected: Arms, feet, hands, joints, knees, legs, musculoskeletal system, tendons

Specialties and related fields: Exercise physiology, family medicine, occupational health, orthopedics, physical therapy, preventive medicine, sports medicine

Definition: An inflammation of a tendon or tendon sheath.

Key terms:

collagen: strengthening protein in tendon tissue

ergonomics: the science of the relationship between the

human form and its biomechanical environment

extracorporeal: pertaining to something occurring outside the body, such as therapy

inflammation: a condition of tenderness and disturbed function of an area of the body, caused by a reaction of tissue to injury or infection

tendinopathy: a general term referring to any type of tendon disorder

Causes and Symptoms

Tendons are fibrous cords that attach muscles to bones. Their function is to transmit force and coordinate the activity between muscles and bones. When too much stress is placed upon the tendons, they may become inflamed (tendinitis), or damaged, or both, from the chronic degeneration of tendon collagen (tendinosis). The cause of such stress is usually poor technique, overuse, or repetitive movements in sports, recreational, and occupational activities. The injury usually follows the progression of multiple microscopic tears in the tendon tissue, eventually leading to acute inflammation and pain. The areas most commonly affected are the rotator cuff of the shoulder, the elbow ("tennis elbow" or "golfer's elbow"), the wrist/thumb (de Quervain's disease), the knee ("jumper's knee"), and the ankle (Achilles tendinitis).

Many athletic activities, such as racquet sports, baseball, running, and weight training, involve repetitive movements that may put excessive stress on the tendons. Many occupations also pose a risk; examples include performing assembly line work, playing a musical instrument, and using a keyboard. Tendinitis may also be caused by infection or by a buildup of calcium deposits (calcific tendinitis) or other materials in a joint as a result of a chronic illness such as diabetes or arthritis.

Pain is the usual complaint. It occurs when the patient moves the affected joint but may sometimes persist when the joint is at rest. In severe cases, simple activities such as raising a coffee cup or brushing teeth may cause pain. There may also be swelling, warmth, and redness in the affected area.

Treatment and Therapy

The term "tendinitis" has traditionally been used as a blanket term for all tendinopathies. However, medical professionals emphasize that tendinitis and tendinosis, while often occurring hand-in-hand, are separate conditions and must be treated accordingly. Tendon overuse conditions have been generally considered inflammatory processes (tendinitis), and therapy has been administered based on that conception. However, it is important to recognize that overuse tendon conditions are frequently caused by collagen damage and degeneration of tendon tissue (tendinosis), eventually leading to an acute inflammatory condition. Tendinosis requires a different approach to therapy once the initial inflammation is treated.

True tendinitis conditions are treated with therapy aimed at reducing inflammation. Rest and avoidance of the causative activity, alternative application of ice and heat, compression and elevation of the affected extremity, and immobi-

---

Information on Tendinitis

Causes: Stress on tendons resulting from poor technique, overuse, or repetitive movements in sports, recreational, or occupational activities; buildup of calcium deposits from chronic illness such as diabetes or arthritis

Symptoms: Pain, swelling, warmth, and redness in affected area

Duration: A few to several weeks; sometimes recurrent

Treatments: Rest, avoidance of causative activity, alternative application of ice and heat, compression and elevation of affected extremity, immobilization with slings and splints, anti-inflammatory drugs (ibuprofen, corticosteroid injections), antibiotics, sometimes surgery

---

lization with slings and splints are all helpful measures. Over-the-counter anti-inflammatory medications such as ibuprofen may be suggested. A method exists for delivering medication to inflamed tissue: iontophoresis, whereby a small electrical current delivers anti-inflammatory medication, such as dexamethasone, through the skin to the inflamed tissue. More severe cases may require corticosteroid injections. Tendinitis caused by infection is treated with antibiotics and sometimes surgery if first-course therapy is not effective. Recovery from tendinitis varies from a few to several weeks.

Tendinosis therapy is aimed at allowing the injured tendon tissue to heal. Rest and avoidance of the offending activity is most important. Icing, ultrasound, and electrical stimulation may enhance collagen production. Once the initial inflammation has been treated, anti-inflammatory medications and corticosteroid injections are not indicated and may actually impede healing. Ergonomic changes in the workplace and the correction of improper technique in sports activities are important. Physical therapy and strengthening exercises play key rehabilitative roles by helping to prevent future injury, and they may also improve collagen formation and thus speed healing. Surgery to remove damaged tissue is used only as a last resort when conservative management has failed. Recovery from tendinosis may take up to several months.

Perspective and Prospects

Tendinopathies have been regarded as conditions that are often recalcitrant to therapy, becoming chronic or frequently reoccurring. It is possible that this difficulty is in part attributable to the lack of distinction between tendinitis and tendinosis. It has been postulated that some of the therapies for tendinitis, when used on tendinosis, may cause further tissue deterioration and thus contribute to the chronic nature of the disorder. Additionally, once the initial inflammation is treated and pain is no longer felt, the injured individual will often begin the offending activity before healing is complete. This leads to further damage and weakened tissue, creating a frustrating cycle. It is therefore crucial that a proper diagnosis is made before treatment begins and that the injured individual follow the full course of therapy and rest to ensure optimal healing.

The investigation of new treatment modalities is ongoing. Extracorporeal shock wave therapy has been shown to have some positive benefits for both tendinosis and calcific tendinitis. The use of ultrasound and electrical stimulation has gained acceptance with some professionals.

Preventive measures can greatly reduce the risk of developing overuse tendinopathies. This approach is becoming more evident in the workplace, where proper ergonomic environments help to decrease employee injury, increase productivity, and reduce injury and absences. Conditioning and emphasis on correct technique in sports and recreational activities will greatly reduce the incidence of tendon overuse disorders.

—*Barbara C. Beattie*

See also Arthritis; Braces, orthopedic; Collagen; Inflammation; Joints; Muscle sprains, spasms, and disorders; Muscles; Orthopedic surgery; Orthopedics; Orthopedics, pediatric; Physical rehabilitation; Rotator cuff surgery; Sports medicine; Tendon disorders; Tendon repair.

For Further Information:

Khan, Karim M., et al. "Overuse Tendinosis, Not Tendinitis: A New Paradigm for a Difficult Clinical Problem." *Physician and Sports Medicine* 28, no. 5 (May, 2000): 38–45.

Khan, Karim M, et al. "Time to Abandon the 'Tendinitis' Myth: Painful, Overuse Tendon Conditions Have a Non-inflammatory Pathology." *British Medical Journal* 324, no. 7338 (March 16, 2002): 626–627.

Leach, Robert E., and Teresa Briedwell. "Tendinopathy." *Health Library*, Mar. 18, 2013.

Porter, Robert S., et al., eds. *The Merck Manual Home Health Handbook*. Whitehouse Station, N.J.: Merck Research Laboratories, 2009.

Standish, William D., Sandra Curwin, and Scott Mandell. *Tendinitis: Its Etiology and Treatment*. New York: Oxford University Press, 2000.

"Tendinitis." *MedlinePlus*, May 9, 2013.

"Tendinitis and Bursitis." *American College of Rheumatology*, Feb. 2013.

"What Are Bursitis and Tendinitis?" *National Institute of Arthritis and Musculoskeletal and Skin Diseases*, Apr. 2011.

TENDON DISORDERS

Disease/Disorder

Anatomy or system affected: Back, bones, legs, ligaments, muscles, musculoskeletal system, tendons

Specialties and related fields: Occupational health, orthopedics, physical therapy, podiatry, sports medicine

Definition: Inflammation or tearing of the tendons.

Tendons are the tough, white, fibrous cords that connect muscles to movable structures such as bone or cartilage. The presence of tendons allows muscles to act at a distance and concentrates the force of the muscle into a small area. Sometimes tendons can change the direction of a muscle's pull, thus allowing the muscle to act around a joint. The structure of a tendon consists of parallel bundles of collagen fibrils, which makes it extraordinarily strong. A sheath, or vagina fibrosa,

surrounds the tendon and is responsible for holding it in place. Between the fibrils and the sheath lie a lymphatic network and a fluid that allow tendon movement without excessive friction. Because of the vital functions of tendons, diseases and injuries to them can be debilitating as well as painful. Damaged tendons tend to heal slower than epithelial tissue, for example, because tendons have a lower blood supply than other soft tissues.

Trauma to tendons usually occurs in conjunction with impact, twisting, overstretching, or the simple overuse of a joint. These actions commonly result in partial or complete tears of the fibrous cord. Only if a tendon has not been stretched more than 4 percent of its original length will it return unchanged to its normal state once the force is released. When it is stretched from 4 to 8 percent of its normal length, the molecular bonds between individual collagen fibers begin to fail and the fibers slide past one another. At 8 to 10 percent strain, the tendon itself is in danger of tearing because individual fibers rupture, placing even more force on the fibers that remain intact. Although Golgi tendon organs send signals to the brain regarding excessive strain on tendons, such tearing usually occurs quickly during physical activities. Pain, swelling, and abnormal motion at the joint follow the damage. Tendinitis is the name given to the inflammation of a tendon.

Tendon disorders of the upper body. Tennis elbow, or lateral epicondylitis, involves the elbow joint and can be attributed to excessive extensor movements in the wrist joint and a sustained gripping of objects such as a tennis racket. There is great diversity in opinion as to the development of this disorder, as well as to its treatment. The latter includes methods such as rest, stretching, icing, heat, ultrasound, bracing, and surgery. Golfer's elbow is less often seen but is a similar tendinitis of the common flexor tendon.

Supraspinatus tendinitis, or swimmer's shoulder, is seen in athletes participating in swimming, tennis, and other activities involving overhead arm movement. Repeated overhead arm swings impinge and sometimes tear the supraspinatus tendon located between the acromion and the proximal end of the humerus. The disorder has also been termed impingement syndrome. Treatments include icing, stretching, modifying stroke technique in swimmers, anti-inflammatory drugs, and surgery.

Bicipital tendinitis usually stems from sports that require throwing or paddling. This type of tendon disorder is similar to the supraspinatus type in that pinching of a tendon is involved. The narrow tendon connecting the long head of the bicep muscle to the scapula lies in a groove and is restrained by a ligament therein. Pain occurring while a physician applies pressure to this groove and moves the patient's arm is diagnostic for this particular tendinitis. Treatments are the same as for supraspinatus tendinitis and are almost always successful.

Vigorous throwing can produce triceps tendinitis. Other tendons prone to injury are those attaching the infraspinatus, teres minor, and teres major muscles. Indeed, any tendon may incur damage depending on the specific activities that an individual undertakes.

```
┌─────────────────────────────────────────────┐
│        Information on Tendon Disorders        │
│                                               │
│  Causes: Disease, trauma, injury, overuse     │
│  Symptoms: Inflammation, pain, abnormal motion│
│  Duration: Acute or recurrent episodes        │
│  Treatments: Rest, appropriate stretching,    │
│     icing, heat, ul-                          │
│     trasound, braces, surgery, anti-          │
│     inflammatory drugs                        │
└─────────────────────────────────────────────┘
```

Synovitis of the wrist extensor tendons is the result of friction between the tendon, its surrounding sheath, and bone processes. Tenosynovitis brings about a thickening of the tendon sheath, and at times a rubbing sound can even be heard during movement. An aching pain develops and may be relieved by methods applied in tendinitis cases. In addition, ultrasound therapy in water is highly successful. The abductor pollicis longus and the extensor pollicis brevis muscles are most often affected.

Tendon disorders of the lower body. Tendons of the lower body undergo greater stress than tendons of the torso because a greater weight is moved and a more continuous motion is involved. Achilles tendinitis often occurs in people participating in sports involving running and jumping. This type of inflammation has become the most common athletic injury. When great tensile strength is needed, the tendon tends to be long compared with the muscle to which it attaches. The Achilles tendon is long and durable but twists as it descends down the lower leg, making certain areas of the tendon vulnerable to the concentration of stress. Quality footwear with slight heel elevation and heel padding can reduce the tearing effect on this tendon. Stretching the gastrocnemius and soleus muscles before athletic exertion ensures that these muscles will absorb a greater portion of the force that would otherwise be transferred to the tendon.

Jumper's knee, or patellar tendinitis, is fairly common in basketball and volleyball players; it is often mistaken for arthritis of the knee. Repetitive extending of the leg at the knee causes microtearing in the kneecap tendon; thus, the torn fibers fray and eventually begin to degenerate. More stress than before is then placed on the remaining intact fibers, resulting in the likelihood of their failing as well.

Many other lower body injuries may involve tendons. Groin pull is most frequent in soccer players because of the sudden stresses involved in kicking and changing direction by planting cleats firmly into the ground and jolting the body into a new configuration. Hamstring pull occurs during bursts of sprinting because the hamstring functions in the forward movement of a leg after a stride is completed. During extremely fast running, the hamstring requires great force to keep pace; thus, damage to the connecting tendon and to the muscle itself is likely to occur if attention is not given to proper stretching techniques before the exertion.

The term "shin splints" refers to several painful injuries to the lower leg. Indicative of shin splints are pain and tenderness along the tibia, or shinbone, and the middle one-third of the leg. The condition develops in athletes who do not use sufficient padding in their shoes or who run and play on hard surfaces. Genuine shin splints do not involve tendons directly; fortunately, tendinitis of the tibial muscles can be differentiated from true shin splints because the pain of tendinitis is located higher up on the leg.

Compartment syndrome is most frequently seen in runners. The leg is divided into three compartments, each encompassed by a tight fascial sheath. When injury occurs to muscles or tendons of a certain compartment, swelling accompanied by a cutting off of the blood supply can cause further problems. Even the sudden growth of muscles as a result of physical activity can impair the function of muscles and nerves deeper in the leg.

—*Ryan C. Horst and Roman J. Miller, Ph.D.*

See also Arthritis; Braces, orthopedic; Collagen; Inflammation; Joints; Muscle sprains, spasms, and disorders; Muscles; Orthopedic surgery; Orthopedics; Orthopedics, pediatric; Osgood-Schlatter disease; Physical rehabilitation; Rotator cuff surgery; Sports medicine; Tendinitis; Tendon repair.

For Further Information:

Delforge, Gary. *Musculoskeletal Trauma: Implications for Sport Injury Management.* Champaign, Ill.: Human Kinetics, 2002.

Józsa, László, and Pekka Kannus. *Human Tendons: Anatomy, Physiology, and Pathology.* Champaign, Ill.: Human Kinetics, 1997.

Leach, Robert E., and Teresa Briedwell. "Tendinopathy." *Health Library*, Mar. 18, 2013.

Stanish, William D., Sandra Curwin, and Scott Mandell. *Tendinitis: Its Etiology and Treatment.* New York: Oxford University Press, 2000.

"Tendinitis." *MedlinePlus*, May 9, 2013.

"Tendinitis and Bursitis." *American College of Rheumatology*, Feb. 2013.

Weintraub, William. *Tendon and Ligament Healing: A New Approach to Sports and Overuse Injury.* 2nd rev. ed. Brookline, Mass.: Paradigm, 2003.

"What Are Bursitis and Tendinitis?" *National Institute of Arthritis and Musculoskeletal and Skin Diseases*, Apr. 2011.

TENDON REPAIR
Procedure

Anatomy or system affected: Bones, feet, hands, joints, knees, legs, ligaments, muscles, musculoskeletal system, tendons

Specialties and related fields: General surgery, occupational health, orthopedics, podiatry, sports medicine

Definition: The surgical repair of tendons, the bands of tissue that attach muscle to bone.

Indications and Procedures

Tendons are straps of collagenous tissue that attach muscles to bone. They are strong and flexible; a tendon approximately 1.3 centimeters (0.5 inch) thick can support a ton. Tendons are most prominently observed in the hand, where they are associated with the muscles that move the fingers and thumbs, and in the heel, where the Achilles tendon joins the muscles and bones of the foot. The Achilles tendon is the longest and thickest tendon in the body.

Tendon injuries can be of several types. If the hand or foot is badly cut, the slice may enter or sever the tendon, resulting in an inability to move the fingers or toes. Tendons have also ruptured during physical activity; the Achilles tendon is at particular risk during certain running or jumping exercises. The sensation that the patient experiences with initial tear has been likened to a kick. Severance of the Achilles tendon is indicated by an inability to stand on tiptoe.

More often, the Achilles tendon may become inflamed by activity. Such inflammation is usually indicated by pain that develops at the beginning and end of a run but that seems to improve during the exercise. Often, the pain becomes worse at night. Treatment of minor inflammation generally involves rest or cessation of the activity. Corticosteroids may be administered to relieve the inflammation.

If a tendon has been cut or severed, surgery is often required for proper repair. Since tendons are under great tension, they may snap or regress from the site of the injury. The surgeon makes an incision through the affected area, whether hand or foot, and sutures the ends of the tendon together.

Uses and Complications

If carried out properly and quickly, tendon repair is generally satisfactory. The patient may be immobilized for weeks, and some permanent stiffness is common. Because the blood supply to tendons is poor, healing may be a problem. One new method for repairing tendons is platelet-rich plasma therapy. Platelets produce growth factors, proteins that take part in the healing process. Blood is drawn from the patient being treated. The blood is spun down using a centrifuge to separate the plasma, which contains platelets, from the red and white blood cells. The resulting platelet-rich plasma is injected into the site of tendon damage, supplying the tendon with healing growth factors. These healing growth factors had been lacking because of the poor blood supply.

—*Richard Adler, Ph.D.*

See also Collagen; Cysts; Exercise physiology; Ganglion removal; Joints; Muscle sprains, spasms, and disorders; Muscles; Orthopedic surgery; Orthopedics; Orthopedics, pediatric; Physical rehabilitation; Rotator cuff surgery; Sports medicine; Tendinitis; Tendon disorders.

For Further Information:

Garrick, James G., and David R. Webb. *Sports Injuries: Diagnosis and Management*. 2d ed. Philadelphia: W. B. Saunders, 1999.

Irvin, Richard, Duane Iversen, and Steven Roy. *Sports Medicine: Prevention, Evaluation, Management, and Rehabilitation of Athletic Injuries*. 2d ed. Boston: Allyn & Bacon, 1998.

"Patellar Tendon Tear." *American Academy of Orthopaedic Surgeons*, August 2009.

"Quadriceps Tendon Tear." *American Academy of Orthopaedic Surgeons*, August 2009.

Scuderi, Giles R., and Peter D. McCann, eds. *Sports Medicine: A Comprehensive Approach*. 2d ed. Philadelphia: Mosby/Elsevier, 2005.

Small, Eric, et al. *Kids and Sports: Everything You and Your Child Need to Know About Sports, Physical Activity, and Good Health*. New York: Newmarket Press, 2002.

"Tendon repair." *MedlinePlus*, August 11, 2012.

Weintraub, William. *Tendon and Ligament Healing: A New Approach to Sports and Overuse Injury*. Rev. ed. Brookline, Mass.: Paradigm, 2003.

TERATOGENS

Disease/Disorder

Anatomy or system affected: All

Specialties and related fields: Embryology, obstetrics

Definition: Agents that alter normal fetal development during pregnancy and cause birth defects.

Types and Effects

Teratogens are agents that cause fetal injury and result in birth defects. Agents such as drugs, chemicals, infections, and environmental contaminants can cause birth defects when a woman is exposed to them during pregnancy. Teratogens can be found at home, in the workplace, or in the environment. The severity of fetal injury and subsequent birth defects that occur are the result of the amount and timing of exposure to a particular agent and the genetic susceptibility of the embryo and mother. At low doses of teratogen, there may be no effect; at intermediate doses, a characteristic pattern of malformations will result; and at high doses, severe malformations will occur that usually result in death of the baby. The first trimester of pregnancy is the most vulnerable time.

Teratogens produce specific abnormalities at specific times during pregnancy. Thalidomide, sold in the late 1950s to help pregnant women with morning sickness, results in babies with phocomelia (lack of long bones and flipper-like hands and feet), while valproic acid and carbamazepine produce spinal cord and brain defects. Other teratogens are also associated with recognizable patterns of birth defects. For example, the antiepileptic drug dilantin/phenytoin results in craniofacial malformations, whereas coumarin anticoagulants, such as warfarin, result in neurological complications.

Teratogenic specificity also applies to individual species. For example, aspirin has been found to be teratogenic in mice and rats but appears to be safe in humans. Thalidomide, on the other hand, was shown not to be teratogenic in rats, cats, dogs, or rabbits but is highly teratogenic in humans, a fact that resulted in approximately ten thousand children born with severe birth defects before it was recognized. The most devastating effects of thalidomide occur when the woman is exposed within the first thirty days of pregnancy.

Classification and Reducing Risk

Known teratogens can be classified as infectious agents, environmental agents, and pharmaceutical drugs. Infectious agents include rubella (German measles), cytomegalovirus (CMV), varicella, herpes simplex, toxoplasmosis, and syphilis. Environmental agents include ionizing agents, radiation therapy, X rays, organic mercury compounds, herbicides, polychlorinated biphenyls (PCBs), and industrial solvents. Pharmaceutical drugs include retinoic acid (isotretinoin, Accutane), aminopterin, steroid hormones, busulfan, angiotensin-converting enzyme (ACE) inhibitors (captopril, enalapril), cyclophosphamide, diethylstilbestrol, diphenylhydantoin (Phenytoin, Dilantin, Epanutin), etretinate, lithium, methimazole, penicillamine, tetracyclines, thalidomide, trimethadione, warfarin, and valproic acid.

Public awareness is essential for the prevention of teratogen exposure during pregnancy. Information about fetal malformations that can be caused by exposure to drugs or environmental agents is important because they are potentially preventable. Women who may become pregnant should be aware of any medications and environmental conditions that might be teratogenic, as severe fetal malformations occur very early before the pregnancy might be discovered.

Awareness of teratogenic agents and potential exposure during pregnancy has led to the development of teratogen information databases in many areas of the country. National databases, such as ReproTox and TERIS, and teratology society organizations, such as the Organization of Teratogen Information Specialists (OTIS), have been established to provide detailed information on numerous potential teratogenic agents.

—*Thomas L. Brown, Ph.D.*

See also Addiction; Alcoholism; Birth defects; Carcinogens; Chickenpox; Childbirth; Childbirth complications; Cytomegalovirus (CMV); DNA and RNA; Embryology; Environmental diseases; Environmental health; Fetal alcohol syndrome; Herpes; Imaging and radiology; Mental retardation; Mercury poisoning; Mutation; Obstetrics; Occupational health; Over-the-counter medications; Pharmacology; Pregnancy and gestation; Premature birth; Radiation therapy; Rubella; Self-medication; Sexually transmitted diseases (STDs); Syphilis; Thalidomide; Toxoplasmosis; Viral infections.

For Further Information:
Barrow, Paul C. *Teratogenicity Testing: Methods and Protocols*. New York: Humana Press, 2012.
Gupta, Ramesh C. *Reproductive and Developmental Toxicology*. Boston: Elsevier, 2012.
Kavlock, Robert J. *Drug Toxicity in Embryonic Development II: Advances in Understanding Mechanisms of Birth Defects*. New York: Springer, 2011.
Ostensen, Monika. "How Safe are Anti-Rheumatic Drugs During Pregnancy?" *Current Opinion in Pharmacology* 13, no. 3 (2013): 470–475.
Shepard, Thomas H., and Ronald J. Lemire. *Catalog of Teratogenic Agents*. 11th ed. Baltimore: Johns Hopkins University Press, 2004.
Shepard, Thomas H. *Catalog of Teratogenic Agents*. 13th ed. Baltimore:Johns Hopkins University Press, 2010.
Shinde, M. U. "Prenatal Exposure to Nitrosatable Drugs, Vitamin C, and Risk of Selected Birth Defects." *Birth Defects Research: Clinical and Molecular Teratology* (2013).
Silverman, William A. "The Schizophrenic Career of a 'Monster Drug.'" *Pediatrics* 110, no. 2 (2002): 404–406.
Wilson, James G., and F. Clarke Fraser, eds. *Handbook of Teratology*. 4 vols. New York: Plenum Press, 1977–1978.

TERMINALLY ILL: EXTENDED CARE

Specialty

Anatomy or system affected: All

Specialties and related fields: All

Definition: The medical, social, and psychological care of patients who are suffering from a terminal illness, the goal of which is to maintain as high a quality of life as possible for the remainder of a patient's life.

Key terms:

adult day care facility: a facility that offers a temporary daytime setting based on either social, maintenance, or rehabilitative services; often used to give the home care provider some time off

extended care facility: a facility that can be found in several settings outside the home, where specialized medical care can be rendered under a physician's orders

home care: the provision of outside services to a person living in a home setting

hospice: a program designed to ease the suffering and grief for terminally ill patients and their families; care can be rendered in the home or in a special hospice setting with special emphasis on the relief of pain

nursing home: a type of extended care facility that can be classified as either skilled or intermediate, depending on the type of care; physicians oversee medical care that is rendered around the clock by a nursing staff

Assessing Patient Needs

Difficult decisions await those trying to care for a patient with a terminal condition. Many families are faced with these decisions soon after the patient leaves the hospital, unable to function alone at home. Physicians and family members are able to choose among several options, depending on the needs and desires of the patient.

The decision process should start when the patient is still in the traditional hospital setting. The decision process should explore all alternatives, based on many factors. The degree of physician involvement is important, since not all doctors make monthly trips to visit patients at other facilities. The possibility of rapid deterioration of health or mental status is a vital concern, and nursing needs and other nonphysician services are also of utmost importance. The patient's desires and the wishes of the family can be addressed through the patient's legal rights to have a living will or durable power of attorney for health care decisions. Both can document, either through the patient's own written directions or through the appointment of a relative as a legal representative, where the patient stands on the issue of being kept alive by artificial means. Specific requests regarding the use of cardiopulmonary resuscitation (CPR) should be made to the physician. These wishes are best discussed long before the patient is near death.

When the terminally ill patient also has a mental illness, such as dementia, the desires of the family members are weighed along with their willingness and ability to care for the person in the home. The problems of mobility, financial constraints, and quality-of-life concerns also enter the picture.

This is a picture that is not clear or easy to visualize. Many questions need to be answered before a suitable arrangement can be made regarding the continued care for a terminally ill person, especially an elderly one. These questions will lead to wiser long-term care decisions.

Extended care includes a wide range of social and support services and can be divided into three categories: in-home services, community-based services, and institutional care. The availability of these long-term care services may vary widely, with differences in eligibility requirements and costs. The choices to be reviewed must fit the family's financial resources. Long-term care should also be based on the medical, personal, and social needs of the patient. Special attention should be paid to the patient's cognitive, psychological/emotional, functional, and economic status. The value system, perspective, beliefs, and goals of the patient are extremely important.

For a terminally ill person, an assessment of the patient's current and potential needs may have to be completed more than once as the illness progresses. A time line showing the patient's current needs and needs within the next year, or even the next five years, should be made. This long-term planning must address physician involvement; nursing coverage; physical, speech, and occupational therapies; social worker and nutrition consultations; dental care; and the need for medical supplies and equipment. Other services that may be necessary include personal care, preparation of meals, transportation, housekeeping and home maintenance, and assistance with daily living skills. The amount of time for which these services must be available and the necessary financial resources may influence early decisions. Unfortunately, financial considerations often dictate the answer before all options can be explored.

The patient's concerns regarding housing are influenced by such things as the amount of importance that is placed on staying in the present home and questions about living with or near family, friends, and religious community and about the availability of social activities. When the terminally ill person is elderly, this issue is even more sensitive. Because of the traumatic aspects of moving an elderly person from the home environment, the easiest transition for the patient should be sought. The choices are having a terminally ill patient remain at home or moving the patient to an extended care facility or a hospice center.

Before family members convene a meeting with the physician to discuss the options, all of them should speak with the patient. The terminal patient should not be given the impression that family members are making decisions for him or her. Such meetings allow patients to inform family members of their wishes, allowing the patients optimum input and providing information that the family may not have. Competent adults, even if they are elderly, have legal rights and privileges that must be honored. Some of these rights present ethical issues to family members trying to decide about long-term care. Unfortunately, such discussions often take place immediately after an older person has an emergency or a patient hears the diagnosis of a terminal illness.

When a patient is in an acute care hospital, the decision process should start before discharge. Many persons within an acute care hospital setting are qualified to assist in these decisions. An attending physician has available many tools to evaluate the patient's needs, especially if the patient is elderly and the doctor has specialized in geriatric care. Questionnaires can determine the daily living needs as well as collect psychological data pertaining to cognitive, emotional, and perceptive functions. The family physician, during the discharge planning, can arrange for the family to speak to the social services area within the hospital.

The family and the patient would be wise to make a checklist to determine the areas of most concern, ranking them by importance so that all persons concerned are able to look at the options more objectively. Although each of the alternative living settings is unique, every person involved in these decisions should visit the actual setting, allowing the patient active involvement to make the transition easier.

Options for Long-Term Care

One of the first options available for a terminally ill patient is to return to his or her own home or to live with relatives. This decision of home health care must be based on the support available from the family: who will help provide care, when, and how. The need for home modifications to make the patient more independent or more comfortable may be a concern. If outside services, such as therapy, are needed, family members must determine how they can be obtained. Another difficult question is identifying responsibility for the financial costs of special care.

These questions are difficult to ask and even more difficult to answer. Families may underestimate the additional stress involved in caring for a terminally ill person in the home. Fortunately, services such as respite care are available to help relieve the additional stresses encountered. Having someone come into the home or having the patient placed in a day care facility can relieve some of the stresses temporarily. One of the first types of stress encountered is one of a physical nature, especially fatigue arising from the additional housekeeping activities of cleaning, laundering, shopping, and cooking for the patient. Additional emotional stress results from trying to balance time, responsibilities, and pressures. Financial worries may also cause stress, even though the costs of home care are often much less than for care in a hospital or other facility.

Home health care does not mean that the family or the patient is alone. Outside professional care, such as part-time nursing or supportive services, can be rendered when a terminal patient is in the home setting. These types of services fall under two headings: skilled care and supportive care. Skilled care involves physicians, nurses, and therapists. Supportive services are those that enable a patient to continue to live independently in the home. These services may meet personal needs (such as bathing and dressing) or involve the performance of chores (such as shopping, meal preparation, and housekeeping). Supportive services may be obtained as often as necessary, but they are not without cost. Moreover, the absence of one needed service may mean that home care is not the best option for the patient, at least at this point in time. Every patient and family member is entitled to make an objective evaluation of which agency is best suited for the homebound patient. An ongoing evaluation should be conducted to ensure that this option remains the best choice. Especially in the case of a terminally ill elder, home care may not remain a viable option for long: As the patient's physical needs change, his or her environment may need to change as well.

One step beyond living independently in the home or with family members would be for the terminally ill patient to arrange for special housing, often called "supportive housing arrangements." This option may include continuing care retirement villages, board-and-care homes, domiciliary care, foster homes, personal care homes, group homes, and congregate care facilities. Board-and-care homes provide regular housekeeping and personal care services. This type of care is called "assisted living," or even "residential care," because the services vary widely, as do the costs. Another possibility is congregate housing, the environment of which is more like an updated version of an old resort hotel, with costs and services greatly variable. Continuing care communities offer independent living arrangements along with twenty-four-hour nursing care. These communities offer what is referred to as "life care," with a wide range of services available, a large entrance fee, monthly charges for services, and a lifetime commitment. They usually cost more than board-and-care homes or congregate housing.

Adult day care, which lies between home care and institutional care, emphasizes either social or medical needs. The three main types of adult day care are social, maintenance, and restorative, with each specializing in addressing the specific needs of the patient. The social model of adult day care emphasizes socialization while also giving families or caregivers some free time. The maintenance model, a mix of social and remedial components, differs from the restorative model, which offers extensive rehabilitation services. These settings may be alternatives to a nursing home. Some specialized adult day care centers, connected to hospitals, teach patients to live independently after discharge, with a special emphasis on daily living skills and the use of community resources.

If extensive care becomes necessary, especially for elderly patients, yet another option would be a nursing home facility, either an intermediate care or a skilled nursing care facility. The skilled nursing home is for the person needing intensive care, twenty-four-hour supervision under a physician's supervision with treatment by a registered nurse. Intermediate care is suitable for those not needing round-the-clock supervision but unable to live alone. This option is expensive, and the costs generally are not reimbursed, placing all the financial responsibility on the patient or on family members. Although nursing homes in the United States are inspected and controlled by the government, the certification status and quality among homes differ greatly. Attention must be given to ensure good medical coverage, provisions for maintaining the patient's individuality and dignity, available activities, nutritious meals, social and recreational activities, and intellectual stimulation.

The hospice setting offers intense medical supervision in comfortable and peaceful surroundings. The philosophy of hospice emphasizes the concept of supportive care and services for the terminally ill and their families in the home or a special center. Although hospices assist in some home health care services and inpatient care, they are designed for terminally ill patients who are no longer being treated for their diseases, with a life expectancy of only weeks or months. Specialized teams composed of a physician, nursing staff, volunteers, social workers, and clergy administer to the physical, spiritual, and emotional needs of each patient through the management of medical symptoms and the control of pain. If the patient is not placed into a hospice center, specialized care from the hospice team is available in the home to meet the needs of terminally ill patients and their families.

Perspective and Prospects

Caring for a terminally ill family member can be a rewarding experience as well as an exhausting one. The location where this care is traditionally given has changed over time and will continue to change in the future. Care in the patient's home or with relatives is the least restrictive and one of the less expensive of the many options available. In fact, care in the home is often the only option because outside care is too expensive. Some family members are motivated to select home care because of a sense of obligation or a fear that no one else can care for the patient as well.

More supplemental resources are available than ever before, allowing home care to be a viable option for some. For many others, however, the additional stresses of responsibility for a terminally ill relative, especially an elderly one, are too high. At this point, tough decisions must be made about where the patient should live. Family members may not be prepared to care for the patient at the home. Despite the high costs of extended care facilities, this option is sometimes the only choice available. An emphasis on quality of life makes placement in the least restrictive environment a common choice. Concerns about pain management and the need for a caring staff may change this choice, however, when the terminally ill face the end of life.

In the United States, the high cost of health care makes such decisions even more difficult. Although the Patient Protection and Affordable Care Act of 2010 states that all insurers must cover palliative care, individual states decide whether and how hospice is covered under this provision. Some provisions have also been enacted to encourage the use of home- and community-based services over placement in nursing homes and other long-term facilities; however, long-term care coverage is not included among the law's provisions. Thus, the financial burden will continue to dictate placement for many of the terminally ill. Although many placement options exist, more will be developed in the future because of the increase in the number of older adults. Some will be suitable and some will not, making this decision process a problem for generations to come. While the final decision about where to live remains with the competent patient, the input of physicians and family members and the influence of financial questions will become larger concerns. Societal influences may also come to the surface as the number of elderly people grows. With improving medical technology, the elderly population will have a greater impact on governmental policy makers and will influence national health care provisions. Advances in medicine may also dictate where and how terminally ill patients are cared for.

Resources for this care are available, but they have specific requirements. Possible benefit providers include the federal government through Medicare and the Social Security Administration's supplemental security income (SSI) program. Qualified persons should contact the Veterans Administration. State programs include Medicaid, the Department of Human Resources, and state supplemental programs. In addition to private insurance coverage, financial help may be sought through community agencies, such as municipal or other local support groups. Several health-related organizations offer some assistance for specific groups of patients, such as the American Cancer Society. Many private agencies, both nonprofit and for profit, offer services. The first and best approach for information when seeking care for a terminally ill patient is through family physicians, hospitals, and local health departments.

—Maxine M. Urton, Ph.D.

See also Acquired immunodeficiency syndrome (AIDS); Aging: Extended care; Allied health; Assisted living facilities; Cancer; Critical care; Critical care, pediatric; Death and dying; Emergency medicine; Ethics; Euthanasia; Geriatrics and gerontology; Home care; Hospice; Hospitals; Law and medicine; Living will; Nursing; Oncology; Palliative medicine; Pediatrics; Pharmacology; Psychiatry; Psychiatry, child and adolescent; Psychiatry, geriatric; Resuscitation.

For Further Information:

A.D.A.M. Medical Encyclopedia. "Hospice Care." *MedlinePlus*, April 4, 2012.

Administration on Aging, Dept. of Health and Human Services. "Home Health Care." *Eldercare Locator*, April 24, 2013.

Appleton, Michael, and Todd Henschell. *At Home with Terminal Illness: A Family Guide to Hospice in the Home*. Englewood Cliffs, N.J.: Prentice Hall Career & Technology, 1995.

Beerman, Susan, and Judith Rappaport-Musson. *Eldercare 911: The Caregiver's Complete Handbook for Making Decisions*. Rev. ed. Amherst, N.Y.: Prometheus Books, 2008.

Corr, Charles A., Clyde M. Nabe, and Donna M. Corr. *Death and Dying, Life and Living*. 6th ed. Belmont, Calif.: Wadsworth/Cengage Learning, 2009.

Forman, Walter B., et al., eds. *Hospice and Palliative Care: Concepts and Practice*. 2d ed. Sudbury, Mass.: Jones and Bartlett, 2003.

Levy, Michael T. *Parenting Mom and Dad: A Guide for the Grown-Up Children of Aging Parents*. New York: Prentice Hall, 1991.

Lieberman, Trudy. *Consumer Reports Complete Guide to Health Services for Seniors*. New York: Crown, 2000.

Lynn, Joanne, and Joan Harrold. "Preparing for the Inevitable." *The Washington Post*, May 30, 1999, p. X03.

Lynn, Joanne, Joan Harrold, and Janice Lynch Schuster. *Handbook for Mortals: Guidance for People Facing Serious Illness*. 2d ed. New York: Oxford University Press, 2011.

Matthews, Joseph L. *Choose the Right Long-Term Care: Home Care, Assisted Living, and Nursing Homes*. 4th ed. Berkeley, Calif.: Nolo, 2002.

National Institute on Aging. *End of Life: Helping with Comfort and Care*. Bethesda, Md.: National Institutes of Health, U.S. Dept. of Health and Human Services, 2012.

Portnow, Jay, and Martha Houtmann. *Home Care for the Elderly: A Complete Guide*. New York: Pocket Books, 1989.

TESTICLES, UNDESCENDED
Disease/Disorder

Also known as: Cryptorchidism
Anatomy or system affected: Genitals, reproductive system
Specialties and related fields: Endocrinology, general surgery, pediatrics, urology
Definition: Testicles that neither reside in nor can be manipulated into the scrotum.

Causes and Symptoms

The testicles, or testes, appear in males by seven weeks of gestation; by eight weeks, they are hormonally active. At eleven weeks, they produce testosterone, which is suppressed by maternal estrogens later in the pregnancy. These estrogens decrease before birth, causing a surge in testosterone production that is indispensable for the descent of the testes at about thirty-six weeks of gestation and for future sperm production.

About 3.4 percent of all male infants born after a full-term pregnancy will have undescended testes, or cryptorchidism. Risk factors include being first born or a twin, having a low birth weight, and/or being born prematurely, as well as being delivered by cesarean section. By three months of age, 1 percent of male infants still have undescended testes, a percentage unchanged by one year of age. In premature infants, most testes will descend by three months after the expected date at which the child should have been born (term).

The tissues of descended and undescended testes are the same for the first year. Thereafter, an undescended testis deteriorates and the chance of infertility increases. Rarely will testes descend spontaneously after six months of age.

Cryptorchidism may be isolated or be part of other conditions such as genetic or endocrine disorders, or intersexuality. Infertility affects about 50 percent of patients with unilateral (one-sided) cryptorchidism. Men with one or more undescended testicles are also at an elevated risk for testicular cancer later in life.

Treatment and Therapy

The American Academy of Pediatric Surgery recommends surgical correction of this condition (called orchiopexy) by the first birthday, thereby decreasing the incidence of infertility and tumors and making the testicle accessible for regular examination. If the testicle is absent, a prosthesis may be inserted for cosmetic purposes. Hormonal treatment is also available, most often with human chorionic gonadotropin

---

Information on Undescended Testicles

Causes: Genetic, hermaphroditic, and endocrine disorders
Symptoms: Testicles that neither reside in nor can be manipulated into scrotum, increased occurrence of cancer, possible infertility
Duration: Typically one to twelve months
Treatments: Surgery, prosthesis for cosmetic purposes, hormonal therapy

(HCG), with varying success rates. A pediatric surgeon or a pediatric urologist will evaluate the child and decide what is best for the individual patient.

—Frances Garcia, M.D.

See also Endocrine system; Endocrinology; Endocrinology, pediatric; Genetic diseases; Genital disorders, male; Glands; Hermaphroditism and pseudohermaphroditism; Hormones; Hydroceles; Men's health; Orchitis; Premature birth; Reproductive system; Sexual differentiation; Sexuality; Surgery, pediatric; Testicular cancer; Testicular surgery; Testicular torsion; Urology; Urology, pediatric.

For Further Information:

Behrman, Richard E., Robert M. Kliegman, and Hal B. Jenson, eds. *Nelson Textbook of Pediatrics*. 19th ed. Philadelphia: Saunders/Elsevier, 2011.

Montague, Drogo K. *Disorders of Male Sexual Function*. Chicago: Year Book Medical, 1988.

Rajfer, Jacob, ed. *Urologic Endocrinology*. Philadelphia: W. B. Saunders, 1986.

Rifkin, Matthew D., and Dennis L. Cochlin. *Imaging of the Scrotum and Penis*. Florence, Ky.: Taylor & Francis, 2002.

Smith, Nathalie. "Undescended Testes." *Health Library*, September 26, 2012.

Swanson, Janice M., and Katherine A. Forrest. *Men's Reproductive Health*. New York: Springer, 1984.

"Undescended Testicle." *MedlinePlus*, September 24, 2012.

Testicular cancer
Disease/Disorder

Anatomy or system affected: Endocrine system, genitals, glands, urinary system

Specialties and related fields: Endocrinology, general surgery, oncology, radiology, urology

Definition: A tumor that appears as a hard lump, often painless, on one or both testicles.

Key terms:

biopsy: the removal and examination of a tissue sample from a living body

hematocele: a swelling of the scrotum that contains blood and may result from an injury to the testes

hydrocele: a collection of fluid in the scrotum

metastasis: the spread of cancer cells from one part of the body to another

orchiectomy: the surgical removal of a testis

orchitis: inflammation of the testis

seminomas: cancers developing from a single cell type, often from the cells that produce sperm

teratomas: cancers developing from multiple cell types

testis: a male sex organ that produces sperm and manufactures the male sex hormone testosterone

Causes and Symptoms

Testicular cancer occurs infrequently and is most often found in Caucasian males between the ages of fifteen and thirty-five. The disorder is virtually unknown among African American males, among boys who have not yet reached puberty, and in men over fifty. The cause of this type of cancer is still unknown, although it has been observed to be more frequent among males with an undescended testicle than it is among the general population.

The most common symptom is a swelling of one testis. This swelling occasionally is accompanied by pain and inflammation, although more frequently than not it will be painless. Many causes trigger swelling in the scrotum, and most such situations prove to be harmless. Among these is a hydrocele, a collection of fluid in the scrotum that typically disappears over a period of several days. Also, injuries to the scrotum, often sustained by young men who are engaged in athletics, may result in a hematocele, a swelling that contains fluid and blood.

Although most swelling in the genital area is not serious, it is wise, especially for those in the fifteen to thirty-five age group, to have such swelling checked by a physician immediately to verify that no malignancy is present. Where orchitis, an inflammation of the testis, is present, it may be accompanied by severe pain, but it usually does not presage cancer, nor is it likely to persist.

Males are encouraged to make periodical digital examinations of the testes to check for any abnormalities. If a hard lump is detected, even though it may not be tender or painful when it is palpated, immediate medical intervention is indicated.

The most common testicular cancers are seminomas, composed of a single cell type, usually sperm-producing cells, or teratomas, which consist of a combination of different cell types. A handful of testicular cancers result from the growth of testicular tissue or lymph tissue within the testis, but these are extremely rare.

Treatment and Therapy

If men regularly examine their testes, any abnormalities should be detected in their earliest stages. If a malignant growth is present, then it is likely to grow quite quickly. Where a malignancy is detected, ultrasound examination can dependably determine the parameters of the growth. This procedure is usually followed by a needle biopsy to check testicular tissue for malignant cells.

Physicians attempt to treat such growths before they have had an opportunity to spread to other parts of the body. The most common treatment is orchiectomy, or removal of the affected testis and the adjacent lymph nodes. Such surgery, while drastic, usually does not limit a man's sexual activity, nor does it typically result in infertility.

Following an orchiectomy, the testis that has been re-

Information on Testicular Cancer

Causes: Unknown; more frequent among males with undescended testicle

Symptoms: Swelling of one testis, occasionally pain and inflammation

Duration: Chronic

Treatments: Removal of affected testis and adjacent lymph nodes, radiation therapy, sometimes chemotherapy

moved is examined closely under magnification to detect malignant cells. The surgery is usually followed by a course of radiation therapy on the remaining testis and the nearby lymph nodes. Such treatment is indicated even if there is no evidence that the malignancy has spread.

Where there is any suggestion that the cancer has spread, however, chemotherapy is usually indicated as well. In such cases, cancerous tissue may also have to be excised from the patient's abdomen and from other nearby areas to limit the spread of the malignancy.

Perspective and Prospects

Testicular cancer is among the easiest cancers to detect, simply by examining the testes digitally at least once every two or three weeks. Digital palpation of both testes will quickly reveal pronounced irregularities. Because the detection process is simpler for this type of cancer than in many other types, early detection is typical. Once an abnormality has been discovered, immediate treatment and follow-up radiation therapy and/or chemotherapy will usually result in a favorable outcome.

In most cases, one of the patient's testes is not affected, so that patients are able to achieve erections and resume a normal sex life. The viability of their sperm usually is not adversely affected by an orchiectomy. The recovery period following surgery is seldom more than a few days, although subsequent radiation therapy and chemotherapy may disable patients for short periods of time following their application.

The cure rate for testicular cancers that are detected early is between 95 and 97 percent. Even in more advanced cases, the cure rate is 80 to 85 percent because of the specificity of treating this disorder surgically and with radiation, especially if the malignancy has not metastasized.

—*R. Baird Shuman, Ph.D.*

See also Cancer; Chemotherapy; Endocrine system; Endocrinology; Endocrinology, pediatric; Genital disorders, male; Glands; Hormones; Men's health; Oncology; Orchiectomy; Orchitis; Radiation therapy; Reproductive system; Testicles, undescended; Testicular surgery; Testicular torsion; Urology; Urology, pediatric.

For Further Information:
Berenberg, Jeffrey L. "Testicular Cancer." In *Oncological Nursing Secrets*, edited by Rose A. Gates and Regina M. Fink. Philadelphia: Hanley & Belfus, 2001.

Gardner, David G. et al., eds. *Greenspan's Basic and Clinical Endocrinology.* 9th ed. New York: McGraw-Hill, 2011.

LaRusso, Laurie. "Testicular Cancer." *Health Library*, February 1, 2013.

LeMone, Priscilla, Karen M. Burke, and Jane E. Bostick. *Clinical Handbook for Medical-Surgical Nursing: Critical Thinking in Client Care.* 5th ed. Boston: Pearson, 2012.

MedlinePlus. "Testicular Cancer." *MedlinePlus*, May 28, 2013.

Reinhart, M. "Testicular Cancer." In *PET in Clinical Oncology*, edited by Helmut J. Wieler and R. Edward Coleman. Berlin: Springer, 2000.

Tamimi, Rulla, and Hans-Olov Adami. "Testicular Cancer." In *Textbook of Cancer Epidemiology*, edited by Adami, David Hunter, and Dimitrios Trichopoulos. 2d ed. New York: Oxford University Press, 2008.

TESTICULAR SURGERY
Procedure

Anatomy or system affected: Endocrine system, genitals, glands, reproductive system

Specialties and related fields: General surgery, urology

Definition: The fixation of a testicle to the scrotum or the removal of a testicle or the veins surrounding a testicle.

Key terms:

orchiectomy: surgical removal of the testicle for benign or malignant conditions

orchiopexy: fixation of the testicle to the internal lining of the scrotum to eliminate the possibility of testicular torsion

testicular torsion: twisting of the testicle in the scrotum, with compromise of the blood supply to the testicle, as a result of spermatic cord rotation

varicocele: an enlarged vein surrounding the testicle as a result of incompetent venous valves; most commonly found surrounding the left testicle

Indications and Procedures

Fixation of a testicle may be performed as treatment for torsion (twisting) of the testicle and undescended testicle (cryptorchidism). Removal of a testicle may be required because of infection, traumatic rupture, pain, necrosis (death of the testicle), or the presence of a testicular tumor.

Testicular torsion occurs most commonly in males under twenty-five years of age. Torsion is usually associated with acute testicular pain that is intense enough to produce nausea, vomiting, and severe discomfort. The testicle is usually firm, tender, and displaced upward in the scrotum. It is frequently difficult to examine the gland because of the severe pain. Manual elevation of the testicle may relieve discomfort in some patients with infections of the epididymis, but it has no effect on patients with torsion. Testicular torsion is considered a surgical emergency. Information regarding this condition can be obtained using scrotal ultrasound or radionucleotide scans, but most patients require surgical exploration to identify this condition. It is important to relieve the torsion as quickly as possible to restore blood supply to the testicle. Prolonged delay before surgical intervention can result in a nonviable, necrotic testicle.

Treatment of testicular torsion is by a surgical procedure called orchiopexy. After an incision in the scrotum, the testicle is untwisted under direct vision. If more than six hours have elapsed before surgery, a necrotic testicle may result and orchiectomy may be required. If the testicle appears viable, orchiopexy is carried out. In orchiopexy, the testis is anchored in the scrotum with a row of three or more absorbable sutures through the lining of the testicle and the dartos muscle layer of the scrotal wall. These sutures fix the testicle to the scrotum to eliminate further torsion. A small plastic drain may be placed to limit swelling and enhance drainage during recovery. The skin is closed with absorbable sutures. Because testicular torsion frequently occurs on both sides, the opposite testicle is similarly fixed with orchiopexy.

Undescended testes are located outside the scrotum, usually in the inguinal canal, but they may also be found in the abdomen. Orchiopexy should be performed at one to two years of age to preserve future testicular function. While rare cases require microsurgery, most orchiopexies are performed using a scrotal incision with testicular fixation similar to that described for torsion.

Varicoceles occur in approximately 15 percent of adult males, usually following puberty. Their importance is the association with infertility in some men with low sperm counts. Varicoceles occur primarily on the left side and result from abnormalities in the veins draining the left testicle. While tying off the veins of the varicocele is important in adolescent males with an associated decrease in testicular size, most varicoceles do not require surgery. If low sperm count, persistent infertility, decreased testicular volume, or prolonged pain occurs from the varicocele, surgical intervention may be appropriate.

Varicocele surgery can be performed through the abdomen, groin, or scrotum. Most surgeons prefer a high ligation, which involves a small incision just above the groin (internal inguinal ring). The vein draining the testicle is identified beneath the abdominal muscles. It is separated from the vas deferens (sperm tube) and arteries supplying the testicle, is ligated with several sutures, and is divided. This method of treatment is the most direct, least complicated, and most effective for varicocele ligation. The procedure is performed on an outpatient basis. Most patients are able to return to normal activity within seven days. Under certain circumstances, with previous failed high ligations, or with very large scrotal varices, a scrotal incision may be selected by the surgeon to remove all dilated veins from around the testicle. This technique is most useful in patients with decreased testicular volume or pain caused by a varicocele.

Orchiectomy, or removal of a testicle, is used to treat an abscess, infection, traumatic rupture, loss of testicular function, prostate cancer, and testicular tumors. Removal of the testicle for testicular tumors is especially important since these tumors are curable if identified and treated early. This procedure is carried out through an incision in the groin and not in the scrotum, a technique that decreases the chance of testicular tumor spread to the scrotum. A small incision in the groin above the scrotum is made, the spermatic cord is clamped, and the testicle is delivered into the incision and inspected. If a testicular tumor is identified, the spermatic cord is tied and the testis removed. The incision is then closed using standard suture techniques. If a testicle is to be removed for other indications, such as infection, prostate cancer, pain, or trauma, a scrotal incision is appropriate. The incision, which is similar to that described for testicular torsion, exposes the testicle and spermatic cord and allows for clamping and ligation of the spermatic cord prior to testicular removal. A drain is not usually necessary for orchiectomy.

Uses and Complications

Rapid identification of testicular torsion is paramount, before compromise of the blood supply results in the death of the testicle. Diagnosis of testicular torsion should be within six to eight hours of onset. Episodic torsion can also occur and is associated with preservation of testicular function and anatomy. Varicocele ligation is carried out for associated decreased testicular volume, pain, and most commonly infertility with diminished sperm count or sperm activity.

The complications associated with testicular surgery include infection in the scrotum, bleeding into the scrotum, and scrotal swelling. Pain, which is usually short-lived and localized, may occur with the inguinal incisions used for the removal of testicular tumors. Bleeding is the most common significant complication of testicular surgery and results in enlargement of the scrotum, significant discoloration, and pain. Bleeding is most often identified within six to twelve hours after testicular surgery. Testicular surgery is usually performed using absorbable sutures in the scrotal skin, and suture removal after surgery is unnecessary.

Perspective and Prospects

Surgical procedures for scrotal abnormalities have been common urologic procedures for centuries. New technologies such as radiographic embolization of testicular veins for varicoceles have been tried, but they are not generally accepted as superior to simple surgical procedures. These procedures, which are expensive and have unique complications, are less likely to be effective than more common, simple surgical intervention. Laparoscopy has been widely used for varicocele ligation, but it has little advantage over high ligation and is more expensive and time-consuming. Orchiopexy for abdominal or other high-lying testes can now be performed using microsurgical techniques. The testis can be removed and transplanted to a scrotal location, or the spermatic cord can be rerouted to permit scrotal placement and to avoid orchiectomy.

—*Culley C. Carson III, M.D.*

See also Circulation; Genital disorders, male; Glands; Hydroceles; Men's health; Orchiectomy; Orchitis; Reproductive system; Surgery, pediatric; Testicles, undescended; Testicular cancer; Testicular torsion; Urology; Urology, pediatric; Vascular system.

For Further Information:
Cockett, Abraham T. K., and Ken Koshiba. *Color Atlas of Urologic Surgery*. Baltimore: Williams & Wilkins, 1996.
Graham, Sam D., Jr., et al., eds. *Glenn's Urologic Surgery*. 7th ed. Philadelphia: Lippincott Williams & Wilkins, 2010.
Kaneshiro, Neil K. "Testicular Torsion Repair." *MedlinePlus*, October 9, 2012.
Kollin, C., et al. "Growth of Spontaneously Descended and Surgically Treated Testes During Early Childhood." *Pediatrics* 131.4 (April 2013): 174–180.
Milsten, Richard, and Julian Slowinski. *The Sexual Male: Problems and Solutions*. New York: W. W. Norton, 2000.
Parker, James N., and Philip M. Parker, eds. *The Official Patient's Sourcebook on Testicular Cancer*. San Diego, Calif.: Icon Health, 2002.
Taguchi, Yosh, and Merrily Weisbord, eds. *Private Parts: An Owner's Guide to the Male Anatomy*. 3d ed. Toronto, Ont.: McClelland & Stewart, 2003.
"Treatment Options for Testicular Cancer by Stage." *American Cancer Society*. January 17, 2013.

Testicular torsion
Disease/Disorder

Anatomy or system affected: Circulatory system, genitals, reproductive system

Specialties and related fields: Family medicine, pediatrics, urology

Definition: A twisting or rotation of the testicle (testis) or spermatic cord on its long axis, causing acute pain and swelling.

Causes and Symptoms

Testicular torsion is most commonly found in infants, adolescents, or young adult males. Roughly half of the cases occur in the early hours of the morning, and cases usually occur on the left side rather than the right. The condition can occur during sleep, rest, game playing, or hard physical activity, but it is more likely to be caused by direct injury. Testicular torsion may also result if the testicle is unusually mobile within its covering in the scrotum because of inadequate connective tissue.

Testicular torsion makes itself known by pain of varying degrees either in the lower part of the abdomen or in the scrotum itself. The pain intensifies rapidly and is occasionally accompanied by nausea as the testicle becomes swollen and very tender and the scrotal skin becomes discolored. A diagnosis can be made by physical examination.

Treatment and Therapy

Immediate treatment of testicular torsion is necessary. The testicle must be untwisted immediately and blood flow restored to the testicle, the epididymis, and other structures. Otherwise, complete blockage of the blood supply (ischemia) for six hours or more may result in gangrene (tissue death) of the testicle. Even a partial loss of circulation can produce atrophy.

Manual untwisting should be followed by surgery within six hours of the onset of symptoms to ensure that the torsion has been undone successfully and that there is no recurrence. An incision is made in the scrotal skin, and the testicle is secured to the scrotum by small stitches. If irreversible damage has been done, the testicle must be removed. The other testicle, which usually remains capable of producing active sperm, is also anchored to prevent torsion on that side. Prompt surgery generally ensures a complete recovery.

—*Keith Garebian, Ph.D.*

See also Genital disorders, male; Glands; Hydroceles; Laparoscopy; Men's health; Orchiectomy; Orchitis; Penile implant surgery; Reproductive system; Testicles, undescended; Testicular cancer; Testicular surgery; Urology; Urology, pediatric; Vasectomy.

For Further Information:

Behrman, Richard E., Robert M. Kliegman, and Hal B. Jenson, eds. *Nelson Textbook of Pediatrics.* 19th ed. Philadelphia: Elsevier/Saunders, 2011.

Montague, Drogo K. *Disorders of Male Sexual Function.* Chicago: Year Book Medical, 1988.

Rajfer, Jacob, ed. *Urologic Endocrinology.* Philadelphia: W. B. Saunders, 1986.

Rifkin, Matthew D., and Dennis L. Cochlin. *Imaging of the Scrotum and Penis.* Florence, Ky.: Taylor & Francis, 2002.

Swanson, Janice M., and Katherine A. Forrest. *Men's Reproductive Health.* New York: Springer, 1984.

Taguchi, Yosh, and Merrily Weisbord, eds. *Private Parts: An Owner's Guide to the Male Anatomy.* 3d ed. Toronto: McClelland & Stewart, 2003.

"Testicular Torsion." *Urology Care Foundation,* Jan. 2011.

Tests. *See* Invasive tests; Laboratory tests; Noninvasive tests.

Tetanus
Disease/Disorder

Also known as: Lockjaw

Anatomy or system affected: Brain, muscles, musculoskeletal system, nervous system

Specialties and related fields: Bacteriology, family medicine, internal medicine, neurology, public health

Definition: An often fatal disease of the nervous system characterized by painful, sustained, and violent muscle spasms; it is almost completely preventable through vaccination.

Key terms:

anaerobic: without oxygen; anaerobic organisms grow in an atmosphere free of oxygen

antibody: a protein found in the blood and produced by the immune system in response to contact of the body with an antigen

antigen: a foreign substance (such as a bacteria, toxin, or virus) to which the body makes an immune response

antitoxin: an antibody against a specific toxin; antitoxins can bind toxins and neutralize them

bacterium: a microscopic single-celled organism that multiplies by means of simple division; bacteria are found everywhere; most are beneficial, but a few species cause disease

endospore: a resistant, dormant structure, formed inside bacteria such as *Bacillus* and *Clostridium*, that can survive adverse conditions

immunity: a capacity to resist a disease caused by an infectious agent

lockjaw: a popular name for tetanus, derived from a symptom associated with the disease

toxin: a poisonous substance produced by some bacteria that cause certain diseases

toxoid: a form of a toxin that can no longer cause the

Information on Testicular Torsion

Causes: Injury, hard physical activity, inadequate connective tissue within scrotum

Symptoms: Acute pain and swelling, discolored scrotal skin

Duration: Acute

Treatments: Manual untwisting, followed by surgery

symptoms of a disease but can cause the body to make anti-bodies against it

vaccination: inoculation with a specific vaccine in order to prevent or lessen the effect of some disease

Causes and Symptoms

Tetanus is a disease of the nervous system caused by the bacterium *Clostridium tetani* (*C. tetani*). Humans and most species of warm-blooded animals are susceptible to tetanus. This disease is not contagious, meaning it cannot be transmitted from one individual to another. It results from the contamination of a natural or surgical wound by spores (endospores) of *C. tetani*. The bacteria grow in the wound and produce a toxin that spreads throughout the body and causes the symptoms of the disease. Neonatal tetanus is the appearance of tetanus in a child less than one month old; it is usually contracted by the infant directly following birth.

C. tetani is an anaerobic, endospore-forming bacterium. Anaerobic bacteria can grow only in an oxygen-free environment. In harsh environments or at times when oxygen is present, all species of Clostridia have the unique ability to form dormant (nongrowing) structures called endospores. These structures develop inside the bacterial cell and serve to protect the genetic material of the cell from harsh environmental stresses that would destroy an actively growing cell. Endospores are very resistant to disinfectants and temperature changes; thus, the bacteria can remain dormant until the surrounding environment becomes better suited for growth. *C. tetani* spores are found throughout the world in soil, human and animal intestines, and especially in soil fertilized with human or animal feces.

A person can get tetanus only if spores from the soil or elsewhere in the environment enter that person under the proper conditions to become living, growing bacteria. The bacteria will grow only if they enter a wound that is free from oxygen, such as a deep puncture wound or a wound that has considerable dead or crushed tissue. There are always a few cases of tetanus, however, that follow no apparent injury. Typical causes of wounds that could be susceptible to tetanus are compound fractures; gunshots; dog bites; punctures caused by glass, thorns, needles, splinters, or rusty nails; "skin popping" by drug addicts; bedsores; outer ear infections; and dental extractions. The most feared form of tetanus, neonatal tetanus, is usually caused by the cutting of the umbilical cord with an unsterile instrument or by improper care of the umbilical stump. In the United States, most cases of neonatal tetanus are found in home deliveries not attended by a health professional.

Spores of *C. tetani* enter the body through a wound or abrasion. In the absence of oxygen, they will germinate (revert from the dormant endospore state to become living, growing cells). The bacteria will grow and multiply but not spread from the initial site of infection. In many cases, the wound hardly appears to be infected at all. As it grows, *C. tetani* produces a toxin called tetanospasmin that can filter through the body. Once the toxin reaches the central nervous system, it binds to nerve cells, causing the beginning stages of symp-

---

Information on Tetanus

Causes: Bacterial infection through wound or abrasion

Symptoms: Restlessness; irritability; stiff neck; difficulty swallowing; stiffness or spasms of jaw muscles (lockjaw); painful, sustained, and violent muscle spasms

Duration: Typically three to twenty-one days

Treatments: Antitoxins; antibiotics; cleaning wound of any dead tissue; control of muscle spasms (barbiturates, Valium, D tubocurarine); positive-pressure breathing apparatus to maintain respiration; possible tracheotomy; dark room to reduce auditory and visual stimuli

---

toms to be seen. Symptoms can appear from one day to several months after infection, with the average incubation period (the time during which symptoms appear after infection) being three to twenty-one days. The wide range of incubation time depends on the amount of time needed for anaerobic conditions to develop and the time required for the toxin to reach the central nervous system.

The tetanus toxin, tetanospasmin, is a simple protein. No one knows why *C. tetani* makes this protein. It has no apparent role in the life of the bacterium, and it is unknown whether this toxin gives the bacterium any selective advantage for survival in the environment. It is unlikely that the bacterium makes this toxin merely to kill people and animals, yet the fact that it does kill them is all that is known about the toxin. Animals vary in their susceptibility to the effects of tetanospasmin; humans and horses are the most susceptible, while birds and cold-blooded animals are resistant. Tetanospasmin is the second most dangerous known toxin, and it is so powerful that an amount of toxin the size of one period on this page could kill thirty people. One milligram of toxin could kill 200 million laboratory mice.

To understand how tetanospasmin works to cause the symptoms of tetanus, one must first understand how muscles function. Most muscles in the body occur in pairs; one muscle in the pair, when contracted, causes that part of the body to move in one direction, and the opposing muscle in the pair, when contracted, causes that part of the body to move in the opposite direction. Normally, the nerves that control the muscle pairs stimulate one muscle in a pair to contract and signal the opposing muscle to relax. In this way, that part of the body is able to move. For example, in using an arm to lift an object, the nerves send a signal to the muscle in the front of the arm to contract and at the same time send a signal to the back of the arm to relax, so that the arm can bend upward at the elbow and lift the object. If the nerves did not signal the opposing muscle to relax, the contraction of the first muscle would cause the opposing muscle to stretch and trigger the "stretch reflex" in that muscle, causing that muscle to contract and counteract the stretch. Tetanus toxin works by binding to the nerve cells at nerve-muscle junctions and somehow blocking the signal of relaxation to the opposing muscle; therefore, when one

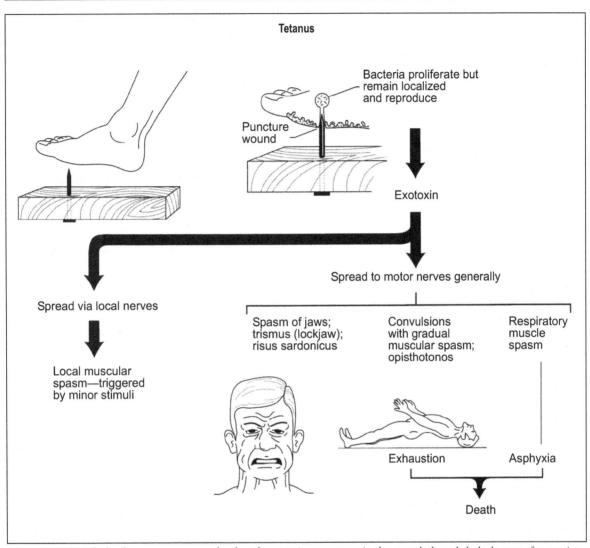

Tetanus is contracted when bacteria enter a wound and produce a toxin, tetanospasmin, that spreads through the body, most often causing death. A program of immunization is nearly 100 percent effective against tetanus.

muscle in a pair of muscles contracts, both muscles contract. The final effect is called spastic paralysis, in which the muscles are in a state of continuous contraction, pulling against each other, causing rigidity in a normally movable part of the body.

The initial symptoms of tetanus include restlessness, irritability, a stiff neck, and difficulty swallowing. In about half of all cases, the initial symptoms include stiffness or spasms of the jaw muscles, known as lockjaw. Gradually, the skeletal muscles (muscles of the arms, legs, back, and stomach) become involved. Muscles move through stages of contractions, from merely twitching to rigid spasms that are brief but may be frequent, painful, and exhausting. Severe stages of the disease are characterized by tetanic spasms (sustained contractions) of some or all of the muscle groups. The slightest disturbance of the victim may cause spasms, generalized seizures, or both. A typical tetanic seizure is characterized by a sudden burst of tetanic spasm of all muscle groups, causing clenching of the jaw to produce a grimace, arching of the back with the neck back, flexion of arms, clenching of fists on the chest, and extension of the lower extremities. The patient is completely conscious during such episodes and experiences intense pain. Some spasms may be severe enough to cause bones to break. Eventually, the muscles of the cardiac and respiratory systems can be affected. Spasms of the throat muscles and respiratory muscles may lead to suffocation or respiratory arrest. The toxin may affect the circulatory system and heart in such a way as to increase the heart rate, increase blood pressure, and cause constriction of blood vessels. Death caused by tetanus is usually a result of circulatory collapse or respiratory failure.

Treatment and Therapy

Tetanus is diagnosed mainly on the basis of the symptoms present and the case history of the patient—the vaccination record and the type of injury sustained. A patient with no recent history of tetanus vaccination who receives a puncture or trauma wound is often treated for tetanus with an injection of antitoxin even before any symptoms appear. Antitoxin is quite effective when given to prevent the symptoms from appearing, but less so when given after the symptoms have already appeared. While other diseases are diagnosed after the organism that causes the disease is isolated from the site of the infection, it is very difficult to diagnose tetanus based on the ability to isolate the *C. tetani* bacteria from the wound, for several reasons. First, Clostridia are present in almost every wound, but they do not always cause disease, so finding them does not necessarily mean that the bacteria are active. Second, there are many other contaminating bacteria in wounds, which makes it difficult to tell which may be causing disease or whether Clostridia are there at all. In addition, the number of *C. tetani* bacteria needed to cause disease is quite small, which makes them harder to isolate. Finally, Clostridia, because of their anaerobic nature, are difficult to grow.

Tetanus may take from a few days to several weeks to run its course. Patients who exhibit certain patterns in the course of the disease usually have a poor chance of recovery. These include patients with a short incubation period between the time of the injury and the onset of seizures, patients who exhibit a rapid development from mild muscle spasms to tetanic spasms, patients with injuries close to the head, patients with a high frequency or strong severity of seizures, and patients who are very young or very old. Patients who do recover usually return to a completely normal state after a variable period of stiffness; except for possible damage to the lungs from pulmonary complications or bone fractures, tetanus leaves no permanent damage. Unfortunately, recovery from the disease does not make the patient immune to future attacks, as with other diseases. The amount of toxin needed to kill a person is not even close to enough toxin to stimulate the patient's immune response to make the patient immune to the disease. Only vaccination with a large dose of inactive toxin can give a person immunity to tetanus.

Tetanus is difficult to treat because no one knows exactly what the toxin does. Doctors know only what kinds of symptoms the toxin causes, so the treatment is mainly symptomatic and is directed at preventing the production of more toxin. Antitoxin is given to block the attachment to the nerve cells of any free toxin that might be circulating in the body. Antitoxin has absolutely no effect on toxin that is already fixed to nerve tissue, but it can fully neutralize any free toxin. Originally, doctors used serum from immunized horses as a source of antitoxin, but this caused serious side effects (namely, serum sickness) in patients, so it is recommended that only pooled hyperimmune human globin (purified serum from immunized humans) be used as a source of antitoxin. Second, large doses of an antibiotic such as penicillin are given to kill any remaining bacteria, in order to prevent the bacteria from producing more toxin. If the patient is allergic to penicillin, tetracycline or clindamycin can be given instead. In addition, the wound may need to be cleansed of any dead tissue, to remove the anaerobic environment necessary for growth of the bacteria.

Third, the muscle spasms need to be controlled. Mild muscle spasms are controlled with barbiturates and diazepam (Valium); severe spasms need a curarelike agent (D tubocurarine is used to poison the paralyzed muscles so that they do not contract) that completely paralyzes the patient. These various muscle relaxants are used to ease the contractions until the toxin already present at the nerve sites wears out. The patient can be put on a positive-pressure breathing apparatus to maintain respiration. A tracheostomy (an operation in which an opening into the trachea, or windpipe, is made) may be necessary to minimize respiratory complications. Also, patients are often kept in quiet dark rooms that reduce auditory and visual stimuli, in order to minimize the frequency and severity of the tetanic spasms. Even with all these treatment measures, three out of five persons who contract tetanus will die.

The best means of controlling tetanus is prevention. In fact, tetanus is nearly 100 percent preventable with active or passive immunization. Active immunization involves stimulating a person's immune system to produce its own antibody to fight off the disease. An injection of tetanus toxoid is given to immunize actively against tetanus. Tetanus toxoid is purified tetanus toxin that has been treated with formaldehyde to be rendered nontoxic (meaning that it will not cause any symptoms of tetanus) but is still capable of stimulating the immune system to produce antitoxin antibody. Active immunization usually lasts a long time, because the cells that make the antibody can keep making more antibody when the first batch runs out or whenever the person comes in contact with tetanus toxin in the future. The tetanus toxoid is usually administered as part of the DPT vaccine. This vaccine protects against diphtheria (D), pertussis (P), and tetanus (T). In the United States, it is recommended that persons be immunized against tetanus at two, four, six, and eighteen months of age, with a booster at four to six years of age and one every ten years after that. Surveys indicate, however, that more than 50 percent of adults over sixty years of age are not protected against tetanus. It is as dangerous to receive too many booster shots for tetanus as it is to receive too few. With too few shots, a person runs the risk of succumbing to the disease and dying. With too many shots, a person runs the risk of developing a potentially fatal allergic reaction to the vaccine. It is best to keep careful records of all vaccinations and to be certain that one receives a tetanus booster every ten years.

Passive immunization involves giving a person antibodies (made in an outside source) that will protect that person from a disease, instead of stimulating the individual to make antibodies. Patients thought to be at risk for tetanus can be given an injection of antitoxin for protection. This type of protection works only for a short period of time, because once the antibody in the injection is used up, the patient cannot make more. The way to immunize infants passively against neonatal tetanus is to immunize their mothers actively. A pregnant patient immunized with tetanus toxoid will produce antitoxin that is passed on to the baby's blood through the placenta. The baby is then born carrying some antitoxin antibodies in its blood that can protect it from neonatal tetanus.

Perspective and Prospects

As early as the fourth century BCE, Hippocrates described tetanus as a common killer of women in childbirth, wounded soldiers, and infants. It was not until 1889, however, that the cause of tetanus, *C. tetani*, was first isolated by Shibasaburo Kitasato. In the early twentieth century, W. T. Glenny and Gaston Ramon paved the way for the development of a tetanus vaccine by discovering tetanus toxoid. War-related cases of tetanus were virtually eliminated by vaccinating soldiers. During World War II, only 12 cases of tetanus were recorded among 2,735,000 hospital admissions for wounds and injuries in soldiers previously immunized. This result led most state legislatures in America to pass laws requiring adequate immunization for tetanus before entering school.

Despite advances in treatment, the mortality rate for tetanus is quite high. The United States has about one hundred cases per year, mostly in the very young, who are in frequent contact with the soil, or in the very old, who have weakened immune systems. Many cases in the United States arise from trivial but fairly deep injuries that are thought to be too minor to bring to a physician. Sporadic cases are most frequently seen in the South, the Southeast, and the Midwest.

Tetanus is relatively rare in developed countries, where routine immunizations are available; it is, however, a common and uncontrolled disease in the developing world. Tetanus is a health problem in developing countries because of the lack of immunization, unsanitary living conditions, and the performance of common wound-causing procedures (such as ear piercing, tattooing, circumcision, and abortion) in an unsanitary manner. Neonatal tetanus is often caused by mothers or midwives who cut the umbilical cord with an unsanitary instrument. In addition, it is a tradition in many developing nations to apply soil, clay, or cow dung to the cut umbilical cord, which can inoculate tetanus spores right into the wound. Throughout the world, nearly 3.5 million children (mostly under five years of age) die yearly of three infectious diseases for which immunization is available. Two million die of measles, eight hundred thousand die of tetanus, and six hundred thousand die of whooping cough; another four million die of various kinds of diarrhea. In parts of some developing nations, 10 percent of deaths within a month of birth are caused by neonatal tetanus. The World Health Organization is making a concerted effort to reduce the incidence of tetanus—especially neonatal tetanus—in developing nations by providing the personnel and resources needed for vaccination. Strategies for reducing the incidence of neonatal tetanus include providing passive immunity to newborns through the immunization of the mothers. Also important are promotion of safe practices, such as clean deliveries and clean cord cutting, and ensuring that unsanitary substances are not applied to cord wounds.

—*Vicki J. Isola, Ph.D.*

See also Asphyxiation; Bacterial infections; Childhood infectious diseases; Gangrene; Immunization and vaccination; Muscle sprains, spasms, and disorders; Muscles; Paralysis; Seizures; Toxicology; Wounds.

For Further Information:
"CDC Report Finds Tetanus Reaching Younger Adults." *Vaccine Weekly*, July 16, 2003, 21–22.

Hollenstein, Jenna. "Tetanus." *Health Library*, November 26, 2012.

Joklik, Wolfgang K., et al. *Zinsser Microbiology*. 20th ed. Norwalk, Conn.: Appleton and Lange, 1997.

Pan American Health Organization. World Health Organization. *Control of Diphtheria, Pertussis, Tetanus, "Haemophilus influenzae" Type B, and Hepatitis B Field Guide*. Washington, DC: Author, 2005.

Pascual, F. B., et al. "Tetanus Surveillance: United States, 1998–2000." *Morbidity and Mortality Weekly Report: Surveillance Summaries* 52, no. 3 (June 20, 2003): 1–8.

"Tetanus." *Mayo Clinic*, April 24, 2013.

"Tetanus." *MedlinePlus*, November 22, 2011.

Traverso, H. P., et al. "A Reassessment of Risk Factors for Neonatal Tetanus." *Bulletin of the World Health Organization* 69, no. 5 (1991): 573–79.

Worf, Neil. "Tetanus—Still a Problem." *RN* 63, no. 6 (June, 2000): 44–49. N

THALASSEMIA
Disease/Disorder
Also known as: Cooley's anemia, hydrops fetalis
Anatomy or system affected: Blood
Specialties and related fields: Family medicine, genetic counseling, hematology, pediatrics
Definition: A group of diverse genetic blood disorders affecting either β or α globin and resulting in decreased amounts of normal hemoglobin.

Causes and Symptoms

Mutations in one or more of the four genes coding for β globin or one or both of the two genes coding for α globin are the causes of thalassemia. The deletions lead to an underproduction of normal hemoglobin, a tetramer of two β and two α globins.

The most severe form of thalassemia is β thalassemia (hydrops fetalis or β thalassemia major), in which all four β globin genes are mutant or deleted and no β globin is produced. Death occurs at or before birth. Milder forms (β thalassemia minor or trait) occur when only two of the β globin genes are nonfunctional or deleted. The mild forms may exhibit mild anemia, but usually no health effects occur. When three β globin genes are deleted or are nonfunctional, the resulting thalassemia is called hemoglobin H disease. Enough β globin is missing in hemoglobin H disease to cause moderate to severe anemia, an enlarged spleen, bone deformities, and fatigue.

In the most severe form of α thalassemia (α thalassemia major or Cooley's anemia), both α globin genes are nonfunctional or deleted and no normal hemoglobin is produced, resulting in severe anemia. Hemoglobin molecules consisting of four β globin chains rather than two β and two α chains are

---

Information on Thalassemia

Causes: Genetic mutation
Symptoms: Depends on type; ranges from mild or no anemia to moderate or severe anemia, spleen enlargement, bone deformities, and fatigue to death at or before birth
Duration: Chronic
Treatments: Blood transfusions every two to three weeks

---

produced, leading to red blood cell aggregates and inclusions that cause red blood cell membrane damage. In milder forms (α thalassemia minor or trait), in which only one α globin gene is nonfunctional or deleted, hemoglobin production is 50 percent of normal, resulting in mild anemia.

Treatment and Therapy

There is no effective treatment for β thalassemia major. Treatment for α thalassemia major involves red blood cell transfusion every two to three weeks. Transfusion therapy results in an iron overload that is controlled using chelators such as Desferal (desferrioxamine).

Perspective and Prospects

The thalassemias constitute the most common single-gene inherited disease in the world. People with mild forms of the disease (thalassemia minor or trait) are usually heterozygotes or carriers. When two carriers have children, there is a one in four chance that the child will have the severe form of the disease (thalassemia major). The frequency of the several forms of thalassemia varies geographically, with β thalassemia most common in Africa, the Middle East, India, Southeast Asia, southern China, and around the Mediterranean, and α thalassemia most common in Italy, Greece, the Arabian Peninsula, Iran, Africa, Southeast Asia, and southern China. It has been estimated that two million people in the United States carry one of the genes for thalassemia. The National Institutes of Health recommends testing for the trait.

—*Charles L. Vigue, Ph.D.*

See also Anemia; Blood and blood disorders; Genetic diseases; Hematology; Hematology, pediatric; Sickle cell disease; Transfusion.

For Further Information:
Cooley's Anemia Foundation. *Cooley's Anemia Foundation*, n.d.
Hollenstein, Jenna. "Thalassemia." *Health Library*, November 26, 2012.
Jorde, Lynn B., et al. *Medical Genetics*. 4th ed. Philadelphia.: Mosby/Elsevier, 2010.
MedlinePlus. "Thalassemia." *MedlinePlus*, May 24, 2013.
Nora, James J., and F. Clarke Fraser. *Nora and Fraser Medical Genetics: Principles and Practice*. 4th ed. Philadelphia: Lea & Febiger, 1994.
Northern California Comprehensive Thalassemia Center. *Northern California Comprehensive Thalassemia Center*, 2012.
Pritchard, Dorian J., and Bruce R. Korf. *Medical Genetics at a Glance*. 3d ed. Hoboken, N.J.: John Wiley & Sons, 2013.

THALIDOMINE

Treatment

Anatomy or system affected: Arms, blood vessels, feet, hands, immune system, legs
Specialties and related fields: Immunology, oncology
Definition: A drug that previously had been used as a sedative and then was banned for many years because of its severe effects on the developing fetus, but is now finding application in the treatment of leprosy and different cancers.

Indications and Procedures

In 1961, a link was established between the use of thalidomide, a mild sedative, and an increase in the frequency of severe defects in newborn babies in Germany, Great Britain, and other countries around the world where the drug had been in use. The "thalidomide babies" had minor defects of the fingers or toes but had major malformations of the limbs, resulting in incomplete or even missing arms and legs. The defects resembled those of a rare genetic disorder known as phocomelia ("seal limb"). Following the tragic discovery that thalidomide is a potent teratogen (a substance that causes a birth defect), use of the drug was discontinued.

In recent years, however, it has been discovered that thalidomide may be a useful therapeutic agent in a number of conditions, including leprosy, several other dermatologic disorders, different types of cancer, and acquired immunodeficiency syndrome (AIDS). The Food and Drug Administration (FDA) in the United States has approved thalidomide for use in the treatment of leprosy. Studies have demonstrated that thalidomide can inhibit in vitro angiogenesis, the process of formation of new blood vessels. Since many types of cancers require development of new blood vessels for their continued growth, thalidomide may be especially useful in cases where conventional treatments have ceased to be effective. Its use may be indicated in patients either relapsing after high-dose chemotherapy or who are developing serious side effects and are not able to tolerate additional chemotherapy.

Indications and Procedures

In 1961, a link was established between the use of thalidomide, a mild sedative, and an increase in the frequency of severe defects in newborn babies in Germany, Great Britain, and other countries around the world where the drug had been in use. The "thalidomide babies" had minor defects of the fingers or toes but had major malformations of the limbs, resulting in incomplete or even missing arms and legs. The defects resembled those of a rare genetic disorder known as phocomelia ("seal limb"). Following the tragic discovery that thalidomide is a potent teratogen (a substance that causes a birth defect), use of the drug was discontinued.

In recent years, however, it has been discovered that thalidomide may be a useful therapeutic agent in a number of conditions, including leprosy, several other dermatologic disorders, different types of cancer, and acquired immunodeficiency syndrome (AIDS). The Food and Drug Administration (FDA) in the United States has approved thalidomide for use in the treatment of leprosy. Studies have demonstrated that thalidomide can inhibit in vitro angiogenesis, the process of formation of new blood vessels. Since many types of cancers require development of new blood vessels for their continued growth, thalidomide may be especially useful in cases where conventional treatments have ceased to be effective. Its use may be indicated in patients either relapsing after high-dose chemotherapy or who are developing serious side effects and are not able to tolerate additional chemotherapy.

Uses and Complications

Since thalidomide is such a powerful angiogenesis inhibitor, it is being used in disorders requiring antiangiogenic therapy. Successful treatments have been made in cases of ovarian cancer, breast cancer, gastrointestinal carcinoma, renal melanoma, chronic graft-versus-host disease, and multiple myeloma. In some cases, the effectiveness of thalidomide increased when accompanied by other treatments, including immunotherapy, chemotherapy, and surgery.

Thalidomide appears to have few side effects in its new applications, but its return to medical respectability has raised again the specter of "thalidomide babies." Adverse effects noted in a few patients have included lethargy, constipation, and peripheral neuropathy. The potential problems associated with thalidomide causing a new round of severe birth defects may be a more serious consequence.

Perspective and Prospects

The outbreak of thalidomide-related birth defects in the 1950s and 1960s led to the creation of birth defect surveillance programs in many countries. Unfortunately, medical standards and safeguards are not uniformly good, and there already appears to be an increase in birth defects associated with the new applications of thalidomide in South America. It will be necessary to regulate and to monitor closely the prescription, dispensing, and use of the drug. Counseling of patients of childbearing age will be an especially critical component if the tragedy of thalidomide's history is not to be repeated.

—*Donald J. Nash, Ph.D.*

See also Birth defects; Cancer; Leprosy; Pharmacology; Pregnancy and gestation; Teratogens.

For Further Information:

Brynner, Rock, and Trent Stephens. *Dark Remedy: The Impact of Thalidomide and Its Revival as a Vital Medicine.* Cambridge, Mass.: Perseus, 2001.

Fanelli, M., et al. "Thalidomide: A New Anticancer Drug?" *Expert Opinion on Investigational Drugs* 12, no. 7 (July 2003): 1211-1225.

Patrias, Karen, Ronald L. Gordner, and Stephen C. Groft. *Thalidomide: Potential Benefits and Risks—January, 1963, Through July, 1997.* Bethesda, Md.: Department of Health and Human Services, 1998.

Perri, A. J., and S. Hsu. "A Review of Thalidomide's History and Current Dermatological Applications." *Dermatology Online Journal* 9, no. 3 (August, 2003): 5.

THORACIC SURGERY
Specialty

Anatomy or system affected: Chest, heart, lungs, respiratory system

Specialties and related fields: Cardiology, general surgery, pulmonary medicine

Definition: The branch of surgery that treats diseases of the chest cavity, especially the heart.

Key terms:

aneurysm: a weakened segment of a heart or blood vessel

balloon catheterization: the use of a balloonlike device on the tip of a catheter to widen blood vessels

cardiac catheterization: the guidance of a catheter into the heart or great blood vessels to measure function, assess problems, and identify solutions

computed tomography (CT) scanning: the use of X-ray computer technology to identify diseases of hard and soft tissues, such as bone and the heart

echocardiography: the use of sound waves to examine heart structures

mitral valve: the valve between the heart's left auricle and ventricle

stenosis: the narrowing of heart valves or blood vessels

Science and Profession

The chest, or thorax, lies between the neck and the abdomen, from which it is separated by the diaphragm. Its side boundaries are the ribs and the muscle that surrounds them, which are attached to the spine and breastbone (sternum) in the back and front of the body, respectively. Overall, the thorax is cone-shaped, with its small and large ends bounded by the neck and diaphragm. Inside this airtight cavity, the lungs are suspended on the right and left sides, covered by the membranous pleura. Between the lungs is the heart, with its covering, the pericardium.

Also located in the chest cavity are the trachea (windpipe), which leads to the lungs; the esophagus, which connects the mouth and stomach; the major blood vessels that enter and leave the heart; and nerves. The chest cavity inflates and deflates as a result of diaphragm and rib muscle movement. This action provides the entry of oxygen to the blood that is circulated around the body through the cardiovascular system.

Thoracic surgeons, sometimes called cardiothoracic/ cardiovascular and thoracic surgeons, handle a wide variety of surgery associated with these organs. Preeminent in many cases is surgery of the heart and major blood vessels. This precise, exacting surgery requires residency training of six years in general surgery and three years in thoracic surgery. In the United States, thoracic surgeons are certified by the American Board of Surgery and the American Board of Thoracic Surgery. Much of the time of thoracic surgeons is spent in hospitals working with critically ill patients whose lives depend on the prompt use of technical and demanding surgical techniques. Most patients are aged fifty-five to sixty-five.

Diagnostic and Treatment Techniques

The diagnostic techniques associated with thoracic surgery are highly refined. They include careful patient histories, laboratory tests, and noninvasive techniques such as echocardiography, computed tomography (CT) scanning, electrocardiography (ECG or EKG), and other types of electrophysiology. Invasive procedures include cardiac catheterization and cineangiography of the heart and surrounding blood vessels with fiber-optic devices. Hence, cardiothoracic surgeons require extensive technical backup and wide expertise. After quick, careful assessment of all information obtained, surgery is carried out. Thoracic surgeons are noted for great surgical dexterity, scientific expertise, and logical, stepwise development of a complete picture that enables them to arrive rapidly at sensible decisions before and during surgery.

Entering the chest cavity, thoracotomy, is required for all thoracic surgery. Patients are given a general anesthetic and concurrently have heart and lung function replaced by a heart-lung machine, which oxygenates the blood and pumps it through the cardiovascular system.

Anterior thoracotomy is used to gain access to the heart and its coronary arteries. First, a vertical incision is made from between the collarbone to the lower end of the sternum, to which the ribs are attached. The sternum is divided with a bone saw and pried apart to expose the surgical area. After surgery, a drain is inserted into the chest, the sternum is wired together, and the muscle and skin are closed.

Lateral thoracotomy uses curved incisions made from between the shoulder blades and around the side of the trunk to just below a nipple. It provides access to the lungs and the great blood vessels. This technique is used by thoracic surgeons, general surgeons, and other specialists who perform lung surgery. After the incision is complete, the ribs are spread apart and surgery is performed. Closure is as with the anterior procedure.

Many different thoracic surgery procedures are carried out on heart and great blood vessels when medical and dietary treatments fail or in cases of congenital and traumatic problems. They can be divided into valve replacement, artery surgery, and heart transplantation. Once, bypass surgery was a major aspect of cardiothoracic surgery. Today, it has been largely replaced by balloon catheterization and related techniques carried out by other specialists.

Three types of important cardiothoracic surgery are heart valve replacement, aneurysm resection, and heart transplantation. Heart valve replacement may be necessitated by severe mitral valve damage, which causes mitral insufficiency or stenosis that can lead to heart failure and death. Aneurysms are weakened portions of the heart or great blood vessels. Heart aneurysms are caused by myocardial infarction (the death of parts of the heart muscle), yielding areas of weak, noncontractile scar tissue. Vessel aneurysms are caused by atherosclerosis or infectious disease. In extreme cases, aneurysms can rupture, and they are always painful and/or life-threatening. They are repaired by resection and replacement with graft materials such as Dacron or Teflon appliances. In the most severe cardiac problems, whole heart transplantation is needed using cadaver hearts. When this is not possible but the heart must be aided, ventricular assist pumps and artificial hearts can be connected temporarily.

Perspective and Prospects

Thoracic surgery was first successful in the United States in the early twentieth century. Development of the New York Thoracic Surgical Society in 1917 began its acceptance as a medical specialty. In the 1930s, the *Journal of Thoracic Surgery* started to describe the area, and treatment methods evolved rapidly. Much impetus came from thoracic injuries that occurred during World War II. By the late 1940s, a Board of Thoracic Surgery was affiliated with the American Board of Surgery. In 1971, it became the independent American Board of Thoracic Surgery, which certifies thoracic surgeons. There are several thousand board-certified thoracic surgeons.

Some firsts in this field were the relief of mitral stenosis, by Elliott Cutler (1923); surgical intervention for cardiac aneurysm, by Ernst Sauerbruch (1931); the successful ligation of an arterial duct, by Robert Gross (1939); the development of a heart-lung machine for humans, by John Gibbon (1954); and the relief of congenital pulmonary defects, by Alfred Blalock (1954).

In current thoracic surgery, the treatment of coronary artery disease, once restricted to surgical bypass, has largely been replaced by techniques performed by cardiologists. Nevertheless, thoracic surgical procedures continue to improve, and the development of ever-better diagnostic tools and appliances is expected, such as a satisfactory artificial heart.

—*Sanford S. Singer, Ph.D.*

See also Aneurysmectomy; Aneurysms; Bypass surgery; Cardiac surgery; Cardiology; Cardiology, pediatric; Chest; Congenital heart disease; Heart; Heart disease; Heart transplantation; Heart valve replacement; Lung surgery; Lungs; Mitral valve prolapse; Pulmonary medicine; Pulmonary medicine, pediatric.

For Further Information:
Beers, Mark H., et al., eds. *The Merck Manual of Diagnosis and Therapy.* 18th ed. Whitehouse Station, NJ: Merck Research Laboratories, 2006.
Crawford, Michael, ed. *Current Diagnosis and Treatment—Cardiology.* 3d ed. New York: McGraw-Hill Medical, 2009.
Doherty, Gerard M., and Lawrence W. Way, eds. *Current Surgical Diagnosis and Treatment.* 12th ed. New York: Lange Medical Books/McGraw-Hill, 2006.
Eagle, Kim A., and Ragavendra R. Baliga, eds. *Practical Cardiology: Evaluation and Treatment of Common Cardiovascular Disorders.* 2d ed. Philadelphia: Lippincott Williams & Wilkins, 2008.
Gersh, Bernard J., ed. *The Mayo Clinic Heart Book.* 2d ed. New York: William Morrow, 2000.
"Heart Surgery Overview." *Texas Heart Institute,* August 2012.
"Lung Surgery." *MedlinePlus,* June 4, 2012.
Pearson, F. Griffith, et al., eds. *Thoracic Surgery.* 2d ed. New York: Churchill Livingstone, 2002.
Taylor, Anita D. *How to Choose a Medical Specialty.* 4th ed. New York: Elsevier, 1999.
"What Is a Heart Transplant?" *National Heart, Lung, and Blood Institute,* January 3, 2012.

THROAT. *See* ESOPHAGUS; PHARYNX.

THROAT, SORE. *See* SORE THROAT.

THROMBOCYTOPENIA
Disease/Disorder
Anatomy or system affected: Blood, circulatory system, liver, spleen
Specialties and related fields: Hematology
Definition: A bleeding disorder in which the blood contains an abnormally low count of functional platelets (thrombocytes).
Key terms:
corticosteroids: a family of adrenal cortex steroids used medically as anti-inflammatory agents
hemorrhage: profuse blood loss from the vessels
megakaryocytes: cells that produce platelets in the bone marrow
petechiae: a skin rash of pinpoint purplish-red spots
platelets: small, disk-shaped cells that circulate in the blood and whose function is to take part in the clotting process; platelets store many molecules inside and on their surface that cause them to stick to one another and to the walls of injured blood vessels

Information on Thrombocytopenia

Causes: Platelet deficiency or increased clearance from blood; may result from autoimmune response, genetic defect, infection, diseases such as leukemia, lymphoma, disseminated intravascular coagulation
Symptoms: Petechiae; rashes; frequent bruising; bleeding from wounds or body cavities; spontaneous bleeding; spleen and liver enlargement; blood in stool, urine, vomit, or sputum; anemia, fatigue; elevated heart rate
Duration: Chronic
Treatments: Depends on cause; may include red blood cell or platelet transfusion, platelet growth factor

Causes and Symptoms

Thrombocytopenia occurs when platelets are lost from the circulation faster than they can be replaced by the bone marrow where they are produced. It may result from either a deficiency in platelet production or an increased clearance rate from the blood. Clinically, thrombocytopenia is defined as a platelet count less than the normal levels of 150,000 to 350,000 per microliter of blood.

There are several specific causes of thrombocytopenia. In artefactual thrombocytopenia, antibodies in a person's blood cause platelets to stick together and cause a falsely low platelet count. In congenital thrombocytopenia, one of several rare genetic diseases causes low platelet counts. Another cause of thrombocytopenia is impaired platelet production, such as in leukemia or lymphoma, where the number of some other cell type in the bone marrow is increased, leaving fewer megakaryocytes for platelet production. Alternatively, the rate of platelet destruction can be increased as in disseminated intravascular coagulation (DIC), in which the blood clotting process is inappropriately activated. Antibodies in the blood, produced because of infections such as human immunodeficiency virus (HIV) or rheumatoid arthritis, can cause platelet removal. Idiopathic or immunologic thrombocytopenic purpura (ITP) causes thrombocytopenia through destruction of platelets by the patient's immune system. Thrombocytopenia can also be attributable to an abnormal distribution of platelets, as when platelets are sequestered in a patient's enlarged spleen. Thrombotic thrombocytopenic purpura (TTP) is a disease resulting in thrombocytopenia. Platelets clump together in areas of clots to the extent that there are fewer platelets in other parts of the body. Finally, a massive transfusion of red blood cells can dilute platelets to thrombocytopenic levels.

Thrombocytopenia can cause excess bleeding and thus has several notable symptoms. Petechiae, rashes, and frequent bruising can appear on the skin, provoked by minor injury or pressure. Bleeding from wounds or body cavities may occur. At extremely low platelet counts, those below 20,000 per microliter, spontaneous bleeding occurs. The spleen and liver may be enlarged and sensitive to the touch if the thrombocytopenia is caused by splenic activity. Impaired clotting may cause blood to appear in the stool, urine, vomit, or sputum. Thrombocytopenic patients may also experience anemia, feel fatigued, or exhibit an elevated heart rate.

Low platelet counts increase the risk of bleeding, which becomes particularly dangerous when the count falls below 10,000 per microliter. Bleeding from the nose and gums is quite common. Serious hemorrhage can occur at the retina in the back of the eye, threatening vision. The most critical bleeding complication posing a risk to life is spontaneous bleeding in the head or in the lining of the gut.

Treatment and Therapy

The primary treatment for thrombocytopenia is to address the underlying cause of the deficiency. This is not always possible. If significant blood loss has occurred, then red blood cell or platelet transfusion may be necessary. However, in the condition of thrombotic thrombocytopenia purpura, the use of platelet concentrates is quite hazardous. Platelet growth factor can be used to stimulate increased platelet production in the bone marrow. Additionally, certain drugs such as aspirin and ibuprofen are to be avoided since they are known to cause antiplatelet activity.

If an infection is suspected as the cause of thrombocytopenia, then treatment such as antibiotics for the specific infection is often initiated. Some viral infections such as glandular fever caused by Epstein-Barr virus have no specific treatment, and only close monitoring is applied. If the thrombocytopenia is caused by the presence of cancer cells in the bone marrow, then treatment such as chemotherapy or radiotherapy is directed at the abnormal cells. In such cases, the bone marrow may become damaged and blood platelet counts further lowered. Platelet transfusions are then given to prevent bleeding, until either the platelet count reaches acceptable levels or the bone marrow recovers its ability to produce sufficient numbers of platelets.

Perspective and Prospects

Prior to the development of plasma exchange as an effective treatment in the 1970s, the mortality from thrombotic thrombocytopenic purpura–hemolytic uremic syndrome (TTP-HUS) was 90 percent. During those times, diagnosis was made using five clinical observations, including thrombocytopenia and fever. The availability of effective plasma exchange treatment has lowered the mortality rate to 20 percent. Early diagnosis is important, with thrombocytopenia and one other criterion the only requirements for initiation of treatment since 1991.

At the start of the twenty-first century, the treatment of children with idiopathic or immunologic thrombocytopenic purpura remained controversial. Platelet counts can be increased by treatment with corticosteroids, but clinical outcomes may not improve. Because most children spontaneously recover from severe thrombocytopenia in several days to weeks, only supportive care is sometimes recommended in this case.

—*Michael R. King, Ph.D.*

See also Bleeding; Blood and blood disorders; Bone marrow transplantation; Hematology; Hematology, pediatric; Plasma; Transfusion; Wiskott-Aldrich syndrome.

For Further Information:

Cattaneo, M. "Inherited Platelet-Based Bleeding Disorders." *Journal of Thrombosis and Haemostasis* 1, no. 7 (July, 2003): 1628–1636.

Chong, B. H. "Heparin-Induced Thrombocytopenia." *Journal of Thrombosis and Haemostasis* 1, no. 7 (July, 2003): 1471–1478.

Dugdale, David C. "Thrombocytopenia." *MedlinePlus*, March 14, 2012.

George, J. N. "Platelets." *The Lancet* 355, no. 9214 (April 29, 2000): 1531–1539.

Goldstein, K. H., et al. "Efficient Diagnosis of Thrombocytopenia." *American Family Physician* 53, no. 3 (February 15, 1996): 915–920.

McCrae, Keith R., ed. *Thrombocytopenia.* New York: Taylor & Francis, 2006.

MedlinePlus. "Platelet Disorders." *MedlinePlus*, May 22, 2013.

National Heart, Lung, and Blood Institute. "What Is Thrombocytopenia?" *NIH: National Heart, Lung, and Blood Institute*, September 25, 2012.

Reid, T. J., et al. "Platelet Substitutes in the Management of Thrombocytopenia." *Current Hematology Reports* 2, no. 2 (March, 2003): 165–170.

Warkentin, Theodore E., and Andreas Greinacher, eds. *Heparin-Induced Thrombocytopenia.* 4th rev. ed. New York: Marcel Dekker, 2007.

THROMBOLYTIC THERAPY AND TPA

Treatment

Anatomy or system affected: Blood, blood vessels, circulatory system, heart, lungs, nervous system, respiratory system

Specialties and related fields: Cardiology, critical care, emergency medicine, hematology, pharmacology, pulmonary medicine, vascular medicine

Definition: The use of drugs to dissolve blood clots blocking an artery or vein (often in the heart, lungs, or brain); TPA is one of the best thrombolytic agents and is frequently administered to patients experiencing heart attacks.

Key terms:

embolism: the blockage of an artery by matter (such as a blood clot) that has broken off from another area

fibrinolysis: the breakdown of fibrin, a major component of blood clots, that occurs after the broken vessel wall has healed; fibrinolytic agents are used to dissolve unwanted clots

hemostasis: a physiological response that arrests bleeding; involves the constriction of the injured blood vessel, the clumping of platelets to form a plug, and the activation of blood-clotting elements such as fibrin

occlusion: the blockage of any vessel in the body, which may be caused by a thrombus or other embolus

plasmin: an enzyme present in the blood that can dissolve clots; plasmin is normally found in its inactive form, plasminogen, until needed

platelets: specialized blood-clotting particles that travel in the blood and become sticky when they come in contact with a damaged blood vessel

thromboembolism: the blockage of a blood vessel by a fragment that has broken off from a thrombus in another blood vessel

thrombolytic drugs: a group of drugs that dissolve blood clots by increasing the level of plasmin in the blood

thrombus: a blood clot that has formed inside an intact blood vessel; a thrombus can be life-threatening if it occludes a vessel that supplies the heart or brain

tissue plasminogen activator (TPA or tPA): a substance produced by the body to prevent abnormal blood clots by stimulating the formation of plasmin from plasminogen; can also be administered to dissolve blood clots

Physiology of Blood Clot Formation

In an undamaged, healthy blood vessel, blood flows smoothly past the lining of the vessel wall. If a blood vessel wall breaks or there is damage to its lining, however, a complex series of biochemical reactions occurs to stop the flow of blood. The blood vessel spasms (vascular spasm), platelets in the bloodstream clump together to form a plug, and proteins form to cause the blood to clot (coagulate). This process is rapid, localized to the area of injury, and carefully controlled. It involves many clotting factors normally present in blood, as well as specialized clotting particles called platelets and some substances that are released by the injured tissues.

The most immediate response to a blood vessel injury is vasoconstriction, a narrowing of a blood vessel. Vasoconstriction decreases the diameter of a vessel, resulting in a decreased flow of blood at the site of damage. Some factors that cause vascular spasm include direct injury, chemicals released by the cells that line a vessel wall, platelets, and nervous reflexes. When the cells that line the interior wall of a blood vessel are damaged, platelets are attracted to the site.

They then swell and become sticky. The platelets adhere to the damaged area and release chemicals called prostaglandins, which attract more platelets to the area. Aspirin, in relatively low doses, is an effective inhibitor of prostaglandin synthesis and therefore an excellent therapy for some individuals who are susceptible to inappropriate blood clotting. The vascular spasm and platelet plug help to stop the bleeding at the injury site. Blood-clotting proteins must be activated, however, in order to seal the damaged area of the blood vessel completely.

Once the platelet plug is formed, coagulation is triggered. Several clotting proteins are produced by the liver and released in their inactive form to the blood. Bacteria within the intestinal tract are responsible for synthesizing vitamin K, which is essential for normal production of the clotting proteins by the liver. Vitamin K is absorbed by intestinal blood vessels and transported to the liver.

The mechanism by which clotting proteins are activated is called a cascade. First, a substance called prothrombin activator is formed. Prothrombin activator converts a protein in the plasma called prothrombin into thrombin, which in turn converts another plasma protein, fibrinogen, into fibrin. Fibrin molecules then combine to form a loose meshwork that fills in the gaps between the cells of the platelet plug, preventing blood loss at the site of injury.

A clot is not meant to be a permanent solution. If the clot completely occludes, or stops the flow of blood to, a tissue, the tissue may die. A process called fibrinolysis removes clots that are no longer needed. Because small clots are continually formed in vessels throughout the body, clot dissolution is essential to reestablishing normal blood flow. Without fibrinolysis, blood vessels would gradually become completely occluded.

One essential component of this natural clot-reducing process is the enzyme plasmin, which is produced when the blood protein plasminogen is activated. A large amount of plasminogen, which binds to fibrin, is incorporated into a blood clot. The plasminogen remains inactive until it receives appropriate signals. Healing of the blood vessel and surrounding tissues will cause the release of a substance called tissue plasminogen activator (TPA or tPA). TPA then converts the plasminogen in the clot to plasmin. It is plasmin that breaks down the fibrin, and thus the clot, through fibrinolysis. Enzymes will quickly destroy any plasmin that escapes into the general circulation. Therefore, most of the fibrinolytic effect of plasmin occurs within the clot itself.

It is important to note that once a clot begins to form, something must limit its growth. A clot that is allowed to grow uncontrollably would eventually fill up all the vessels in the body. Several factors regulate the extent of clot formation. Any tendency toward clot formation in rapidly moving blood is usually unsuccessful because the activated coagulation factors are diluted and washed away, preventing them from accumulating to a concentration necessary for clotting. The second mechanism restricting clot formation is that as a clot forms, almost all the thrombin produced is absorbed into the fibrin. Therefore, fibrin effectively acts as an anticoagulant to prevent enlargement of the clot by holding onto thrombin so that it cannot act elsewhere. Any thrombin that escapes is bound by a substance in the blood called antithrombin III. Antithrombin III can be activated by a substance called heparin, a natural anticoagulant produced by some white blood cells and other undamaged cells that line blood vessels. Heparin acts to inhibit thrombin activity, and thus clotting, by stimulating antithrombin III.

Additional factors prevent clotting in undamaged blood vessels. The factors that normally ward off unnecessary clotting include both structural and chemical characteristics of the lining of blood vessels. As long as the cells lining the vessels remain undamaged, there is no vasospasm, no platelet plug forms, and no clot results. The cells on the wall lining can repel platelets using specialized chemicals on their surfaces. They also secrete heparin and a substance known as prostacyclin, both of which prevent platelet activation.

Despite the body's protective mechanisms to prevent inappropriate blood clots, clotting sometimes does occur. A clot that forms in an undamaged vessel is called a thrombus. If the thrombus is large, it may block blood flow to the tissue beyond the occlusion and starve the tissue to death. This starvation process is called ischemia, and the result is infarction, or cell death. A relatively common site for a thrombus to occlude a vessel is in the heart. If the blockage occurs in a coronary artery, a vessel that supplies the heart with blood, the consequences may be death of this tissue and even death of the affected individual.

A thrombus (or any other type of matter, such as lipids) that breaks away from a vessel and floats freely in the bloodstream is called an embolus. An embolus becomes a problem if it enters a blood vessel that is too narrow for it to pass through. For example, emboli that become trapped in a blood vessel going to the lungs can significantly alter an individual's ability to obtain oxygen. An embolus that occludes a vessel feeding the brain will cause a stroke.

What would cause a clot to form in the body when there is no trauma to a vessel? Several factors are known to cause clot formation even when there is no bleeding. Anything that causes the lining of a blood vessel to become roughened or irregular will allow platelets to gain a foothold and cling to the vessel wall, starting the clotting process.

Arteriosclerosis, in which there is an abnormal accumulation of fatty plaques in the wall of an artery, and blood vessel inflammation are the most common causes of irregularities in the lining of blood vessels. Anything that causes the flow of blood to slow and pool enhances clot formation. In this case, clotting factors are not washed away and diluted, so they tend to accumulate until their concentrations are high enough to initiate clotting. Conditions in which this may occur include atrial fibrillation, aneurysms, and varicose veins. Atrial fibrillation is the abnormally rapid beating of the upper chambers (atria) of the heart. Because the contractions that normally force blood into the lower chambers (ventricles) are inefficient, blood pools and clots may form. Aneurysms occur when there is a weakening of an artery wall. This causes the blood vessel wall to bulge out and form a pocket where blood can pool. Thus, aneurysms provide a potential site for inappropriate clotting. Varicose veins are relatively common and usually occur in the veins returning blood from the legs. When the valves in a vein weaken, the flow of returning blood slows and the vein swells. As a result, clotting factors may accumulate in the vein and be returned to the heart or forced into the lungs.

Indications and Procedures

If inappropriate clotting occurs in blood vessels supplying critical tissues, such as the brain, heart, lungs, or kidneys, the resulting tissue damage can be debilitating or even life-threatening. Fortunately, physicians have a few options in treating patients with clotting problems.

A blood clot in the arteries supplying oxygen and nutrients to the heart can cause numerous symptoms. Sudden pain, pressure, squeezing, and fullness in the chest that last longer than fifteen minutes may indicate a heart attack. The pain may be excruciating; it may also be mild, resembling heartburn or indigestion. In general, the elderly tend to have less pain during a heart attack. Heart attack pain does not go away with rest and may radiate across the chest to the shoulders (usually on the left side), neck, arms, jaw, or even the middle of the back. Because the pumping mechanism and efficiency of the heart have been impaired, patients often feel dizzy or light-headed. They may even faint, become nauseated or vomit, have difficulty breathing, or begin to sweat.

A number of drugs are used to prevent undesirable clotting in persons at risk for a heart attack. Aspirin is a common drug whose action blocks the production of chemicals called prostaglandins, which cause platelets to adhere to one another. Heparin helps to prevent clot formation. Warfarin is a drug that interferes with the action of vitamin K in the formation of clotting proteins. If a clot has already formed, some drugs are available that will dissolve clots, including TPA, streptokinase, and urokinase. These drugs are known as thrombolytic agents and are often administered in an emergency room to people experiencing heart attacks.

In 2003, researchers announced a breakthrough in the treatment of persons prone to blood clots. Since the 1950s, warfarin has been given to patients for a period of three to six months. Studies showed an increased risk of severe bleeding with longer use of warfarin, thus preempting its use after six months. However, without warfarin, nearly one-third of patients will form another blood clot within eight years. The 2003 findings showed that after several months of full doses of warfarin, moderate doses of the medicine can follow and can reduce the risk of further clots without introducing the risk of hemorrhage.

The time period for which thrombolytic agents are effective is relatively brief; the sooner these drugs are given, the greater is the benefit. To be effective, these potent drugs must be given before irreversible damage occurs. For heart attack victims, this means within six hours after the onset of symptoms. Most studies indicate that thrombolytic therapy can be given safely and effectively before heart attack victims reach the emergency room and that early treatment reduces the like-

lihood of death. Therefore, it is important for individuals to contact a physician or emergency medical team promptly after experiencing suspicious symptoms that may indicate a heart attack.

Uses and Complications

Most patients who are thought to be experiencing a heart attack are given TPA or streptokinase intravenously to reverse or at least halt damage. Like all drugs, however, the thrombolytic agents have potentially adverse effects. Because these medications can increase bleeding, patients are not given thrombolytic therapy if they are at high risk for hemorrhage (abnormal bleeding). Some of the factors that may increase the risk of bleeding include surgery within the past six weeks, severe hypertension, diabetic eye disease, recent head trauma, recent stroke, stomach or duodenal ulcers, or recent cardiopulmonary resuscitation.

If the thrombolytic drug is administered and bleeding becomes a significant problem, a drug called aminocaproic acid can be used to help correct the problem. Aminocaproic acid inhibits the thrombolytic effects of TPA, streptokinase, and urokinase by preventing their action and inhibiting plasmin. In life-threatening situations, the physician may have to give the patient blood transfusions or fibrinogen infusions to reverse the effects of thrombolysis. The adverse effects of thrombolytic agents are relatively rare, however, and should not discourage physicians from the appropriate use of these agents.

Thrombolytic therapy is used in nearly 300,000 patients in the United States each year. Tissue plasminogen activator is the fastest-acting thrombolytic agent. It is produced naturally in the body but can be manufactured in large amounts using genetic engineering techniques. Streptokinase, on the other hand, is produced by bacteria and at about one-tenth the cost of TPA. When these two thrombolytic agents were compared in 41,000 heart attack patients, TPA showed a slightly better effectiveness. In a one-month follow-up study, researchers found that there were 14 percent fewer deaths among heart attack patients given TPA and intravenous heparin (to help keep blood clots from re-forming) than among heart attack patients treated with streptokinase and heparin.

In addition to their use as therapeutic agents for heart attacks, thrombolytic drugs are also used to treat abnormal blood clots in the blood vessels of the lungs. These clots, known as pulmonary emboli, usually originate in a leg vein, a condition called venous thrombosis. Part or all of the thrombus breaks away, forms an embolus, and travels to the heart, which then pumps it into the pulmonary arteries. If the embolus is large enough to block the main pulmonary artery leading from the heart to the lungs, or if there are many clots, the condition can be life-threatening. Pulmonary embolism is responsible for more than 50,000 deaths in the United States each year.

The symptoms that a patient may experience depend on the size of the obstructing clot. If an embolus is so large that it blocks the main pulmonary artery, an affected individual will die. Smaller emboli may cause severe shortness of breath, rapid heart rate, dizziness, sharp chest pains when breathing, and coughing up of blood.

Physicians treat pulmonary emboli with similar medical therapy as that used for heart attacks. Anticoagulant drugs such as heparin and warfarin are usually administered to reduce the clotting ability of the blood and to reduce the chance of more clots occurring. Thrombolytic agents, including urokinase and streptokinase, can also be used to destroy the clot in much the same way that they are used in heart attack victims.

The third major use of thrombolytic agents is to clear intravenous catheters of blood clots. A catheter may be placed into a person's vein if health care workers need to draw frequent blood samples or administer drugs at frequent intervals. Because the catheter is in direct contact with the blood, it is a site for potential clot formation. Urokinase can be used to reopen an occluded catheter.

Perspective and Prospects

Each year 1.2 million Americans experience a heart attack. An attack lasts longer than most people realize. It is actually a four to six-hour process that starts when one of the arteries supplying the heart muscle becomes blocked, usually by a blood clot. The pain that one experiences is partially attributable to a cramping of the heart muscle from lack of oxygen and an accumulation of waste products. As a result, heart muscle is destroyed, which interferes with the heart's function. If the amount of muscle destruction is severe, it can lead to the patient's death.

Studies show that individuals treated within one to two hours of the onset of heart attack symptoms have significantly less heart damage than those treated later. Yet, half of all heart attack patients wait more than two hours before getting medical attention. The American Heart Association estimates that 300,000 Americans die of heart attacks each year before reaching a hospital. This number could be greatly reduced if people responded more quickly to the symptoms of a heart attack.

Recent studies have shown that women are even less likely to receive initial medical care within the required four to six-hour time interval. Women frequently see to other responsibilities such as child or elder care before seeking medical help. Many women believe the myth that they are not likely to have a heart attack. This is true before the menopause, but, within five years of the menopause, women have the same risk of heart attacks as men. In addition, physicians are more likely to misdiagnose heart attack symptoms in women, attributing them to anxiety or stress.

The goal in treating a heart attack is to stop it and, if possible, reverse the clotting process. Treatment with thrombolytic agents helps to minimize or even reverse the damage to heart tissue. As with most diseases, however, it is better to prevent heart attacks entirely. Individuals who exercise regularly, who eat a diet relatively low in fat, and who do not smoke have a low incidence of heart attacks and may never need drug therapy to unclog their arteries. Yet, it is comforting to know that these agents are available if the need ever arises.

Because of the success of thrombolytic agents in the treatment of coronary artery disease, these agents are also being tried in patients showing early symptoms of stroke. Strokes and heart attacks occur for similar reasons. In a stroke, blood clots in the arteries that supply the brain prevent the delivery of oxygen and nutrients to the sensitive nerve cells and cause an accumulation of waste products. As a result, these sensitive brain cells die. As in heart attack treatment, timing is critical. In heart attack patients, agents that dissolve clots work best when given within six hours after the onset of symptoms. For stroke patients, it appears that treatment with a thrombolytic drug must begin within three hours to have maximal effectiveness. Therefore, awareness of the early symptoms of stroke is even more important. These symptoms develop rapidly and depend on the region of the brain that is damaged. Some common symptoms include muscle weakness, loss of touch sensations, speech disturbances, and visual disturbances.

If thrombolytic agents are found to be effective in treating strokes, up to 80 percent of all stroke victims may be helped. As with heart attack patients, these drugs cannot be used in stroke patients with hemorrhagic (bleeding) strokes or other disorders in which the risk of bleeding is greater than the potential benefits from such therapy.

—Matthew Berria, Ph.D.;
L. Fleming Fallon, Jr., M.D., Ph.D., M.P.H.;
updated by Bradley R. A. Wilson, Ph.D.

See also Angiography; Angioplasty; Arteriosclerosis; Bleeding; Blood and blood disorders; Blood vessels; Brain; Bypass surgery; Cardiac arrest; Cardiology; Catheterization; Circulation; Echocardiography; Embolism; Emergency medicine; Endarterectomy; Enzymes; Heart; Heart attack; Heart disease; Heart valve replacement; Hematology; Ischemia; Lungs; Pharmacology; Pulmonary medicine; Strokes; Thrombosis and thrombus; Transient ischemic attacks (TIAs); Varicosis; Vascular medicine; Vascular system.

For Further Information:
American College of Chest Physicians. *A Patient's Guide to Antithrombotic and Thrombolytic Therapy.* [N. p.]: Author, 2012.
American Medical Association. *American Medical Association Family Medical Guide.* 4th rev. ed. Hoboken, N.J.: John Wiley & Sons, 2004.
Bick, Roger L. *Disorders of Thrombosis and Hemostasis: Clinical and Laboratory Practice.* 3d ed. Philadelphia: Lippincott Williams & Wilkins, 2002.
Hales, Dianne. *An Invitation to Health Brief.* Updated ed. Belmont, Calif.: Wadsworth/Cengage Learning, 2010.
Katzung, Bertram G., et al., eds. *Basic and Clinical Pharmacology.* 12th ed. New York: McGraw-Hill Medical, 2012.
Loscalzo, Joseph, and Andrew I. Schafer, eds. *Thrombosis and Hemorrhage.* 3d ed. Philadelphia: Lippincott Williams & Wilkins, 2003.
McCance, Kathryn L., and Sue M. Huether. *Pathophysiology: The Biologic Basis for Disease in Adults and Children.* 6th ed. St. Louis, Mo.: Mosby/Elsevier, 2010.
Mikati, Issam. "Thrombolytic Therapy." *MedlinePlus,* June 1, 2010.

Thrombosis and thrombus
Disease/Disorder

Anatomy or system affected: Blood, blood vessels, brain, circulatory system, head, heart, lungs, respiratory system

Specialties and related fields: Cardiology, hematology, internal medicine, vascular medicine

Definition: Thrombosis is an abnormal blood condition in which blood cells called thrombocytes (platelets) produce clots that move through the bloodstream and eventually clog blood vessels; a thrombus is such a clot.

Key terms:

artery: a blood vessel that transports blood away from the heart to the cells and tissues of the body

clot: a clumping of platelets, blood, fibrin, and clotting factors that normally accumulates in damaged tissue as part of the body's healing process

embolus: an object, air bubble, or other material moving through the bloodstream that is capable of creating a blockage to circulation

fibrin: a critical protein produced by platelets during the clotting process in bleeding, damaged tissue; the fibrin seals openings in damaged blood vessels

myocardial infarction: a condition in which the blood and oxygen supply to the cells of the heart muscle is cut off, thereby causing heart cell death; commonly called a heart attack

shock: a situation in which the body or a region of the body is not receiving an adequate supply of blood and oxygen, thereby leading to collapse of the organism

thrombocytes: white blood cells that secrete the proteins thrombin and fibrin in response to chemical signals from damaged tissue in the body; also called platelets

thrombus: an abnormal clumping of platelets and platelet proteins that moves through the bloodstream and may act as an embolus to block circulation through key arteries

vein: a blood vessel which returns blood to the heart from various regions of the body

Causes and Symptoms

Clotting is a critical process in the maintenance of damaged bodily tissue and the prevention of blood loss leading to conditions of shock within the organism. Shock involves the disorientation and collapse of major organ systems within the body when excessive blood has been lost; it can be fatal if it is not treated immediately.

When the body is damaged from a cut or other breach of the body's epithelial and connective tissue defense layers in the skin, chemical signals called chemoattractants stimulate a white blood cell type called a thrombocyte to secrete proteins, leading to the sealing of the damaged tissue region. Thrombocytes, also called platelets, are versatile cells floating in the approximately 10 to 12 liters of blood flowing through roughly 100,000 kilometers of blood vessels within the average human body. There are roughly 500,000 thrombocytes per cubic millimeter of blood. Their clotting response to tissue damage is rapid and efficient, although

---

Information on Thrombosis and Thrombus

Causes: Heart attacks, strokes, blood-clotting abnormalities, compromised immune system, bone marrow abnormalities, phlebitis (from surgery or prolonged confinement)

Symptoms: Sudden pain or tenderness along course of vein, skin discoloration, swelling and edema below obstruction, rapid pulse, mild fever

Duration: Acute

Treatments: Anticoagulants, compression stockings

---

very intricate in the chemical signaling between cells.

Once activated by alarmones, emergency chemical-signaling hormones released from the damaged tissue, the thrombocytes are activated to respond at the site of tissue damage. Each thrombocyte releases the proteins thrombin and fibrinogen. The thrombin modifies the fibrinogen to produce fibrin, the principal sealant protein for the damaged region. The fibrin is secreted massively from thousands of thrombocytes within only a few minutes of the initial tissue damage. Fibrin protein is put down by the cells in intricately connected layers from the outer edges of the tissue damage progressively inward, eventually forming a plug.

Following the sealing of the damaged tissue by the clotting thrombocytes, other white blood cells of the immune system, called leukocytes, move into the region to immobilize and destroy contaminating bacteria and viruses, as well as to break down damaged cells. Surrounding healthy cells initiate mitotic cell divisions to grow into the damaged region, thereby regenerating the missing tissue. White blood cells such as leukocytes and thrombocytes are termed "white" because they do not produce hemoglobin and hence are not "red." The two white blood cell types work intricately in the maintenance of body tissue primary defense layers.

When the clotting process of thrombocytes and other related cells does not occur properly, problems can arise. Normally, a clot will form at a breach in a blood vessel, whether that vessel is an artery carrying blood away from the heart to the body or a vein returning blood to the heart from the body. Abnormal clotting of thrombocytes and fibrin proteins, however, can form masses that break off from a blood clot and float through the bloodstream. Such a floating blood clot is called a thrombus.

A thrombus is a type of embolism, an object that floats through the bloodstream and can cause a blockage in small arteries, veins, and capillaries. Emboli can be pockets of air or solid clots such as thrombi. Both air emboli and thrombus emboli can cause serious blockages of important vessels supplying blood to particular body regions. As a thrombus or other embolus flows along with blood, it will eventually float through a vessel that becomes progressively smaller in diameter. The thrombus blocks the vessel so that nothing can pass any farther through it—not the thrombus, not blood, and not the oxygen and nutrients within the blood.

As a result, cells downstream from the blockage will be starved for essential oxygen, sugar, and other nutrients necessary for carrying out the cellular chemical reactions of life. Most cells have only about a ten-minute supply of chemical and oxygen reserves needed for life. These cells depend on a continuous supply of blood to provide oxygen, sugar, and other nutrients and to carry away carbon dioxide and other waste products. The blood clot occludes the artery going to a cell region, thereby preventing blood flow and causing the death of these cells. In many parts of the body, these dead cells cannot be replaced, particularly within the heart, brain, and spinal cord.

The existence of thrombi within the circulatory system is a serious medical condition known as thrombosis. The five principal types of thrombi are agonal, ball, hyaline, laminated, and white thrombi. An agonal thrombus is a type of blood clot that forms from clumping blood cells when a person is dying. A ball thrombus is a spherically shaped blood clot composed of platelets, red blood cells, and fibrin. A hyaline thrombus is a mass of depigmented, hemoglobinless, clumped red blood cells. A laminated thrombus is an array of clumped cell types accumulated at differing times, creating a snowball effect. A white thrombus is a clump of leukocytes of varying types. Regardless of type, all thrombi can seriously impede efficient blood flow and thereby contribute to localized cellular and tissue death, damage that is often irreparable.

Two of the most serious cases of localized cellular and tissue death brought about by thrombi are myocardial infarctions and strokes. A myocardial infarction, also called a heart attack, occurs when the muscular layer of cells within the heart (the myocardium) is starved for oxygen and nutrients, and dies, because of a blockage to one of the branches of the coronary arteries supplying blood to the heart. If only a small branch of the coronary artery is blocked by a thrombus or other occlusion, then only a few hundred myocardial cells will die and the heart attack will be mild.

If the thrombus blockage is to a major coronary artery, however, then many thousands of cells in the myocardium will die, and a major heart attack will occur. It should be emphasized that the death of myocardial cells is permanent; they cannot be replaced. Therefore, a thrombus-induced heart attack causes permanent death of a region of heart muscle, whether large or small. In many cases, the heart attack is so severe that the normal, rhythmic contraction of the heart is disrupted, thereby leading to cardiac arrest and death.

In the same manner, a stroke, also called a cerebrovascular accident, occurs when an artery transporting blood to a region of brain cells is blocked by a thrombus or other embolus. Brain cells downstream from the blockage are starved for oxygen and nutrients; they die within minutes. If a small artery or capillary is blocked, only a few brain cells will die and the stroke will be minimal, perhaps not even noticeable to the individual. It is possible that many people have such "microstrokes" repeatedly during the course of their lives, although the effects of these small strokes are cumulative over time. Decreased and impaired neurological and motor functioning throughout the body ensue from damaged brain regions in stroke victims.

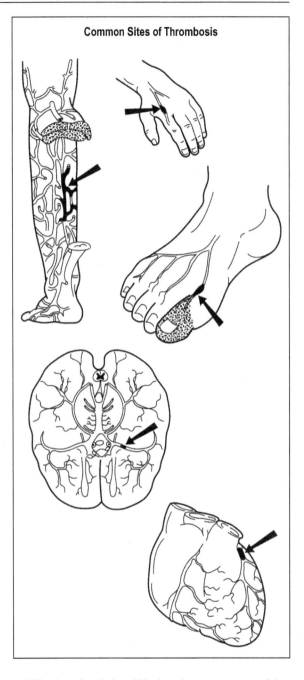

Common Sites of Thrombosis

If the thrombus-induced blockage is to an artery supplying blood to a large brain cell region, however, then millions of brain cells will die. The stroke is severe, perhaps deadly, if the affected brain region is essential for certain bodily life processes. If the severe stroke victim survives, then the effects will be noticeable as sluggish neuromuscular motor activity on the opposite side of the body from the affected brain region. Heart attacks and strokes are manifestations of the same problem: arteries occluded by thrombi and other emboli.

Treatment and Therapy

Thrombosis is a problem of major concern for the physician facing patients with certain types of medical conditions and patients who recently have had major internal surgery. Furthermore, individuals with blood-clotting abnormalities, compromised immune systems, and bone marrow abnormalities also are prone to forming thrombi and other solid emboli. Phlebitis is an inflammation of a vein brought about by surgery, prolonged confinement to bed, or prolonged sitting, in which blood clots form in deep veins, a condition called deep vein thrombosis (DVT). These blood clots can break off and flow through the general blood circulation, eventually clogging an artery or vein leading to a critical bodily region.

Consequently, thrombi and thrombosis are of major concern to medical doctors because they represent potential complications and side effects from other medical conditions and certain needed surgical treatments. People who have had abdominal or pelvic surgery (such as the removal of certain organs such as the spleen and portions of the stomach because of cancer) or individuals who have been bedridden with leg fractures are prone to forming thrombi and emboli.

The elderly are particularly prone to thrombi because of the gradual decline of the immune system and the breakdown of bone development that accompany the aging process. Moreover, the natural chemical substances in the blood that dissolve floating blood clots are not as prevalent in the elderly. As a result, more cases of thrombi are seen in elderly patients, particularly individuals above the age of seventy.

Once thrombi and other solid emboli have formed, they may float for a long time through an individual's blood vessels. They usually can pass through the heart unimpeded without causing any serious disruptions of cardiac rhythm. Occasionally, large thrombi can become lodged in one of the four valves of the heart, creating an occlusion and triggering a heart attack, but this is very rare. More commonly, the thrombi become trapped in the general circulation in progressively smaller arteries and capillaries going to a localized tissue region.

Within the body, oxygenated blood leaves the left ventricle of the heart through the largest artery in the body, the aorta, and subsequently branches and subbranches through thousands of successively smaller arteries, arterioles, and capillaries until reaching each of the quadrillion cells of the body. These cells extract oxygen and nutrients from the blood and deposit carbon dioxide and waste products into the bloodstream. Small capillaries combine to produce small venules that combine to produce small veins, which in turn combine into larger veins. These veins eventually come together into the inferior and superior vena cavae, returning blood to the right atrium of the heart for eventual delivery to the lungs. Once in the heart, blood flows from the right atrium to the right ventricle and then through the pulmonary arteries branching to the tissues of the lungs, where the blood is oxygenated through breathing. Oxygenated blood returns to the left atrium of the heart via the pulmonary veins and then flows through the left ventricle to the aorta to make another trip through the body.

Thrombi can flow through this system repeatedly. They usually become caught, however, in the progressively smaller arteries and capillaries transporting blood to the tissues. The resulting blockage and starvation of cells downstream from the blockage leads to the death and decay of the affected tissue region, resulting in a localized tissue infarction. The two most serious types of infarctions are the myocardial infarction and the stroke, but both of these infarctions can be caused by other types of blockages, including arterial rupture and fatty clogging of arteries from the conditions atherosclerosis and arteriosclerosis. Nevertheless, thrombi are a major contributory factor to the occurrences of strokes and heart attacks, two leading killers in the United States and other stressful, technological Western nations. In both strokes and heart attacks, thrombal blockages to key cellular regions lead to localized cellular death. Heart cells and brain cells cannot be regenerated. The tissue death is permanent, and the resulting physiological effects will remain with the victims for the rest of their lives if they survive the stroke or heart attack.

Another serious thrombal blockage can occur in the pulmonary arteries and arterioles transporting blood to lung tissue for oxygenation. Such blockages lead to the localized death of lung tissue and sudden shortness of breath in affected individuals. About 10 percent of cases of pulmonary thrombosis and embolism end in death, resulting in a fatality figure much smaller than the hundreds of thousands of deaths from heart attacks and strokes in the United States each year.

Scuba divers who spend excessive periods of time at great depths and then ascend rapidly are prone to decompression sickness, or "the bends," in which nitrogen bubbles form emboli that create the same blockages as thrombi in localized tissue spaces. Nitrogen bubble emboli can accumulate in the heart, lung, and brain tissue and are fatal if not immediately treated in a decompression chamber.

Perspective and Prospects

Thrombi and thrombosis are serious problems that can arise in any individual, although the likelihood increases with age and the corresponding decline in individuals" immune systems. Care must be taken with various surgical procedures, particularly abdominal and pelvic surgery and the treatment of leg fractures, to reduce the chances of thrombi forming. Any severe cut has the potential to form thrombi, but the status of an individual's immune system is an important factor in determining whether these thrombi are captured and dissipated.

In many surgical procedures, including open heart surgery, physicians and surgeons will administer anticlotting agents to minimize the risk of thrombi forming during and following the surgery and in the recovery phase of the operation. These anticlotting agents are administered intravenously and diffuse throughout the patient's circulatory system so that any thrombi and other blood clots dissolve before they can occlude various tissue regions. Medical doctors are versed in the science of thrombi and thrombosis because these conditions often are associated with other medical conditions. Physicians are aware of contributory factors to thrombosis and can take action to guard against thrombal occurrence early in the medical treatment process.

Since the 1950s, the drug warfarin has been given to patients for a period of three to six months. Studies showed an increased risk of severe bleeding with longer use of warfarin, thus preempting its use after six months. However, without warfarin, nearly one-third of patients will form another blood clot within eight years. In 2003, findings showed that after several months of full doses of warfarin, moderate doses of the medicine can follow and can reduce the risk of further clots without introducing the risk of hemorrhage. A study published in the International Journal of Cardiology in May 2013 reported that the drug Pradaxa (dabigatran) was comparably effective against stroke.

—David Wason Hollar, Jr., Ph.D.

See also Arteriosclerosis; Behçet's disease; Blood and blood disorders; Blood vessels; Cardiac arrest; Cardiology; Cholesterol; Deep vein thrombosis; Disseminated intravascular coagulation (DIC); Echocardiography; Embolism; Heart; Heart attack; Heart disease; Hyperlipidemia; Hypertension; Infarction; Ischemia; Phlebitis; Plaque, arterial; Strokes; Transient ischemic attacks (TIAs); Varicosis; Vascular medicine; Vascular system; Venous insufficiency.

For Further Information:

Bick, Roger L. *Disorders of Thrombosis and Hemostasis: Clinical and Laboratory Practice*. 3d ed. Philadelphia: Lippincott Williams & Wilkins, 2002.

Cohen, Barbara J. *Memmler's The Human Body in Health and Disease*. 11th ed. Philadelphia: Wolters Kluwer Health/Lippincott Williams & Wilkins, 2009.

Lichtman, Marshall A., et al., eds. *Williams Hematology*. 7th ed. New York: McGraw-Hill, 2006.

Marder, Victor J., and William C. Aird. Â *Hemostasis and Thrombosis: Basic Principles and Clinical Practice*. 6th ed. New York: Lippincott Williams & Wilkins, 2012. Print.

Kitchens, Craig S. Â *Consultative Hemostasis and Thrombosis* . New York: Elsevier, 2013. Print.

Limmer, Daniel, et al. *Emergency Care*. 11th ed. Upper Saddle River, N.J.: Pearson/Prentice Hall Health, 2009.

Loscalzo, Joseph, and Andrew I. Schafer, eds. *Thrombosis and Hemorrhage*. 3d ed. Philadelphia: Lippincott Williams & Wilkins, 2003.

Wistreich, George A., and Max D. Lechtman. *Microbiology*. 5th ed. New York: Macmillan, 1988.

THUMB SUCKING

Development

Anatomy or system affected: Mouth, teeth

Specialties and related fields: Dentistry, pediatrics, speech pathology

Definition: A common oral behavior among young children that may cause physical, psychological, and social problems if it is continued past a certain age.

Physical and Psychological Factors

It has been estimated that 45 percent of all two-year-olds, 36 percent of four-year-olds, 21 percent of six-year-olds, and 5 percent of eleven-year-olds suck their thumbs. As children grow older, by age five, the occurrence of thumb sucking generally begins to fade during the daytime. If children continue to suck their thumbs, it is generally limited to nighttime.

Thumb sucking seems to be reinforcing to children because of its soothing property. For example, it is often observed among children when they are tired, frustrated, hungry, or uncomfortable, such as when teething causes discomfort. Furthermore, thumb sucking tends to increase the level of independence in infants. This becomes evident when observing an infant who is occupied by this self-stimulating behavior.

Disorders and Effects

Although thumb sucking is relatively harmless among children younger than three years of age, problems can develop if the behavior persists. Negative consequences may consist of dental problems, inhibited speech development, and critical peer and parental reactions.

One of the main problems associated with thumb sucking is dental problems, especially if this behavior persists after the age of four or five. Thumb sucking can also inhibit speech development in formal and informal settings at school or day care. For example, when children are sucking their thumbs during formal group activities, they are less likely to respond to adult questions. Also, during free-play time, children who are sucking their thumbs are less likely to speak spontaneously.

In addition to causing problems for speech and physical development, thumb sucking can create social difficulties for children. According to the *Pediatrics* article "Influence of Thumb Sucking on Peer Social Acceptance in First-Grade

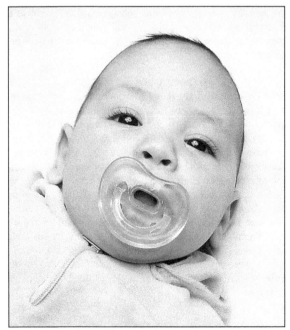

A thumb or pacifier fulfills some infants' strong need for sucking in the early months of life but can become a difficult habit to break. (PhotoDisc)

Children," by P. C. Friman and colleagues, "Social acceptance is lower among children who suck their thumb, and they are viewed by their peers as being less intelligent, happy, attractive, likable, or fun, and less desirable as a friend, playmate, seatmate, classmate, or neighbor." Furthermore, thumb sucking can create negative interactions between the parents and children. Because parents are often troubled by thumb sucking, children are routinely asked to stop. These requests can be positively reinforcing to the child and can increase the frequency of the behavior.

Given the problems associated with thumb sucking, many parents wonder at what point in time a child should be treated for this behavior. In their 1989 article "Thumb Sucking: Pediatricians" Guidelines" in *Clinical Pediatrics*, Friman and B. D. Schmitt provide some guidelines to answer this question. As a simple rule, thumb sucking should not be treated until the potential negative consequences outweigh the benefits, which is seldom before the age of four. When children do suck their thumbs, often it is not frequent enough to warrant treatment. They also point out that at times the potential benefits may outweigh the risks, such as when a child uses thumb sucking as a means of coping with fear, pain, or a significant loss. As suggested by these authors, another indication for treatment is chronic thumb sucking, which they define as occurring "across two or more settings (e.g., home and school) and when it occurs day and night."

Both positive and negative reinforcement techniques have been used to treat persistent thumb sucking. These include offering other types of stimulation or comfort (depending on whether the cause is boredom or stress), rewarding the child for not sucking his or her thumb, involving the child in breaking the habit, and applying bitter substances to the thumb as a deterrent. As with reprimands, the utility and ethics of other negative reinforcements such as bitter coatings continue to be debated.

Perspective and Prospects

Attitudes toward oral behavior in children have fluctuated over the years. It has been viewed as both indulgent and detrimental. There have been high and low attempts to prohibit the activity. Sigmund Freud and his colleagues did much to draw attention to the oral drive in the first year of life, and over the years, many writers have made observations about oral habits and psychological health.

The advent and wide use of pacifiers has done much to neutralize concern over oral behaviors. Pacifiers are generally seen as preferable to the thumb, from a dental perspective. Thumb sucking tends to arouse more anxiety for both parents and medical specialists than does the use of the pacifier; however, pacifier use beyond age four can lead to the same types of dental problems as those caused by prolonged thumb sucking.

—*Jay D. Schvaneveldt, Ph.D.*

See also Anxiety; Cognitive development; Dental diseases; Dentistry; Dentistry, pediatric; Developmental stages; Phobias; Psychiatry, child and adolescent; Reflexes, primitive; Separation anxiety; Teeth; Teething; Weaning.

For Further Information:

American Academy of Pediatrics. "Pacifiers and Thumb Sucking." *HealthyChildren.org*, May 11, 2013.
A.D.A.M. Medical Encyclopedia. "Thumbsucking." *MedlinePlus*, January 24, 2011.
Berk, Laura E. *Child Development*. 8th ed. Boston: Pearson/Allyn & Bacon, 2009.
Friman, P. C., K. M. McPherson, W. J. Warzak, and J. Evans. "Influence of Thumb Sucking on Peer Social Acceptance in First-Grade Children." *Pediatrics* 91, no. 4 (April, 1993): 784–86.
Leach, Penelope. *Your Baby and Child: From Birth to Age Five.* Rev. ed. London: Dorling Kindersley, 2010.
Nathanson, Laura Walther. *The Portable Pediatrician: A Practicing Pediatrician's Guide to Your Child's Growth, Development, Health, and Behavior from Birth to Age Five*. 2d ed. New York: HarperCollins, 2002.
"Thumb Sucking and Teeth." *Pediatrics for Parents* 19, no. 12 (2002): 1–2.
"Thumb Sucking: Help Your Child Break the Habit." *Mayo Foundation for Medical Education and Research*, September 20, 2012.
Van Norman, Rosemary. *Helping the Thumb-Sucking Child*. Garden City Park, N.Y.: Avery, 1999.
Walker, C. Eugene, and Michael C. Roberts, eds. *Handbook of Clinical Child Psychology*. 3d ed. New York: John Wiley & Sons, 2001.

THYMUS GLAND
Anatomy

Anatomy or system affected: Blood, cells, endocrine system, glands, immune system, lymphatic system
Specialties and related fields: Biochemistry, endocrinology, immunology, oncology
Definition: A gland that produces types of white blood cells for maintaining the immune system.

Structure and Functions

The thymus gland is a pinkish-gray organ that lies in front of the ascending aorta, beneath the top of the sternum. It consists of two lobes that are divided into lobules by a septum, or wall. Each thymic lobule is made of connective tissue, which consists of a densely packed outer cortex and less-dense center (medulla). The thymus is relatively large in infants and typically grows to its maximum size around the age of two. After puberty, it gradually decreases in size until it blends in with surrounding tissue.

The major cells of the thymus are morphologically indistinguishable from small, circulating lymphocytes. Lymphocytes (white blood cells) divide, differentiate, and mature in the thymic cortex to become T cells, a heterogeneous group of cells that are essential in protecting the body against infections that can be produced by invading foreign organisms. Once T cells mature, they migrate into the thymic medulla and eventually enter the bloodstream and travel to other lymphatic organs, where they bolster the immune system against disease. The thymus also produces a hormone, thymosin, which stimulates the maturation of lymphocytes in other lymphatic organs.

Disorders and Diseases

The thymus is critical in developing the immune system in

children. If it malfunctions or is surgically removed, then a child has little to no ability to fight off disease. Signs and symptoms of thymus dysfunction include shortness of breath, facial swelling, muscle weakness, blurred vision, double vision, flushing, diarrhea, and neck pain and swelling. Myasthenia gravis, a neuromuscular disease that causes fluctuating muscle weakness, has been linked to thymus dysfunction. Proper diagnosis is critical so that appropriate treatment can be administered.

Although uncommon, thymic cancer can occur. Thymomas are generally slow-growing tumors that are most often found in middle-aged people. A much rarer condition is thymic carcinoma, which develops more quickly than thymoma and is more likely to spread to other parts of the body. If a thymic tumor is found from images produced by chest X rays, computed tomography (CT) scanning, or magnetic resonance imaging (MRI), then the tumor may be surgically removed or treated with radiation.

Perspective and Prospects

The first description of the thymus gland was reported in the early sixteenth century by Italian anatomist Giacomo da Capri. The functions of the thymus were not well understood until the 1960s, when its role in the immune system was discovered. In 2007, it was reported that natural killer T (NKT) cells, a type of regulatory T cells that mature in the thymus, help regulate insulin-dependent diabetes mellitus. Research is focused on the development of NKT cell-based approaches for immunotherapeutic treatment of this disease.

—*Alvin K. Benson, Ph.D.*

See also Blood and blood disorders; Connective tissue; Diabetes mellitus; Glands; Immune system; Immunology; Immunology, pediatric; Lymphatic system; Myasthenia gravis.

For Further Information:

Anastasiadis, Kyriakos, and Chandi Ratnatunga, eds. *The Thymus Gland: Diagnosis and Surgical Management.* New York: Springer, 2007.

Dabrowski, Marek P., and Barbara Dabrowska-Bernstein. *Immunoregulatory Role of Thymus.* Boca Raton, Fla.: CRC Press, 1989.

Lavini, Corrado, et al., eds. *Thymus Gland Pathology: Clinical, Diagnostic, and Therapeutic Features.* New York: Springer, 2008.

THYROID DISORDERS
Disease/Disorder
Anatomy or system affected: Endocrine system, glands, neck
Specialties and related fields: Endocrinology
Definition: Underactivity (hypothyroidism) or overactivity (hyperthyroidism) of the thyroid gland.

Causes and Symptoms

The thyroid gland normally weighs about twenty to thirty-five grams and is located in the neck just below the larynx, or voice box. The gland is named for the shield-shaped "thyroid" cartilage that forms the front of the larynx. The thyroid has two lateral lobes that are connected by an isthmus that crosses in front of the trachea. By placing a finger on the trachea below the larynx it is possible to feel the ridge-like isthmus pass under the finger after swallowing. The bilobed (two-lobed) shape of the rest of the gland can be felt just under the skin of the neck on either side of the midline, although its boundaries are normally indistinct except to a trained examiner.

The thyroid produces two major hormones. Thyroxine, a product of the follicular cells, is the major hormone produced by the thyroid that helps regulate metabolism. Within the thyroid are also parafollicular cells that produce calcitonin, an essential hormone involved in calcium metabolism. In the tissue of the thyroid are also embedded two pairs of parathyroid glands. The parathyroid glands produce parathyroid hormone, which is required to maintain normal levels of blood calcium. In the case of thyroid surgery, it is important that the parathyroid glands are not damaged or removed; otherwise, there may be life-threatening tetanus—the sustained contraction of muscles, including those needed for breathing.

The normal functioning of the thyroid results from an elaborate physiological control system involving the hypothalamus of the brain, the anterior lobe of the pituitary gland, and the thyroid gland. The hypothalamus produces thyrotropic-releasing hormone (TRH), which is passed by special blood vessels to the anterior lobe of the pituitary, the adenohypophysis. The TRH-stimulated cells in the adenohypophysis produce thyroid-stimulating hormone (TSH), which is released into the general circulation. When it reaches the thyroid gland, it stimulates the gland to produce thyroxine. Normally, thyroxine has a negative feedback effect on its own production; that is, thyroxine can inhibit the activity of the hypothalamus and the pituitary to maintain its concentration in the blood. Various thyroid disorders, which

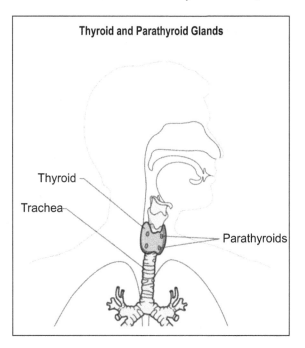

Thyroid and Parathyroid Glands

Thyroid

Trachea

Parathyroids

Information on Thyroid Disorders

Causes: Tumors, iodine deficiency, autoimmune disorders

Symptoms: In hypothyroidism, intolerance of cold, low body temperature, tendency to sleep longer, lack of energy, infrequent bowel movements, constipation, possible weight gain, puffy face and hands; in hyperthyroidism, bulging eyes, intolerance of heat, weight loss, nervousness, increased or decreased skin pigmentation, more frequent bowel movements, hair loss, rapid heart rate

Duration: Several months to chronic

Treatments: Thyroxine, antithyroid drugs (propylthiouracil, methimazole), radioactive iodine, surgery

are more common in women than in men, can develop from tumors that either increase or decrease the hormones produced in these three interdependent structures.

The normal thyroid (or euthyroid state) produces mainly thyroxine, which is converted into triiodothyronine in the tissues of the body before it has its effects, which are generally to increase the metabolic rate of the body. Some triiodothyronine is directly produced by the thyroid. The thyroxine molecule contains iodide, the negative ion of iodine; iodine is therefore an essential component of one's diet. If iodine is not available in the diet—as in the case of vegetables grown in geographical areas glaciated in the past, such as mountainous terrain and the American Midwest—then the body cannot produce thyroxine. Industrialized countries have iodine added to table salt to ensure an adequate supply of this element in the diet. A lack of iodine, and therefore a lack of thyroxine, prevents the functioning of the negative feedback effect of thyroxine on the hypothalamus and pituitary, resulting in very low thyroxine levels and high TSH levels in the blood. High levels of TSH cause substantial growth of the thyroid, which will bulge from the neck as a goiter. A person with such a condition would be hypothyroid (that is, have lower-than-normal thyroxine levels in the blood) and may be affected by cretinism (mental impairment and stunted physical growth) if this condition occurs early in childhood.

Hypothyroidism can arise in other ways as well. Hashimoto's thyroiditis is a common type of hypothyroidism that is caused by an autoimmune reaction whereby white blood cells known as lymphocytes infiltrate the thyroid and gradually destroy its tissue. The presence of antibodies against normal thyroid proteins can be detected with this condition. The usual signs of hypothyroidism are an intolerance of cold, a low body temperature, a lower rate of metabolism, a tendency to sleep longer, a general lack of energy, infrequent bowel movements, constipation, possible weight gain, a puffy face and hands, a slow heart rate, cold and scaly skin, a lack of perspiration, and possible emotional withdrawal and depression.

Graves' disease, the most common type of hyperthyroid-

ism, is an autoimmune disorder in which antibodies mimic the action of TSH and therefore stimulate the thyroid to produce excessive thyroxine. Sometimes, nodules develop in the thyroid that may produce the excessive thyroxine. Although the presence of a nodule in the thyroid may cause a person to suspect cancer, the nodules are usually benign. Hyperthyroidism may be associated with bulging eyes, but this orbitopathy does not always occur. Generally, there is an intolerance of heat, a loss of body weight, a high degree of nervousness, increased or decreased skin pigmentation, more frequent bowel movements, loss of hair, and a very rapid heart rate.

Treatment and Therapy

Patients suspected of having hypothyroidism or hyperthyroidism will have their blood tested for levels of TSH and thyroxine. Ultrasonography can be used to detect tumors and serve as an anatomical guide for potential surgery. Hypothyroidism patients are prescribed a small oral dose (less than 1 milligram per day) of thyroxine, which is adjusted until a euthyroid state is obtained within a few months. Then the patient is maintained on thyroxine, with perhaps yearly checkups by a physician. For hyperthyroidism patients, several modes of treatment are possible. Antithyroid drugs, such as propylthiouracil (PTU) or methimazole, can be given to inhibit thyroxine synthesis. Radioactive iodine is commonly given to destroy part of the thyroid gland and thus reduce its thyroxine output. Second or even third doses of radioactive iodine may be given if the blood thyroxine levels remain high. Radioactive iodine is not used during pregnancy because damage to the fetal thyroid is likely. Additionally, surgery can be performed to remove enough thyroid tissue to restore normal thyroxine levels. Following any of the treatments, a hypothyroidism may be induced that will require that the patient receive thyroxine supplements. Finally, surgery can be used to reduce the bulging of the eyes caused by hyperthyroidism.

—*John T. Burns, Ph.D.;*
updated by Matthew Berria, Ph.D.

See also Congenital hypothyroidism; Endocrine disorders; Endocrine glands; Endocrinology; Endocrinology, pediatric; Glands; Goiter; Hashimoto's thyroiditis; Hormones; Hyperparathyroidism and hypoparathyroidism; Metabolic disorders; Metabolism; Parathyroidectomy; Thyroid gland; Thyroidectomy; Vitamins and minerals.

For Further Information:

Bar, Robert S. *Early Diagnosis and Treatment of Endocrine Disorders.* Totowa, N.J.: Humana Press, 2003.

Braverman, Lewis E., ed. *Diseases of the Thyroid.* 2d ed. Totowa, N.J.: Humana Press, 2003.

Health Library. "Hyperthyroidism." *Health Library,* November 26, 2012.

Health Library. "Hypothyroidism." *Health Library,* March 15, 2013.

Hershman, Jerome M., ed. *Endocrine Pathophysiology: A Patient-Oriented Approach.* 3d ed. Philadelphia: Lea & Febiger, 1988.

Kovacs, William J.., and Sergio R. Ojeda, eds. *Textbook of Endocrine Physiology.* 6th ed. New York: Oxford University Press, 2012.

MedlinePlus. "Thyroid Diseases." *MedlinePlus,* May 30, 2013.

Melmed, Shlomo, and Robert Hardin Williams, eds. *Williams Textbook of Endocrinology.* 12th ed. Philadelphia: Elsevier/Saunders, 2011.

Ruggieri, Paul, and Scott Isaacs. *A Simple Guide to Thyroid Disorders: From Diagnosis to Treatment.* Omaha, Nebr.: Addicus Books, 2010.

Surks, Martin I. *The Thyroid Book.* Rev. ed. Yonkers, N.Y.: Consumer Reports Books, 1999.

THYROID GLAND

Anatomy

Anatomy or system affected: Endocrine system, glands, neck
Specialties and related fields: Endocrinology
Definition: A gland found in the neck that secretes the hormones responsible for the synthesis and breakdown of proteins and the metabolism of carbohydrates.

Key terms:

cretinism: a severe hypothyroidism in which infants are born with insufficiently developed thyroid tissue

endocrine system: a series of ductless glands that deliver hormones to target cells directly through the bloodstream

Graves' disease: a common type of hyperthyroidism in which the thyroid gland produces an oversupply of hormone

hormones: chemicals, usually proteins or steroids, that carry messages regulating the body's chemical balance, responses to stimuli, and development

hypothyroidism: a condition in which the thyroid gland produces an insufficient supply of hormone

parathyroid: one of four small endocrine glands physically close to the thyroid that control the calcium balance of the body

pituitary: the endocrine gland responsible for the functioning of the thyroid, along with many other central control activities

thyroxine: the chief hormone of the thyroid gland, an iodine-containing derivative of the amino acid tyrosine

Structure and Functions

The human body is, to an extraordinary extent, under the metabolic control of chemical secretions called hormones. These molecules are produced by the ductless, or endocrine, glands and carry messages that regulate the rate of production of necessary substances in remote parts of the organism. The endocrine glands in turn are largely controlled by the nervous system, which also uses chemical messengers to manage the multiple and interrelated systems of the body.

The thyroid gland was one of the earliest glands to be studied in detail. It synthesizes, stores, and secretes two principal hormones, thyroxine and triiodothyronine. These substances stimulate carbohydrate metabolism and protein synthesis or breakdown.

The first description of the thyroid that has been accepted as definite was given by Thomas Wharton in 1656; he also named the gland. In his studies of all the glands, he performed animal dissections and human autopsies. Although his written accounts were widely reprinted, it was more than two hundred years later before any serious further work was undertaken.

Nineteenth century clinical studies of goiter (swelling of the thyroid) and hyperthyroidism (the gland's overproduction of hormones) contributed little to an understanding of the thyroid. An exception is found in the study of the insufficient production of hormone by the thyroid, called hypothyroidism. English and Swiss physicians made discoveries that are considered by some medical historians to be as important as the demonstration that the element iodine is associated with thyroid action.

In the 1870s, the Swiss surgeon Emil Theodor Kocher began to describe the significance of the thyroid gland and its role in goiter formation. He was awarded the 1909 Nobel Prize in Physiology or Medicine for providing a fuller appreciation of the thyroid and associated glands. Kocher was neither a physiologist nor a pathologist by training or disposition, but he recognized that to be an effective surgeon it was essential to understand well the function of the thyroid and its role in the goiters so common in Bern. In this region, 80 to 90 percent of schoolchildren had a malfunctioning thyroid gland and the often-associated goiter. Kocher's drawings in books and papers show that such enlargements are extremely disfiguring and often interfere with normal breathing and speech.

In Kocher's day, little was known about any of the endocrine glands, of which the thyroid is the first to have been

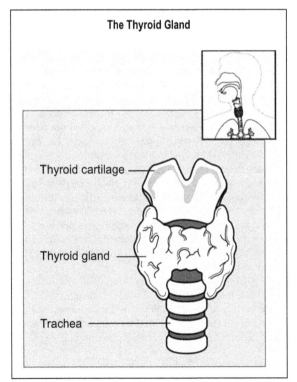

The Thyroid Gland

Thyroid cartilage

Thyroid gland

Trachea

The thyroid is an important gland that produces thyroid hormone, the proper level of which is crucial to health; the inset shows the location of the thyroid gland.

studied surgically. Such glands deposit chemical regulatory substances called hormones directly into the bloodstream, which carries them to the sites of their activity.

Later clinical observations provided evidence that the thyroid gland produces some material essential for good health. In 1896, Eugen Baumann made the key discovery that the thyroid contains an unusual amount of iodine. He also showed that this excess iodine is present in a protein that he could decompose with water to yield a new substance. During the next twenty-five years, technical progress was made to the point that the hormone thyroxine could be produced in a pure, crystalline form.

With the new tool of radioactive iodine, a powerful method for the study of thyroid functions and malfunctions became available. For example, overactive and underactive thyroid glands can be easily determined through the ingestion of a tiny amount of one of the radioactive isotopes of iodine and the later determination of the amount of the tracer present in the thyroid.

Disorders and Diseases

It is possible for the thyroid to produce either too much (hyperthyroidism) or too little (hypothyroidism) of the hormone thyroxine, which plays a role in controlling metabolism and body growth. If an insufficient quantity of it is produced, the condition called Gull's disease results. In children, this condition limits both physical and mental growth and is known as congenital hypothyroidism or cretinism. In Graves' disease and related conditions, the overactive thyroid gland produces too much hormone. Either of these conditions can produce an enlarged thyroid gland, or goiter. This imbalance existed in many different countries, but physicians designated it by various names, thus causing much misunderstanding and confusion. Emil Kocher's studies presented the first organization of the field in the form of these basic definitions.

In his first one hundred operations carried out between 1872 and 1883, Kocher completely removed the thyroid gland in thirty-four cases. After a report by his colleague Jacques Louis Reverdin indicating that removal of the thyroid was a causal factor in cretinism, Kocher made as detailed a follow-up of these patients as possible. His conclusion was that if the entire gland was removed, cretinlike symptoms almost always appeared. If at least some of the gland was left, it appeared to regenerate itself and supply the required hormone. He vowed never to remove a thyroid completely again except in the case of malignancy.

Only in the twentieth century did reliable diagnoses and treatments become available for thyroid disorders. Because of the variety of these conditions and their causes, accurate diagnosis is indispensable. Modern approaches that supplement radioactive iodine include ultrasound and the needle biopsy.

The principal difficulty in the treatment of a malfunctioning thyroid gland is the several variations often displayed. Hyperthyroidism can occur in forms that appear quite unrelated to the most common form, Graves' disease. For example, there may not be a heredity basis, the condition may not

spread over the entire gland, the production of antibodies may not be involved, and there may be no progressive failure of the thyroid.

The causes of hypothyroidism are also less than uniform. The age at which the disorder begins is significantly related to its cause. Newborn children with this condition may have never developed the required amount of thyroid tissue. Others may have inherited a defect that prevents the thyroid from producing sufficient hormone. In developing countries, iodine deficiency remains a problem (although an overabundance of that element in the diet of expectant mothers can lead to infants with hypothyroidism and a goiter). Later in life, infection can be the cause of Hashimoto's disease and the loss of thyroid tissue. Finally, the treatment of an overactive thyroid places a person at risk of later underproduction of hormone.

The most common symptoms associated with thyroid problems are a too rapid or too slow heartbeat, nervousness or a tired and run-down feeling, frequent bowel movements or constipation, and weight loss or weight gain. An excess of the hormones that direct the use of food and the production of energy might reasonably be expected to produce the first of each pair of contrasting observations, while a deficiency would lead to the opposite effects.

The treatment of Graves' disease falls into three distinct classes, and in modified application these techniques are employed with the other forms of hyperthyroidism. Since the early 1940s, a series of antithyroid drugs have been synthesized. They function by preventing the gland from making hormone, and the symptoms lessen in a short time. Unfortunately, only about 30 percent of patients remain well when the medication is stopped after six to twelve months.

If antithyroid drugs fail to control the overactive thyroid, a radioactive isotope of iodine is often successful. Since the iodine goes directly to the thyroid and remains there for a period of time, it is able to irradiate and destroy a portion of the tissue. It is a demanding task to calculate the proper amount of iodine to administer, but a surprising 80 percent of patients find their condition under control after a single treatment.

Surgical treatment of Graves' disease and related hyperthyroid conditions became practical with Kocher's efforts, and it remains the method of choice in many cases. Kocher began his Nobel Prize lecture by describing the crucial importance of the work of Louis Pasteur, Joseph Lister, and others in making surgery on internal organs possible, and he suggested the future of thyroid research when he examined the effective use of extracts and the search for chemical means of providing substitutes for the gland's secretions.

The standard treatment of hypothyroidism is oral thyroid hormone tablets. Typically, a synthetic form of thyroxine, called Levothyroxine, is given to compensate for low thyroid hormone levels. As is the case with Graves' disease, good follow-up is essential because the prescribed dosage will likely change with the patient's age. The administration of too much thyroxine can lead to hyperthyroidism.

Two notes should be made in concluding this discussion of malfunctions of the thyroid. First, there is a tendency to believe that iodine prevents and cures goiter. Statements to that effect, found in many general reference books, are both misleading and dangerous. Second, publications for laypersons tend to minimize the importance of thyroid blood tests, which is a serious disservice. Regular and complete physical examinations are essential in maintaining good health.

Perspective and Prospects

Historians of medical history have attributed knowledge of the thyroid gland and the treatment of goiter to many significant figures. The works of Galen, Paracelsus, ancient Chinese writers, and other classical Roman and Greek authors, as well as medieval manuscripts, have been studied. In the twentieth century, the study of the thyroid and goiter illustrates central themes in the evolution of medical practice; these are shown clearly in the career of Emil Kocher. His being chosen as an early Nobel laureate is prophetic—first for his role in creating modern surgery, with its total reliance on a germ-free environment and its demand for detail, and second for successful synthesis of the roles of clinician and research scientist. He both possessed the necessary surgical skill to develop such a delicate procedure as thyroidectomy (removal of the thyroid gland) and appreciated the importance of understanding the role played by the thyroid in controlling distant and seemingly unrelated functions. Finally, Kocher kept abreast of any new discovery that might, in any way, be of significance to his surgical goals.

The study of the thyroid in many ways unlocked the secrets of other endocrine glands. As in many areas of scientific research, new medical knowledge follows quickly after the discovery of materials and techniques. At the same time, the search for knowledge provides both motivation and information driving the discovery of materials and techniques.

The identification of iodine as an elemental substance by the French chemist Bernard Courtois in 1811 rapidly led to its indiscriminate use as a treatment for goiter, along with a wide variety of related conditions. Important work in the mid-nineteenth century by A. Chatin demonstrated the high correlation between goiter and low levels of iodine in the food and water supplies throughout central Europe. In the 1930s, with the creation of radioactive isotopes, including those of iodine, a vital and productive new phase of thyroid research began.

A similar pattern is seen during World War II, when four independent research groups showed that sulfa drugs were capable of exerting a strong influence on the behavior of the thyroid. All these studies were conducted within a two-year period, and it was less than a year later that the therapeutic use of sulfa drugs was demonstrated.

While much knowledge and technical skill concerning the thyroid has been gained, the number of conferences and publications devoted to endocrinology attests to the continued importance of that general field of study. For example, while malignant tumors are rare in the thyroid, benign lumps or nodules are common. The reasons for this pattern and the role of endocrine glands in the development and spread of cancerous cells warrant detailed and continuing study.

In 2013, researchers analyzing data from the U.S. National Health and Nutrition Examination Survey linked exposure to perfluorinated chemicals (PFCs) to changes in thyroid function. PFCs are often found in fabrics, cosmetics, and carpets.

—K. Thomas Finley, Ph.D.

See also Congenital hypothyroidism; Endocrine disorders; Endocrinology; Endocrinology, pediatric; Glands; Goiter; Growth; Hashimoto's thyroiditis; Hormone therapy; Hormones; Metabolic disorders; Metabolism; Systems and organs; Thyroid disorders; Thyroidectomy.

For Further Information:

Bayliss, R. I. S., and W. M. Tunbridge. *Thyroid Disease: The Facts.* 4th ed. New York: Oxford University Press, 2008.

Burman, Kenneth D., and Derek LeRoith, eds. *Thyroid Function and Disease.* Philadelphia: Saunders/Elsevier, 2007..

Dallas, Mary Elizabeth. "Thyroid Disorders Tied to Complications in Pregnancy." *MedlinePlus.* May 29, 2013.

DeGroot, Leslie J., P. Reed Larsen, and Georg Hennemann. *The Thyroid and Its Diseases.* 6th ed. New York: Churchill Livingstone, 1996.

Holt, Richard I. G., and Neil A. Hanley. *Essential Endocrinology and Diabetes.* 5th ed. Malden, Mass.: Blackwell, 2007.

Marieb, Elaine N. *Essentials of Human Anatomy and Physiology.* 9th ed. San Francisco: Pearson/Benjamin Cummings, 2009.

Melmed, Schlomo, et al. *The Pituitary.* 2d ed. Boston: Blackwell Science, 2002.

Moore, Elaine A., and Lisa Moore. *Graves' Disease: A Practical Guide.* Jefferson, N.C.: McFarland, 2001.

Preidt, Robert. "Chemicals in Carpets, Cosmetics Tied to Thyroid Problems." *MedlinePlus.* May 29, 2013.

Preidt, Robert. "Iodine Supplements May Be Too Much of a Good Thing." *MedlinePlus.* June 12, 2013.

Rosenthal, M. Sara. *The Thyroid Sourcebook.* 5th ed. New York: McGraw-Hill, 2009.

Ruggieri, Paul, and Scott Isaacs. *A Simple Guide to Thyroid Disorders: From Diagnosis to Treatment.* Omaha, Nebr.: Addicus Books, 2004.

Wood, Lawrence C., David S. Cooper, and E. Chester Ridgway. *Your Thyroid: A Home Reference.* 4th rev. ed. New York: Ballantine Books, 2005.

THYROIDECTOMY

Procedure

Anatomy or system affected: Endocrine system, glands, neck
Specialties and related fields: Endocrinology, general surgery
Definition: The surgical removal of all or a portion of the thyroid gland.

Indications and Procedures

A thyroidectomy is performed in order to remove thyroid tumors, to treat thyrotoxicosis (whereby the thyroid gland excretes very large amounts of thyroid hormone), to evaluate a mass, or to excise an enlarged thyroid that is causing problems with breathing, swallowing, or speaking.

The thyroid gland is located at the base of the neck. It is composed of two lobes that straddle the trachea (throat) and a third lobe that is in the middle of the neck. Surgery on the thyroid is usually performed under general anesthesia. The patient's neck is extended, and an incision along a natural fold or crease is made through the skin, platysma muscle, and fascia that lie over the thyroid. The muscle is cut high up to minimize damage to the nerve that controls it.

The thyroid is then carefully freed from surrounding structures (blood vessels, nerves, and the trachea). One at a time, the upper portion of each lobe is freed to allow identification of the veins that take blood from the thyroid. The veins are ligated (tied) in two places and cut between the ties. The ligaments that suspend the thyroid are cut next. It is important for the surgeon to avoid damaging the superior laryngeal nerve. Once the nerve has been protected, other blood vessels are clamped, tied, and cut. A similar procedure is followed for the lower lobes: ligating and cutting veins, protecting the inferior and recurrent laryngeal nerves, and freeing the remainder of the thyroid lobes.

Four parathyroid glands, each about the size of a pea, are embedded in the thyroid gland. At least one of these must be preserved since they play a vital role in regulating calcium. Once these glands are identified, the tissue of the thyroid is cut away, leaving the parathyroids intact.

The remnants of the thyroid gland are folded in and sutured to the trachea to control bleeding. A final inspection for bleeding is made. The fascia is sutured closed over the thyroid; any muscles that were cut are sewn back together. Finally, the edges of skin are carefully brought together and sutured with very fine material; occasionally, clips are used. The instruments needed for a tracheostomy are left nearby to cope with any emergency that might occur during the next twenty-four hours.

Uses and Complications

Approximately one week after a thyroidectomy, the patient returns for a postoperative checkup, and sutures or clips are removed. Many, but not all, individuals having this procedure must take a synthetic thyroid hormone to make up for the tissue removed during the thyroidectomy.

Thyroid surgery is not uncommon. In the past, radiation was used to shrink the thyroid, but this procedure led to many cancers and has been discontinued. Laser techniques may reduce the size of the incision, thus reducing the size of the resulting scar in the neck.

Complications that may occur as a result of a thyroidectomy include bleeding into the neck, causing difficulty breathing; a surge of thyroid hormones into the blood, called thyroid storm or thyrotoxic crisis; and injury to the vocal cords, which can result in changes in voice pitch.

—*L. Fleming Fallon, Jr., M.D., Ph.D., M.P.H.;*
updated by Sharon W. Stark, R.N., A.P.R.N., D.N.Sc.

See also Endocrine disorders; Endocrinology; Endocrinology, pediatric; Glands; Goiter; Hashimoto's thyroiditis; Hormone therapy; Hormones; Parathyroidectomy; Thyroid disorders; Thyroid gland.

For Further Information:

Bayliss, R. I. S., and W. M. Tunbridge. *Thyroid Disease: The Facts.* 4th ed. New York: Oxford University Press, 2008.
Bhimji, Shabir. "Thyroid Gland Removal." *MedlinePlus*, May 6, 2011.
Burman, Kenneth D., and Derek LeRoith, eds. *Thyroid Function and Disease*. Philadelphia: Saunders/Elsevier, 2007.
Doherty, Gerard M., and Lawrence W. Way, eds. *Current Surgical Diagnosis and Treatment*. 12th ed. New York: Lange Medical Books/McGraw-Hill, 2006.
Kronenberg, Henry M., et al., eds. *Williams Textbook of Endocrinology*. 12th ed. Philadelphia: Saunders/Elsevier, 2011.
Miccoli, Paolo, et al., eds. *Thyroid Surgery: Preventing and Managing Complications*. Hoboken, N.J.: 2013.
Rosenthal, M. Sara. *The Thyroid Sourcebook: Everything You Need to Know*. 5th ed. New York: McGraw-Hill, 2008.
Ruggieri, Paul, and Scott Isaacs. *A Simple Guide to Thyroid Disorders: From Diagnosis to Treatment*. Omaha, Nebr.: Addicus Books, 2010.
Wood, Lawrence C., David S. Cooper, and E. Chester Ridgway. *Your Thyroid: A Home Reference*. 4th ed. New York: Ballantine Books, 2006.

TIAs. *See* TRANSIENT ISCHEMIC ATTACKS (TIAs).

TICKS. *See* LICE, MITES, AND TICKS.

TICS
Disease/Disorder
Also known as: Habit spasm
Anatomy or system affected: Brain, muscles, musculoskeletal system, nerves, nervous system, psychic-emotional system
Specialties and related fields: Neurology, psychology
Definition: Small, brief, recurrent, inappropriate, compulsive jerking movements or twitches, sometimes called habit spasms, often set off by stressful events and including tic douloureux, involving the trigeminal nerve, and Tourette's syndrome, a lifelong disorder associated with a large variety of tics.

Key terms:

neuralgia: pain in one of the peripheral nerves

paroxysm: an uncontrolled spasm or convulsion that may sometimes be violent

psychogenic: psychological in origin; set off by psychologically stressful events

stereotyped: performed exactly the same way from one occasion to the next, or from one individual performer to the next

tic douloureux (trigeminal neuralgia): painful tics of the fifth cranial nerve (trigeminal nerve)

Tourette's syndrome: a neurological disorder characterized by bizarre or unusual tics, compulsive swearing, strange facial gestures, and animal-like noises

Causes and Symptoms

Tics are small, inappropriate, involuntary, compulsive jerking or twitching movements that recur uncontrollably and appear to be nonrhythmic (erratic) in pattern. Tics are stereotyped movements of small portions of the body that last only briefly but may be repeated often. They are often set off by psychologically stressful events. In many cases, tics can be voluntary and temporarily suppressed, but often with the result that the same movements occur more forcefully afterward. The term "habit spasm" is often used for tics that occur among children. A tic is a symptom rather than a disease. Many tics are believed to be of psychogenic origin, and certain others seem to be related to epilepsy, encephalitis, or diseases of unknown origin.

Motor tics commonly involve coarse muscle movements of small magnitude, including movements of the face (such as eye blinks, grimaces, or sniffing movements), shrugging of the shoulders, jerks of the neck, or twitches of the body parts. Many motor tics (and also vocal tics) are easily imitated by others but are performed involuntarily and uncontrollably by the patient. Distracting the patient's attention may stop certain tics. In most cases, the tic does not interfere with the patient's use of the hands or feet, even in delicate movements. Several neurologists distinguish simple motor tics (eye winking, head twitching, shoulder shrugs, or facial grimaces) from complex motor tics using more muscles and requiring coordination. Complex motor tics may include touching oneself or other people, jumping, hitting, or throwing things.

Vocal or phonic tics include the making of sounds, which may include grunts, coughs, sniffs, clearings of the throat, animal noises (especially barking and yelping), or understandable words. The words may simply be repeated utterances of the patient's own words (palilalia), repetition of words spoken to the patient (echolalia), or obscene and offensive words (coprolalia). Although coprolalia is one of the more striking symptoms of Tourette's syndrome and has been vividly portrayed in many popular accounts of this disorder, it is usually a mild or transient symptom and appears in only a minority of cases.

Sensory tics are unusual sensations of pressure, cold, warmth, tickling, or other common sensations that are generally brief in duration. Some otherwise inexplicable movements may be interpreted as actions taken by the patient to alleviate these sensory tics. Sensory tics are reported to be present in about 40 percent of patients with Tourette's syndrome.

Tic disorders can be classified into four types: tic douloureux, transient tic disorder of childhood, chronic tic disorder, and Tourette's syndrome. One of the most common forms of tic is trigeminal neuralgia, also called tic douloureux, a disorder that affects about fifteen thousand individuals annually in the United States. Tic douloureux is a disorder of the trigeminal or fifth cranial nerve, the nerve that supplies motor stimulation to the jaw muscles and sensory innervation to much of the skin of the face. Tic douloureux usually begins with a very brief but very intense, sharp pain, often described as feeling like an electric shock or a stabbing, swiftly spreading in many cases along the course of the affected nerve. The pain is usually accompanied by uncontrolled spasms or paroxysms that last less than a second but continue to recur for several minutes. These episodes may be separated from one another by tic-free periods lasting from weeks to more than a year. The pain and twitching are generally confined to one side of the face, often to one of the three divisions of the trigeminal nerve, usually the maxillary or mandibular division, or, much less often, the ophthalmic division. In addition to the uncontrollable tics, patients suffering from tic douloureux often wince visibly from the pain; this

---

Information on Tics

Causes: Stressful events, disease (e.g., epilepsy, encephalitis), tumors, psychological disorders, Tourette's syndrome

Symptoms: Small, brief, recurrent, and compulsive jerking movements or twitches; unusual vocalizations (grunting, coughing, throat clearing, animal noises) or word repetition

Duration: Acute to chronic with recurrent episodes

Treatments: Surgery, drug therapy, injection of ethyl alcohol into trigeminal nerve ganglion, vitamin supplements, psychotherapy

---

habit is responsible for the term "tic douloureux," meaning "painful tic."

The immediate event precipitating an attack of tic douloureux is usually a mild stimulation or irritation of a "trigger zone" on or about the face, lips, tongue, or gums. The trigger zone is often a small area that is constant for a particular patient; some patients can trigger an episode by stimulating the trigger zone themselves. The most common locations for the trigger zone are along the cheek or the attached parts of the lips; less common locations include the gums or the floor of the mouth beside the tongue. Some patients suffering an attack of tic douloureux will apply pressure to their faces, but the pain usually goes away by itself. Attacks generally occur during the day rather than at night, and they typically increase in intensity and become more frequent and exhausting to the patient until treatment is sought.

The stimulus that normally evokes an attack of tic douloureux may be an exposure to touch or pressure, to cold, to food in the mouth, or even to a puff of air. Because an attack can be precipitated by touching or otherwise stimulating the trigger zone, many victims of tic douloureux avoid touching the region in which the trigger zone is located. When the trigger zone is on the outside of the face, patients may become very fearful of touching the affected part, and men may avoid shaving. Some patients avoid brushing their teeth and remain unwashed for weeks or even months in the vicinity of their trigger area, with social consequences that often contribute to pessimistic feelings and even depression.

When tongue or cheek movements precipitate attacks, patients suffering from tic douloureux may develop the habit of holding the affected side of their face motionless, which sometimes restricts talking, eating, or similar everyday movements. In some cases, certain chewing movements or the presence of food in certain locations in the mouth may precipitate an attack; in these cases, patients are often very careful to avoid eating or chewing on the affected side, and in extreme cases they may so often avoid eating or drinking that they become dehydrated and emaciated. Some physicians advise such patients to modify their diet and drink only liquids, fortified with vitamins, that can be consumed without chewing. Malnutrition and physical inactivity are in many cases reinforced by the social consequences of facial uncleanliness and lack of hygiene, or by the fear of such consequences. The lack of social contact may result in pessimistic or negative feelings, feelings of inadequacy or lack of worth, preoccupation with loss and with past events, feelings of rejection or powerlessness, and other symptoms of clinical depression in many patients.

Dental disease or trauma may sometimes be associated with tic douloureux, but in most cases the tic has no apparent cause. Tic douloureux is more common after the age of forty and is slightly more common in women than in men. Some researchers believe that infection with a herpesvirus (especially herpes simplex) may be causally related to trigeminal neuralgia, but other researchers doubt this connection. Tumors of the trigeminal (Gasserian) ganglion, brain-stem tumors, multiple sclerosis, or localized damage to the brain stem tissue can sometimes give rise to conditions that closely resemble tic douloureux, but the majority of tics occur among patients having none of these conditions.

The remaining forms of tic disorder are considered by at least some researchers to be related to one another, or to form a spectrum of conditions from mild or imperceptible to severe. The mildest types are the tics or "habit spasms" of children. These tics are usually considered psychogenic in origin because they occur more often under conditions of stress or tension. Tics of this kind are more common in boys than in girls. Common types of childhood tics include eye blinks or other facial movements, as well as occasional vocal tics such as throat-clearing noises. In some children—perhaps many—tics of this kind may disappear (or be "outgrown") spontaneously if no attention is drawn to them.

Chronic tics can be of either the motor or the vocal type. Chronic motor tics are uncommon tics in which three or more muscle groups are usually involved at the same time. Chronic vocal tics are also uncommon and consist of uncontrolled sounds that are more often animal sounds than words of articulate speech. Either kind of chronic tic can originate either in children or in adults, even beyond the age of forty. In either case, they usually last for the remainder of the patient's life. The disorder is equally prevalent in both sexes. Some researchers think that these chronic tics, and possibly also the transient habit spasms of childhood, may result from the same (as yet unidentified) cause as Tourette's syndrome, but in much milder form.

Tourette's syndrome is a neurological disorder characterized by bizarre or unusual tics, compulsive swearing or cursing, strange facial gestures, and sudden barking or other animal-like sounds. The spectrum of these tics and other symptoms is broad, which has complicated earlier attempts to describe the disease or to find its cause. The disease usually first appears in children between five and ten years of age and continues throughout life.

The variability of symptoms is one of the characteristic features or highlights of Tourette's syndrome. According to the American Psychiatric Association's *Diagnostic and Statistical Manual of Mental Disorders: DSM-IV-TR* (4th ed., 2000), among the diagnostic criteria for Tourette's syndrome are that both motor and vocal tics must occur and that the number, frequency, complexity, severity, and anatomical lo-

cation of these tics must change over time. The tics must occur many times a day, usually in bouts, and they must recur "nearly every day or intermittently throughout a period of more than one year." The disease must appear before the age of twenty-one to be considered Tourette's syndrome (although in many cases symptoms are so mild as to escape attention).

Associated with Tourette's syndrome are a number of other conditions, including obsessive-compulsive behaviors, attention-deficit disorder, hyperactivity, school phobias, test anxiety, conduct disorders, depression, dyslexia, poor socialization skills, and low self-esteem, though many of these symptoms can also appear by themselves. Several experts consider Tourette's syndrome and attention-deficit disorder to be variable manifestations of a common underlying disorder that may relate to a chemical imbalance in the brain. About half of Tourette's patients also show symptoms of attention-deficit disorder, such as frequent inattention, impulsiveness, and hyperactivity.

The association between Tourette's syndrome and attention-deficit disorder should be regarded as provisional. The two disorders may have an underlying cause in common, such as a common genetic basis. In many cases, however, the motor and vocal tics are made worse by the administration of stimulants such as methylphenidate, which is commonly used for the treatment of the hyperactivity that so often accompanies attention-deficit disorder. Thus it is possible that the presence of Tourette's syndrome in such cases may be attributable not to the attention-deficit disorder, but to the drugs used to treat the disorder. In certain cases, these drugs may have caused a transient or chronic tic disorder to progress to the more severe Tourette's syndrome. Clearly, more research is needed to clarify the exact nature of the relationship between Tourette's syndrome and attention-deficit disorder, both in the presence and in the absence of various drugs.

There are several other aspects of Tourette's syndrome that are being examined. For example, a number of researchers now suspect that the factors that predispose a patient to develop Tourette's syndrome may also predispose male patients to one form of alcoholism. Other researchers believe that the brain disorder responsible for Tourette's syndrome is related to the endorphins, the brain's natural opiates.

Some promising research involves the connection between this disorder and the neurotransmitter dopamine. Neurologists suspect that Tourette's syndrome results from increased sensitivity of certain parts of the brain to dopamine. Some of the evidence for the hypersensitivity of dopamine receptors derives from the observation that drugs such as haloperidol, which is known to inhibit the dopamine receptors, are effective in reducing the symptoms of Tourette's syndrome, while amphetamines and other drugs that enhance dopamine neurotransmission make the symptoms worse. Also, the cerebrospinal fluid of patients with Tourette's syndrome contains reduced levels of homovanillic acid, a breakdown product of dopamine. The corpus striatum in the brain is considered to be the most likely location for the supersensitive dopamine receptors. One researcher has found a total absence of a brain peptide called dynorphin in fibers of the corpus striatum, where this peptide normally occurs. The fibers in question project to the globus pallidus at the base of the cerebral hemispheres.

One theory that attempts to explain the relationship of the several symptoms in Tourette's syndrome is that they all stem from a loss of the inhibition that normally controls involuntary movements. The obscene or offensive words, normally inhibited, are expressed more often than other types of words because the inhibition has been removed. This theory supposes that children who find that they have expressed "bad" words that should not have been said out loud become obsessed with these words and thus (in the absence of inhibitions) say them more often, making the problem worse.

Studies of the families of Tourette's syndrome patients show that there are familial inheritance patterns, with many family members having at least some symptoms of tic disorders, attention-deficit disorders, or both. In many or most cases, the tic disorders of affected family members are so mild that they never caused any problems and were never mentioned to any physician. This finding leads many researchers to conclude that the underlying disorder is variable in the extent of its expression and that it is much more common than medical records show. One expert has even estimated that nearly 1 percent of the population has some form of tic disorder.

If all forms of tic disorder are included, it becomes clear that tics run in families and that Tourette's syndrome is simply one end of a spectrum of variable expression. Studies on identical twins confirm that the trait has a genetic basis. Additional studies of family histories suggest that everyone with the gene experiences symptoms of the disorder. The penetrance of the gene is somewhat greater in males than in females, meaning that more males have symptoms while females are more often symptom-free. Among those family members who have symptoms, the expression of those symptoms is highly variable.

Mimicking some of the symptoms of Tourette's syndrome are the so-called tardive tics that appear during adolescence or adult life. Tardive tics are considered by many researchers to be iatrogenic (drug-induced), arising from the prolonged use of neuroleptic drugs (tranquilizers) such as phenothiazines (Thorazine, Compazine, and Mellaril). Symptoms include isolated, short, quick, uncoordinated jerking movements. The mechanism by which tardive tics appear is unclear, but the same dopamine pathways may be involved as in genuine cases of Tourette's syndrome.

Treatment and Therapy

Various treatments are available for tic douloureux, both medical and surgical. Partial relief may be afforded by medical treatments, which include carbamazepine (tegretol), trichloroethylene, anticonvulsants such as phenytoin or phenylhydatoin (Dilantin), vasodilators such as tolazoline (Priscoline), analgesic (pain-killing) drugs, vitamin B$_{12}$, or the repeated injection of 95 percent ethyl alcohol directly into the trigeminal nerve ganglion.

None of these treatments is successful in all cases, however, and some, such as trichloroethylene, have toxic side effects. Surgical treatments include neurotomy (cutting of the affected branch of the trigeminal nerve), decompression of the posterior nerve root, or the cutting of one or more of the trigeminal tracts in the brain stem, either in the midbrain or in the medulla. The most frequently performed surgical procedures include destruction, or partial destruction, of the trigeminal ganglion, either by electrocoagulation, by radio frequency therapy, or by mechanical means. The facial paralysis or partial paralysis that follows nerve destruction often resembles Bell's palsy except that the damage is usually permanent, with minimal possibility of recovery.

Treatment of childhood transient tic disorders usually consists of psychological intervention to control or reduce the level of stress. Many cases of transient or chronic tic disorder are so mild that they do not require any treatment.

For Tourette's syndrome, haloperidol (Haldol) is most often prescribed, and it is said to be effective in 50 to 90 percent of the cases, depending on the authority consulted. Other drugs occasionally prescribed include clonidine, penfluridol, and pimozide. These drugs can reduce the severity and frequency of tics and may reduce impulsive or aggressive behavior. They also have side effects, however, causing sedation, depression, and weight gain in many patients.

Perspective and Prospects

Because tics are highly noticeable, suggestions regarding their cause have been made throughout history. It was not until the eighteenth century, however, that scientific studies were conducted on patients exhibiting these movements. Thus, while there are indications that tic douloureux was known and recognized in ancient times, James Fothergill (1712–1780) is usually credited with the first modern description of the disorder in 1773.

Georges Gilles de la Tourette (1857–1904) was a French physician who, in 1885, first described the medical syndrome that bears his name. Tourette described the disorder, which he considered to be heritable, on the basis of eight patients whose symptoms included jerking movements, noises, coprolalia, and echolalia. Tourette was shot three times by one of his patients in 1893; he never recovered from the resulting brain injury. Tourette's syndrome was usually ignored in medical literature or described as a rare disorder until the 1980s, when several researchers studying the families of Tourette's syndrome patients began to notice that many of the family members had mild forms of the same disorder that had previously escaped attention. When they looked more closely for tic symptoms, they discovered that such disorders were much more common than had previously been thought. Connections with obsessive-compulsive disorders and with alcoholism were first noticed from the discovery of these conditions among the relatives of Tourette's syndrome patients.

—*Eli C. Minkoff, Ph.D.*

See also Anxiety; Attention-deficit disorder; Encephalitis; Epilepsy; Huntington's disease; Motor neuron diseases; Muscle sprains, spasms, and disorders; Muscles; Nervous system; Neuralgia, neuritis, and neuropathy; Neurology; Neurology, pediatric; Palsy; Seizures; Speech disorder; Stress; Tourette's syndrome.

For Further Information:

American Psychiatric Association. *Diagnostic and Statistical Manual of Mental Disorders: DSM-IV-TR*. 4th ed. Arlington, Va.: Author, 2000.

Behrman, Richard E., Robert M. Kliegman, and Hal B. Jenson, eds. *Nelson Textbook of Pediatrics*. 18th ed. Philadelphia: Saunders/Elsevier, 2007.

Bloom, Floyd E., M. Flint Beal, and David J. Kupfer, eds. *The Dana Guide to Brain Health*. New York: Dana Press, 2006.

Brill, Marlene Targ. *Tourette Syndrome*. Brookfield, Conn.: Millbrook Press, 2002.

Chipps, Esther M., Norma J. Clanin, and Victor G. Campbell. *Neurologic Disorders*. St. Louis, Mo.: Mosby Year Book, 1992.

Nicholls, John G., A. Robert Martin, and Bruce G. Wallace. *From Neuron to Brain*. 4th ed. Sunderland, Mass.: Sinauer, 2007.

Victor, Maurice, and Allan H. Ropper. *Adams and Victor's Principles of Neurology*. 9th ed. New York: McGraw-Hill, 2009.

Waxman, Stephen G. *Correlative Neuroanatomy*. 25th ed. New York: Lange Medical Books/McGraw-Hill, 2002.

Woods, Douglas W., and Raymond G. Miltenberger, eds. *Tic Disorders, Trichotillomania, and Other Repetitive Behavior Disorders: Behavioral Approaches to Analysis and Treatment*. New York: Springer, 2006.

TINGLING. *See* NUMBNESS AND TINGLING.

TINNITUS
Disease/Disorder

Anatomy or system affected: Brain, ears, head, nerves, nervous system, psychic-emotional system

Specialties and related fields: Audiology, family medicine, neurology, otorhinolaryngology, psychiatry

Definition: An auditory sensation originating in the head without external stimulation. This common disorder (often considered a symptom) affects up to 10 percent of the general population in the United States, with the highest prevalence in persons between forty and seventy years old.

Key terms:

acoustic neuroma: a benign tumor of the auditory nerve

auditory cortex: an area of the cerebral surface gray matter where auditory information is ultimately processed

auditory nerve: a sensory nerve (eighth cranial) that conducts hearing and equilibrium impulses

brain stem: a part of the brain that connects the cerebral hemispheres with the spinal cord

cerumen: earwax; secreted by glands at the outer third of the ear canal

cochlea: the coiled part of the inner ear containing the hearing receptors (hair cells with fine cilia)

Eustachian tube: an auditory tube extending from the middle ear to the nasopharynx

Ménière's disease: an inner-ear fluid imbalance resulting in recurrent episodes of hearing loss, tinnitus, severe dizziness, and ear pressure

oto-: a combining form indicating "ear"

otosclerosis: an abnormal bone growth in the middle ear

Causes and Symptoms

One proposed classification of tinnitus distinguishes two main categories. Subjective tinnitus, the most common type, is perceived only by the patient, usually as a continuous "phantom" sensation. Objective tinnitus, the second type, can be heard through a stethoscope placed over head and neck structures and is frequently perceived as a pulsatile sound.

Continuous subjective tinnitus occurs in a multitude of ear conditions. It is most often encountered in the context of hearing loss due to aging, excessive noise exposure, or ototoxic medication (such as salycilates, aminoglycoside antibiotics, chemotherapeutics, and diuretics). The auditory sensation can be induced or worsened by ear infections or an excess of cerumen.

Other otologic causes are Ménière's disease, otosclerosis, and acoustic neuroma. Neurologic conditions (multiple sclerosis, stroke, head injury), temporomandibular joint (TMJ) disorder, and metabolic and psychogenic factors can also lead to tinnitus.

The causes of continuous tinnitus are often difficult to pinpoint, and the pathophysiology is still poorly understood. Prominent theories include repetitive discharge from injured cochlear hair cells that generate continuous impulses in the auditory nerve, spontaneous auditory nerve activity, hyperactive brain stem auditory nuclei, and decreased suppression of peripheral nerve impulses by the auditory cortex. A neurobiological model that has gained acceptance includes two essential events: initial damage to peripheral auditory structures, which triggers the tinnitus, and subsequent (maladaptive) plastic changes in the central auditory pathway, with increased activity in brain stem and cortical areas.

Pulsatile tinnitus is caused by blood flow perturbations (through either normal or abnormal blood vessels near ear structures) and mechanical factors. Atherosclerosis, vascular tumors, arteriovenous malformations, aneurysms, and vascular loops often lead to unilateral tinnitus and can be identified using imaging techniques. Vascular inflammation and thrombosis are additional causes of pulsatile tinnitus. Conditions associated with high cardiac output, such as pregnancy, anemia, or an overactive thyroid, can result in tinnitus. Mechanical causes of pulsatile tinnitus are represented by open Eustachian tubes and middle-ear muscle spasms.

Patients with tinnitus report a disturbing noise localized in

---

Information on Tinnitus

Causes: Various otologic, neurologic, vascular, and metabolic conditions

Symptoms: Sound sensations without external physical stimulus

Duration: Acute (days to weeks) or chronic (more than six months)

Treatments: Pharmacotherapy, surgical intervention, hearing support, cognitive and behavioral therapy

one or both ears and sometimes in the head. They describe it as ringing, whistling, hissing, swishing, roaring, buzzing, or clicking. Ear fullness or pain can be present. The severity ranges from an occasional awareness of the noise to a frustrating, even unbearable sound. Epidemiologic studies indicate that 25 percent of patients with tinnitus experience a pronounced discomfort, while the rest do not report significant distress. Sensations perceived as severe can result in attention deficit, anxiety, and depression. In general, pulsatile tinnitus, unilateral tinnitus, and tinnitus associated with additional ear symptoms should be investigated carefully because they can signal a potentially serious underlying disorder.

Treatment and Therapy

The assessment of a patient with tinnitus includes physical examination, blood pressure measurements, audiometric profile, complete blood chemistry, hematocrit and lipid levels, thyroid studies, and brain imaging. Most cases of tinnitus should be evaluated by an ear, nose, and throat (ENT) specialist.

Therapeutic steps vary according to the type of tinnitus diagnosed and how the symptoms affect a patient's life. Specific treatment should be provided for any underlying illness. Inflammatory ear disease is treated with antibiotic and anti-inflammatory medication. Conditions such as tumors, vascular abnormalities, otosclerosis, and Ménière's disease may warrant surgical intervention. If the tinnitus is caused by hearing damage, then reassurance is often sufficient. Hearing aids, noise-masking devices, and cognitive and behavioral therapy are sometimes recommended. Patients should avoid ototoxic medication, loud noise, and stress.

Many treatments are still in the experimental phase or have variable efficacy. Proposed pharmacologic therapies for severe cases include antianxiety and antidepressant agents, lidocaine, and carbamazepine. Drugs that improve brain metabolism (nootropics) and neurotransmitter-directed agents might prove beneficial. Additional approaches focus on neck exercises, sound therapy, acupuncture, and electrical brain stimulation.

Perspective and Prospects

Tinnitus has been considered a disease entity for centuries. It was only in the second half of the twentieth century that physicians were able to discriminate between various types of tinnitus and their underlying pathology. Tinnitus remains a perplexing disorder, both for the sufferer and for the physician. No single treatment is truly efficacious, especially in subjective tinnitus. Many variables are associated with this "phantom" sensation, and a multitude of biological mechanisms can cause it. Nevertheless, the neurobiology of tinnitus has become less mysterious. A growing body of research continues to unveil striking neural changes. Animal models are employed to elucidate brain activity patterns in tinnitus and to explore therapeutic avenues. As a result of this complexity, it is likely that successful therapeutic strategies will have to target multiple factors simultaneously.

—*Mihaela Avramut, M.D., Ph.D.*

See also Audiology; Ear infections and disorders; Ears; Hearing;

Hearing loss; Ménière's disease; Nervous system; Neurology; Otorhinolaryngology; Sense organs; Signs and symptoms.

For Further Information:
"About Tinnitus." *American Tinnitus Association*, 2013.
Claussen, Claus F. "Tinnitus." In *Conn's Current Therapy 2013*, edited by Edward T. Bope and Rick D. Kellerman. Philadelphia: Saunders/Elsevier, 2013.
Crummer, Richard W., and Ghinwa A. Hassan. "Diagnostic Approach to Tinnitus." *American Family Physician* 69, no. 1 (January 1, 2004): 120.
"Tinnitus." *MedlinePlus*, May 7, 2013.
Tyler, Richard S., ed. *The Consumer Handbook on Tinnitus*. Sedona, Ariz.: Auricle Ink, 2008.
Wood, Debra, and Kari Kassir. "Ringing in the Ears." *Health Library*, Sept. 10, 2012.

TIREDNESS. *See* FATIGUE.

TOENAIL REMOVAL. *See* NAIL REMOVAL.

TOILET TRAINING
Development

Anatomy or system affected: Bladder, gastrointestinal system, genitals, intestines, kidneys, psychic-emotional system, urinary system

Specialties and related fields: Family medicine, gastroenterology, pediatrics, psychiatry, psychology, urology

Definition: Toilet use is a complex skill that children usually master within the first four years of life.

Key terms:
encopresis: defecating outside the toilet
enuresis: urinating outside the toilet

Physical and Psychological Factors

Toilet use may seem simple, but it is a complex skill. Children must learn to produce both urine and bowel movements on the toilet, stay dry when not on the toilet, clean themselves, dress and undress, initiate going to the toilet without being reminded, and stay dry while asleep. Most children are fully toilet trained—dry all day and night with complete independence in cleaning and dressing—by the age of four. All successful toilet training methods have three things in common: timing, consistency, and a positive approach.

Two kinds of timing are important. First, training should begin when the child is ready. The child is physically ready when voluntary control over the urethral and anal sphincters is established, usually between twelve and twenty-four months of age. Behavioral signs of physical readiness include a reduction in the frequency of urination. Another sign of readiness is seeking out privacy, often under or behind furniture, before defecating.

The child may indicate psychological readiness by showing awareness of being wet, revulsion or irritation when soiled, or interest in watching parents and older children in the bathroom. Some children show these signs of readiness as early as twelve months of age; others never do. Most children can begin toilet training successfully by twenty-four to thirty-six months of age.

The second type of timing is in visiting the toilet. Children need to use the toilet after meals, every one or two hours between meals, and before bedtime or long car trips, much as adults do. Encouraging the child to sit on the toilet at these times for a few minutes each visit usually produces results.

Consistency is also important. A consistent schedule for meals and visits to the toilet is helpful, as is a consistent place for the child to use the toilet, such as a child-sized toilet (or potty), in the bathroom. Training pants help children to recognize when they are wet and may be worn every day once toilet training starts; diapers, plastic mattress covers, or training pants may be used at night, which is the most difficult time for the child to master elimination. Finally, parents should respond consistently, showing pleasure every time that the child is successful and remaining calm when accidents occur.

A positive approach includes giving children encouragement and affection regardless whether they succeed, discussing toilet use with the child in a calm and encouraging manner, and potentially providing small treats or special activities to celebrate successes. Picture books for toddlers can provide an easy way for parents to talk to their child about toilet use.

Methods for toilet training children with disabilities or developmental delays are similar to those for children without disabilities, but the onset of training, timing of toilet use, and other factors must be tailored to the individual child's needs, abilities, and preferences.

Disorders and Effects

Children who have developmental delays or physical disabilities may have difficulty with toilet use. Sometimes, mild developmental delays or health problems are first discovered because of problems with toilet training. Special training methods for these children include positive reinforcement; liquid intake, food intake, and bathroom trips scheduled to maximize the chance of success; high-fiber diets; timers to remind children to use the bathroom; and sensors in clothing that trigger an alarm when wet. In some cases of physical malformation or disease, biofeedback, medication, or surgery may be attempted. Even children with very severe disabilities can learn to use the toilet, although they may continue to need reminders or physical assistance.

Toilet use problems of typically developing children include enuresis; fear of the toilet, urine, or feces; encopresis (involuntary movement of bowels) and hiding or playing with feces; retention of feces or urine; and frequent tantrums and accidents. It is normal for children under the age of four occasionally to have any of these problems, stressful as they are for parents. Such problems are especially likely during times of high stress for the child, such as a move, birth of a younger sibling, or other transition, and may resolve on their own as the child adjusts. Constipation and urinary tract infections can occur in children during and after toilet training, so parents should seek medical care if they notice or suspect these conditions.

For older children, medical causes should be ruled out. Family therapy directed at both toilet use and discipline problems is often helpful. Nighttime enuresis, or bed-wetting, is the most common toilet use problem experienced by older children and adults. The cause of most cases of bed-wetting is probably developmental immaturity and may be inherited; it is rarely caused by mental illness, as many once believed. Effective treatments are available for this common problem.

Perspective and Prospects

In European history, toilet training recommendations have ranged from sitting the child on the toilet at three months to giving no training at all. Punitive methods such as tying the child on the toilet, forcing food or drink, or hitting the child were common. By the early twentieth century, two schools of thought on toilet training had developed. Sigmund Freud, the founder of psychoanalysis, believed toilet training that was too early, punitive, indulgent, or sexualized would cause lifelong personality problems. The behaviorist school of thought held that with the right technique, children could be toilet trained quickly at any age in as little as a day. Neither camp had any direct evidence in support of its position.

Freudian ideas dominated popular advice on child care in the United States from the 1940s through the 1960s, leaving many parents anxious about ruining their children's lives with the wrong toilet-training methods. During the 1960s, researchers discovered the variety of actual toilet-training practices around the world. They found that toilet training before thirteen months was not effective and that training after thirteen months through age three was typical and rarely led to problems. Often, children who were punished during toilet training not only developed toilet-use problems but also had nightmares, tantrums, and discipline problems throughout childhood. In addition, they found that children and adults with disabilities—previously thought to be untrainable—could be toilet trained using positive methods. By the early 1980s, developmental psychologists concluded that consistency, encouragement, and patience produce the best long-term results.

—*Kathleen Zanolli, Ph.D.*

See also Anxiety; Bed-wetting; Developmental stages; Emotions: Biomedical causes and effects; Motor skill development; Phobias; Psychiatry, child and adolescent; Soiling; Stress.

For Further Information:

American Academy of Family Physicians. "Toilet Training Your Child." *FamilyDoctor.org*, November, 2010.

American Academy of Family Physicians. "Toilet Training Children with Special Needs." *HealthyChildren.org*, May 11, 2013.

Berk, Laura E. *Child Development*. 8th ed. Boston: Pearson/Allyn & Bacon, 2009.

Faull, Jan. *Mommy, I Have to Go Potty! A Parents" Guide to Toilet Training*. Seattle: Parenting Press, 1996.

Frankel, Alona. *Once upon a Potty*. Buffalo, N.Y.: Firefly Books, 2007.

National Center for Infants, Toddlers and Families. "Learning to Use the Toilet." *ZeroToThree.org*, 2012.

"Potty Training: How to Get the Job Done." *Mayo Foundation for Medical Education and Research*, November 16, 2011.

Preidt, Robert. "Potty-Training Pitfalls and How to Avoid Them." *HealthDay*, June 21, 2013.

Rogers, June. "Child Centered Approach to Bed-Wetting." *Community Practitioner* 76, no. 5 (May, 2003): 163–65.

Schaefer, Charles, and Theresa Foy DiGeronimo. *Ages and Stages: A Parent's Guide to Normal Childhood Development.* New York: Wiley, 2000.

"Toilet Training: Is Your Child Ready?" *Health News* 18, no. 3 (June/July, 2000): 8.

Warner, Penny, and Paula Kelly. *Toilet Training without Tears or Trauma.* Minnetonka, Minn.: Meadowbrook Press, 2003.

TONSILLECTOMY AND ADENOID REMOVAL
Procedures

Anatomy or system affected: Lymphatic system, respiratory system, throat

Specialties and related fields: General surgery, otorhinolaryngology, pediatrics

Definition: The removal of the palatine tonsils (tonsillectomy) or the palatine tonsils and the adenoids (pharyngeal tonsils), in adenotonsillectomy.

Key terms:

abscess: a painful, localized collection of pus in any part of the body; caused by tissue infection and deterioration

antibody: a blood protein that provides immunity against a disease-causing microorganism

crypt: a pit or cavity in the surface of a body organ (such as a tonsil)

lymphocyte: a white blood cell that produces antibodies

lymphoid tissue: tissue that can make lymphocytes; any portion of the lymphatic system

pharynx: the throat

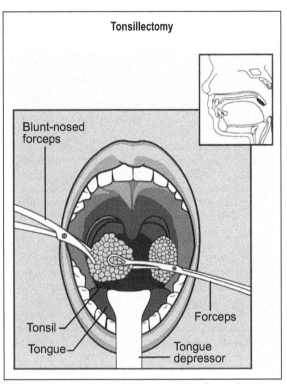

Although this procedure is performed less often than in the past, the removal of the tonsils may still be required by chronic or severe infections; the inset shows the location of the tonsils.

Indications and Procedures

In common use, the term "tonsils" indicates two pinkish palatine tonsils, almond-shaped masses of soft lymphatic tissue located on either side of the back of the mouth. There are two other tonsil types: the lingual tonsils, positioned at the back of the tongue, and the pharyngeal tonsils (adenoids), found in the pharynx and near the nasal passages. Together, the three types of tonsils constitute an irregular band of lymphatic tissue that roughly encircles the throat at the back of the mouth. This tissue band is called Waldeyer's ring. The surface of each tonsil is composed of many deep crypts that, in the case of the palatine tonsils, often become the sites where food debris lodges or sites of bacterial and viral infections. The resulting inflammation of the tonsils is called tonsillitis.

In many cases, acute tonsillitis causes severe throat pain that is easily cured by antibiotic treatment, without recurrence. In others, it returns repeatedly, leading to chronically infected palatine tonsils. Infection of the pharyngeal tonsils (adenoids) causes nasal congestion, and it sometimes produces hearing loss as a result of the obstruction of the Eustachian tubes, which lead from the ear to the throat. This obstruction of the Eustachian tubes may also predispose a person to ear infections.

Severe, chronic tonsillitis is most often treated by surgery to remove the palatine tonsils. When such surgery is carried out, physicians often elect to remove the infected adenoids as well. This double surgery is called adenotonsillectomy. The lingual tonsils are rarely removed because they do not often become infected. While the exact function of the components of Waldeyer's ring is not clear, they are seen as important to the production of bacteria-killing lymphocytes and antibodies, which protect the throat and digestive system from infection. For this reason, unlike in the past, the tonsils are removed only when absolutely necessary, and tonsillitis (or adenoid infection) is most often treated with antibiotics; penicillins and cephalosporins are the drugs of choice.

Usually, the onset of acute tonsillitis is signaled by sudden and severe throat pain, high fever, headache, chills, and diffuse pain in the lymph glands of the neck. These symptoms will normally clear up in five to seven days. The most dangerous form of tonsillitis is caused by streptococcal bacteria, usually the *Streptococcus pyogenes* species. Associated complications increase with the severity of the infection.

Especially severe cases of tonsillitis may lead to a deep infection of the throat involving peritonsillar abscess (quinsy). Many cases of quinsy must be treated by lancing the infected region, causing it to drain. The most severe complications of inappropriately or incompletely treated streptococcal tonsillitis are acute nephritis (kidney disease) and rheumatic fever, which may lead to serious heart problems. Both glomerulonephritis and rheumatic fever are due to autoimmune processes triggered by the infection.

When tonsillectomy is carried out, the adenoids are not removed unless they too cause frequently recurring health problems. The removal of the adenoids alone (adenoidectomy) is sometimes deemed necessary in children when repeated blockages of the nasal passages have caused excessive breathing through the mouth. Prolonged mouth breathing in children can lead to facial deformities because of stress on the developing facial bones.

The tonsils of children are removed under general anesthesia. With adults, local anesthesia is used whenever possible. Tonsillitis in children is much more severe and frequent than in adults because the tonsils decrease in size as one gets older. Similarly, the surgery is more difficult and severe in children because of larger tonsil size.

Uses and Complications

In most cases, tonsillectomy, adenotonsillectomy, and adenoidectomy are simple surgeries with few complications. The entire recovery period from such a procedure is usually several weeks. Most patients experience severe throat pain during the first few days of the recovery period, but this pain diminishes rapidly with time. It is important for the patient to eat soft food during recovery in order to prevent bleeding, which can become dangerous in some cases. Palatine tonsils do not grow back after surgery, although adenoids may sometimes reappear. The secondary adenoids, however, rarely become troublesome. Tonsillectomy, adenotonsillectomy, and adenoidectomy do not lead to freedom from sore throats. They do usually result, however, in a decreased frequency and severity of throat infections.

—Sanford S. Singer, Ph.D.

See also Abscesses; Adenoids; Antibiotics; Bacterial infections; Ear infections and disorders; Hearing loss; Lymphatic system; Otorhinolaryngology; Pediatrics; Pharynx; Quinsy; Sore throat; Strep throat; Streptococcal infections; Tonsillitis; Tonsils.

For Further Information:

Beers, Mark H., et al., eds. *The Merck Manual of Diagnosis and Therapy.* 18th ed. Whitehouse Station, N.J.: Merck Research Laboratories, 2006.

Ferrari, Mario. *PDxMD Ear, Nose, and Throat Disorders.* Philadelphia: PDxMD, 2003.

Icon Health. *Tonsillectomy: A Medical Dictionary, Bibliography, and Annotated Research Guide to Internet References.* San Diego, Calif.: Author, 2004.

"Surgery offers mixed benefits for kids' sleep apnea." *MedlinePlus,* May 21, 2013.

Tierney, Lawrence M., Stephen J. McPhee, and Maxine A. Papadakis, eds. *Current Medical Diagnosis and Treatment 2007.* New York: McGraw-Hill Medical, 2006.

"Tonsil and adenoid removal " discharge." *MedlinePlus,* November 9, 2012.

"Tonsillectomy Might Be Worth It for Some Adults." *MedlinePlus,* April 2, 2013.

Townsend, Courtney M., Jr., et al., eds. *Sabiston Textbook of Surgery.* 18th ed. Philadelphia: Saunders/Elsevier, 2008.

TONSILLITIS

Disease/Disorder

Anatomy or system affected: Ears, lymphatic system, throat

Specialties and related fields: Family medicine, general surgery, otorhinolaryngology, pediatrics

Definition: Inflammation, infection, and enlargement of the palatine tonsils, two small masses of lymphoid tissue located on either side of the back of the throat, and frequently of the pharyngeal tonsils, or adenoids, which are located high in the throat above the soft palate.

Causes and Symptoms

Four small pairs of lymphatic tissue called tonsils together form a ring that circles the nasal cavity and mouth. In children, these tonsils help filter and protect the respiratory and alimentary tracts from infection. As children grow, however, this function dwindles and the tonsils shrink. Tonsillitis, or an infection of these tissues, can be either viral or bacterial in origin. Viral infections are more common in children under three, while older children usually suffer from bacterial infections. A throat culture can determine whether bacteria are present, thus indicating antibiotic treatment.

The two pairs of tonsils most often infected and inflamed are the palatine tonsils, which are those removed in a tonsillectomy, and the adenoids. Symptoms of infected and enlarged tonsils include a sore throat, difficulty swallowing, fever, chills, bad breath, and breathing exclusively through the mouth.

Treatment and Therapy

Viral tonsillitis is self-limiting and typically lasts for five days or less. In these cases, treatment should be symptomatic and includes a soft or liquid diet, warm saltwater or mild antiseptic gargles, throat lozenges, rest, and an analgesic drug such as acetaminophen. If a throat culture indicates bacterial causes, treatment should also include a ten-day course of penicillin or other appropriate drug and a second culture to determine the effectiveness of the treatment.

Occasionally, tonsillectomy (removal of the palatine tonsils) and adenoidectomy (removal of the adenoids) may also be indicated. Because the tonsils play an important role in the development of the immune system, children under three should not be surgically treated. Before the discovery of peni-

---

Information on Tonsillitis

Causes: Bacterial or viral infection

Symptoms: Sore throat, difficulty swallowing, fever, chills, bad breath

Duration: Acute

Treatments: Alleviation of symptoms (soft or liquid diet, warm saltwater or mild antiseptic gargles, throat lozenges, rest, analgesics); antibiotics; tonsillectomy if needed

cillin and other antibiotics, a tonsillectomy was the treatment of choice for children who suffered recurrent tonsillitis. Because of the inherent risks of even minor surgery, however, tonsillectomies are now performed only if infected and enlarged tonsils are so problematic that they threaten to obstruct breathing.

—*Jane Marie Smith, M.S.L.S.*

See also Abscess drainage; Abscesses; Adenoids; Antibiotics; Bacterial infections; Immune system; Inflammation; Nasopharyngeal disorders; Otorhinolaryngology; Pharyngitis; Quinsy; Sore throat; Strep throat; Streptococcal infections; Tonsillectomy and adenoid removal; Tonsils; Viral infections.

For Further Information:

Beers, Mark H., et al., eds. *The Merck Manual of Diagnosis and Therapy.* 18th ed. Whitehouse Station, N.J.: Merck Research Laboratories, 2006.

"The Difference Between a Sore Throat, Strep, and Tonsillitis." *HealthyChildren.org. American Academy of Pediatrics*, May 11, 2013.

Icon Health. *Tonsillitis: A Medical Dictionary, Bibliography, and Annotated Research Guide to Internet References.* San Diego, Calif.: Author, 2004.

Kemper, Kathi J. *The Holistic Pediatrician: A Pediatrician's Comprehensive Guide to Safe and Effective Therapies for the Twenty-five Most Common Ailments of Infants, Children, and Adolescents.* 2d. ed. New York: Quill, 2007.

Lewy, Jennifer, and Brian Randall. "Sore Throat." *Health Library*, Sept. 30, 2012.

Litin, Scott C., ed. *Mayo Clinic Family Health Book.* 4th ed. New York: HarperResource, 2009.

Silverstein, Alvin, Virginia B. Silverstein, and Laura Silverstein Nunn. *Sore Throats and Tonsillitis.* New York: Franklin Watts, 2000.

"Tonsillitus." *HealthyChildren.org.* American Academy of Pediatrics, May 11, 2013.

"Tonsillitis." *KidsHealth.* Nemours Foundation, May 2013.

"Tonsils and Adenoids." *MedlinePlus*, May 22, 2013.

Woolf, Alan D., et al., eds. *The Children's Hospital Guide to Your Child's Health and Development.* Cambridge, Mass.: Perseus, 2002.

TONSILS

Anatomy

Anatomy or system affected: Immune system, lymphatic system

Specialties and related fields: Family medicine, oncology, otorhinolaryngology, pediatrics

Definition: The palatine tonsils are two compact bodies of lymphoid tissue located laterally between the opening of the mouth and the pharynx.

Key terms:

B lymphocytes: immunologically active lymphocytes predominantly found in tonsil tissue

group A streptococcus: the most common bacterial infection of the tonsils

human papillomavirus (HPV): a common virus affecting skin and mucosal surfaces

tonsillar fossa: the bed in which the tonsil sits

tonsillectomy: the common operative procedure used to remove diseased or hypertrophic tonsils

tonsilloliths: small white plugs or stones that form within the crypts of tonsil tissue

Waldeyer's ring: the ring of lymphoid tissue at the upper end of the pharynx consisting of the palatine tonsils laterally, the adenoids superiorly, and the lingual tonsils at the back of the tongue

Structure and Functions

The palatine tonsils are the largest bodies of lymphoid tissue in Waldeyer's ring. In contrast to the adenoid and lingual tonsil tissues, which are diffuse and adherent to the nasopharynx and the base of the tongue, the palatine tonsils are encapsulated by a specialized fascia and are easily dissected from their muscle beds. The tonsil tissues have ten to thirty deep crypts that extend into each tonsil and are lined by stratified squamous epithelium. Each tonsil sits in a tonsillar fossa in the lateral wall of the opening between the mouth and the pharynx. This tonsil bed is composed of three muscles that hold the tonsil in place. The anterior pillar of the tonsil is formed by the palatoglossus muscle, the posterior pillar is formed by the palatopharyngeal muscle, and the floor of the tonsil bed is formed by the superior constrictor muscle of the pharynx. The tonsils get their blood supply primarily at their lower pole from branches of the dorsal lingual and facial arteries. The tonsils" main nerve supply is from the tonsillar branches of the glossopharyngeal nerve.

The tonsils are immunologically active lymphatic organs. The lymphocytes of tonsil tissues are approximately composed of 60 percent B lymphocytes and 40 percent T lymphocytes. The location of the tonsils in the upper part of the aerodigestive tract exposes them to many airborne allergens. Tonsil crypts are able to trap foreign material and transport it to lymphoid follicles. When stimulated by antigens, B cells can proliferate in the germinal centers of the tonsils and produce all five major antibody classes. It has been shown that the immunologic activity of the tonsils and the adenoids in Waldeyer's ring helps protect the entire upper aerodigestive tract. Tonsils are most immunologically active between the ages of four and ten. Although it has been a point of controversy over the years, there is no evidence that removing the tonsils results in any immunologic deficiency.

Disorders and Diseases

Acute tonsillitis is commonly caused by both virus and bacteria. Enlargement of the tonsils without exudates is common with the common cold virus. Epstein-Barr virus may cause mononucleosis with high fever, dysphagia, and tonsillitis characterized by thick gray exudates. The most common bacterial infection of the tonsils is group A streptococcus, which is most commonly seen in children at age five to six years. Before antibiotics, acute streptococcal tonsillitis was a frequent precursor of rheumatic fever.

Recurrent tonsillitis and chronic tonsil hypertrophy are the most common reason for performing tonsillectomy in children. Enlarged tonsils can contribute to airway obstruction and sleep apnea. A peritonsillar abscess is more likely to be seen in young adults. The abscess usually forms between the tonsil and the anterior pillar, causing pain, dysphagia, and drooling, and requires drainage. The combination of exudates and bacteria in the crypts of the tonsils can lead to the formation of plugs or stones called tonsilloliths that can cause pain and bad breath. In severe cases, this condition may also be an indication for tonsillectomy.

Cancer of the palatine tonsil accounts for less than 1 percent of all cancers. Men are affected four times more frequently than women, with an age range between fifty and seventy. More than 70 percent of malignancies are squamous cell carcinomas, with lymphoma accounting for most other tonsil malignancies. Risk factors for squamous cell carcinoma include smoking, drinking alcohol, and infection from HPV.

Perspective and Prospects

Tonsillectomy is one of the oldest recorded surgical procedures, with the first removal of tonsils being described by the Roman surgeon Aulus Cornelius Celsus in 30 CE. Between 1911 and 1917, Samuel J. Crowe, professor of otolaryngology at Johns Hopkins, reviewed one thousand tonsillectomies performed. His description of sharp dissection with low incidence of complications opened the way to common use of this procedure. By the middle part of the twentieth century, there were more than two million tonsillectomies being performed every year in the United States. Between 1915 and 1960, tonsillectomy and adenoidectomy was the most frequently performed surgery in the United States. Today that number has dropped to about 600,000 cases per year in the United States, according to the American Academy of Otolaryngology. The introduction of new techniques such as electrocautery, laser surgery, and high-frequency ablation have further contributed to lowering the complication rate associated with tonsillectomy to the point that about 80 percent of procedures are now done as outpatient surgery.

Recent research regarding cancers of the oral cavity including squamous cell tonsillar cancers has centered on the emerging role of HPV. HPV is one of the most common viruses in the world. In most cases, these viruses are relatively harmless. However, sexually transmitted types HPV 16 and 18 have been strongly linked to cervical cancer, and they are increasingly being recognized as a cause of oral cancer as well. Smoking and drinking alcohol may promote the invasive ability of these viruses in the oral cavity. Recent studies suggest that as many as 25 percent of oral cancers may be positive for HPV. Some studies suggest that HPV-positive oral cancers have a better prognosis than HPV-negative cancers. Another recent study suggests that HPV-positive tumors are more likely to begin within the tonsillar crypts. Understanding the relationship and effect of HPV on tonsil cancer may lead to novel approaches for prevention, targeted therapy, and improved ability to predict the prognosis of these tumors.

—*Chris Iliades, M.D.*

See also Abscess drainage; Abscesses; Antibiotics; Bacterial infections; Head and neck disorders; Immune system; Inflammation; Nasopharyngeal disorders; Otorhinolaryngology; Pharyngitis; Quinsy; Sore throat; Strep throat; Streptococcal infections; Tonsillectomy and adenoid removal; Tonsillitis; Viral infections.

For Further Information:

"Adenoid Removal." *MedlinePlus*. November 9, 2012.

Cummings, W. Charles, et al. *Cummings Otolaryngology: Head and Neck Surgery*. 4th ed. Philadelphia: Mosby/Elsevier, 2005.

Emery, Gene. "Surgery Offers Mixed Benefits For Kids' Sleep Apnea." *MedlinePlus*. May 21, 2013.

"Enlarged Adenoids." *MedlinePlus*. November 12, 2012.

Lalwani, K. Anil. *Current Diagnosis and Treatment in Otolaryngology—Head and Neck Surgery*. 2d ed. New York: McGraw-Hill, 2008.

Luginbuhl, A., et al. "Prevalence, Morphology, and Prognosis of Human Papilloma Virus in Tonsillar Cancer." *Annals of Otology, Rhinology, and Laryngology* 118, no. 10 (October, 2009): 742-749.

Pasha, Raza. *Otolaryngology: Head and Neck Surgery—A Clinical and Reference Guide*. 2d ed. San Diego, Calif.: Plural, 2005.

"Tonsillectomy Facts In The U.S.: From ENT Doctors." *American Academy of Otolaryngology–Head and Neck Surgery*. July 22, 2013.

TOOTH DECAY. *See* CAVITIES.

TOOTH EXTRACTION
Procedure
Anatomy or system affected: Gums, mouth, teeth
Specialties and related fields: Dentistry, orthodontics
Definition: The surgical removal of a tooth because it is damaged by decay, disease, or trauma; threatening the health of other teeth; or near the site of significant disease.

Indications and Procedures

A tooth may have to be extracted for one of several reasons. Impaction is a condition in which a developing tooth is forced into an adjacent tooth, blocking its progress; the impacted tooth can threaten the health and proper alignment of nearby teeth if it is not extracted. The occurrence of crooked or misaligned teeth may also require surgical removal. In tooth decay, dental tissue weakens in a gradual process and can eventually be destroyed. Decay usually begins in the outer layer of the tooth, penetrates to the underlying dentin, and kills the innermost tissue (pulp) of the tooth. Tooth extraction is necessary if this process of decay cannot be halted.

The extraction of teeth is one of the most common procedures in dentistry. Dentists usually perform simple extractions, but they often refer patients needing more complicated procedures to oral surgeons.

In simple extractions, the dentist first applies a local anesthetic to deaden the area surrounding the tooth that is to be pulled. Then, the dentist uses forceps and short levers to loosen the tooth in its socket. The tooth is removed in one piece by breaking the ligaments that hold the tooth in place. Once the tooth has been extracted, the dentist cleans the empty socket and ensures that the blood flowing from the socket is clotting properly. The socket is dressed to protect it and help it heal.

The oral surgeon may use a general anesthetic with a patient needing a complex extraction. The surgeon may need to cut through gum and bone to gain access to the tooth requiring extraction. The tooth may be cut into small pieces before it can be removed. Sutures may be required to close the wound.

The pain caused by extraction usually peaks a few hours after the procedure. Patients are given analgesics (painkillers) and are encouraged to keep the head elevated and to use an ice pack.

—Russell Williams, M.S.W.

See also Braces, orthodontic; Cavities; Dental diseases; Dentistry; Endodontic disease; Gum disease; Oral and maxillofacial surgery; Orthodontics; Periodontal surgery; Periodontitis; Root canal treatment; Teeth; Toothache.

For Further Information:

Christensen, Gordon J. "When It Is Best to Remove a Tooth." *Journal of the American Dental Association* 128, no. 5 (May, 1997): 635–636.

Chwistek, Marcin. "Tooth Extraction." *Health Library*, Mar. 15, 2013.

Columbia University College of Dental Medicine. "Tooth Extraction." *Simple Steps to Better Dental Health*. Aetna, Jan. 18, 2011.

Diamond, Richard. *Dental First Aid for Families*. Ravensdale, Wash.: Idyll Arbor, 2000.

Klatell, Jack, Andrew Kaplan, and Gray Williams Jr., eds. *The Mount Sinai Medical Center Family Guide to Dental Health*. New York: Macmillan, 1991.

Langlais, Robert P., and Craig S. Miller. *Color Atlas of Common Oral Diseases*. 4th ed. Philadelphia: Lippincott Williams & Wilkins, 2009.

Morant, Helen. "NICE Issues Guidelines on Wisdom Teeth." *British Medical Journal* 320, no. 7239 (April 1, 2000): 890.

Smith, Rebecca W. *The Columbia University School of Dental and Oral Surgery's Guide to Family Dental Care*. New York: W. W. Norton, 1997.

"Tooth Disorders." *MedlinePlus*, May 14, 2013.

"Your Dental Health: A Guide for Patients and Families." *Healthnet: Connecticut Consumer Health Information Network*. University of Connecticut Health Center, Nov. 27, 2012.

TORTICOLLIS

Disease/Disorder

Also known as: Spasmodic torticollis

Anatomy or system affected: Muscles, neck

Specialties and related fields: Neurology, physical therapy

Definition: A form of dystonia (muscle rigidity) in which the neck muscles contract involuntarily, causing spasms, abnormal movements, and posture of the neck and head backward (retrocollis), forward (antercollis), or sideways (torticollis).

Causes and Symptoms

Torticollis occurs equally in the sexes and may develop in childhood or adulthood. Its causes are unknown, but some cases seem to be genetic, while others are acquired from secondary damage to the nerves affecting the head or neck muscles. Congenital torticollis may be caused at birth by malpositioning of the head in the uterus or by prenatal injury of the muscles or blood supply in the neck. Torticollis results from abnormal functioning of the basal ganglia, situated at the base of the brain, which control all coordinated movements.

Information on Torticollis

Causes: Unknown; possibly genetic

Symptoms: Muscle spasms, abnormal movements and posture of neck and head, tingling and numbness, headaches

Duration: Short-term to chronic

Treatments: Drug therapy, physical therapy

The first symptoms may appear gradually as the head tends to rotate or turn to one side involuntarily. Other symptoms may involve asymmetry of an infant's head from sleeping on the affected side, enlargement or stiffness of the neck muscles, limited range of head motion, neck pain, and even headaches.

Treatment and Therapy

Because the cause of torticollis is unknown in most cases, presently no certain cure exists. Drug therapy is frequently employed, but these medications often produce only unpredictable, short-term benefits. Some patients experience relief when treated by physiotherapists, who may use local moist heat, ice, ultrasonography, or a custom-fitted soft collar. Surgery is not recommended as an initial treatment, but it has proven helpful in cases unresponsive to medication.

Perspective and Prospects

Torticollis is easiest to correct in infants and children and in adults who receive early treatment. With chronic conditions, tingling and numbness may develop as nerve roots in the cervical spine become depressed. Recent innovative surgical procedures are helpful, but they are not a complete cure for chronic spasmodic torticollis. Patients with long-term torticollis will probably retain some degree of head tilt or rotation.

—John Alan Ross, Ph.D.

See also Botox; Head and neck disorders; Headaches; Muscle sprains, spasms, and disorders; Muscles; Neurology; Neurology, pediatric; Numbness and tingling.

For Further Information:

American Medical Association. *American Medical Association Family Medical Guide*. 4th rev. ed. Hoboken, N.J.: John Wiley & Sons, 2004.

"Dystonias Fact Sheet." *National Institute of Neurological Disorders and Stroke*, February 1, 2013.

Litin, Scott C., ed. *Mayo Clinic Family Health Book*. 4th ed. New York: HarperResource, 2009.

Moore, Keith L., and Arthur F. Dalley II. *Clinically Oriented Anatomy*. 6th ed. Philadelphia: Kluwer/Lippincott Williams & Wilkins, 2010.

Nagler, Willibald. "Rehabilitating a Stiff Neck." *Family Practice News* 36, no. 3 (February 1, 2006): 38.

Noback, Charles R., et al. *The Human Nervous System: Structure and Function*. 6th ed. Totowa, N.J.: Humana Press, 2005.

Pathak, Mayank, Karen Frei, and Daniel Truong. *The Spasmodic Torticollis Handbook: A Guide to Treatment and Rehabilitation*. New York: Demos Health, 2003.

Savitsky, Diane. "Torticollis." *Health Library*, November 26, 2012.

Tomczak, Kinga K., and N. Paul Rosman. "Torticollis." *Journal of Child Neurology* 28, no. 3 (March 2013): 365–78.

TOUCH
Biology

Anatomy or system affected: Nerves, nervous system, skin
Specialties and related fields: Dermatology, neurology
Definition: One of the five special senses; nerve endings and specialized structures in the skin and other tissues send the brain data about the organism's environment, both internal and external.

Key terms:

adaptation: a decreased sensitivity to a stimulus, even though the stimulus may still be present, ultimately resulting in an ever-slowing release of nerve impulses until the impulses stop entirely

exteroceptors: sensory receptors generally located on the skin or body surfaces that supply the brain with information about the external environment in which the body is located

mechanoreceptors: sensory receptors that, when mechanically deformed (such as being pressed on), send nerve impulses causing sensations of pressure and touch

Meissner's corpuscles: receptors at which the sense of a light touch or low-frequency vibrations are detected; also called corpuscles of touch

Merkel's disks: sensory receptors located in deeper layers of epidermal (skin) cells; also called tactile disks

modality: the ability to distinguish one sensation from another; the ability to discriminate light or heavy touch, pain, pressure, vibratory, or hot and cold sensations from one another

Pacinian corpuscles: receptors at which the sensations of heavy touch or deep pressure originate; also called lamellated corpuscles

projection: the process whereby the cerebral cortex determines where the point of a stimulus is located

root hair plexus: a network of sensory receptors located at hair roots that generates an impulse when hairs are moved

Ruffini endings: sensory receptors that respond to heavy and continuous touch and pressure; also called type II cutaneous mechanoreceptors or the end organs of Ruffini

Structure and Functions

An essential attribute of the survival of a species is the ability to detect both the internal and external environment. This is necessary so that appropriate and life-sustaining actions can be taken at all times. When changes or modifications of these environments take place, many responses can occur within an individual, ranging from rolling over during sleep to restore blood flow to an arm to avoiding contact with a prickly pear cactus. This kind of monitoring occurs within the general and special sense organs or structures found in humans and many other species.

One way in which the body monitors its internal and external environments is through the general senses. General sensations include temperature, pain, touch, pressure, vibration, tickle, and proprioception (internal sensations relating to how one's body is situated in space). Sensations of touch usually originate at or very near the skin surface; some originate from receptors found in deeper, subcutaneous (below the skin) layers. Many of the general senses are collectively called the "tactile senses"—notably, those of touch, pressure, vibration, and tickle. In addition, the term "somatic senses" refers to the sensory receptors associated with skin, muscles, joints, and visceral organs. Receptors in the muscles or joints are essential for the awareness of body movement. Visceral receptors play important roles in monitoring changes in body pain, as in stomach pain, hunger, and thirst. The somatic senses provide a means by which the internal and external environments are monitored with regard to touch, pressure, stretch, pain, and temperature. While these terms are not precisely interchangeable, there is overlap in the sensations of touch, pressure, vibration, and tickle with all three categories: general, tactile, and somatic sensations.

Another means whereby a human interacts with the environment is controlled by the special senses. Special senses include taste, vision, smell, hearing, and body equilibrium in space (or balance). Special senses involve relatively large and specialized structures of the tongue, eyes, nose, and ear and inner ear, in contrast to the general senses, in which the structures are relatively simple but are more widely dispersed throughout the entire body. The neurological pathways are also simplified relative to the neurological events that occur in the special senses" organs and pathways. Combined, the general and special senses form an intricate and elegant system that allows for an individual's survival.

Sensations occur when a receptor receives a stimulus from the external or internal world. The result is a neural impulse that can be utilized in the brain to provide some awareness of the body and its immediate environment. Perception results from the interpretation of the sensory information at a conscious level. Conscious awareness of sensory stimulation generally occurs only when a sufficiently large, or sometimes abrupt, change in the status quo happens in either the internal or external environment. At that point, the perception of a sense will be registered and noted in the cerebral cortex.

An untold number of sensory receptors are stimulated at any given second, including receptors that note where each body part is placed—from the tiniest portion of each finger and toe, to the position of the body in a chair. Other receptors respond to inhalation and exhalation pressure changes or feel air brushing past. All receptors work simultaneously and in harmony in a healthy person, but most of this activity is on a subconscious level. Only if a sufficient change in either the internal or external world occurs will a sensation no longer be simply monitored but instead cause a conscious response. An example is feeling the hard coolness of a bench when being seated: at first, the perception of the hard and cold surface is pronounced, but this perception will decrease over time until one seemingly "forgets" about being seated on an uncomfortable bench. This kind of decreased sensitivity to a stimulus is called "adaptation."

The Sense of Touch

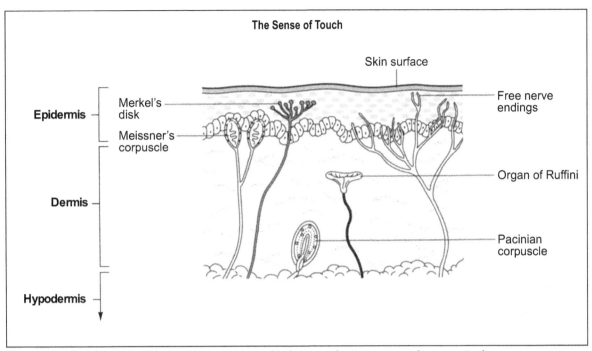

The sensation of touch is produced by special receptors in the skin that respond to temperature and pressure stimuli.

It appears that adaptation prevents the conscious mind from being overloaded with "meaningless" data or data that require no particular response. Adaptation may also allow for new, perhaps more important, stimuli to be noted at the receptor sites. Thus, the adaptation mechanism acts as a "reset" button. Consider the bench example again: in spite of one's "forgetfulness" about the bench being beneath the body, the stimulus is not, in fact, gone. Rather, the mind conveniently elects to ignore the stimulus unless a change occurs that reminds the brain of the bench's presence. This new perception of the bench might recur if a shift in body position causes new receptors to receive stimuli from new contact places between the body and the bench. Eventually, these new sensations will undergo the adaptation process and the bench will once again be "forgotten." (Although thermal equilibrium will be reached between the bench and the person, this process is slow and does not account for the quick rate of adaptation.)

There are four necessary components of sensation: a stimulus, which is generally caused by a change in the environment; a receptor, which can experience a stimulus and produce a generator potential to initiate a nerve impulse; an impulse, which carries the signal from the point of stimulation of the receptor to the brain; and a translation of the impulse within the brain, so that a meaningful interpretation of the kind of sensations experienced, such as a tickle or a floral fragrance, can be made.

All sense receptors are very excitable, but only if stimulated by the specific sensation that they are designed to monitor. This means that sensory receptors are highly specialized in their function. Sense receptors have a low threshold of re-

sponse to the type of stimuli to which they are designed to respond, while having a high threshold of response to other kinds of stimuli. (Pain receptors are an exception to this rule, perhaps because of the variety of stimuli that can include a sense of pain.) An example of specialization of the receptors is seen in the fact that certain regions of the body are more susceptible to sensing a tickle than others. Specialization of receptors is attributed to the unique structures of the receptors, even though all sense receptors contain dendrites from sensory neurons.

At a receptor site, a stimulus may induce a generator potential, which sometimes is called the "receptor potential." The generator potential is a localized and graded response that may reach its threshold if enough depolarization of the dendrites occurs. In other words, if threshold potential is achieved at the receptor, then a nerve impulse will ensue. This kind of response is an all-or-none response, the landmark characteristic of nerve cells.

The cerebral cortex is essential in the perception (interpretation) of a sensation. All different impulses arriving at the cerebral cortex are chemically the same; the only difference between an impulse carrying a message of a soft touch or of a heavy pounding is where the impulse arrives within the cerebral cortex. Impulses arriving at different locations of the cortex allow the brain to identify, classify, and locate the origins of a stimulus. The ability to distinguish one sensation from another is called "modality"; the ability to locate precisely the point at which the stimulus is applied is called "projection". Modality and projection are functions of the cerebral cortex. In addition, the cortex can prompt many shifts in body position (such as stretching after reading) or body chemistry (such as the release of epinephrine to increase heart rate and blood flow in a crisis) if a response to the stimulus is deemed necessary.

Receptors can be classified according to the location or type of stimuli that cause the receptors to respond. Touch receptors can be classified as exteroceptors by virtue of the fact that these sensory receptors are externally located, mainly on the skin surface. Other classes of somatic receptors are located internally. Visceroreceptors monitor internal organs for data on hunger, thirst, pressure, and nausea. Proprioceptors monitor the muscles, tendons, joints, and inner ear for exacting knowledge of body position and body movement.

"Mechanoreceptors" are an alternative classification for touch receptors. This label is based on the type of stimulus—a mechanical displacement or disfiguring, for which touch receptors have a low threshold. Light touch is felt when the skin is very gently touched and no indentation or distortion of the skin results. Touch pressure is felt when a heavy touch causes a distortion of the skin surface, either laterally, as in a tugging sensation, or vertically, as in a depression of the skin surface.

Six types of touch receptors have been identified in the human anatomy: root hair plexuses, free nerve endings, tactile disks (or Merkel's disks), corpuscles of touch (or Meissner's corpuscles), type II cutaneous mechanoreceptors (or end organs of Ruffini), and Pacinian corpuscles (or lamellated corpuscles). At these structures, a mechanical stimulus can be transformed into a sensation, provided that the stimulus is sufficiently strong to bring about a threshold potential.

Root hair plexuses are located in networks at the hair roots. On the scalp, these generate a sensation of touch when the hair is being pulled, brushed, or stroked. On the body surface, these receptors are sensitive to movement of the hair, as can occur if a small breeze passes over the skin or if a silk scarf is dragged lightly over the skin hairs. Root hair plexuses are not structurally supported, nor are they protected by any surrounding structure.

Free nerve endings are everywhere on the skin surface and seem to be responsive to many kinds of stimuli. These little dendritic processes of sensory neurons are not protected or supported by surrounding structures.

Made of disklike formations of dendrites, Merkel's disks, or tactile disks, are found in the deeper layers of the skin. Merkel's disks are particularly abundant on the fingertips, palms, soles of the feet, eyelids, lips, nipples, clitoris, tip of the penis, and tip of the tongue. Merkel's disks are particularly suited to receiving stimuli of fine touch and pressure.

Meissner's corpuscles, or corpuscles of touch, are egg-shaped dendritic masses that are sensitive to light touch and vibrations of a low frequency. Found in the hairless portions of the skin, these receptors are also used in making judgments about the textures of whatever the skin may contact. Two or more sensory nerve fibers enter each corpuscle of touch; the nerve fibers terminate as tiny knobs within the corpuscle. In addition, Meissner's corpuscles contain dendritic extensions. The entire mass is enclosed in connective tissue, which offers some support and protection to the disks. Corpuscles of touch

are found in the external genitalia, tip of the tongue, eyelids, lips, fingertips, palms and soles, and nipples of both sexes.

The end organs of Ruffini, or type II cutaneous mechanoreceptors, are found all over the body but especially in the deep dermis (skin) and deeper tissues below the dermis. These are also called "corpuscles of Ruffini" and are responsive to heavy and continuous touch and pressure.

Finally, the Pacinian corpuscles are relatively large ellipses that are found in the subcutaneous tissue (below the skin) and deeper subcutaneous tissues. Also known as "lamellated corpuscles," these touch receptors are found under tissues that contain mucous membranes, serous membranes, joints and tendons, muscles, mammary glands, and external genitalia. Pacinian receptors are sensitive to deep and heavy pressure and vibrations of low frequency. As such, these receptors detect pulsating, vibrating stimuli. There is an abundance of Pacinian receptors in the penis, vagina, feet and hands, clitoris, urethra, breasts, tendons, and ligaments. Inside each ellipsoid are dendrites from sensory nerves; the bundle itself is wrapped in connective tissue that can serve as a protective support.

Disorders and Diseases

Loss of tactile senses is a symptom rather than a disease. In general, a lost ability to sense touch, pressure, vibration, or tickle is a result of physical damage to a group of nerves or of a disease of the nervous system. Sensory receptors are not themselves targets of disease, but they can be physically or chemically impaired, especially if the skin is severely damaged.

An example of severe damage to the skin that will cause a loss of tactile sensations is a third-degree burn of the body. Third-degree burns are marked by the total destruction of the full thickness of the skin. This destruction includes the epidermis, the dermis, and any associated skin structures, such as secretion glands, hair, and the general sensory receptors. No pain is sensed when regions of the body that have received a third-degree burn are touched, because the nerve fibers that innervate the touch receptors and the free nerve endings, as well as nerves located in the subcutaneous layers, have been destroyed by the burn. In such cases, total destruction of the nerve fibers and the skin has occurred. Third-degree burns can have a charred, dry appearance or a mahogany or ash-white color. Regeneration of the dermis and the subcutaneous structures is slow and painful as the healing occurs. Although skin grafting can facilitate the regeneration process, it is not uncommon for scarring to result from the rapid contraction of the wounded area as it heals.

The sense of touch is largely lost in scar tissue, since new nerve fibers cannot be formed. (Nerve cells are formed only during gestation and early life and are designed to last a lifetime.) Some tactile senses can return to scarred regions through a process called "sprouting." This process involves the branching forth, or the sprouting, of dendritic processes originating in undamaged nerve cells near to, but removed from, the injured site. In this kind of recovery, the healthy nerves assist in restoring tactile senses, to a limited degree, in the damaged regions.

Aside from a total loss of sensation, a sense of numbness can indicate a loss of proper blood circulation to a body region. For example, if one sits or folds oneself into a position so that a leg is receiving pressure from other body parts, the sensation of touch and pressure on the leg will eventually cause a sense of numbness; a form of pain ensues that feels like a tingling sensation that is often described as "pins and needles" all over the leg. The loss of blood circulation to the numbed region actually triggers pain receptors, sending an impulse to the cerebral cortex that warns of an odd feeling. The cerebral cortex will perceive the problem and command responses of the skeletal and muscular systems to change body position. Proprioceptors will sense the new body position, and as blood circulation restores a normal environment, the tingling decreases until it disappears. Numbness can also be a symptom of nerve damage or can result from the use of certain drugs, such as Novocain, that are used in dental and medical applications.

Changing of body position is an important outcome of the touch, pressure, and pain senses. Without the ability to change the position of the body, as can happen in some elderly or quadriplegic persons, damage to the areas on which the whole of the body is resting can occur. Neglect of these persons in home care or in health care facilities will result in bedsores (pressure ulcers) developing at these pressure points. If left unchecked, these bedsores will grow and can lead to gangrene. As a part of their care, such individuals require physical therapy or physical aid in moving body parts and in changing sitting and sleeping positions several times each day.

Damage to the right lobe of the brain may cause abnormalities in the senses of touch and pressure, which in turn can cause a deficit in the ability to locate precisely where a tactile sensation originates on the body surface (the ability to project tactile sensations), making adjustment to and interaction with the external environment challenging. Right lobe damage, therefore, may give rise to a condition called "passive touch deficit." Passive touch deficits are revealed by an impaired ability to discriminate touch sensations and by altered thresholds of touch and pressure that cause a sensation to be perceived.

Damage to the right lobe may also lead to deficits in active touch, meaning that such descriptors as size, shape, and texture cannot be readily discerned in touch tests. Generally, right lobe damage also leads to the loss of fine motor control of the fingers, which is especially challenging for musicians, authors, computer operators, visual artists, surgeons, and others who require exacting motor control of the fingers.

Sometimes, lesions in the right lobe of the cerebral cortex will lead to a condition called "tactile agnosia." Tactile agnosia will occur only in the left hand, given the contralateral arrangement of the hands and neurological pathways to the cortex. The symptom of tactile agnosia is the diminished ability, or the inability, to identify common items (such as a key, pencil, or comb) when it is placed in the left hand. Fortunately, this condition is not common.

Another interesting form of loss of touch can occur in an odd behavior called "neglect." Again, the problem with this loss of sensation originates from damage to the cerebral cortex, not to the touch receptors of the body. In neglect, lesions of the right parietal lobe are generally present but the contralateral neural pathway results in lost sense on the left side of the body. The ability to perceive a left-side stimulus is lost; patients may not notice anything in the internal or external environments on the left side of the body. In left-side neglect, patients may step into the right leg of a pair of pants but not the left leg and will not know that anything is wrong. Left-side neglect can also result in only right turns being made in walking patterns, and stimuli from the visual, auditory, and tactile sensations are not at all perceived. The sensation is traveling from the point of stimulation, but the cerebral cortex cannot process the sensation.

Finally, the issue of the phantom limb has significance in the medically related aspects of the sense of touch. "Phantom limb" is the term used to describe a sensation that seems to arise from a limb that has been amputated. Patients who have lost body parts to amputation, either surgically or mechanically (as a result of trauma such as a car accident or an accident while operating a meat-processing machine), often describe sensations of itching, burning, or heat or cold, as well as other general sensations in the limb that is missing.

Although the limb—such as a finger, toe, or part of a leg or arm—may be absent, general sensations seem to arise from these absent body parts because of the neurological pathways that would normally connect the limbs to the cerebral cortex. In addition, a sensation is only as accurate as the cortex's ability to locate and identify the stimulus. This recall is called "perception." Perception, however, is not an exact science; it results from experiences and associations that teach the cortex how to sort and analyze sensory data. Much information comes into the brain on common pathways, as if only a few streets led into a special city and all cars wanted to travel those streets to get there. An index finger may have had priority access to the paths during the training days of a young concert pianist. If, however, the pianist loses that index finger, neurological activity along the pathway to which the finger was once connected has not stopped. In fact, during the adjustment and recovery period immediately following the amputation, neurological activity may be heightened. As these sensory receptors and neurons send impulses along the avenues as before, these impulses will now be dominant in the absence of the index finger. Although the conscious mind is fully aware that the finger is absent, the subconscious mind has not yet acclimated itself to the change. Thus, a false association is made before the conscious mind can "correct" the perception and realize that the stimulus must be originating from a place other than the absent body part.

Perspective and Prospects

Responsiveness to different kinds of touch at different locations on the body reveals a relationship between receptor structures and their subsequent function. Specifically, the hands of the human body are exquisitely sensitive to touch.

The calculated innervation (number of nerve connections) for touch alone on the palms of the hands is seventeen thousand units.

On the palms, the most abundant type of touch receptors are Meissner's corpuscles. Accounting for 43 percent of all the touch receptors of the palms, they are responsible for the sensations of texture, light touches, and low-frequency vibrations and clearly play an important role in the human experience. Meissner's corpuscles are particularly abundant on the tips of all fingers and both thumbs. Although these receptors adapt at a moderately rapid pace, they are not so fast at adapting that the pleasure of stroking a cat or caressing a baby's head is lost.

After Meissner's corpuscles, Merkel's disks are second most abundant on the palms. Constituting 25 percent of the touch innervation density, these cells are suited for fine touch and pressure. Mainly confined to the digits" and thumbs" full length, Merkel's disks are important in tactile pursuits such as painting, drawing, sewing, writing, and dentistry. They are equally important in the expression of loving gestures to other people, animals, and plants via touch. Merkel's disks are slow to adapt; thus, these sensations are somewhat sustained.

Constituting 19 percent of the palms" innervation are the Ruffini endings. These are scattered throughout the palm surface area and are not localized. Ruffini endings are receptive to heavy and continuous touch and are slow adaptors. While a person is carrying a stack of books, for example, these endings are "firing" the nerves that connect to them.

Finally, making up only 13 percent of the palms" innervation to touch are the Pacinian corpuscles. Having a slight clustering in the fingertips, these are very quick at adapting to stimuli. They are receptive to deep and heavy pressure, such as the sensations that can be felt while massaging the hands.

Hairless regions of the skin, such as the palms, soles, penis, and vagina, contain Merkel's disks, Ruffini endings, Meissner's corpuscles, and Pacinian corpuscles. The combinations of receptors within these regions make these body parts acutely aware of and sensitive to light or heavy touch, rough or velvety textures, and pulsating or vibratory stimuli. These areas are also associated with pleasure centers of the body, in part because of their heightened tactile sensitivity.

Hairy skin, such as on the legs, chest, and arms, contains tactile disks, Ruffini endings, root hair plexuses, and Pacinian corpuscles. These body parts are sensitive to vibratory stimuli, breezes and other forms of displacement of body hairs, and pressure and tugging or pulling of the skin.

People are often willing to go to extra lengths to take care of their special sensory organs—the eyes, ears, mouth, and nose—because of their unique and important functions in the human body, but rarely do the general senses receive such attention. In spite of being largely overlooked, the general senses provide humans and other species with something so fundamental to life that it is often forgotten: touch. Offering a means of experiencing the most intimate communication and connection between self and others or between self and the environment, touch is an integral aspect of life.

—*Mary C. Fields, M.D.*

See also Acupressure; Amputation; Burns and scalds; Grafts and grafting; Nervous system; Neuralgia, neuritis, and neuropathy; Neurology; Neurology, pediatric; Numbness and tingling; Physical rehabilitation; Sense organs; Skin.

For Further Information:
Møller, Aage R. *Sensory Systems: Anatomy, Physiology, and Pathophysiology.* 2d ed. Richardson, Tex.: Author, 2012.
National Institute of Dental and Craniofacial Research. "NIH Scientists Discover Molecule Triggers Sensation of Itch." *National Institutes of Health*, May 23, 2013.
National Institute of Neurological Disorders and Stroke. "Pain: Hope Through Research." *National Institutes of Health*, July 10, 2013.
Piergrossi, Joseph. "Untangling the Source of Ouch and Itch." *National Institute of General Medical Sciences, National Institutes of Health*, June 12, 2013.
Schmidt, Robert F., ed. *Fundamentals of Sensory Physiology.* Translated by Marguerite A. Biederman-Thorson. Rev. 3d ed. Berlin: Springer, 1986.
Shier, David N., Jackie L. Butler, and Ricki Lewis. *Hole's Essentials of Human Anatomy and Physiology.* 11th ed. Boston: McGraw-Hill, 2011.
Tortora, Gerard J., and Bryan Derrickson. *Principles of Anatomy and Physiology.* 13th ed. Hoboken, N.J.: John Wiley & Sons, 2012.
Wolfe, Jeremy M., et al. *Sensation and Perception.* 2d ed. Sunderland, Mass.: Sinauer, 2009.

Tourette's syndrome
Disease/Disorder

Also known as: Gilles de la Tourette syndrome

Anatomy or system affected: Brain, muscles, musculoskeletal system, nerves, nervous system, psychic-emotional system

Specialties and related fields: Biochemistry, family medicine, genetics, neurology, psychiatry, psychology

Definition: A disorder characterized by recurrent, multiple motor tics and one or more vocal tics that causes stress and impairs social functioning.

Key terms:
coprolalia: involuntary vocalization involving the uttering of obscenities or other socially inappropriate comments
copropraxia: a complex motor tic that involves involuntary, obscene gestures
echolalia: repetition of the words or gestures of others
palilalia: repetition of one's own words
tic: a sudden, rapid, recurrent, irresistible, nonrhythmic, and stereotyped movement; tics may involve motor movements, sudden vocalizations, or a combination of both

Causes and Symptoms

Tourette syndrome is a disorder marked by multiple motor tics, involuntary vocalizations, and significant impairment of social functioning, often resulting in low self-esteem. For a diagnosis of Tourette syndrome, the symptoms must persist for a period of at least one year, although they may decrease or subside during that time for brief periods of three months or less. Onset must be prior to eighteen years of age. The motor and vocal tics manifested must not be a consequence of drug use or the result of a previously existing medical condition such as Huntington's chorea.

Definitive causes for Tourette syndrome remain under investigation. Research in the late 1990s and early 2000s included an exploration of genetic factors that might cause a susceptibility to the disorder and studies of the frequency of the disorder in subsequent generations within families. Studies in brain chemistry were also conducted.

Tourette syndrome differs from a disease in that sufferers manifest a number of symptoms that occur together. Symptoms may be seen in sequence or in combination. Simple motor or vocal tics are most often first noticed in children between the ages of two and seven, but initial symptoms may not be seen until the teenage years. Typically, the first symptoms noticed are simple motor tics such as eye blinking, tongue protrusion, facial grimacing, or other movements in the head area, such as grunting, coughing, throat clearing, or unusual vocalizations.

Complex motor tics include such behaviors as involuntary touching, knee bends, touching of objects in sequence, or other repetitive behaviors. Although many patients first display eye blinks, the anatomical location, severity, and frequency of the tics may change over time. As a child matures, the tics may involve other areas of the body, such as the torso or the limbs.

The social implications of this disorder are as important as the physical ones for a child with Tourette syndrome. Such motor tics as touching inappropriately and involuntary utterances and outbursts can be disastrous to both self-image and social standing. Palilalia, echolalia, coprolalia, copropraxia, and bizarre behaviors brought about by involuntary compulsions cause affected children much anxiety. That their symptoms may mimic or coexist with other disorders is another concern. Although some children may outgrow the disorder in their twenties, generally Tourette syndrome is a lifelong disorder. With concentration and relaxation techniques, tics may be delayed or suppressed for brief periods, but they present ongoing problems for those living with Tourette syndrome.

Treatment and Therapy

By the turn of the twenty-first century, physical treatment for Tourette syndrome involved a combination of relaxation techniques and medication therapy. Counseling has also proven useful in conjunction with other treatments, by helping patients to deal with the social and emotional effects of this disorder. Relaxation techniques such as visualization of a calm setting and a variety of related therapies have proven successful in reducing the number and severity of the tics. Touch therapy and related techniques such as stroking and rocking have been helpful in reducing stress, as have some forms of massage.

Music is another effective means of relaxing the mind and the body. Some researchers have recommended that musical selections with a beat close to one's resting heartbeat are the most effective in reducing stress levels. Musical instruments

---

Information on Tourette's Syndrome

Causes: Unknown; possibly genetic
Symptoms: Repetitive eye blinking, tongue protrusion, facial grimacing, or other head movements; unusual vocalizations (grunting, coughing, throat clearing); involuntary touching, knee bends, touching of objects in sequence, or other repetitive behaviors
Duration: Chronic
Treatments: Relaxation techniques, drug therapy, counseling, touch therapy, music therapy

---

and other forms of creative expression have proved to be effective tools against stress and associated tics. Hobbies, diaries, written expression, and counseling have all been used effectively to treat the physical and emotional symptoms of Tourette syndrome.

A number of medication therapies are also being used. The blood-pressure medication clonidine has been helpful in the treatment of tics, with some side effects. Antiseizure medications have also had success, but with undesirable side effects. Children also suffering from related disorders such as attention-deficit disorder (ADD) have been treated successfully with Ritalin. Drugs such as Anafinil and Prozac have proven useful in treating obsessive-compulsive disorder and other anxiety disorders sometimes seen in conjunction with Tourette syndrome. Dopamine blockers such as fluphenazine and haloperidol have also been shown to reduce tics, but these medications can also cause unwanted side effects.

Perspective and Prospects

Treatment and understanding have evolved substantially since 1885 when Georges Gilles de la Tourette first identified Tourette syndrome, which was thought to be a psychological disorder influenced by environmental factors. Many significant gains have been made since the 1980s in the clinical and scientific understanding of this complex disorder. Research in the late 1990s and early 2000s explored connections between brain chemistry and Tourette syndrome, with some studies indicating that abnormal dopamine and serotonin levels in the brain may be a factor. The role of genetics in the transmission and manifestation of the disorder has also been studied extensively, although the specific genes involved in Tourette syndrome are still being identified. Promising new medications continue to be developed as well.

—*Kathleen Schongar, M.S., M.A.*

See also Antianxiety drugs; Anxiety; Attention-deficit disorder (ADD); Learning disabilities; Motor skill development; Nervous system; Neurology; Neurology, pediatric; Obsessive-compulsive disorder; Psychiatric disorders; Psychiatry; Psychiatry, child and adolescent; Tics.

For Further Information:

American Psychiatric Association. *Diagnostic and Statistical Manual of Mental Disorders: DSM-IV-TR*. 4th ed. Arlington, Va.: American Psychiatric, 2000.

Brill, Marlene Targ. *Tourette Syndrome*. Brookfield, Conn.:

Millbrook Press, 2002.

Cohen, Donald J., Ruth D. Bruun, and James F. Leckman, eds. *Tourette's Syndrome and Tic Disorders*. New York: John Wiley & Sons, 1988.

Conelea, Christine, et al. "The Impact of Tourette Syndrome in Adults: Results from the Tourette Syndrome Impact Study." Community Mental Health Journal 49, no. 1 (2013): 110–120.

Koplewicz, Harold S. "Tourette Syndrome." In *It's Nobody's Fault: New Hope and Help for Difficult Children and Their Parents*. New York: Three Rivers Press, 1997.

Kushner, Howard I. *A Cursing Brain? The Histories of Tourette Syndrome*. Rev. ed. Cambridge, Mass.: Harvard University Press, 2000.

Parker, James N., and Philip M. Parker, eds. *The Official Parent's Sourcebook on Tourette Syndrome*. San Diego, Calif.: Icon Health, 2002.

Rosenblum, Laurie. "Tourette Syndrome." *Health Library*, April 3, 2013.

Shimberg, Elaine Fantle. *Living with Tourette Syndrome*. New York: Simon & Schuster, 1995.

"Tourette Syndrome." *Mayo Clinic*, August 10, 2012.

TOXEMIA

Disease/Disorder

Also known as: Preeclampsia, eclampsia

Anatomy or system affected: Blood vessels, circulatory system, reproductive system

Specialties and related fields: Obstetrics

Definition: A common disorder of pregnancy characterized by hypertension and proteinuria (protein in the urine). When severe, toxemia can affect multiple organ systems and even lead to seizures.

Causes and Symptoms

The precise cause of toxemia is unknown. Multiple theories exist, the leading ones pointing to an immunologic or vascular cause. Toxemia occurs after twenty weeks of gestation and is associated with a number of risk factors, including nulliparity, twin gestation, family history of toxemia, diabetes, antiphospholipid syndrome, chronic hypertension, and renal disease.

Symptoms and signs that are required for a diagnosis of toxemia are systolic blood pressure over 140 and diastolic blood pressure over 90 across a span of six hours and urine with protein in excess of 300 milligrams over twenty-four hours. Other symptoms may be present, such as facial edema. In severe cases, headache, visual changes, upper abdominal pain, decreased urine output, hyperreflexia (overactive reflexes), or fluid in the lungs may be present. These symptoms may be accompanied by laboratory abnormalities indicating liver, kidney, red blood cell, or platelet disorders. Toxemia may also manifest as seizures, with the risk of concomitant stroke, which is termed eclampsia. In women with prolonged preeclampsia, uteroplacental insufficiency (decreased blood supply to the fetus) may occur, leading to oligohydramnios (too little amniotic fluid) and/or restriction in fetal growth.

Treatment and Therapy

The treatment of toxemia depends on the severity of the

Information on Toxemia

Causes: Unknown; risk factors include first pregnancy, more than one fetus, family history of toxemia, diabetes, antiphospholipid syndrome, chronic hypertension, renal disease

Symptoms: Elevated blood pressure and facial edema; in severe cases, headache, visual changes, upper abdominal pain, decreased urine output, overactive reflexes, fluid in lungs

Duration: Chronic during pregnancy

Treatments: Depends on severity and gestational age of fetus; may include blood pressure medications (hydralazine, labetalol), bed rest, delivery of baby

---

disease and the gestational age of the fetus. High blood pressure can be controlled with medications such as hydralazine or labetalol. The patient is placed on bed rest, and the patient's fluid status is monitored. Delivery of the infant and placenta is curative. While this is the treatment of choice when the infant is full term, the treatment plan in preterm pregnancies is more complex.

In a preterm pregnancy, ultrasonography and fetal heart tone monitoring are carried out to check for any adverse effects of toxemia on the fetus. If toxemia becomes severe or there is evidence of fetal compromise, then the decision for delivery may be made, even if the infant is preterm. If delivery is anticipated, then the patient will receive intravenous magnesium to decrease the risk of seizures. If the fetus is less than thirty-four weeks of gestation, then the patient also receives steroid injections to facilitate fetal lung maturity. If seizures occur, a bolus of magnesium can be given to stop the seizures, and stabilization measures are taken to maximize maternal and fetal safety.

—*Anne Lynn S. Chang, M.D.*

See also Blood pressure; Childbirth; Childbirth complications; Embryology; Hypertension; Obstetrics; Preeclampsia and eclampsia; Pregnancy and gestation; Premature birth; Seizures; Vascular medicine; Vascular system; Women's health.

For Further Information:

Brewer, Thomas H. *Metabolic Toxemia of Late Pregnancy: A Disease of Malnutrition*. Rev. ed. New Canaan, Conn.: Keats, 1998.

Cunningham, F. Gary, et al, eds. *Williams Obstetrics*. 23d ed. New York: McGraw-Hill, 2010.

Gabbe, Steven G., et al, eds. *Obstetrics: Normal and Problem Pregnancies*. 6th ed. Philadelphia: Churchill Livingstone/Elsevier, 2012.

"High Blood Pressure in Pregnancy." *MedlinePlus*, May 28, 2013.

"High Blood Pressure in Pregnancy." *National Heart, Lung, and Blood Institute*, May 29, 2013.

"Preeclampsia and Eclampsia." *National Institute of Child Health and Human Development*, Apr. 3, 2013.

Savitsky, Diane, and Andrea Chisholm. "Pre-Eclampsia." *Health Library*, Mar. 14, 2013.

Sibai, Baha M. "Treatment of Hypertension in Pregnant Women." *New England Journal of Medicine* 335, no. 4 (July, 1996): 257–265.

Toxic shock syndrome

Disease/Disorder

Anatomy or system affected: All

Specialties and related fields: Critical care, emergency medicine, general surgery, gynecology, internal medicine, microbiology

Definition: A potentially fatal infection causing failure of multiple organs of the body, most notably associated with tampon use.

Causes and Symptoms

Toxic shock syndrome, an overwhelming and potentially life-threatening infection, is most commonly known for its association with tampon use in young women. Although this is still the most commonly affected population, toxic shock syndrome can affect nonmenstruating women and men as well.

Two distinct organisms can be responsible for toxic shock syndrome, each associated with a different constellation of symptoms. The bacteria *Staphylococcus aureus* (staph) causes all cases of menstrual toxic shock syndrome, and some nonmenstrual cases as well. Nonmenstrual cases can arise from an infected surgical wound or infections elsewhere in the body. The bacteria *Streptococcus pyogenes* (strep) is re-

---

In the News: Sinus Infections Leading to Toxic Shock Syndrome in Children

A retrospective study at The Children's Hospital of Denver found that rhinosinusitis (infection of the nose and paranasal sinuses) can be a primary cause of toxic shock syndrome in young children. The study published in the June, 2009, issue of *Archives of Otolaryngology—Head and Neck Surgery* describes data from seventy-six pediatric patients admitted between 1983 and 2000 who were identified through medical records as having toxic shock syndrome. Of these patients, 21 percent had rhinosinusitis. Study authors, including Kenny Chan, chief of Pediatric Otolaryngology at Children's Hospital of Denver and professor of otolaryngology at the University of Colorado, suggest that physicians consider rhinosinusitis a primary cause of toxic shock syndrome when another site of infection cannot be identified. Because toxic shock syndrome can be fatal, quick treatment and identification of the source are critical.

Sinus infections have not been well reported as a potential primary source of toxic shock syndrome. A study published by Paul D. Gittelman from New York University Medical Center and colleagues found an association between toxic shock syndrome and rhinologic surgery and medical devices. The study, published in *Laryngoscope* in 1991, included 140 adult patients. Toxic shock syndrome was linked to circulating exotoxin of a toxogenic strain of *Staphylococcus aureus*. About 30 percent of patients in the study selected for surgery were *S. aureus* carriers, with toxin-capable isolates identified in 40 percent of those tested. The study also found users of cocaine, topical decongestants, and steroid sprays had a statistically higher rate of *S. aureus* compared to nonusers.

—*Sandra Ripley Distelhorst*

Information on Toxic Shock Syndrome

Causes: Bacterial infections with staphylococci (menstrual cases, associated with tampon use) or streptococci (nonmenstrual cases, as from injuries, surgical wounds, infections elsewhere in body)

Symptoms: In staph cases, high fever, lightheadedness, low blood pressure, diffuse rash, redness and irritation of eyes, mouth, and vagina, vomiting, diarrhea, muscle aches, jaundice, kidney failure, confusion; in strep cases, severe pain and swelling at injury site, fever, confusion, low blood pressure, tissue death (necrotizing fasciitis)

Duration: Acute

Treatments: Hospitalization, intravenous fluids, antibiotics, removal of cause (tampon, bandages or packing), sometimes surgery to remove infected tissue

---

sponsible for nonmenstrual toxic shock syndrome only.

All patients with staph toxic shock syndrome have high fevers, light-headedness associated with low blood pressure, and a diffuse rash resembling a sunburn. The eyes, mouth, and vagina can become red and irritated, and several weeks following the initial illness, the skin on the palms and soles begins to slough. Other symptoms may include vomiting, diarrhea, muscle aches, jaundice, kidney failure, and confusion.

Strep toxic shock syndrome typically arises at a site of minor trauma to the skin, either an injury or a recent surgical wound. Severe pain at the site is the most common finding. The patient may have a fever, confusion, and low blood pressure. Severe swelling at the site of infection can lead to major damage to the skin and underlying tissues; this necrotizing fasciitis (so-called flesh-eating bacteria) is a well-known manifestation of strep toxic shock syndrome.

Treatment and Therapy

Because of the severity of the illness, almost all patients with toxic shock syndrome require hospitalization. Intravenous fluids and other medications are administered to improve the blood pressure, and antibiotics are used to kill the bacteria and to decrease production of the toxins that they release.

In cases of menstrual toxic shock syndrome, removal of the tampon is critical. For infected surgical wounds, removal of bandages and packing is required, as well as occasional removal of infected tissue with surgery.

In cases of necrotizing fasciitis, surgical removal of infected tissue is necessary and may involve a loss of a significant amount of skin and underlying muscle.

Perspective and Prospects

The initial association of toxic shock syndrome with highly absorbent tampons in the 1980s led to a withdrawal of such products from the market. Consequently, the number of cases of menstrual toxic shock syndrome has significantly declined; however, extended tampon use remains a risk factor for toxic shock syndrome. Frequent tampon changes and tampon use only on the heaviest days of bleeding should reduce this risk. Women who have had menstrual toxic shock syndrome or other problems with staph infections should avoid tampon use.

—*Gregory B. Seymann, M.D.*

See also Antibiotics; Bacterial infections; Bacteriology; Genital disorders, female; Gynecology; Menstruation; Methicillin-resistant *Staphylococcus aureus* (MRSA) infections; Necrotizing fasciitis; Staphylococcal infections; Streptococcal infections; Wounds; Women's health.

For Further Information:

Beers, Mark H., et al., eds. *The Merck Manual of Diagnosis and Therapy*. 19th ed. Whitehouse Station, N.J.: Merck, 2011.

Icon Health. *Toxic Shock Syndrome: A Medical Dictionary, Bibliography, and Annotated Research Guide to Internet References*. San Diego, Calif.: Icon Health, 2004.

Mandell, Gerald L., John E. Bennett, and Raphael Dolin, eds. *Mandell, Douglas, and Bennett's Principles and Practice of Infectious Diseases*. 7th ed. New York: Churchill Livingstone/ Elsevier, 2010.

Parker, James N., and Philip M. Parker, eds. *The Official Patient's Sourcebook on Toxic Shock Syndrome*. San Diego, Calif.: Icon Health, 2002.

Sheen, Barbara. *Toxic Shock Syndrome*. San Diego, Calif.: Lucent Books, 2006.

Vorvick, Linda J., Jatin M Vyas, and David Zieve. "Toxic Shock Syndrome." *Medline Plus*, August 15, 2012.

Wood, Debra. "Toxic Shock Syndrome." *Health Library*, November 26, 2012.

TOXICOLOGY

Specialty

Anatomy or system affected: All

Specialties and related fields: All

Definition: The scientific study of the effects of poisonous substances (also known as toxicants or toxins) on organisms. Poisons interfere with physiological functions and are typically chemicals generated either naturally (such as poisonous plants, venomous snakes, pathogenic microorganisms, and geochemical cycling) or artificially (industrial products such as PCBs, tetraethyl lead, and certain pharmaceutical or personal care products).

Key terms:

acute toxicity: rapid development of disease symptoms following exposure of an organism to toxic agents (ranging from a few minutes to several hours; typically less than fourteen days)

chronic toxicity: slow or cumulative expression of disease symptoms following exposure of organisms to toxic agents (typically more than one year)

poison: a chemical substance that can cause injury, sickness, or death to organisms; may be from natural or artificial sources

toxicant: the preferred term used to denote a poisonous substance strictly from artificial sources that has been introduced into the environment and has a capacity to adversely affect humans, wildlife, and ecosystem processes

toxin: the preferred term used to denote a poisonous substance strictly from biological sources, such as toxic algae or the tetanus toxin from the bacterium *Clostridium tetani*

Science and Profession

Since its inception, toxicology has gone through many paradigmatic shifts and has developed several subdisciplines, each with their own approaches and techniques but united by the fundamental challenge of understanding and controlling the interaction between toxic agents and physiological processes. The scale of analysis in which toxicological questions are investigated ranges from molecules to ecosystems, and toxicologists study all kinds of organisms, from the smallest viruses to the largest terrestrial and aquatic organisms.

The popular expression "the dose makes the poison" is one of the key principles of toxicology. It refers to the fact that adverse physiological effects can be produced by practically any substance if given at a dose large enough to overwhelm the body's natural capacity to process it. Extremely toxic chemicals impart their effects at very small doses. A key measure of toxicity is the lethal dose (LD), which is defined as the amount of a toxic substance that kills an organism. Because the individuals in a group of organisms do not exhibit identical responses, the actual quantitative measure is termed "LD-50," which is the dose that kills 50 percent of the individuals in an exposed population.

There are three major branches of toxicology: descriptive, mechanistic, and regulatory toxicology. All three branches contribute to risk assessment, which is the main societal application of toxicological knowledge. Mechanistic toxicology is concerned with elucidating the biochemical mechanisms underpinning the expression of toxic effects of poisons at the cellular and/or molecular levels. Assessing the potential toxicity risks associated with new chemicals depends largely on the work of mechanistic toxicologists, who are able to determine whether toxic effects observed in laboratory species are relevant to human exposure levels and physiological attributes. Mechanistic toxicologists also study dose-response relationships that are important for establishing safety thresholds of exposure for industrial chemicals used in manufacturing products and for pharmaceuticals used to treat diseases.

Regulatory toxicology involves the study of how best to protect people from toxic chemicals through the formulation of regulatory policies that govern the manufacture of commercial products, the use and disposal of potentially toxic chemicals, and the protection of workers from toxic exposures at occupational settings. The final responsibility for rejecting or approving specific chemicals for use in commerce rests with regulatory toxicologists, who are trained to evaluate data generated by mechanistic and descriptive toxicologists in light of federal and regional policies designed to protect public and environmental health. Regulatory toxicologists must make judgments following an evaluation of risks associated with short-term exposures and immediate effects (acute toxicity) as well as longer-term exposures and small doses that may result in symptoms long after the initial exposure occurs (chronic toxicity).

Descriptive toxicology forms the bridge between mechanistic and regulatory toxicology. Descriptive toxicologists are responsible for using toxicity testing for comparative risk assessment. For example, the US Food and Drug Administration (FDA) is charged with protecting public health through rigorous evaluation of toxicity levels of drugs and food additives, and descriptive toxicologists employed by the FDA are experts in selecting the best toxicity tests for that purpose. Descriptive toxicologists in the service of the US Environmental Protection Agency (EPA) or the US Department of Agriculture (USDA) collaborate in the comparative toxicity assessment of pesticides used on crops or to control disease vectors. Industrial toxicologists perform similar roles for chemicals used in manufacturing, to minimize adverse impacts on people and the environment.

Toxicologists are usually trained at graduate-level institutions that award master's or doctorate degrees following specialization in one or more subdisciplines. Clinical toxicology is typically studied and practiced in the hospital setting to quickly recognize the symptoms of toxic exposure, usually in an uncommunicative patient, and to identify the responsible poison, followed by administration of an antidote or other forms of therapy.

Environmental toxicology is the study of the sources, transportation, transformation, and sinks of toxicants in the environment, and how humans come into contact with, and suffer from, exposure to these toxicants. Ecotoxicology is a subspecialty of environmental toxicology that deals strictly with the study of the effects of toxicants on wildlife and ecosystems.

Forensic toxicology is the study of how poisons kill people and how to measure residual levels of poisons in corpses in order to determine the cause and time of death. The practice of forensic toxicology is essential in cases of suicide or homicide involving poisons.

Molecular toxicology is the study of the effects and metabolism of toxic materials in the body at the level of molecules, typically involving molecular genetic analysis and biochemical enzymology. Molecular toxicologists also study how variability in individual genetic characteristics affects human sensitivity to toxic agents, just as age, gender, and body size can all influence human exposure and sensitivity to toxic substances.

Pharmacotoxicology is the study of the toxic effects of pharmaceutical products intended for human or animal consumption. This discipline is aimed at finding the appropriate dose of a chemical that has a healing effect without overwhelmingly toxic side effects.

Most practicing toxicologists belong to the professional Society of Toxicology, an organization that defines the responsibilities of toxicologists. The first is to develop new and improved ways of determining the potentially harmful effects of chemical and physical agents and the dose that will cause these effects. This responsibility requires a thorough understanding of the molecular, biochemical, and cellular processes responsible for diseases caused by exposure to toxic substances. The second responsibility is to study commercial chemicals and products using carefully designed and controlled empirical analyses and modeling to determine the conditions under which they can be used with minimum or no adverse effects on human health, wildlife, and ecosystems. The third is to conduct toxicological risk assessments, including estimating the probability that specific chemicals or processes pose significant risks to human health and/or the environment. The risk assessments form the basis for establishing rules and regulations that underpin government policies designed to protect public health and the environment.

Diagnostic and Treatment Techniques

The diagnostic and treatment techniques used by toxicologists depend largely on the branch of toxicology in which they practice. For example, clinical toxicologists in the hospital setting must be proficient at rapid diagnostic techniques for implementing emergency response to acute exposure to poisons. According to data published by the American Association of Poison Control Centers (AAPCC), which operates the National Poison Data System, 10,830 calls are made to poison centers in the United States each day; these poison response centers deal with a new poisoning case approximately every thirteen seconds.

More than half of all poisoning cases occur in children younger than six years of age, although these incidents are rarely fatal. A major challenge for toxicologists is to quickly diagnose poisoning events in children who typically may not have the vocabulary or level of consciousness to describe the exposure event to their caregivers or to the emergency response staff when they are brought to the hospital. Most poisonings occur in the home from domestic items such as cosmetics and personal care products, cleaning fluids, medications, and pest control chemicals. Therefore, the first step in diagnosis is to identify as precisely as possible the specific chemical(s) that caused the poisoning; this can most easily be achieved through perusing the list of ingredients on the suspected container but is not always possible. It is more difficult if the poison is gaseous with a remote source. Therefore, body fluid samples (saliva, urine, or blood) can be tested using rapid techniques to identify major categories of common poisons, their known physiological effects, or biomarkers of exposure.

Application of first aid techniques is the first line of treatment for poisonings after ensuring that the patient is removed completely from the source of exposure. Follow-up treatment of poisoned patients involves three major steps. The first is to facilitate the elimination of ingested or injected poison from the body. Stomach pumping is sometimes effective for ingested poisons if applied within a time frame that occurs before a fatal dose is absorbed in the stomach. Typically, in a gastric lavage process, a siphon tube is inserted into the stomach through the mouth to repeatedly flush and empty the contents.

The second step is the application of effective antidotes that aid the excretion or inactivation of the poison either through natural liver functions or through specific biochemical reactions. Activated charcoal may be given, preferably to conscious patients through the mouth, for the purpose of absorbing the poison, thereby reducing the biologically available dose. In serious situations in which poisons are injected into the bloodstream or when poisons have been absorbed extensively from the stomach or lungs, hemodialysis may be performed to filter the blood directly through the use of artificial kidneys. Where artificial kidneys are not available, charcoal may be used for blood filtration (hemoperfusion). For poisoned patients exhibiting respiratory distress, breathing support through ventilators is an essential treatment strategy.

The third step is the treating of symptoms and the aiding of recovery. Depending on the nature of the poison, treatment may involve controlling seizures, correction of irregular heartbeat, regulation of blood pressure, and repair or replacement of damaged organs, including the kidneys and liver.

Posttreatment counseling is recommended to prevent further poison exposures through educational programs, drug rehabilitation, or mental health referrals in cases of suicide attempts. Poisoning cases may also involve substantial legal proceedings for forensic toxicologists or in cases of potential homicide.

Perspective and Prospects

Poisons and their effects on human health have been known since antiquity, but the scientific study of poisons and systematic information on their synthesis and mode of action is a relatively recent development. The German scientist Auroleus Phillipus Theostratus Bombastus von Hohenheim (1493–1541), popularly known as Paracelsus, is considered by many to be the world's first authority on and founder of toxicology as a scientific discipline. Among his several notable accomplishments, Paracelsus is credited with introducing the use of mercury and arsenic into medical practice for curative purposes. Furthermore, he is the source of the famously paraphrased maxim "the dose makes the poison." His exact statement in German translates as, "All things are poison and nothing is without poison; only the dose makes a thing not be poison."

Toxicology is a rapidly evolving specialty, driven by innovations in chemical manufacturing and the growing number of toxic substances accessible to the general population. Progress in toxicology is also driven by discoveries in human genomics and proteomics. The more that is learned about the variability in the nucleotide sequences of individuals in a population, the better understood are the differences in human response to toxic chemicals. Additional work in mechanistic toxicology and descriptive toxicology remains to be done to understand adequately the interactions among genetics, age, gender, body size, and behavioral traits that mediate human exposure and response to poisons. Furthermore, the human body is exposed to a large number of chemicals on a daily basis. Very little is known about how these chemicals interact to make people more or less vulnerable to the toxic effects of poisons.

It is important to create a seamless strategy for translating laboratory data, including those based on animal or microbial model systems, into regulatory policies designed to protect the most vulnerable members of society. It is also important to create a seamless strategy for understanding the interactions of toxic chemicals in ecosystems and how these interactions influence human vulnerability and sensitivity to toxic exposures at the workplace, on the streets, and at home. Finally, toxicology has been neglected for too long by the engineering professions that create the products upon which society relies. Toxicology must be engaged as much as possible in the product design stage, before large-scale manufacturing of consumer products that end up endangering the public and ecosystems through the expression of toxicity at various stages of the product life cycle.

—*Oladele A. Ogunseitan, Ph.D., M.P.H.*

See also Asbestos exposure; Biological and chemical weapons; Bites and stings; Blood testing; Botulism; Carcinogens; Critical care; Critical care, pediatrics; Dermatitis; Eczema; Emergency medicine; Environmental diseases; Environmental health; Enzyme therapy; Food poisoning; Forensic pathology; Hepatitis; Herbal medicine; Homeopathy; Insect-borne diseases; Intoxication; Itching; Laboratory tests; Lead poisoning; Liver; Mercury poisoning; Occupational health; Pathology; Pharmacology; Pharmacy; Poisoning; Poisonous plants; Rashes; Snakebites; Teratogens; Toxoplasmosis; Urinalysis.

For Further Information:

Agency for Toxic Substances and Disease Registry. Centers for Disease Control and Prevention, 1 Aug. 2013.

"Common Toxicology Terms." *Society of Toxicology*, 2013.

Hodgson, Ernest, and Robert C. Smart, eds. *Introduction to Biochemical Toxicology.* 3d ed. New York: Wiley Interscience, 2001.

Hoffman, David J., et al. *Handbook of Ecotoxicology.* Boca Raton, Fla.: CRC Press, 1995.

Klaassen, Curtis D., ed. *Casarett and Doull's Toxicology.* 8th ed. New York: McGraw-Hill, 2013.

Landis, Wayne G., Ruth M. Sofield, and Ming-ho Yu. *Introduction to Environmental Toxicology.* 4th ed. Boca Raton, Fla.: CRC Press, 2011.

Malachowski, M. J., and Arleen F. Goldberg. *Health Effects of Toxic Substances.* 2d ed. Rockville, Md.: Government Institutes, 1999.

Smart, Robert C., and Ernest Hodgson, eds. *Molecular and Biochemical Toxicology.* 4th ed. Hoboken, New Jersey: Wiley, 2008.

TOXOPLASMOSIS
Disease/Disorder

Anatomy or system affected: Gastrointestinal system, immune system, nervous system, skin

Specialties and related fields: Family medicine, pediatrics

Definition: A widespread, infectious disease caused by a protozoan parasite.

Causes and Symptoms

The parasite *Toxoplasma gondii*, which causes toxoplasmosis, is fairly common and can infect warm-blooded animals as well as reptiles, but the ordinary domestic cat is the only known animal that sheds the toxoplasma parasite in its feces. Humans can also be infected by coming into contact with cat feces in a litter box or by eating raw or undercooked meat from infected animals.

The parasite may be acquired or congenital. Both forms seem to have a wide variety of clinical outcomes, ranging

Information on Toxoplasmosis

Causes: Parasitic infection; may be acquired or congenital
Symptoms: Often asymptomatic; may include swollen glands, headaches, sore throat, jaundice, fever, anemia, spleen or liver enlargement
Duration: Two to twelve weeks
Treatments: Pyrimethamine, sulfa drugs

from a mild, asymptomatic state to an infection with fatal results. Congenital infection may manifest in jaundice, fever, anemia, convulsions, inflammation of the retina (chorioretinitis), an enlarged liver or spleen, and lymphadenopathy.

Acquired toxoplasmosis infection may be mild or severe. The vast majority of people who contract the disease have no or few symptoms, while others may have swollen glands, headaches, or a sore throat. These symptoms generally appear within ten to fourteen days after infection and subside within two to twelve weeks. Severe toxoplasmosis manifests in a possible fever, rash, pneumonia, encephalitis, myocarditis, pericarditis, hepatitis, and muscle inflammation (polymyositis).

When toxoplasmosis is acquired during pregnancy, it may badly harm the fetus, even if the mother does not have any symptoms. The degree to which the infection damages the fetus depends upon the stage of pregnancy. The parasite can be passed to the fetus in 15 percent of women infected during the first trimester, in approximately 25 percent infected during the second trimester, and in up to 65 percent of those infected during the last trimester. It is possible for the pregnant woman to suffer a spontaneous abortion or a stillbirth or to deliver a premature or a full-term child in whom birth defects are present.

Toxoplasmosis can occur when the immune system is impaired. Reactivation of previously acquired toxoplasma organisms has become a serious problem for HIV-infected persons. Improved HIV treatment and prophylaxis for toxoplasmosis with trimethoprim-sulfamethoxazole have reduced the incidence of disease. Similar reactivation of toxoplasma has also occurred in immunologically suppressed solid-organ and bone-marrow transplant patients.

Treatment and Therapy

Pyrimethamine and sulfa drugs have reduced the complications from toxoplasmosis. When pyrimethamine is given to a pregnant woman during her first trimester, however, birth defects may occur. Physicians will prescribe sulfa drugs alone for infections occurring during pregnancy.

Perspective and Prospects

The protozoan *Toxoplasma gondii* was first isolated from an African rodent and was eventually described as a new species in 1909. In 1940, it was established as a factor for human disease.

It is possible to prevent toxoplasmosis by feeding cats only well-cooked meat or commercial cat food; keeping cats indoors, so that they cannot hunt and eat birds or mice; staying away from cats and having someone else clean the litter box during pregnancy; washing one's hands after touching uncooked meat; and cooking meat to a minimum of 150 degrees Fahrenheit (66 degrees Celsius), or 165 degrees Fahrenheit (74 degrees Celsius) for poultry.

—Earl R. Andresen, Ph.D.

See also Birth defects; Blindness; Brain damage; Encephalitis; Eye infections and disorders; Eyes; Fever; Glands, swollen; Headaches; Hepatitis; Parasitic diseases; Pneumonia; Pregnancy and gestation; Protozoan diseases; Rashes; Sore throat; Vision disorders; Zoonoses.

For Further Information:
Ambroise-Thomas, Pierre, and Eskild Petersen, eds. *Congenital Toxoplasmosis: Scientific Background, Clinical Management, and Control*. New York: Springer, 2000.
Despommier, Dickson D., et al. *Parasitic Diseases*. 5th ed. New York: Apple Tree, 2006.
Joynson, David H. M., and Tim G. Wreghitt, eds. *Toxoplasmosis: A Comprehensive Clinical Guide*. Rev. ed. New York: Cambridge University Press, 2005.
Martin, Richard J., Avroy A. Fanaroff, and Michele C. Walsh, eds. *Fanaroff and Martin's Neonatal-Perinatal Medicine: Diseases of the Fetus and Infant*. 2 vols. 9th ed. Philadelphia: Mosby/Elsevier, 2011.
"Parasites—Toxoplasmosis (*Toxoplasma* Infection)." *Centers for Disease Control and Prevention*, January 10, 2013.
Parker, James N., and Philip M. Parker, eds. *The Official Patient's Sourcebook on Toxoplasmosis*. San Diego, Calif.: Icon Health, 2002.
Roberts, Larry S., and John Janovy, Jr., eds. *Gerald D. Schmidt and Larry S. Roberts" Foundations of Parasitology*. 8th ed. Boston: McGraw-Hill Higher Education, 2010.
Rosenblum, Laurie. "Toxoplasmosis." *Health Library*, November 26, 2012.
"Toxoplasmosis." *Mayo Clinic*, June 24, 2011.

TRACHEA
Anatomy
Also known as: Windpipe
Anatomy or system affected: Chest, neck, respiratory system
Specialties and related fields: General surgery, otorhinolaryngology, pulmonary medicine
Definition: The cartilaginous tube that conducts air from the larynx to the bronchi and into the lungs.
Key terms:
bronchi: the right and left branches from the trachea which supply air into the lungs
hyaline cartilage: the most common type of human cartilage
larynx: the organ of voice placed at the upper part of the air passage
respiratory mucosa: the mucous membrane that lines the respiratory tract
tracheal stenosis: a narrowing of the tracheal lumen
tracheomalcia: a weakening of the tracheal lumen that allows collapse during respiration
tracheostomy: a surgical opening into the trachea

Structure and Functions

The trachea, also commonly referred to as the windpipe, is the part of the airway that connects the larynx to the two main bronchi. The trachea is made up of sixteen to twenty hyaline cartilage rings that maintain the airway lumen width at about 2.5 centimeters. The cartilage rings are incomplete and flattened posteriorly, where they are completed by fibrous tissue and muscle fibers. The first cartilage ring is thicker than the others and connected by the cricotracheal ligament to the lower edge of the cricoid cartilage of the larynx. At its lower end, the trachea bifurcates into the right bronchus, which is wider, shorter, and more vertical, and the left bronchus which is narrower. This explains why aspirated foreign bodies are more likely to lodge in the right bronchus. The length of the trachea from top to bottom in an adult is 10 to 12 centimeters.

The anatomical relations of the trachea include the esophagus posteriorly and the great vessels of the neck laterally. The thyroid gland lies over the anterior surface in the lower neck. As the trachea enters the thorax, it is protected by the bony manubrium sterni. The cartilaginous structure is enclosed by an elastic fibrous membrane, and supported by nonstriated longitudinal muscle externally. Internally, transverse fibers of the trachealis muscle form a connection between the posterior ends of the cartilage rings.

In addition to its function of maintaining a patent (open) airway, the trachea also has the function of trapping foreign particles and of warming and moistening the air that flows to the lungs. It accomplishes this function by virtue of the lining of the tracheal lumen. The ciliated, respiratory mucosa of the tracheal lumen contains goblet cells that produce mucus. In the submucosa are numerous blood vessels that give warmth and seromucous glands that contribute to the lubrication of the airway. Blood supply to the trachea is from the inferior thyroid arteries. Nerve supply is from branches of the vagus and recurrent laryngeal nerves.

Disorders and Diseases

The most serious disorders of the trachea are those that cause interference with the airway. Tracheal stenosis can develop from trauma, tumors, radiation therapy, autoimmune diseases, and infection. The most common cause is prolonged intubation. Symptoms include shortness of breath, cough, and stridor. Treatment involves correcting any underlying medical condition, laser surgery, reconstructive surgery, dilation, and airway stenting. In 2008, the first tracheal transplant using patient stem cells was reported; in 2011, doctors implanted the first synthetic trachea.

Tracheomalacia occurs when the lumen of the trachea collapses inward, obstructing the airway during breathing or coughing. The most common cause of tracheomalacia is chronic obstructive pulmonary disease (COPD). Other causes include prolonged intubation, recurrent infection, injury from tracheostomy, and tumors or abnormal blood vessels that press against the trachea. A form of congenital tracheomalacia also exists. Symptoms are due to a compromised airway and are similar to tracheal stenosis. Management is also similar, including short- and long-term stenting

and reconstructive surgery.

Acute inflammation of the trachea is usually the result of bacterial infection. Symptoms may resemble croup or epiglottitis, with cough, fever, and stridor. Bacterial tracheitis has become more common than acute epiglottitis as a cause of airway distress from bacterial infection. It is much less common than croup, occurring in only 0.1 cases per 100,000 children. Bacterial infection may follow trauma during intubation or a viral infection and is more common in pediatric patients. Treatment is usually successful with airway support and appropriate antibiotics, although mortality rates have been reported at 4 to 20 percent.

Perspective and Prospects

Tracheostomy is the most common surgical procedure performed on the trachea. The term "tracheotomy" implies a surgical opening made in the trachea. The term "tracheostomy" refers to an opening into the trachea that is kept open with a cannula (a tube) or made permanent. In most medical literature, however, the term "tracheostomy" is used to describe both procedures. The purpose of tracheostomy is to gain access to the tracheal airway in order to bypass a respiratory obstruction or to facilitate breathing. This potentially lifesaving procedure has been known since ancient times. There is a description of a healed tracheotomy incision in the Sanskrit hymns of the *Rigveda*, dating to 2000 BCE. The physician Chevalier Jackson (1865–1958) of Philadelphia is the founder of the modern tracheostomy, having described the indications, complications, and the basics of the modern surgical procedure. In the nineteenth century, the procedure was commonly done to relieve airway obstruction in diphtheria patients, and in the twentieth century polio was a frequent indication. Today, the most common indication is for prolonged ventilator-assisted breathing.

Tracheal surgery made history in 2008 when the first tracheal transplant using a patient's own stem cells was successfully performed. This milestone was accomplished by a team of doctors in Barcelona, Spain. The patient was a thirty-year-old woman who had scarring of her trachea from tuberculosis. A donor trachea was obtained and stripped of living cells. Stem cells from the woman's bone marrow were then seeded into the trachea prior to transplantation. This procedure took yet another step forward in 2011, when scientists crafted an artificial trachea and seeded it with stem cells from a cancer patient, into whom it was then implanted by doctors in Sweden. This was considered a significant advance, because artificial organ transplantation does not require a donor and carries no risk of rejection by the recipient's body.

—*Chris Iliades, M.D.*

See also Asphyxiation; Bronchi; Cartilage; Choking; Critical care; Critical care, pediatric; Emergency medicine; Paramedics; Pulmonary medicine; Pulmonary medicine, pediatric; Respiration; Resuscitation; Tracheostomy.

For Further Information:

Cummings, W. Charles, et al. *Otolaryngology: Head and Neck Surgery.* 4th ed. Philadelphia: Mosby/Elsevier, 2005.

Drake, L. Richard, et al. *Gray's Anatomy for Students*. 2d ed. New York: Churchill Livingstone/Elsevier, 2009.

Engels, P. T., et al. "Tracheostomy: From Insertion to Decannulation." *Canadian Journal of Surgery* 52, no. 5 (October, 2009): 427–433.

Lalwani, K. Anil. *Current Diagnosis and Treatment in Otolaryngology: Head and Neck Surgery*. 3d ed. New York: McGraw-Hill, 2012.

Macchiarini, P., et al. "Clinical Transplantation of a Tissue-Engineered Airway." *The Lancet* 372 (2008): 2023–2030.

"Tracheotomy." *Health Library*, November 26, 2012.

TRACHEOSTOMY

Procedure

Anatomy or system affected: Neck, respiratory system, throat

Specialties and related fields: Critical care, emergency medicine, general surgery

Definition: The creation of a hole in the trachea, thus providing an alternative source for getting air into the lungs.

Indications and Procedures

A tracheostomy is the surgical creation of an opening into the trachea through the throat. It is done to relieve upper airway obstruction, decrease the effort of breathing, provide access for mechanical ventilation, and improve patient comfort. It is uncommonly used in an emergency except in the field; the preferred method of establishing an airway is to pass a tube through the trachea via the mouth.

Local anesthesia is used to deaden the skin of the front of the neck. A horizontal incision is made over the space between the second and third tracheal rings. If the thyroid gland is encountered, it is divided. Bleeding must be carefully controlled throughout the procedure. The trachea is entered through an incision that will divide the second and third rings of cartilage. In an adult, a small portion of the third ring may be removed. A previously tested tracheostomy tube with a cuff is inserted within the interior of the trachea. The wound is loosely closed, and a gauze dressing is applied. An X ray is taken after the procedure to ensure that the tube has been correctly placed and that there is no free air in the mediastinum or thorax.

Uses and Complications

Once a tracheostomy has been performed, ambient air in a patient's room must be humidified and warmed. If any secretions develop, the tracheostomy site must be suctioned in a sterile manner. If shortness of breath is observed, the tracheostomy site should be examined for a mucus plug. The tracheostomy tube should be removed and the opening closed at the earliest possible time that is consistent with the condition of the patient.

Some potential problems are associated with a tracheostomy. The most common is bacterial contamination of the lungs or adjacent tissues. Air may enter the space between the lungs and the tissue that lines the cavity containing the lungs, a condition known as pneumothorax. The tube may also become displaced. Attempting to replace the tube blindly can result in obstruction.

Perspective and Prospects

Although dramatic when portrayed on television programs, a tracheostomy is a delicate surgical procedure that requires skill and training. With the invention of modern laryngoscopes, tracheostomies are uncommon, being used primarily in cases of fracture of the anterior neck.

—L. Fleming Fallon, Jr., M.D., Ph.D., M.P.H.

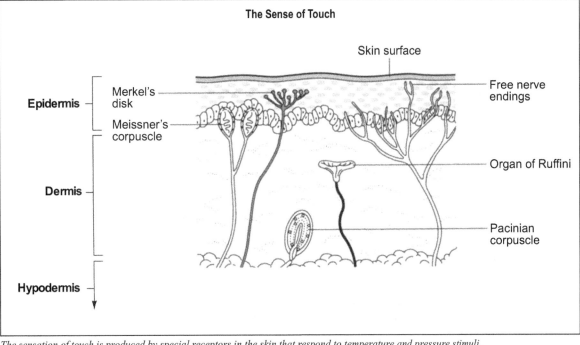

The sensation of touch is produced by special receptors in the skin that respond to temperature and pressure stimuli.

See also Asphyxiation; Choking; Critical care; Critical care, pediatric; Emergency medicine; First aid; Paramedics; Pulmonary medicine; Pulmonary medicine, pediatric; Respiration; Resuscitation; Trachea.

For Further Information:
Kertoy, Marilyn. *Children with Tracheostomies: Resource Guide.* Albany, N.Y.: Singular/Thomson Learning, 2002.
Kittredge, Mary. *The Respiratory System.* Edited by Dale C. Garell. Philadelphia: Chelsea House, 2000.
Levitzky, Michael G. *Pulmonary Physiology.* 7th ed. New York: McGraw-Hill Medical, 2007.
Mason, Robert J., et al., eds. *Murray and Nadel's Textbook of Respiratory Medicine.* 5th ed. Philadelphia: Saunders/Elsevier, 2010.
Myers, Eugene N., and Jonas T. Johnson, eds. *Tracheotomy: Airway Management, Communication, and Swallowing.* 2d ed. San Diego, Calif.: Plural, 2008.
Parker, Steve. *The Lungs and Breathing.* Rev. ed. New York: Franklin Watts, 1991.
"Speech for People With Tracheostomies or Ventilators." *American Speech-Language-Hearing Association,* June 26, 2013.
"Tracheostomy." *Mayo Clinic,* June 26, 2013.
"What Is a Tracheostomy?" *National Heart, Lung, and Blood Institute,* March 19, 2012.

Trachoma
Disease/Disorder
Anatomy or system affected: Eyes
Specialties and related fields: Environmental health, family medicine, ophthalmology, pediatrics
Definition: An infectious disease of the eyes that causes blindness.

Causes and Symptoms
Trachoma is caused by the *Chlamydia trachomatia* bacteria. It is carried primarily by children throughout the developing world, where water is scarce and washing is difficult. Combined with a general lack of hygiene, blowing dust and smoke from cooking fires provide a perfect environment for *Chlamydia trachomatia* bacteria to take hold.

Flies from refuse areas crawl on faces of children who sleep in crowded conditions. The insects touch those children with the bacteria, then infect and reinfect others rapidly throughout an entire village. The eyes become red, painful, and sticky, causing irritation to the underside of the eyelid. Infection easily spreads as children touch the faces of their mothers and other children.

Left untreated, the eyelid and eyelashes turn in, damaging the cornea. The disease becomes more painful and injurious to adults as the eyelashes break off. This bristle-like effect lacerates the cornea and opaque scarring builds (a condition called trichiasis). Blindness is inevitable, usually by the age of forty to fifty.

Treatment and Therapy
Tetracycline eye ointment, twice a day for six weeks, gets rid of the infection. Face cleansing, especially for children, is the best way to prevent infection, along with environmental improvement and education. After the disease has advanced, the

Information on Trachoma
Causes: Bacterial infection
Symptoms: Red, painful, and sticky eyes; irritation to underside of eyelid; turning in of eyelid and eyelashes with corneal damage; eventual blindness
Duration: Typically six weeks
Treatments: Tetracycline eye ointment, face cleansing, surgery if prolonged

last hope is a surgical procedure to rotate the eyelid to its original position. The procedure is relatively simple. Nurses, medical assistants, and technicians can be trained to perform it at local clinics. Efforts to eliminate *Musca sorbens*, the aggressive flies in Africa and Asia, are also effective in controlling trachoma.

Perspective and Prospects
The World Health Organization (WHO) estimates trachoma has blinded 6 million of the 38 million blind people in the world. Active infectious trachoma affects 150 million children. Areas most affected are Mexico, Brazil, Burkina Faso, Egypt, Kenya, China, Myanmar, and interior Australia.

In 1997, WHO launched a concerted effort to control trachomatous blindness by forming a consortium, the Global Elimination of Trachoma by 2020 (GET 2020). Strategy for GET 2020 is summarized by the acronym "SAFE," which refers to the four field-tested activities for control of trachoma; *s*urgery, *a*ntibiotics (tetracycline), clean *f*aces, and *e*nvironmental change. Trachoma control is one of the most affordable health interventions.

Education of the peoples involved is difficult. Because the disease is not fatal, they have little concern, accepting the disease as a fact of life. Mothers are being educated to find time to retrieve well water for washing their children's faces even when drought and poverty make feeding their families a trial. Mothers are being taught to understand the relationship between dirt on children's faces and the eye diseases making their own eyes red and sore. As such environmental improvement techniques are taught, villages are motivated to cooperate with worldwide and local agencies in the interest of curing trachoma.

—*Virginiae Blackmon*

See also Bacterial infections; Blindness; Childhood infectious diseases; Epidemiology; Eye infections and disorders; Eyes; Insect-borne diseases; Vision; Vision disorders; World Health Organization; Zoonoses.

For Further Information:
Buettner, Helmut, ed. *Mayo Clinic on Vision and Eye Health: Practical Answers on Glaucoma, Cataracts, Macular Degeneration, and Other Conditions.* Rochester, Minn.: Mayo Foundation for Medical Education and Research, 2002.
Dawson, Chandler. "Flies and the Elimination of Blinding Trachoma." *The Lancet* 353, no. 9162 (April 24, 1999): 1376.
Hertle, Richard, David B. Schaffer, and Jill A. Foster, eds. *Pediatric Eye Disease: Color Atlas and Synopsis.* New York: McGraw-Hill, 2002.

Johnson, Gordon J., et al., eds. *The Epidemiology of Eye Disease.* 2d ed. New York: Oxford University Press, 2003.

Mayo Clinic. "Trachoma." *Mayo Clinic,* October 3, 2012.

Miller, Stephen J. H. *Parsons" Diseases of the Eye.* 19th ed. New York: Elsevier, 2002.

Schachterm, J., et al. "Azithromycin in Control of Trachoma." *The Lancet* 354, no. 9179 (May, 1999): 630.

Sutton, Amy L., ed. *Eye Care Sourcebook: Basic Consumer Health Information About Eye Care and Eye Disorders.* 3d ed. Detroit, Mich.: Omnigraphics, 2008.

Vorvick, Linda J. "Trachoma." *MedlinePlus,* September 3, 2012.

World Health Organization. "Global Health Observatory: Trachoma." *World Health Organization,* 2013.

TRANSFUSION
Procedure

Anatomy or system affected: Blood, circulatory system, immune system

Specialties and related fields: Critical care, emergency medicine, general surgery, hematology, immunology, neonatology, serology, vascular medicine

Definition: The introduction of whole blood or blood components (such as platelets, red blood cells, or fresh-frozen plasma) directly into the bloodstream.

Key terms:

allogeneic: of the same species; in allogeneic blood transfusion, recipients are transfused with blood from another human being

alloimmunization: immunization by means of antibodies that react against substances from another person (such as blood)

apheresis: the removal of whole blood from a donor, followed by its separation into components, the retention of the desired component, and the return of the recombined remaining elements

autologous: self-derived; in autologous blood transfusion, recipients are transfused with their own blood

plasma: the liquid portion of blood in which the particulate components, such as proteins, are suspended; plasma is the origin of the blood components fresh-frozen plasma and cryoprecipitate

platelets: small, disk-shaped structures in blood that play a key role in blood clotting

red blood cells: blood cells that contain hemoglobin; the role of red blood cells is to transport oxygen

white blood cells: blood cells involved in the defense systems of the body; granulocyte components consist of white blood cells and are used to combat infections

whole blood: blood from which none of the elements has been removed

Indications and Procedures

Blood transfusion is the introduction of whole blood or blood components directly into the bloodstream. Human blood has been transfused with success since the early nineteenth century. Modern transfusion therapy, however, is largely the result of scientific advances made during the twentieth century and is, therefore, a young discipline. Blood transfusion plays a critical role in modern medical practice by enabling physicians to provide care, both surgical and nonsurgical, which is not feasible in its absence. Until relatively recent times, transfusion options were limited to two items: whole blood and plasma. The introduction of blood component therapy in the 1960s had a major impact on transfusion practice.

Physicians are now able to choose from a large variety of specific blood products. Some products are the result of manufacturing processes that concentrate a portion of blood (blood derivatives), such as factor VIII concentrates for the treatment of hemophilia A. Other products, such as red blood cells or platelet concentrates (blood components), are separated, produced, and distributed by blood collection facilities for transfusion purposes. The cardinal principle of modern transfusion therapy is to administer the specific blood products that patients require. Portions of blood not required by the patient should not be transfused. Therefore, indications for the use of whole blood are very limited and its use is considered, in general, to be wasteful. The two major categories of transfusion are autologous and allogeneic. Autologous transfusion is the infusion of an individual with his or her own blood. Allogeneic transfusion is the infusion of blood collected from a person or people other than the transfusion recipient.

Autologous transfusion. There are four distinct types of autologous blood transfusion services available: preoperative donation, intraoperative hemodilution, intraoperative blood collection and reinfusion, and postoperative collection and reinfusion.

Patients scheduled for surgical procedures in which blood transfusion is likely are candidates to donate and store their own blood in advance for use at the time of surgery. This is preoperative donation. It may be possible to collect and store multiple units of blood with this technique. Close communication between patient and physician is critical in preoperative donation because the number of autologous units required must be determined and a donation schedule must be established. Usually, the last donation occurs no later than seventy-two hours before the scheduled operation. For surgical procedures in which the likelihood of transfusion is remote, preoperative donation has not proven to be cost-effective.

Intraoperative hemodilution is the removal of one or more units of blood from a patient at the beginning of an operation for reinfusion during or at the end of the procedure. The volume of blood removed is replaced by the infusion of solutions that contain no blood cells and no risk of infection, such as Ringer's lactate or albumin. Intraoperative hemodilution is considered beneficial for a number of reasons. First, this technique lowers blood viscosity (that is, it thins the blood), which may improve blood flow to vital organs. Second, the amount of actual blood loss during the operation is decreased because the patient's blood is diluted at the start of the surgery. Third, a supply of fresh, normal autologous blood for transfusion is available during and at the end of the surgery.

Intraoperative blood collection and reinfusion refers to the collection and return of blood recovered from the operative field or from machines used for the performance of an operation, such as a return of blood from the cardiopulmonary bypass machine used in cardiovascular surgery. Intraoperative autologous transfusion has proven to be an effective form of blood conservation in a number of surgical procedures, including cardiac, vascular, orthopedic, urologic, trauma, gynecologic, and transplantation surgeries.

Postoperative blood collection and reinfusion refers to the collection and return of blood recovered from surgical drains following an operation. This technique has been used predominantly following cardiac or orthopedic surgery.

The different types of autologous transfusion should not be considered independently of one another. A coordinated approach using multiple techniques offers the greatest opportunity to maximize the value of autologous transfusion and minimize the chance that allogeneic transfusion will be required.

Allogeneic transfusion. This type of therapy begins with blood collection from informed, healthy donors. The allogeneic blood supply in the United States has never been as safe as it is at present. Blood donors are selected according to criteria designed to maximize donor safety and minimize recipient risks. Donor selection criteria are based on a high standard of medical practice and must comply with federal, state, and local regulations concerning blood collection. Facilities that collect and/or process blood and blood components for transfusion must comply with the United States Public Health Service's "Current Good Manufacturing Practice for Blood and Blood Components." These manufacturing practices are defined by the Code of Federal Regulations and are administered by the Food and Drug Administration (FDA). State and local laws often govern blood donor age requirements and the filing of reports, such as to state and county health departments, pertaining to donors whose laboratory tests reveal the presence of infectious diseases. There are similar procedures in countries other than the United States as well.

Blood donor selection starts with education regarding donor qualifications. Prior to every donation, potential blood donors are given information about human immunodeficiency virus (HIV) and acquired immunodeficiency syndrome (AIDS). Information is provided on the potential of HIV transmission to individuals receiving blood and on risk behaviors associated with HIV infection. Potential donors are informed of the absolute necessity of refraining from donation if they are at risk for HIV infection. Honest donor self-exclusion is a critical step in maintaining a safe blood supply.

The next phase of the donation process is the health history interview. Confidential interviews, often consisting of both a self-administered questionnaire and direct questioning, are conducted prior to every blood donation. Prospective donors are also tested for hemoglobin level (to check for the presence of anemia), temperature, pulse, and blood pressure. Some individuals are excluded because it is determined that blood donation poses an unacceptable health risk for the donor. Some exclusions, such as when a donor has a history of infectious disease or risk factors for HIV infection, are designed to pro-

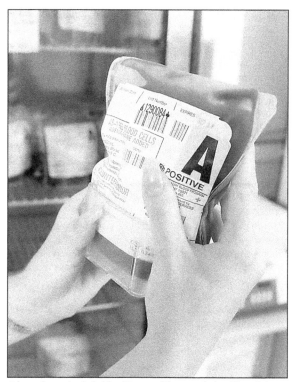

A bag of type A whole blood is stored for transfusion if needed. (Digital Stock)

tect blood recipients. Prospective donors are allowed to terminate the blood donation process at any time. Prior to the start of the actual blood donation, eligible donors are given the opportunity to ask additional questions and provide additional information. They are then asked to sign an informed consent statement. Some individuals may feel obligated to donate blood despite the realization that they do not qualify as safe donors. In this situation, donors are provided another opportunity to disqualify themselves through confidential unit exclusion (CUE). In CUE, blood donors choose "Transfuse" or "Do Not Transfuse" by marking a form or selecting a bar code label following the blood donation.

Laboratory testing of donor blood is required before whole blood or blood components can be made available for routine transfusion. A blood sample from every donation must pass an FDA-licensed test and be found to be negative for hepatitis B surface antigen (HBsAg) and for antibodies to HIV viruses types 1 and 2 (anti-HIV 1/2), hepatitis B core antigen (anti-HBc), hepatitis C virus (anti-HCV), human T-cell lymphotropic viruses types I and II (anti-HTLV-I/II), and West Nile virus. Other tests routinely performed with every donation include a test for syphilis and a test for liver function called the alanine aminotransferase (ALT) level; these tests must be negative and normal, respectively.

Units of blood collected for "Autologous Use Only" at blood centers are ordinarily tested for syphilis, anti-HIV 1/2, HBsAg, anti-HCV, and anti-HBc. Blood units remain acceptable for autologous transfusion despite positive results in one or more tests. Some health care facilities collect Autologous Use Only blood components for transfusion within the institution. Such blood components drawn, stored, and infused at one facility may have not been tested for all the above-mentioned infectious diseases. If autologous blood donors have been screened and tested in a manner identical to allogeneic blood donors, unused autologous blood may be used for allogeneic blood transfusions. Most transfusion services, however, opt to destroy unused autologous blood.

The transfusion process begins with a physician's assessment of patient need and a formal order, clearly identifiable in the patient record, specifying the blood product to be transfused, the quantity, and any special administration requirements. This order is then transcribed to a special transfusion request form; computer-transmitted requests are acceptable as long as the required information is present. Forms requesting blood or blood components and forms accompanying blood samples from the patient must contain sufficient information for positive identification of the recipient. The first and last name and unique identification number of the patient are required. With the exception of extreme emergencies, such as patients who will bleed to death if there is any delay in transfusion of blood or blood components, the ABO (A, B, AB, or O) and Rh (positive or negative) types of the intended recipient must be determined before blood or blood components are issued for transfusion.

If the patient is to receive whole blood, red blood cells, granulocytes, or platelet components containing more than five milliliters of red cells (red cell–containing components), the recipient's serum (plasma lacking coagulation factors) must also be tested for the presence of clinically significant unexpected antibodies and for compatibility with the donor red blood cells. The only expected antibodies in a patient's serum are those directed at the A and/or B groups. Individuals who are in blood group O have antibodies directed toward the A and B groups, those who are in group A have anti-B antibodies, and group B individuals have anti-A antibodies. People who are in group AB do not have antibodies directed toward the A or B groups. There is no anti-O antibody. If the serum of a prospective transfusion recipient contains a clinically significant unexpected red cell antibody, red cell-containing components chosen for transfusion must lack the corresponding antigen (the determinant to which the antibody is directed).

With the exception of emergencies, the recipient's serum is usually tested with red blood cells from the donor prior to the release of red cell–containing components for transfusion. This procedure is known as the major crossmatch, and if recipient serum does not react with donor red cells, the red cell–containing unit is termed crossmatch compatible. It is now acceptable to use properly functioning computer systems to select compatible red cell units for transfusion in the place of a major crossmatch for recipients who do not have clinically significant unexpected antibodies. Blood components that do not contain five milliliters or more of red blood cells, such as fresh-frozen plasma, cryoprecipitate, and most platelet components, do not have to be crossmatched.

Patients should receive blood and blood components of their own ABO group whenever possible. For red cell–containing components, with the exception of whole blood, alternative choices exist when ABO identical components are not available. For red cell–containing components, the donor red cells must be compatible with the recipient's plasma. For example, group A recipients may receive group O red blood cells. When transfusing components that contain plasma (whole blood, fresh-frozen plasma, cryoprecipitate, or platelets), it is best to transfuse blood products that are compatible with the recipient's red blood cells. For example, group A recipients may receive group AB fresh-frozen plasma since the plasma from group AB donors does not contain anti-A. Whole blood transfusion should be ABO identical because donor red cells and plasma must be compatible with the recipient.

For whole blood, red blood cells, platelets, and granulocytes, Rh-identical products should be provided whenever possible. Rh-negative units are acceptable for transfusion into Rh-positive individuals, but Rh-negative units should be reserved for Rh-negative recipients because of the limited supply of Rh-negative blood. The transfusion of Rh-positive blood into Rh-negative recipients will likely result in the formation of antibodies to the Rh antigen and therefore should be avoided in all but emergency situations. Rh type is not a consideration when transfusing fresh-frozen plasma or cryoprecipitate.

When there is a desperate requirement for blood, there may be a need to transfuse uncrossmatched red blood cells. If the recipient ABO group and Rh type are unknown, group O red cells should be transfused, and it is preferable that they be Rh negative. If there has been time to determine the recipient's ABO and Rh types with a current blood sample, then appropriate ABO and Rh type blood can be issued uncrossmatched (that is, uncrossmatched A-positive red cells can be provided to a recipient determined to be A positive). Previous records must not be used to determine which blood group to issue, nor may the recipient's blood type be taken from other records such as credit cards, dog tags, or a driver's license.

Whole blood. A unit of whole blood contains approximately 450 milliliters of blood and 63 milliliters of anticoagulant/preservative solution. All the elements that make up human blood are in whole blood. Whole blood stored for more than twenty-four hours, however, contains few functional platelets or white blood cells. In addition, the levels of two proteins in whole blood necessary for normal blood clotting, known as coagulation factors V and VIII, decrease with storage. Stored whole blood, therefore, cannot be considered a source of functional platelets, functional white cells, or therapeutic levels of coagulation factors V and VIII. Whole blood provides oxygen-carrying capacity and blood volume expansion. Oxygen-carrying capacity is accomplished through the red blood cells present in whole blood. Red blood cells carry oxygen, which they deliver to vital organs and tissues. The approximately 500-milliliter volume of a unit of whole blood

In the News:
The Development of Blood Substitutes

Red blood cell (RBC) substitutes were initially developed both to address the needs of the military by providing an improved resuscitation fluid and to avoid concerns about blood safety among the general population. A blood substitute with a long shelf life that is pathogen-free and universal in type would find wide clinical use: Human blood used for transfusions is sensitive to periodic blood shortages and cannot be used on patients with religious convictions against RBC transfusion. Blood substitutes can be classified into two general categories: hemoglobin-based oxygen carriers (HBOCs) and perfluorochemicals (PFCs).

The first HBOC to reach advanced Phase III clinical trials was a tetramer made of four connected hemoglobin molecules called Hemassist. Development of Hemassist was terminated after an interim review of data showed that twenty-four of fifty-two patients receiving the product had died, giving a mortality rate of 46.2 percent; the control group experienced a mortality rate of 17.4 percent. As of 2007, no HBOC had been approved for use in the United States. However, one HBOC based on bovine hemoglobin, Hemopure, had been approved for use in general surgery in the Republic of South Africa. Moreover, by 2003, at least ten HBOCs were under development and were being studied in either preclinical, Phase II, or Phase III clinical trials.

The other category of blood substitutes under development is PFCs. PFCs are synthetic, highly fluorinated, inert organic compounds that can dissolve large volumes of oxygen and other gases. They are unreactive in the body and are excreted as vapor by exhalation. PFCs can be safely injected into the bloodstream as microscopic drops, with one such product, Oxygent, in advanced clinical trials in Europe and China.

—*Michael R. King, Ph.D.*

may make a significant addition to the total blood volume of a patient. The maintenance of a normal blood volume is vital to maintaining a proper level of pressure within the vascular system to get blood to and from vital organs and tissues. Patients lacking in blood volume may benefit from the volume provided by whole blood. Whole blood transfusions may be used, therefore, when there is a need for blood volume support combined with oxygen-carrying capacity, such as in patients experiencing severe acute hemorrhage.

For patients requiring oxygen-carrying capacity only, such as patients who have a normal blood volume but are anemic, red blood cell transfusion is recommended. When blood volume support is the sole need, such as in the early stages of acute blood loss when oxygen-carrying capacity has not yet become compromised but the blood volume is diminished, blood volume expanders that pose no risk of infectious disease—for example, normal saline (a salt and water solution)—are favored. Whole blood and other red cell components should not be used in patients with anemias that can be treated safely with specific medications such as iron, vitamin B_{12}, recombinant erythropoietin, or folic acid. Coagulation factor deficiencies, such as hemophilia, are more effectively treated with other blood components or derivatives. The storage period for whole blood varies from twenty-one to thirty-five days, based on the type of anticoagulant/preservative solution. As a result of time constraints posed by prerelease testing, whole blood that is less than twenty-four hours old is not routinely available. Whole blood stored less than seven days is often considered a desirable blood product for exchange transfusions in neonates (newborn children).

Red blood cell components. These components are pro-

duced when centrifugal or gravitational separation of red cells from plasma in whole blood is followed by the removal of 200 to 250 milliliters of plasma. The storage period of red cells collected and stored in an anticoagulant/preservative solution known as CPDA-1 is thirty-five days. Many red cell components contain a supplemental additive solution in addition to the anticoagulant/preservative. Additive systems extend the storage period for red blood cells to forty-two days. Red cell transfusions increase oxygen-carrying capacity by increasing the circulating red blood cell mass. Increasing oxygen delivery to the body's organs and tissues with red cell transfusions may correct or prevent the manifestations of anemia. Red cell transfusions should be administered to patients with symptomatic anemia when other treatments are unavailable or ineffective and to those patients for whom rapid replacement of red cell mass is of critical importance. A unit of red blood cells contains essentially the same number of red cells as a whole blood unit. The volume of a red cell unit, however, is approximately 50 to 66 percent of whole blood. Thus, the use of red cells allows for the delivery of more red cells per milliliter transfused than whole blood, and smaller volume transfusions are required to achieve desired increases in oxygen-carrying capacity. When red blood cell components are used for exchange transfusion, it is common to use units that are less than seven days old. Stored red blood cells do not contain functional platelets or white blood cells.

In adults, a hemoglobin value of seven grams per deciliter or less is commonly used as a guideline for red cell transfusion. (An example of a normal range for hemoglobin is 13.5 to 16.5 grams per deciliter in adult men and 12.0 to 15.0 grams per deciliter in adult women.) This is a useful guideline; however, the decision to transfuse red cells should be based on patient clinical status. Laboratory data should be utilized as part of overall patient assessment and not as a sole indicator for transfusion therapy. Signs and symptoms reflecting a possible need for red cell transfusion include fainting, shortness of breath, a drop in blood pressure when sitting up or standing up, rapid heart rate, chest pain, and transient neurologic deficits. In rapid acute blood loss, the hemoglobin value may not reflect circulating red cell mass. Red cell transfusion decisions in this setting are based on assessments of blood loss, cardiorespiratory status, and oxygen delivery to tissues. Certain diseases compromise oxygen delivery to tissues or the adequate oxygenation of red blood cells, such as heart disease, lung disease, and disease of the blood vessels supplying the brain. Such patients may need to be transfused at higher hemoglobin levels than other patients in order to maintain adequate organ and tissue oxygenation. In summation, the decision to transfuse red cells should be based on patient symptoms, laboratory data, underlying diseases, and the urgency of need for oxygen-carrying capacity.

In neonates, red cell transfusions are usually small in volume (five to ten milliliters per kilogram) and administered frequently. The most common indication for red cell transfusion in neonates is to replace blood drawn for laboratory studies. Blood losses caused by laboratory sampling are proportionately large in neonates because of their small blood volumes. Usually, red cells are transfused following the removal of 5 to 10 percent of the estimated blood volume from sick neonates requiring frequent monitoring. Neonates with severe respiratory disease, particularly those requiring oxygen and/or respiratory support, are usually transfused to maintain a hematocrit level (a laboratory test used as a marker for anemia) above 40 percent. An example of a normal range for hematocrit values in children is 40 to 50 percent. Similar transfusion guidelines have been established for neonates with congenital heart disease. In neonates without severe respiratory or heart disease, it has been recommended that red cell transfusions be given to maintain hematocrit levels above 30 percent for infants with shortness of breath, rapid breathing, episodes of no breathing, rapid heart rate, and abnormal heart rhythms. Some physicians advocate red cell transfusions to maintain hematocrit levels above 30 percent for infants experiencing poor weight gain.

Red cell components may be modified by centrifugation, filtration, washing, sedimentation, or freezing/thawing to remove white blood cells. White cell removal procedures must result in a component that contains fewer than 5×10^8 residual white blood cells while maintaining at least 80 percent of the original red cells. Many white cell filters achieve much higher levels of white cell removal. White cell–depleted blood components are used to prevent febrile transfusion reactions (fever), to prevent or delay alloimmunization to white blood cell antigens, to prevent poor responses to platelet transfusions as a result of alloimmunization, and to prevent the transmission of white blood cell–associated viruses, such as cytomegalovirus, by cellular blood components.

Automated techniques are available for the washing of red cell units with sterile saline. This is less effective than filtration for white blood cell removal. The washing of red cells, however, does remove as much as 99 percent of the plasma from the red cell unit. Washed red cells may be indicated for patients requiring minimal plasma exposure. Examples include patients with a disease known as paroxysmal nocturnal hemoglobinuria, patients with IgA antibodies, and patients who have experienced recurrent or severe allergic transfusion reactions. Signs and symptoms of allergic reactions include hives, wheezing, low blood pressure, swelling of the throat, and fluid in the lungs.

Frozen red cells are prepared through the addition of glycerol, a cryoprotective (cold-protecting) agent, to red cells that are usually less than six days old, followed by freezing. The storage period for frozen red cells is up to ten years from the date that the unit was collected. When needed for transfusion, frozen red cells are thawed and washed with a series of saline-glucose solutions to remove glycerol. The unit is resuspended in sterile saline or a saline-glucose mixture. After thawing, washing, and resuspension, the storage period is twenty-four hours at one to six degrees Celsius. Frozen/thawed red cells are virtually devoid of plasma, anticoagulant, and platelets. The degree of white cell removal with this procedure is comparable to current filtration methods. Freezing is useful for the storage of rare red cell units and for the long-term preservation of autologous red cells. Because frozen/thawed red cells contain minimal amounts of plasma and white blood cells, they may be used when leukocyte-depleted and/or plasma-depleted red cell units are indicated.

Platelets. Platelet concentrates are prepared from whole blood by centrifugation. Most platelet concentrates contain at least 5.5×10^{10} platelets. The usual storage period for platelet concentrates is five days at twenty to twenty-four degrees Celsius. Platelets are often administered as a pool of concentrates.

Apheresis platelets are the second type of platelet component available. They are collected from a donor through the use of a blood cell separator in a procedure known as plateletpheresis. Most apheresis platelets contain at least 3×10^{11} platelets. An apheresis platelet (collected from one donor) is the equivalent of six to eight units of platelet concentrates. Apheresis platelets are sometimes beneficial in patients who are not responding satisfactorily to platelet concentrates because of antiplatelet antibodies (alloimmunization). Antiplatelet antibodies often arise in response to human leukocyte antigens (HLAs) present on donor platelets; these antigens aid the immune system in recognizing "self" or "nonself" material. Donors possessing HLAs that are identical or similar to those of the recipient may be selected to provide platelets for transfusion. Such components are known as HLA-matched platelets. Apheresis platelets can be used to decrease the number of blood donor exposures for a recipient and to reduce or delay the development of alloimmunization.

A low number of platelets (less than fifty thousand per cubic millimeter) is known as thrombocytopenia; the normal range for platelets is 150,000 to 400,000 per cubic millimeter of blood. Thrombocytopenia may result from disease processes, such as leukemia or aplastic anemia, or from the medical treatment of diseases, such as the use of chemotherapy for the treatment of cancer. Thrombocytopenia can lead to bleeding problems. Patients with functionally abnormal platelets may experience bleeding and have normal platelet counts. Platelet transfusions may be indicated to treat significant active bleeding or to protect against bleeding prior to invasive procedures, such as major surgery, in patients with platelet dysfunction or thrombocytopenia. Prophylactic platelet transfusions are commonly administered to prevent bleeding in patients with thrombocytopenia caused by decreased platelet production, as with cancer therapy. A commonly accepted threshold for prophylactic platelet transfusion in such patients is a platelet count of less than twenty thousand per cubic millimeter. Platelet transfusions are usually not effective in the setting of rapid platelet destruction, such as in a condition known as idiopathic (or autoimmune) thrombocytopenic purpura (ITP). Platelets are also not recommended for routine use in a condition known as thrombotic thrombocytopenic purpura (TTP). In the event of life-threatening hemorrhage in ITP or TTP, however, platelet transfusions may be necessary.

Prophylactic platelet transfusions are recommended for all neonates with a platelet count less than twenty thousand per cubic millimeter. In the presence of active bleeding or prior to invasive procedures, platelet transfusions are recommended to keep the platelet count above fifty thousand per cubic millimeter. In stable premature neonates, prophylactic platelet transfusions are recommended to maintain a platelet count above fifty thousand per cubic millimeter. In sick premature neonates, platelet transfusions are given to maintain a platelet count above 100,000 per cubic millimeter.

Fresh-frozen plasma. The fluid portion of whole blood is called fresh-frozen plasma (FFP). It can be separated and frozen at -18 degrees Celsius or colder within eight hours of whole blood collection. FFP may be stored for up to one year at -18 degrees Celsius or colder. It contains all plasma proteins present in normal blood.

FFP may be used to treat isolated deficiencies of coagulation proteins (factors II, V, VII, IX, X, and XI) when more specific components are not available or appropriate. Patients on oral anticoagulant therapy, such as warfarin, may require FFP to reverse anticoagulant effect rapidly prior to emergency invasive procedures or because of active bleeding. Depletion of multiple coagulation factors may occur in patients who have developed a deficiency of vitamin K, in those patients receiving massive blood replacement, or with a condition known as disseminated intravascular coagulation (DIC). The use of FFP may be necessary to treat such problems. FFP may be required for patients with liver disease who are actively bleeding or who face invasive procedures. FFP contains antithrombin III (AT-III), a naturally occurring anticoagulant, and it may be used in patients requiring AT-III. Plasma components, either through simple transfusion or as part of plasma exchange procedures, have become a vital aspect of therapy for TTP.

Indications for FFP in neonates include liver failure, inherited coagulation factor deficiencies, bleeding caused by vitamin K deficiency, the treatment of DIC, protein C deficiency (another naturally occurring anticoagulant), and AT-III replacement therapy.

FFP is not recommended for coagulation abnormalities that can be treated more effectively or safely with specific therapy such as vitamin K (in less serious situations, vitamin K deficiency is treated with vitamin K replacement instead of FFP), cryoprecipitate, or specific coagulation factor concentrates. FFP should not be used as a volume expander or as a nutritional source.

Cryoprecipitate. A concentrated source of certain plasma proteins, cryoprecipitate is a white precipitate that forms when FFP is thawed at between one and six degrees Celsius.

The cryoprecipitate is removed and refrozen at -18 degrees Celsius or colder. A single bag of cryoprecipitate has a volume of ten to fifteen milliliters. Cryoprecipitate has a storage period of one year when stored at -18 degrees Celsius or colder. Several proteins necessary for normal blood clotting are present in cryoprecipitate, including factor VIIIc, von Willebrand factor (vWF), fibrinogen, and factor XIII.

Cryoprecipitate is used in the treatment of hemophilia A (a deficiency or abnormality of factor VIIIc), von Willebrand disease (a deficiency or abnormality of vWF), inherited or acquired fibrinogen deficiency or dysfunction, and factor XIII deficiency. Cryoprecipitate has been beneficial in some kidney disease patients with abnormal bleeding. It is used to prepare fibrin glue, a material with adhesive and hemostatic properties that has been shown to be of value as a sealant in many operative procedures.

Granulocytes. Units of white blood cells (granulocytes) may be obtained by apheresis or by removal from units of fresh whole blood. Granulocytes collected by apheresis have a volume of two hundred to three hundred milliliters and should contain more than 1.0×10^{10} granulocytes. To maximize therapeutic effect, granulocytes should be transfused as soon as possible following preparation. If storage is necessary, granulocytes may be stored for twenty-four hours at twenty to twenty-four degrees Celsius.

Granulocyte transfusions have been used to aid in the treatment of serious infections in patients with dysfunctional or very low numbers of white blood cells who are not responding to conventional therapies. Neonates with blood infections (sepsis) may receive granulocyte transfusion as a supplement to antibiotic therapy.

Uses and Complications

The use of autologous transfusion has increased markedly since the mid-1980s. This increase is largely the result of concerns of patients and physicians about the transmission of certain diseases, such as AIDS and hepatitis. In addition to minimizing the risk of transmitting such diseases, autologous transfusion provides numerous other advantages. Alloimmunization, the formation of antibodies to substances (alloantigens) present in allogeneic blood, will not occur when autologous blood is used. Some patients requiring blood transfusion are already alloimmunized from previous allogeneic transfusion or from pregnancy. The provision of compatible allogeneic blood to such patients can sometimes be difficult. Therefore, the availability of autologous blood in these situations, when possible, is advantageous.

A number of transfusion reactions may result from exposure to allogeneic blood—allergic reactions, fever, hemolytic reactions, graft-versus-host disease (GVHD)—which are prevented with autologous blood. Allogeneic blood appears to suppress the immune systems of transfusion recipients. Although there is still much to be learned about this phenomenon, the effect may adversely influence recurrence rates and mortality following some forms of cancer surgery and may lead to increased susceptibility to viral and bacterial infections. Autologous blood usage avoids these potential immunosuppressive effects. The use of autologous blood also leads to the conservation of vital blood resources. In the absence of the availability of autologous blood, transfusion needs must be met through the use of a volunteer allogeneic blood supply. For practical purposes, transfused autologous blood can be thought of as conserving a like amount of allogeneic blood. The availability of autologous blood may also lessen patient anxiety regarding the need for transfusion.

The overall risk of HIV infection from allogeneic blood transfusion is estimated at one in 225,000 per unit of blood (whole blood and blood components). The transfusion-transmitted infection rates for hepatitis B virus, HTLV-I/II, and HCV are estimated to be one in 200,000, one in 60,000, and one in 3,300 per unit, respectively. Although fear of HIV infection is a primary concern of transfusion recipients, transfusion-transmitted HCV infection is the principal infectious disease risk. The incidence of other transfusion-transmitted infections is very low in countries such as the United States. The current estimate of risk is less than one in one million per unit for transfusion-transmitted yersiniosis (*Yersinia enterocolitica* infection), malaria, babesiosis, and Chagas disease (trypanosomiasis).

Transfusion-associated GVHD is a rare but severe complication of transfusion therapy. While patients with underdeveloped or impaired immune systems are at the greatest risk for developing this disease, it can occur in patients with normal immune systems. The transfusion of blood and blood components donated by blood relatives may put a recipient at risk for transfusion-associated GVHD. Gamma irradiation of whole blood and cellular blood components is the only acceptable method to reduce the risk. Fresh-frozen plasma and cryoprecipitate have not been implicated in this disease.

It is an absolute necessity that proper identification of recipients be obtained prior to any transfusion procedure. Transfusing facilities must have strict policies to guarantee that the appropriate types of blood or blood components are transfused to the correct patients. Blood and blood components are visually inspected prior to their release for transfusion. If their fitness is questioned upon inspection, they will not be released. Visual abnormalities include hemolysis (evidence of red cell breakage), follicular material, cloudy appearance, or a deviation from the usual color of the blood or blood component. Blood and blood components are prepared by techniques designed to safeguard sterility through their expiration date. Once the seal of a blood component has been broken for any reason, the expiration time is four hours if maintained at room temperature (twenty to twenty-four degrees Celsius) or twenty-four hours if refrigerated (one to six degrees Celsius). All transfusions must be administered through a filter. Transfusion recipients should be observed carefully during the first fifteen minutes of a transfusion. If a life-threatening transfusion reaction occurs, such as from the mistaken transfusion of incompatible red blood cells, it usually develops following the infusion of only a small volume of the blood or blood component. Blood transfusion must be completed prior to the expiration time of the component or within four hours, whichever is sooner. All adverse reactions to transfusion, including possible bacterial contamination or suspected disease transmission, must be reported to the transfusion service.

Perspective and Prospects

The first well-documented transfusion of human blood to a patient was administered by James Blundell on September 26, 1818. For most of the first hundred years of human blood transfusion, blood was transfused from donor to recipient by means of a direct surgical communication between the donor and recipient blood supplies. Numerous transfusion-related fatalities resulted, probably from the infusion of incompatible blood. A landmark event in the history of transfusion medicine occurred in 1901 when Karl Landsteiner published his observations that the sera of some individuals causes the red cells of others to agglutinate (clump). This led to the discovery of the ABO blood group system and set the stage for safe transfusion therapy. Reuben Ottenberg and David J. Kaliski subsequently published their key observations on the importance of pretransfusion compatibility testing in 1913.

Despite these advances, blood transfusion remained a cumbersome technique until the value of blood anticoagulants was noted by multiple investigators in 1914 and 1915. For the first time, blood donation could be separated, in time and place, from blood transfusion. Blood could be drawn and set aside for use at a later time. This led to the development of blood banks for the storage and distribution of blood. The first hospital blood bank in the United States was established at Cook County Hospital in Chicago in the mid-1930s. Blood was collected in glass bottles that were washed, sterilized, and reused following transfusion. The introduction of plastic containers for blood in 1952 led to the development of disposable plastic systems for the collection, separation, and preservation of blood products. The advent of such plastic systems allowed whole blood to be separated easily into multiple blood components, thus setting the stage for modern blood component therapy.

Transfusion medicine has become a vital aspect of modern medical practice. Patients with cancer may be treated more aggressively because of the support provided by blood products. Organ and tissue transplantation (such as liver, kidney, and bone marrow transplants) and other complex surgical procedures have become possible because of blood and blood component therapy.

The use of blood and components is constantly evolving. Continual efforts are being made to maximize the safety and availability of the blood supply. Indications for blood and blood component transfusions continue to be analyzed and clarified. Alternatives to allogeneic blood transfusion, such as autologous transfusion, the use of blood growth factors (such as recombinant erythropoietin), and manufactured blood substitutes (such as oxygen-carrying perfluorochemical solutions), continue to be explored and are expected to receive more widespread application.

—*James R. Stubbs, M.D.*

See also Anemia; Bleeding; Blood and blood disorders; Blood banks; Blood testing; Catheterization; Circulation; Critical care;

Critical care, pediatric; Emergency medicine; Hematology; Hematology, pediatric; Immune system; Immunology; Immunopathology; Phlebotomy; Plasma; Rh factor; Serology; Surgery, general; Surgery, pediatric; Surgical procedures; Transplantation; Vascular medicine; Vascular system.

For Further Information:

American Association of Blood Banks, American Red Cross, and Council of Community Blood Centers. *Circular of Information for the Use of Human Blood and Blood Components*. Arlington, Va.: Author, 2002.

"Blood Transfusion." *National Heart, Lung, and Blood Institute*, Jan. 30, 2012.

"Blood Transfusion and Donation." *MedlinePlus*, May 31, 2013.

Brecher, Mark, ed. *Technical Manual*. 15th ed. Bethesda, Md.: American Association of Blood Banks, 2005.

Hillyer, Christopher D., et al., eds. *Blood Banking and Transfusion Medicine*. 2d ed. Philadelphia: Churchill Livingstone/Elsevier, 2007.

McCullough, Jeffrey. *Transfusion Medicine*. 3d ed. Philadelphia: Churchill Livingstone/Elsevier, 2012.

Petz, Lawrence D., et al., eds. *Clinical Practice of Transfusion Medicine*. 3d ed. New York: Churchill Livingstone, 1996.

Schaub Di Lorenzo, Marjorie, and Susan Strasinger. *Blood Collection in Healthcare*. Philadelphia: F. A. Davis, 2002.

Starr, Douglas P. *Blood: An Epic History of Medicine and Commerce*. New York: Perennial, 2002.

Woods, Michael. "Blood Transfusion." *Health Library*, Mar. 26, 2013.

Transient ischemic attacks (TIAs)
Disease/Disorder

Also known as: Ministrokes

Anatomy or system affected: Blood vessels, brain, circulatory system

Specialties and related fields: Neurology, vascular medicine

Definition: Temporary interference with blood flow to the brain, resulting in transient strokelike symptoms.

Causes and Symptoms

A transient ischemic attack (TIA) is very similar to a stroke. Most physicians define a TIA as an episode of strokelike symptoms that fully resolves within twenty-four hours. A stroke, on the other hand, is defined as an episode that produces neurological symptoms that are permanent.

Strokes and TIAs are caused when the blood supply to the brain is interrupted. This interruption may occur because of a hemorrhage in an artery in the brain. Other causes of stroke or TIA may include a blood clot or piece of plaque that breaks loose from somewhere else in the body and eventually lodges in an artery that feeds the brain, or from severe narrowing in an artery that feeds the brain. Symptoms from a stroke or TIA that originates in the carotid arteries (the main arteries in the front of the neck) include weakness or numbness on one side of the body, temporary loss of vision in one eye, and difficulty speaking. When the back of the brain is damaged, symptoms such as dizziness, difficulty walking, or a drop attack (sudden loss of leg strength) may occur.

One might think that since the symptoms of a TIA go away, such an attack is not a serious condition. However, a TIA is

---

Information on Transient Ischemic Attacks (TIAs)

Causes: Temporary interruption of blood supply to brain from hemorrhage, embolism, severe narrowing in artery; risk factors include high blood pressure, high cholesterol, smoking, diabetes, advancing age, cardiac disease, stress, lack of physical activity, genetics

Symptoms: In carotid arteries, weakness or numbness on one side, temporary loss of vision in one eye, difficulty speaking; in back of brain, dizziness, difficulty walking, drop attacks

Duration: Acute episodes that resolve within twenty-four hours

Treatments: Emergency care, sometimes surgery to remove narrowed section, medications (anticoagulants, antiplatelet drugs, clopidogrel, ticlopidine, dipyridamole)

---

often a warning signal of an impending stroke. For this reason, anyone suffering a TIA should immediately seek medical attention.

The risk factors for TIA and stroke are similar. They include high blood pressure, high cholesterol, smoking, diabetes mellitus, advancing age, cardiac disease (especially irregular heart rhythm problems), stress, and lack of physical activity. Genetics can make one more likely to have a stroke or a TIA as well.

Treatment and Therapy

A person experiencing symptoms of a TIA should call paramedics in order to be seen in an emergency room immediately. Doctors can assess the patient's situation and determine whether treatment can be initiated that will limit the amount of time that the brain is starved of oxygen. A stroke has been referred to as "brain attack" to underscore the need to seek prompt medical attention quickly, as one would for a heart attack.

Diagnostic tests will likely include magnetic resonance imaging (MRI) of the brain to check for hemorrhage or damage. Other tests may include magnetic resonance angiography (MRA) of the arteries or an ultrasound of the arteries that serve the brain. If these studies show a narrowing of the carotid arteries, then surgery can be done to remove the narrowed section before it causes more damage.

In some cases, medications will be used to lessen the risk of a full-blown stroke. They may include anticoagulants (blood thinners) and antiplatelet drugs such as aspirin, clopidogrel (Plavix), ticlopidine, and dipyridamole (Aggrenox). Drugs that lower cholesterol may also be prescribed.

—*Steven R. Talbot, R.V.T.*

See also Angiography; Arteriosclerosis; Brain; Brain damage; Brain disorders; Carotid arteries; Cholesterol; Circulation; Embolism; Hyperlipidemia; Hypertension; Ischemia; Numbness and tingling; Paralysis; Plaque, arterial; Speech disorders; Strokes; Subdural hematoma; Thrombolytic therapy and TPA; Thrombosis and thrombus; Vascular medicine; Vascular system.

For Further Information:

Adams, Harold P., Jr., Vladimir Hachinski, and John W. Norris. *Ischemic Cerebrovascular Disease.* New York: Oxford University Press, 2001.
American Stroke Association. http://www.stroke association.org.
Chaturvedi, Seemant, and Steven R. Levine, eds. *Transient Ischemic Attacks.* Malden, Mass.: Blackwell Futura, 2004.
Kikuchi, H., ed. *Strategic Medical Science Against Brain Attack.* New York: Springer, 2002.
Parker, James N., and Philip M. Parker, eds. *The Official Patient's Sourcebook on Transient Ischemic Attack.* Rev. ed. San Diego, Calif.: Icon Health, 2004.
"Transient Ischemic Attack (TIA)." *Mayo Clinic*, March 3, 2011.
"Transient Ischemic Attack (TIA)." *National Stroke Association*, 2013.
Wood, Debra. "Transient Ischemic Attack." *Health Library*, September 30, 2012.

TRANSITIONAL CARE
Specialty
Anatomy or system affected: All
Specialties and related fields: All
Definition: A set of actions designed to ensure the coordination and continuity of healthcare as patients transfer between locations or different levels of care in the same location.

Transitional care is a generally compact period of healthcare in which its principal focus is a smooth transition among various healthcare settings or from one level of care to another. Examples of this transition of care can be seen when a patient transfers from different floors within a hospital or a patient is discharged from an inpatient hospital setting to a rehabilitation center or skilled nursing facility (SNF).

Key Components
During a transition of care, there are several key components of patient information that must be communicated. This data is crucial to ensure a smooth transition for both patient and providers. The communication of this vital information can be transmitted through face-to-face communication, a telephone conversation, a secured electronic medical record, or by the patient's paper medical record. The following is essential information needed in a transition of care:
- Current diagnoses
- Past medical history
- Past surgical history
- Medications
- Allergies
- Advanced directives
- Baseline physical and cognitive assessments
- Lab and imaging results

It is also important to note that contact information for both caregivers and providers should be included whenever possible to ensure that any gaps in information can be filled. There may be situations where other pertinent patient information may need to be included to ensure a transition of care is not fragmented and missing significant components.

Challenges
Patient care has changed immensely over the past decade. It is rare that one practitioner cares for a patient across the continuum of medical settings. It is now more common for a practitioner to care for their patients in a single, specific setting. For example, a primary care provider may only see their patients in a clinical outpatient setting. If their patient is admitted to the hospital, a provider within the hospital will then most likely take over the patient's care. Furthermore, this patient may then be transferred to an outpatient setting such as a SNF, where another provider then takes over the patient's care. This is a common example of transitional care across healthcare settings. Each of these transfers has the potential to leave out crucial patient information. This can lead to medical oversights and mistakes including repeat lab tests, unnecessary diagnostic imaging, and medication errors.

Transitional care that is well executed can reduce unnecessary healthcare costs and mistakes. This transition of care must include several key components of the patient's current medical state and past medical history. Cooperation among providers and clear communication between all of those involved in the patient's care can create a more optimal transition of care for patients, caregivers, and providers.

—*Carly A. Gray and Geraldine Marrocco, Ph.D.*

For Further Information:
Coleman, E.A. "Falling Through the Cracks: Challenges and Opportunities for Improving Transitional Care for Persons with Continuous Complex Care Needs." *Journal of the American Geriatrics Society,* 51 (2003): 549-555.
Coleman, E.A., and R. Berenson. "Lost in Transition: Challenges and Opportunities for Improving the Quality of Transitional Care." *Annals of Internal Medicine,* 140 (2004): 533-536.
Naylor, Mary. "A Decade of Transitional Care Research with Vulnerable Elders." *Journal of Cardiovascular Nursing,* 3 (2000): 88-89.

TRANSPLANTATION
Procedure
Anatomy or system affected: Blood, circulatory system, eyes, heart, immune system, kidneys, liver, lungs, pancreas, respiratory system, spleen, urinary system
Specialties and related fields: Cardiology, emergency medicine, general surgery, genetics, immunology, nephrology, oncology, urology
Definition: The transfer of tissue or organs from one individual to another, usually from cadavers or living related donors.
Key terms:
acute rejection: the rejection of a transplanted organ by cells of the immune system; acute rejection is common days to weeks after cadaveric organ transplants and can usually be treated successfully with antilymphocytic drugs
allotransplantation: the transplantation of tissue or organs between unrelated individuals
chronic rejection: the rejection of a transplanted organ months or years after the procedure because of mechanisms that are poorly understood; most long-term graft

losses are caused by chronic rejection, and no effective therapy exists

distributive justice: allocating transplanted organs to recipients based on need

hematopoietic stem cell transplantation (HSCT): transplantation of the bone marrow cells to a recipient

human leukocyte antigens (HLAs): structures located on the surface of each cell that are unique to an individual; also called transplantation antigens

material justice: allocating transplanted organs to recipients based on who would most benefit

orthotopic: the placement of a transplanted organ in the position occupied by the original organ

tissue typing: the process of identifying a person's transplantation antigens

utilitarianism: an ethical theory in which individuals make moral decisions based on the likelihood of benefitting the maximum number of people

vascularized transplant: transplanted tissue or organs that must have blood vessels reattached in the recipient in order to function (such as a kidney); corneal or bone marrow transplants are examples of nonvascularized transplants

xenotransplantation: the transplantation of tissue or organs between different species (such as baboon to human)

The Immune System and Transplantation

Transplantation antigens are proteins expressed on the surface of an individual's cells. Every individual has a unique set of these proteins, called human leukocyte antigens (HLAs), which are encoded on chromosome 6. Each parent contributes one HLA-containing chromosome, and both chromosomes are expressed in the offspring. The purpose of these antigens is to help the body recognize what is "self" and what is not. In this manner, bacteria and other pathogens harmful to the individual can be sensed as "nonself" and destroyed by the immune system.

When an organ is transplanted between unrelated people (allotransplantation), it will not be recognized as self in the recipient's body, and the immune system will start to attack it in a process called rejection. In the same way, transplants between identical twins, with the same HLA proteins on their cells, will be recognized as self and not be rejected.

White blood cells (lymphocytes) are intimately involved in the body's immune response. They protect the individual from invading bacteria, viruses, and fungi. Lymphocytes can be divided into two subsets: B and T cells. The T cell is the main cell involved in the recognition and destruction of allotransplants. Receptors found on the T lymphocyte cell surface are stimulated by the foreign antigens found on allotransplants. With T-cell stimulation, events are initiated that lead to the allotransplant's destruction.

With the knowledge that T cells are responsible for rejection, methods of modulating T-cell activity were developed. One of the first approaches was to destroy them using total-body irradiation. This method had only limited success, and the side effects of the radiation were severe. Attention then turned toward drugs that acted directly on T cells.

Azathioprine was one of the first drugs to be used successfully. By preventing the biosynthesis of essential components of cell growth, azathiaoprine inhibits T cells from replicating. Steroids were next found to have immunosuppressive properties. Azathiaoprine and steroids at one time were used in combination to prevent rejection in human kidney allografts. Although these drugs were effective, they were not specific for T cells. Other cells were affected, and both immunosuppressive drugs had serious side effects in high doses. In 1978, a T-cell-specific inhibitory drug was tried clinically for kidney allotransplants. This drug, named cyclosporine, has since become the mainstay of immunosuppressive therapy for all vascularized allotransplants. In most transplant centers, patients who have received allotransplants are given a combination of the above three drugs, since each drug works differently on T-cell function. The harmful side effects of these drugs can be minimized by using all three in smaller amounts, thus preventing the side effects from larger doses.

With the advent of cyclosporine, patients receiving kidneys without matching HLAs do almost as well in the short term (one to five years) as those receiving HLA-matched kidneys. Transplanted kidneys with HLAs in common, however, function significantly longer (ten years). Therefore, physicians try to match HLAs between donor and recipient. Most organs available for transplantation are from cadavers. It takes days to tissue-type the cadaver, find a compatible recipient, and transport the organ to him or her. Kidneys are the only organ that can be stored this long and still function. Therefore, only kidneys are matched for HLAs. With the liver, heart, and pancreas, only blood type is matched between donor and recipient. Currently, kidneys may be stored up to three days. The liver and pancreas must be transplanted within eighteen to twenty hours.

Indications and Procedures

With the advent of dialysis in 1960, renal failure is no longer fatal and patients can live by having their blood filtered several times per week. Kidney transplantation, however, offers a significant improvement in the quality of life compared with dialysis. Unfortunately, while more than 16,000 patients in the United States receive kidney transplants each year, another 93,000 patients remain on waiting lists. There is much room for greater success.

Two donor options are available to the recipient awaiting a kidney transplant: living related and cadaveric. The first option involves removing a kidney from a willing family member and transplanting it into the recipient. Removing one of two donor kidneys does not significantly affect a healthy individual. The second option is for the recipient to be placed on a waiting list for a cadaveric kidney. When a cadaveric kidney that is of a compatible blood type for a particular recipient becomes available, arrangements are made to admit this patient to the hospital for transplant.

Approximately 30 percent of all kidney transplants are living related. The advantages of a living related transplant are twofold. First, the waiting period for a cadaveric kidney is

In the News:
Donor Bone Marrow Instead of Rejection Drugs

Transplantation using bone marrow cells has dramatically increased over the past four decades. Bone marrow transplantation is used as treatment for certain types of cancer, including lymphoma and leukemia. Two types of bone marrow transplantation are termed allogenic (nonself) or autologous (self). Allogenic transplant requires blood cells from a donor, while autologous transplant requires only a patients own cells.

In autologous transplant, the bone marrow or blood cells are taken from a patient, frozen, and subsequently given back to that patient (transplanted) after chemotherapy has been given. After the autologous stem cells are given back to a patient, the cells can mature into one of three types: red blood cells, which carry oxygen; white blood cells, which fight infection; or platelets, which help blood clotting.

Despite efforts to match a donor's blood cells to a recipient, complications often occur in allogenic transplants. For instance, a complication known as graft-versus-host disease (GVHD) develops in about 50 percent of patients undergoing allogenic bone marrow transplant with related matched donors. To prevent this complication, the patient may receive medications that suppress the immune system (antirejection drugs). In contrast, autologous transplants have a lower incidence of GVHD, which sometimes allows for less antirejection medication. Despite this benefit, autologous transplants do have a higher incidence of cancer relapse causing death (73 percent in autologous transplants versus 33 percent of allogenic transplants).

Autologous transplants do have other benefits, including better results when used instead of chemotherapy alone in certain advanced brain cancers, such as neuroblastoma. For example, the three-year disease-free survival rate is higher for patients that undergo autologous transplant for advanced stage neuroblastoma; however, the patient survival rate does not exceed 35 percent.

—*Jesse Fishman, Pharm.D.*

the place of the liver during surgery, and speed is vital. The liver is the largest organ in the body, weighing about 5 pounds in an adult. Because the liver is so large, and its blood supply complex, it is necessary to remove the patient's own liver during the transplant. The average time for a liver transplant varies, ranging from five to thirty hours. The worst complication of liver transplant is failure to function after surgery. The only treatment is to find another liver for transplantation before the patient dies.

Pancreas transplants are done exclusively for patients with complications of insulin-dependent diabetes mellitus (IDDM). Around half of the new cases of IDDM per year will develop complications such as renal failure and blindness. There is no way to predict which patients will develop these complications. Currently, combined pancreas-kidney transplants are done for diabetics who experience renal failure. The transplanted pancreas prevents damage

eliminated, as the operation can be scheduled as soon as the recipient has been evaluated. Second, kidneys from living related donors tend to work immediately and have better long-term results. Because of organ shortages, some medical centers will allow unrelated volunteers to donate a kidney to a recipient. Such transplants usually occur between spouses.

A typical kidney transplant operation takes three hours to perform. Usually, the patient's own kidneys are not removed, and the transplanted kidney is placed in the pelvis. The vessels of the new kidney are sewn into the iliac blood vessels of the leg. After the transplant procedure, patients stay in the hospital ten days before returning home. They must take medications every day to prevent rejection but otherwise are independent.

Orthotopic liver transplantation is now considered the optimal form of therapy for end-stage liver disease in adults and children. Since no machine exists to take the place of the liver, transplantation is the only alternative in patients with liver failure. Cadaveric livers are the source for transplants because individuals have only one liver. Because of a shortage in cadaveric organs, many patients die each year waiting for a liver transplant. For this reason, a few medical centers have experimented with living related liver transplants, usually from parent to child. In this operation, one of the two lobes of the donor's liver is removed and transplanted to the recipient. The remaining liver in the donor will grow back to normal size in one week.

A liver transplant is one of the most difficult operations to perform. Unlike heart operations, there is no machine to take

from recurring in the new kidney and also makes the individual insulin-independent. Pancreas transplants are not performed for diabetics without complications because the risk of immunosuppression is not worth the benefit of insulin independence.

Unlike with liver transplants, short operative time for pancreas-kidney transplantation is not essential to patient survival. Both the pancreas and the kidney are placed into the pelvis, and the pancreas is anastomosed (sewn) to the right iliac vessels and the kidney to the left. Operative time is about ten hours. As with kidney transplants, the patient's own pancreas and kidneys are left in place because there is no advantage to removing them.

The transplantation of bone marrow, sometimes called hematopoietic stem cell transplantation (HSCT), is less demanding than transplantation of vascularized organs. The bone marrow is composed of stem cells that are primarily responsible for developing into red and white blood cells. A stem cell is any cell from which a whole population of different cells may develop. Transplant recipients, who usually have a blood disease such as leukemia, undergo a process of chemoradiotherapy to destroy their own stem cells. Once it is certain that all their own cells are destroyed, the donor cells are injected into the long bone of the leg. Following HSCT, the recipient may be immunologically incompetent for some time. The functioning of the immune system is vital to the success of this type of transplant. The white blood cells begin to reappear in the blood during the second or third week after the transplant. Although many lymphocytes begin functioning as soon as they are generated, the T and B cells do not become active until later. This is primarily due to the suppression of WBC function due to the presence of immunosuppressive drugs.

Fetal tissue transplantation therapy is related to stem cell therapy in that vascularized organs are not transplanted. Fetal tissue cell lines, sometimes called pluripotent stem cells, have the ability to develop into any cell types found in the adult human body: brain cells for Alzheimer sufferers, pancreas cells for diabetics, heart cells for cardiac patients, and more. There are four sources for pluripotent stem cells: preimplanted human embryos from in vitro fertilization (IVF), umbilical cord blood, cadaveric human fetal tissue, and human germ cell tumors. Although potentially very valuable, research in this area has become an ethical firestorm due to the embryonic source of the tissues. There is the worry that to obtain these cells researchers may actively begin aborting human embryos. Despite this controversy, the stem cell treatment holds such therapeutic promise that no one has yet abandoned the concept.

In 2011, researchers at the University of Wisconsin announced they had successfully transplanted into a mouse brain neurons made from human embryonic stem cells. These neurons could both send and receive nerve impulses, proving that when neurons derived from human embryonic stem cells were transplanted, they could fully integrate and behave like any other neuron, which in turn makes treating neurological disorders such as Parkinson's disease, ALS, and epilepsy more feasible. Use of embryonic stem cells is a controversial issue, which resulted in a ban on federal funding of embryonic stem cell research during the early 2000s. In 2009, the federal position was reversed by President Barack Obama. The ethical debate surrounding embryonic stem cell research, however, continues.

Perspectives and Prospects

There are a number of ethical problems connected to organ transplantation. Primary among these is the problem of donor selection. Cadaverous donors sometimes present the problem of whether sufficient permission was given to donate organs. Without full consent of the donor, it is considered unethical to harvest tissues. In cases where the potential donor died without giving consent, very often relatives who knew of their wish will give consent in their stead. In the case of living donors who are donating kidneys or bone marrow, questions will sometimes arise of their ability to give full consent; for example, whether the donor is fully competent and informed of what consent means. These questions of competence will usually arise with the mentally ill, but often arise when the donor potentially has been coerced by physicians or relatives. Coercion on anyone's part eliminates full consent from the donor.

Another ethical dilemma is the use of human newborns or late stage embryos as organ donors. Is it ethically permissible to use a fetus as an "organ farm"? There have been reports in the last several years of parents with a terminally ill child conceiving another child to act as an organ donor. Although most

often these donor infants become family members, they are sometimes aborted because the needed organ can only be obtained in that way. The bioethicist Mary Anne Warren has argued that the mere "potential to become a person"—unaccompanied by awareness, consciousness, and perception—does not entitle one to life compared to that of a person who needs a transplant. Warren finds no ethical objection to killing a fetus, an "entity below the level of personhood," in order to save the life of a grown human being. Whether or not there is abortion involved in the harvesting process, the ethicist Daniel C. Maguire submits that "person" is a relative term and even baby persons are intrinsically related to other persons. Maguire argues that using the uterus as an organ farm or the "objectified" fetus as an organ bank is intrinsically wrong at the level of consent. What right does anyone have to presume the permission of the baby to donate an organ to a sibling or even a parent? He suggests that the privacy and autonomy of the baby be protected until it grows and can itself consent to an organ donation.

Maguire's argument has also been applied to the harvest and use of embryonic stem cells. When the cells are harvested directly from an embryo, whether that embryo was discarded from IVF or conceived for that specific purpose, the question of consent still remains unanswered.

Finally, allocation of transplanted organs has become increasingly difficult in recent years as the number of available organs has become overwhelmed by the number of potential recipients. A series of ethical questions has arisen in organ transplant allocation. Will the young or old recipient better benefit from a transplant? Should countries limit organ donations from their citizens to non-immigrant aliens? Should organ recipients of particular note, such as film stars and athletes, be moved ahead of "commoners" who are already on the waiting list? Should the location of the recipient affect the decision to provide an organ?

One principle that has been suggested as a guide to allocation is called "distributive justice." Distributive justice suggests that donor organs should go to those most in need. Most countries have now devised rules by which available organs go to those who are the most critically ill. The problem with this selection strategy is that the patients who are in the greatest need are the least likely to survive long term. If the goal is to maximize the overall benefit to society, as the ethical theory of utilitarianism suggests, then this method reduces the overall advantage to society compared to a system that would donate to patients with a better prognosis.

The opposing theory, called "material justice," suggests that patients who are likely to benefit most from transplantation get the organs first. This would maximize the benefit to society, which is risking less on a recipient with a better prognosis. One interpretation of this principle is that children with longer lives ahead of them would get preference for transplantation over adults or the elderly.

These two principles seem at odds with one another. Although the individual will benefit most from distributive justice, society may suffer, and the opposite might be true of material justice where society will benefit, but the individual may suffer. To make allocation as just as possible, the United Network for Organ Sharing (UNOS), the primary body which coordinates organ donors and recipients worldwide, has utilized a point system since August 1995. This point system creates a value for determining the suitability of a recipient for a particular donor based on number of years waiting, rank on the waiting list, HLA tissue mismatches, immune reactivity, and age.

Additionally, the geographic profile of the recipient can be problematic. If a potential transplant recipient has come to the United States from the developing world, where organ donors are rare, in the hope of more easily getting a transplant, should he or she be considered a serious candidate? Should that person be placed ahead of native or naturalized citizens on the waiting list? Should an American citizen and potential recipient living in an isolated geographic location be placed lower on a waiting list because of his or her isolation? These questions are difficult to answer because they bring geography and politics into the equation with medicine and human needs. In September, 2000, the US Department of Health and Human Services (DHHS) proposed rules to reduce the importance of geographic and political boundaries on organ allocation. The prime selection criterion—especially in heart and lung transplantation—would be altered by the DHHS primarily to reflect waiting time. Under these criteria, it would not matter where the candidate resided or where they originated. The only basis for selection would be their need and how long they had been waiting for a transplant.

It has been proposed that organ donors be allowed to sell transplanted organs to the highest bidder. This concept has been defended as "allowing the free market economy to flourish" and letting the poor have the right to "do with their bodies as they see fit." One ethical difficulty with the idea of commercializing human organ sales is that those who are richest will tend to receive the "best" organs. Organ allocation would suffer from these sales, and just distribution would become meaningless. No longer would the most needful recipient get an organ, but rather those who could most afford it would benefit. Furthermore, the poor would be victimized, become commodities, and would be dehumanized as they potentially become organ farms.

—Edmund C. Burke, M.D.,
and Peter N. Bretan, M.D.;
updated by James J. Campanella, Ph.D.

See also Bone marrow transplantation; Cancer; Cirrhosis; Corneal transplantation; Diabetes mellitus; Dialysis; Eye surgery; Eyes; Facial transplantation; Fetal tissue transplantation; Grafts and grafting; Hair loss and baldness; Hair transplantation; Heart; Heart transplantation; Hepatitis; Immune system; Immunology; Kidney transplantation; Kidneys; Leukemia; Liver; Liver transplantation; Renal failure; Systems and organs; Xenotransplantation.

For Further Information:

Brunicardi, F. Charles, et al., eds. *Schwartz's Principles of Surgery.* 9th ed. New York: McGraw-Hill, 2010.

Chen, Yi-Bin. "Bone Marrow Transplant." *MedlinePlus*, February 7, 2012.

Chopra, Sanjiv. *The Liver Book: A Comprehensive Guide to Diagnosis, Treatment, and Recovery.* New York: Simon & Schuster, 2002.

Mulholland, Michael W., et al., eds. *Greenfield's Surgery: Scientific Principles and Practice.* 4th ed. Philadelphia: Lippincott-Raven, 2006.

National Research Council. Institute of Medicine. *Stem Cells and the Future of Regenerative Medicine.* Washington, D.C.: National Academy Press, 2002.

Organ Donor. http://www.organdonor.gov.

"Pancreas Transplant." *Mayo Clinic*, September 22, 2011.

Sacks, Kevin. "Kidney Transplant Committee Proposes Changes Aimed at Better Use of Donated Organs." *New York Times*, September 21, 2012.

Stewart, Susan K. *Autologous Stem Cell Transplants: A Handbook for Patients.* Highland Park, Ill.: Blood and Marrow Transplant Information Network, 2000.

Toouli, James, et al., eds. *Integrated Basic Surgical Sciences.* New York: Oxford University Press, 2000.

Townsend, Courtney M., Jr., et al., eds. *Sabiston Textbook of Surgery.* 19th ed. Philadelphia: Saunders/Elsevier, 2012.

Trzepacz, Paula T., and Andrea F. Dimartini, eds. *The Transplant Patient: Biological, Psychiatric, and Ethical Issues in Organ Transplantation.* New York: Cambridge University Press, 2011.

Welsh, Jennifer. "Growing Brains in Bio Labs, One Cell at a Time." *FoxNews*, May 23, 2011.

TRAUMATIC BRAIN INJURY
Disease/Disorder
Anatomy or system affected: Brain
Specialties and related fields: Neurology, neuroscience, psychiatry, psychology, neuropsychology, rehabilitation
Definition: Injury to the brain that usually results from an accident.

Key terms:

amnesia: a condition exhibited by memory problems

aphasia: a condition exhibited by language problems

brain herniation: brought about by an increase in intracranial pressure, brain structures can stop functioning normally by being shifted, dislocated, and squeezed

edema: abnormal swelling of the brain

intracranial pressure: the amount of pressure inside the cranium; when this reaches abnormally high levels, it can damage brain cells

Causes and Symptoms

Every year, there are over 1.5 million instances of traumatic brain injury (TBI) in the United States with most of those cases affecting young people between the ages of 15-24 years. The most common known causes of TBI are falls (approximately 35 percent), motor vehicle accidents (17 percent), colliding with a stationary or moving object such as common with a sports injury (over 16 percent), and injuries due to assault (10 percent). However, the leading cause of TBI-related deaths is motor vehicle accidents (17.3 percent of TBI, 31.8 percent of deaths). The next most common cause of TBI-related death is being struck by an object (16.5 percent, including collisions in sports-related injuries), followed by assault (10 percent). Although the incident rate for TBI is disproportionally young males under the age of 30 years, around 20 percent are older adults over the age of 75 years.

Brain injuries can be classified according to several different criteria. One common system is to refer to them as either a "penetrating" or "closed-head" TBI. Penetrating head injuries occur when the skull has been compromised by a foreign object such as a gunshot wound. This type of injury is particularly destructive to the brain since not only are brain cells damaged by an object, but bleeding occurs along with the possibility of infection. This is why penetrating head injuries product the highest morbidity and mortality rates. Closed-head injuries, on the other hand, are typically acceleration-deceleration injuries, caused by the brain hitting an object, such as with a severe fall.

Symptoms of TBI often result from primary (or focal) injuries as well as secondary (diffuse) injuries. Brain damage associated with primary injuries results from the initial impact of the brain hitting another object, such as with a fall. The head striking the ground causes the brain to move within the cranium, which can cause bruising, tearing, and shearing injuries (referred to as the "shear-strain effect") as it makes contact with the bony skull. The end result is that brain cells expire. Secondary injuries can occur within minutes or hours after the initial TBI. Symptoms include increased intracranial pressure (ICP) due to edema. Severe edema needs to be controlled or it can lead to death. Brain herniation can occur as a result of hemorrhages or an infection that has set in. This can also contribute to rising ICP that causes brain structures to get displaced and squeezed to a point that they no longer function properly. Compromising lower brain stem structures is serious, since these areas control several components of the autonomic nervous system that keep us alive.

TBI not only produces symptoms for the tissues of the brain that can lead to additional injuries, it can also bring about cognitive, emotional, and behavioral symptoms. Cognitive changes such as language production and comprehension deficits can emerge (aphasia). Experiencing memory problems for past events is frequent, along with a diminished ability to form new memories (amnesia). Overall, TBI sufferers may experience mental clouding and have difficulty making decisions that allow them return to their job and manage their affairs. Besides the emergence of cognitive problems, emotional changes can occur that can lead to experiencing mood swings, irritability, depression, and anxiety. In instances of repeated concussions (a mild TBI), postconcussion syndrome can occur that brings about symptoms such as headaches, irritability, dizziness, lack of concentration, and impaired memory.

Treatment and Therapy

Assessing the severity of traumatic brain injury is often associated with corresponding scores on the Glasgow Coma Scale (GCS). This scale provides a quick measure of the severity of TBI to medical professionals. The scale ranges from 3-15, with 3 being the most severe and 15 being the mildest form of TBI. People who have been assessed a score of below 9 are referred to being in a coma with a diminished level of conscious awareness regarding their surroundings.

Intracranial monitoring has been praised as the cornerstone for medical therapy for TBI. Keeping intracranial pressure within normal levels is the most effective way to reduce the risk of developing additional injuries. One way ICP is managed is by ventilating cerebrospinal fluid that is building up within the brain cavity. This is done by drilling a small hole into the skull and inserting a tube usually into a lateral ventricle. In terms of medicines, Mannitol is an osmotic diuretic and can have significant effects on ICP, cerebral blood flow, and brain metabolism. The drug has two primary mechanisms of action. It expands circulating volume and decreases blood viscosity, which increases cerebral blood flow and cerebral oxygen delivery.

The range of therapeutic needs for a TBI sufferer can vary greatly. A neuropsychologist will be brought in to conduct neuropsychological testing to assess cognitive and behavioral deficits. Once an assessment has been completed, a treatment plan is developed to help the individual progress as far as he or she is capable. Since a brain injury can influence several systems in the body, it is common for an interdisciplinary team to work with TBI patients to provide not only cognitive therapy, but sensory-motor therapy, occupational therapy, speech and language therapy, and physical therapy, among others.

Perspective and Prospects

The study of TBI has helped neuroscientists learn more about the relationship between brain structures and their respective functions. Brain injury, in some instances, can be focused and lead to specific deficits. Back in 1861, Paul Broca, a French surgeon, treated a patient who had been unable to speak for several decades. After the patient's death, Broca performed an autopsy and discovered a lesion in the left frontal lobe near the lateral fissure, which demarcates the frontal lobe from the temporal lobe of the brain. After studying several additional cases of patients with a similar language disturbance, Broca published his results in 1865. This paper supported the theorizing that language processes were localized to specific brain structures. What is now known as Broca's aphasia, which is a form of nonfluent aphasia, is characterized by problems associated with the production of speech. However, if damage is only limited to Broca's area, speech comprehension remains intact. Additional language centers of the brain have been discovered. Depending on the extent of the TBI, multiple language problems can emerge.

Investigators continue to study TBI using the clinical autopsy; however, what has become more common is to use some of the new brain imaging technologies that can look at the structure of the brain while at the same time study its functional properties in vivo. These new imaging technologies, such functional magnetic resonance imaging (fMRI) and positron emission tomography (PET), have revolutionized research into TBI. These technologies provide neuroscientists with a window into the living brain to understand the relationship between brain structures and function. They also provide medical doctors the ability to more accurately diagnose and treat several forms of head injury while the patient is still living.

One major development that has emerged within the literature on recovery and rehabilitation for those who suffer from TBI is the concept of plasticity-the ability of the brain to reorganize itself after an injury has occurred. Plasticity enables brain tissue that was genetically programmed to take charge of a particular set of responsibilities to take on new functions. Brain damage as the result of a TBI could be mitigated by the recruitment of nearby healthy tissue.

—*Bryan C. Auday, Ph.D., and Erika A. Abrahamsen*

See also Concussion, Edema; Glasgow Coma Scale; Neuropsychology; Neuroscience

For Further Information:

Brain Injury Association of America: http://www.biausa.org.

Horton Jr., Arthur MacNeill, and Danny Wedding. *The Neuropsychology Handbook.* 3rd ed. New York: Springer Publishing Company, 2008.

Kolb, Bryan, and Ian Q. Whishaw. *Fundamentals of Human Neuropsychology.* 6th ed. New York: Worth Publishers, 2009.

Lambert, Kelly G., and Craig H. Kinsley. *Clinical Neuroscience: Psychopathology and the Brain.* 2nd ed. New York: Oxford University Press, 2011.

Zillmer, Eric A., Mary V. Spiers, and William C. Culbertson. *Principles of Neuropsychology.* 2nd ed. Belmont, CA: Thomson Wadsworth, 2008.

TREMORS

Disease/Disorder

Also known as: Trembling, shaking

Anatomy or system affected: Arms, feet, hands, head, legs, muscles, nerves, nervous system, throat

Specialties and related fields: Genetics, geriatrics and gerontology, internal medicine, neurology, pharmacology, psychiatry, serology, toxicology

Definition: Rhythmic, oscillating, and involuntary movements that vary with respect to frequency, amplitude, pattern, and anatomical site.

Causes and Symptoms

A very fine physiological tremor is present in the limbs of all people and may be noticeable when the hand is outstretched. This normal tremor is aggravated by fear and anxiety, cold, stress, fatigue, caffeine, alcohol withdrawal, toxin exposure, and a variety of drugs. For example, enhanced physiological tremor is a side effect of antipsychotic drugs that interfere with dopamine uptake in the brain.

The immediate cause of tremor is the repeated contraction and relaxation of muscles. This muscular pattern may be the consequence of neurological damage to the extrapyramidal structures of the brain, including the basal ganglia, or may be an inherited condition.

Two major types are rest and action tremor. The former occurs when a person is resting and typically disappears or is reduced by voluntary movement, whereas the latter occurs when the person is active.

A "pill-rolling" rest tremor in the hand is usually the first noticeable sign of Parkinson's disease; later, the arms and then the legs may become tremulous. If the rest tremor be-

---

Information on Tremors

Causes: Repeated contraction and relaxation of muscles; may result from neurological damage, inherited condition, or Parkinson's disease and be aggravated by fear and anxiety, cold, stress, fatigue, caffeine, alcohol withdrawal, toxin exposure

Symptoms: Involuntary movement, either with rest or with activity

Duration: Acute or chronic and progressive

Treatments: Depends on type and cause; may include anxiety management with cognitive-behavioral therapy, treatment of alcoholism, reduction of caffeine intake, sleep improvement, medications (dopamine receptor agonists, beta-blockers, anticonvulsants, benzodiazepines), stereotactic brain surgery, deep-brain stimulation

---

comes severe enough, then a postural tremor occurs when maintaining a position against gravity. Hence, rest and action tremors may be present at the same time.

Essential tremor is hereditary and is erroneously called senile tremor. It typically affects one hand and then the other, progressing to the arms, and may involve the head and voice. Essential tremor tends to worsen with age and is most visible during slow movements.

Cerebellar tremor is a slow tremor that is visible with targeted, voluntary movements. The probable cause is damage to a cerebellar pathway. This damage may be the result of disease, such as multiple sclerosis, stroke, or trauma to the brain.

Psychogenic tremor is subconsciously controlled by the person. The symptoms and signs point to both rest and action tremors, complicating the diagnosis. The onset may be sudden. The tremor may diminish or disappear when the person is distracted, and there may be a history of somatization disorder. Metabolic disorders and liver or kidney failure resulting in brain damage can also manifest themselves as tremors, known as flapping tremors, which are characterized by oscillations of the hand between dropping and rising positions.

Treatment and Therapy

The treatment of tremor depends on the type. For example, nondrug interventions are sometimes appropriate for enhanced physiological tremor and may include managing anxiety with cognitive-behavioral therapy, treating alcoholism, reducing caffeine intake, improving sleep, and so on.

A variety of drugs can be used for the treatment of tremor, including dopamine receptor agonists, beta-blockers, anticonvulsants, and benzodiazepines. For example, propanolol, a common beta-blocker, may reduce essential tremor as well as Parkinsonian tremors. Drug therapy is less effective for cerebellar tremor. Stereotactic brain surgery (involving spatial coordinates for precision) to destroy part of the thalamus and thus interrupt the circuitry generating tremors or deep-brain stimulation via an electric probe implanted in the thalamus may provide relief.

—*Tanja Bekhuis, Ph.D.;*
updated by W. Michael Zawada, Ph.D.

See also Aging; Alcoholism; Anxiety; Brain; Brain damage; Brain disorders; Caffeine; Fatigue; Multiple sclerosis; Muscle sprains, spasms, and disorders; Muscles; Nervous system; Neurology; Palsy; Parkinson's disease; Psychosomatic disorders; Seizures; Stress; Strokes; Toxicology.

For Further Information:

"About ET." *International Essential Tremor Foundation*, Apr. 2013.

Beers, Mark H., et al., eds. *The Merck Manual of Diagnosis and Therapy*. 18th ed. Whitehouse Station, N.J.: Merck Research Laboratories, 2006.

Owens, D. G. Cunningham. *A Guide to the Extrapyramidal Side-Effects of Antipsychotic Drugs*. New York: Cambridge University Press, 2000.

Stuart, Annie, Rimas Lukas, and Brian Randall. "Benign Essential Tremor." *Health Library*, May 22, 2013.

"Tremor." *MedlinePlus*, May 24, 2013.

"Tremor Fact Sheet." *National Institute of Neurological Disorders and Stroke*, Feb. 21, 2013.

Velickovic, Miodrag, and Jean-Michel Gracies. "Movement Disorders: Keys to Identifying and Treating Tremor." *Geriatrics* 57, no. 7 (July, 2002): 32–37.

Vorvick, Linda J., and David Zieve. "Drug-Induced Tremor." *MedlinePlus*, July 15, 2012.

Zieve, David, David R. Eltz, and Luc Jasmin. "Parkinson's Disease." *MedlinePlus*, Sept. 26, 2011.

TRICHINOSIS
Disease/Disorder
Also known as: Trichinellosis
Anatomy or system affected: Gastrointestinal system, intestines, muscles, musculoskeletal system
Specialties and related fields: Microbiology, public health
Definition: A parasitic disease of humans caused by nematodes of the *Trichinella* genus and acquired by eating contaminated, undercooked meat.

Causes and Symptoms

Trichinosis is a zoonosis (disease acquired from animals) caused by nematodes (roundworms) belonging to the *Trichinella* genus, most commonly *T. spiralis. Trichinella* are parasites of carnivores that show little host specificity, infecting pigs, bears, horses, and humans among other mammals. Undercooked, contaminated pork and bear meat are the most significant sources of human infection. While food processing requirements in developed parts of the world have resulted in decreases in trichinosis, other areas, particularly Latin America (Argentina, Mexico, Chile) and Thailand, continue to experience outbreaks of this disease.

The worms are ingested as larvae that are encysted in the muscle of the infected animal. Once ingested, the larvae hatch from the cysts and mature as adults in the upper intestine. There, the worms mate. Gravid female worms penetrate the intestinal mucosa and deposit larvae that migrate in the bloodstream, eventually becoming encapsulated in the muscle of the infected individual.

Information on Trichinosis

Causes: Parasitic infection transmitted through ingestion
Symptoms: Nausea, vomiting, diarrhea or dysentery, fever, sweating, swelling in face and hands, muscle inflammation and pain, coughing, hoarseness
Duration: Chronic
Treatments: Antihelminthic agents (e.g., mebendazole), corticosteroids

---

Ingesting large numbers of larvae results in gastrointestinal symptoms such as nausea, vomiting, diarrhea or dysentery, fever, and sweating that begin seventy-two hours after infection and may last two weeks. As the larvae migrate, edema (swelling) may be observed around the eyes, side of the nose, temples, and hands. Encysted larvae often result in muscle inflammation and pain, and respiratory symptoms such as cough and hoarseness may be observed late in the infection.

Diagnosis is difficult because of the number of body systems affected and the variety of symptoms. Changes in blood, including an increase in the number of eosinophils (eosinophilia), can be monitored. Because the nematodes are highly antigenic, the human immune response is strong, and antibodies in the blood indicate infection. Sensitive tests involving fluorescently labeled antibodies and enzyme-linked immunosorbent assay (ELISA) can be used to detect circulating antigens in blood serum. Definitive diagnosis is made by examining muscle biopsies for the presence of encysted larvae.

Treatment and Therapy

Trichinosis is usually treated using antihelminthic compounds. Early in the infection, mebendazole (Vermox) may be used. Treatment with these compounds is often accompanied by the administration of corticosteroids to prevent hypersensitivity reactions. The effectiveness of treatment depends on a variety of factors, including the stage of infection, the nature of the infected individual's immune response, the species of nematode, and the initial number of larvae ingested.

Control of the disease is primarily through control of feeding and processing of meat food products, especially pork. In Europe, feeding garbage to pigs has been banned, and in the United States, any garbage-fed pigs and hogs must be pretreated. Inspectors examine animals at slaughter, and in the United States freezing, heating, or freeze-drying of meat products is required during processing. Educating the public to cook pork thoroughly to a temperature of 71 degrees Celsius (161 degrees Fahrenheit) is an important focus of control and prevention efforts.

—*Michele Arduengo, Ph.D.*

See also Food poisoning; Insect-borne diseases; Intestinal disorders; Intestines; Parasitic diseases; Worms; Zoonoses.

For Further Information:

Centers for Disease Control and Prevention. "Parasites—

Trichinellosis (also known as Trichinosis)." *Centers for Disease Control and Prevention*, August 8, 2012.

Doyle, Michael P., Larry R. Beuchat, and Thomas J. Montville, eds. *Food Microbiology: Fundamentals and Frontiers*. 3d ed. Washington, D.C.: ASM Press, 2007.

Forbes, Betty A., Daniel F. Sahm, and Alice S. Weissfeld. *Bailey and Scott's Diagnostic Microbiology*. 12th ed. St. Louis, Mo.: Mosby/Elsevier, 2007.

Jay, James M., Martin J. Loessner, and David A. Golden. *Modern Food Microbiology*. 7th ed. New York: Springer, 2005.

Moorhead, A., et al. "Trichinellosis in the United States, 1991–1996: Declining but Not Gone." *American Journal of Tropical Medicine and Hygiene* 60 (1999): 66–69.

Ray, Bibek and Arun Bhunia. *Fundamental Food Microbiology*. 4th ed. Boca Raton, Fla.: Taylor & Francis, 2008.

Vyas, Jatin M. "Trichinosis." *MedlinePlus*, November 11, 2012.

TRICHOMONIASIS
Disease/Disorder

Also known as: Trich

Anatomy or system affected: Genitals, reproductive system, urinary system

Specialties and related fields: Epidemiology, gynecology, neonatology, obstetrics, perinatology, public health, urology

Definition: A sexually transmitted disease in which motile *Trichomonas vaginalis* protozoans become established in the genitourinary tract of men and women.

Key terms:

asymptomatic: infected but with no discernable symptoms of disease

carrier: a person infected by an organism who can transmit that organism to other people but who is asymptomatic

Centers for Disease Control and Prevention (CDC): a government facility, located in Atlanta, that coordinates investigations of disease occurrence in the United States

protozoan: a unicellular organism with an organized nucleus

sexually transmitted disease (STD): a disease that is usually transmitted from person to person through contact between the vaginal or urethral discharges from an infected person and the genital mucous membranes of a person susceptible to infection

urethritis: inflammation and infection of the urinary tract

vaginitis: inflammation and infection of the vagina

Causes and Symptoms

Flagellated motile protozoans known as *Trichomonas vaginalis* cause trichomoniasis, one of the most widespread and common of sexually transmitted diseases (STDs). The disease is common among people with multiple sex partners, those who engage in unprotected sex, and those who seek services at STD clinics. Trichomoniasis in pregnant women is a leading cause of premature birth in the United States.

Some estimates suggest that 180 million people a year are infected with trichomoniasis worldwide. The most common population found to be infected is females sixteen to thirty-five years old, which is prime childbearing age. This is an important epidemiological group, as trichomoniasis infections

---

Information on Trichomoniasis

Causes: Protozoan infection transmitted via sexual contact or congenitally

Symptoms: In sexually transmitted form, ranges from asymptomatic to frothy yellow or green vaginal discharge, urethritis, vaginitis, itching, red patches on cervix and vaginal walls (in women) and frothy or purulent urethral discharge, urethritis, dysuria, and scrotal pain (in men); in congenital form, placental rupture, premature birth, low birth weight

Duration: Chronic

Treatments: Metronidazole

---

are a leading cause of premature rupture of the placenta, premature birth, and low birth weight.

After infection, there is an incubation period of about seven days, with a range from about four to twenty days. Although up to 70 percent of infected women may remain asymptomatic, *T. vaginalis* infections may sometimes produce a frothy yellow or green vaginal discharge. Women's symptoms may also include urethritis, vaginitis, and itching of the vulva. Sometimes, vaginal inspection shows a distinctive "strawberry cervix" (red patches on the cervix) and red spots on the vaginal walls. Men's symptoms sometimes include urethritis, dysuria, a frothy or purulent urethral discharge, and, in rare cases, scrotal pain as the tube connecting the testicle with the vas deferens becomes inflamed.

The symptoms of infection by *T. vaginalis* are of questionable value in diagnosing the infection. In addition, many infected people remain asymptomatic for many years, and most existing tests, such as microscopic viewing of wet mounts, Pap tests, and polymerase chain reaction (PCR), often fail to show the infectious agent in people with symptoms. Culture of vaginal and urethral smears is considered to be the most effective way of detecting *T. vaginalis* infection. These factors add to the difficulty in reducing infection rates.

Treatment and Therapy

The CDC's *Sexually Transmitted Diseases Treatment Guidelines 2006*, which includes trichomoniasis, focuses on microbiological cure, alleviation of signs and symptoms, prevention of sequelae, and prevention of transmission.

The infection is treated with a single oral dose of either metronidazole or tinidazole. Any sex partner should be treated simultaneously even if he or she is asymptomatic. Treatment is successful in 90 to 100 percent of cases. Treatment during pregnancy is controversial, but no case of fetal malformation has been attributed to metronidazole. Studies have shown that trichomoniasis is associated with low infant birth-weight, premature rupture of the membranes, and preterm births. However, studies of pregnant women with trichomoniasis who are treated failed to show an improvement in preterm deliveries and even trended toward more preterm deliveries; therefore, treatment remains controversial.

Perspective and Prospects

Many men and women infected by the organism remain asymptomatic for years, spreading the disease to other people through sex. Safer sex practices help prevent transmission. People with multiple sex partners should use latex or polyurethane condoms to help curtail the spread of this disease. It is crucial that sex education programs emphasize that people with any unusual genital symptoms, including urethritis and vaginal discharge, seek medical treatment.

People infected by *T. vaginalis* may also be infected by other STD organisms, especially the bacterium that causes gonorrhea. Medical professionals believe that infection by the *Trichomonas* protozoan predisposes a person to infection by the human immunodeficiency virus (HIV) upon exposure through unprotected sex with infected partners.

Trichomoniasis in young children may indicate sexual abuse, and health professionals may be obligated to report such infections, if local regulations require it.

—*Anita Baker-Blocker, M.P.H., Ph.D.*

See also Acquired immunodeficiency syndrome (AIDS); Epidemiology; Genital disorders, female; Genital disorders, male; Gonorrhea; Gynecology; Human immunodeficiency virus (HIV); Men's health; Preventive medicine; Protozoan diseases; Sexually transmitted diseases (STDs); Urethritis; Urinary disorders; Urinary system; Women's health.

For Further Information:

Boston Women's Health Collective. *Our Bodies, Ourselves: A New Edition for a New Era.* 35th anniversary ed. New York: Simon & Schuster, 2005.

Centers for Disease Control and Prevention. *Sexually Transmitted Diseases Treatment Guidelines.* http://www.cdc.gov/std/treatment.

Heymann, David L., ed. *Control of Communicable Diseases Manual.* 19th ed. Washington, D.C.: American Public Health Association, 2008.

Scharbo-DeHaan, Marianne, and Donna G. Anderson. "The CDC 2002 Guidelines for the Treatment of Sexually Transmitted Diseases: Implications for Women's Health Care." *Journal of Midwifery and Women's Health* 48 (February, 2003): 96-104.

Sommers, Michael.Â *Yeast Infections, Trichomoniasis, and Toxic Shock Syndrome (Girls' Health).* New York: Rosen Publishing Group, 2007. Print.

Sutton, Amy L., ed. *Sexually Transmitted Diseases Sourcebook.* 3d ed. Detroit, Mich.: Omnigraphics, 2006.

TUBAL LIGATION

Procedure

Anatomy or system affected: Abdomen, reproductive system, uterus

Specialties and related fields: Gynecology, obstetrics

Definition: A surgical procedure that closes the Fallopian tubes and causes permanent sterilization.

Indications and Procedures

Tubal ligations are performed strictly for sterilization of a female patient. While there has been some success with reversing the procedure, it must be considered permanent. The woman must be well informed and certain that she does not want additional children under any circumstances.

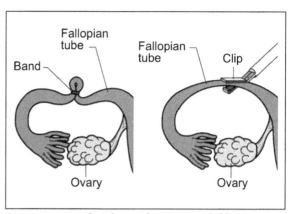

A common means of sterilization for women is tubal ligation, in which the Fallopian tubes through which eggs must pass to reach the uterus are severed or interrupted with clips or bands.

The most common technique for tubal ligation is laparoscopy. As an outpatient, the woman receives local anesthetic and a light sedative. A small incision is made in the navel, and gas is used to inflate the abdomen, allowing easy visibility of the patient's Fallopian tubes. An instrument called an intrauterine cannula is inserted through the vagina, and a clamp called a tenaculum is positioned on the cervix. Both are used to manipulate the tubes into position. A laparoscope, a thin tube containing a camera and light, is inserted through the incision in order to view the tubes. An instrument to block the tubes is inserted through the laparoscope. The tubes may be blocked by burning, cutting, or applying rings or clips. The incision is sewn closed.

In a minilaparatomy, a small incision is made above the woman's pubic bone. The tubes are brought through the incision and are tied and cut. Tubal ligations can also be performed through a woman's vagina (culdoscopy or colpotomy).

Many tubal ligations are done immediately, or within a day, following the delivery of a baby. If a patient has a cesarean section, then tubal ligation is often done as part of the same surgical procedure. Following a vaginal delivery, a woman desiring a tubal ligation is usually brought to the operating room the next day. In cases in which there is a problem with the baby (including extreme prematurity, anomalies, or sepsis), the sterilization procedure is often delayed, pending a good outcome for the infant.

Uses and Complications

The only purpose of tubal ligation is sterilization. It is highly effective (with a 0.2 percent failure rate) and largely irreversible. Depending on the type of blockage used, it is about 30 percent reversible; however, only 10 percent of women become pregnant after undergoing tubal reconstruction. Other forms of birth control are recommended for any patient who is not absolutely certain about the procedure.

Tubal ligations take only thirty minutes to perform, and there is only minor postsurgical pain. A rare complication may be an ectopic pregnancy within the Fallopian tube, which could rupture. Other potential problems are those associated with any abdominal surgery, including unintentional damage to other internal organs, bleeding, and infection. One recent study indicated that there is no change in the level of hormones produced by women prior to or following tubal ligation.

—*Karen E. Kalumuck, Ph.D.;*
updated by Robin Kamienny Montvilo, R.N., Ph.D.

See also Contraception; Gynecology; Hysterectomy; Laparoscopy; Pregnancy and gestation; Reproductive system; Sterilization; Women's health.

For Further Information:
Ammer, Christine. *The New A to Z of Women's Health: A Concise Encyclopedia*. 6th ed. New York: Checkmark Books, 2009.
Berek, Jonathan S., ed. *Berek and Novak's Gynecology*. 15th ed. Philadelphia: Lippincott Williams & Wilkins, 2012.
Connell, Elizabeth B. *The Contraception Sourcebook*. Chicago: Contemporary Books, 2002.
Cunningham, F. Gary, et al., eds. *Williams Obstetrics*. 23d ed. New York: McGraw-Hill, 2010.
Gentile, Gwen P., et al. "Hormone Levels Before and After Tubal Sterilization." *Contraception* 73, no. 5 (May, 2006): 507–511.
Health Library. "Tubal Ligation—Laparoscopic Surgery." *Health Library*, April 22, 2013.
Manassiev, Nikolai, and Malcolm I. Whitehead. *Female Reproductive Health*. New York: Parthenon, 2004.
MedlinePlus. "Tubal Ligation." *MedlinePlus*, May 13, 2013.
Quilligan, Edward J., and Frederick P. Zuspan, eds. *Current Therapy in Obstetrics and Gynecology*. 5th ed. Philadelphia: W. B. Saunders, 2000.
Zite, Nikki, Sara Wuellner, and Melissa Gilliam. "Barriers to Obtaining a Desired Postpartum Tubal Sterilization." *Contraception* 73, no. 4 (April, 2006): 404–407.
Zollinger, Robert M., Jr., and Robert M. Zollinger, Sr. *Zollinger's Atlas of Surgical Operations*. 9th ed. New York: McGraw-Hill, 2011.

TUBERCULOSIS
Disease/Disorder
Anatomy or system affected: Chest, lungs, respiratory system
Specialties and related fields: Bacteriology, microbiology, public health, pulmonary medicine
Definition: A chronic, highly infectious lung disease that can destroy tissue.
Key terms:
BCG: a weakened version of *Mycobacterium bovis* that is used in vaccines to protect against tuberculosis
PPD (purified protein derivative): proteins from mycobacteria used in the tuberculin test; exposure to tuberculosis will result in the sensitization of the immune system to these proteins
primary tuberculosis: a form of tuberculosis that often does not produce symptoms and that develops after exposure to tuberculosis-causing bacteria
sanatorium: an institution designed for the treatment of chronic illnesses, such as tuberculosis
secondary tuberculosis: the recurrence of tuberculosis in individuals who chronically carry the bacterium; a more severe form of the disease in which the lungs are usually damaged
tuberculin test: a skin test used to detect exposure to tuberculosis; a useful test in countries in which vaccines against tuberculosis are not routinely administered
tuberculosis bacilli: bacteria that belong to the genus and species *Mycobacterium tuberculosis*; sometimes called tubercle bacilli, these organisms are the causative agents of tuberculosis

Causes and Symptoms
Tuberculosis derives its name from the Latin word *tubercle*, which means "little lump." Tubercles, or small nodules of diseased tissue, are often found in the lungs of infected individuals. In humans, bacteria that belong to the genus *Mycobacterium* cause tuberculosis. In the vast majority of cases, *Mycobacterium tuberculosis*, often referred to as the tuberculosis bacillus or the tubercle bacillus, is the responsible organism. Other species within the genus may also cause tuberculosis or tuberculosis-like diseases. For example, *M. avium*, a disease-causing organism, or pathogen, is found in birds and swine; it can cause a tuberculosis-like disease in humans. Before it was common to pasteurize milk, *M. bovis*, a pathogen found in cattle, was responsible for cases of human tuberculosis of the digestive tract. In most cases of tuberculosis in humans, the lungs are the major organs affected, but other tissues and organs such as the bones, skin, and digestive tract may also be sites of infection.

Poverty, overcrowding, unsanitary conditions, poor health, and poor nutrition provide ideal conditions for the spread of tuberculosis. It is found at a high frequency in the developing areas of the world, such as parts of Africa, Asia, and Oceania. Immigrants from these countries present a serious public health concern when they enter other countries. Other individuals who have a greater risk for developing tuberculosis infection are inmates of correctional institutions, alcoholics, intravenous drug users, the homeless, and the elderly.

People at a particularly high risk of developing tuberculosis after exposure are those whose immune systems are compromised or suppressed, such as cancer patients receiving chemotherapy, organ transplant recipients, or people with acquired immunodeficiency syndrome (AIDS). Diabetics and individuals with a lung condition known as silicosis are also at high risk of developing tuberculosis as a result of exposure to the disease. Silicosis is an occupational disease that develops as a result of exposure to silica. Silica is found in sand and is a crystalline material encountered by miners, tunnel diggers, stonecutters, glassmakers, and those involved in

---

Information on Tuberculosis

Causes: Bacterial infection
Symptoms: Ranges with severity; may include low-grade fever, fatigue, chest pain, appetite loss, weight loss
Duration: Chronic
Treatments: Antituberculosis drugs, antibiotics

sandblasting operations.

Under a microscope, tuberculosis bacilli appear as straight or slightly curved, rod-shaped organisms. Their widths vary from 0.3 to 0.6 of a micrometer, and their lengths vary from 1 to 4 micrometers. Mycobacteria have unique properties that appear to be linked to their abilities to cause tuberculosis. The cell wall, a protective layer that surrounds all bacteria, is unique in mycobacteria because it contains some unusual lipids. These lipids, which include mycolic acid, give the bacteria special staining properties. Mycobacteria are the only bacteria that resist decolorization with a solution of acid and alcohol (hydrochloric acid and ethyl alcohol) and are thus termed acid-fast. Acid-fastness is the most important characteristic of mycobacteria because it can be used to differentiate them from other types of bacteria. The acid-fast staining procedure can be used to identify mycobacteria and to visualize them in clinical specimens such as lung tissue and sputum.

Mycobacteria populations grow very slowly compared to other bacteria. Under optimal conditions, typical mycobacteria will divide every twelve to eighteen hours, while many other bacteria will divide in twenty to thirty minutes. Mycobacteria require oxygen for growth and are very resistant to drying, most likely because of the lipids in their cell walls. Mycobacteria also resist many chemical and physical agents that would normally kill bacteria. This resistance allows them to survive both in the body and in the exterior environment. Cultures of *M. tuberculosis* maintained in a laboratory usually remain viable for many years. These bacteria can also remain viable outside both a laboratory and the human body. They can retain their pathogenic properties in dried sputum for many months. They are sensitive to ultraviolet light, however, and are killed in about two hours after exposure to direct sunlight.

The mycobacteria that cause tuberculosis are found in the droplets released when a person with active tuberculosis coughs, sneezes, or even talks. This mist of tiny droplets can remain aloft for hours. The manner by which a person becomes infected with tuberculosis usually involves the inhalation of these droplets. The tuberculosis bacilli can then be carried to the lungs. It is fortunate that most individuals who are exposed to tuberculosis will not develop the disease. Tuberculosis is less contagious than the common childhood diseases (such as measles, chickenpox, and mumps) and is usually contracted only after long exposure to an infectious individual who has an active case of tuberculosis. Of all newly infected individuals, approximately 5 percent will show symptoms of tuberculosis within a year. The remaining infected individuals continue to have some risk of developing the disease at any time.

When tuberculosis infection does occur, the initial period is referred to as the primary infection. During this period, an infected individual may not experience any symptoms of illness, or the symptoms may be nonspecific, such as low fever and tiredness. Tuberculosis bacilli in the lung become the focus of an attack by the body's immune system. Primary tuberculosis may also involve the lymph nodes and the pleural cavity. This reaction may lead to the accumulation of fluid within the pleural cavity, accompanied by fever or chest pain. As a result of activities of the immune system and the ingestion of tuberculosis bacilli by white blood cells known as macrophages, the primary infection will often spontaneously subside without medical intervention. Yet, although healing occurs, the tuberculosis bacilli can remain in a somewhat dormant state, walled up in the primary lesions. They live within the cells of the immune system but do not divide. The bacilli can remain in this state for years or decades without producing further symptoms of the disease. Untreated individuals will remain infected throughout their lifetimes even though the disease is in remission.

Most individuals recover from primary tuberculosis. In a small percentage of cases, however, the disease progresses and lung destruction occurs. The reactivation of the disease is referred to as secondary tuberculosis and most frequently occurs when the immune system is weakened. Destruction of lung tissue is a hallmark of this phase of the disease. Much of the damage produced in the lung is the result of efforts by the immune system to destroy the tuberculosis bacilli. Parts of the lung suffer tissue death (necrosis) and soften. These lesions can merge, enlarge, liquefy, and discharge their contents of tuberculosis bacteria into the bronchi. The bacteria can spread to other parts of the lung and be coughed up in sputum, where they contaminate the environment and serve as a source of infectious organisms that will spread the disease. Secondary tuberculosis, if untreated, is a chronic condition in which the symptoms worsen progressively to include fever, fatigue, loss of appetite, and weight loss.

If the bacteria spread to other parts of the body, a condition known as miliary tuberculosis results. Multiple small lesions that resemble millet seeds are found throughout the body. The most common sites in which these lesions are found are the bones and joints, the urogenital system, lymph nodes, the meninges (membranes surrounding the brain and spinal cord), and the peritoneum. Individuals with AIDS are at an increased risk for contracting tuberculosis outside the lungs (extrapulmonary tuberculosis).

Treatment and Therapy

On a global basis, close to ten million new cases of tuberculosis are diagnosed each year, and approximately 1.5 million deaths are attributable to this disease. Since tuberculosis presents a serious public health concern, many countries have employed strategies to prevent its spread. Control of the spread of tuberculosis could decrease the numbers of new cases seen each year. Improvements in living conditions, sanitation, and general standards of living have, in the past, been associated with the decreased incidence of tuberculosis in populations. These goals cannot easily be met in impoverished regions of the world. The medical approaches designed to inhibit the further transmission of tuberculosis include vaccination, rapid diagnosis, and the development of effective drug treatments.

In the United States after the mid-twentieth century, measures were developed to diagnose tuberculosis and prevent its transmission. This program resulted in a marked decrease in death rates from tuberculosis. Total death rates declined dramatically until the mid-1980s. Believing that the disease was one of the past, New York City officials dismantled the entire public tuberculosis health infrastructure of hospitals, sanatoriums, and diagnosis centers during the 1970s. Only a decade later, the city was forced to rebuild that system at a cost of $1 billion to contain a new tuberculosis outbreak that included deadly drug-resistant strains. By the 1990s, tuberculosis was once again on the rise, but the distribution pattern of the disease had changed. One prominent change was that tuberculosis began to be seen more in individuals with AIDS; the rate of tuberculosis infection became much higher in patients with AIDS than in any other group in the population. The immunocompromised nature of AIDS patients renders them highly susceptible to tuberculosis. An illustration of the extent of this phenomenon is the fact that individuals newly diagnosed with tuberculosis are also presumed to have AIDS until laboratory tests prove otherwise.

The tuberculin skin test is a safe and reliable diagnostic test for tuberculosis. When some of the proteins from the tubercle bacilli, in a preparation known as purified protein derivative (PPD), are injected into the skin of an individual who has been exposed to tuberculosis, a characteristic skin reaction will occur. The reaction is characterized by redness and swelling around the injection site, which appears in forty-eight to seventy-two hours. The accumulation and activities of cells of the immune system that recognize the bacterial protein cause this reaction. This type of immune response is referred to as a delayed hypersensitivity reaction and will be seen only in persons who have been previously exposed to these bacterial proteins, usually following infection with tuberculosis bacilli. A positive test does not necessarily mean that a person has an active case of tuberculosis and could therefore be contagious; it merely indicates that at some time, past or present, a tuberculosis infection occurred, even if the individual did not display symptoms of the disease.

The tuberculin skin test is not useful in those parts of the world where many individuals in the population have been vaccinated against tuberculosis with a vaccine composed of Bacillus Calmette-Guérin (BCG). The BCG vaccine contains proteins that sensitize the immune system to PPD. After this occurs, a tuberculin skin test will be positive in an individual who has been vaccinated, even though the individual has never been exposed to live tuberculosis bacilli. All individuals who may become exposed to tuberculosis, such as medical personnel, are advised to receive the tuberculin skin test at regular intervals. If an individual should have a positive skin test, it is common practice to begin treatment with antituberculosis drugs.

In 2005, a new blood test for the diagnosis of tuberculosis was approved by the Food and Drug Administration (FDA). The test, QuantiFERON-TB-Gold, is an enzyme-linked immunosorbent assay (ELISA) that can be used in all instances where the PPD skin test is used; no follow-up visit is required for skin-test reading. The test also can be used in individuals who have had prior BCG vaccination.

Other methods for the diagnosis of tuberculosis include

the detection of acid-fast mycobacteria in sputum, chest X-rays to examine the lungs, and the laboratory culture and examination of mycobacteria grown from clinical specimens. The latter procedure may take from four to six weeks because mycobacteria grow so slowly. The growth and examination of these organisms in the laboratory is necessary, however, to confirm diagnosis when tuberculosis is suspected because of the patient's history and the lung damage seen on X-ray, but microscopic examination fails to show the presence of mycobacteria.

The treatment of tuberculosis changed drastically in the last half of the twentieth century. In the place of quarantine in a sanatorium—a common practice to prevent the spread of the disease—or surgery to remove portions of the diseased lung tissue, tuberculosis patients are now treated with antituberculosis drugs and antibiotics on an outpatient basis. Once treatment is begun, individuals can no longer transmit the disease and are therefore not contagious.

The most effective antituberculosis drugs include isoniazid, pyrazinamide, ethambutol, and the antibiotics rifampicin and streptomycin. The prescribed antituberculosis medications must be used for a long period, usually about nine months, to ensure the destruction of all live tuberculosis bacilli. An ever-increasing problem in the treatment of tuberculosis is the appearance of tuberculosis bacilli that are resistant to drug therapy. These bacteria develop resistance as a result of genetic mutation, and when such drug-resistant bacteria are present in a patient, the disease will not respond to that particular drug. For this reason, most treatment procedures involve the use of three to four different antituberculosis drugs. The probability of the development of two or more separate mutations is much less than the development of a single mutation.

Even though tuberculosis bacilli are less likely to be resistant to more than one drug, multiple-drug-resistant bacteria are emerging in populations throughout the world. Combined drug therapy is ineffective because these organisms can withstand exposure to several of the antituberculosis drugs at once. Without an effective means of treatment, patients who harbor these multiple-drug-resistant organisms are a continued source of infection to the community unless they are kept in isolation.

Because of the long treatment period, some tuberculosis patients stop taking their medication before the destruction of all tuberculosis bacilli. Some of these patients discontinue their medication because their symptoms have disappeared and they believe that they are cured. A recurrence of the disease is highly probable when the full course of treatment is not followed.

In some countries, the BCG vaccine is widely used as a preventive measure. This vaccine is prepared from live bacteria that belong to a strain of *M. bovis* that has lost its pathogenic properties. The effectiveness of the vaccine is not absolute; studies show that in countries where the vaccine is employed, there may be a 60 to 80 percent decrease in the incidence of tuberculosis. The BCG vaccine is not used in the United States because the incidence of tuberculosis in the general population is quite low compared to other countries. In addition, if the BCG vaccine were widely used, it would negate the utility of the tuberculin skin test as a reliable and valuable diagnostic tool.

Perspective and Prospects

Throughout the ages, tuberculosis has been a scourge of humankind. Human fossils, excavated from a Neolithic burial ground dated about six thousand years ago, show evidence of tuberculosis of the spine. Egyptian mummies from 1000 BCE with signs of tuberculosis suggest that the disease was widespread in ancient Egypt. Symptoms of tuberculosis such as fever, excessive weight loss, night sweats, breathlessness, pain in the side and chest areas, and coughing up of sputum and blood are described in the writings of ancient Hindu, Greek, and Roman writers. The widespread nature of the disease appears in accounts from early European history, from the fifth to eighteenth centuries, which refer to a "touching" ceremony that was performed by English and French monarchs and believed to cure scrofula (tuberculosis of the lymph glands in the neck region).

One of the greatest causes of disease and death in the world, tuberculosis has been known by many names, including scrofula, phthisis, and consumption. In writings, it has been referred to as "the white plague" and "the captain of all the men of death." During the nineteenth century, tuberculosis was widespread in Europe. The symptoms of tuberculosis were not thought to represent a disease but rather hallmarks of an especially sensitive personality—the ideal for an artist, musician, poet, or writer. At that time, it was somewhat fashionable to be pale and thin, and to have a slight cough.

Although tuberculosis has been a serious health threat for such a long period of human history, the disease and its cause were poorly understood until the 1880s. Robert Koch is credited with discovering the tuberculosis bacillus. His masterful treatise, published in 1882 and translated under the title "The Etiology of Tuberculosis," presents convincing experimental evidence for implicating a bacterium that came to be known as *M. tuberculosis* as the causative agent of tuberculosis. Despite this great breakthrough, a rational effective treatment for the disease could not be found. One type of therapy that became popular was simply rest and fresh air. Edward Livingston Trudeau, an American physician who suffered from tuberculosis, observed that he regained his health when he traveled to Saranac Lake in the Adirondack Mountains in the state of New York. He attributed his recovery to the restful environment and clean air. Trudeau later founded a sanatorium at Lake Saranac that became popular for tuberculosis patients.

It was not until the discovery of the antibiotic streptomycin in 1943 by Selman A. Waksman that a truly potent antituberculosis agent was found. The tuberculosis bacilli, however, proved to be quite resistant to a multitude of other antibiotics and antibacterial drugs. Fortunately, several antibiotics and antibacterial drugs, especially when used in combination and for the full duration of their prescription, can cure many tuberculosis patients.

The disease's spread seemed to slow again by the early 1990s. Over an eight-year period, from 1992 to 2000, the number of new tuberculosis cases decreased an average of 7 percent per year. However, from 2000 to 2001, this rate of decrease slowed to 2 percent, reflecting transmission in foreign-born patients; in crowded shelters and prisons where people are weakened by poor nutrition, drug addiction, and alcoholism; and in long-term care facilities such as nursing homes where residents develop active tuberculosis from infections with *M. tuberculosis* that occurred much earlier in life because their general health has declined. Despite the slowed pace, the number of cases has increasingly dropped since 2006; new cases fell at a rate of 2.2 percent in 2011. Overall, the mortality rate for tuberculosis has dropped 41 percent since 1990. Thus, in today's world, while the major problems presented by tuberculosis have been the increasing incidence of the disease, the increasing prevalence of cases that display multiple-drug resistance, and the association with AIDS—which make these cases of tuberculosis difficult to treat and further the possibilities for widespread transmission of the disease—effective measures to prevent and treat the disease have helped decrease the incidence rate and save millions of lives.

—Barbara Brennessel, Ph.D.; updated by
L. Fleming Fallon, Jr., M.D., Ph.D., M.P.H.

See also Acquired immunodeficiency syndrome (AIDS); Antibiotics; Bacillus Calmette-Guérin (BCG); Bacterial infections; Bacteriology; Coughing; Drug resistance; Epidemics and pandemics; Epidemiology; Immunization and vaccination; Lungs; Pulmonary diseases; Pulmonary medicine; Respiration; Wheezing.

For Further Information:

Badash, Michelle, and Michael Woods. "Tuberculosis." *Health Library*, Nov. 26, 2012.
Daniel, Thomas M. *Captain of Death: The Story of Tuberculosis*. Rochester, N.Y.: University of Rochester Press, 1997.
Dormandy, Thomas. *The White Death: A History of Tuberculosis*. New York: New York University Press, 2000.
Gandy, Matthew, and Alimuddin Zumla, eds. *Return of the White Plague: Global Poverty and the "New" Tuberculosis*. New York: Verso, 2003.
Levitzky, Michael G. *Pulmonary Physiology*. 8th ed. New York: McGraw-Hill Medical, 2013.
Lutwick, Larry I., ed. *Tuberculosis: A Clinical Handbook*. Chicago: Chapman and Hall, 1995.
Mazurek, Gerald H., et. al. "Guidelines for Using the QuantiFERON-TB Gold Test for Detecting Mycobacterium Tuberculosis Infection, United States." *Morbidity and Mortality Weekly Report (MMWR)* 54 (December 16, 2005): 49–55.
Rom, William N., and Stuart M. Garay, eds. *Tuberculosis*. 2d ed. Philadelphia: Lippincott Williams & Wilkins, 2004.
Scharer, Lawrence, and John M. McAdam. *Tuberculosis and AIDS: The Relationship Between Mycobacterium TB and the HIV Type 1*. New York: Springer, 1995.
"Tuberculosis." *American Lung Association*, Mar. 21, 2013.
"Tuberculosis." *MedlinePlus*, May 24, 2013.
"Tuberculosis (TB)." *Centers for Disease Control and Prevention*, Apr. 12, 2013.
"Tuberculosis: WHO Global Tuberculosis Report 2012." *World Health Organization*, 2012.
West, John B. *Pulmonary Pathophysiology: The Essentials*. 8th ed.

Philadelphia: Wolters Kluwer/Lippincott Williams & Wilkins, 2013.

TULAREMIA
Disease/Disorder

Anatomy or system affected: Abdomen, joints, lymphatic system, muscles, respiratory system, skin

Specialties and related fields: Bacteriology, emergency medicine, environmental health, epidemiology, immunology, public health

Definition: A highly infectious bacterial disease, caused by *Francisella tularensis*, that is of concern as a potential biological weapon.

Key terms:

biological warfare: also called biowarfare; warfare using biological agents or toxins produced by biological agents

biological weapon: also called a bioweapon; a biological agent or toxin produced by a biological agent used as a weapon

zoonoses: a disease that can be transmitted from animals to humans and vice versa

Causes and Symptoms

Tularemia is a bacterial disease, caused by *Francisella tularensis*, that is of significant concern as a potential biological weapon because it is easily spread via airborne routes and is highly infectious—inhaling as few as ten bacterial cells is enough to cause disease in humans. If the bacteria were released in a densely populated area, then large numbers of people could fall ill within days.

The bacterium *F. tularensis* was discovered following a plaguelike disease that swept through ground squirrels in Tulare County, California, in 1911. Shortly after its initial discovery, it was demonstrated to cause disease in humans. The organism is common throughout North America and Eurasia. The disease is transmitted via a number of routes: bites of infected insects, contact with the carcasses of infected animals, eating contaminated food or drinking contaminated water, and breathing in the bacteria. The disease is not spread via person-to-person contact.

After infection, symptoms typically appear within two weeks. They include fever, chills, aches, pain, headaches, diarrhea, coughing, and, as the disease progresses, increasing weakness. Some individuals develop skin ulcerations and swollen lymph nodes, as well as pneumonia with accompanying chest pain, bloody sputum, and difficulty breathing—sometimes leading to respiratory failure.

Treatment and Therapy

Tularemia can be treated with a number of antibiotics, but preventing infections is ideal. Infection may be prevented by controlling exposure to insect and animal carriers of the bacterium, eating thoroughly cooked food, and drinking clean water.

Vaccines may also be used to prevent the disease. Russia has used a tularemia vaccine in areas where the disease naturally occurs since the 1930s. A vaccine has been under review

---

Information on Tularemia

Causes: Infection with *Francisella tularensis* bacteria through insect bites, contact with infected animals, contaminated food or water, inhalation

Symptoms: Fever, chills, aches, headache, diarrhea, coughing, progressive weakness, skin ulcerations, swollen lymph nodes, pneumonia

Duration: Acute

Treatments: Antibiotics

---

by the Food and Drug Administration (FDA) but is not yet available in the United States.

Perspective and Prospects

Since tularemia is easily contracted via inhalation of a small number of bacterial cells, it has been tested by some countries as a weapon to be released via the air. Japanese germ warfare units researched the use of tularemia as a weapon in Manchuria from 1932 through 1945. Tens of thousands of German and Russian troops were sickened by the disease on the Eastern Front in World War II, and some researchers suspect that the infections were intentional rather than natural. The United States and other countries have continued to research tularemia as a weapon since the war.

—*David M. Lawrence*

See also Bacterial infections; Bacteriology; Biological and chemical weapons; Environmental diseases; Environmental health; Epidemiology; Food poisoning; Insect-borne diseases; Plague; Pulmonary diseases; Zoonoses.

For Further Information:
Farlow, Jason, et al. "*Francisella tularensis* in the United States." *Emerging Infectious Diseases* 11, no. 12 (December, 2005): 1835-1841.

Henderson, Donald A., Thomas V. Inglesby, and Tara Jeanne O'Toole. *Bioterrorism: Guidelines for Medical and Public Health Management*. Chicago: American Medical Association, 2002.

Sidell, Frederick R., and Ernest T. Takafuji. *Medical Aspects of Chemical and Biological Warfare*. Washington, D.C.: Borden Institute, Walter Reed Army Medical Center, 1997.

Siderovski, Susan Hutton.Å *Tularemia (Deadly Diseases and Epidemics)*. New York: Chelsea House Publishers, 2006. Print.

TUMOR REMOVAL
Procedure

Anatomy or system affected: All (primarily brain, breasts, gastrointestinal system, intestines, lungs, respiratory system)

Specialties and related fields: General surgery, histology, oncology

Definition: The removal-through surgery, chemotherapy, or radiotherapy-of any neoplasm.

Key terms:

computed tomography (CT) scanning: a medical imaging technique which involves the X-ray observation of cross sections of tissue

magnetic resonance imaging (MRI): a medical imaging

technique in which the image is produced by the scanning of a magnetic field

metastasis: the spread of cancer cells from the primary tumor to other sites in the body

neoplasm: an uncontrolled growth of cells which can develop into a tumor; may be malignant (cancerous) or benign

oncogene: a regulatory gene in a cell which, when mutated, may cause that cell to become cancerous

Indications and Procedures

The uncontrolled, progressive growth of cells, termed a neoplasm, usually results in a mass or tumor. The tumor may be malignant (cancerous) or benign. Generally, benign tumors remain localized, are often encapsulated, and contain cells that remain well differentiated. Since the cells of a benign tumor do not metastasize, the tumor is usually less of a threat to life. The site of the tumor, however, can be as critical as its malignant or nonmalignant state: tumors within inoperable portions of the brain may pose a threat regardless of whether they are malignant.

Most tumors are initially observed as localized masses of cells, or lumps. Any symptoms that occur result from tumor growth in this particular tissue. While any tissue or cell is at risk for the development of a tumor, most such forms of uncontrolled growth are found in the female breasts, the colon, and the lungs, the latter a result of the increased use of cigarettes in the twentieth century.

When a tumor is observed, several options exist for its elimination. Surgery remains the method of choice when applicable. This method poses two advantages: under ideal circumstances, surgery can result in complete removal of the tumor and total cure; in addition, the removal of the tissue allows for proper diagnosis, and subsequent prognosis, of the form of tumor. Surgery may also play a palliative role, allowing for elimination of some of the tumor mass, temporary relief of symptoms, and a greater chance for alternative forms of therapy to effect a cure.

While alternative methods of noninvasive diagnosis were developed during the latter half of the twentieth century, most notably computed tomography (CT) scanning and magnetic resonance imaging (MRI), surgery remains the best method for both tumor diagnosis and cure. The procedure for diagnosis of most tumors is relatively straightforward. When the patient is examined, a complete analysis of symptoms is carried out. The tumor, though not necessarily its prognosis, may be directly observable, such as a lump in the breast. Sometimes, symptoms may be secondary, such as blood in the feces resulting from a tumor in the colon or a cough associated with lung cancer. Biopsy of the material, often in conjunction with surgery, may be necessary to determine whether the tumor is malignant; many tumors are not. If the tumor is determined to be malignant, the material obtained in the biopsy may also be useful in determining the staging of the tumor, a classification system used to identify the extent of the tumor, its degree of spread, and the likely prognosis. Though several methods of staging are used, the most popular is the TNM system. T refers to the size of the tumor (T0 to T4, depending on its size),

N refers to the extent of lymph node involvement (N0 to N2), and M indicates whether metastasis has occurred (M0 or M1).

If the tumor is localized, surgical removal remains the best chance for a cure. In general, the patient is anesthetized and the region of the tumor is surgically removed. For a tiny breast tumor, this may involve a lumpectomy (removal of the lump only). For larger tumors, extensive amounts of tissue may have to be excised. Surgery usually involves the use of a knife, though alternative forms such as laser surgery or electrosurgery may be used under specific circumstances. The surgeon will attempt to remove the area of cancer or, when warranted, the entire organ and a margin of adjacent normal-looking tissue, in the event that a few cells have spread beyond the visible tumor. Localized lymph glands may also be removed, both to estimate the chance of metastasis and to improve the chance of removing all the tumor since the local lymph nodes are generally the sites to which cancer cells initially spread.

When the tumor is too large, or if metastasis has occurred, additional forms of treatment to effect tumor removal may be needed. Radiation therapy, the use of beams of high-energy X-rays or radioactivity, may be used to reduce the size of a tumor or to eliminate any cancer cells that remain in the vicinity of an excised tumor. Chemotherapy, the use of metabolic poisons, is often employed when the tumor has spread beyond its initial site.

Tumor removal may also be palliative, a procedure employed for the reduction of symptoms or for the restoration of normal organ function. For example, the removal of a tumor on the colon may reduce pain and restore function temporarily, even if the tumor has spread and the prognosis is poor. Common benign tumors may also cause discomfort, even if not life-threatening. Nearly one-quarter of women over the age of thirty develop fibroid tumors on the wall of the uterus, a condition which is more of a nuisance than dangerous; surgical removal of such tumors may be necessary to eliminate pain or bleeding.

The decision regarding the methodology of tumor removal often depends on the site and extent of the tumor. The biopsy of the material may be immediately followed by surgical removal of the tumor while the patient remains under anesthesia. This is often the method of choice if the tumor is small or confined to a single organ. After surgery, any additional options can be discussed with the patient. If various options exist for tumor removal, the results of the biopsy may first be discussed with the patient, and a decision on specific forms of treatment may follow.

The most convenient procedure for biopsy during surgery is needle aspiration, the insertion of a small needle into the tumor for the removal of a small number of cells. If more tissue is needed, a larger needle may be used. If the tumor is small enough, the entire tumor may be removed at this stage.

When the tumor has been removed, the entire tissue is given to a pathologist. Analysis of this gross specimen allows for a firmer diagnosis of the form of tumor, its staging, and a possible prognosis.

Uses and Complications

Two strategies are associated with tumor removal: First is the attempt to effect a cure. Ideally, complete elimination of a malignant tumor will result in a cure for the disease. The assumption in this case is that metastasis has not occurred. If the tumor is benign, removal should alleviate any symptoms associated with its growth. As indicated above, fibroid tumors of the uterus, while common in middle-aged women, rarely pose a threat to life; it is their very presence that results in discomfort or other symptoms. Likewise, parotid tumors, growths in the salivary gland, may result in unsightly lumps in the region of the jaw, as well as pain or discomfort; on some occasions, there may be facial paralysis. Removal of the tumor, generally through surgery but with radiation or chemotherapy if the condition warrants, may be indicated.

Colon cancer is one of the more common forms of cancer among adults. Symptoms include rectal bleeding, diarrhea, loss of weight, and loss of appetite. If a patient complains of such symptoms, the physician will likely recommend a rectal examination, including the removal of tissue for biopsy, generally as part of a colonoscopy (the visual examination of the colon with a flexible fiber-optic tube).

Treatment for colon cancer depends on the results of the biopsy and the general health of the patient. Surgical removal, however, is the most common treatment. If the tumor is small and confined, as in the form of a polyp, the removal of the polyp (polypectomy) is usually sufficient to effect a cure. If the tumor is relatively large, both the tumor and surrounding tissue must be removed (wedge resection). The extent of tissue removal depends on the size and stage of the tumor. Complete removal often includes supplementary treatments such as chemotherapy or radiation therapy. Since metastasis has often occurred by the time that symptoms appear, the prognosis for colon cancer is often poor.

Surgical procedures for smaller, more accessible tumors in other parts of the body are more straightforward. In the case of a parotid tumor, diagnosis often includes a CT scan or MRI, along with a biopsy. If the tumor is benign, removal of the lump is relatively simple. In rare instances in which the tumor is malignant, radiation therapy may be included as part of the treatment.

Breast cancer is one of the more common forms of cancer in women. In addition to its life-threatening potential, the disease can result in disfigurement as a result of treatment.

Breast cancer often is first observed as a lump in the breast. If the biopsy shows it to be malignant, several courses of action may be considered, usually associated with surgical removal of the tumor along with healthy surrounding tissue. If the tumor is very small, removal of the lump may be sufficient; if the tumor has spread, complete removal of the breast is often the choice (mastectomy). Radical mastectomy, which also involves the removal of surrounding muscle, may be necessary if the cancer has spread into that tissue. Nearby lymph nodes from the armpit (axillary nodes) are often included in order to evaluate whether the cancer has metastasized.

Perspective and Prospects

The first attempts at the surgical removal of tumors date to as early as 1600 BCE in Egypt. These procedures were obviously crude and limited. Modern surgical treatment for tumor removal is credited to the American surgeon Ephraim MacDowell, who in 1809 removed a twenty-two-pound tumor from a patient. (The patient survived and lived another three decades.) Two complications limited such forms of surgery, even for localized, readily accessible tumors: pain and infection. Though extracts from the poppy and the drinking of alcohol were both used to deaden pain in earlier centuries, it was not until the routine use of ether in the mid-nineteenth century that pain could be eliminated from surgery. In 1846, William T. G. Morton demonstrated the use of ether as a general anesthetic, first in the extraction of a tooth and later in a public demonstration in which a vascular tumor of the jaw was removed from a young patient. The pain-free operation lasted nearly thirty minutes and ushered in the era of general surgery.

Though pain during surgery could now be eliminated, there was still the problem of infection. Tumor removal in the mid-nineteenth century was confined to those of the breast or superficial areas of the body. It remained for Joseph Lister in the 1860s and 1870s to develop the antiseptic procedures necessary to reduce the chances for infection and subsequent mortality associated with surgery as a means of tumor removal.

Surgical procedures continued to improve in the twentieth century. Following the discovery of radioactivity by Wilhelm Conrad Röntgen, the use of X-rays was added to the repertoire for the elimination of tumors. By damaging the genetic material of cells, radiation was demonstrated to be capable of reducing the size of tumors or of eliminating localized tumors altogether. The discovery in the mid-twentieth century of chemicals that interfere with the growth or metabolism of cancer cells resulted in the development of chemotherapy as a method of treatment.

Technological advances have resulted in better methods both for the diagnosis of tumors and in their elimination. Both CT scanning and MRI have the advantage of being noninvasive, though surgical biopsy remains the method of choice for diagnosis and staging of a tumor. Along with the development of these techniques have come more aggressive forms of treatment. Until the 1970s, tumor removal generally involved surgery, chemotherapy, or radiation therapy, but not often in combination. It became apparent that the elimination of the tumor was more effective when these procedures were used together: radiation therapy could be used first to shrink the tumor, allowing for more effective surgical removal. As knowledge of the immunology of cancer (and the immune system in general) developed, physicians began to apply the immune system itself as a form of therapy. Interleukins and other chemicals secreted by the body's immune cells were seen to boost the immune response, aiding in the killing of tumor cells.

Many of the future goals in this medical field center on the prevention of tumor formation, as well as their elimination. It is known that certain carcinogens such as cigarette ingredients are involved in the induction of tumors. Reduction in the number of persons smoking would have a significant impact on the prevalence of smoking-related tumors of the mouth and respiratory system. In addition, many tumors have been found to have a genetic basis; specific forms of cancer are associated with oncogenes in the cell. Through periodic screening, it is possible to observe whether such genes have undergone mutation and to remove any tumors that occur while they are still small and before they have undergone metastasis.

—*Richard Adler, Ph.D.*

See also Biopsy; Bladder cancer; Brain tumors; Breast biopsy; Breast cancer; Breasts, female; Cancer; Cervical, ovarian, and uterine cancers; Chemotherapy; Colonoscopy and sigmoidoscopy; Colorectal cancer; Colorectal polyp removal; Cryosurgery; Electrocauterization; Gallbladder cancer; Gastroenterology; Gastrointestinal disorders; Gastrointestinal system; Gynecology; Kidney cancer; Lung cancer; Lung surgery; Lungs; Malignancy and metastasis; Mammography; Mastectomy and lumpectomy; Melanoma; Mouth and throat cancer; Myomectomy; National Cancer Institute (NCI); Oncology; Plastic surgery; Prostate cancer; Prostate gland; Prostate gland removal; Pulmonary diseases; Pulmonary medicine; Radiation therapy; Stomach, intestinal, and pancreatic cancers; Testicular cancer; Tumors.

For Further Information:

Brunicardi, F. Charles, et al., eds. *Schwartz's Principles of Surgery.* 9th ed. New York: McGraw-Hill, 2010.

"Cancer." *MedlinePlus*, June 10, 2013.

"Chemotherapy—What It Is, How It Helps." *American Cancer Society*, Mar. 25, 2013.

Doherty, Gerard M., and Lawrence W. Way, eds. *Current Surgical Diagnosis and Treatment.* 13th ed. New York: Lange Medical Books/McGraw-Hill, 2010.

Dollinger, Malin, et al. *Everyone's Guide to Cancer Therapy.* Rev. 5th ed. Kansas City, Mo.: Andrews McMeel, 2008.

Griffith, H. Winter. *Complete Guide to Symptoms, Illness, and Surgery.* Revised and updated by Stephen Moore and Kenneth Yoder. 6th ed. New York: Perigee, 2012.

Mulholland, Michael W., et al., eds. *Greenfield's Surgery: Scientific Principles and Practice.* 5th ed. Philadelphia: Lippincott Williams & Wilkins, 2011.

"Radiation Therapy—What It Is, How It Helps." *American Cancer Society*, Nov. 26, 2012.

Sarg, Michael J., and Ann D. Gross. *The Cancer Dictionary.* 3d ed. New York: Checkmark Books, 2007.

"Treatment Types." *American Cancer Society*, n.d.

"Understanding Cancer Surgery: A Guide for Patients and Families." *American Cancer Society*, Aug. 25, 2011.

Zollinger, Robert M., Jr., and Robert M. Zollinger, Sr. *Zollinger's Atlas of Surgical Operations.* 9th ed. New York: McGraw-Hill, 2011.

TUMORS

Disease/Disorder

Anatomy or system affected: All

Specialties and related fields: Endocrinology, histology, internal medicine, oncology, pulmonary medicine

Definition: Abnormal growths of bodily tissues caused by genetic changes within normal cells; tumors may be benign (noninvasive) or malignant (invasive).

Key terms:

benign tumor: a tumor that grows rapidly within a localized area without invading other tissue regions; noncancerous

cancer: a malignant tumor that grows rapidly and uncontrollably, starting with a transformed cell and spreading throughout the affected body, causing organ damage, failure, and death

carcinogen: a mutagenic substance that triggers cellular biochemical events causing normal cells to become cancerous

cellular transformation: the biochemical process by which a normal body cell becomes tumorous, especially cancerous

differentiation: the physiological event in all multicellular organisms by which identical cells with identical genetic information specialize to become different tissue types

gene regulation: the control of whether a gene is active (that is, encoding messenger RNA and protein) or inactive (that is, not encoding RNA or protein), a process often affected by hormones

malignant tumor: a cancerous mass of cells that invades various body regions, contributing to tissue and organ failure as well as to the eventual death of the entire organism

metastasis: the breaking off and movement of cancer cells from one body tissue region to another, with transport being facilitated by the organism's bloodstream

mutagen: a substance (usually chemicals or ionizing radiation) that penetrates body cells and alters the nucleotide sequence of deoxyribonucleic acid (DNA), thus generating a mutation

virus: an obligate intracellular parasite, composed of genetic information protected by protein, that reproduces within living cells

Causes and Symptoms

Tumors, also called neoplasms, are caused by a variety of factors—including mutations, improper hormonal signaling, viruses, and environmental influences—which cause certain normal body cells to deviate from a genetically determined developmental pattern for that particular organism. Tumors arise in all multicellular eukaryotic organisms, such as animals, plants, and fungi, where colonies of cells are intricately connected and are dependent on one another.

A tumor arises when a mistake is made in the cellular expression of a given gene. At a certain point in the cell's development, a gene may be activated when it should not produce protein, or it may be inactivated when it should be producing protein. In either case, a cascade of subsequent developmental changes within the cell may be initiated. The cell may function inefficiently, die, or start to grow and divide at a faster rate than normal. In this latter scenario, the cell has become tumorous.

Many developmental biologists view the tumorous state as a throwback to the early embryonic development of the organism, when cells are undifferentiated and do not reveal the effects of specific hormonal genetic controls. Therefore, tumors reflect a dedifferentiated state of the cell. Tumors may be benign or malignant. A benign tumor grows as an enlarged tissue region without spreading elsewhere; often, it is only an inconvenience or irritant to the organism without harming the individual. A malignant tumor is invasive, spreading rapidly throughout many tissues, draining the organism of various resources, and eventually destroying key tissues and killing the individual. The breaking off and rapid spread of malignant tumors is termed metastasis.

The changes within genes and the subsequent gene expression or cellular dedifferentiation associated with tumors are brought about by mutations, changes within the nucleotide sequence (the genetic code) of the genes. Mutations can be caused by a number of agents called mutagens. Two major classes of mutagens are chemical mutagens (including benzene, carbon tetrachloride, and diethylstilbestrol) and radiation such as ultraviolet light, X radiation, and gamma radiation. Some mutagens also are carcinogens, causing malignant tumors. Not all mutagens, however, are also carcinogens. Caffeine, for example, is mutagenic but not carcinogenic.

Tumors can arise within cells of any of the five principal tissue types: epithelia, endothelia, connective tissue, nerve, and muscle. Epithelial tissue lines the organs outside and inside the body, including the skin, exocrine glands (such as oil and sweat glands), the digestive tract, and the reproductive organs. Endothelial tissue includes blood cells, blood vessels, and lymph nodes and glands. Connective tissue includes bone, fat cells, and cartilage. Nerve tissue includes the billions of nerves that compose the brain, spinal cord, and peripheral sensory and motor nerves. Muscle tissue includes the heart, more than six hundred skeletal muscles, and tens of thousands of smooth muscles.

Epithelial tissue cancers collectively are called carcinomas; they include adenocarcinomas, basal cell carcinomas, melanomas, malignant melanomas, squamous cell carcinomas, cervical cancer, uterine cancer, prostate cancer, colorectal cancer, and lung cancer. Whereas benign tumors of the skin such as freckles, moles, and warts are not serious, cancers of the skin and internal organ membranes can be fatal. Adenocarcinomas affect glands. Basal cell carcinomas, melanomas, and squamous cell carcinomas are serious cancers of the skin that can arise from prolonged sun exposure. Malignant melanoma is a rapidly invasive skin cancer that can penetrate other body tissues and cause death within two or three months. Cervical and uterine cancers are serious tumors of the female reproductive tract. Prostate cancer is prevalent among males and is a leading cause of cancer deaths. Colon and rectal cancers, believed to be triggered by the lack of roughage in diets, are also relatively common. Lung cancer may result from exposure of lung tissue to cigarette smoke and air pollution.

Endothelial tissue cancers include leukemias, which affect blood cells, and lymphomas, which affect lymphatic tissue. Most leukemias affect the immune system's white blood cells (leukocytes) or the stem cells from which they are derived. Leukemias include acute lymphoblastic leukemia, acute myeloblastic leukemia, acute monoblastic leukemia, chronic lymphocytic leukemia, and chronic granulocytic leukemia. Lymphatic cancers attack the lymph nodes and glands that

---

Information on Tumors

Causes: Genetic and environmental factors, disease, improper hormonal signaling, viruses
Symptoms: Varies with affected region and severity; may include discomfort, pain, swelling, bloating, diarrhea, vomiting, constipation, skin lumps or lesions
Duration: Short-term to recurrent
Treatments: Removal through surgery, lasers, freezing, chemotherapy, radiation therapy

---

serve as blood reservoirs for the circulatory system. Lymphatic cancers include lymphosarcomas, Hodgkin disease, and Burkitt lymphoma, which is induced by the Epstein-Barr virus.

Connective tissue tumors include benign varieties such as osteomas and osteochondromas affecting bone, chondromas affecting cartilage, and lipomas affecting adipose (fat) tissue. Connective tissue cancers are called sarcomas. Chondrosarcomas are cartilaginous tissue cancers affecting joints. Osteosarcomas are bone cancers. Liposarcomas are fatty tissue cancers that attack a variety of bodily regions. Fibrosarcomas are cancers of the dense, fibrous tissue that holds together many bodily structures, including the skin.

Benign muscle tissue tumors are called myomas, whereas malignant muscle cancers are called myosarcomas. Leiomyosarcoma is a malignancy of smooth, visceral muscle. Rhabdomyosarcoma is a malignancy of cardiac and skeletal muscle.

Benign tumors of the central nervous system are called neuromas and neurofibromas. They include multiple neurofibroma, a condition in which numerous nerve tumors develop throughout the body, thereby causing a severely distorted physical appearance; multiple neurofibroma (or neurofibromatosis) is also known as the "Elephant Man" syndrome after the term used to describe Joseph Merrick, a nineteenth-century Englishman who suffered from this disease. Nervous system cancers include brain cancer and neurogenic sarcoma, glioblastoma, neuroblastoma, and malignant meningioma.

The formation of tumors is probably triggered by many factors. For example, the stress associated with living in a fast-paced technological society causes severe disturbances to the normal homeostatic balance within the body, particularly with reference to the nervous and endocrine systems. The nervous system activates many organ systems and tissues throughout the body. Even more potent in its effects is the endocrine system, which directly controls gene expression in various body cells and tissues via chemical messengers called hormones. When these hormones are hyperactivated by stress, they may activate or inactivate certain genes and their protein products at the wrong time in an individual's development, thereby causing drastic changes in cellular functioning, often accompanied by abnormal growth of tissue into a tumor.

Virus infections may also result in cancer. In 1908, cell-free extracts prepared from leukemia in mice were shown to transmit the disease. In 1910, Peyton Rous discovered that a similar filterable agent would transmit a solid tumor, a sarcoma, in chickens. However, it was felt at the time that cancers in animals represented special circumstances, and that the work was not directly applicable to human cancer. The existence of the Rous sarcoma virus (RSV) was corroborated later by other researchers, culminating in the awarding of the 1966 Nobel Prize in Physiology and Medicine to Rous. Most human cancers are of endogenous (genetic) origin and not associated with viral infection, but there are a number of notable exceptions. Hepatitis B virus infection is associated with a hepatocarcinoma, or cancer of the liver. The Epstein-Barr virus, the etiological agent of infectious mononucleosis, is associated with both Burkitt lymphoma and nasopharyngeal carcinoma.

Treatment and Therapy

Oncologists and other medical researchers study both benign and malignant tumors. Studies are devoted to the occurrence of these tumors, improved means of diagnosis, and the development of effective treatments. Cancer is the second-leading cause of death in many Western nations. Stress, viruses, pollution, and an individual's everyday exposure to hazardous materials increase the chance of developing tumors.

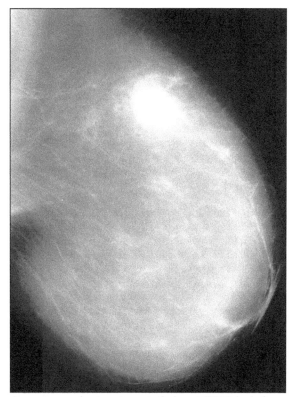

A mammogram showing a tumor in the breast. (SIU School of Medicine)

Regardless of a tumor's cause, it is important that it be identified and treated. The American Cancer Society's seven warning signs for cancer serve as an important model for tumor and cancer prevention. The warning signs are a sore that does not heal, persistent coughing, a lump anywhere on the body, unusual bleeding, a change in a wart or mole, a change in bladder or bowel movements, and difficulty swallowing.

Tumors may be benign or malignant. Benign tumors are less severe in most cases because they continue to grow within a localized region without invading other tissue regions. Benign tumors may press on critical organs and cause discomfort, however, thereby necessitating their surgical removal or inactivation using lasers, freezing, cytotoxic chemicals, or radiation. Warts represent a good example of a benign tumor. Warts are caused by a papillomavirus that infects skin cells of the dermis and enters a lysogenic phase, where it lays dormant in the host cell DNA but accelerates cell growth into a small tumor. A person can contract a papillomavirus merely by shaking an infected individual's hand. Some warts may become malignant.

Malignant tumors are invasive cancers that multiply rapidly, break off into the bloodstream, and colonize other body regions, where they destroy tissues, organs, and sometimes the entire organism. Malignant cancer cells are immortal in the sense that they reproduce without any developmental barriers. Many malignant colonies can manipulate available blood supplies away from normal tissue, thereby promoting their own growth. Malignant cancers are classified according to tissue type. Any tissue is subject to cancerous growth, given the appropriate stimuli.

Genetic and biochemical research focuses heavily on the study of neoplastic cellular transformation. The prime emphasis is upon gene regulation, the ultimate control point that determines whether a cell will function properly. Mutations in gene regulatory regions, improper hormonal signaling, or viral interference via lysogeny may contribute to abnormalities in cellular growth.

Benign and malignant tumors can be induced and studied in laboratory animals. The application of a chemical mutagen to a localized tissue region in a mouse usually gives rise to a tumor. Female mice infected with the mouse mammary tumor virus pass the virus to their young via milk during suckling; this virus generates grotesquely large tumors that are often as big as the mouse itself. Tumors or sections of tumors removed from humans are studied by biopsy and subsequent biochemical analysis. Human cells are grown in tissue culture in flasks and roller bottles containing fetal calf serum so that medical researchers can study the nature of the neoplastic tumorous cells.

Perspective and Prospects

The study of tumors is of critical importance to medicine because tumor formation is a major cause of illness in millions of people yearly. An understanding of the genetic mechanisms underlying tumor formation is directly applicable to both the study of cancer and the understanding of mechanisms that regulate cell growth in general.

Critical to understanding the genetic basis of cancer was the discovery of retroviruses, RNA viruses that replicate using a DNA intermediate. These viruses were discovered to carry oncogenes, cancer-causing genes that the viruses originally acquired from the cells they infected. It was discovered that oncogenes actually encode a variety of proteins that regulate cell growth, including growth factors and DNA regulatory proteins. The genetic basis behind most human cancers seems to involve mutations in these genes. The study of the mechanism by which these proteins function may eventually lead to a fuller understanding of how cancers develop.

Since most cancers have a genetic origin, the ability to screen for certain genetic patterns allows clinicians to observe patients most at risk for the disease. For example, women who carry certain forms of the genes *BRCA1* and *BRCA2* are at greater risk for developing ovarian or breast cancer.

Developing cancers in certain tissues may also secrete unique forms of proteins, allowing for detection of the disease at an early stage. For example, prostate tumors, the leading form of cancer in men (other than skin cancer), secrete a prostate specific antigen (PSA); elevated levels of PSA in the blood suggest a possible tumor in the prostate.

Oncofetal proteins, normally found on fetal cells, may also be reexpressed by certain tumors. Elevated levels of alpha-fetoprotein and carcinoembryonic antigen in serum may indicate liver or colorectal cancer. The increasing sensitivity of such screening methods holds out the prospect that the most common forms of cancer may be detected in a "curable" stage.

—*David Wason Hollar, Jr., Ph.D.;*
updated by Richard Adler, Ph.D.

See also Anal cancer; Biopsy; Bladder cancer; Bone cancer; Brain tumors; Breast biopsy; Breast cancer; Cancer; Carcinoma; Cervical, ovarian, and uterine cancers; Colorectal cancer; Cysts; Endometrial biopsy; Gallbladder cancer; Hodgkin's disease; Kidney cancer; Leukemia; Liver cancer; Lung cancer; Lymphadenopathy and lymphoma; Malignancy and metastasis; Mammography; Mastectomy and lumpectomy; Mouth and throat cancer; Mutation; National Cancer Institute (NCI); Neurofibromatosis; Oncology; Ovarian cysts; Prostate cancer; Sarcoma; Skin cancer; Stomach, intestinal, and pancreatic cancers; Testicular cancer; Tumor removal; Warts.

For Further Information:
Alberts, Bruce, et al. *Molecular Biology of the Cell.* 5th ed. New York: Garland, 2008.
"Benign Tumors." *MedlinePlus*, May 9, 2013.
"Cancer." *MedlinePlus*, May 28, 2013.
Chiras, Daniel D. *Biology: The Web of Life.* St. Paul, Minn.: West, 1993.
Dollinger, Malin, et al. *Everyone's Guide to Cancer Therapy.* Rev. 5th ed. Kansas City, Mo.: Andrews McMeel, 2008.
Eyre, Harmon J., Dianne Partie Lange, and Lois B. Morris. *Informed Decisions: The Complete Book of Cancer Diagnosis, Treatment, and Recovery.* 2d ed. Atlanta: American Cancer Society, 2002.
Janes-Hodder, Honna, and Nancy Keene. *Childhood Cancer: A Parent's Guide to Solid Tumor Cancers.* 2d ed. Cambridge, Mass.: O'Reilly, 2002.
Kindt, Thomas J., Richard A. Goldsby, and Barbara A. Osborne. *Kuby Immunology.* 6th ed. New York: W. H. Freeman, 2007.
"Learn about Cancer." *American Cancer Society*, Feb. 6, 2013.
Ross, Michael H., and Wojciech Pawlina. *Histology: A Text and Atlas.* 6th ed. Baltimore: Lippincott Williams & Wilkins, 2011.
Stark-Vance, Virginia, and M. L. Dubay. *One Hundred Questions and Answers About Brain Tumors.* 2d ed. Sudbury, Mass.: Jones and Bartlett, 2011.
"Understanding Cancer Series: Cancer." *National Cancer Institute*, Sept. 30, 2009.
Varmus, Harold, and Robert Weinberg. *Genes and the Biology of Cancer.* New York: W. H. Freeman, 1993.

TURNER SYNDROME
Disease/Disorder
Also known as: Gonadal dysgenesis, Bonnevie-Ullrich syndrome, monosomy X
Anatomy or system affected: Cells, endocrine system, reproductive system
Specialties and related fields: Endocrinology, genetics, gynecology, obstetrics
Definition: A genetic condition in which cells are missing all or part of an X chromosome.

Causes and Symptoms
Turner syndrome affects an estimated one out of every 2,500 girls born. The disorder is congenital, which means that it begins at conception. Normal males have one X and one Y chromosome. Normal females have two X chromosomes. Females with Turner syndrome have only one X chromosome (an XO pattern) in each of their cells or two X chromosomes with one being incomplete. Although the exact cause is unknown, scientists believe that the disorder may result from an error during the division of the parent's sex cells.

Shortness is the most common feature of Turner syndrome. The average height of a woman with this condition is 4 feet, 8 inches. Other physical features associated with the syndrome include puffy hands and feet at birth, a webbed neck, prominent ears, a low hairline at the back of the neck, drooping eyelids, dry eyes, flat and broad chest, soft fingernails that turn up at the end, and vaginal dryness.

Ovaries may or may not develop in those with Turner syndrome, and most patients experience ovarian failure. Since the ovaries normally produce estrogen, girls and women with Turner syndrome lack this essential hormone, resulting in infertility, incomplete sexual development, and increased risk of osteoporosis.

Cardiovascular disorders are the single source of increased mortality in patients with Turner syndrome. Women with Turner syndrome are at higher risk of hypertension, renal abnormalities, type 2 diabetes, hypothyroidism, ear infection, diabetes, obesity, cataracts, and celiac sprue.

Treatment and Therapy
No treatment is available to correct the chromosome abnormality that causes this condition. Nevertheless, early injections of human growth hormone can restore much of the growth deficit. Unless they take hormone therapy, women and girls with Turner syndrome will not menstruate or develop breasts and pubic hair. Hormone therapy also reduces

---

Information on Turner Syndrome

Causes: Genetic defect
Symptoms: Short stature, puffy hands and feet at birth, webbed neck, prominent ears, soft fingernails that turn up at end, ovarian failure leading to infertility and incomplete sexual development, cardiovascular problems
Duration: Chronic
Treatments: Hormonal therapy for some symptoms

---

the risk of bone loss. Although infertility cannot be altered, pregnancy may be possible through in vitro fertilization. Girls and women with Turner syndrome should be monitored and treated for associated conditions.

Perspective and Prospects

Turner syndrome was first identified by Henry Turner in 1938. In 1959, C. E. Ford discovered that a chromosomal abnormality involving sex chromosomes causes the syndrome.

—Fred Buchstein; updated by
Sharon W. Stark, R.N., A.P.R.N., D.N.Sc.

See also Dwarfism; Endocrine system; Endocrinology; Endocrinology, pediatric; Genital disorders, female; Genetic diseases; Genetics and inheritance; Growth; Hormone therapy; Hormones; Infertility, female; Menstruation; Ovaries; Puberty and adolescence; Reproductive system; Sexual differentiation; Women's health.

For Further Information:

A.D.A.M. Medical Encyclopedia. "Turner Syndrome." *MedlinePlus*, March 30, 2012.

Henry, Helen L., and Anthony W. Norman, eds. *Encyclopedia of Hormones*. 3 vols. San Diego, Calif.: Academic Press, 2003.

Kronenberg, Henry M., et al., eds. *Williams Textbook of Endocrinology*. 12th ed. Philadelphia: Saunders/Elsevier, 2011.

Lewis, Ricki. *Human Genetics: Concepts and Applications*. 10th ed. Dubuque, Iowa: McGraw-Hill, 2012.

Milunsky, Aubrey, ed. *Genetic Disorders and the Fetus: Diagnosis, Prevention, and Treatment*. 5th ed. Baltimore: Johns Hopkins University Press, 2004.

Money, John. *Sex Errors of the Body and Related Syndromes: A Guide to Counseling Children, Adolescents, and Their Families*. 2d ed. Baltimore: Paul H. Brookes, 1994.

National Institute of Child Health and Human Development. "Turner Syndrome: Condition Information." *U.S. Department of Health and Human Services, National Institutes of Health*, November 30, 2012.

Pinsky, Leonard, Robert P. Erickson, and R. Neil Schimke. *Genetic Disorders of Human Sexual Development*. New York: Oxford University Press, 1999.

Rosenblum, Laurie, and Kari Kassir. "Turner Syndrome." *Health Library*, September 12, 2012.

Rosenfeld, Ron G., and Melvin M. Grumbach, eds. *Turner Syndrome*. New York: Marcel Dekker, 1990.

"What is TS?" *Turner Syndrome Society of the United States*, 2011.

TWINS. *See* MULTIPLE BIRTHS.

TYPHOID FEVER
Disease/Disorder

Anatomy or system affected: Circulatory system, gallbladder, gastrointestinal system, intestines, kidneys, liver, skin, spleen
Specialties and related fields: Bacteriology, environmental health, epidemiology, internal medicine, public health
Definition: An acute, systemic, febrile disease caused by bacteria that are transmitted through contaminated food or water.

Causes and Symptoms

Typhoid fever, a serious disease with the potential to become epidemic under conditions of poor sanitation, is caused by the bacterium *Salmonella enterica*, serotype Typhi (formerly *Salmonella typhi*). These bacteria are transmitted to humans through the consumption of water or food contaminated with the feces from individuals who carry the serotype Typhi but who most often remain asymptomatic.

An infective dose of bacteria in susceptible individuals is estimated to be quite small, generally less than one thousand cells. The ingested bacteria pass through the stomach to the small intestines, where they establish an initial site of infection. These intestinal lesions usually ulcerate, and the bacteria spread to other body tissues via the bloodstream and lymphatic system. The organs most often affected by these secondary infections include the liver, spleen, kidneys, bone marrow, and especially the gallbladder. Symptoms include headache, abdominal pain, general malaise, and a generalized rash with rose-colored spots. If no complications ensue, then the fever will abate after about three weeks, but mortality rates average about 15 percent in untreated cases.

Treatment and Therapy

The first drug with demonstrable effectiveness in treating typhoid fever was chloramphenicol, which became generally available in 1948. Other antibiotics, notably ampicillin and ciprofloxacin, have largely replaced chloramphenicol as the treatment of choice, and their use has reduced the death rate to approximately 1 percent. Improved sanitation and living conditions since the 1920s have drastically reduced the incidence of this disease in the United States, although worldwide it remains a major public health concern. The World Health Organization estimates that at least 16 million cases and more than 200,000 deaths can be attributed to typhoid fever each year.

Information on Typhoid Fever

Causes: Bacteria transmitted through contaminated food or water
Symptoms: Fever, headache, abdominal pain, malaise, rash with rose-colored spots
Duration: Three weeks
Treatments: Antibiotics

Development of Typhoid Fever

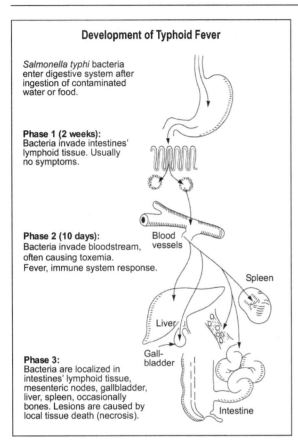

Salmonella typhi bacteria enter digestive system after ingestion of contaminated water or food.

Phase 1 (2 weeks):
Bacteria invade intestines' lymphoid tissue. Usually no symptoms.

Phase 2 (10 days):
Bacteria invade bloodstream, often causing toxemia. Fever, immune system response.

Blood vessels

Spleen

Liver

Gall-bladder

Phase 3:
Bacteria are localized in intestines' lymphoid tissue, mesenteric nodes, gallbladder, liver, spleen, occasionally bones. Lesions are caused by local tissue death (necrosis).

Intestine

Vaccines are available to prevent typhoid fever, but their effectiveness is suboptimal. Temporary immunity is acquired by about 60 to 75 percent of vaccinated individuals. Individuals who recover from the disease often become healthy carriers of the bacteria, and surgical removal of the gallbladder may be necessary to rid them of their carrier status.

Perspective and Prospects

The most famous case of a healthy carrier of the typhoid fever bacteria was a cook by the name of Mary Mallon, called "Typhoid Mary," who worked in several establishments in New York during the period from 1902 to 1915. In those years, she was linked to several different outbreaks of typhoid fever, resulting in fifty-one cases of illness and three deaths. When she repeatedly refused to cooperate with public health authorities, she was eventually taken into custody and confined in a state hospital. After almost three years, she was released, but she soon skipped parole and disappeared. Four years later, she was apprehended again as the source of a typhoid fever outbreak that involved twenty-five cases and two deaths. She was returned to the secure hospital in 1915, where she remained until her death in 1938. The important legal issues generated by her case, including incarceration for having an infectious disease and forced surgery, were the driving forces behind the founding of the American Civil Liberties Union (ACLU).

—Jeffrey A. Knight, Ph.D.

See also Antibiotics; Bacterial infections; Bacteriology; Epidemics and pandemics; Fever; Food poisoning; Gallbladder diseases; Immunization and vaccination; Microbiology; Salmonella infection.

For Further Information:
Badash, Michelle, and Michael Woods. "Typhoid Fever." *Health Library*, Nov. 26, 2012.
"Diarrhoeal Diseases: Typhoid Fever." *World Health Organization*, Feb. 2009.
Lock, Stephen, John Last, and George M. Dunea, eds. *The Oxford Companion to Medicine.* 3rd ed. New York: Oxford University Press, 2006.
Murray, Patrick R., Ken S. Rosenthal, and Michael A. Pfaller. *Medical Microbiology.* 7th ed. Philadelphia: Mosby/Elsevier, 2013.
"Salmonella Infections." *MedlinePlus*, Apr. 19, 2013.
Tortora, Gerard J., Berdell R. Funke, and Christine L. Case. *Microbiology: An Introduction.* 11th ed. San Francisco: Pearson Benjamin Cummings, 2013.
"Typhoid Fever." *Centers for Disease Control and Prevention*, May 14, 2013.
Vorvick, Linda J., Jatin M. Vyas, and David Zieve. "Typhoid Fever." *MedlinePlus*, June 9, 2011.

TYPHUS

Disease/Disorder

Also known as: Epidemic typhus, rickettsiosis

Anatomy or system affected: Circulatory system, kidneys, nervous system, respiratory system, skin

Specialties and related fields: Bacteriology, environmental health, epidemiology, internal medicine, public health

Definition: An acute, systemic, febrile disease caused by bacteria that are transmitted through the bite of a body louse.

Causes and Symptoms

The causative agent of epidemic typhus is the bacterium *Rickettsia prowazeckii*, an obligate intracellular parasite. These bacteria are transmitted to humans following the bite from an infected body louse, *Pediculus humanus corporis*. The pathogen is excreted with the louse feces and invades the site of a louse bite when the bitten host scratches the bite. The onset of the disease is marked by a high and prolonged fever with accompanying headache and rash. The bacteria are spread throughout the body through the bloodstream and can cause secondary lesions in many tissues, including the kidneys, heart, and brain. Mortality can be as high as 40 to 60 percent in untreated cases.

Treatment and Therapy

Antibiotic treatment is essential for reducing the severity of the disease, and chloramphenicol, tetracycline, and doxycycline are the antibiotics of choice. Improved sanitation and living conditions since the 1920s have virtually eliminated this disease in countries such as the United States. The last US epidemic was in 1922. Since then, there have been sporadic reports of isolated cases involving transmission from flying squirrels, indicating a possible animal reservoir; however, there is no real evidence to support this. Epidemic typhus still persists in some regions of Africa, Central America, and South America. The best course of action for

---

Information on Typhus

Causes: Bacteria transmitted through lice bites
Symptoms: Fever, headache, rash
Duration: Acute
Treatments: Antibiotics

---

prevention is to practice good hygiene and sanitation, and to avoid areas where there might be rat fleas and lice.

Perspective and Prospects

Epidemic typhus, also known as jail fever, is primarily a disease of crowded, substandard living conditions and poor sanitation. Millions of cases occurred in the trenches of World War I and in the concentration camps of World War II. Anne Frank, the noted teenage diarist, died of typhus contracted while at a concentration camp. It has been said that Napoleon's retreat from Russia was started by a louse, and that lice have defeated the most powerful armies of Europe and Asia.

The pioneering investigations of Howard Taylor Ricketts and Stanislas von Prowazeck in the early twentieth century paved the way for the discovery of both the bacteria and the louse vector, although both men died from the disease that they studied. They were honored posthumously when the bacterium was named *Rickettsia prowazeckii*.

—*Jeffrey A. Knight, Ph.D.*

See also Antibiotics; Bacterial infections; Bacteriology; Bites and stings; Epidemics and pandemics; Fever; Insect-borne diseases; Lice, mites, and ticks; Microbiology; Parasitic diseases; Zoonoses.

For Further Information:

Dugdale, David C. III, Jatin M. Vyas, and David Zieve. "Typhus." *MedlinePlus*, Oct. 6, 2012.

Eremeeva, Marina E., and Gregory A. Dasch. "Rickettsial (Spotted and Typhus Fevers) and Related Infections (Analplasmosis and Ehrlichiosis." *Centers for Disease Control and Prevention*, July 1, 2011.

Lock, Stephen, John Last, and George M. Dunea, eds. *The Oxford Companion to Medicine*. 3d ed. New York: Oxford University Press, 2006.

Murray, Patrick R., Ken S. Rosenthal, and Michael A. Pfaller. *Medical Microbiology*. 7th ed. Philadelphia: Mosby/Elsevier, 2013.

Tortora, Gerard J., Berdell R. Funke, and Christine L. Case. *Microbiology: An Introduction*. 11th ed. San Francisco: Pearson Benjamin Cummings, 2013.

"Typhus Fever (Endemic Louse-Borne Typhus)." *World Health Organization*, 2013.

Zinsser, Hans. *Rats, Lice, and History*. New York: Black Dog & Leventhal, 1996.

ULCER SURGERY

Procedure

Anatomy or system affected: Gastrointestinal system, intestines, stomach

Specialties and related fields: Gastroenterology, general surgery, nutrition

Definition: The removal of areas of the stomach or duodenum that are ulcerated; a procedure often avoided by nonsurgical treatment.

Key terms:

duodenum: the first part of the small intestine

metastasis: the transfer of disease-producing cells to other parts of a body

partial gastrectomy: the removal of part of the stomach

pepsin: a substance in the stomach that breaks down most proteins

peritonitis: inflammation of the peritoneum or stomach lining

pyloric stenosis: a narrowing of the passageway between the stomach and the duodenum

Indications and Procedures

Many people who are host to peptic ulcers have no symptoms. As these ulcers—which may occur as single or multiple eruptions having a diameter between 0.75 centimeter (0.3 inch) and 2.5 centimeters (1 inch) and a depth of about 0.02 centimeter (0.01 inch)—enlarge and multiply, however, symptoms often become apparent. These symptoms include a burning or gnawing pain in the abdominal region, particularly when the stomach is empty. Therefore, people who are asymptomatic during the day when they are ingesting food at regular intervals may become symptomatic at night. One way to allay symptoms, particularly those caused by a duodenal ulcer, is to eat so that the gastric juices feed on the food rather than on the lining of the stomach or duodenum. Symptoms often reappear, however, a few hours after eating.

In some cases, patients experience a loss of appetite. If the ulcer is in the duodenum, however, the opposite may occur, in which case it is best to eat small quantities of food that is not overly spicy. Belching often accompanies ulcer problems, although, and in and of itself, this is not categorically indicative of ulcers. People suffering from ulcers sometimes lose weight, largely because they feel bloated and therefore tend to eat less. Nausea and vomiting accompany some ulcer problems.

In extreme cases, an ulcer may start to bleed, in which case the patient may vomit blood. Black, tarry stools are also an indication of bleeding in the stomach, although elements in one's diet, particularly iron, can also produce darkened stools. Where bleeding is profuse, the patient may require a blood transfusion. On rare occasions, an ulcer may eat through the back wall of the digestive tract and involve the pancreas, causing a pain that reaches as far as the patient's back. When ulcers eat through the front of the duodenum, the result may be peritonitis, a life-threatening inflammation of the abdominal lining that requires immediate attention.

If ulcers persist and go untreated, they can cause dangerous scarring of the stomach lining and duodenum. As a result, the passageway between the stomach and duodenum narrows. When this condition, called pyloric stenosis, occurs, patients usually experience vomiting and weight loss.

Some ulcers are malignant (cancerous) and must be removed surgically. Follow-up radiation and/or chemotherapy may be indicated in such cases. The surgical removal of ulcers involves making an incision in the abdomen and removing the portion of the stomach or duodenum that is ulcerated. The area affected is then joined and sutured. Large portions of the stomach may be removed if necessary and will, in time, regenerate.

Uses and Complications

Except where a malignancy is suspected, ulcer surgery is a treatment of last resort. Often, changes in diet can control the situation, as can discontinuing smoking and the drinking of alcoholic beverages or beverages that contain caffeine. Aspirin and nonsteroidal anti-inflammatory drugs (NSAIDs) can irritate the stomach and are usually not advised for people with ulcers. The appearance of ulcers has been linked to stress, so changes in lifestyle can result in considerable improvement.

The most common early treatment is with nonprescription antacids or with similar prescription drugs that coat the stom-

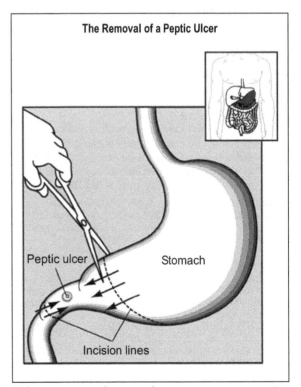

The Removal of a Peptic Ulcer

Peptic ulcer Stomach

Incision lines

With a severe peptic ulcer, it may be necessary to remove a section of the stomach and join the remaining ends; the inset shows the location of the stomach.

ach lining and neutralize the acids that are causing the problem. Prescription drugs such as H2 blockers and proton pump inhibitors, as well as antimicrobial treatment of the ulcerogenic bacteria *Helicobacter pylori*, can almost invariably cure gastric and duodenal ulcers, leaving surgery for removal of malignancies and control of bleeding that cannot be stopped by endoscopic cautery. Ulcer patients are also generally advised to eat several small meals a day rather than two or three large ones. Doing so helps to keep food in the stomach, and even nibbling through the night produces favorable results in some patients.

Because ulcer surgery is major and is usually done under general anesthesia, it carries the risks associated with any major surgery. The recovery rate after ulcer surgery is good, however, particularly as the areas around the excision begin to return to normal through regeneration. Where a malignancy has been detected early and removed surgically, metastasis can usually be prevented, particularly if follow-up radiation or chemotherapy is employed.

Perspective and Prospects

Ulcers were once treated by bed rest and a bland, boring diet, mostly of soft foods as boiled eggs, toast, and custards accompanied by plenty of milk, which supposedly lined the stomach and protected it from damage by gastric juices. Such treatment is now generally considered unnecessary. Most ulcer patients can remain active and can eat sensibly but relatively normally. Extremely spicy food, which can irritate an ulcer, should be avoided if ulcer symptoms are present.

In the past, another method of ulcer treatment was to freeze the affected area, which seemed to produce immediate, favorable results. In time, however, many of the ulcers treated in this way returned. This treatment, although appealing for its short-term results, is now uncommon because its benefits do not appear to be lasting.

In recent years, the management of ulcers has become increasingly conservative, with surgery the least frequent and most extreme treatment of all. In the foreseeable future, it is likely that ulcer surgery will become an increasing rarity.

—*R. Baird Shuman, Ph.D.*

See also Digestion; Endoscopy; Food biochemistry; Gastrectomy; Gastroenterology; Gastrointestinal disorders; Gastrointestinal system; Intestinal disorders; Intestines; Peritonitis; Small intestine; Stress; Stress reduction; Ulcers; Vagotomy.

For Further Information:

Chan, F. K. L., Lau, J. Y. W. "Peptic Ulcer Disease." In *Sleisenger & Fordtran's Gastrointestinal and Liver Disease*, edited by Feldman M, Friedman, L. S., Brandt L. J. 9th ed. Philadelphia: Saunders Elsevier; 2010.

Griffith, H. Winter. *Complete Guide to Symptoms, Illness, and Surgery*. 6th ed. New York: Perigee, 2012.

Herlong, H. Frank. *Digestive Disorders*. Baltimore, Md.: Johns Hopkins Medicine, 2011.

Longstreth, George F. "Peptic Ulcer." *MedlinePlus*, August, 11, 2011.

Margolis, Simeon, and Sergey Kantsevoy. *Johns Hopkins White Papers 2002: Digestive Disorders*. New York: Rebus, 2002.

Swabb, Edward A., and Sandor Szabo, eds. *Ulcer Disease: Investigation and Basis for Therapy*. New York: Marcel Dekker, 1991.

Szabo, Sandor, and Carl J. Pfeiffer, eds. *Ulcer Disease: New Aspects of Pathogenesis and Pharmacology*. Boca Raton, Fla.: CRC Press, 1989.

Tytgat, G. N. J., ed. *Peptic Ulcer Disease*. Orlando, Fla.: W. B. Saunders, 2000.

Zakim, David, and Andrew J. Dannenberg, eds. *Peptic Ulcer Disease and Other Acid-Related Disorders*. Armonk, N.Y.: Academic Research Associates, 1991.

Zinner, Michael. *Atlas of Gastric Surgery*. New York: Churchill Livingstone, 1992.

Zollinger, Robert M., Jr., and Robert M. Zollinger, Sr. *Zollinger's Atlas of Surgical Operations*. 9th ed. New York: McGraw-Hill, 2011.

ULCERATIVE COLITIS
Disease/Disorder

Anatomy or system affected: Abdomen, anus, gastrointestinal system, immune system, intestines

Specialties and related fields: Gastroenterology, general surgery

Definition: An inflammatory bowel disease that causes open sores in the colon.

Key terms:

antibodies: specialized proteins that bind to those foreign substances in the body that triggered their production, and neutralize them

B-lymphocytes: special white blood cells that make and secrete antibodies in response to stimulation by foreign substances known as antigens

monoclonal antibodies: antibodies made by a single B-lymphocyte clone that are homogeneous and recognize only one antigen

mucosae: the innermost, mucous-secreting layer that lines the gastrointestinal tract

T-lymphocytes: a group of closely related white blood cells that develop in the thymus and regulate the immune system's response to infections and tumors

Causes and Symptoms

Crohn's disease and ulcerative colitis (UC) are the two types of inflammatory bowel diseases (IBDs). UC only affects the large intestine (colon) and its upper mucosal layer, but Crohn's disease can cause lesions anywhere in the gastrointestinal tract and affects all layers of it. The incidence of UC varies widely and ranges from 0.2-24.5 / 100,000 persons.

The exact cause of UC remains unknown, but studies with identical twins and families with a history of UC have estab-

---

Information on Ulcerative Colitis

Causes: Autoimmune response against the colon

Symptoms: Abdominal pain, bloody diarrhea with mucus for extended period of time, fever, nausea

Duration: A chronic disease that lasts for the remainder of the patient's life, unless the colon is removed

Treatments: Aminosalicylates, corticosteroids, immunomodulators, surgery

lished a strong genetic component to it. However, environmental and behavioral factors definitely contribute to the severity of the disease. Psychological stress, diet, smoking, the use of nonsteroidal anti-inflammatory drugs, breastfeeding, and isotretinoin (Accutane) have all been implicated as factors that influence the course and onset of UC.

UC presents as an autoimmune disease of the colon, since white blood cells called T-lymphocytes accumulate at the bottom of the mucosal epithelium, attack it, and damage it. Yet another type of white blood cell, B-lymphocytes, which produce and secrete antibodies, release antibodies that bind to the colonic tissues and damage them. The continuous damage to the colon causes ulcers, which are replaced by granulation tissue (a mass of new connective tissue and capillaries that form on the surface of a healing wound). Accumulation of granulation tissue leads to the formation of pseudopolyps.

UC is graded as mild (rectal bleeding and fewer than four bowel movements a day), moderate (rectal bleeding and more than four bowel movements a day), severe (bleeding from the rectum, more than four bowel movements a day and the symptoms of systemic illness, e.g., fever, elevated heart rate, and low blood cell counts), or fulminant (more than ten bowel movements a day, continuous bleeding and a vastly enlarged colon or megacolon).

Another classification scheme for UC depends on the parts of the colon affected by the disease. Proctitis is limited to the rectum; proctosigmoiditis extends from the rectum to the sigmoid colon; left-sided colitis involves the rectum, sigmoid colon, ascending colon and the beginning of the transverse colon; and pancolitis involves the entire colon.

UC patients typically complain of rectal bleeding, frequent bowel movements with mucous discharge, lower abdominal pain, and a constant feeling of needing to pass a stool even though the colon is empty (tenesmus). In the case of severe disease, the patient also shows fever, severe diarrhea, cramps, and abdominal distension. Complete blood counts reveal an elevated white blood cell count (leukocytosis).

Some UC patients show symptoms outside the colon. These include inflammation of the iris of the eye (uveitis), arthritis, skin lesions (erythema nodosum), clubbing at the ends of the fingers, inflammation of the bile ducts (cholangitis), ulcers in the mouth, and blood clots (deep vein thrombosis).

Diagnosis of UC requires a colonoscopy or flexible sigmoidoscopy to rule out Crohn's disease, intestinal cancer, or diverticulitis. The gastroenterologist inserts a colonoscope through the anus and into the colon to view the colon. A colon from a UC patient contains continuous ulcers without the scarring normally observed in Crohn's disease. Biopsies of the colon reveal involvement of the mucosae and not the lower layers.

Treatment and Therapy

Patients with active UC may require hospitalization and treatment with high-dose corticosteroids (e.g., prednisone). These drugs can relieve symptoms and induce remission. Because corticosteroids have significant side effects, they are typically not used long term.

The first-line treatments for managing UC include anti-inflammatory drugs that quell inflammation in the colon. Sulfasalazine (Azulfidine), mesalamine (Asacol, Delzicol, and others), balsalazine (Colazal), and olsalazine (Dipentum) come in oral forms specially formulated so that they release their medicine primarily in the colon, and liquid forms for enemas. Anti-inflammatory drugs have few side effects, but if they do not control the patient's disease, then immunomodulators are added. These drugs include azathioprine (Azasan, Imuran), 6-mercaptopurine (Purinethol), and cyclosporine (Gengraf, Neoral, and Sandimmune). Because they suppress the immune response, immunomodulators cause severe side effects. Biological immunomodulators, monoclonal antibodies that bind to and inactivate the pro-inflammatory protein tumor necrosis factor-alpha, include infliximab (Remicade), adalimumab (Humira), and golimumab (Simponi). Because of their severe side effects and high cost, these drugs are a last resort.

If medications do not properly manage UC, then surgical options remain. Surgical removal of the colon (colectomy) or colon and rectum (proctocolectomy) can cure UC. A surgical procedure called ileoanal anastomosis reattaches the severed end of the small intestine to the anus and eliminates the need for a colostomy bag. Because UC increases the risk of colon cancer, some long-term UC patients have their colons removed as a preventative measure or when routine colon biopsies show signs of colon cancer.

Perspective and Prospects

Although historical accounts contain several probable descriptions of UC, Sir Samuel Wilks first referred to UC by name in 1859. Some years after Wilk's discovery, the Surgeon General of the Union Army directly referred to UC, and showed microscopic pictures of tissue sections from the colon of a UC patient. In the decades that followed, detailed clinical and pathological descriptions of UC sealed its place as a recognized condition.

Alicaforsen is a first-generation antisense oligonucleotide that binds to the messenger ribonucleic acid (mRNA) for the ICAM-1 gene and inhibits the synthesis of ICAM-1 protein. Increased ICAM-1 expression in the colon correlates with the severity of the disease and inhibition of ICAM-1 decreases inflammation. In the future, antisense oligonucleotide treatments that specifically bind to and inactivate the messenger RNAs expressed by particular pro-inflammatory genes might be used to successfully treat UC.

—*Michael A. Buratovich, Ph.D.*

See also Gastroenterology; Histology; Immunology; Immunopathology; Oncology

For Further Information:

Ali, Tauseef. *Crohn's and Colitis for Dummies.* Hoboken, NJ: For Dummies, 2013.

Sabil, Fred. *Crohn's Disease and Ulcerative Colitis: Everything You Need to Know.* 3rd ed. Cheektowaga, NY: Firefly Books, 2011.

Zinser, Stephanie. *The Good Gut Guide: Help for IBS, Ulcerative Colitis, Crohn's Disease, Diverticulitis, Food Allergies and Other Gut Problems.* New York: Thorsons, 2012.

ULCERS
Disease/Disorder

Anatomy or system affected: Gastrointestinal system, mouth, stomach

Specialties and related fields: Family medicine, gastroenterology, internal medicine, nutrition

Definition: Ulcers, specifically those referred to as peptic ulcers, are open sores that develop on the mucous membranes that line the gastrointestinal tract and are caused by excessive secretion of gastric juices, particularly from the pancreas into the intestine.

Key terms:

acid pump inhibitors: a group of drugs that block the stomach cells' mechanism for producing hydrochloric acid

histamine II blockers: the general term used to describe various drugs that block the hormonal stimulation of histamine, one inducer of stomach acid

nonulcerous dyspepsia: a condition that exhibits many of the symptoms of peptic ulcers but does not involve actual lesions in the linings of the stomach or intestines

pepsin: the first component of gastric juice to be discovered, in the 1830s; the term "peptic ulcer" derives from the name of this digestive fluid

prostaglandins: chemical substances in the stomach lining that help fight ulceration by increasing blood flow to the lesion area

Zollinger-Ellison syndrome: a rare condition in which secretions of acid are so sudden and excessive that normal gastric defenses cannot prevent the immediate ulceration of stomach membranes

Causes and Symptoms

In the most general of terms, an ulcer is an open sore that does not respond readily to the normal processes of healing. It may occur on the skin itself or on internal mucous membranes. A corneal ulcer, for example, may occur as a result of infections stemming from local injuries of, or foreign objects lodged in, the eye. Circulatory disturbances associated with varicose veins or long periods in bed without sufficient body exercise can also cause skin ulcers. The latter form is sometimes referred to as bedsores.

The most commonly occurring ulcer, however, is the peptic ulcer, which occurs at various points in the gastrointestinal tract. Specifically, such ulcers affect the lower portion of the esophagus, the stomach (in which case the term "gastric" ulcer may be employed), and two locations in the small intestine: the duodenum and the jejunum. Approximately 10 percent of the general population in the United States and Western Europe is thought to suffer from peptic ulcers. A substantially higher percentage of the population may suffer from a condition that resembles ulcers in its symptomatic levels of discomfort and pain but that does not actually involve lesions. This condition is called nonulcerous dyspepsia.

When ulceration of the stomach or intestinal tissue advances past a certain stage, internal bleeding usually occurs. Reaction to this stage of deterioration may involve vomiting,

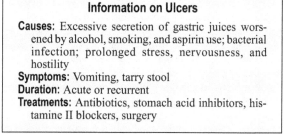

Information on Ulcers

Causes: Excessive secretion of gastric juices worsened by alcohol, smoking, and aspirin use; bacterial infection; prolonged stress, nervousness, and hostility

Symptoms: Vomiting, tarry stool

Duration: Acute or recurrent

Treatments: Antibiotics, stomach acid inhibitors, histamine II blockers, surgery

in which case the granular bloody material that is expulsed resembles partially digested food and is brownish rather than red in color. This condition stems from the effect of acidic gastric juices on the blood that has been released. If bleeding from ulcers becomes evident through the presence of blood in the stools, the effect is different: the fecal material is black in color, a condition that was referred to in past generations as "tarry stool."

Although modern medical science has identified the hydrochloric acid content of the gastric juice as the corrosive agent that causes ulcer sores in all these regions of the digestive system, the term "peptic ulcer" is still commonly used to refer to all ulcers. This label was first applied following the discovery, in 1836, of the enzyme pepsin, one of the first subcomponents of the gastric juice to be isolated in the laboratory.

In the twentieth century, the original contributions of physicians to the understanding of what ulcers are were combined with equally scientific observations of social and psychological factors that can bring about ulcers. Increasingly, many of these causes were associated with environmental and nervous emotional factors.

The likelihood of ulcers forming in the gastrointestinal tract is increased if an imbalance occurs in the normal functioning of a specific phase of the digestive process. That phase begins when, at the time that foods are taken into the mouth and swallowed, the body secretes gastric juice containing both acid and pepsin. The essential acid in gastric juice is hydrochloric acid, which is highly dangerous in its pure state and poisonous if swallowed directly. Pepsin is an enzyme produced in the lining of the stomach that has proteolytic, or protein-degrading, characteristics. Both these components in gastric juices are essential in the first stages of digestion to break down the foodstuffs in the stomach and to facilitate their passage into the small intestine, where other secretions from the liver and pancreas continue the process of digestion. In the case of the enzyme pepsin, it is secreted in an inactive chemical state; it therefore requires the presence of hydrochloric acid (also secreted in the stomach lining) to convert it chemically to an active state and an optimum degree of acidity (pH 1 to 3) for the digestive function it fulfills. If the chemical conversion of pepsin into an active digestive agent does not make use of all the hydrochloric acid that has been secreted, the excess acid is free to do damage to the sensitive tissue of the stomach or intestinal lining.

Ulcers can occur in any of several areas of the gastrointestinal tract when excessive amounts or imbalanced component proportions of gastric juice are secreted. In recent times, doctors established that a continuing state of nervousness or hostility can cause gastric juice to flow almost continuously. Such hypersecretion will damage the mucous membranes lining the digestive tract unless a more-or-less constant supply of food is taken in by the organism. Thus, the nervous eater who is constantly consuming foods may be unconsciously trying to control the potential development of ulcers in his or her gastrointestinal tract. The side effects on the body of constant nervous eating may be potentially as harmful as the localized effects associated with ulcers.

In essence, what happens when an ulcer begins to form is that the acid and pepsin in the gastric juice begin to digest membrane tissue in the gastrointestinal tract itself. Normally, the stomach has a series of internal defenses to combat localized attacks by active gastric juice against its own sensitive membranes. In the first place, the mucous lining of the internal organs themselves forms a sort of barrier between membrane tissue and the combined food-gastric juice content of the functioning organ.

The cells of the stomach lining also secrete a natural antacid in the form of bicarbonate of soda. If the normal presence of these two protective agents is insufficient to prevent deterioration of the stomach or intestinal lining, a more active struggle ensues in the area where an ulcer has begun to develop. Surface cells begin to constrict to form a more resistant surface area around the nascent lesion. If the process does not proceed too rapidly, damaged cells may be replaced by healthy cells in the immediate area of the lesion.

Even more specialized reactions in the area of ulceration are associated with prostaglandins, which are chemical agents in the stomach lining that stimulate increased blood flow to nourish besieged cells. Prostaglandins can also bring about higher levels of antacid production and mucus accumulation where they are needed most.

With one notable and fairly rare exception, known as the Zollinger-Ellison syndrome (excessive production of acid), almost all cases of stomach ulcers (gastric ulcers) occur as a result of dysfunction in the defensive systems described

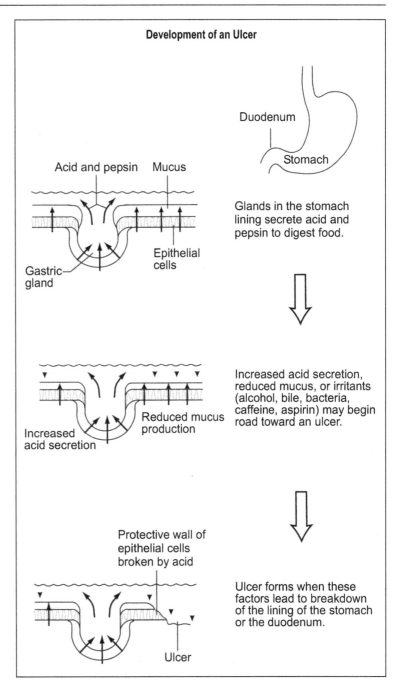

Development of an Ulcer

Duodenum

Stomach

Acid and pepsin   Mucus

Epithelial cells

Gastric gland

Glands in the stomach lining secrete acid and pepsin to digest food.

Increased acid secretion

Reduced mucus production

Increased acid secretion, reduced mucus, or irritants (alcohol, bile, bacteria, caffeine, aspirin) may begin road toward an ulcer.

Protective wall of epithelial cells broken by acid

Ulcer

Ulcer forms when these factors lead to breakdown of the lining of the stomach or the duodenum.

above. As for duodenal (upper small intestine) ulcers, it appears that only about a third of all cases stem from higher-than-normal secretions of acid.

Doctors are not in full agreement regarding the way in which certain externally introduced substances may cause, or seriously contribute to, ulcers. Most have concluded, however, that a "big three" of clearly abusive substances—cigarettes, alcohol, and some over-the-counter drugs, especially aspirin—play a significant role. Cigarette smoking has been linked with the slowing down of essential body functions that either provide defenses against ulcers or contribute to their healing. One such function is the rate of blood flow itself, which is vital for the nourishment of cells that may be under attack by ulcers. Other side effects of smoking may include reduced production of prostaglandins, which make important contributions to the defensive reaction of the body against ulcerations.

As for the other potentially abusive agents, alcohol and certain over-the-counter or otherwise common drugs, it is the latter that are almost universally condemned for their negative effects on the proper functioning of the gastrointestinal system.

Alcohol, for its part, apparently does nothing to stimulate excessive acid production in the stomach. It does, however, interfere with the healing processes that are so vital in combating ulcers.

While caffeine is not usually considered to be an over-the-counter drug, it is known to be an important stimulator of acid secretions. Some doctors consider it to be second only to aspirin as a negative "foreign agent" affecting the sensitive mechanism of digestion in the stomach and small intestine.

Another common drug, aspirin, shares a dubious reputation in this respect with a number of other drugs classified as nonsteroidal anti-inflammatory drugs (NSAIDs) that are used to treat arthritis and other muscular or joint inflammations.

There is a widespread consensus that the occurrence of ulcers may be linked to external agents that are taken into the body. The simplest evidence of this hypothesis revolves around associations that have been established between the bacillus *Helicobacter pylori* and ulcerous conditions in the stomach and intestines.

Doctors had observed the presence of this bacillus (along with many others) in the human stomach for at least a century. Studies by the Australian researchers Bernard Marshall and J. R. Warner, however, noted that a very high percentage (nearly 100 percent) of patients diagnosed as having ulcers also had substantial traces of *H. pylori*.

Treatment and Therapy

As the debate over the role of *H. pylori* in causing ulcers took form in the early 1990s, those researchers who wanted to find proof that medicine was on the verge of a major breakthrough organized a full campaign to prescribe drugs that were known to kill the suspect bacillus.

It is now clear that *H. pylori* is a major contributing factor not only in ulcer development but also in the extremely high recurrence rate of relapse in healed patients. Because of the inflammation that the infecting organism causes in the stomach and duodenal linings, normal protective mechanisms break down. Once these barriers that protect the lining from damage by the acid and enzymes used in digesting food are gone, the process of ulceration begins. Even after the ulcer has healed, very high rates of recurrence are found unless the bacterial infection is eradicated.

Because so many people are infected with these common bacteria but not everyone develops ulcers, other contributing factors are clearly present. In the vulnerable patient, a combi-

nation of the well-known risk factors along with infection work together to bring about ulcers. It is now a routine treatment to administer antibiotics and stomach acid inhibitors simultaneously. Cure rate times and relapse rates have improved significantly.

Whatever the ultimate explanation concerning the causes of this surprisingly common ailment may be, the medical world remained, in the late twentieth century, devoted to the necessary use of a number of drugs to control the effects of gastric and peptic ulcers by fighting the flow of gastric juices that do the physical damage of ulceration. On the whole, these drugs, which are called histamine II blockers, aim at one objective: to block the formation of stomach acid. A similar effect is produced by several widely used (and markedly expensive) medicines that are prepared under commercial labels: Tagamet, Zantac, Pepcid, and Axid. Drugs in the class called acid pump inhibitors, such as Prilosec, also block stomach acid, but by a different and nearly complete method: they prevent the stomach cells from actually making the acid, in the final step before it is secreted into the stomach. These drugs are effective even in the most difficult cases of ulceration.

Much more complicated than the problem of treating normal cases of ulcers is the technical question of how to guard against the further deterioration of ulcers into different forms of gastrointestinal cancer. New forms of technology were being tested in the late twentieth century that allowed physicians to examine the inner mucous membranes of the intestines directly. One such device, called the fiber-optic endoscope, consists of a long tube that is passed through the esophagus and stomach to penetrate the upper portions of the small intestine. The fiber-optic endoscope not only views and photographs the surface areas affected by ulcers but also allows the physician to biopsy the tissue at the same time. This and other methods of diagnosis, although not available to all hospitals and clinics, and not mastered by all physicians who were trained in the pre-fiber-optic generation, represent enormous potential advances over the rather basic therapies developed during the previous century.

Perspective and Prospects

Long before modern scientific research techniques provided the medical world with a relatively precise idea of what causes ulcers and how to treat them, an entire literature on the disease had accumulated. It was apparently Hippocrates himself, in the fifth century BCE, who first studied the gastric hemorrhaging that can result from a peptic ulcer. Others, including the first century CE Roman Celsus, noted the favorable effect of prescribing a nonacid diet to patients suffering from ulcers. It was not until the eighteenth and nineteenth centuries, however, that doctors prepared the first clinical accounts of the effects of ulcers based on pathological studies.

Not much had changed by the early twentieth century regarding the attitude of physicians toward the role of acids in the stage-by-stage degenerative process of ulceration. The American doctor Bertram W. Sippy was often quoted after his famous 1912 statement to medical students that "where there is no acid, there is no ulcer." The question of what caused the presence of excess acid in the intestines aside, medical science would try to come closer to being able to detect the actions of the "culprit at work." To the general public, the advanced process of fiber-optic endoscopy gives the appearance of having been developed overnight in the last decades of the twentieth century. In fact, a number of necessary prestages had been pioneered all over the globe for more than a century.

As early as 1868, nearly thirty years before X-rays were discovered, German physician Adolf Kussmaul performed experiments that involved inserting a hollow lighted tube into patients" stomachs. He was actually able to see the interior surface of the stomach with the naked eye. Later, also in Germany, in 1908, a doctor named Hammeter was able to display a gastric ulcer by using barium meal X-ray technology. At a certain point, still well before the advent of fiber-optic endoscopy, a technique called arteriography was employed to explore the extent of ulcer damage when hemorrhaging occurred. This method, which still complemented fiber-optic endoscopy into the 1990s, involves the injection, through a fine tube passing through key arteries, of a dye whose movement in the intestinal tissue is then traced by means of a rapid series of X-ray images.

—Byron D. Cannon, Ph.D.;
updated by Connie Rizzo, M.D., Ph.D.

See also Abdomen; Abdominal disorders; Acid reflux disease; Acidosis; Alcoholism; Bacterial infections; Behçet's disease; Canker sores; Cold sores; Endoscopy; Esophagus; Gastrectomy; Gastroenterology; Gastrointestinal disorders; Gastrointestinal system; Heartburn; Indigestion; Intestinal disorders; Intestines; Lesions; Small intestine; Ulcer surgery.

For Further Information:

Goldman, Lee, and Dennis Ausiello, eds. *Cecil Textbook of Medicine*. 23d ed. Philadelphia: Saunders/Elsevier, 2007.

Janowitz, Henry D. *Indigestion: Living Better with Upper Intestinal Problems, from Heartburn to Ulcers and Gallstones*. New York: Oxford University Press, 1994.

Janowitz, Henry D. *Your Gut Feelings: A Complete Guide to Living Better with Intestinal Problems*. Rev. ed. New York: Oxford University Press, 1995.

Kapadia, Cyrus R., James M. Crawford, and Caroline Taylor. *An Atlas of Gastroenterology: A Guide to Diagnosis and Differential Diagnosis*. Boca Raton, Fla.: Parthenon, 2003.

Litin, Scott C., ed. *Mayo Clinic Family Health Book*. 4th ed. New York: HarperResource, 2009.

Margolis, Simeon, and Sergey Kantsevoy. *Johns Hopkins White Papers 2002: Digestive Disorders*. New York: Rebus, 2002.

McCoy, Krisha, Daus Mahnke, and Brian Randall. "Gastric Ulcer." *Health Library*, Apr. 29, 2013.

Monroe, Judy. *Coping with Ulcers, Heartburn, and Stress-Related Stomach Disorders*. New York: Rosen, 2000.

Parker, James N., and Philip M. Parker, eds. *The 2002 Official Patient's Sourcebook on Peptic Ulcer*. San Diego, Calif.: Icon Health, 2002.

"Peptic Ulcer." *MedlinePlus*, May 20, 2013.

"Ulcers." *FamilyDoctor.org*. American Academy of Family Physicians, Jan. 2011.

Wood, Debra, Daus Mahnke, and Brian Randall. "Peptic Ulcer." *Health Library*, Apr. 29, 2013.

ULTRASONOGRAPHY

Procedure

Anatomy or system affected: Abdomen, bladder, blood, gallbladder, heart, kidneys, reproductive system, urinary system, uterus

Specialties and related fields: Cardiology, embryology, gynecology, internal medicine, obstetrics, radiology, urology, vascular medicine

Definition: A technique that directs ultrasonic waves into body tissues and uses the reflections to create visual images, making it possible to view the anatomy of organs and blood vessels and to evaluate the dynamics of blood flow.

Key terms:

Doppler effect: the relationship of the apparent frequency of waves, such as sound waves, to the relative motion of the source of the waves and the observer or instrument; the frequency increases as the two approach each other and decreases as they move apart; an effect also known as the Doppler shift

duplex scan: an ultrasound representation of echo images of tissues and blood vessels combined with a Doppler representation of blood flow patterns

frequency: the number of complete cycles, such as sound cycles, produced by an alternating energy source; sound is measured in cycles per second, and one cycle per second is equal to 1 hertz

oscilloscope: an instrument that displays a visual representation of electrical variations on the fluorescent screen of a cathode-ray tube

transducer (probe): a device designed to transfer ultrasound waves into the body noninvasively, receive the returning echoes, and transform those echoes into electrical voltages

ultrasonic: referring to any frequency of sound that is higher than the audible range-that is, higher than 20,000 cycles per second (20 kilohertz)

Indications and Procedures

Sound waves are mechanical pressure waves that can propagate through liquids, solids, and, to some extent, gases. A sound wave is composed of cyclic variations that occur over time; one cycle per second is called 1 hertz (Hz). Ultrasound waves have a frequency of oscillation that is higher than 20,000 hertz, placing ultrasound above the audible range for humans. The useful frequency range for medical diagnostic ultrasound is between 1 and 10 megahertz (10 million hertz), although surgical instruments often use carrier frequencies greater than 20 megahertz.

The basic ultrasound system has two principal components. The first, and perhaps more important, component is the transducer, or probe. The transducer converts electrical pulses into mechanical pressure (sound) waves that are transmitted into the tissues. It then detects the echoes that are reflected from the tissues and transforms those echoes into electrical voltages. The second component is the audiovisual electronic component, which processes and displays the reflected echoes in the form of an image of internal organs and structures or an image of the movement of red blood cells.

Ultrasound waves are created when the crystalline material within the transducer is excited by an electrical voltage produced by the instrument's oscillator. The application of an electrical charge causes the crystalline particles to expand and contract, producing mechanical waves and pulses. These pulses of sound pass from the face of the transducer into the body, where they strike the organs, bones, and blood vessels. The reflected echoes in turn strike the face of the transducer, again causing the crystalline particles to vibrate and produce an electrical charge. Such crystalline material is said to have piezoelectric (a combination of the Greek word *piesis*, meaning "pressure," and the word "electric") properties.

Ultrasound systems commonly employ sound in two modalities. The transducer uses sound waves to create an echo image of body structures. The audiovisual component uses the Doppler shift theory to analyze the range of velocities over which red blood cells are moving.

To create an echo image, millions of pulses of sound must be transmitted into the body each second. For each transmitted pulse, one line of echo information is received by the transducer crystal. To build up an image rapidly and depict the real-time motion of body structures, the pulses are sent into the body from many angles as the sound beam is moved over the body surface. The depth of the echoes is displayed as a function of time, and a two-dimensional image is created by relating the sound's direction of propagation to the direction of the echo-image trace that appears on the instrument's oscilloscope.

The time required for a sound pulse to travel from the transducer to its target within the body, reflect, and return to the transducer can be used to measure the distance to the target, as radar does. In body tissues, sound travels at a speed of 1,540 meters per second. It takes approximately thirteen microseconds for a sound pulse to travel 1 centimeter into the body and return to the transducer. The depth and orientation of echoes may be determined by using this information.

As a sound beam travels through tissues, it is attenuated, or reduced in amplitude and intensity. Attenuation occurs as the energy from the beam is absorbed by the tissues and transformed into heat. Additionally, a part of the beam may be reflected into the surrounding tissues at an angle away from the incident angle or backscattered as the long wavelength of the sound beam strikes the smaller red blood cells. Only a small fraction of the returning echoes reach the face of the transducer.

Because the attenuation of the sound beam increases as the depth of penetration increases, the echoes that return from the deepest part of the image field will be reduced in intensity when compared to the echoes that return from the structures nearer the skin surface. The echo intensity is dependent on the degree of change and impedance of each tissue through which the echo passes, the strength of the incident sound beam, and the degree of attenuation of the beam. To equalize the intensity of the echoes from all depths of the image field, the echoes that travel farthest, and therefore take the longest time to reach the transducer, are amplified over time by using time-gain compensation methods.

For medical imaging applications, the returning echoes may be displayed in several ways. The amplitude mode (A-mode) depicts the returning echoes as deflections on the instrument's oscilloscope; the height of the deflection depends on the strength of the returned signal, and the distance between the deflections depends on the depth of the signal. The brightness mode (B-mode) depicts the strength of the echoes as shades of gray, with the strongest echoes appearing the brightest. The B-mode display makes it possible to differentiate tissue texture characteristics. The time-motion mode depicts movement over time by moving the B-mode trace across the face of a high-persistence oscilloscope, showing the depth, orientation, and strength of echoes with respect to time.

The transducer crystal determines the shape and focus of the sound beam and the frequency of the sound waves, features that are important in resolving echo information into complex images. The beam may be divided into three parts: the near field, the focal zone, and the far field. The beam width, close to the face of the transducer, is equal to the width of the transducer. The beam converges as it travels away from the transducer and then diverges at its narrow focal zone. In order for tissue targets to be resolved into discrete image points, both the lateral and the axial planes of the beam must be narrow. The focusing of the beam is facilitated by placing convex acoustic lenses in front of the transducer crystal to shorten the near field to a narrow focal point, thereby increasing the lateral resolution.

Axial resolution is the ability to distinguish targets along the sound beam. If a single pulse is emitted from the transducer, echo sources lying close together in the axial path of the beam may not be separated. Multiple short bursts of sound are used to separate the echo sources; each echo is captured as a discrete burst. Because axial resolution is inversely proportional to the duration of the ultrasound pulse (and the resonant frequency of the crystal is inversely proportional to its diameter), small-diameter, high-frequency crystals are used to obtain maximum axial resolution.

Ultrasound may be used to determine the velocity of blood flow. This velocity is determined in relation to the frequency of the incident sound beam according to the Doppler theory. Several different techniques may be used to process and display the echoes from moving red blood cells. The ultrasound system's computers may be programmed to perform fast Fourier transform analysis, a complex mathematical method for ranking the speed of the echoes returning over time. The signals may be displayed either as spectral tracings of the range of Doppler frequency shifts, represented in the returned echoes recorded throughout the cardiac cycle, or as color-coded Doppler-shifted signals from within the blood vessels, superimposed on a gray-scale image of the surrounding tissues.

Uses and Complications

High-resolution abdominal ultrasonography is a valuable technique for the visualization of intra-abdominal organs and disease processes. For example, liver conditions such as parenchymal abnormalities, abscesses, hematomas, cysts, and cancerous lesions can be identified easily by means of this technique. B-mode and Doppler color-flow imaging are particularly valuable technologies that can be used to evaluate the tissue characteristics and blood flow patterns of transplanted organs. An ultrasound examination of the gallbladder may reveal gallstones, obstruction of the common bile duct, or inflammatory disease. Ultrasound imaging of the pancreas is used to identify pancreatitis, pancreatic pseudocysts, and carcinoma of this organ. An ultrasound examination of the spleen may reveal splenomegaly, or enlargement of the spleen in response to disease or trauma.   Additionally, ultrasonography can be used to evaluate splenic volume and to identify hematomas, congenital cysts, infarctions, and tumors within the organ. The technology is particularly well suited for the study of tumors and abscesses within the abdomen. Ascites and other fluid collections

A pregnant woman undergoes ultrasound to check the health of her baby. (PhotoDisc)

may be recognized, and primary tumors and lymph node metastases within the abdominal cavity may be identified by means of pulse-echo imaging.

Ultrasound has certain characteristics that make it particularly valuable for examining the kidneys and the genitourinary tract. The ability to image both native and transplanted kidneys noninvasively from the longitudinal and transverse planes provides additional diagnostic information in uremic patients for whom the injection of contrast agents is undesirable or may fail to provide sufficient information. Urologic ultrasonography may be used to determine renal size and position or to identify cysts and masses, kidney or bladder stones, obstruction of the ureters, and bladder contour.

Transabdominal scanning of the pelvic organs, which is used to determine the presence or absence of suspected lesions, makes possible the precise localization and quantitative mapping of pelvic abdominal masses, facilitating the determination of disease stages and the positioning of radiation ports. The technology is used to differentiate cysts from solid tumors and to determine if pelvic tumors are of uterine, ovarian, or tubal origin.

The sonographic resolution of deep abdominal structures is achieved by internal scanning; endorectal or endovaginal approaches are used to reduce the distance between the transducer and the target organ. During these procedures, the transducer probe either is in direct contact with the genital organs or prostate gland or is separated from them by the thin walls of the bladder or rectum. The information obtained with these techniques is thought to be submacroscopic, observed

at approximately twenty to thirty times light magnification.

Ultrasonography plays a major role in the evaluation of obstetrical cases. Ultrasonic imaging is used to study earlypregnancy and high-risk cases, as well as to confirm ectopic pregnancy (development of the fetus outside the uterus). In cases of spontaneous abortion, ultrasound procedures are used to indicate whether the fetus and placenta have been retained. Ultrasonography is often used to determine fetal growth rate and placental development and to confirm intrauterine fetal death, threatened abortion, and fetal abnormalities. It is the best method for guidingamniocentesis (the sampling of placental fluids). A study published in the *Journal of the American Medical Association* in 2013 confirmed that ultrasound is the best detector of ectopic pregnancies.

Echocardiography, the ultrasound evaluation of the heart, is a reliable and useful tool for the study of patients with congenital and acquired heart disease. The role of cardiac ultrasound in the investigation of cardiac dysfunction, tetralogy of Fallot, transposition of the great vessels, and atrial septal defect has been well defined. Echocardiology is used to detect pericardial effusion; is coupled with Doppler ultrasound to evaluate the pulmonic, mitral, tricuspid, and aortic valves; and is used to investigate primary myocardial disease and atrial tumors. Improved resolution of cardiac structures and patterns of blood flow can be achieved by using endoesophageal (transesophageal) imaging and Doppler color-flow technology.

The vascular system of the body can be studied by combining pulse-echo imaging of the blood vessels and Doppler ultrasound detection of red blood cell movement. This combined technology, known as duplex scanning, not only offers information that is relevant to the anatomy and morphology of blood vessels but also—and this is most important—provides the opportunity to evaluate the dynamics of blood flow and the pathophysiology of vascular disease. Duplex technology is used to demonstrate the presence and characteristics of atherosclerotic disease and to define the severity of vascular compromise resulting from the progression of disease or the presence of blood clots in vessels (thrombosis).

Applications of the technology have been extended to the evaluation of arteries and veins of the extremities, the abdomen, and the brain. Advances in computer technology have made it possible to color-code the Doppler-shifted signals returning from moving red blood cells within the vessels. Doppler color-flow imaging has facilitated the investigation of vascular disorders that result in slow or reduced blood flow (venous thrombosis or preocclusive narrowing of vessels) or that affect the vascularity of organs and tissues (tumors or transplanted organs). Therefore, vascular ultrasonography plays a major role in the evaluation of patients with arterial occlusive disease and those suspected of having thrombosis of the deep or superficial venous systems.

Perspective and Prospects

Ultrasonic techniques have assumed a preferred role in the diagnosis of many diseases and have become an essential component of quality medical care. In contrast to the rapid development and use of x-ray technology in medical diagnosis, the application of diagnostic ultrasound has been relatively slow. Progress depended in large part on the development of high-resolution electronic devices and transducers. Early research into medical applications involved the adaptation of instruments that had been designed for industrial or military purposes.

The first attempts to locate objects with ultrasound probably occurred following the sinking of the *Titanic* in 1912. Improvements in the technology led to the widespread industrial and military use of ultrasound for the detection of flaws in metals, for the determination of range and depth information, and for navigation. The first application of ultrasound to medical diagnosis occurred in 1937, when K. T. Dussik attempted to image the cerebral ventricles by measuring the attenuation of a sound beam transmitted through the head. In 1947, Douglas H. Howry pioneered the ultrasonic imaging of soft tissues and constructed a pulse-echo system that utilized a transducer submerged in water. The system utilized surplus Navy sonar equipment, a high-fidelity recorder power supply, and a metal cattle-watering trough in which the patient and the transducer were immersed.

In the 1960s, Howard Thompson and Kenneth Gottesfeld performed obstetric and gynecologic examinations using the first contact scanner, which had been produced in 1958 by Tom Brown, an engineer, and Ian Donald, a professor of midwifery, at Glasgow University in Scotland. The first commercial scanner marketed in the United States was designed by William L. Wright, an engineer at the University of Colorado.

The two-dimensional scanning system was developed in 1953 by John Reid, an engineer, in cooperation with John Wild, a physician who demonstrated that ultrasound could detect differences between normal tissues, benign tumors, and cancers. The collaboration between medicine and engineering has propelled diagnostic ultrasonography forward at a phenomenal rate of development since that time.

The field of echocardiography was pioneered by Inge Edler, who discovered in the 1950s that echoes from the moving heart could be received and displayed by using a time-motion ultrasonic flow detector. Using this technology, Edler diagnosed mitral stenosis, pericardial effusion, and thrombus in the left atrium.

The use of ultrasound to evaluate blood flow was first described by S. Satomura in 1959. This investigator observed that ultrasound could be transmitted through the skin to derive information about the velocity of blood flow by using the Doppler effect to analyze the reflected signals from the moving blood cells. The first transcutaneous continuous-wave Doppler system was developed at the University of Washington in the 1960s. The instrument was first used to detect fetal life by demonstrating the fetal heartbeat. This application of Doppler ultrasound spurred research under the guidance of Eugene Strandness Jr. that ultimately led to the development of duplex scanners, instruments that combine pulse-echo imaging with analysis of blood flow patterns derived from the Doppler effect. As a result of the efforts of these early investigators and others, diagnostic medical ultrasonography has evolved into a highly useful tool with diverse clinical applications.

—Marsha M. Neumyer

See also Abdomen; Abdominal disorders; Abscesses; Amniocentesis; Blood vessels; Cholecystitis; Circulation; Echocardiography; Ectopic pregnancy; Embryology; Gallbladder diseases; Heart; Heart disease; Imaging and radiology; Lithotripsy; Noninvasive tests; Obstetrics; Pancreas; Pancreatitis; Pregnancy and gestation; Stone removal; Stones; Tumors; Uterus; Vascular medicine; Vascular system.

For Further Information:

Bates, Jane A. *Abdominal Ultrasound: How, Why, and When*. 3d ed. New York: Churchill Livingstone/Elsevier, 2011.

Bernstein, Eugene F., ed. *Vascular Diagnosis*. 4th ed. St. Louis, Mo.: Mosby, 1993.

Griffith, H. Winter. *Complete Guide to Symptoms, Illness, and Surgery*. Revised and updated by Stephen Moore and Kenneth Yoder. 6th ed. [N. p.]: Perigee/Penguin Group, 2012.

Hagan, Arthur D., and Anthony N. DeMaria. *Clinical Applications of Two-Dimensional Echocardiography and Cardiac Doppler*. 2d ed. Boston: Little, Brown, 1989.

Kremkau, Frederick W. *Diagnostic Ultrasound: Principles and Instruments*. 7th ed. St. Louis, Mo.: Saunders/Elsevier, 2006.

MedlinePlus. "Ultrasound." *MedlinePlus*, May 28, 2013.

Pagana, Kathleen Deska, and Timothy J. Pagana. *Mosby's Diagnostic and Laboratory Test Reference*. 11th ed. St. Louis, Mo.: Mosby/Elsevier, 2013.

Voyatzis, Diane. "Doppler Ultrasound." *Health Library*, November 19, 2012.

Umbilical Cord

Anatomy
Anatomy or system affected: Blood vessels, skin
Specialties and related fields: Neonatology, perinatology
Definition: The cord connecting the developing fetus to the placenta.

Structure and Functions

The umbilical cord is composed of a thickened fibrous covering over a gelatinous material that protects three blood vessels. Two umbilical arteries carry blood from the baby to the placenta and coil around the single umbilical vein. Blood containing oxygen and other essential nutrients returns from the placenta through the umbilical cord.

At term, the umbilical cord measures approximately 20 inches. The cord may be short if there is little amniotic fluid and if the baby has a muscular weakness, limiting movement inside the uterus. Umbilical cord lengths of less than 14 inches have a high incidence of traumatic separation and fetal blood loss at the time of a vaginal delivery.

Disorders and Diseases

Normally, the umbilical cord dries rapidly after birth, with most of its fluid content evaporating in two days. The base of the cord is then colonized by bacteria. An immune system response to the bacteria and chemicals released by white blood cells are required for the final shedding of the dried cord. The untreated umbilical cord is shed approximately seven to ten days after birth. Any treatment (such as alcohol) used to dry or delay cord bacterial colonization allows the cord to persist for nearly twice as long as in the untreated condition.

Persistence of an umbilical cord beyond three weeks after drying may be caused by a persistent blood supply and may require evaluation by a pediatric surgeon. Conditions that are associated with a persistent cord blood supply include a hemangioma, a connection from an artery in the skin to the vein of the umbilical cord, a small outpouching of the lining of the abdominal cavity, or retained elements of tissue connected to the bladder.

Once the cord has been fully shed, a reactive overgrowth of tissue may occur at the base of the cord. This is termed an umbilical granuloma and is readily managed by the application of silver nitrate, which cauterizes the tissue. There should be no further drainage from the base of the umbilicus beyond six weeks after birth.

During normal embryonic development, the umbilical cord is associated with a portion of two extraembryonic membranes, the yolk sac and the allantois. In late embryonic stages, the umbilical region normally herniates out of the embryo's body wall and is then fully retracted. If part of the herniated bowel is not returned to its normal position, then a connection between the base of the umbilical cord and the small intestine may occur. This is known as a Meckel's diverticulum of the ileum. Similarly, if the allantois does not completely degenerate, then it can leave a connection between the umbilical cord and the top of the bladder, known as a patent urachus. Both conditions are usually easily corrected by surgery.

Perspective and Prospects

Within the last decades, the umbilical cord has taken on new significance as the source of embryonic stem cells. Blood from the umbilical cord taken immediately after the infant has been born can be isolated and cryoprotected for many years. Should the infant (or even individuals who are not perfectly matched immunologically) require new blood stem cells to repopulate the immune system after chemotherapy or radiation therapy, then the cord blood stem cells can be thawed and injected into the recipient. A host of diseases have been successfully treated using cord blood, including many genetic diseases, and thousands of parents have opted to bank their infant's cord blood. The cost of harvesting and maintaining cord blood, however, is a source of controversy. Harvesting and storing cord blood is expensive, and the chances of an individual spontaneously acquiring a childhood neoplasm or serious genetic disease that would require cord cell therapy is not high. In addition, alternative therapies, such as bone marrow transplants, are sometimes available. On the other hand, parents in which such diseases run in the family may seriously consider cord blood banking.

The hope of stem cell technology in the future lies in the possibility that specific differentiated cell lineages can be stimulated to cure disease and not simply to reconstitute the immune system. For example, diabetic patients might have stem cells in cord blood engineered to produce insulin-secreting cells under appropriate control of circulating glucose concentration. Using the patient's own cord blood to produce such differentiated stem cells would avoid the problem of host-graft rejection.

In July 2013, the *New York Times* reported on a study suggesting that doctors clamp umbilical cords too soon following birth. According to the study, waiting at least one minute before cutting the cord improves iron and hemoglobin levels in newborns.

—David A. Clark, M.D.;
updated by Alexander Sandra, M.D.

See also Blood vessels; Childbirth; Childbirth complications; Circulation; Embryology; Hernias; Hypertrophy; Neonatology; Pediatrics; Perinatology; Placenta; Pregnancy and gestation; Stem cells; Uterus; Vascular medicine; Vascular system.

For Further Information:
Cunningham, F. Gary, et al., eds. *Williams Obstetrics.* 23d ed. New York: McGraw-Hill, 2010.
Kurtzberg, J., A. D. Lyerly, and J. Sugarman. "Untying the Gordian Knot: Policies, Practices, and Ethical Issues Related to Banking of Umbilical Cord Blood." *Journal of Clinical Investigation* 115 (October, 2005): 2592-2597.
Moore, Keith L., and T. V. N. Persaud. *The Developing Human.* 8th ed. Philadelphia: Saunders/Elsevier, 2008.
Oppenheimer, Steve B. *Introduction to Embryonic Development.* 4th ed. Upper Saddle River, N.J.: Pearson Education, 2004.
Patten, Bradley M. *Patten's Human Embryology.* Edited by Clark Edward Corliss. Rev. ed. New York: McGraw-Hill, 1982.
Preidt, Robert. "Later Clamping of Umbilical Cord May Benefit Newborns: Study." *MedlinePlus.* July 11, 2013.
Reynolds, Karina, Christoph Lees, and Grainne McCarten. *Pregnancy and Birth: Your Questions Answered.* Rev. ed. New York:

DK, 2007.

Simkin, Penny, Janet Whalley, and Ann Keppler. *Pregnancy, Child-birth, and the Newborn: The Complete Guide*. 3d ed. Minnetonka, Minn.: Meadowbrook Press, 2008.

Tsiaras, Alexander, and Barry Werth. *From Conception to Birth: A Life Unfolds*. New York: Doubleday, 2002.

"Umbilical Cord Abnormalities." *March of Dimes*. February 2008.

"Umbilical Cord Care: Do's and Don'ts For Parents." *MayoClinic*. February 22, 2013.

UNDESCENDED TESTICLES. *See* TESTICLES, UNDESCENDED.

UPPER EXTREMITIES
Anatomy

Anatomy or system affected: Arms, bones, hands, lymphatic system, muscles, musculoskeletal system, nerves, nervous system, skin

Specialties and related fields: Neurology, orthopedics, physical therapy

Definition: The arms (upper arms, forearms, and hands), which are attached to the shoulder blade at the shoulder joint and which consist of muscles, bones, blood vessels, lymph vessels, nerves, skin, and fingernails.

Key terms:

carpus: the wrist

distal: farther away from the base or attached end

elbow: the joint between the upper arm and the forearm

forearm: the region from the elbow joint to the wrist; also called the antebrachium

humerus: the bone that forms the structural beam of the upper arm

proximal: closer to the base or attached end

radial: toward the edge of the forearm and hand containing the radius and thumb

radius: the shorter of the two forearm bones, on the thumb side

ulna: the larger of the two forearm bones, forming the principal part of the elbow joint with the humerus

ulnar: toward the edge of the forearm and hand containing the ulna and little finger

upper arm: the region from the shoulder joint to the elbow joint; also called the brachium

Structure and Functions

The upper extremities consist of the upper arms, forearms, and hands. Each extremity is attached to the shoulder blade (or scapula) at the shoulder joint. The upper extremity is made mostly of bones and muscles, but it also contains blood vessels, lymphatics, nerves, skin, fingernails, and other associated structures. Important directional terms associated with the upper extremity include proximal (closer to the base or attached end), distal (farther from the base or attached end), radial (on the same side as the radius and the thumb), and ulnar (on the same side as the ulna and the little finger). Along the forearm and hand, the surface bearing the palm is called palmar; the opposite surface is called dorsal.

The bones and muscles of the shoulder provide support structures for the upper extremity. Beyond the shoulder, the major parts of the upper extremity include the upper arm (or brachium), from the shoulder joint to the elbow; the forearm, from the elbow to the wrist; the carpus, or wrist; and the manus, or hand. Beginning with the thumb, the five fingers of the hand are numbered one through five. Digit two is also called the index finger, digit three the middle finger, digit four the ring finger, and digit five the little finger.

Like other parts of the body, the upper extremity is clothed in skin, or integument. The skin covering the armpit (or axilla) has more hair and also more glands (especially the apocrine sweat glands) than most other parts of the body. The palm of the hand is unusual, along with the sole of the foot, in being completely hairless and in having a very thick outermost layer, called the stratum corneum. The ridges on the palm and fingers form individually characteristic patterns called dermatoglyphics, both fingerprints and palm prints. Each finger also has on its dorsal surface a fingernail; the thin crescent of semitransparent skin covering the base of the fingernail is called the eponychium.

The bones of the upper extremity include the scapula, clavicle, humerus, radius, ulna, carpals, metacarpals, and phalanges. The scapula, or shoulder blade, develops as part of the skeleton of the upper extremity and remains more strongly attached to the upper arm than to the trunk of the body. The outer (superficial) surface of the scapula is marked by a ridge called the spine, perpendicular to the scapular blade; the outer tip of this blade is called the acromion. The sculpted area above the spine is called the supraspinous fossa; the larger sculpted area below the spine is called the infraspinous fossa. The flat undersurface of the scapula is the subscapular fossa. The superior border of the scapula is marked by a hooklike coracoid process. At the shoulder joint itself, the scapula has a nearly spherical glenoid cavity into which the head of the humerus fits. The clavicle, or collarbone, runs from the upper end of the sternum (the manubrium) to the edge of the glenoid cavity of the scapula. It strengthens the shoulder region and provides additional support to the upper extremity.

The humerus runs from the shoulder joint to the elbow. At the shoulder joint, it attaches to the scapula by means of a rounded head that fits into the glenoid cavity of the scapula. The head is flanked by two protruding structures, the greater and lesser tuberosities, to which various muscles attach. At the elbow joint, the humerus attaches to the ulna by means of a pulleylike structure called the trochlea. The humerus also attaches to the radius by a smaller, rounded structure called the capitulum. Areas for muscle attachment on the lower end of the humerus include the lateral epicondyle (on the outer side) and the medial epicondyle (on the inner side).

The forearm contains two bones, the radius and ulna. The ulna is the larger of the two and forms the principal attachment with the humerus by means of a semilunar notch. Part of the ulna extends proximally beyond this semilunar notch to form a projection called the olecranon process (the hard structure on which one rests the elbows). The smaller of the

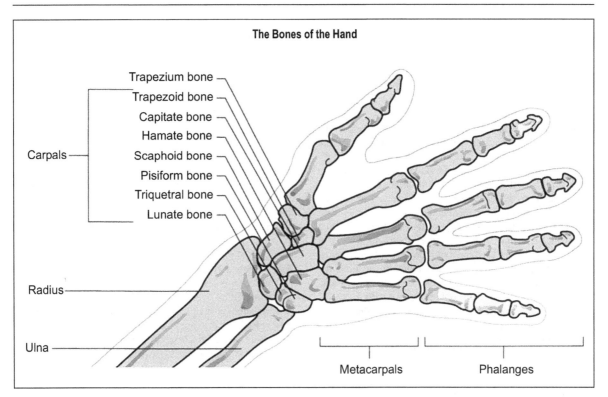

The Bones of the Hand

Trapezium bone
Trapezoid bone
Capitate bone
Hamate bone
Scaphoid bone
Pisiform bone
Triquetral bone
Lunate bone

Carpals

Radius

Ulna

Metacarpals

Phalanges

two forearm bones is the radius, which articulates loosely with the humerus and more strongly with the wrist and hand.

The carpus, or wrist, includes two rows of small bones. The proximal row includes (in order from the radial side to the ulnar) the scaphoid, lunate, cuneiform (triquetrum), and pisiform bones. The distal row includes the trapezium, trapezoid, capitate, and hamate bones, also in order from radial to ulnar. The trapezium supports the thumb, the trapezoid supports the index finger, the capitate supports the middle finger, and the hamate supports the two remaining digits. An important ligament called the transverse carpal ligament (or flexor retinaculum) runs across the palmar side of the wrist, forming a tunnel through which the tendons of the flexor muscles run. A similar ligament, the dorsal carpal ligament (or dorsal retinaculum) crosses the back of the wrist, forming a similar tunnel through which the tendons of the extensor muscles run. Beyond the wrist, the palm of the hand is supported by five bones called metacarpals, numbered one through five. The thumb contains two finger bones, or phalanges; each of the remaining fingers contains three phalanges.

The muscles of the upper extremity are divided into extensors (which straighten joints) and flexors (which bend joints). The shoulder muscles attaching the upper extremity to the trunk of the body include the trapezius, pectoralis major, pectoralis minor, deltoideus, coracobrachialis, subscapularis, supraspinatus, infraspinatus, teres major, teres minor, and latissimus dorsi. Of these, the trapezius, deltoideus, and supraspinatus are extensors; the coracobrachialis, latissimus dorsi, and the two pectoralis muscles are flexors; and the re-

maining muscles are primarily responsible for rotational movements. The trapezius originates from the cervical and thoracic vertebrae, including the adjoining ligaments and the adjacent part of the skull; its fibers converge mostly onto the spine and acromion of the scapula, but some also insert onto the clavicle. The pectoralis major is triangular; it originates from the sternum, costal cartilages, and a portion of the clavicle, from which its fibers converge toward an insertion on the greater tuberosity of the humerus. The pectoralis minor originates from the third through fifth ribs and inserts onto the coracoid process of the scapula. The deltoideus is a triangular muscle that originates from the clavicle and from the spine and acromion of the scapula; its fibers converge to insert by means of a strong tendon onto the shaft of the humerus. The coracobrachialis runs from the coracoid process to an insertion along the shaft of the humerus. The subscapularis originates from the subscapular fossa and inserts onto the lesser tuberosity of the humerus. The supraspinatus originates along the supraspinous fossa and inserts onto the greater tuberosity of the humerus. The infraspinatus originates from the infraspinous fossa and inserts onto the greater tuberosity of the humerus. The teres major and teres minor originate from the lower (inferior) border of the scapula; the teres major inserts onto the lesser tubercle of the humerus, and the teres minor inserts onto the greater tubercle. The latissimus dorsi is a broad, flat muscle that originates from the lower half of the vertebral column (and part of the ilium) by way of a tough tendinous sheet (the lumbar aponeurosis); it inserts high on the humerus.

The major flexors of the upper arm include the biceps brachii and the brachialis. The biceps brachii originates in two heads, one from the coracoid process of the scapula and one from the capsule of the shoulder joint. Both heads insert by means of a strong tendon onto a raised tuberosity of the radius. The brachialis originates from the shaft of the humerus and inserts high on the ulna.

The major extensor of the upper arm is the three-part triceps brachii, but a smaller anconeus and an epitrochlearis are sometimes present as well. The long head of the triceps originates from the scapula just below the armpit; the other two heads originate along the shaft of the humerus. All three heads insert onto the olecranon process by means of a strong tendon. The anconeus (or subanconeus) is not always present; its fibers run directly from the shaft of the humerus to that of the ulna. The epitrochlearis (or dorsoepitrochlearis), also variably present, may be viewed as a connecting band of muscle tissue from the latissimus dorsi onto the triceps brachii.

Flexors of the forearm include the flexor carpi radialis, palmaris longus, flexor carpi ulnaris, pronator teres, flexor digitorum superficialis, flexor digitorum profundus, flexor pollicis longus, and pronator quadratus. Many of these muscles have long, thin tendons that run in the tunnel formed beneath the transverse carpal ligament. The first five of these muscles originate from the medial epicondyle of the humerus. The pronator teres runs at an angle and inserts onto the shaft of the radius. The flexor carpi radialis inserts by a long, thin tendon onto the base of the second metacarpal. The palmaris longus ends in a broad tendon that spreads out over the palm of the hand to form the palmar aponeurosis, a sheet that sends tendinous branches into the fingers. The flexor carpi ulnaris inserts by a tendon onto the pisiform bone; the tendon then continues onto the hamate bone. The flexor digitorum superficialis originates from parts of the radius and ulna as well as the humerus; its strong tendon passes beneath the transverse carpal ligament, then divides into four branches to each of digits two through five. Each of these branches splits and then reunites to allow a tendon of the flexor digitorum to penetrate. The flexor digitorum profundus originates mostly from the shaft of the ulna; it gives rise to four strong tendons that run beneath the transverse carpal ligament, separate from one another over the palm of the hand, run into the second through fifth fingers, penetrate through the openings in the tendons of the flexor digitorum superficialis, and insert onto the base of the terminal phalanx of each finger except the thumb. The flexor pollicis longus arises from the radius alongside the previous muscle; its tendon runs beneath the transverse carpal ligament and inserts onto the base of the distal phalanx of the thumb. The pronator quadratus consists of a muscular sheet running between the distal portions of the radius and ulna.

The more superficial (shallower) extensors of the forearm include the brachioradialis, extensor carpi radialis longus, extensor carpi radialis brevis, extensor carpi ulnaris, extensor digitorum communis, and extensor digiti minimi. The brachioradialis originates from a ridge on the shaft of the humerus and inserts onto the radius at its distal end. The extensor carpi radialis longus originates from the shaft of the humerus; its tendon passes beneath the dorsal carpal ligament to insert near the base of the second metacarpal. The next four muscles originate together from the lateral epicondyle of the humerus. The extensor carpi radialis brevis gives rise to a tendon that passes beneath the dorsal carpal ligament to insert onto the base of the third metacarpal. The extensor carpi ulnaris gives rise to a tendon that passes beneath the dorsal carpal ligament and inserts onto the base of the fifth metacarpal. The extensor digitorum communis gives rise to four tendons that pass beneath the dorsal carpal ligament, then diverge to run into each finger except the thumb, where they each insert onto the base of the second phalanx, the base of the terminal phalanx, and a tendinous sheath covering the first phalanx. The extensor digiti minimi gives rise to a tendon that runs beneath the dorsal carpal ligament and unites over the first phalanx of the fifth finger with the tendon to that digit of the extensor digitorum communis.

The deeper extensors of the forearm include the supinator, abductor pollicis longus, extensor pollicis brevis, extensor pollicis longus, and extensor indicis. The supinator originates mostly from the proximal end of the ulnar shaft, but some of this muscle also originates from the capsule of the elbow joint and from the lateral epicondyle of the humerus. Its fibers spiral toward the midline of the body and insert onto the shaft of the radius. The abductor pollicis longus originates beneath the supinator from the shaft of the radius; it inserts by means of a tendon onto the base of the first metacarpal. The extensor pollicis brevis originates from the shaft of the radius and inserts by means of a tendon onto the base of the first phalanx of the thumb. The extensor pollicis longus originates from the middle portion of the shaft of the ulna; it gives rise to a tendon which runs beneath the dorsal carpal ligament to insert onto the base of the distal phalanx of the thumb. The extensor indicis arises beside the preceding muscle from the shaft of the ulna; its tendon passes beneath the dorsal carpal ligament and eventually attaches to the tendon going to the index finger from the extensor digitorum communis.

The flexor muscles that are "intrinsic" to the hand—that is, those confined to the hand—include the flexor pollicis brevis, abductor pollicis brevis, adductor pollicis, opponens pollicis, palmaris brevis, flexor digiti minimi, abductor digiti minimi, opponens digiti minimi, the lumbricales, and the interossei. There are no intrinsic extensor muscles in the hand.

The upper extremity can move in various ways. At the shoulder joint, possible movements include extension (or protraction) of the shoulder, which raises the arms; flexion (or retraction) of the shoulder, which lowers the arms; adduction of the arms, bringing them closer together; and abduction of the arms, pulling them farther apart. The two movements possible at the elbow joint are extension (straightening) and flexion (bending). Two special movements are possible within the forearm: Pronation is an inward rotation of the radius upon the ulna in such a way that the palms face downward; supination is an outward rotation of the radius upon the ulna in such a way that the palms face upward. Various movements are possible at the wrist, including flexion (bending), extension (straightening), hyperextension (bending the hand upward), radial abduction (twisting the hand toward the thumb side), and ulnar abduction (twisting the hand toward the little finger side). Movements of the phalanges include flexion (bending), extension (straightening), abduction (spreading the fingers), and adduction (bringing the fingers back together).

Blood vessels of the upper extremity include both arteries and veins. The brachial artery is the major continuation of the subclavian and axillary arteries into the upper arm; as it approaches the elbow, it divides into the radial and ulnar arteries, which supply most of the forearm. Near the wrist, each of these last two arteries divides into a branch that runs closer to the palm and another that runs closer to the back of the hand. The two palmar branches then connect with each other to form a loop called the palmar digital arch; the other two branches also connect, forming a loop called the dorsal digital arch. From these two digital arches arises a secondary digital arch running into each finger, connecting in each case to the palmar arch at one end and to the dorsal arch at the other end. This type of arrangement, called collateral circulation, uses multiple alternate routes to permit blood flow even if one of the routes is temporarily blocked.

There are several important veins draining the upper extremity. Several of these run just beneath the skin: the cephalic vein, running along the radial margin of the forearm and upper arm; the median antebrachial vein, draining the palmar surface of the hand and forearm; and the basilic vein, continuing the median antebrachial vein along the inner side of the upper arm. The deep veins of the arm all drain into the brachial vein. As it flows into the shoulder, the brachial vein joins with the basilic vein to form the axillary vein, which then becomes the subclavian vein when it reaches the rib cage.

The major nerves to the upper extremity arise from a series of complex branchings known as the brachial plexus, originating mostly from the fifth through eighth cervical nerves and the first thoracic nerve. The major nerves of the brachial plexus are a lateral cord (formed from branches of the fifth, sixth, and seventh cervical nerves), a medial cord (formed from branches of the last cervical and first thoracic nerves), and a posterior cord (formed from branches of the sixth, seventh, and eighth cervical nerves). The major nerves of the arm include a musculocutaneous nerve arising from the lateral cord, an axillary nerve and a radial nerve arising from the posterior cord, an ulnar nerve and a medial antebrachial cutaneous nerve arising from the medial cord, and a median nerve arising from both the lateral and the medial cords. The musculocutaneous, ulnar, and median nerves constitute the main nerve supply to the flexor muscles of the arm and hand, while the axillary nerve supplies the deltoid muscle and the radial nerve supplies the remaining extensor muscles. In addition, the radial nerve supplies sensory branches to the skin of the dorsal side of the forearm and hand (except for the fifth finger and part of the fourth), while the musculocutaneous and medial antebrachial cutaneous nerves supply sensory branches to the skin over the palmar or flexor side of the arm and forearm. The median nerve sends sensory branches to the

skin over most of the palmar surface of the hand from the thumb up to the middle of the fourth finger, while the ulnar nerve sends sensory branches to the skin on both the palmar and dorsal sides of the fifth finger and the ulnar half of the fourth. At the elbow, the ulnar nerve passes around the olecranon process just under the skin, where it is easily subject to accidental pressure; the tingling that results from such pressure is the source of the term "funny bone."

Disorders and Diseases

Many types of medical conditions and disorders can affect the upper extremities. For example, many types of contact dermatitis, from poison ivy to "dishpan hands," are first noticed on the surface of the hands and forearms. Other medical problems of the upper extremity include animal bites, injuries, and an assortment of neuromuscular disorders.

Neuromuscular disorders involving the upper extremity include nerve paralyses, uncontrolled shaking (choreic) movements, muscular atrophies, and muscular dystrophies. Nerve paralyses may arise from traumatic injury, but the most common type of paralysis is cerebral palsy. Cerebral palsy is actually a group of paralytic disorders that begin at birth or in early childhood. The extent of the paralysis may vary, often involving large groups of muscles while sparing others. In addition to the lack of muscular control of the limbs, other symptoms may include spasms, athetoid (slow, rhythmic, and wormlike) movements, or muscular rigidity. Some types of cerebral palsy may result from injuries received at birth or in early infancy.

Uncontrolled, purposeless, and irregular shaking movements of the extremities are called choreic movements. These disorders, which involve the upper extremities more often than the lower, include both Sydenham's chorea and Huntington's chorea. Sydenham's chorea (true chorea) typically begins in children and young adults, with maximum disability occurring two to three weeks after symptoms begin. Choreic symptoms typically diminish and disappear in a few months, but they may recur at a later time. The movements can be controlled with drugs. Huntington's chorea, also called Huntington's disease, seldom begins before the age of forty. It typically begins with uncontrolled choreic movements of the hands. The disease progressively worsens and ultimately causes death about fifteen years after onset. The disease is caused by a single dominant gene.

Muscular atrophies are a variety of diseases in which muscle tissues become progressively weaker and smaller, usually beginning between forty and sixty years of age. Spastic movements may sometimes occur. The small muscles of the hands are usually affected sooner and more severely in comparison to the large muscles of the arms and shoulders. Amyotrophic lateral sclerosis (ALS), commonly called Lou Gehrig's disease, is a progressive muscular atrophy that usually begins with weakness and deterioration of the hand muscles. The disease proceeds to affect the rest of the extremities, then other parts of the body; it is usually fatal within three to five years after onset. A more rare type of atrophy, myelopathic muscular atrophy (or Aran-Duchenne atrophy), also begins in the small hand muscles and slowly spreads to the arms, shoulders, and trunk muscles, in that order. A degenerative lesion of the gray matter in the cervical region of the spinal cord is usually responsible. Weakness and wasting of the muscles of the hands and forearms also characterize syringomyelia, a disorder of the glial cells in the cervical region of the spinal cord. Impairment of the cutaneous senses often occurs with this disease and frequently results in burns and other injuries to the hand when the patient, unaware of a threat, fails to withdraw or take other countermeasures.

Muscular dystrophy is an inherited disease—actually several related diseases—that usually begins in early childhood and affects males more often than females. The most common type, Duchenne muscular dystrophy, is believed to be caused by a sex-linked recessive trait. Spastic movements do not occur, and the disease affects the large muscles of the shoulder, arm, and thigh more than the small muscles of the hand. The affected muscles become very weak but remain approximately normal in size or increase as fatty and fibrous tissue replaces muscle. Progressive weakening makes walking impossible, but patients can live for decades with proper care.

Repetitive motion injuries of the upper extremity may occur at the elbow joint (tennis elbow) or in the vicinity of the wrist. Some repetitive wrist movements are capable of producing carpal tunnel syndrome, an injury of the tendons running through the tunnel beneath the transverse carpal ligament.

Perspective and Prospects

The first well-illustrated anatomical texts were produced by Belgian physician Andreas Vesalius (1514–1564); along with the rest of the human body, they showed the major muscles and bones of the upper extremities. An accurate medical understanding of the circulatory system began with the studies of the English physician William Harvey (1578–1657), who examined the veins in the arms of many patients. Harvey noticed the valves in the veins and was able to prove that the blood circulates outward from the heart, throughout the body, and then back again to the heart.

Injuries to the arm are generally treated surgically. Whenever possible, broken bones are set in place, immobilized in a cast, and then allowed to heal. Torn muscles (or tendons) must be sewn together, and nerve endings must be placed in their former positions for them to grow back correctly. If the whole hand is severed at the wrist, many tendons and blood vessels must be reattached; such an operation is very difficult. When a portion of the upper extremity must be amputated, the stump is generally covered with a flap of skin. Sometimes an artificial hand is attached to the muscles that are still usable.

—*Eli C. Minkoff, Ph.D.*

See also Amputation; Arthritis; Arthroplasty; Arthroscopy; Bone disorders; Bone grafting; Bones and the skeleton; Carpal tunnel syndrome; Casts and splints; Fracture and dislocation; Fracture repair; Frostbite; Grafts and grafting; Lower extremities; Marfan syndrome; Muscle sprains, spasms, and disorders; Muscles; Nail removal; Orthopedic surgery; Orthopedics; Orthopedics, pediatric; Osteopathic medicine; Prostheses; Rheumatoid arthritis; Rheumatology; Warts; Wounds.

For Further Information:
Agur, Anne M. R., and Arthur F. Dalley. *Grant's Atlas of Anatomy.* 13th ed. Philadelphia: Wolters Kluwer Health/Lippincott Williams & Wilkins, 2013.
"Arm Injuries and Disorders." *MedlinePlus*, July 10, 2013.
"Hand Injuries and Disorders." *MedlinePlus*, July 19, 2013.
Marieb, Elaine N. *Essentials of Human Anatomy and Physiology.* 10th ed. San Francisco: Pearson/Benjamin Cummings, 2012.
Rosse, Cornelius, and Penelope Gaddum-Rosse. *Hollinshead's Textbook of Anatomy.* 5th ed. Philadelphia: Lippincott-Raven, 1997.
Standring, Susan, et al., eds. *Gray's Anatomy.* 40th ed. New York: Churchill Livingstone/Elsevier, 2008.

Uremia
Disease/Disorder

Anatomy or system affected: Bladder, blood, circulatory system, heart, kidneys, urinary system

Specialties and related fields: Cardiology, hematology, nephrology, urology

Definition: A condition that occurs when an excess of urea and other waste elements accumulate in the blood as the result of reduced or inadequate kidney function, or both.

Key terms:

amino acids: any of a number of nitrogen-rich compounds used by the body for the production of protein

antihypertensive drugs: medicines designed to reduce and control elevated blood pressure

diuretics: drugs used to increase urination and eliminate wastes from the bloodstream

edema: an abnormal accumulation of watery fluid in the connective tissues, resulting in swelling

hemolytic uremia: a type of uremia that afflicts mostly young children and infants

renal failure: the failure of the kidneys, making it impossible for them to function efficiently

urea: the waste product when proteins and other nitrogen-rich compounds are broken down

Causes and Symptoms

Uremia is a condition that results when the waste products in the blood, notably urea and creatinine, build up in the bloodstream and are not excreted, as would normally be the case by being transported to the liver and subsequently expelled in the urine. In some patients suffering from uremia, a marked reduction or absence of vitamin B_6 is noted. Often, there is inadequate blood supply to the kidneys, especially in cases where hemorrhaging or shock have occurred.

Congestive heart failure may accompany uremia or may be, at least in part, an initial cause of it. Renal azotemia is a disease affecting the kidneys and may lead to kidney failure. Postrenal azotemia occurs when the flow of urine in the area below the kidneys is blocked. This condition may be attributed to several causes, including kidney stones, pregnancy, compressed ureters, enlargement of the prostate, or bladder stones, often associated with gallbladder problems. When the amino acids that the body uses to produce protein get out of control, uremia may result. In such cases, there is usually no underlying kidney disease, but a heightened resistance to the

Information on Uremia

Causes: Excessive levels of nitrogen compounds in blood, resulting in decreased cardiac output
Symptoms: Lethargy, pale skin color, deposits of solid uric compounds resembling frost on skin, rapid pulse, markedly acute thirst, dry mouth, edema in mouth, mental confusion, fluctuations in blood pressure, exhaustion, nausea, vomiting
Duration: Indefinite; extreme cases may result in death
Treatments: Dietary changes, hemodialysis, kidney transplantation, diuretics, antihypertensive medication, vitamin B_6 therapy when deficiency exists

flow of urine can result in its backing up into the kidneys, which leads to a condition known as hydronephrosis. This condition can lead to dangerous toxicity and, in extreme cases, may prove fatal.

A unique kind of uremia that is found largely in infants and young children is hemolytic uremia. The origins of this disorder are not fully understood, but it appears to result from damage to the red blood cells in the kidneys. Hemolytic uremia is accompanied by excessively high blood pressure. Many specialists in the field believe that the disorder has viral or bacterial origins.

Treatment and Therapy

Patients suffering from uremia sometimes become disoriented and confused. They lose energy and tire easily. They may become nauseated and lose interest in food and in eating. They may also experience some outward manifestations including eruptions on the skin, sores and/or edema in the mouth, and excessive thirst. Medications to deal with nausea and to help the patient return to more normal eating habits are indicated where nausea is a continuing factor.

In relatively mild cases, therapy with vitamin B_6 may partially or wholly eliminate the condition. Patients may also respond well to changes in their diet, strongly reducing the protein content of what they consume. This solution, however, must be adhered to strenuously and continued throughout one's life span unless such treatment as a kidney transplant is successful and permits the patient to experience better health overall.

Extreme cases may require hemodialysis to cleanse the blood of its impurities or may indicate the removal of uric toxins by modified blood separation and absorption therapies. Such treatments can make serious inroads on one's normal life because treatment in sixty- to ninety-minute sessions is often indicated three or more times a week. In cases of renal failure, a kidney transplant may offer the most effective long-term solution.

When uremia elevates the blood pressure to dangerous levels, particularly in hemolytic uremia, treatment with antihypertensive medications is essential and is usually successful. Dialysis may be necessary so that impurities can be removed, giving the kidneys a chance to recover.

In such cases, the patient may find it virtually impossible to urinate and what urine is excreted may be streaked with blood. Despite such disturbing manifestations, most patients suffering from hemolytic uremia make a full recovery, often in as little as two weeks.

Perspective and Prospects

Uremia exists in varying degrees, but much of it can be managed successfully and controlled to the point that it appears to be cured. With adequate care during the acute stages of the disorder, some patients recover in anywhere from seven to fifteen days, although they may incur some kidney damage, either temporary or permanent.

Uremia is most dangerous when it is accompanied by acute pancreatitis, as it often is. In cases involving this complication, the prognosis is not encouraging, although with adequate care, the death rate is substantially reduced.

—*R. Baird Shuman, Ph.D.*

See also Dialysis; Diuretics; Edema; End-stage renal disease; Hemolytic uremic syndrome; Incontinence; Kidney disorders; Kidney transplantation; Kidneys; Lithotripsy; Nephrectomy; Nephritis; Nephrology; Nephrology, pediatric; Polycystic kidney disease; Proteinuria; Pyelonephritis; Renal failure; Stone removal; Stones.

For Further Information:

Brenner, Barry M. *Brenner and Rector's The Kidney.* Philadelphia: Saunders/Elsevier, 2008.

Chen, Shuang. *The Guide to Nutrition and Diet for Dialysis Patients.* Coral Springs, Fla.: Metier Books, 2008.

Gennan, F. John. *Medical Management of Kidney and Electrolyte Disorders.* New York: Dekker, 2001.

Gurland, Hans J., ed. *Uremia Therapy: Perspectives for the Next Quarter Century.* 1st ed. New York: Springer, 2012. Print.

Massry, Shaul G., and Richard J. Glassock, eds. *Massry and Glassock's Textbook on Nephrology.* Philadelphia: Lippincott Williams & Wilkins, 2001.

Nissenson, Allan R., and Richard N. Fine, eds. *Dialysis Therapy.* Philadelphia: Hanley and Belfus, 2002.

Tamparo, Carol D. *Diseases of the Human Body.* Philadelphia: Davis, 2000.

URETHRITIS

Disease/Disorder

Anatomy or system affected: Bladder, genitals, urinary system

Specialties and related fields: Bacteriology, family medicine, internal medicine, urology

Definition: An infection or inflammation of the urethra, which may be caused by infective organisms, ingested irritants, or trauma.

Causes and Symptoms

Urethritis is most often contracted through intercourse with a partner infected with a sexually transmitted disease (STD), particularly gonorrhea and chlamydia. It will usually appear a few days after sex. Urethritis may also be caused by a variety of other organisms, including *Escherichia coli* (*E. coli*) and *Mycoplasma genitalium* bacteria, *Trichomonas vaginalis* protozoa, and herpes simplex viruses. Another source of the disease is irritation of the urethra produced by soaps, lotions,

---

Information on Urethritis

Causes: Infection with STDs, bacteria, protozoa, or viruses; irritation from soaps, lotions, or spermicides; trauma from catheters or cystoscopes; kidney stones; weakened immune system; urinary tract malformations

Symptoms: Burning or pain with urination, frequent urination, chills or fever; pus-filled and cloudy penile discharge in men and vaginal discharge, rectal discomfort, pain or bleeding during intercourse in women

Duration: One to two weeks with treatment; sometimes recurrent

Treatments: Antibiotics (doxycycline, azithromycin, erythromycin, roxithromycin, tetracycline); increased fluid intake rate (especially cranberry juice)

---

or spermicides. Trauma produced by medical instruments, such as urinary catheters or cystoscopes, can also generate urethritis. Complicated urethritis may be associated with kidney stones, a weak immune system, or malformations of the urinary tract. There are cases of nonspecific urethritis that have no known cause.

General symptoms for males and females include burning or pain when urinating, unusually frequent urination, and chills or fever. In males, pus and cloudy discharges may come from the penis, and the opening to the penis may stick together from dried-up secretions and may be red, sore, and itchy. In females, vaginal discharge may be present, as well as discomfort in the rectal area and pain or bleeding during sexual intercourse. In some cases, no accompanying symptoms are associated with urethritis.

Treatment and Therapy

To assess possible bacterial sources of urethritis, urinalysis and urine culture laboratory tests are performed. Abnormal genital discharges and, in some cases, urethral swabs are also examined. If urethritis is diagnosed, then antibiotics are usually administered. The most common ones used are doxycycline, azithromycin, erythromycin, roxithromycin, and tetracycline. Even for cases of nonspecific urethritis, antibiotics have provided an effective treatment. Drinking copious fluids can help dilute bacteria and flush the urinary system. Acupuncture and homeopathic therapies sometimes help relieve the effects of urethritis.

If symptoms of urethritis are present, then the urethra should be rested by abstaining from sexual intercourse and masturbation until medical treatment has been received. When treated quickly and correctly, the symptoms are usually resolved in one to two weeks. Without proper treatment, serious complications might include infection spreading into the bladder or kidneys, as well as transmission of the causative organism to a sexual partner.

When it is not associated with a general urinary tract infection, urethritis is more common in males than females, probably because males have a longer urethra. In some individuals,

nonspecific urethritis can have a high recurrence rate. Burning during urination can be reduced by adding a small amount of baking soda to drinking water to reduce the acidity of urine. Cranberry juice contains a compound that prevents bacteria from sticking to the urethra and growing there.

—*Alvin K. Benson, Ph.D.*

See also Bacterial infections; Chlamydia; Cystitis; *E. coli* infection; Genital disorders, female; Genital disorders, male; Gonorrhea; Men's health; Reproductive system; Sexually transmitted diseases (STDs); Trichomoniasis; Urinalysis; Urinary disorders; Urinary system; Urology; Urology, pediatric; Women's health.

For Further Information:

Beers, Mark H., et al., eds. *The Merck Manual of Diagnosis and Therapy.* 18th ed. Whitehouse Station, N.J.: Merck Research Laboratories, 2006.

Kasper, Dennis L., et al., eds. *Harrison's Principles of Internal Medicine.* 16th ed. New York: McGraw-Hill, 2005.

Schmitt, Barton D. *Your Child's Health: The Parents'' One-Stop Reference Guide to Symptoms, Emergencies, Common Illnesses, Behavior Problems, Healthy Development.* Rev. ed. New York: Bantam Books, 2005.

URETHROPLASTY. *See* HYPOSPADIAS REPAIR AND URETHROPLASTY.

URINALYSIS

Procedure

Anatomy or system affected: Bladder, kidneys, urinary system

Specialties and related fields: Biochemistry, microbiology, nephrology, toxicology, urology

Definition: The chemical, microscopic, and/or physical examination of urine.

Key terms:

dipstick: a chemically treated paper strip used for the chemical analysis of urine

ketones: the by-products of fat metabolism; their presence may be indicative of diabetes mellitus

pH: a value that represents the relative acidity or alkalinity of a solution; values below pH 7 are acidic, while values above pH 7 are basic

specific gravity: the density of a solution relative to that of water; abnormal values can be indicative of elevated sugar or protein levels in urine

Indications and Procedures

Urinalysis is one of the oldest and most useful of noninvasive clinical tests. In addition to aiding in the diagnosis of urinary tract or kidney disease, the procedure may be applied to the analysis of most metabolic by-products that pass through the kidneys. Thus it may be applied to observations of kidney or liver abnormalities and metabolic diseases such as diabetes mellitus.

For routine analysis, approximately 10 to 15 milliliters of urine are collected in a clean jar, though larger volumes are preferable. Initial examination involves the physical appearance of the urine sample: color, turbidity, and possible odor.

Normal urine is generally pale yellow in appearance, though variation from such color is not necessarily abnormal. Bacteria may cause alterations in this color, as can simple by-products of the diet. Normal urine is generally clear, though as with color, turbidity (cloudiness) may be associated with a variety of causes. Fresh urine also has a characteristically mild odor.

The specific gravity of the urine may be analyzed at this time, though the usefulness of this test is limited to those circumstances in which the water intake of the patient is known. Generally, the only specimen of use for this test is one utilizing the first urine output of the day. The pH is most accurately determined using a pH meter, though dipstick pads impregnated with colored pH indicators can be used when frequent (or inconvenient) monitoring is necessary.

Hematuria, the presence of blood in the urine, is never normal, though its detection need not indicate a significant pathology. Hemoglobin may be detected using a dipstick method with follow-up necessary to determine the specific cause.

The microscopic examination of urine consists of centrifugation of a volume of urine under specified conditions followed by resuspension of the sediment in a standard volume of liquid. The presence of any blood cells, bacteria, yeast, or other types of sediment can then be determined.

Chemical analysis can be utilized for determination of the presence of a wide variety of chemicals or drugs. Routinely, chemical procedures are used to detect sugar, protein, or by-products of fat metabolism such as ketones. Dipsticks are available for routine analysis.

Uses and Complications

Diagnosis of urinary or metabolic problems cannot necessarily be made from a single abnormal test result, as a variety of factors have a potential impact on test results. Rather, analysis of a combination of tests is often necessary in diagnosis of a problem.

Urinalysis involves the physical, chemical, and microscopic analysis of urine. Physical examination centers on the color, turbidity, and odor of urine. A pink or red color can be indicative of the presence of blood, though microscopic or chemical examination is needed for confirmation. (For example, a red color may simply indicate that the patient recently ate beets.) An increase in turbidity can result from the presence of yeast or mucus, indicating infection, or from diet by-products such as lipids. Likewise, abnormal odors can result from urinary tract infection (elevated levels of ammonia) or certain metabolic diseases; however, ingestion of asparagus may also result in unusual odors.

Chemical analysis of urine ranges from the determination of pH to the detection of any of a variety of chemicals. On a routine basis, this usually involves examination for sugar, protein, or ketones. Normal urine is usually acid (pH 6), though the patient's diet will often affect such values as well. A high pH may be indicative of urinary tract infection; microscopic detection of microorganisms may be used to confirm this diagnosis.

Small quantities of protein in the urine are normal. Elevated levels of proteinuria, however, can result from kidney disorders, particularly those associated with glomerular damage, or from urinary tract disease. Likewise, small quantities of sugar in the urine are generally of no clinical significance. In the case of diabetes, however, with resultant high levels of glucose in the bloodstream, significant quantities of glucose may be found in the urine. Persons with severe diabetes are unable to remove and utilize glucose from the blood; metabolism in such individuals will switch to the utilization of fat, with resultant breakdown products such as ketones being secreted in the urine. Such products are volatile and may disappear from urine if the sample is not analyzed within sufficient time. Since fat metabolism is employed as a source of energy in the absence of carbohydrates, severe dieting may also result in the excretion of ketones.

Perspective and Prospects

Analysis of urine for diagnosis of disease was among the earliest of medical procedures. Greek physicians at the time of Hippocrates observed the color of urine and its taste. Pouring urine on the ground to see if insects were attracted to it could be used to test for sugar.

Until the mid-twentieth century, chemical tests on urine utilized a variety of liquid reagents. The introduction of dipsticks significantly improved the efficiency and convenience of such analysis. The dipstick consists of a thin strip of plastic with a cellulose pad attached. Impregnated in the pad are the chemicals necessary to carry out the specific test. For example, the dipstick used in the analysis of pH contains an indicator that will change color depending on the degree of acidity or alkalinity.

Instrumentation is available that allows the analysis of a combination of tests simultaneously, much as a blood sample can be analyzed. Either the dipstick or the urine sample itself may be inserted into a machine for urinalysis. For simple home analysis in which only a single test is necessary, commercial production began in the 1980s of analogous materials for detection of urinary chemicals. For example, home pregnancy kits are available and are home drug testing kits, and in theory, similar kits could be used for the detection of any substance in urine.

—*Richard Adler, Ph.D.*

See also Bladder cancer; Bladder removal; Cystoscopy; Cytology; Cytopathology; Hematuria; Laboratory tests; Noninvasive tests; Pathology; Pregnancy and gestation; Proteinuria; Urethritis; Urinary disorders; Urinary system; Urology; Urology, pediatric.

For Further Information:

Boston Women's Health Collective. *Our Bodies, Ourselves: A New Edition for a New Era*. Rev. ed. New York: Touchstone, 2011.

Griffith, H. Winter. *Complete Guide to Symptoms, Illness, and Surgery*. 6th ed. New York: Perigee, 2012.

Humes, H. David, et al., eds. *Kelley's Textbook of Internal Medicine*. 4th ed. Philadelphia: Lippincott Williams & Wilkins, 2000.

Pagana, Kathleen Deska, and Timothy J. Pagana. *Mosby's Diagnostic and Laboratory Test Reference*. 4th ed. St. Louis, Mo.: Mosby/Elsevier, 2010.

Simon, Harvey. *Staying Well: Your Complete Guide to Disease Prevention*. Boston: Houghton Mifflin, 1992.

Strasinger, Susan J., and Marjorie Schaub Di Lorenzo. *Urinalysis and Body Fluids*. 5th ed. Philadelphia: F. A. Davis, 2008.

Vorvick, Linda J. "Urinalysis." *MedlinePlus*, February 1, 2011.

URINARY DISORDERS

Disease/Disorder

Anatomy or system affected: Abdomen, bladder, kidneys, urinary system

Specialties and related fields: Gynecology, nephrology, urology

Definition: Diseases or pathologies associated with any organs of urine production or secretion, such as the kidneys, ureters, urinary bladder, and urethra.

Key terms:

bacteriuria: the presence of bacteria in the urine

cystitis: inflammation of the urinary bladder, often characterized by pain and dysuria

dysuria: painful or difficult urination, often the result of urinary tract infection or obstruction

urethra: the tubular structure that drains the urine from the bladder

urethritis: inflammation of the urethra, often characterized by dysuria

urinary bladder: the muscular organ that stores urine to be discharged through the urethra

urinary tract infection: infection involving any organs associated with the urinary system

Causes and Symptoms

Diseases of the urinary tract represent one of the most common forms of infection by microorganisms. In the United States, the prevalence of urinary tract infections is a reflection of both gender and age. By the age of five, bacteriuria is found in approximately 4 to 5 percent of girls, which is about ten times the rate among boys. Infections are far more common among female adolescents and young women than among men, with a yearly prevalence of approximately 20 percent of American women in the age group of sixteen to thirty-five years accounting for approximately six million reported cases each year. Data regarding prevalence of infection varies depending on what definition of infection is used. The prevalence of infection among both men and women rises sharply among the elderly, often reflecting problems with aging, including enlargement of the prostate in men. Most infections are self-limiting, particularly among the young. If not treated properly, however, such infections have the potential to be more serious.

Normally, urine is free of microbial contamination. The much higher incidence of urinary tract infections in women reflects, to a large degree, the anatomical differences between males and females. In women, the close proximity of the urethra to the rectum permits relatively easy access of intestinal flora to the urinary tract. Not surprisingly, most urinary infections are caused by enteric bacteria. The most common infectious agent, *Escherichia coli*, represents approximately 80 percent of the acquired infections of the urinary tract. Other bacterial genera of importance include *Enterobacter*, *Klebsiella*, and *Proteus*. *Proteus* infections may be of particular significance because colonization by that organism may lead to the deposition of urinary calculi (stones). Less often, *Streptococcus faecalis* or *Pseudomonas aeruginosa* may be involved; the latter can be a particular problem because of its high level of drug resistance.

Urinary tract infections usually begin with entry of the organisms into the distal end of the urethra; the migration of microorganisms into the vagina may occur in a similar manner. Most bladder infections result from ascending movement of the microbial agents along the urethra into the urinary bladder. Inflammation of the urethra (urethritis) or urinary bladder (cystitis) results from a combination of microbial colonization and the host's immune response to the infection. Often, such inflammation may be the first symptom of these infections.

Various factors appear to predispose certain individuals to urinary tract infections. Strains of *E. coli* that colonize the urethra appear to have a greater ability to adhere to the surface tissue. In particular, those strains that frequently ascend into the ureters or kidneys often possess unique types of fimbriae (filamentous structures), which promotes adherence to the epithelial cells that line the surface of the urinary tract; this bacterial structure may be of particular importance to the course of the infection, since the flushing action of urinary flow is a mechanism by which the body maintains the sterility of the urinary tract. Likewise, anything with the potential to interrupt micturition (urination), such as the presence of calculi or tumors, may predispose an individual to a urinary tract infection. Enlargement of the prostate gland in older men is a frequent cause of such problems. Among children, congenital abnormalities at the site of ureter entry into the bladder may result in a vesicoureteral reflux, or urine backflow, which may interfere with normal urine flow. Such abnormalities, which are not uncommon, are found in equal numbers among both young boys and girls; they frequently disappear naturally by the time of puberty. Nevertheless, such problems may contribute to infections among those in this age group.

Certain forms of birth control, in addition to the act of intercourse itself, may contribute to urinary infections. The term "honeymoon cystitis" is often applied, reflecting the bacteriuria often found following intercourse. The colonization of *E. coli* may be associated with the use of diaphragms or spermicides. The reasons for this connection are unclear, but both appear to represent an alteration in the normal flora of the periurethral area and vagina.

Clinical manifestations of urinary tract infections vary with age and are often nonspecific. The infiltration of leukocytes (white blood cells), resulting in inflammation, accounts for many of the symptoms. Among children, abdominal pain is often present, accompanied by fever and sometimes vomiting. Among adults, cystitis and urethritis are often accompanied by difficulty in urination (dysuria), including painful urination and frequent urination, particularly in women. A sensation of abdominal heaviness or lower back pain, in addition to low-grade fever, is often observed. The urine may be bloody or turbid, reflecting a mixture of microbial agents and white blood cells. Bacteriuria is detected by the collection of a sample of voided urine and inoculation of an appropriate culture dish; the presence of at least 100,000 colony-forming units per milliliter of sample constitutes "significant bacteriuria."

Infection of the urinary tract may also result from a variety of sexually transmitted organisms. Chlamydial infections are common in both males and females, and they represent one of the most commonly observed forms of sexually transmitted disease (STD). *Chlamydia trachomatis* causes urethritis in both males and females; though many chlamydial infections are asymptomatic, they can lead to severe complications. Urethritis may also result from other microbial STDs, both viral and bacterial.

The use of catheters, particularly among hospitalized elderly persons, is a frequent cause of urinary infections. An estimated 40 percent of nosocomial (hospital-acquired) infections result from the use of catheters. Despite attempts to maintain sterility through the use of closed, sterile drainage systems, by two weeks after catheterization 50 percent of both men and women have developed a urinary tract infection, and with longer or permanent catheterizations, nearly all persons will develop some degree of infection. In most cases, these infections are inapparent, but such persons remain predisposed to cystitis or urethritis.

The urinary tract is also subject to other disorders, including cancer. The most common form of neoplasm of the urinary tract is bladder cancer. Such cancers tend to be highly aggressive, often occur as multiple growths, and are difficult to cure once metastasis has begun. Approximately two-thirds of cases of bladder cancer are diagnosed in men, perhaps in part a reflection of risk factors. Exposure to both cigarette smoke and carcinogens, particularly those used in the petrochemical industry, has been linked to an increased incidence of bladder cancers. The symptoms of bladder cancer resemble those of urinary tract infections: dysuria, cystitis, and the frequent need to urinate. If the tumor is diagnosed early enough, electrosurgery or resection may be sufficient to remove the lesion. If the tumor has begun to infiltrate the bladder tissue, complete removal of the bladder may be necessary. Radiation and chemotherapy are also commonly used in the treatment of certain forms of urinary tract cancers.

In May 2013, the journal *Science Translational Medicine* published a report suggesting that repeat urinary tract infections may be caused by a strain of *E. coli* bacteria present in the stomach or bladder. According to a study, an adaptable strain of *E. coli* that can survive repeated treatment efforts may be the cause of recurrent infections.

Treatment and Therapy

Standard treatment for urinary tract infections consists of a regimen of antimicrobial drugs. Ideally, the antibiotics of choice are secreted in the urine over a prolonged period, rather than achieving high concentrations in the blood serum. In this manner, the drug is directed at the infection itself, with minimal effect on the normal flora elsewhere in the body.

Depending on whether the infection is limited to the lower urinary tract (urethra or bladder) or has spread to the upper tract (ureters or kidneys), the period of regimen may last for several days or up to two weeks. Generally, infections of the upper urinary tract require more prolonged treatment and may be subject to recurrence.

Standard therapy of conventional lower-tract infections routinely consists of a three-day regimen of trimethoprim-sulfamethoxazole (TMP-SMX), or TMP alone. Since most of the drug combination is excreted in the urine, there is a minimum of side effects and little danger to the normal flora

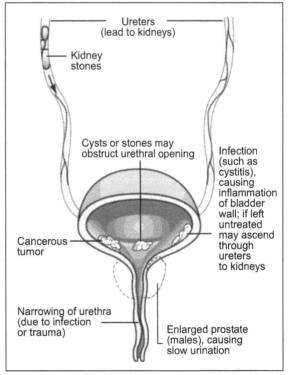

In addition to the variety of infections that may attack the urinary system, urinary disorders may be caused by cancerous tumors, cysts, stones that cause obstruction, reactions to trauma, and in males pressure from an enlarged prostate.

within the body. The short duration of treatment also minimizes the chances of encouraging the growth of resistant populations of bacteria. Elderly patients or persons with diabetes mellitus may require longer treatment. If the person shows evidence of upper-tract infection, treatment is generally given over a two-week period.

If there is evidence of kidney involvement or inflammation (pyelonephritis), the patient is often hospitalized in order to monitor treatment, which usually involves a fourteen-day course of TMP-SMX. Severe illness or evidence of spreading may require more intensive therapy with other antibiotics.

Since the flushing action of urine is itself a nonspecific means of removing bacteria from the bladder or urethra, patients are usually advised to drink as much water as possible. In this manner, weakly adherent or nonadherent bacteria may be flushed from the site of infection, reducing the number of bacteria and supplementing the course of antimicrobial therapy. In some cases, this action is sufficient to relieve symptoms or even cure the infection.

In situations in which the infection is asymptomatic, unless the situation warrants treatment (such as impending surgery), antimicrobial therapy may not be necessary, as the infection is self-limiting. Given the large proportion of persons, particularly women, who develop bacteriuria, forgoing therapy may minimize the chances for the artificial selection of resistant strains. In individuals with heart disease, renal failure, or diabetes, however, such therapy may be necessary as a preventive measure for later problems.

Bacteriuria during pregnancy represents a special situation. During early pregnancy, from 4 to 7 percent of women develop bacteriuria, which is probably related to such physiological changes as the dilation of the bladder and uterus, along with vesicoureteral (bladder and urethra) reflux. Even though the infection may be asymptomatic, urinary tract infection is associated with increased risk of both pyelonephritis and loss of the fetus; about one-third of women with untreated bacteriuria during pregnancy develop infections within the upper urinary tract by the third trimester. For this reason, it is generally recommended that pregnant women be screened for such infections and undergo treatment if bacteriuria is present. Pregnant women generally undergo a three-day treatment regimen, though with alternative antibiotics considered safer in the presence of a developing fetus: ampicillin, nitrofurantoin, or cephalexin. Patients should be monitored at intervals during the pregnancy to prevent recurrence. If pyelonephritis should develop, the woman is routinely hospitalized to allow close monitoring of both the mother and the fetus during therapy.

Bacteriuria associated with catheterization is generally treated only when it is symptomatic, since recurrence of the infection is common; long-term treatment presents no advantage and may select for antibiotic-resistant strains. Since the catheter may harbor bacteria, it usually is removed at the start of therapy.

The treatment of sexually transmitted diseases follows much the same pattern. Fortunately, most STDs can be treated or controlled. Both chlamydial infections and gonorrhea are generally treated with doxycycline, a derivative of tetracycline.

Perspective and Prospects

Urinary tract infections are notoriously difficult to prevent. Because in most cases the associated etiological agents are the normal intestinal flora, vaccination or prophylactic use of antibiotics would be impractical. Proper hygiene appears to be the most effective means of prevention among young adults.

STDs can be a source of urinary tract disease. Either a decrease in sexual promiscuity or more effective use of physical barriers (such as condoms) is necessary to reduce the level of such forms of infection. While vaccines against some of the more prevalent forms of STD (gonorrhea, chlamydia) remain a possibility, antibiotic therapy continues to be the most reliable means to treat urinary infections within the individual.

Catheters represent an important source of infection among the elderly, particularly those who are hospitalized. Since a single catheterization results in infection among less than 1 percent of patients, limiting catheterization, or avoiding it entirely, would appear to be the most effective preventive measure. The use of closed drainage systems has also reduced significantly the incidence of such infections. Antiseptic solutions and ointments have had limited success in the prevention of urinary tract infections. The use of antibiotic therapy has been effective in the short term, but over time such therapy may simply select for resistant mutants among the microorganisms. Development of catheters that do not lend themselves to microbial colonization, or that actively inhibit microbial growth (such as silver-impregnated catheters), may reduce the chances of such types of urinary tract infections.

—*Richard Adler, Ph.D.*

See also Abscess drainage; Abscesses; Adrenalectomy; Bed-wetting; Bladder cancer; Bladder removal; Candidiasis; Catheterization; Cystitis; Cystoscopy; Cysts; Dialysis; Diuretics; Endoscopy; Fistula repair; Genital disorders, female; Genital disorders, male; Hematuria; Hemolytic uremic syndrome; Hypertension; Incontinence; Internal medicine; Kidney cancer; Kidney disorders; Kidney transplantation; Kidneys; Laparoscopy; Lithotripsy; Nephrectomy; Nephritis; Nephrology; Nephrology, pediatric; Proteinuria; Pyelonephritis; Renal failure; Reye's syndrome; Sexually transmitted diseases (STDs); Stone removal; Stones; Ultrasonography; Urethritis; Urinalysis; Urinary system; Urology; Urology, pediatric; Women's health.

For Further Information:

Ammer, Christine. *The New A to Z of Women's Health: A Concise Encyclopedia*. 6th ed. New York: Checkmark Books, 2009.

Boston Women's Health Collective. *Our Bodies, Ourselves: A New Edition for a New Era*. 35th anniversary ed. New York: Simon & Schuster, 2005.

Gorbach, Sherwood L., John G. Bartlett, and Neil R. Blacklow, eds. *Infectious Diseases*. 3d ed. Philadelphia: W. B. Saunders, 2004.

Hooton, T.M. "Uncomplicated Urinary Tract Infection." *New England Journal of Medicine*. 366. (2012): 1028-1037.

Humes, H. David, et al., eds. *Kelley's Textbook of Internal Medicine*. 4th ed. Philadelphia: Lippincott Williams & Wilkins, 2000.

Parker, James N., and Philip M. Parker, eds. *The Official Patient's*

Sourcebook on Urinary Tract Infection. San Diego, Calif.: Icon Health, 2002.

Schrier, Robert W., ed. *Diseases of the Kidney and Urinary Tract.* 8th ed. Philadelphia: Wolters Kluwer Health/Lippincott Williams & Wilkins, 2007.

Stamm, W. E., and T. M. Hooton. "Current Concepts: Management of Urinary Tract Infections in Adults." *New England Journal of Medicine* 329. (1993): 1328-1334.

URINARY SYSTEM

Anatomy

Anatomy or system affected: Abdomen, bladder, kidneys

Specialties and related fields: Nephrology, urology

Definition: A system, composed of the kidneys, ureters, urinary bladder, and urethra, that removes body waste, maintains the proper amount of body water, and regulates the acid-base balance of the blood.

Key terms:

glomerular filtration: the first step in urine formation; passive filtration in which fluids and solids dissolved in the fluid (solutes) are forced through a membrane, resulting in the filtration of the blood

nephron: tiny blood-processing unit located in the kidneys that carries out the processes that form urine; each kidney contains approximately one million nephrons

tubular reabsorption: the process of returning important solutes that were filtered out of the blood back into the blood; these important solutes include glucose, amino acids, vitamins, and most ions

tubular secretion: the process of tubular reabsorption in reverse; important solutes moved from the filtrate to the urine include hydrogen and potassium ions, organic acids, ammonia, and creatine

ureters: slender, expandable tubes that carry urine from the kidney to the urinary bladder

urethra: a muscular tube that transports urine from the urinary bladder out of the body

urinary bladder: a stretchable, muscular sac that functions to store urine

Structure and Functions

The urinary system consists of two kidneys, two ureters, a urinary bladder, and a urethra. The kidneys function to remove metabolic waste from the blood, maintain proper water balance for the body, and maintain the proper acid-base balance in the blood. The ureters, urinary bladder, and urethra are involved in the moving of the urine formed in the kidneys to the external environment. The kidneys play the major role in the function of the urinary system.

Most people have two kidneys, located at the lower end of the rib cage and lying against the back of the body wall. Typically, the right kidney is positioned a little lower than the left kidney because the right kidney is pushed down by the liver. An adult kidney is about 12.5 centimeters long, 7.5 centimeters wide, and 2.5 centimeters thick and is shaped like a kidney bean. Each kidney is surrounded by a thick layer of fat, which is important for holding the kidneys in their normal body position.

Inside each kidney is a lighter outer region called the renal cortex. Deep in the cortex is a darker layer called the renal medulla. Within the cortex and medulla are found tiny structures called nephrons. Each kidney contains approximately one million nephrons, most of which are in the renal cortex. Nephrons are the functional units of the kidney, carrying out the processes involved in urine formation.

Each nephron consists of two main parts, the glomerulus and the renal tubule. The glomerulus is composed of a knot of capillaries that fit inside the Bowman's capsule, the cup-shaped head of the renal tubule. The rest of the renal tubule is about 2.5 centimeters long. The neck of the renal tubule undergoes a high degree of coiling and twisting just before it makes a hairpin loop. This part of the renal tubule is called the proximal convoluted tubule. The hairpin loop of the renal tubule is termed the loop of Henle. After coming out of this loop, the renal tubule again undergoes a high degree of coiling and twisting and is called the distal convoluted tubule. The distal convoluted tubule then enters another tube, the collecting duct. Surrounding and encasing the renal tubule is the peritubular capillary bed.

Urine formation occurs in the nephron and is the result of three processes: glomerular filtration, tubular reabsorption, and tubular secretion. The glomerulus acts as a filter. This process of glomerular filtration occurs as a result of the capillaries in the glomerulus being somewhat leaky as compared to other capillaries in the body. This process of filtration is a passive process that does not require any metabolic energy. High pressure in the glomerular capillaries causes the formation of a filtrate that consists primarily of blood, except that it lacks the red blood cells and blood proteins. (Both red blood cells and blood proteins are too large to pass through the leaky glomerular capillaries.) The filtrate contains the metabolic waste as well as the many useful substances found in the blood, including glucose, amino acids, vitamins, and water. This filtrate will be continually formed as long as the systemic blood pressure is normal.

The filtrate that is formed is caught in the Bowman's capsule of the renal tubule. From here, the filtrate will pass into the proximal convoluted tubule. Rather than losing the useful substances in the urine, the nephron works to put them back into the blood through the process of tubular reabsorption. Tubular reabsorption begins as soon as the filtrate enters the proximal convoluted tubule. Cells within the tubule take up needed substances from the filtrate and pass them out to the space between the proximal convoluted tubule and the surrounding peritubular capillaries. Once these useful substances are brought into this space, termed the extracellular space, they can be absorbed back into the blood contained within the peritubular capillaries. Some of this reabsorption is passive, not requiring any metabolic energy; water is an example of a substance that is reabsorbed passively. Most substances, however, depend on membrane transporters to carry them out to the extracellular space. These membrane transporters require metabolic energy in the form of adenosine triphosphate (ATP). There are a large number of membrane transporters for those substances that need to be reabsorbed, and few if any transporters for those substances that do not need to be transported. This imbalance helps to explain why substances such as glucose and amino acids are almost completely reabsorbed back into the blood while metabolic waste products such as urea and uric acid are not.

The process of tubular secretion occurs in the loop of Henle and is essentially opposite to that of tubular reabsorption, with substances taken from the blood and put back into the filtrate. Some substances that are secreted from the blood

and into the filtrate include hydrogen and potassium ions, ammonium ions, and certain drugs (for example, penicillin). It is the process of tubular secretion that allows the kidneys to remove toxins and drugs from the body, as well as to maintain the acid-base balance of the blood.

The regulation of the volume of urine secreted is controlled by the distal convoluted tubules and the collecting ducts to which they attach. After the filtrate has gone through the proximal convoluted tubules and the loop of Henle, it is fairly concentrated and therefore does not contain a large amount of water. The distal convoluted tubule and collecting duct are impermeable to water when a substance called vasopressin, or antidiuretic hormone (ADH), is present, in which case the filtrate will contain little water and the final urine volume will be small. If ADH is not present, the distal convoluted tubule and collecting ducts become permeable to water and, because the concentration of solutes is higher in the distal convoluted tubule and collecting duct, water enters into these two structures from the blood. The result is a dilution of the filtrate, with an increased water content and a large volume of urine. The role of ADH in determining urine volume can be seen with the ingestion of alcohol or coffee, both of which inhibit ADH release from the pituitary gland: The distal convoluted tubule and collecting duct become permeable to water, and the urine volume and the frequency of urination increase. It is by this mechanism that the kidneys regulate the body's water balance.

Once the urine is formed in the kidney, it will flow into a tube, the ureter. The ureters, one for each kidney, are passageways that carry urine from the kidney to the urinary bladder. Because the ureters run downward from the kidney, it might seem that the movement of urine to the urinary bladder is created by gravity. In reality, the ureters, which are stretchy and muscular tubes, contract at a rate of one to five times per minute to force the urine toward the bladder, a process termed peristalsis (the same type of contractions that move food through the digestive system). Where the ureters enter the urinary bladder, small, valvelike folds prevent the backflow of urine from the urinary bladder toward the kidneys.

The urinary bladder is a muscular, collapsible sac located in the pelvic cavity. When the bladder is empty, it is only 5.0 to 7.5 centimeters long and its walls are thrown into folds. As urine enters the bladder, it causes the organ to expand. A moderately full bladder is about 12.5 centimeters long and will contain approximately one-half of a liter of urine. A completely full bladder is capable of holding approximately 1 liter of fluid. The kidneys are continually forming urine. Thus, the bladder acts as a temporary storage unit for urine, allowing the individual to empty the bladder when it is convenient.

The urethra is a thin-walled tube that carries urine from the urinary bladder to the exterior of the body. Near where the urethra exits the urinary bladder is a band of smooth muscle that makes up the internal urethral sphincter. This sphincter, which is not under conscious control, acts to keep the urethra shut when urine is not being voided. A second sphincter, the external urethral sphincter, is found farther down the length of the urethra and is composed of skeletal muscle. This

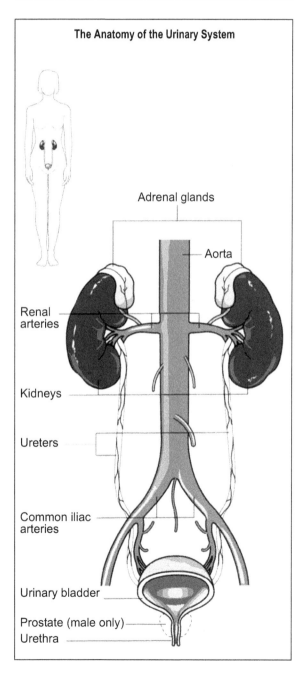

The Anatomy of the Urinary System

Adrenal glands

Aorta

Renal arteries

Kidneys

Ureters

Common iliac arteries

Urinary bladder

Prostate (male only)

Urethra

sphincter is under voluntary control: when it is not convenient to void the urine, this sphincter is used to prevent urination.

The urge to urinate is brought about by the stretching of the bladder. Ordinarily, the urge to urinate occurs when the bladder contains about 200 milliliters (almost 7 ounces) of urine. This amount of urine causes a stretching of the bladder that sends impulses to the spinal cord initiating the contraction of the urinary bladder. The contractions of the urinary bladder force urine past the internal urethral sphincter. At this time, a person will feel the need to void the urine, a process termed urination or micturition.

Disorders and Diseases

Renal and urinary disorders can be categorized based on their mechanism of action and the portion of the urinary system that they affect. These disorders include obstructive disorders that interfere with normal urine flow anywhere within the urinary tract, urinary tract infections, and glomerular disorders, which affect the glomeruli in the kidneys.

Obstructive disorders of the urinary system can be caused by many different factors. Obstruction of the passage of the urine will usually cause a backing up of the urine into the kidney or kidneys. The result is a swelling of the kidney termed hydronephrosis.

Perhaps the most common obstruction is caused by kidney stones, also referred to as renal calculi. Kidney stones consist of crystallized minerals such as calcium, magnesium, or uric acid salts that form hard stones in the distal end of the collecting ducts. If the stones are small, they will pass through the remainder of the urinary tract. Larger stones, however, get caught in the ureters, thus blocking the passage of urine from the kidneys to the urinary bladder. This blockage usually results in intense pain as the ureters rhythmically contract in an effort to dislodge the stone; this condition is sometimes referred to as renal colic. If the stone does not move from its position of blockage, a buildup of urine in the kidney may occur; if this continues, damage may be done to the kidneys.

Damage to the nerves that innervate the bladder, termed neurogenic bladder, can also result in an obstructive disorder. Damage to these nerves results in the loss of normal control over the voiding of urine from the bladder. Consequently, there is a retention of urine in the bladder since there is no signal telling the bladder to contract.

Tumors of the urinary system may also cause obstruction of urine flow. Another cause of obstruction is the loss of the fat surrounding the kidney. When this occurs, one or both kidneys may drop from their normal position, a condition referred to as renal ptosis. When the kidneys drop, there is a chance that the ureters exiting the kidney may become kinked and prevent the normal flow of urine from the kidneys to the urinary bladder.

Urinary tract infections are usually caused by bacteria and can involve the urethra, ureters, urinary bladder, kidneys, or all the above. Urinary infections in the urethra are termed urethritis and result in the inflammation of the urethra. The two most common bacterial infections involved in urethritis are

gonorrhea and chlamydia. Males are more likely than females to have urethritis.

Cystitis refers to any inflammation of the urinary bladder. This condition usually results from bacterial infections, but it may also be caused by tumors or by the presence of stones in the bladder. Cystitis occurs more frequently in women than in men and is characterized by pelvic pain, a frequent urge to urinate, and possibly blood in the urine.

Nephritis is a general term used to describe inflammatory kidney diseases. The inflammation of the nephrons within the kidney is referred to as pyelonephritis. Pyelonephritis is often attributable to bacterial infection but may also be caused by viral infections, tumors, kidney stones, or pregnancy.

Glomerulonephritis is a term that refers to any type of glomerular disorder. It can be further subdivided into two categories: acute glomerulonephritis and chronic glomerulonephritis. Acute glomerulonephritis is the most common form and may be caused by bacterial infection. Chronic glomerulonephritis refers to noninfectious kidney disorders. It commonly occurs when the immune system reacts to and destroys the body's own glomeruli. This type of glomerulonephritis eventually leads to kidney failure. Acute glomerulonephritis, if it is left untreated or it does not respond to treatment, can become chronic glomerulonephritis.

Renal (kidney) failure is simply the inability of the kidneys to form urine. Renal failure can be classified as either acute or chronic. Acute renal failure is the abrupt loss of kidney function, which may result from excessive loss of blood, severe burns, pyelonephritis, glomerulonephritis, or infection or obstruction of the urinary tract. Chronic renal failure is the slow destruction of the nephrons in the kidney. This form of renal failure may result from infections, glomerulonephritis, tumors, obstructive disorders, or autoimmune diseases. Unless the progression of nephron loss is stopped, chronic renal failure will eventually lead to death.

Diabetes insipidus is a disease that does not directly attack the urinary system, but it has a profound effect on the urinary system through its influence on the pituitary gland and the hypothalamus. With diabetes insipidus, the pituitary gland fails to release antidiuretic hormone, as a result of an injury or tumor of the posterior portion of the pituitary gland or hypothalamus. Because of the decreased amount of antidiuretic hormone, large amounts of urine, and thus water, are flushed from the body daily. If left untreated, diabetes insipidus can lead to dehydration and electrolyte imbalances. To offset the loss of water in the urine, individuals with diabetes insipidus must drink large amounts of water.

Perspective and Prospects

The complexity of the human kidney can be seen in science's inability to build an artificial kidney that is continuously functional and can be inserted into the body in place of the normal kidney. Until the development of tubing that contained miniature holes (dialysis tubing), kidney failure nearly always resulted in death. Dialysis tubing allowed the development of renal dialysis, which cleanses the blood of toxic substances and helps to regulate electrolyte balance. The process of renal dialysis is carried out using a thin membrane that is permeable to only a few select substances. The tubing is immersed in a bathing solution that is very similar to normal blood plasma. As blood circulates through the tubing, toxic substances and someelectrolytes move out of the blood and into the bathing solution. This dialysis tubing and the bathing solution are often referred to as an artificial kidney. Dialysis is usually done three times a week, with each session requiring about four to eight hours. Although effective, dialysis is a far cry from the functioning of the human kidney and is no cure for chronic renal failure. When the kidneys are no longer functioning, the only hope is a kidney transplant.

Because the kidneys are so effective at filtering unneeded substances out of the blood, the urine formed by the kidney is the principal fluid used for drug testing and drug screening. Furthermore, the kidney also secretes some white blood cells into the urine. As techniques continue to develop, it will be possible to perform genetic tests on these white blood cells to determine genetic traits such as sex and the color of hair and eyes, as well as the possibility of the presence of genetic diseases or personality traits. Such technology could have considerable impact on the future of individual privacy, as many companies and employers require a mandatory analysis of urine, primarily for the presence of drugs in the urine, prior to the possibility of employment. Thus, with a simple urine sample, the company could know not only the possible drug use of prospective employees but also their genetic makeup.

—*David K. Saunders, Ph.D.*

See also Abdomen; Abdominal disorders; Abscess drainage; Abscesses; Adrenalectomy; Bed-wetting; Bladder cancer; Bladder removal; Candidiasis; Catheterization; Circumcision, male; Cystitis; Cystoscopy; Cysts; Dialysis; Diuretics; *E. coli* infection; Endoscopy; Fistula repair; Fluids and electrolytes; Geriatrics and gerontology; Hematuria; Hemolytic uremic syndrome; Host-defense mechanisms; Hypertension; Incontinence; Internal medicine; Kidney cancer; Kidney disorders; Kidney transplantation; Kidneys; Laparoscopy; Lithotripsy; Nephrectomy; Nephritis; Nephrology; Nephrology, pediatric; Pediatrics; Penile implant surgery; Proteinuria; Pyelonephritis; Renal failure; Reye's syndrome; Schistosomiasis; Stone removal; Stones; Systems and organs; Transplantation; Ultrasonography; Uremia; Urethritis; Urinalysis; Urinary disorders; Urology; Urology, pediatric.

For Further Information:

Greenberg, Arthur, et al., eds. *Primer on Kidney Diseases*. 5th ed. Philadelphia: Saunders/Elsevier, 2009.

Guyton, Arthur C., and John E. Hall. *Guyton and Hall Textbook of Medical Physiology*. 12th ed. Philadelphia: Saunders/Elsevier, 2011.

Marieb, Elaine N. *Essentials of Human Anatomy and Physiology*. 10th ed. San Francisco: Pearson/Benjamin Cummings, 2012.

Marieb, Elaine N., and Katja Hoehn. *Human Anatomy and Physiology*. 9th ed. San Francisco: Pearson/Benjamin Cummings, 2010.

O'Callaghan, C. A., and Barry Brenner. *The Kidney at a Glance*. Malden, Mass.: Blackwell Science, 2000.

Patt, Gail R. *Carola Human Anatomy and Physiology*. 3d ed. New York: McGraw-Hill, 1995.

Thibodeau, Gary A., and Kevin T. Patton. *Anatomy and Physiology*. 8th ed. St. Louis, Mo.: Mosby/Elsevier, 2013.

"Your Urinary System and How It Works." *National Kidney and Urologic Diseases Information Clearinghouse*, June 29, 2012.

UROLOGY

Specialty

Anatomy or system affected: Abdomen, bladder, genitals, kidneys, reproductive system, urinary system

Specialties and related fields: Family medicine, gynecology, microbiology, nephrology, obstetrics, proctology

Definition: The branch of medicine that deals with the physiology and disorders of the urinary system (kidneys, ureters, bladder, and urethra) and the male genital tract.

Key terms:

-otomy: combining form meaning an opening or incision in an organ or structure; for example, a ureterotomy is an opening in the ureter

ureter: either of the two tubes that carry urine from the kidneys to the bladder

urethra: the tube that carries urine from the bladder, voiding the liquid from the body

-uria: combining form meaning the presence of a substance in urine; for example, hematuria refers to blood in the urine

urinalysis: the physical, chemical, and microscopic analysis of urine

urinary system assessment: the evaluation of the complete urinary tract, including kidneys, bladder, ureters, and urethra; also includes an analysis of the patient's personal medical history

urine: fluid collected in the kidneys that contains metabolic wastes, including urea and salts

urogram: the injection of a radiopaque substance, followed by X rays of the urinary tract as the substance passes through it

Science and Profession

The urinary system is a complex series of structures that includes the kidneys, ureters, urinary bladder, and urethra. Since in males the urinary tract is closely associated with the genital tract, urology properly deals with disorders of the male genitourinary tract and the female urinary tract. Urologists may also study disorders of the adrenal glands, which are closely associated with the kidneys.

Urine production begins in the kidneys, a pair of bean-shaped organs found within the abdomen. Urine is produced through a complex system of units called nephrons; approximately one million nephrons are found within each kidney. Each nephron consists of a ball-shaped capillary network called the glomerulus, which is surrounded by a capsule (Bowman's capsule) through which the actual filtration of blood takes place. Blood enters the glomerulus under high pressure, forcing the liquid and dissolved material through the basement membrane into the renal tubules that extend from the capsule.

The long, convoluted tubule that extends from each capsule follows a circuitous route through the kidney. As it emerges from the capsule, the proximal convoluted tubule is found within the outer region, or cortex, of the kidney. The tubule then passes through the inner portion, or medulla, of the kidney, forming an extended loop called the loop of Henle.

The tubule winds its way back to the cortical region as the distal convoluted tubule. Blood circulates completely through the kidneys about twenty times each hour. Approximately 20 percent of the plasma (liquid portion of the blood) is filtered through the Bowman's capsules during this time, the equivalent of some 180 liters of fluid per day. Much of the plasma and nearly all the nutrient material found within the liquid that passes through the tubules are reabsorbed into the capillary network surrounding the tubules. Approximately 80 percent is absorbed within the proximal convoluted tubule, with the remainder being absorbed as it flows through the tubule system. The rest of the fluid, approximately one liter per day for the average person, contains nitrogenous material such as urea, salts, and other metabolic wastes, which are voided.

The distal tubules emerge from the cortex of the kidney and again pass into the medulla, where they now merge into increasingly larger collecting ducts. The collecting ducts form clearly visible pyramids, or papillae, within the medulla. The merging of the largest ducts within the renal pelvis, the lowest portion of the kidney, results in the formation of a single tube, the ureter. One ureter emerges from each kidney to empty the urine into the bladder.

The ureters are thick-walled tubes that extend through the pelvic region. They enter the bladder in a slanted manner, which helps prevent backup of the urine from the bladder when it is full. Urine is pumped through the ureters by means of peristaltic, or rhythmic, contraction of the smooth muscle that lines the ureters.

The urinary bladder is a membranous organ in the pelvis that serves to store and discharge urine. The average individual's bladder is capable of holding approximately one-third to one-half of a liter of liquid. When full, it can cause the lower abdomen to bulge visibly. Since the structure is adjacent to the uterus in women, conditions such as pregnancy may significantly lower the carrying capacity of the bladder.

The musculature in the lower portion of the bladder is thickened, forming the bladder neck, and serves to retain the liquid within the organ. The muscle, in turn, is continuous with that of the urethra, the tubular structure that drains the urine from the bladder.

In women, the urethra is three to four centimeters in length and emerges just in front of the vagina. In men, the tube is approximately twenty centimeters long. Emerging from the bladder in the male, it passes through the prostate gland and into the penis, where it serves as a passage both for the elimination of urine and for semen during ejaculation.

Since urine formation begins in the kidney, urology may overlap with nephrology at times. Strictly speaking, however, nephrology deals with the kidney as a regulatory organ for fluid and salt levels in the body, in addition to its role as an endocrine gland; urology deals with disorders of the urinary tract, in addition to problems associated with the genitourinary tract in males, since the two systems are so closely associated.

Approximately 20 percent of adult visits to a physician involve problems associated with the genitourinary tract. Urinalysis—the physical, chemical, and microscopic evaluation of collected urine—thus becomes an important diagnostic tool. The process begins with proper collection of urine in a sterile specimen container. The sample initially undergoes a macroscopic examination in which color and appearance are evaluated. Since recent ingestion of food may result in the discoloration of urine or alteration in its pH, it is best to obtain the sample several hours after the patient has eaten. Generally, the odor is unimportant; for example, by-products of asparagus ingestion may produce a rather characteristic odor in urine that is of no medical significance. Nevertheless, a pungent aroma may signify an infection. Metabolic diseases may also lead to by-products that have characteristic smells.

Macroscopic examination of urine also involves a determination of the specific gravity, or density, of the solution and its pH. Densities outside the normal density range for urine may be indicative of diabetes mellitus or renal dysfunction. The pH is a measurement of hydrogen ion concentration in the fluid. A pH of 7.0 is neutral. Normal levels in urine vary considerably, from an acid level of 4.6 to an alkaline pH of 8.0. Generally, urine samples obtained soon after a meal will be slightly alkaline, but a consistently alkaline level may be indicative of a urinary tract infection. Other macromolecules that may be observed in urine as a result of various pathologies include elevated levels of protein or sugar and the presence of blood (hematuria).

Microscopic analysis of urine is a necessary part of a thorough urinalysis. The urine sample is centrifuged, or spun at high speed, to concentrate material in a smaller volume. The pellet from the centrifugation is then stained and observed for bacteria or blood cells. Normally, the number of bacteria and white blood cells in urine is low, and some bacterial contamination of the specimen during collection is common. Large numbers of either may be indicative of an infection. The presence of red blood cells in urine is always considered abnormal and may signify inflammation or bleeding within the urinary system.

Diagnostic and Treatment Techniques

A thorough urinary system assessment involving the examination of the kidneys, ureters, bladder, and urethra may be necessary for an accurate diagnosis of certain pathologies. In addition to the normal urinalysis, including the use of a catheter for obtaining a urine sample, the study includes the patient's medical history and vital signs. The diagnosis of urinary problems may include procedures for obtaining images of the urinary tract, such as x-rays of the kidneys or urinary tract, as well as excretory or intravenous urography. The latter involves the injection of a radiopaque solution into the system, followed by x-ray analysis as the solution passes through the tract. Direct observation through cystoscopy may also be carried out. Other methodologies developed during the 1980s includes computed tomography (CT) scanning and magnetic resonance imaging (MRI).

Depending on the problem, treatment may be as simple as prescribing antibiotics. Urologic surgery becomes necessary if diagnostic procedures reveal a tumor or obstruction. Such circumstances may require surgical removal, reconstruction, or relocation. For example, damage to the urinary system as a result of neurologic or neoplastic (cancerous) conditions may require the diversion of urine through an opening in the abdomen, a ureteroileostomy, instead of through normal channels.

Pathologic conditions of the urinary tract may take a variety of forms, such as an obstruction that interferes with urinary flow or an infection by any of a wide array of bacteria. Either condition may lead to inflammation and subsequent urinary problems. Damage may also result from external forces, such as injuries caused by falling or blunt force.

Urinary obstructions are generally classified on the basis of several characteristics: the etiology or source of the obstruction, the length of time over which the obstruction takes place (acute or chronic), and the site of the obstruction. The source of the obstruction may be congenital, often resulting from a stenosis, or narrowing, of the meatus (opening or tunnel) within the urethra. An additional congenital abnormality may result from the inability of the ureterovesical junction, the site at which the ureters enter the bladder, to prevent urine reflux, or backflow, into the ureter. The result of any such obstruction is frequently pyelonephritis, an infection within the urinary system. Since any infection may ascend to the kidney, damage can occur at any site in the urinary tract.

Obstructions may result from injury to the urinary tract, from benign or malignant tumors, or from the formation of stones. In women, extension of the uterus during pregnancy may impinge on the ureters, interfering with normal flow. The obstructions may develop anywhere along the urinary tract. An obstruction in the lower urinary tract (the region along the urethra) may cause ballooning or dilation of the urethra; in men, this dilation may extend into the prostate gland. The weakening of the urethral wall may result in the formation of diverticula, pouchlike herniations in the muscle wall. If the region becomes infected, a likely possibility, the increased hydrostatic pressure coupled with the weakening of the wall may cause the urethra to rupture.

Midtract obstructions are associated with the bladder. To compensate for increased resistance to urine flow, the muscle of the bladder may initially thicken, sometimes increasing in thickness by a factor of two or three. The increased size of the musculature of the bladder may in turn actually decrease the urine flow from the ureter as a result of the downward pull on these tubes. The resulting backflow may cause damage to the ureters or kidneys.

The increased pressure within the bladder may also force the tissue, or mucosa, between bundles of musculature, resulting in pockets called cellules. Continued pressure may result in larger pockets, or diverticula, being formed within the bladder wall. Since these regions tend to retain urine, infections are common, and surgery may be necessary to remove the diverticula.

Obstructions of the upper urinary tract are associated with the ureters and kidneys. Increased pressure from backflow may cause dilation of the ureter wall, with an increase in muscle development as compensation. This stage is generally followed by one of decompensation, in which the ureters lose their ability to contract and maintain urine flow. Likewise, the kidneys may be subjected to increased pressure. Normally, the pressure on the kidneys from within the urinary tract is very low. When the pressure is increased on the kidney pelvis, the regions in which the collecting ducts form, the pelvis becomes subject to pressure, which ultimately has an impact on blood flow. The result is ischemia, or lack of oxygen to the region. The kidney itself may atrophy, followed by renal failure.

Generally, obstructions can be visualized through a variety of procedures. Tumors or calcified stones within the tract will show on x-rays. An excretory urogram, a technique in which the urinary tract is x-rayed following injection of a radiopaque substance, may reveal the precise site of the obstruction. The urogram is preferred for observation of certain forms of urinary tract stones that may not appear on conventional x-rays. It can also be used to observe sites of both dilation and stenosis.

Depending on the source of obstruction, urologic surgery may become necessary for its removal. If kidney function is significantly reduced, temporary or permanent dialysis or even transplantation may be necessary. However, temporary urinary diversion may provide relief to the system, allowing natural healing to repair dilated tubes once the obstruction has been removed. Ureteroileostomy, in which a portion of the ureter is diverted through an opening, or stoma, in the intestine, has been used under such circumstances.

Urinary stones remain the most common cause of obstructions. The formation of stones is related to a variety of factors, including the diet and metabolic state of the patient, genetics, and the anatomic features of the urinary tract. The result is increased deposition of salts such as calcium around an initial foreign body in the urine. Eventual crystallization leads to steady increases in the size of the stone and, unless it is passed naturally within the urine, eventual obstruction. Stones may form anywhere in the tract, but they tend to be less common in the urethra. In general, stones are crystals of either calcium salts or, less often, uric acid.

A variety of techniques exists for the elimination of urinary stones. Stone dissolution, including lithotripsy (the breaking up of the stone with a surgical instrument or shock waves), is preferred, since it requires minimal invasiveness and hospitalization. Hemiacidrin, a magnesium-containing solution, has been used successfully in dissolving certain stones. Ultrasonographic lithotripsy, which uses ultrasonic vibrations to dissolve the stone, has also proved successful. Some stones, however, particularly those composed of calcium, may not respond adequately to these forms of treatment. If the obstruction is significant, and particularly if an infection is present, surgical removal may become necessary.

Infections of the urinary tract may be primary (a direct result of contamination) or secondary (the result of other pathological conditions, such as obstructions). Infections may be confined to a single site or may spread to other organs or areas. Since the clinical signs of infection may resemble those of other conditions, recognition of the microbial cause is necessary for proper treatment. Infections that spread to the kidneys may cause significant damage or organ failure.

Infections are categorized as being either specific or nonspecific. Specific infections are those in which a disease is manifested as a result of a particular agent. For example, sexually transmitted diseases (STDs) are specific in the sense that gonorrhea is caused only by *Neisseria gonorrhoeae* and urinary tuberculosis by *Mycobacterium tuberculosis*. Nonspecific infections are diseases in which the pathology or manifestation may be similar but the symptoms may be caused by any of a variety of bacteria. For example, common causes of nonspecific urinary infection include *Escherichia coli* (*E. coli*) and members of the genera *Proteus* and *Staphylococcus*.

The most common cause of urinary tract infections is *E. coli*, a natural colon bacillus. Secondary problems may also result from specific agents. For example, members of the genus *Proteus* produce urease, an enzyme capable of splitting urea to form ammonia. The result is a rise in pH, an alkaline condition that may cause precipitation of magnesium or calcium salts and subsequent stone formation.

The specific physical manifestation of the infection is generally related to the site within the urinary tract. Urethritis, accompanied by reduced or painful urination, often results from STDs. Infection may spread as far up as the kidney, with resulting pyelonephritis. Both *E. coli* and STDs are common causes, though other bacteria may also cause similar types of infections. Proper diagnosis of bacterial infections generally requires the isolation and identification of the organism, if possible, and the ruling out of other possible causes of the symptoms, such as diabetes. The agent may be isolated from pus, from urine, or through the insertion of a needle into the lesion itself. Treatment usually involves antimicrobials (antibiotics) suited to the particular etiological agent. Abscesses, particularly those in the kidney, may require surgical drainage. If the abscess is too large or does not respond to treatment, then nephrectomy (the surgical removal of a kidney) may be necessary.

Damage from external sources may also result in injury to the urinary tract. Depending on the damage, surgical repair or realignment of the urethra, bladder, or ureters may be necessary. Observations via x-rays, cystograms, or urethrograms are routinely used for such assessment.

Perspective and Prospects

The understanding of urine formation and excretion has its roots in the work of the Roman physician Galen during the second century CE. Though observations had been carried out before this period, it remained unclear whether the source of urine was the kidney or the bladder. Galen settled the issue by tying off the ureters in animals, demonstrating that no urine would be found below the stricture, and thus urine formation began in the kidney.

Urology as a branch of medicine, and indeed clinical interest in urine formation, arguably began in the early decades of the nineteenth century. In 1827, English physician Richard Bright described a form of chronic nephritis, which became known as Bright's disease, in which progressive kidney failure generally resulted in the death of the individual. Bright demonstrated that as a result of kidney failure, instead of urine being secreted from the body, its constituents are retained in body fluids. It was also in 1827 that German chemist Friedrich Wöhler chemically synthesized urea, the first demonstration of the synthesis of an organic compound from inorganic materials.

Beginning in 1844, Carl Ludwig attempted to explain urine formation on the basis of a purely physical process. He suggested the hydrostatic pressure of the blood is sufficiently high that a protein-free filtrate is forced through the kidney glomeruli, followed by passage through the tubules, and ultimately into the ureters. The first definitive work on urine secretion was Arthur Robertson Cushny's 1917 monograph *The Secretion of Urine*. Cushny believed that urine secretion involves both an active and a passive process: mechanical filtration and movement through the urinary tract, and active tubular reabsorption of most nutrients before the liquid leaves the kidney. He was subsequently proved to be essentially correct in this belief, though Cushny's mechanics of reabsorption were less than accurate and were later refined by others.

The development of noninvasive techniques for the elimination of stones and improved surgical methods for urinary diversion marked much of the progress in urology in the 1970s and 1980s. Extracorporeal shock-wave lithotripsy (ESWL), the use of ultrasonic vibration for the disintegration of stones, eliminated the need for the surgical removal of these obstructions in most cases. The use of ureterosigmoidostomy (implantation of the ureter into the intestinal tract) dates to the nineteenth century. It was replaced with alternate methods of bladder augmentation. The ureter itself could be replaced with segments of intestinal ileum, or it could be joined to the other ureter (ureteroureterostomy).

—*Richard Adler, Ph.D.*

See also Abdomen; Bed-wetting; Bladder cancer; Bladder removal; Catheterization; Chlamydia; Circumcision, male; Cystitis; Cystoscopy; Dialysis; Diuretics; *E. coli* infection; Endoscopy; Fluids and electrolytes; Gender reassignment surgery; Genital disorders, female; Genital disorders, male; Geriatrics and gerontology; Gonorrhea; Hematuria; Hemolytic uremic syndrome; Human papillomavirus (HPV); Hydroceles; Hypospadias repair and urethroplasty; Incontinence; Infertility, male; Kidney cancer; Kidney disorders; Kidney transplantation; Kidneys; Laser use in surgery; Lithotripsy; Nephrectomy; Nephritis; Nephrology; Nephrology, pediatric; Pediatrics; Pelvic inflammatory disease (PID); Penile implant surgery; Prostate cancer; Prostate gland; Prostate gland removal; Proteinuria; Pyelonephritis; Reproductive system; Schistosomiasis; Sexual differentiation; Sexual dysfunction; Sexually transmitted diseases (STDs); Sterilization; Stone removal; Stones; Syphilis; Testicular surgery; Transplantation; Ultrasonography; Uremia; Urethritis; Urinalysis; Urinary disorders; Urinary system; Urology, pediatric; Vasectomy; Warts.

For Further Information:

Albala, David M., et al. *Oxford American Handbook of Urology*. New York: Oxford University Press, 2011.
Chisholm, Geoffrey D., and William R. Fair, eds. *Scientific Foundations of Urology*. 3d ed. Chicago: Year Book Medical, 1990.
Gillenwater, Jay Y., et al., eds. *Adult and Pediatric Urology*. 4th ed. Baltimore: Lippincott Williams & Wilkins, 2002.
McAninch, Jack W., and Tom F. Lue, eds. *Smith and Tanagho's General Urology*. 18th ed. New York: McGraw-Hill, 2013.
Reynard, John, Simon Brewster, and Suzanne Biers. *Oxford Handbook of Urology*. 3d ed. Oxford: Oxford University Press, 2013.

Stamm, W. E., and T. M. Hooton. "Current Concepts: Management of Urinary Tract Infections in Adults." *New England Journal of Medicine* 329 (October 28, 1993): 1328–1334.

Tomasini, J. M., and B. R. Konety. "Urinary Markers/Cytology: What and When Should a Urologist Use." *Urologic Clinics of North America* 40, no. 2 (May 2013): 165–173.

Wagenlehner, F. M., et al. "Prevention of Recurrent Urinary Tract Infections." *Minerva urologica e nefrologica* 65, no. 1 (March 2013): 9–20.

Wallace, Robert A., Gerald P. Sanders, and Robert J. Ferl. *Biology: The Science of Life*. 4th ed. New York: HarperCollins, 1996.

Wan, J. "Adolescent Urology Update." *Adolescent Medicine: State of the Art Reviews* 24, no. 1 (April 2013): 273–294.

Wein, Alan J., et al., eds. *Campbell-Walsh Urology*. 10th ed. 4 vols. Philadelphia: Saunders/Elsevier, 2012.

UTERINE CANCER. *See* CERVICAL, OVARIAN, AND UTERINE CANCERS.

UTERUS
Anatomy
Also known as: Womb

Anatomy or system affected: Genitals, reproductive system

Specialties and related fields: Embryology, gynecology, obstetrics, oncology, perinatology

Definition: The organ, located in the pelvis of the female, in which a fetus develops after conception.

Structure and Functions

The uterus provides a space for a fetus to grow. Situated in the pelvis, in front of the rectum and behind the bladder, the uterus is a bulb-shaped pouch about 3 inches (8 centimeters) in length that has heavily muscled walls and is held firmly in place by several ligaments. The uterus has two main parts: the body (corpus) includes the area above the opening to the two Fallopian tubes, while the fundus is the larger area below the Fallopian tubes to the cervix, all positioned at about a ninety-degree angle to the vagina; the cervix is a funnel that connects the body to the vagina. During a woman's reproductive years, the body is about double the size of the cervix, but that proportion reverses after menopause. The thick muscle (myometrium) of the uterus is lined with mucous membrane, the endometrium.

During ovulation, sperm can enter the body through the cervix on its way to fertilize an egg in a Fallopian tube. During menstruation, blood and excess endometrium exit the uterus through the cervix. During gestation, the uterus expands to accommodate the growth of the fetus, and during labor the walls contract to impel the fetus through the cervix and vagina.

Disorders and Diseases

Among common disorders specific to the uterus are various noncancerous growths. Fibroids are masses of muscle and fibrous tissue, of unknown cause, in the uterine wall that occur in about 20 percent of women more than thirty-five years old. If small, they are seldom noticed, but large fibroids can affect urination and menstruation and cause pain. Adenomyosis involves enlargement of the uterus after glandular tissue obtrudes into the myometrium; it can result in heavy, painful periods, sensations of pressure, and bleeding between periods. Endometriosis occurs when bits of the endometrium grow outside the uterus, which may produce pain in the lower abdomen or pelvis. The uterus is also subject to abnormal bleeding and vaginitis, inflammation caused by chemical irritants, bacteria, or yeast (candidiasis). Sometimes, because of pregnancy or birth, the uterus sags and protrudes into the vagina, a condition known as prolapsed uterus.

Two cancers in the uterus are among the most common to afflict women. Endometrial cancer grows in the membrane lining the body. It usually develops between the ages of fifty and sixty and has a high cure rate if detected early. Cervical cancer usually develops between the ages of thirty-five and fifty-five, following infection by the human papillomavirus, and is also curable if detected early. Untreated, both penetrate the uterine wall and spread to nearby organs.

—*Roger Smith, Ph.D.*

See also Abortion; Amenorrhea; Amniocentesis; Assisted reproductive technologies; Cervical, ovarian, and uterine cancers; Cervical procedures; Cesarean section; Childbirth; Childbirth complications; Conception; Culdocentesis; Dysmenorrhea; Ectopic pregnancy; Endometrial biopsy; Endometriosis; Gamete intrafallopian transfer (GIFT); Genital disorders, female; Gynecology; Hysterectomy; In vitro fertilization; Infertility, female; Menopause; Menorrhagia; Menstruation; Miscarriage; Multiple births; Obstetrics; Pap test; Pelvic inflammatory disease (PID); Pregnancy and gestation; Premature birth; Premenstrual syndrome (PMS); Puberty and adolescence; Sexual differentiation; Sexually transmitted diseases (STDs); Sterilization; Stillbirth; Systems and organs; Tubal ligation; Ultrasonography; Women's health.

For Further Information:

Beers, Mark H., ed. *The Merck Manual of Medical Information*. 2d ed. Whitehouse Station, N.J.: Merck Research Laboratories, 2003.

Fortner, Kimberley B., ed. *The Johns Hopkins Manual of Gynecology and Obstetrics*. Philadelphia: Lippincott Williams & Wilkins, 2007.

Parker, Steve. *The Human Body Book*. New York: DK Adult, 2001.

Thibodeau, Gary A., and Kevin T. Patton. *Structure and Function of the Body*. 14th ed. St. Louis: Mosby/Elsevier, 2012.

"Uterine Diseases." *MedlinePlus*, May 28, 2013.

VACCINATION. *See* **IMMUNIZATION AND VACCINATION.**

VAGOTOMY
Procedure
Anatomy or system affected: Gastrointestinal system, nerves, nervous system, stomach
Specialties and related fields: Gastroenterology, general surgery, neurology, nutrition
Definition: The surgical cutting of the vagus nerve or nerves as part of the treatment for gastric ulcers.

Indications and Procedures

The vagus nerves, the longest nerves in the body, pass from the head through the neck, chest, and abdominal regions. They regulate such processes as speech, coughing, swallowing, heart rate, and the hunger sensation. Branches of the vagus nerve also stimulate gastric acid secretions and gastric movements.

Vagotomy is generally carried out in conjunction with treatments for gastric (stomach) and duodenal (intestinal) ulcers. Such peptic ulcers are characterized by the loss of mucous membranes in regions exposed to such stomach secretions as hydrochloric acid and the digestive enzyme pepsin. Mild ulcers may heal on their own, but chronic ulceration may result in significant damage or scarring to the stomach or intestinal wall. In addition to the pain and discomfort associated with an ulcer, under some circumstances the ulcer may become cancerous. While the formation of peptic ulcers is poorly understood, it is known that acid secretion by the stomach can aggravate the condition.

Since the vagus nerve serves to stimulate acid secretions by the parietal cells of the stomach, cutting of the nerve is an effective way to reduce such secretions. Since cutting of the vagus nerve will also reduce or eliminate peristalsis, the

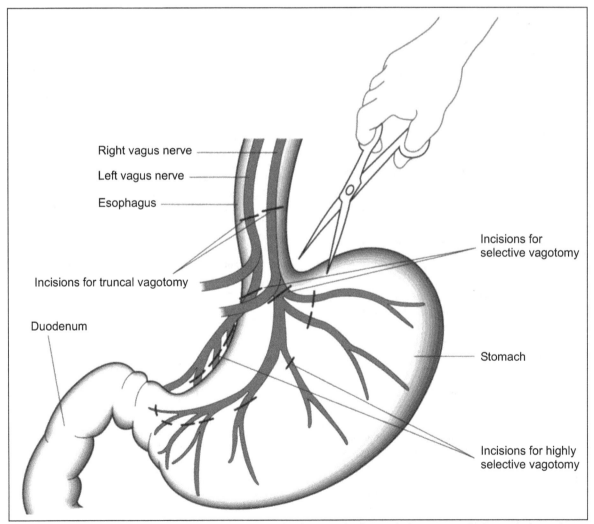

Right vagus nerve
Left vagus nerve
Esophagus
Incisions for truncal vagotomy
Duodenum
Incisions for selective vagotomy
Stomach
Incisions for highly selective vagotomy

Vagotomy, the severing of the vagus nerve, is a radical treatment for chronic acid reflux, in which gastric juice backs up into the esophagus.

rhythmic contraction of muscle that forces food through the stomach, additional procedures are often carried out in combination with vagotomy. For example, an artificial opening between the stomach and small intestine may be created (gastroenterostomy) in order to allow the food to move directly from the stomach to the intestine without the necessity of stomach peristalsis.

The specific region of the vagus nerve on which the vagotomy will be carried out depends on the site of the ulcer. For example, in the case of a duodenal ulcer, the most common form of ulcer, the branch innervating the parietal area of the stomach is severed, reducing the amount of acid produced by the cells in that outer portion of the stomach. Recovery is similar to that for any other general surgical procedure. Medication is provided for pain, and food is reintroduced gradually.

—*Richard Adler, Ph.D.*

See also Acid reflux disease; Digestion; Enzymes; Gastroenterology; Gastrointestinal disorders; Gastrointestinal system; Nervous system; Neurology; Peristalsis; Sympathectomy; Ulcer surgery; Ulcers; Vagus nerve.

For Further Information:

Abrahams, Peter H., Sandy C. Marks, Jr., and Ralph Hutchings. *McMinn's Color Atlas of Human Anatomy.* 6th ed. St. Louis, Mo.: Mosby/Elsevier, 2008.

Baron, J. H., et al., eds. *Vagotomy in Modern Surgical Practice.* Boston: Butterworths, 1982.

Margolis, Simeon, and Sergey Kantsevoy. *Johns Hopkins White Papers 2002: Digestive Disorders.* New York: Rebus, 2002.

Monroe, Judy. *Coping with Ulcers, Heartburn, and Stress-Related Stomach Disorders.* New York: Rosen, 2000.

Tortora, Gerard J., and Bryan Derrickson. *Principles of Anatomy and Physiology.* 13th ed. Hoboken, N.J.: John Wiley & Sons, 2012.

Zollinger, Robert M., Jr., Robert M. Zollinger, Sr., et al. *Zollinger's Atlas of Surgical Operations.* 9th ed. New York: McGraw-Hill, 2011.

VAGUS NERVE
Anatomy

Also known as: Tenth cranial nerve

Anatomy or system affected: Brain, neck, tongue

Specialties and related fields: Gastroenterology, neurology

Definition: The tenth cranial nerve, which starts in the brain stem within the medulla oblongata and sends sensory information about the function or state of the body parts to the central nervous system.

Structure and Function

The vagus nerve is actually two nerves that run from the brain stem and exit from the skull at its base through the jugular foramen and descend the neck through the carotid sheath between the internal carotid artery and the internal jugular vein. The vagus nerve passes not only through the neck and head but also through the chest and abdomen, where it contributes to the innervation of the viscera. The superior laryngeal nerve is the first branch that travels with the superior thyroid artery, whereby this nerve innervates the cricothyroid muscle

through its external branch, thus supplying sensation to the supraglottic larynx. The facial nerve, the glossopharyngeal nerve, and the vagus nerve can all recognize flavor. The swallowing reflex is connected to the vagus nerve as well.

Activation of the vagus nerve lowers blood pressure and reduces the heart rate, which typically occurs with gastrointestinal illness (acute cholecystitis or viral gastroenteritis) or in response to other stimuli such as the Valsalva maneuver or pain in having blood drawn.

Disorders and Diseases

The vagus nerve can be tested by a clinician through the gag reflex, usually with a tongue depressor or observing the uvula and the back of the throat when the patient speaks. If anything about these processes is unusual, then further examination of the ninth and tenth cranial nerves is warranted. Some people who suffer from a congenital vagus nerve disorder may have trouble breathing and may need a breathing apparatus or even a pacemaker to keep the heart regular. Fainting can possibly be related to a vagus nerve problem.

A particular disorder related to the vagus nerve is called gastroparesis or delayed gastric emptying, in which the stomach takes a longer time than usual to empty food into the small intestines for the digestion process. This disease occurs when the vagus nerve is damaged and the muscles of the intestines and stomach do not function correctly. The food slows down or completely stops in the digestive tract. The most common cause of gastroparesis is diabetes. When the blood sugar is high, a chemical reaction occurs in the nerves that damages blood vessels that carry nutrients and much-needed oxygen.

Perspective and Prospects

Vagotomy is the cutting of the vagus nerve to reduce acid buildup to the stomach. Vagotomy is being researched as a less invasive procedure for weight loss than gastric bypass surgery. Another procedure, vagus nerve stimulation (VNS), is sometimes used to treat conditions such as epilepsy and drug-resistant depression. Wider applications for VNS are under study.

—*Marvin Morris, L.Ac., M.P.A.*

See also Blood pressure; Digestion; Dizziness and fainting; Gastroenterology; Gastrointestinal disorders; Gastrointestinal system; Nervous system, Neurology; Otorhinolaryngology; Vagotomy.

For Further Information:

"Cranial Nerve X—Vagus." *Yale University School of Medicine,* January 8, 1998.

Flint, Paul W., et al., eds. *Cummings Otolaryngology: Head and Neck Surgery.* 5th ed. Philadelphia: Mosby/Elsevier, 2010.

"Motor Speech and Swallowing Disorders." In *Neurology and Clinical Neuroscience,* edited by Anthony H. V. Schapira et al. Philadelphia: Mosby Elsevier, 2007.

"Sarcoidosis of the Nervous System." In *Neurology and General Medicine,* edited by Michael J. Aminoff. 4th ed. Philadelphia: Churchill Livingstone, 2008.

"VNS." *Epilepsy Foundation,* 2012.

VARICOSE VEIN REMOVAL

Procedure

Anatomy or system affected: Blood vessels, circulatory system, legs

Specialties and related fields: General surgery, plastic surgery, vascular medicine

Definition: A surgical procedure that is used to rid the body of swollen blood vessels.

Indications and Procedures

Varicose veins are caused by an expansion of a superficial vein that is associated with incompetence of the valves within the vein. Conditions such as pregnancy and tumors that increase intra-abdominal pressure contribute to varicose vein formation. Initial treatment involves compression with support stockings.

Sclerotherapy is a more invasive treatment option. In this technique, several injections of a small amount of a solution are made into the affected vessels over an extended period of time. This solution irritates and destroys the inner lining of the blood vessel. The vein subsequently ceases to carry blood, and circulation is improved by the elimination of this diseased blood vessel. Each vessel usually requires one to six treatments at intervals of three to four weeks. Although the procedure is relatively painless, the fading of vessels is a slow process that can take one to six months.

The traditional method of treating varicose veins is surgery, which is usually performed on an outpatient basis. The most common site of varicose veins is in the lower extremities. The varicose veins are marked out on the surface of the leg. The leg is prepared with iodine and draped from the groin to the toes. A local anesthetic is injected in the skin overlying the ends of the varicose veins. A transverse incision is made over each end. The most distant (distal) end is freed, and a suture is tied around the vein. The surgeon must take care to avoid nearby sensory nerves. The near (proximal) end of the vein is similarly located and tied off. The vein is then cut, and a thin wire is passed from the distal to the proximal incision. A bullet-shaped stripper is tied to the wire; the vein is secured to the stripper. The stripper is slowly pulled out, removing the varicose vein. If a branch prevents the vein from moving, an incision is made, a suture is placed around the branch, and the branch is cut.

After the stripper passes through the entire vein, the varicosity has been removed. The path of the vein is then compressed with warm towels for several minutes to stop small branches from bleeding. Other marked branches are removed. The incisions are closed with sutures or tape. Dressings are placed over the path of the vein, and the leg is wrapped from the toe to groin with rolled, soft gauze and elastic bandages. The patient is instructed to walk but not to sit for prolonged periods of time for at least two days.

Several newer and less invasive techniques for treating varicose veins include radio frequency ablation, ambulatory phlebectomy, laser surgery, and intense pulsed light therapy. Radio frequency ablation or closure is a nonsurgical technique that uses heat in the form of radio frequency energy to collapse and seal varicose veins. The problem vein is essentially shut down, and other, healthy veins take over the blood flow. This procedure is much less invasive than vein stripping. In the closure technique, a thin catheter (flexible tube) is inserted into the vein through a small opening. The catheter delivers the radio frequency energy to the vein wall, causing it to heat up and seal shut. The vein is eliminated by placing the catheter in the lower portion of the vein and then advancing the catheter up the vein using ultrasound guidance. There is no bleeding. After this one-day procedure, patients with little trauma can ambulate more quickly and wear compression dressings for a shorter period of time than in traditional vein stripping.

Ambulatory phlebectomy is a minimally invasive technique in which a varicose vein is removed through small punctures or stab incisions along the path of the vein. Through these tiny holes, the surgeon uses a surgical hook to remove the varicose vein.

In laser surgery, a high intensity laser beam focuses a single wavelength of light at a tiny point on the vein. The light heats the vein but passes through the skin with only minimal surface damage. The underlying vein, however, is damaged by the heat and is then slowly reabsorbed by the body over a period of a few weeks. As opposed to laser surgery, intense pulsed light therapy focuses a broad spectrum of light in a

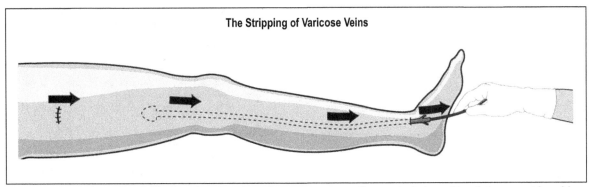

The Stripping of Varicose Veins

Varicose veins, which are identified by their characteristic swollen appearance, usually occur in the legs; although they are not harmful, many patients wish to have them stripped for cosmetic reasons.

range of wavelengths that are adjustable through the use of filters and computer-guided parameters of energy delivery. This adjustability allows the physician to customize precisely the characteristics of the light energy according to the needs of each patient, thereby minimizing damage to surrounding tissue and reducing recovery time.

Uses and Complications

Nonabsorbable sutures are removed after a week during a postoperative visit to the surgeon; elastic bandages are used for at least two weeks. Medication for pain may be needed for two to four days. The patient is instructed to walk increasing distances over the next few weeks. Patients who walk rarely experience complications.

Perspective and Prospects

The prevention of varicose veins is preferable to surgical removal. Removing excess weight, exercising, and avoiding articles of clothing that constrict the top of the thighs will help. Varicose veins affect men as well as women, although they are more common among the latter.

—*L. Fleming Fallon, Jr., M.D., Ph.D., M.P.H.;*
updated by Genevieve Slomski, Ph.D.

See also Blood vessels; Circulation; Deep vein thrombosis; Laser use in surgery; Lower extremities; Plastic surgery; Varicose veins; Vascular medicine; Vascular system.

For Further Information:
Carson-DeWitt, Rosalyn. "Varicose Veins." *Health Library*, March 13, 2013.
Goldman, Mitchel P., John J. Bergan, and Jean-Jérôme Guex. *Sclerotherapy: Treatment of Varicose and Telangiectatic Leg Veins*. 5th ed. Edinburgh: Saunders/Elsevier, 2011.
Hamdan, Allen, Edward H. Livingston, and Cassio Lynm. "Treatment of Varicose Veins." *Journal of the American Medical Association Patient Page*, March 27, 2013.
Hobbs, J. T. *The Treatment of Venous Disorders: A Comprehensive Review of Current Practice in the Management of Varicose Veins and the Post-thrombotic Syndrome*. Philadelphia: J. B. Lippincott, 1977.
MedlinePlus. "Varicose Veins." *MedlinePlus*, June 19, 2013.
Narins, Rhoda, and Paul Jarrod Frank. *Turn Back the Clock Without Losing Time: Everything You Need to Know About Simple Cosmetic Procedures*. New York: Three Rivers Press, 2002.
National Heart, Lung, and Blood Institute. "How Are Varicose Veins Treated?" *NIH National Heart, Lung, and Blood Institute*, February 1, 2011.
Saltin, Bengt, et al., eds. *Exercise and Circulation in Health and Disease*. Champaign, Ill.: Human Kinetics, 2000.
Townsend, Courtney M., Jr., et al., eds. *Sabiston Textbook of Surgery*. 19th ed. Philadelphia: Saunders/Elsevier, 2012.
Weiss, Robert A., Craig Feied, and Margaret A. Weiss, eds. *Vein Diagnosis and Treatment: A Comprehensive Approach*. New York: McGraw-Hill, 2001.

VARICOSE VEINS
Disease/Disorder

Anatomy or system affected: Blood vessels, circulatory system
Specialties and related fields: Cardiology, plastic surgery, vascular medicine

Definition: The distension of superficial veins, usually affecting the legs and causing the appearance of twisted, swollen, blue veins, especially on the backs of the calves.

Causes and Symptoms

The main task of normal leg veins is to return blood to the heart and lungs. This is difficult because the blood must be pushed upward, against the constant force of gravity. The force that propels the blood up the leg comes from the contraction of the calf muscles surrounding the deep veins that occurs during the act of walking. This forward momentum is quickly lost as gravity pulls the blood back down; however, one-way valves attached to the inside of the vein wall allow blood to pass up the leg freely, then close before the blood can be pulled back down. With each step taken, the column of blood moves up the leg until it eventually reaches the heart.

The system works well until one of the valves fails. Valves may fail because of congenital defect or because of damage from venous thrombosis (blood clots in the veins of the leg). As one ages, long periods of sitting or straining eventually cause even normal veins to become stretched and dilated, causing the valve leaflets to close improperly. When a vein valve does not close correctly, blood leaks backward, placing extra pressure on the valve beneath it. This increased pressure causes the vein to become dilated and twisted. Such veins are said to be "varicose." If this vein is near the skin, it will bulge out and become visible. These unsightly veins become more pronounced while standing and disappear or become less noticeable when lying down.

Once damaged, the valve cannot repair itself. The increased pressure continues to damage valve after valve until the small bump eventually becomes a large, bluish rope. Varicose veins are frequently accompanied by an aching sensation or a feeling of heaviness in the legs. These symptoms are aggravated by sitting or standing. People who must be on their feet all day usually experience severe discomfort. As the condition worsens, the legs and feet swell. These symptoms, which are often absent upon arising from bed in the morning, usually become more severe as the day progresses.

Although varicose veins are sometimes painful, they are not always a serious condition. Most people experience only minor inconvenience from them. If allowed to progress, however, varicose veins lead to more serious conditions. One of the most common—and most serious—of these complications is a

---

Information on Varicose Veins

Causes: Aging process; damage from venous thrombosis; long periods of standing, sitting, or straining; pregnancy; congenital valve or vessel defects; obesity

Symptoms: Twisted, swollen, blue, or bulging veins; achiness or heaviness in legs; swollen feet and legs

Duration: Short-term to chronic

Treatments: Compression stockings, surgery, sclerotherapy

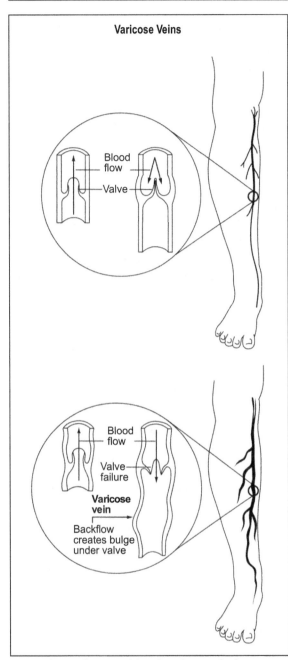

Varicose Veins

Blood
flow
Valve

Blood
flow
Valve
failure

**Varicose
vein**

Backflow
creates bulge
under valve

In normal veins, the wings of the valves shut completely, preventing backflow of blood; in varicose veins, backflow creates a bulge in the vein that leads to the characteristic appearance of branched blue veins on the legs.

blood clot within the varicose vein. As long as blood is moving quickly in a vessel, it is very difficult for it to clot. When a vein becomes varicose, the dilated portion of the vein allows blood to pool. If blood stagnates, it can become a solid mass of blood called a thrombus, or a blood clot. This blood clot may continue to grow up the vein. It can fill the entire vein from the foot

to the groin and enter the deep veins of the leg.

A clot in a deep vein is a potentially life-threatening condition, as it may break loose, pass through the heart, and lodge in the arteries that take blood to the lungs. This condition is referred to as a pulmonary embolism. If this happens, and the blood clot is small, the patient experiences shortness of breath and chest pain. If the clot that breaks loose is big and lodges in a larger lung artery, it can result in sudden death. Blood clots limited to the superficial veins (near the skin) are far less likely to break loose and result in a major pulmonary embolism. The symptoms of clot in the superficial veins are pain and redness directly over the vein involved. The varicose vein may also become hard. This is called a superficial cord. As the clot grows, the redness, pain, and cord move up the leg. This is a serious condition and requires immediate medical attention.

Other complications associated with varicose veins relate to the impact of having increased venous pressure in the legs over a long period of time. When the valves are working, the pressure in the tissue at the ankle is kept at a low level. When varicose veins are severe, the pressure in the tissue becomes so high that blood flow to the skin decreases. If this occurs over a long period of time, the skin becomes discolored and hardens. Ultimately, the skin breaks down, and venous ulcers occur. These open, weeping sores can become infected and become a chronic problem.

Treatment and Therapy

Minor varicose veins are managed quite effectively—if caught early—with well-fitting elastic compression stockings. These place pressure over the superficial veins, giving them support and preventing additional damage to them. This also forces blood into the deep veins. Assuming the deep veins have functioning valves in them, this provides relief and slows progression of the problem. Another popular approach is to surgically remove the damaged vein. This operation, called stripping, removes the veins with damaged valves, forcing blood to go through healthy veins. This can resolve the symptoms of varicose veins altogether. However, other veins may eventually become varicose.

Another intervention to get rid of varicose veins is injection therapy, or sclerotherapy, in which the patient is injected with a material that irritates the varicose vein, causing a clot to form in it. The clot is carefully controlled so that it stays only in the vein being treated. The clot attaches to the vein wall, causing the vein to shrink. This shrinking of the vein makes it seem to disappear. Sclerotherapy is not appropriate in more serious cases of varicose veins.

Perspective and Prospects

Although varicose veins can occur at any time, they are particularly predominant among the elderly; 50 percent of all individuals can expect to develop varicose veins by the age of fifty.

Nothing can be done to change congenital or inherited factors that cause varicose veins. Simple measures, however, can prevent the development of varicose veins before they occur or can slow their progression once they have developed. These preventive measures all have a common theme: avoiding long periods of sitting or standing and keeping the calf muscle active. Doctors advise people who must sit or stand for any length of time to flex and relax their calf muscles by pulling their feet up and pushing them back down. This keeps the blood moving and keeps it from pooling. Other measures include breaking up long periods of inactivity by walking a few minutes every hour, elevating the legs from time to time, wearing loose clothing that does not restrict blood flow, and avoiding high-heeled shoes. Some doctors also recommend eating a high-fiber diet since some varicose vein problems result from straining during difficult bowel movements. Patients with varicose veins who are overweight or obese will ease the symptoms of the varicose veins with weight loss. Strength-training exercises for the muscles of the leg, especially the calf, can also help to relieve some of the symptoms of varicose veins.

—*Steven R. Talbot, R.V.T.*

See also Blood vessels; Circulation; Deep vein thrombosis; Embolism; Lower extremities; Plastic surgery; Thrombosis and thrombus; Varicose vein removal; Vascular medicine; Vascular system; Venous insufficiency.

For Further Information:
Baron, Howard C., and Barbara A. Ross. *Varicose Veins: A Guide to Prevention and Treatment.* New York: Facts On File, 1997.

Goldman, Lee, and Andrew I. Schafer, eds. *Cecil Textbook of Medicine.* 24th ed. Philadelphia: Saunders/Elsevier, 2011.

"How Are Varicose Veins Treated?" *National Heart, Lung, and Blood Institute,* February 1, 2011.

Kumar, Vinay, et al., eds. *Robbins Basic Pathology.* 8th ed. Philadelphia: Saunders/Elsevier, 2007.

Narins, Rhoda, and Paul Jarrod Frank. *Turn Back the Clock Without Losing Time: Everything You Need to Know About Simple Cosmetic Procedures.* New York: Three Rivers Press, 2002.

Nath, Ronald L. "Treatment of Varicose Veins of the Leg." *Health Library,* September 24, 2012.

Townsend, Courtney M., Jr., et al., eds. *Sabiston Textbook of Surgery.* 19th ed. Philadelphia: Saunders/Elsevier, 2012.

"Varicose Veins." *Mayo Clinic,* January 31, 2013.

Weiss, Robert A., Craig Feied, and Margaret A. Weiss, eds. *Vein Diagnosis and Treatment: A Comprehensive Approach.* New York: McGraw-Hill, 2001.

VAS DEFERENS
Anatomy
Also known as: Ductus deferens
Anatomy or system affected: Genitals, reproductive system
Specialties and related fields: Urology
Definition: The tube that conveys sperm from the epididymis to the urethra in the male reproductive system.

Structure and Functions
In the male reproductive system, the testes make sperm, which is then stored in an adjacent structure, the epididymis. The epididymis is connected to the urethra via the vas deferens (plural, vasa deferentia), a smooth tube about 18 inches (45 centimeters) in length with thick, muscular walls that forms part of the spermatic cord along with various nerves, muscles, and blood vessels.

A male has two vasa deferentia. From the epididymis, located to the rear of each testis, a vas deferens leads up into the abdominal cavity through the inguinal canal (a passageway through the abdominal wall). It curves around behind the bladder and, via an enlargement called the ampulla, merges with the seminal vesicle near the base of the bladder. From there it passes through the prostate gland into the urethra.

During sexual intercourse, the walls of the vas deferens contract to move sperm out of the epididymis. The sperm mixes with seminal fluids from the seminal vesicle, prostate gland, and bulbourethral glands (Cowper's glands). The ampulla and duct of the seminal vesicle together are the ejaculatory duct through which sperm is propelled into the urethra for ejaculation from the penis.

Disorders and Diseases
Congenital defects of the male reproductive system that cause infertility include malformation or absence of one or both of the vasa deferentia. The exact mechanisms behind the defects are unknown, although there is a correlation with the genetic markers for cystic fibrosis. Obstructions in the vas deferens also occur, or an inguinal hernia may pinch it.

A principal means of contraception by sterilizing men involves the vas deferens. This is the vasectomy (also, deferentectomy), in which the vasa deferentia are either cut and sealed, clipped, or injected with a material to block them. Urologists perform the procedure, usually during an office visit, and it takes about twenty minutes. Possible complications include reduced sexual desire, bleeding, inflammation, sperm leakage, and spontaneous reopening. Postvasectomy pain syndrome is a condition of chronic pain in some men because of pressure, inflammation, or physical changes in the vas deferens. In some cases, a vasectomy can be reversed surgically so that the man is again fertile.

—*Roger Smith, Ph.D.*

See also Conception; Contraception; Erectile dysfunction; Genital disorders, male; Glands; Infertility, male; Masturbation; Men's health; Orchitis; Penile implant surgery; Prostate cancer; Prostate enlargement; Prostate gland; Prostate gland removal; Puberty and adolescence; Reproductive system; Semen; Sexual dysfunction; Sexuality; Sexually transmitted diseases (STDs); Sterilization; Testicles, undescended; Testicular cancer; Testicular surgery; Testicular torsion; Vasectomy.

For Further Information:
Beers, Mark H., ed. *The Merck Manual of Medical Information.* 2d ed. Whitehouse Station, N.J.: Merck Research Laboratories, 2003.

Denniston, George C. *Vasectomy.* Victoria, B.C.: Trafford, 2002.

Parker, Steve. *The Human Body Book.* New York: DK Adult, 2001.

Thibodeau, Gary A., and Kevin T. Patton. *Structure and Function of the Body.* 14th ed. St. Louis: Mosby/Elsevier, 2012.

"Vasectomy." *Urology Care Foundation,* January 2011.

VASCULAR MEDICINE
Specialty

Anatomy or system affected: Blood vessels, circulatory system, lymphatic system

Specialties and related fields: Cardiology, family medicine, hematology

Definition: The diagnosis and management of diseases of the arteries, veins, and lymphatic system, exclusive of the heart and lungs.

Key terms:

aneurysm: an abnormal area of an artery (or, less commonly, a vein) that enlarges for a variety of reasons and produces a focal ballooning

atherosclerosis: hardening of the arteries; a nonspecific term for the buildup of fatty material in the wall of any artery; over time, this buildup can obstruct the flow of blood through the artery and lead to adverse consequences in the organ it supplies

bypass graft: a surgical procedure that reroutes blood around an obstruction, usually caused by atherosclerosis; the "new" artery can be either plastic or constructed from an expendable, healthy section of vein in another part of the patient's body

embolus: any particle in the arterial or venous system that travels with the flow of blood and eventually lodges in the lungs, brain, or other organ or blood vessel

endarterectomy: a surgical procedure during which an artery is opened and the atherosclerotic material is manually removed, effectively cleaning out the artery and restoring more normal blood flow

ischemia: a state of blood deprivation of any organ in the body; ischemia may occur as a result of atherosclerosis in the main artery that supplies the organ, decreasing the amount of blood that can reach the organ

plaque: the fatty material composed of cholesterol, degenerating cells, and proteinaceous substances that can build up in the wall of any artery

thrombosis: the act of complete clotting of an artery or vein, through which no blood can then flow

Science and Profession

Vascular medicine, especially peripheral vascular surgery, has become an important specialty of general surgery. In the past, general surgeons performed surgery on the arteries and veins, but technical advances have led to the creation of vascular surgery as a field of its own.

Western society has produced an older population because of its high level of primary care, but with this older population come the ravages of atherosclerosis. The modern lifestyle is ideally suited to the formation of atherosclerosis in many arteries as a result of cigarette smoking, stress and high blood pressure, a fatty diet, and a sedentary lifestyle. Peripheral vascular surgeons can contribute in a positive way and help many patients with these diseases. This help may come in the form of stroke prevention, the restoration of blood flow to a leg that might otherwise not be saved, or occasionally the saving of a life through repair of a ruptured aortic aneurysm.

One of the most common arteries affected by atherosclerosis is the carotid artery, in the neck. This artery branches high in the neck near the jawline. One branch continues up into the brain, supplying a large part of the area that controls motor and sensory function. Atherosclerosis tends to occur at areas of branching arteries, and the carotid bifurcation is no exception. The buildup of material in this location is especially hazardous, because small pieces of the material, called emboli, can break off the arterial wall, travel up the artery, and lodge in the brain.

When an embolus lodges in the small arteries of the brain, it blocks the flow of blood to the area of brain tissue supplied by those arteries. This results in ischemia, or restricted blood flow, and the body functions controlled by that part of the brain may be altered. If the ophthalmic artery is involved, then blindness can ensue. If the middle cerebral artery is involved, then symptoms of motor and sensory dysfunction, such as abnormal sensation, numbness, weakness, or paralysis of one side of the body, can occur. Fortunately, very small emboli often do not cause permanent loss of neurological function, and a complete recovery is possible. They are, however, warning signs that atherosclerotic debris resides in the carotid artery, and if treatment is not begun and the brain tissue is irreversibly damaged, a permanent stroke might occur. If this happens, the patient will lose some neurologic function and may be unable to see to his or her own daily needs. The patient also may need extensive and expensive rehabilitation. Strokes can be prevented if the warning signs are properly interpreted and acted upon.

Atherosclerosis also results in stenoses, or blockages, in other arteries. Depending on the location of these blockages, various symptoms can result. If the arteries to the intestines are involved, patients can feel abdominal pain that is very difficult to diagnose, given that there are many other causes of abdominal pain, such as ulcer disease, gallbladder problems, and colitis. Intestinal ischemia is somewhat rare and often is not thought of as a cause of abdominal pain. These patients may have to endure this pain for a long period of time and may experience severe eating problems, weight loss, and addictions to painkillers. If the problem is properly diagnosed, many patients can be helped with nonsurgical and surgical techniques, resulting in the cessation of pain, the regained ability to eat, and the maintenance of proper nourishment.

One form of atherosclerotic arterial disease is called renovascular hypertension. In this syndrome, plaque builds up in the renal (kidney) arteries. Patients with renovascular hypertension exhibit a type of high blood pressure, or hypertension, that is somewhat different from the kind of high blood pressure that affects most patients. The majority of patients with hypertension have what is called essential hypertension, for which there is no known cause. For the minority of patients whose hypertension results from pathology in the renal arteries, the blood flow in these arteries is decreased because of atherosclerotic plaques in the arterial walls that severely limit the space through which blood can flow. When this happens, the kidney "senses" this decreased flow and releases a variety of chemical hormones that serve to increase the blood flow. These hormones indirectly raise the blood pressure by trying to preserve blood flow to the kidney.

Renovascular hypertension is often difficult to diagnose and treat. Many patients need to take up to five kinds of blood-pressure pills to keep their pressure under reasonable control; such patients should be screened for renovascular hypertension. A variety of treatments can be offered to these patients once a diagnosis is made, although the medicines they must take all have significant side effects.

The arteries that supply the muscles and nerves of the extremities also can be affected by atherosclerotic disease. Peculiarly, the upper extremities are usually spared of this disease, whereas the lower extremities are not. The mildest form of lower-extremity disease manifests itself in the form of *claudication*, a term that describes the specific symptoms that develop in an ischemic limb. Most of the time, there are no symptoms when a patient is at rest, but when the patient undergoes the physical stress of walking or other exercise, pain develops in the limb in certain areas that correspond to the areas of muscle tissue supplied by the blocked artery. A characteristic pain syndrome develops after a certain amount of exercise and repeats itself regularly. The pain stops after exercise, and this cessation of pain also follows a pattern.

Claudication is the classic example of arterial occlusive disease. If the disease is severe enough, it may cause resting pain. Such patients have profound ischemia of their leg(s), which is limb threatening and requires intervention. People afflicted with ischemia of the leg have difficulty healing small scrapes and cuts on the feet, sometimes causing them to turn into large lesions that do not heal. If these lesions become secondarily infected, they can also become limb threatening and ultimately necessitate amputation. In many patients, however, amputation can be avoided by timely intervention with either surgery or other techniques.

A rather curious phenomenon occurs in some patients whereby there is a focal dilatation of a portion of an artery. The mechanism by which this occurs is largely unknown, but it may be related in some way to the atherosclerotic process. Instead of a buildup of debris in the arterial wall resulting in a blockage in the artery, aneurysms are characterized by a thinned-out wall. They enlarge over time and can cause problems. They may clot off entirely or become a source of emboli, giving rise to problems farther down the arterial tree. The most devastating complication of an aneurysm, however, is acute rupture. Laplace's law of hemodynamics states that wall tension in a tube of fluid is related to the fourth power of the radius. Accordingly, as an aneurysm enlarges, the wall tension increases in exponential fashion. If rupture does occur, it can lead to rapid blood loss if expert medical and surgical care is not readily available.

Aneurysms can form anywhere in the body, but they most commonly occur in the aorta (the main artery coming out from the heart) directly beneath the umbilicus. Because this location is surgically accessible, repair of these aneurysms is a common operation. In this location, most aneurysms will not cause a problem until they measure approximately five centimeters in diameter, at which size the risk of rupture becomes significant. Smaller aneurysms are usually monitored with serial examinations over time, and if they do enlarge, then the appropriate therapy can be instituted. Other, less common areas of aneurysm formation include the splenic, renal, iliac, femoral, and popliteal arteries. Similar complications can ensue with these aneurysms.

The majority of peripheral vascular surgery practice deals with the diseases of the arteries, but venous disease is a very common problem that many physicians in many specialties must address. Patients with simple phlebitis of the superficial veins of the leg usually require no more than supportive care until they feel better, but if the clots are in or extend into the deep veins of the leg, much more aggressive treatment is necessary. A clot in this location has a chance of migrating into the lungs (pulmonary embolus) and can be fatal. Therefore, intensive treatment with intravenous and then oral blood thinners (anticoagulants) is mandatory. There are some patients who then have chronic venous problems because the clots in their legs can damage the valves in the veins. This results in severe pain, swelling, and even ulceration of the legs that can be very difficult to treat.

Diagnostic and Treatment Techniques

Many patients who suffer from vascular diseases are not treated with surgery right away. They may ultimately need an operation, but often long periods of time elapse before surgery is undertaken. Nonoperative therapy, such as quitting smoking, lowering serum cholesterol, or starting an exercise program, is often all that is needed to control certain aspects of the patient's symptoms. Vascular surgeons provide guidelines for patients who need this sort of therapy.

Atherosclerosis may appear in many forms and affect patients differently. For example, a forty-five-year-old postal carrier complains of pain in his or her thighs in the same location whenever he or she walks more than a few hundred feet. This person may have been a heavy smoker for many years, his or her cholesterol levels may be elevated, and there may be many relatives in his or her family with hardening of the arteries. Such a person has a classic case of claudication resulting from atherosclerotic occlusive disease of the arteries that supply the thigh muscles. The patient has several options. Other causes of leg pain must be ruled out, such as nerve problems or back conditions, but when this is accomplished, the field of vascular surgery can help this patient maintain his or her lifestyle. If the patient would like to investigate options for intervention, an arteriogram is performed next. In this procedure, specially trained radiologists insert a small tube into the arteries and take pictures after dye has been injected. This allows an exact replica of the patient's arterial anatomy to be projected in two dimensions. The arteriogram allows the surgeons and radiologists to determine the best course of action for this patient.

Some atherosclerotic plaques are in particular locations that may allow their treatment with balloon angioplasty rather than open surgery. In this procedure, again performed by trained radiologists or some vascular surgeons, a catheter with a balloon at its end is inserted into the artery, and the balloon is inflated in the area of the offending plaque in an effort to open the clogged artery. This procedure is often performed on the arteries of the heart, but it can also be performed on other arteries, such as those in the kidneys, intestines, or legs. A vascular surgeon usually oversees the care of the patient, as not all the balloon procedures are completely successful and open surgery is sometimes necessary. Open surgery might include a bypass graft with a woven or knitted prosthetic artery or a graft made with an expendable vein in the patient's leg, using the same vein as for heart bypass surgery. The postal worker described above could be a candidate for either a balloon procedure or a surgical bypass graft, but in either case, he or she should be restored to almost normal walking capability and be able to return to work.

Another common scenario might involve a more serious situation. A person may have an open sore on his or her foot that has been there for more than six months and is getting bigger, perhaps infected. This person may also be a heavy smoker with cholesterol problems and severe diabetes mellitus. He or she has not walked more than a block in the past few years because this causes his or her feet to hurt. The problem may be related to poor blood flow to the legs and feet, and the diabetes certainly does not help. Before vascular surgery techniques became popular, this patient ultimately would have required an amputation of the leg, either below or above the knee. It is physically and emotionally difficult for patients to cope with such a loss, and the long, expensive period of rehabilitation includes learning to walk with a prosthetic extremity. This patient would be a good candidate for an arteriogram and would undoubtedly need some surgery. This would most likely be in the form of a bypass graft, which could stretch from the groin all the way to the foot, crossing the knee and the ankle. Ultimately, a successful outcome would be healing of the open sore and control of the infection; the patient would then be able to continue walking with his or her own leg.

Another situation that might involve vascular surgery is as follows. A patient has a history of deep vein clots following prior major surgery. Treatment consisted of long-term blood thinners, and the patient may have had no major problems since that time. The patient now needs a hip operation, however, and hip operations carry a high risk of blood-clot formation in the deep veins of the leg. Because deep-vein thrombosis carries risks of a pulmonary embolus as well as chronic problems in the leg, a vascular surgeon is called upon to help design a program that can prevent these complications from occurring. The usual methods of prophylaxis do not necessarily apply to this patient, and as the patient is labeled high risk, it might be most prudent to place a device in the body to catch any pulmonary emboli if they occur. The theory behind this management is that, in this high-risk patient, the formation of blood clots in the legs is almost unavoidable, and the majority of effort should be aimed at preventing the most serious, potentially fatal complication: the pulmonary embolus. In this case, vascular surgeons could place a filter device in the main vein that carries blood to the heart and lungs, which would effectively trap any free-floating emboli that could cause a problem.

Perspective and Prospects

Peripheral vascular surgery has assumed a paramount role in medical practice. By 1900, significant contributions had been made regarding the basic reconstructive techniques needed to sew arteries together. The work of Alexis Carrel in the early twentieth century is considered the most important contribution to the technical art of vascular surgery. His techniques for transplanting organs and sewing arteries together are still routinely performed. By the 1950s, synthetic materials were introduced as arterial replacements, which became acceptable treatment for many patients.

In addition to balloon angioplasty, nonsurgical or minimally invasive surgical techniques for opening blocked arteries and veins to improve blood flow include the use of a stent, or a small mesh tube, which can be expanded inside a blocked blood vessel to increase its diameter and then remain there to hold it open; an atherectomy, in which a thin tube is inserted into the vessel to cut away the plaque; and thrombolysis, which is the use of either traditional pharmaceuticals or biopharmaceuticals to break down blood clots. Although technically performing a bypass graft is feasible, the graft cannot approach the durability and performance of a native artery and typically does not last longer than fifteen years. Research involving the transplantation of human arteries may solve some of these problems and allow more patients to benefit from surgery.

Vascular surgery can benefit large numbers of people simply because of the nature of atherosclerosis. It may be a product of habits, the environment, or genetic makeup, but it is widely accepted that as the population ages, more and more people will suffer from diseases that can be helped by vascular surgery, allowing them to maintain lifestyles that are as productive as possible. Basic scientific research into the mechanisms of atherosclerosis may yield important answers and lead to new therapies for patients with vascular disease.

—Mark Wengrovitz, M.D.

See also Amputation; Aneurysmectomy; Aneurysms; Angiography; Angioplasty; Arteriosclerosis; Behçet's disease; Biofeedback; Bleeding; Blood and blood disorders; Blood pressure; Blood vessels; Bypass surgery; Carotid arteries; Catheterization; Cholesterol; Circulation; Claudication; Deep vein thrombosis; Diabetes mellitus; Dialysis; Embolism; Endarterectomy; Exercise physiology; Glands; Healing; Hematology; Hematology, pediatric; Hemorrhoid banding and removal; Hemorrhoids; Histology; Hypercholesterolemia; Hyperlipidemia; Ischemia; Klippel-Trenaunay syndrome; Lipids; Lymphatic system; Mitral valve prolapse; Phlebitis; Phlebotomy; Podiatry; Shunts; Stents; Strokes; Sturge-Weber syndrome; Systems and organs; Thrombolytic therapy and TPA; Thrombosis and thrombus; Transfusion; Transient ischemic attacks (TIAs); Varicose vein removal; Varicose veins; Vascular system; Vasculitis; Venous insufficiency.

For Further Information:

Ancowitz, Arthur. *Strokes and Their Prevention: How to Avoid High Blood Pressure and Hardening of the Arteries.* New York: Jove, 1980.

Cissarek, Thomas, et al., eds. *Vascular Medicine: Therapy and Practice*. New York: McGraw-Hill Medical, 2011.

Cronenwett, Jack L., and K. Wayne Johnston, eds. *Rutherford's Vascular Surgery*. 7th ed. Philadelphia: Saunders/Elsevier, 2010.

Ernst, Calvin B., and James C. Stanley, eds. *Current Therapy in Vascular Surgery*. 4th ed. St. Louis, Mo.: Mosby, 2001.

Jaff, Michael, and Corey Goldman. *Handbook of Vascular Medicine for the Cardiologist: The Basics of Vascular Diagnosis and Therapy*. Boston: Blackwell, 2003.

Marieb, Elaine N. *Essentials of Human Anatomy and Physiology*. 10th ed. San Francisco: Pearson/Benjamin Cummings, 2012.

Rooke, Thom W., Timothy M. Sullivan, and Michael R. Jaff, eds. *Vascular Medicine and Endovascular Interventions*. Columbia, Md.: Society for Vascular Medicine and Biology, 2007.

Society for Vascular Medicine. http://www.vascularmed.org

Tortora, Gerard J., and Bryan Derrickson. *Principles of Anatomy and Physiology*. 13th ed. Hoboken, N.J.: John Wiley & Sons, 2012.

"Vascular Diseases." *MedlinePlus*, September 3, 2013.

VASCULAR SYSTEM

Anatomy

Anatomy or system affected: Blood vessels, circulatory system, legs

Specialties and related fields: Cardiology, exercise physiology, hematology, vascular medicine

Definition: The pipeline through which every cell of the body receives oxygen, vitamins, hormones, and the metabolic fuels necessary to sustain life.

Key terms:

arteries: the vessels that carry blood from the heart to all parts of the body

atherosclerosis: the buildup of lipid-containing (fatty) materials beneath or within the inner wall of an artery, which can lead to narrowing or occlusion of the artery

capillaries: minute blood vessels that connect the smallest arteries (arterioles) to the smallest veins (venules); they allow passage of oxygen and nutrients from the arteries into the tissue and passage of waste products from the tissues into the veins

collaterals: small vessels that enlarge to compensate for the obstruction or narrowing of another vessel

heart attack: sudden and permanent damage to a part of the heart muscle as a result of impaired blood flow through the coronary arteries

metabolism: the chemical changes that occur when the body transforms oxygen and nutrients into energy or heat

stroke: permanent damage to part of the brain as a result of impaired blood flow

veins: blood vessels that carry blood from the cells back to the heart

venous thrombosis: the presence of blood clots in the veins, usually in the legs or arms

Structure and Functions

The vascular system is faced with the enormous task of supplying every cell of the human body with a constant supply of the oxygen and nutrients needed to sustain life. This elaborate system circulates more than 2,000 gallons of blood per day through more than 12,000 miles of arteries, veins, and capillaries. Moreover, the job of the vascular system is not finished when the nutrients arrive at the cell. After the cell uses the nutrients, waste products that are left over from metabolism must be carried away and disposed of before they damage the cell. For this reason, several kinds of vessels exist within the human body that differ in structure and function. They can be broken into three categories: arteries, veins, and capillaries.

The term "artery" comes from the Greek word *arteria*, meaning "windpipe," because arteries were thought to be filled with air. (This misconception evolved because after death, much of the blood usually pumped through the arteries had been pumped out, leading observers to conclude that air, rather than blood, was circulated within them.) Arteries are thick-walled blood vessels that carry oxygen-rich blood from the left side of the heart to all parts of the body. The blood circulating within them is usually moving at high velocities and exerts pressure against the artery walls, creating an expansion of the artery during the contraction of the heart. This expansion, called a pulse, can be palpated in areas where the arteries are large and close to the surface of the skin: in the neck (the carotid artery) or in the wrist (the radial artery). The pressure being exerted against the artery varies greatly. A doctor taking a blood pressure reading is measuring this variation in pressure. A blood pressure of 120/80, for example, would mean that the force from the heart is exerting 120 millimeters of mercury pressure against the artery wall while the heart is contracting (the systolic pressure) and 80 millimeters of mercury when the heart is at rest (the diastolic pressure). Clearly, the artery has to be a very strong structure.

Veins, on the other hand, are thin-walled, almost transparent vessels that return blood to the heart after it has visited the cells. There are far more veins in the body than there are arteries. The blood moving in the veins is under very little pressure and usually is moving quite slowly in comparison to the flow in the arteries. The flow in the veins is slow because much of the force from the contraction of the heart is dissipated by the time the blood passes by the cells of the body. For this reason, the flow in the veins must be helped along by contraction of the muscles around these blood vessels. For example, with each step, the muscles in the calves of the legs propel the blood in the calf veins upward with great force. For this reason, the calf of the leg is sometimes referred to as the "venous heart." If this pump is not active, blood flow in the veins can stagnate and life-threatening clots can form in the veins.

Another problem for the venous circulation is that its blood is often moving against gravity. If veins were built like arteries (simple hollow tubes), the blood would flow upward toward the heart with the contraction of the muscles but would fall back down as soon as the contraction stopped. Fortunately, the veins are equipped with one-way valves not found in arteries. These valves open when blood is moving toward the heart and close when blood starts to fall backward. Veins are also different from arteries in that they can expand to several times their normal size. This allows the veins to be used as a storage area for blood. When the body's need for blood is low, such as during a resting state, the veins enlarge

In the News: Treating Vascular Disease with Therapeutic Angiogenesis

Many diseases of the vascular system are associated with decreased perfusion, or the passage of blood through organ vessels; restoration of blood flow is the most effective means to limit damage to ischemic tissue. Therapeutic angiogenesis as related to cardiovascular disease refers to the improvement of myocardial and extremity blood flow and function within ischemic regions where traditional methods of restoring blood vessel structure are not feasible. Angiogenesis refers to the chemical promotion of new vessel growth.

Fibroblast growth factors (FGFs) and vascular endothelial growth factors (VEGFs) have been the most widely studied protein families capable of inducing new vessel growth. Two modes of introducing FGF to the body have been explored: direct injection or implantation of the FGF protein and the induction of individual cells to produce increased amounts of FGF by the incorporation of appropriate deoxyribonucleic acid (DNA) fragments, called gene therapy. The FGF-2 Initiating Revascularization Support Trial (FIRST), described in the *Journal of the American College of Cardiology* in 2000, compared a single intracoronary dose of FGF-2 with placebo in 337 patients. After ninety days, patients receiving FGF did not differ significantly from the placebo group in total exercise time possible, a commonly used indirect measure of restored blood flow. Frequency of angina was also similar in the two groups, indicating that this recombinant (engineered) protein treatment was ineffective. Gene transfer therapies, in which a patient's own cells internally produce new FGF protein, are viewed as holding more promise in eventually translating into a clinically accepted treatment for ischemia. Human studies of FGF gene therapy are ongoing.

—*Michael R. King, Ph.D.*

particular cell of the calf muscle in the leg. Here the nutrients are delivered to the cell. The waste products are dumped back into the capillaries. From the capillaries, one travels into venules. These tiny veins become continually larger until one is finally moving up through a large vein just behind the knee called the popliteal. Soon one is back in the abdomen in the large vein called the vena cava, which enters the heart at the right atrium. The blood then travels through the right ventricle and eventually into another large vessel called the pulmonary artery (the only artery that carries blood that is not oxygenated). This artery leads into the lungs, where the waste products of metabolism are released and exchanged for oxygen. With a new load of oxygen, one travels through the pulmonary veins (the only veins that carry oxygenated blood), into the left atrium of the heart, and into the left ventricle, where the journey began. In a normal person, this entire voyage takes only eighteen to twenty-four seconds.

and fill with the blood that is not being actively circulated. When the need for blood increases, as during strenuous activity, the stored blood is forced back into active circulation. Because veins have such thin walls and stretch so easily, one might think they are not as strong as arteries. In reality, veins are strong enough to be used as surgical substitutes for failed arteries and hold up quite well under arterial pressure.

Capillaries are extremely small vessels with very thin walls. These vessels connect the smallest arteries (arterioles) with the smallest veins (venules). Although their size can vary, the average diameter of a capillary is about 8 microns (0.008 millimeter), which is about the size of a single red blood cell. The nutrients carried in the blood pass through tiny pores in the vessel wall directly into the body's other cells, which use the nutrients to produce energy and heat. During this process, waste products are created that are poisonous to the cells; they must be removed quickly or the cells will die. The waste products therefore pass from the cells into the capillaries and then into tiny veins that will carry the waste products away.

A trip through the system of arteries, capillaries, and veins—to deliver nutrients to one cell in a calf muscle, for example—would begin in the left ventricle of the heart, where blood is pumped through the aorta (the largest artery) with great force. The aorta has branches that serve the structures of the head and neck (which includes the most important organ—the brain), the upper extremities, the abdomen, and the lower extremities. On this imaginary trip, one passes through the aortic arch and travels down the main artery in the abdomen, called the abdominal aorta. This artery eventually branches into two arteries (at about the level of the navel) that send blood to each leg. This artery continues to branch into smaller and smaller arteries until one reaches the capillaries serving the

Disorders and Diseases

When the vascular system is functioning correctly, all the cells of the body are receiving the right amount of blood at all times. Many problems can arise, however, in the complex functioning of the human organism, and the vasculature must have ways of meeting these challenges. Such problems include the obstruction of vital vessels by plaque formation (a buildup of fatty deposits called atherosclerosis), thrombus (blood clot) formation, and vasospasm (a closing down of a blood vessel in response to cold or trauma). Moreover, some organs in the body cannot survive for more than a few minutes without oxygen before damage occurs. For example, the brain can survive for only a few minutes without oxygen, while the cells in the arms and legs can be deprived of oxygen for a matter of hours without irreversible damage. For this reason, whenever there is a problem the vascular system must be able to set priorities about which systems receive blood flow and which systems do not. When there is a life-threatening problem, the vessels in the arms and legs contract, forcing blood out of the extremities; this allows more flow to reach the brain, where it is most urgently needed. When an artery is narrowed by plaque, the vascular system will compensate by enlarging smaller vessels in the area to help maintain flow. If the artery is totally obstructed, this system of collateral vessels takes over.

While these and other mechanisms work quite well, sudden obstruction or other disease processes involving an artery or vein can result in major problems. The major problems that can result from arterial disease include stroke, myocardial infarction (heart attack), and peripheral artery disease. Problems involving the veins may include deep vein thrombosis, pulmonary embolism, and varicose veins.

A stroke is a condition in which part of the brain is deprived of oxygen long enough to cause permanent damage. The medical term for such an event is a cerebrovascular accident, or CVA. The symptoms may include one-sided weakness or numbness, headache, difficulty in speaking, or transient blindness in one eye. If these symptoms completely resolve within twenty-four hours, the event is referred to as a transient ischemic attack, or TIA. The difference between a TIA and a CVA is that the damage done by the TIA is not permanent. TIAs, however, are often precursors of impending full-blown strokes. Therefore, patients who experience them should see a doctor immediately so that steps can be taken to prevent another, perhaps more severe, episode. The treatment for patients who experience a TIA may include surgery to remove plaque buildup from the carotid artery, bypass surgery (in which another vessel is used to bypass a narrowed area), the use of blood-thinning drugs, or the use of antiplatelet drugs (such as aspirin). Rehabilitation, the use of blood-thinning or antiplatelet drugs, and lifestyle modification are often prescribed for those who have already suffered major strokes.

Myocardial infarction is one of the leading killers in Western societies. A heart attack occurs when blood flow is inadequate to the heart muscle and part of the heart muscle dies. The symptoms include pain in the chest (especially pain that is brought on by exertion), shortness of breath, sweating, nausea, and fatigue. Similar, although usually less severe, symptoms may be present with a condition called angina, in which blood flow to the heart muscle is impaired but there is no permanent damage. Acute treatment for heart attacks can include rest (to reduce additional damage to the heart muscle), treatment with blood-thinning drugs, treatment with drugs that dissolve blood clots, balloon catheters (to help open narrowed arteries), or coronary bypass surgery.

Peripheral artery disease—the narrowing or blockage of arteries in the arms or legs—is also quite common. Symptoms may include pain in the limb, loss of feeling, coolness, and discoloration; in severe cases, tissue loss may result. This disease process is usually progressive. A patient may first notice pain in the calf of the leg that comes on only with walking and goes away as soon as the exercise stops. This condition, called intermittent claudication, indicates that there is minimal narrowing of the arteries in the leg. As more of the artery narrows, the pain occurs even without exercise. Finally, blood flow to the limb is not sufficient to maintain the cells, and tissue begins to die. Treatment of peripheral artery disease may include medication and exercise (during the early stages) and progress to the surgical bypass of narrowed arteries (in later stages). Sometimes arteries in the extremities become clogged by a thrombus instead of plaque. If this is the case, drugs that dissolve blood clots or surgical operations to remove the clot may be used. If treatment for severe peripheral disease is unsuccessful, amputation may be necessary.

The risk factors for developing arterial disease—of the coronary, carotid, or peripheral arteries—include high blood pressure, smoking, diabetes, elevated cholesterol levels, stress, a family history of arterial disease, obesity, and advancing age.

Veins do not develop plaque as do arteries; instead, blood can stagnate and form clots that can obstruct them. When this happens, a condition called venous thrombosis, blood stagnates in the veins behind the clot and a larger clot forms. It is not unusual for clots to fill all the major veins in the leg once this process begins. These clots cause swelling and pain in the leg but do not usually threaten the leg as obstruction of the arteries does. Instead, the danger lies in the possibility of a clot breaking loose and traveling to the lungs. This clot, called a pulmonary embolism, can be fatal. The risk factors for developing venous thrombosis include anything that can slow blood flow in the veins, such as prolonged sitting or standing, a long airplane trip or car trip, a surgical operation, or pregnancy. Injury to the vein can also trigger clots, as can an imbalance of clotting factors in the blood. The best way to prevent venous thrombosis is to keep active.

Another venous problem that strikes as many as one of every four women and one of every five men is a condition most commonly known as varicose veins, in which the veins become stretched out and elongated to the point where they bulge out when the patient is sitting or standing. Although this is mostly a cosmetic problem, severe cases can lead to blood pooling in the leg and tissue damage.

Perspective and Prospects

The vasculature of the human body has not always been understood, even in recent times. The ancient Egyptians knew about the importance of the heart and the pulse, but this knowledge was not passed on to more modern civilizations. The Greek physician Hippocrates (c. 460–c. 370 BCE) had serious misconceptions about the functions of the circulatory system: he thought that the pulse was caused by movements of the blood vessels. Other great thinkers, such as Aristotle and Galen, made similar errors in their study of the vascular system, errors that influenced medicine for many years.

In 1628, a doctor in London named William Harvey published a paper introducing radical theories about how the blood circulates. He changed the way medical people thought about this system by describing it as a closed circuit, with blood being forced through it via contractions of the heart. He postulated that blood passed from the arteries into the veins at the cellular level. It was not until the 1660s, when early microscopes were developed, that this theory could be confirmed.

In 1733, a clergyman named Stephen Hales became the first person to measure blood pressure within the arterial system. He inserted a large glass tube into the neck artery of a horse. To his amazement, the blood rose 9 feet up the tube. This method of measuring blood pressure was not practical, however, and it was not until the late nineteenth century that the sphygmomanometer was developed to measure blood pressure, utilizing blood pressure cuffs and air pressure.

Another pioneer in the understanding of the vascular system was German physician and biologist Rudolf Virchow

(1821–1902), who theorized about how blood clots formed in veins. He concluded that clots formed when the blood flow was slowed down, the vein wall was injured, or an imbalance of clotting factors in the blood existed. These observations were astonishingly correct considering that, at this time, many people still thought blood clots in the veins were composed of pus. Understanding of these principles makes possible modern treatments and prevention techniques.

In the late nineteenth century, modern vascular surgery began with development of techniques to repair blood vessels. By the early twentieth century, methods for connecting the ends of vessels with a watertight suture became commonplace. In 1948, a surgeon in Paris took a saphenous vein and used it to bypass a blockage in an artery in the leg. In the 1950s, the technology necessary to support sustained heart surgeries was introduced, and heart surgery has since become routine. Blood vessels can now be surgically repaired, bypassed, or cleaned out. Laser surgery and clot-dissolving drugs are also becoming routine.

—Steven R. Talbot, R.V.T.

See also Amputation; Aneurysmectomy; Aneurysms; Angiography; Angioplasty; Arteriosclerosis; Behçet's disease; Biofeedback; Bleeding; Blood and blood disorders; Blood pressure; Blood vessels; Bypass surgery; Carotid arteries; Catheterization; Cholesterol; Circulation; Claudication; Deep vein thrombosis; Diabetes mellitus; Dialysis; Embolism; Endarterectomy; Exercise physiology; Glands; Healing; Hematology; Hematology, pediatric; Hemorrhoid banding and removal; Hemorrhoids; Histology; Hypercholesterolemia; Hyperlipidemia; Ischemia; Klippel-Trenaunay syndrome; Lipids; Lymphatic system; Mitral valve prolapse; Phlebitis; Phlebotomy; Podiatry; Shunts; Stents; Strokes; Sturge-Weber syndrome; Systems and organs; Thrombolytic therapy and TPA; Thrombosis and thrombus; Transfusion; Transient ischemic attacks (TIAs); Varicose vein removal; Varicose veins; Vascular medicine; Vasculitis; Venous insufficiency.

For Further Information:

Hershey, Falls B., Robert W. Barnes, and David S. Sumner, eds. *Noninvasive Diagnosis of Vascular Disease.* Pasadena, Calif.: Appleton Davies, 1984.

Loscalzo, Joseph, and Andrew I. Schafer, eds. *Thrombosis and Hemorrhage.* 3d ed. Philadelphia: Lippincott Williams & Wilkins, 2003.

Mohrman, David E., and Lois Jane Heller. *Cardiovascular Physiology.* 7th ed. New York: Lange Medical Books/McGraw-Hill, 2010.

Standring, Susan, et al., eds. *Gray's Anatomy.* 40th ed. New York: Churchill Livingstone/Elsevier, 2008.

Strandness, D. Eugene, Jr. *Duplex Scanning in Vascular Disorders.* 4th ed. London: Lippincott Williams & Wilkins, 2009.

"Vascular Diseases." *MedlinePlus,* June 26, 2013.

VASCULITIS
Disease/Disorder

Anatomy or system affected: Abdomen, blood vessels, chest, circulatory system, ears, eyes, gastrointestinal system, hands, immune system, intestines, kidneys, legs, lungs, nerves, nose, respiratory system, skin

Specialties and related fields: Cardiology, dermatology, gastroenterology, nephrology, neurology, ophthalmology, otolaryngology, pulmonary medicine, rheumatology

Definition: A number of conditions characterized by inflammation of blood vessels, both arteries and veins, that leads to decreased circulation in the affected tissue or organ, which can damage the tissue or organ. Inflammation may be continuous or spotty and can result in damage to the walls of the blood vessel, leading to destruction of the blood vessel or the formation of an aneurysm.

Causes and Symptoms

There is no definite cause of vasculitis. Some types may be autoimmune in nature, in which the body attacks its own tissues. Some types of vasculitis may be caused by an allergic reaction to a medication, exposure to a toxic chemical, or a virus, such as the hepatitis B and hepatitis C viruses. Vasculitis may occur with connective tissue disease such as rheumatoid arthritis, Sjögren's syndrome, and lupus, or with a blood cell cancer such as leukemia or lymphoma.

These conditions are often classified by the size of the blood vessels involved in the condition or by the type of cells involved in the inflammation of the blood vessels. Large vessel vasculitis includes Takayasu arteritis, Behçet's syndrome, polymyalgia rheumatica, and giant cell arteritis. Medium vessel vasculitis includes Buerger's disease, polyarteritis nodosa, Kawasaki disease, cutaneous vasculitis, and primary central nervous system vasculitis. Small vessel vasculitis includes Wegener's granulomatosis, Churg-Strauss arteritis, microscopic polyarteritis/angiitis, hyperallergic vasculitis, Henoch-Schonlein purpura, essential cryoglobinemic vasculitis, hypersensitivity vasculitis, and vasculitis secondary to connective tissue disorders. The types of cells that may be observed in the various vasculitis types are neutrophils, lymphocytes, leukocytes, eosinophils, or granulomatous cells. The two classification systems tend to overlap, and the cell type can change in a type of vasculitis as the condition progresses.

The first symptoms that are reported are usually systemic. They include fatigue, fever, night sweats, weakness, weight loss, anorexia, muscle and joint pain, and numbness. More specific symptoms depend on the type of vasculitis. Some of the types demonstrate only skin lesions, which can be purple spots (purpura), areas of necrosis, or skin ulcers. They include hypersensitivity vasculitis, Buerger's disease, and cutaneous vasculitis. Each type of vasculitis then has its own symptoms based on the part of the body that is affected. Symptoms can include a skin rash, joint or extremity pain, neuropathy, ulcerations of the skin, headache, visual problems, abdominal pain, vomiting, diarrhea, anemia, coughing up blood, muscle pain, conjunctivitis, weakness, heart failure, palpitations, sinus problems, bleeding into the lungs, and abnormal kidney function. Some types of vasculitis are self-limiting, but most are chronic conditions. The damage that vasculitis can cause can be life-threatening.

Vasculitis is diagnosed by blood tests, including a complete blood count (CBC), general chemistry, liver function tests, and kidney function tests. These tests demonstrate what body organs are affected by the vasculitis. Some tests that are

Information on Vasculitis

Causes: Body attacking its blood vessels as result of autoimmunity, certain viral infections, some cancers, some connective tissue diseases (rheumatoid arthritis), allergies to some medications

Symptoms: Depends on type; fatigue, fever, night sweats, weakness, weight loss, anorexia, muscle and joint pain, numbness, skin rash, skin ulcers, headache, visual problems, abdominal pain, vomiting, diarrhea, anemia, coughing up blood, muscle pain, heart failure, sinus problems, kidney problems

Duration: Some self-limiting, others chronic

Treatments: Drugs suppressing inflammation or immune system, particularly corticosteroids (prednisone, cytoxan)

commonly abnormal with vasculitis are erythrocyte sedimentation rate (ESR), C-reactive protein (CRP), antinuclear antibody (ANA), and antineutrophil cytoplasmic antibody (ANCA). These tests indicate the presence of inflammation in the body, which is a sign of vasculitis. The most specific test for vasculitis is a biopsy of an affected area of the body, such as the skin or a kidney. The biopsy actually demonstrates the presence of vasculitis. Sometimes, angiograms (X-rays of the blood vessels) are performed to look for vasculitis. If kidney problems are suspected, then urine is tested for the presence of microscopic blood and protein.

Treatment and Therapy

The treatment for vasculitis is based on the type of disease. The most common treatment is the administration of corticosteroid drugs, such as prednisone or solumedrol. They can be given orally or intravenously. Corticosteroids are used to control the inflammation in the blood vessels. Often, other immune system suppressant drugs are administered with the corticosteroids. They include cyclophosphamide, azathioprine, and methotrexate. These medications can also be administered orally or intravenously. Both of these groups of medications have a number of side effects. Corticosteroids can cause weight gain, diabetes, osteoporosis, insomnia, hypertension, increased risk of infection, mood changes, stomach upset, and cataracts. The immune system suppressant drugs are cytotoxic substances that are also used to treat some types of cancer and to prevent the rejection of transplanted organs. They, too, have many side effects. They can cause hair loss, fatigue, bladder cancer, hemorrhagic cystitis, increased risk of infections, nausea, vomiting, diarrhea, and liver damage.

Usually, vasculitis responds well to one or both of these medications, particularly if it is diagnosed early. If vasculitis does not respond well to this treatment, plasmapheresis can be performed or the medication interferon alpha can be given. Plasmapheresis is a procedure in which plasma is removed from blood previously taken from the body. Removal is done by centrifuging the blood, which is separated into plasma with other immune cells and the red blood cells. The red blood cells are then returned to the patient. Eliminating many of the white blood cells can interfere with the immune response. Interferon alpha is a biologic drug that can affect the immune response. This drug is still being studied for its role in treating vasculitis.

Prospective and Prospects

Although symptoms of conditions that sound like vasculitis have appeared in ancient medical writings, vasculitis was not identified until 1866 by Adolf Kussmaul. Kussmaul noted that the affected patient had nodules under his skin, but on autopsy, he was able to see that there were nodules on the patient's arteries. He called this condition periarteritis nodosa. Kussmaul attributed the arterial nodules to inflammation of the blood vessels, and he considered it to be a novel condition that had not been described previously.

After Kussmaul's description of periarteritis nodosa, other cases of apparent vasculitis were compared to it. However, many of these conditions were actually different types of vasculitis. There are approximately twenty different types of vasculitis. Giant cell arteritis was described in 1890. Giant cell arteritis is inflammation of the large temporal arteries of the head. It causes localized pain and tenderness, and it can lead to blindness if untreated. It is diagnosed by biopsy of a temporal artery. Polymyalgia rheumatica was first described in 1957, and it occurs in roughly 50 percent of those who develop giant cell arteritis. Polymyalgia rheumatica affects the large arteries of the shoulders and hips and causes muscle pain in the arms and legs.

Takayasu's arteritis, first described in 1908, is inflammation of the aorta and its major branches, the optical arteries. This vasculitis affects young women and can lead to heart failure. Buerger's disease was also described in 1908. It is characterized by severe lack of blood flow to the hands and feet, causing severe pain, blue fingers and toes, and tissue death. Buerger's disease is caused by cigarette smoking. Kawasaki disease was described in 1939. It demonstrates inflammation of the medium-sized arteries of the mucous membranes, lymph nodes, and coronary arteries. This condition occurs only in young children and causes swollen glands in the neck, conjunctivitis, inflammation around the mouth and on the palms of the hands and the bottom of the feet, a skin rash, and aneurysms of the coronary arteries.

Three of the more serious forms of vasculitis are Wegener's granulomatosis, Churg-Strauss syndrome, and microscopic polyarteritis. These conditions can be rapidly fatal unless treated aggressively. All three are associated with the presence of antineutrophil cytoplasmic antibodies in the blood. Wegener's granulomatosis was first described in 1936, and it affects the small blood vessels of the skin, lungs, eyes, sinuses, and kidneys. Churg-Strauss syndrome was described in 1951. It begins with the development of asthma and then progresses to affect the nerves, skin, heart, lungs, gastrointestinal tract, and kidneys. Microscopic polyarteritis was first described in 1948. It affects the smallest blood vessels of the lungs and kidneys. All three conditions can lead to bleeding by the small

blood vessels in the lungs and lead to kidney failure.
—*Christine M. Carroll, R.N., B.S.N., M.B.A.*

See also Aneurysmectomy; Aneurysms; Behçet's disease; Bleeding; Blood and blood disorders; Blood vessels; Circulation; Claudication; Inflammation; Varicose vein removal; Varicose veins; Vascular medicine; Vascular system.

For Further Information:

Qontro Medical Guides. *Vasculitis Medical Guide*. Minneapolis: Author, 2008.
Schwar, Sheri Lyn. *Vasculitis: Sick and Tired of Being Sick and Tired*. Lincoln, Nebr.: iUniverse, 2006.
Swart, Myrna. *There Must Be a Reason: My Daughter's Battle With Wegener's Granulomatosis*. Lincoln, Nebr.: iUniverse, 2008.
"Vasculitis." *MedlinePlus*, May 16, 2013.
"Vasculitis Syndromes of the Central and Peripheral Nervous Systems Fact Sheet." *National Institute of Neurological Disorders and Stroke*, Feb. 7, 2012.
"What Is Vasculitis?" *The Johns Hopkins Vasculitis Center*, 2013.
"What Is Vasculitis?" *National Heart, Lung, and Blood Institute*, Apr. 1, 2011.

VASECTOMY

Procedure

Anatomy or system affected: Genitals, reproductive system
Specialties and related fields: Family medicine, general surgery, urology
Definition: A surgical means of birth control for males that involves the interruption of the tubes that transport sperm to the semen.

Key terms:

ejaculation: the expulsion from a man's erect penis at the time of orgasm of a fluid made up of semen and sperm

elective surgical sterilization: a voluntary operation that is intended to produce permanent birth control

local anesthesia: the injection of medication into the body that renders the immediate area free of pain

scrotum: the genital skin sac that holds the testicles and related structures

semen: fluid produced by a man's prostate gland, which makes up 95 percent of the fluid that is ejaculated

sperm: a man's reproductive cells, made in the testicles; they carry the man's genetic traits to a woman's egg

*vas (*pl. *vasae):* the small, muscular tube that carries sperm from the testicle to the prostate gland

Indications and Procedures

The term *vasectomy*, literally meaning "cutting the tubes," describes a minor surgical procedure performed on a man who desires a permanent form of birth control. Vasectomy results in sterilization because it obstructs the passageway through which sperm travel to reach the female ovum. A man's testicles produce both male hormones (that stimulate male characteristics and sex drive) and sperm. A collection of small tubes called the epididymis along each testicle mature and deliver sperm to a single tube called the vas (or vas deferens), which is about the width of a spaghetti noodle. Each vas runs through the scrotum, up the groin on each side, and through the wall of the abdomen, ending in a storage area called the seminal vesicle, which is next to the prostate gland near the base of the penis. From there, the sperm mix with semen from the prostate gland and are expelled from the penis during ejaculation.

Vasectomy occludes (closes off) the vas to block the passage of sperm without affecting the important hormonal functions of the testicle. The surgery is done in the first, straight part of the vas, above the testicle and through the skin of the scrotum, making the procedure relatively easy and safe to perform.

Physicians performing vasectomy come from the specialties of urology, family medicine, general practice, or general surgery. Since the procedure is relatively simple, in comparison with other surgeries, physicians" expertise usually depends more on specific training and interest in performing vasectomies and following up on the procedure than on their particular specialty training.

Vasectomies are usually done on an outpatient basis, either in a physician's office or in a hospital-based or freestanding ambulatory surgery facility. Local anesthesia of the skin and the vasae is produced by an injection into the scrotum, which can be briefly uncomfortable until the medication has taken its full effect (usually after several seconds). Because of anxiety on the part of many men about having any discomfort in this area, many patients and physicians also choose to use sedation in the form of either tranquilizer pills or an injection for both mental and physical relaxation during vasectomy.

A number of techniques can be used safely and effectively by a physician performing a vasectomy, but the procedure can be thought of in terms of accomplishing three basic goals: The first is anesthesia, or the placement of numbing or freezing medication into the scrotum; the second is to gain access to the vas; and the third is its occlusion to prevent the passage of sperm.

Vasectomy can be made almost completely painless when local anesthesia in the form of medication such as lidocaine is used; this drug is similar to the anesthesia commonly used for dental procedures. By blocking the local nerves that send pain messages to the brain, normally painful procedures can be performed with little or no discomfort. A man having a vasectomy will feel the needle used to inject the medication into the skin and then a brief stinging sensation until it takes effect. The rest of the injection into the tubes themselves may or may not cause further discomfort, what some men describe as a pulling sensation.

The standard access procedure that the physician uses can vary with training and experience. It involves making either one incision into the scrotum in the middle of the front side or two incisions, one on either side. The incisions are made after the physician positions the vas directly under the skin, and then the other layers of tissue are separated to expose the vas itself. After each vas is occluded, the incision, which is between 1 and 1.5 centimeters long, must be closed with stitches, usually the type that dissolve and do not have to be removed.

A refinement of the access procedure, called the "no-scalpel" vasectomy, was introduced into the United States in the late 1980s. It originated in China in 1974, and a study comparing it with a standard technique found a more than 80 percent reduction in postoperative complications. It is being adopted only gradually by United States physicians, however, because performing it requires two simple but specially designed surgical instruments and because some physician retraining is required. Many physicians with experience in the new procedure believe that it should become the new standard for the vasectomy access procedure.

The occlusion of the vas is important because it determines the success of the vasectomy in preventing pregnancy. The physician can choose to occlude the vas ends by simple tying, folding back and tying, applying small metal clips, or cauterizing (burning with heat or special electrical current). In addition, one of the vas ends can be covered with a layer of the tissue that surrounds it to form a further barrier to sperm. Although all occlusion methods have been effective, cautery of the opening of the vasae may be the most reliable because it depends less on the technical precision of the physician doing the vasectomy than do the other methods, which can fail if applied too loosely or too tightly.

Finally, some physicians perform an open-ended technique, in which the end of the vas coming from the testicle is left open while only the outgoing end is occluded. This is thought to reduce the amount of backed-up sperm that can cause later complications and to make it easier to perform a

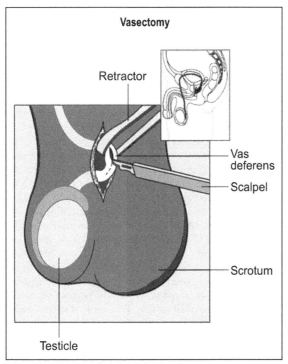

Vasectomy

Retractor

Vas deferens

Scalpel

Scrotum

Testicle

The most popular method of sterilization for men is vasectomy, which involves the severing of the vas deferens, the tube that transports sperm from the testes; the inset shows the location of the vas deferens in the male reproductive system.

vasectomy reversal. Some physicians believe, however, that the rate of vasectomy failure is higher with this technique.

Men from all over the world choose to have vasectomy performed, including about one-half million Americans every year. Vasectomy has been commonly available in the United States since the 1960s and is the fourth most commonly used birth control method overall, with one in eight women stating that they rely on this contraceptive method.

Some men who have undergone vasectomies choose, for various reasons, to reverse them. In such a reversal procedure, the patient, under general anesthesia, has a one- to two-inch incision made in the scrotum over the site of the previous vasectomy. The ends of the vas deferens are located and cut free of the surrounding scar tissue. A drop of fluid from the testicular end of the vas is placed on a glass slide and examined under an electronic microscope to determine precisely what kind of microsurgery is most appropriate.

Uses and Complications

Most physicians make recommendations to the patient about what should be done, or not done, following a vasectomy, including activity restriction, pain control strategies, and follow-up. A period of rest for about forty-eight hours after a vasectomy helps to prevent pain and complications such as postoperative bleeding into the scrotum, which causes swelling. All sexual activity should be avoided for up to a week. Many men find more relief from an ice pack applied to the scrotum for the first few days following the surgery than from any medication, although acetaminophen (such as Tylenol) or mild prescription narcotics are often helpful as well. Aspirin and ibuprofen, although effective for pain, are generally best avoided in the first few days following a vasectomy because they have a blood-thinning effect that may increase the tendency to bleed. Because aspirin has a longer-lasting blood-thinning effect on platelets (the small blood cells that initiate normal blood clotting and stop minor bleeding), it should also not be taken for about ten days prior to the vasectomy.

Follow-up with a physician should be available in case complications occur in the period immediately following the vasectomy. The physician must also check the semen to ensure that no sperm are present. If sperm remain, it may indicate that one or both vasae remain open or have grown back together, meaning that the procedure has failed and the man remains fertile. If there are no sperm in the semen three to six months after the vasectomy, then it is extremely unlikely that a failure can still occur. Most doctors do not recommend any further follow-up unless a problem arises.

Informed consent means that the patient who will undergo a treatment has been given the opportunity to understand the risks and benefits of that treatment. In the case of vasectomy, the risks are pain, complications, the chance that it will fail, and the possibility that there will be a change of heart and that the man will want to father more children. The benefit is having very reliable, safe, and permanent birth control without ongoing costs or effort required.

The complications of vasectomy are best thought of in

terms of those occurring early and late. Early complications include infection and hematoma. Infection is fairly uncommon but can include symptoms of pain, swelling, fever, redness, and abnormal drainage from the vasectomy wound. Treatment consists primarily of antibiotic medication. A hematoma is a collection of blood in a localized area such as the scrotum. Blood vessels in the scrotum that are cut or torn during vasectomy and not tied, clipped, or cauterized can ooze a small or large amount of blood. In the worst case, surgery to remove the blood may be considered to relieve pain and pressure. Fortunately, small hematomas resolve without surgery in a few weeks" time, and the more serious ones are rare, probably occurring in far less than 1 percent of vasectomies.

Later complications include problems with the area between the vasectomy incision and the testicles. Because the sperm are blocked from leaving the vas, and therefore the testicle, they can accumulate and cause three possible problems. First, sperm may back up at the site of the vasectomy and form a knot of sperm and inflamed scar tissue known as a sperm granuloma. It can be a painless lump, tender to pressure, or in rare cases it may be painful enough to require surgery to remove it. If swelling occurs because of accumulated sperm along the collecting area between the straight vas and the testicle (called the epididymis), the area can become tender or painful; this is known as congestive epididymitis. If this process extends backward to the testicle, it is known as orchitis. Fortunately, it is also rare for surgical removal of the entire epididymis to be required for relief of pain; sperm production slows in response to the pressure, and the body reabsorbs old sperm, eventually eliminating the pressure. Therefore, it is usually recommended that congestive epididymitis be treated with anti-inflammatory pain relievers such as ibuprofen, as well as with soaking in a warm bath.

Since there are many misconceptions about the risks and complications of vasectomy, it is useful to point out some problems that are not associated with the procedure. The complications of vasectomy are relatively minor and very rarely require hospitalization. Deaths and major surgical complications are largely unheard of. Impotence, loss of sexual drive, and changes in male characteristics such as beard growth, body hair, and voice do not occur. An apparent link between vasectomy and the hardening of the arteries that causes heart attacks has been disproven since the only such study was publicized in the late 1970s. Although a slight statistical association between vasectomy and cancer of the prostate gland was noted in two studies published in 1993, experts do not believe that vasectomy causes or contributes to prostate cancer because there is no reasonable mechanism for it to do so. Many men with milder forms of prostate cancer never die from it, and the statistics can be misleading because men who have seen a doctor for a vasectomy are also more likely to see a doctor for a prostate examination. Therefore, vasectomy may lead not to a greater risk of prostate cancer but to better detection of this disease.

Perspective and Prospects

Vasectomy has been performed to cause sterility since 1925, but its common use for that purpose started in the 1960s. The concepts of birth control and the desirability of limiting family size became increasingly valued in industrialized countries. Some states in the United States removed legal barriers to sterilization around this time, and the oral contraceptive or birth control pill became available to large numbers of women. These developments and the increased openness to discussion of sexual topics helped to form the basis for what was labeled the sexual revolution. In this environment, vasectomy became quite popular. It exceeded female sterilization by the early 1970s, driven in part by reports of the side effects of birth control pills. Sterilization for women (also called tubal ligation, literally "tying the tubes") is more invasive than vasectomy because the surgeon must enter the woman's abdomen to occlude the tubes that enable eggs to pass into her uterus. Therefore, vasectomy is somewhat safer when seen in the perspective of family planning. The women's movement of the 1960s placed a new emphasis on the control that women have over their bodies, especially in relation to health and medical decisions. Because the man can assume some of the reproductive responsibility and undergo a safer procedure, vasectomy also has a philosophical advantage for many couples.

Technological innovation by the mid-1970s had produced the first laparoscopic instruments, which enabled a gynecologic surgeon to enter a women's abdomen through two pencil-sized openings and identify and occlude her Fallopian tubes. This procedure, safer than the old one, with visibly smaller scars, and performed by obstetrician-gynecologists (the physicians whom women see most often), quickly became more popular than vasectomy and has remained so ever since. In spite of its high degree of safety, laparoscopic tubal ligation still occasionally results in deaths from general anesthesia and abdominal complications necessitating major surgery. Yet, even though tubal ligation costs three to five times more than vasectomy, it is still done more than twice as often. There are probably several reasons for this discrepancy, one of the most important being that when a woman has to make the sterilization decision alone, only tubal ligation can be chosen. When a woman is single or in a relationship with a lower level of commitment, or when there is a lack of consensus or support for the decision between the two partners, it is often easier for the woman to choose a tubal ligation. When a decision is made by a couple together, however, the risks and benefits give a comparative advantage to the male sterilization procedure.

When a couple makes a well-informed and mutual decision to choose vasectomy, the feelings in the months following the procedure most commonly include an increased sense of relaxation about sex because of lack of fear of unwanted pregnancy and an absence of anxiety and/or side effects related to contraceptive methods. On the other hand, if one of the partners was not ready and feels pressured into acceptance, the vasectomy decision can create irreconcilable conflict in the relationship.

Most doctors and clinics that counsel men about vasectomy emphasize the fact that vasectomy should be regarded

2350 • VENOUS INSUFFICIENCY

as permanent. Every year, thousands of men seek the reversal of their vasectomies. Although the vasae can be surgically "spliced" back together in a safe and minor operation called vasovasostomy, sometimes years after a vasectomy, there are many reasons not to expect a simple reversal of the procedure. Reversal is expensive and often not covered by medical insurance, and the chances of restored fertility (as measured by later pregnancy) are only about 50 percent. The odds of reversal can be improved if the surgeon (usually a urologist) has substantial experience in the procedure, a microsurgical technique is used, and the vasectomy was relatively recent, and perhaps if the open-ended technique was used as well.

Some highly experienced urologists claim a 95 percent success rate in reversals, so patients should be cautioned to seek out a urologist who has extensive experience in performing the procedure. Reversal certainly offers hope to someone who has undergone a divorce or personal tragedy and wants to start a new family, but an ambivalent couple should not be reassured that after vasectomy they can change their minds and easily reverse the procedure.

The decision process by a man or a couple to pursue a vasectomy for family planning reasons often begins years before the procedure is actually done. First, they must feel that they have completed their family and be aware of vasectomy as a birth control option. Dissatisfaction with other birth control methods because of inconvenience and real or feared side effects often presses the decision. Discussion about vasectomy with one or more patients who have had one is a very common prerequisite to the decision for many men. Finally, a scare that an unwanted pregnancy can occur—such as a late period or a broken condom discovered too late—or even an actual unplanned pregnancy itself may be the last straw for many couples. The high rates of satisfaction with vasectomy may be attributable to the strong sense of comfort that follows this long and thorough decision process.

—*John J. Seidl, M.D.;*
updated by R. Baird Shuman, Ph.D.

See also Contraception; Electrocauterization; Men's health; Reproductive system; Sterilization; Testicular surgery; Vas deferens.

For Further Information:

Connell, Elizabeth B. *The Contraception Sourcebook.* Chicago: Contemporary Books, 2002.

Denniston, George C. *Vasectomy.* Victoria, B.C.: Trafford, 2002.

Haldar, N., et al. "How Reliable Is a Vasectomy? Long-Term Follow-up of Vasectomised Men." *The Lancet* 356, no. 9223 (July 1, 2000): 43–44.

Health Library. "Vasectomy." *Health Library*, October 26, 2013.

MedlinePlus. "Vasectomy." *MedlinePlus*, May 20, 2013.

Miller, Karl E. "No-Scalpel Technique vs. Standard Incision." *American Family Physician* 61, no. 5 (March 1, 2000): 1464.

Parker, James N., and Philip M. Parker, eds. *The Official Patient's Sourcebook on Vasectomy.* [N. p.]: ICON Group, 2007.

Paulson, David. "Diary of a Vasectomy." *American Health* 12 (July, 1993): 70–75.

VENEREAL DISEASES. *See* **SEXUALLY TRANSMITTED DISEASES (STDs).**

VENOUS INSUFFICIENCY

Disease/Disorder

Anatomy or system affected: Blood vessels, circulatory system, legs

Specialties and related fields: Cardiology, vascular medicine

Definition: An abnormality characterized by decreased blood return from the legs to the trunk that is caused by inefficient valves in the veins.

Causes and Symptoms

Venous insufficiency can be either reversible (acute) or irreversible (chronic). It is caused by conditions that increase the amount of circulating blood combined with a decrease in venous flow and is most commonly manifested by thrombophlebitis, varicose veins, and leg ulcers. Thrombophlebitis and varicose veins may be reversible in acute insufficiency.

Thrombophlebitis is an inflammation of the vein, commonly occurring in the legs. It may impede blood flow, resulting in pain, tenderness, redness, warmth along the vein, and edema (swelling). Thrombi (clots) may also form, enlarge, break off, and produce an embolus (dislodged clot), obstructing circulation and causing death. Varicose veins are large, protruding, and painful veins unable to return blood adequately to the trunk as a result of inefficient valves. They may be caused by pregnancy, congenital valve or vessel defects, obesity, pressure from prolonged standing, and poor posture. Leg ulcers are open, draining, painful wounds resulting from an inadequate supply of oxygen and other nutrients. They may also develop on skin surrounding varicose veins because of the stasis (slowing or halting) of the blood flow.

Information on Venous Insufficiency

Causes: Conditions that increase amount of circulating blood and decrease venous flow (e.g., thrombophlebitis, varicose veins, leg ulcers)

Symptoms: Vary; may include achiness, swelling, blue or bulging veins

Duration: Acute or chronic

Treatments: Leg elevation, warm and moist heat, anticoagulants, elastic stockings or bandages, surgery, debridement

---

Treatment and Therapy

The treatment for thrombophlebitis includes rest; leg elevation; warm, moist heat to decrease pain and discomfort; and anticoagulant (blood-thinning) therapy to assist with circulation and to impede clot formation. Elastic stockings or bandages assist the return of blood to the heart. Drugs may be used to dissolve clots and to dilate vessels, improving circulation.

The conservative treatment of varicose veins includes the use of elastic stockings or bandages and rest. Aggressive treatment may include injecting the vein with sclerosing agents to occlude it and stop blood flow, thereby collapsing it.

Surgical treatment may include ligating (tying off) the vein and then stripping and removing it.

Leg ulcer treatment includes debridement (the chemical or surgical removal of dirt or dead cellular tissue), cleansing and dressing the wound with ointments, pressure bandages, and the application of medicated castlike (unna) boots. Skin grafting may be attempted if other measures are not effective.

—*John A. Bavaro, Ed.D., R.N.*

See also Circulation; Deep vein thrombosis; Edema; Embolism; Phlebitis; Thrombosis and thrombus; Ulcer surgery; Ulcers; Varicose vein removal; Varicose veins; Vascular medicine; Vascular system.

For Further Information:

Bergan, John J., and Jeffrey L. Ballard, eds. *Chronic Venous Insufficiency: Diagnosis and Treatment.* New York: Springer, 2000.

Carson-DeWitt, Rosalyn, and Michael J. Fucci. "Varicose Veins." *Health Library,* Mar. 13, 2013.

"Chronic Venous Insufficiency." *Vascular Disease Foundation,* Mar. 15, 2012.

Cohen, Barbara J., et al. *Memmler's The Human Body in Health and Disease.* 12th ed. Philadelphia: Wolters Kluwer Health/ Lippincott Williams & Wilkins, 2013.

Dugdale, David C. III, and David Zieve. "Deep Venous Thrombosis." *MedlinePlus,* Feb. 19, 2012.

Ernst, Calvin B., and James C. Stanley, eds. *Current Therapy in Vascular Surgery.* 4th ed. St. Louis, Mo.: Mosby, 2001.

Grossman, Neil, and David Zieve. "Venous Insufficiency." *MedlinePlus,* June 27, 2012.

Hershey, Falls B., Robert W. Barnes, and David S. Sumner, eds. *Noninvasive Diagnosis of Vascular Disease.* Pasadena, Calif.: Appleton Davies, 1984.

Loscalzo, Joseph, and Andrew I. Schafer, eds. *Thrombosis and Hemorrhage.* 3d ed. Philadelphia: Lippincott Williams & Wilkins, 2003.

Mohrman, David E., and Lois Jane Heller. *Cardiovascular Physiology.* 7th ed. New York: Lange Medical Books/McGraw-Hill, 2010.

VERTIGO

Disease/Disorder

Anatomy or system affected: Brain, ears, nervous system

Specialties and related fields: Audiology, neurology, otorhinolaryngology

Definition: A sensation of motion or spinning when not moving.

Key terms:

ataxia: coordinated movement difficulties

auditory nerve: the eighth cranial nerve, which conveys information from the ear to the brain

disequilibrium: off-balance sensation

dizziness: non-specific term that includes vertigo, fainting, and disequilibrium

electronystagmography: specialized eye movement measurements

endolymph: inner-ear fluid

labyrinth: mazelike system of canals in the inner ear

Ménière's disease: a disorder affecting endolymph

nystagmus: rhythmic involuntary movements of the eyes

oscillopsia: the sensation of bouncing vision

otoliths: granular bones of the inner ear

otorhinolaryngologist: the ear, nose, and throat (ENT) specialist

proprioception: the ability to locate the body in space

tinnitus: ringing in the ear

vestibular: the inner ear, vision, and nervous systems responsible for balance

Causes and Symptoms

Vertigo is a sensation of spinning or movement. Dizziness and disequilibrium are broader terms that include vertigo in some cases.

Vertigo results from disorders of the inner ear or central nervous system. Inner-ear causes include vestibular injury, labyrinthitis, vestibular neuritis, acute or recurrent vestibulopathy, benign positional vertigo, Ménière's disease, perilymphatic fistula, and vestibular toxicity from drugs. Labyrinthitis or vestibular nerve dysfunction can result from trauma, cancer (acoustic neuroma), benign tumor, infection, connective tissue disorders, autoimmune disorder, otosclerosis, or middle-ear infection. Central nervous system causes of vertigo include brain stem stroke, cervical vertigo, tumors adjacent to the brain stem, migraines, multiple sclerosis, cranial nerve injury or degeneration, seizure disorders, hereditary familial ataxia, and inflammatory paraneoplastic syndromes. Problems with peripheral nerves and vision can contribute to vertigo.

Three systems work together to provide balance. The first is the inner-ear labyrinth system of tiny canals filled with a fluid called endolymph and tiny bones called otoliths. These canals contain tiny hair cells that sense endolymph movement. Information from the inner ear is conveyed to the brain through the eighth cranial nerve (auditory nerve) as well as branches of the seventh cranial nerve (facial nerve). The second system, vision, provides information to the brain via the optic nerve. The third system is proprioception, the ability to orient the body in space using input from the musculoskeletal system and from peripheral nerves. Specialized areas of the brain process information from these three systems to provide balance and maintain the vestibular ocular reflex and the vestibular spinal reflex. Adaptation to variations in input from these systems allows for activities such as figure skaters being able to tolerate high-speed spins. Balance is also possible with just two of three balance systems, allowing normal individuals to stand with eyes closed and not lose balance.

Disruption of one or more balance systems causes vertigo.

Information on Vertigo

Causes: Inner ear or central nervous system disorders

Symptoms: Sensation of movement or spinning, sometimes accompanied by tinnitus, nausea, disequilibrium, clumsiness, ataxia

Duration: Varies depending on cause; may be episodic

Treatment: Depends on cause; may include otolith repositioning, inner ear surgery, low-salt diet, medications, vestibular rehabilitation therapy, treatment of underlying diseases

Additional symptoms may include tinnitus, disequilibrium, hearing loss, sensitivity to sound, nausea, blurred vision, oscillopsia, nystagmus, ataxia, clumsiness, or headaches. Symptoms of underlying disease may be present.

Onset and additional symptoms; examination of the ear, nose, and throat; and a general neurological examination will help in diagnosis. Specialized techniques include the Hallpike maneuver (tilting the head over the edge of the examination table) and the fistula test, done by plugging one ear. Testing may include complete eye examination, computed tomography (CT) scan, magnetic resonance imaging (MRI), electronystagmography, hearing test, and rotational chair testing. Diagnosis of the underlying disorder is necessary for treatment.

Treatment and Therapy

Treatment of vertigo depends on the cause. Ménière's disease and other inner-ear conditions such as vestibular neuronitis may be treated with a salt-restricted diet, diuretics, motion sickness medication, antinausea medication, steroid injections, lifestyle modification including stress reduction, or inner-ear surgery. Otolith repositioning involves specialized physical therapy maneuvers that may be helpful for benign positional vertigo. Perilymphatic fistula may respond to bed rest. Middle-ear infections are treated with antibiotics.

Vertigo requires treatment aimed at correcting the underlying disorder. For example, acoustic neuromas may be treated with surgery and radiation. Symptoms from multiple sclerosis may respond to oral or intravenous steroids.

Diagnosis and treatment of vertigo will require a team of specialists, including a family physician, otorhinolaryngologist, neurologist, audiologist, internist, physical therapist, and occupational therapist.

Vestibular rehabilitation treats vertigo and other balance and dizziness problems through adaptation. Because vision is an important part of the balance system, significant vision impairment might limit rehabilitation effectiveness. Exercises prescribed by a physical or occupational therapist target activities that are problematic and may be done at home, in a rehabilitation center, or both. Exercises include targeted movements such as bending over, walking with one foot in front of the other, or walking with the head turned. Rehabilitation can take several weeks to several months.

Perspective and Prospects

Vertigo and dizziness are common symptoms. Because of the variety of causes, some otolaryngologists and neurologists focus solely on the diagnosis and treatment of vertigo and dizziness.

Ménière's disease is the best-known cause of vertigo, first presented by Prospère Ménière to the French Academy of Medicine in 1861. Other inner-ear problems cause similar symptoms, but Ménière's disease specifically affects the endolymph fluid, causing vertigo and tinnitus. With modern diagnosis, Ménière's disease is now known to be less common than once thought.

Several famous people may have suffered from Ménière's disease or other forms of vertigo. Julius Caesar was said to have "falling disease" attributed to Ménière's disease or epilepsy. Other famous sufferers include artist Vincent Van Gogh, poet Emily Dickinson, and film star Marilyn Monroe.

Fortunately, vertigo does not usually indicate serious or life-threatening disease; however, it can take time and numerous tests to pinpoint the cause. With patience and persistence, most people can find a treatment or combination of treatments to reduce or eliminate their symptoms.

—E. E. Anderson Penno, M.D., M.S., FRCSC

See also Balance disorders; Brain; Brain disorders; Dizziness and fainting; Ear infections and disorders; Ears; Eye infections and disorders; Eyes; Hypotension; Ménière's disease; Vision; Vision disorders.

For Further Information:

Alan, Rick, and Kari Kassir. "Meniere's Disease." *Health Library*, Sept. 10, 2012.
"Causes of Dizziness." *Vestibular Disorders Association*, 2012.
"Dizziness and Vertigo." *MedlinePlus*, May 17, 2013.
Fauci, Anthony, et al. *Harrison's Principles of Internal Medicine*. 18th ed. New York: McGraw-Hill. 2012.
Jasmin, Luc, et al. "Vertigo-Associated Disorders." *MedlinePlus*, Nov. 2, 2012.
Poe, Dennis. *The Consumer Handbook on Dizziness and Vertigo*. Sedona, Ariz.: Auricle Ink, 2005.
Schroeder, Karen, and Rimas Lukas. "Vertigo." *Health Library*, Apr. 25, 2013.
West, John. *Best and Taylor's Physiological Basis of Medical Practice*. 12th ed. Baltimore: Williams & Wilkins, 1991.

VIRAL HEMORRHAGIC FEVERS

Disease/disorder

Anatomy or system affected: All
Specialties and related fields: Epidemiology, virology
Definition: Acute zoonotic diseases caused by viruses.
Key terms:

epidemiology: the study of the occurrence, frequency, causes, and distribution of diseases within a population

hemorrhagic: referring to a disease or disorder characterized by abnormal bleeding, often from internal organs, although bleeding may also occur under the skin, in the mucous linings of the nose and throat, and in tear ducts

reservoir species: animals that can carry a virus or bacterium that causes a disease in other species without suffering serious or fatal illness themselves

zoonoses: disorders carried by animal hosts that can be transmitted to humans

Causes and Symptoms

Viral hemorrhagic fevers are caused by a variety of viruses, including members of the *Arenaviridae, Bunyaviridae, Flaviviridae,* and *Filoviridae* families, with the last mentioned being the one associated with diseases such as Ebola hemorrhagic fever and Marburg hemorrhagic fever. Many of the hemorrhagic diseases are zoonoses that exist in reservoir species, such as bats, and are transmitted to humans through various modes; others are vector-borne. Crimean-Congo

Information on Viral Hemorrhagic Fevers

Causes: Viral infection
Symptoms: Fever, sore throat, generalized body aches, headache, vomiting, diarrhea, rash, red eyes
Duration: Varies depending on specific disease, from few days to several weeks
Treatments: Primarily supportive care to minimize suffering and alleviate symptoms

hemorrhagic fever, for example, is carried by ticks; humans become infected when they are bitten. In contrast, Ebola hemorrhagic fever, caused by a filovirus, is suspected of making the leap from animals to humans through the handling and eating of infected wild game, while Lujo fever, which is caused by an arenavirus, apparently infects humans when they inhale dust from rodent droppings. However, some viral hemorrhagic fevers may have the ability to aerosolize and thus may be transmitted person-to-person from an infected patient to caregivers or family members when an infected person sneezes or coughs. Contact with body fluids, such as blood or vomit, from an infected person can also cause the disease to spread.

The initial clinical signs and symptoms for viral hemorrhagic fevers are similar to those of many common illnesses, such as influenza or dysentery, with the patient complaining of a fever, headache, generalized aches and pains, or nausea. In the case of Ebola hemorrhagic fever, clinical signs may include a skin rash or red eyes. It is usually not until several days after the onset of the illness that the hemorrhagic signs, such as bloody diarrhea indicating internal bleeding, appear. Because the symptoms for many hemorrhagic fevers are similar to those of common tropical diseases, initial diagnosis and quarantine efforts may be delayed.

The virulence of the hemorrhagic fevers varies, depending both on the specific viral strain involved and how quickly medical treatment is obtained. Despite the name hemorrhagic fever, it is rarely the blood loss associated with the diseases that causes death but instead the failure of organs such as the kidneys. Some Ebola hemorrhagic fevers have resulted in death rates of close to 90 percent of infected patients, while others have been as low as 20 percent. Similarly, incubation periods vary for the different diseases, from only a few days for some diseases to as long as three weeks for others. The best-known hemorrhagic fever, Ebola, has an incubation period of two to twenty-one days.

Treatment and Therapy

Treatment for viral hemorrhagic fever varies from disease to disease. In many cases, the only care that can be given is that of relieving the suffering of the patient by treating the symptoms—giving liquids intravenously to replace fluids lost through vomiting or diarrhea, trying to keep electrolytes balanced, and giving drugs that may reduce the patient's fever or body aches. In some cases, patients have been successfully treated with blood transfusions from persons who have

survived a similar illness.

Because the exact transmission routes for many hemorrhagic fevers remain unclear, once patients are diagnosed, a strict quarantine must be instituted, with health care workers and family members alike wearing protective clothing to prevent becoming contaminated with any infectious material. When a patient dies, the body must also be handled carefully. In the case of Ebola, the World Health Organization (WHO) recommends burial or cremation as quickly as possible following death.

Perspective and Prospects

As the population has expanded globally and humans have encroached upon formerly isolated wildlife habitats, more viral hemorrhagic fevers have been discovered, sometimes through the case of just one or two persons becoming infected by a previously unknown pathogen and sometimes through devastating outbreaks resulting in many deaths. Despite many years of research, many of these diseases still remain scientific mysteries.

The best-known example, Ebola hemorrhagic fever virus, exists in multiple locations in Africa. Some strains are comparatively mild; some are extremely virulent, spreading quickly and causing high numbers of deaths within a population. Researchers now know that, as is true with many viruses, patients who have been infected by Ebola and survive retain antibodies to that strain of virus for decades. They do not yet know if that means those people are effectively immune to Ebola.

Theoretically, it should be possible to develop vaccines against the viral hemorrhagic diseases, but several factors mitigate such work. First is the reality that although many can be quite devastating in terms of death rates, outbreaks that have occurred to date have been in remote areas or have affected very low numbers of persons. It is easy to argue for funding vaccine research work when a disease is widespread, as in the historical example of polio; it becomes much more difficult for researchers when the disease in question is localized in a nonindustrialized country such as the Sudan or Uganda. In recent years, the threat of viruses such as Ebola being utilized for bioterrorism, however, has led to more effort being put into finding effective vaccines and treatments, but for most of the viral hemorrhagic diseases any vaccines or treatments developed to date remain classified as experimental.

—Nancy Farm Mannikko, Ph.D.

See also Bleeding; Centers for Disease Control and Prevention (CDC); Dengue fever; Ebola virus; Emerging infectious diseases; Epidemics and pandemics; Epidemiology; Hemorrhage; Marburg virus; Tropical medicine; Viral infections; Zoonoses.

For Further Information:
"Ebola Haemorrhagic Fever." *World Health Organization*, Aug. 2012.
"Hemorrhagic Fevers." *MedlinePlus*, May 20, 2013.
"Haemorrhagic Fevers, Viral." *World Health Organization*, Jan. 2013.
Hewlitt, Barry S., and Bonnie L. Hewitt. *Ebola, Culture, and*

Politics: The Anthropology of an Emerging Disease. Belmont, Calif.: Thomson Higher Education, 2008.

Shors, Teri. *Understanding Viruses.* 2d ed. Sudbury, Mass.: Jones and Bartlett, 2013.

Strauss, James H., and Ellen G. Strauss. *Viruses and Human Disease.* 2d ed. San Diego, Calif.: Academic Press, 2008.

"Viral Hemorrhagic Fevers." *Centers for Disease Control and Prevention,* Nov. 22, 2011.

VIRAL INFECTIONS

Disease/Disorder

Anatomy or system affected: All

Specialties and related fields: Epidemiology, family medicine, internal medicine, virology

Definition: A wide range of diseases, from mild (such as the common cold) to fatal (such as rabies, smallpox, and AIDS), caused by viruses, life-forms that function as intracellular parasites.

Key terms:

capsid: the protein coat of a virus, composed of subunits known as capsomeres

envelope: an additional covering found on animal viruses; it is composed of lipids and proteins and surrounds the genome and the protein coat of the virus

genome: the genetic material of a virus; in a virion, the genome consists of deoxyribonucleic acid (DNA) or ribonucleic acid (RNA) and is protected by the capsid

lysogenic (temperate) virus: a virus that integrates its genome into the genome of the host cell; such viruses exist in a latent state and do not produce progeny viruses

lytic virus: a virus that guides the production of progeny viruses and that ultimately causes the death and lysis (disintegration) of the host cell

virion: the form of the virus as it exists outside the host cell

How Viruses Work

Viruses are entities that infect the cells of all organisms. Some scientists classify viruses as living organisms based on their ability to reproduce inside an appropriate host cell. Yet, viruses lack cellular structure and have no metabolic capability of their own. They are completely dependent on host cells to reproduce. In addition, some viruses can be crystallized and thus have properties of complex molecules rather than of living organisms.

Viruses can be visualized only with an electron microscope. They are small in size, ranging from approximately 10 to 300 nanometers in either length or diameter. Because viruses cannot easily be seen within the host cells that they infect, studies of viral structure often utilize the extracellular form of the virus, called the viral particle or virion.

Viruses are quite variable with respect to size, shape, and biological properties, but they do have some common features. All viruses contain a genome, which is genetic material in the form of either deoxyribonucleic acid (DNA) or ribonucleic acid (RNA). A protein coat known as a capsid that is composed of protein subunits called capsomeres protects the genome of a virus. The capsid is arranged either into a symmetrical structure with spherical (round) or up to twenty-sided (icosahedral) symmetry. Alternatively, the capsid can assume a helical shape.

Some viruses contain additional protein structures that aid in their attachment and penetration of host cells. Other viruses, especially the ones that infect animal cells, are surrounded by a complex membrane structure known as the envelope. While the lipids in the envelope are derived from host cells, the proteins and glycoproteins contained in the envelope are usually viral-specific structures that are encoded by the genetic material of the virus. In animal viruses, the genetic material and protein coat, together called the nucleocapsid, constitute the core of the virus. In addition to these features, some viruses carry enzymes that are necessary for the virus to infect a host cell or to replicate.

Most viruses can infect only one type of host; that is, they display species specificity. The virus that causes rabies is a notable exception since it can infect a variety of mammalian species. All types of organisms—bacteria, protozoa, fungi, plants, and animals—are known to be hosts to viruses. Viruses that infect bacteria are called bacteriophages, or phages. The elucidation of many of the aspects of viral structure and the stages of viral infection was derived from the study of the mechanism by which phages infect their specific bacterial hosts.

Slow virus diseases are a class of viruses that reproduce very slowly, often over months or years. They are difficult to study. A common result of slow virus infections is a condition called spongiform encephalopathy, which is a degeneration of brain cells that ultimately causes death. Recent research has shown that slow viruses cause such diseases as kuru and Creutzfeldt-Jakob disease (CJD) in humans and scrapie in sheep.

Several steps have been identified in the process by which viruses infect host cells. Because they lack motility, viruses must come into contact with host cells by chance. They are transmitted from host to host in the same ways as other microorganisms: through air, water, or food or by physical contact. A common mode of transmission is by aerosols produced when an infected individual coughs, sneezes, or breathes. Virions in the aerosols gain access to the host by means of the respiratory system. Common cold and influenza viruses are transmitted in this manner, as are the viruses that cause common childhood diseases such as chickenpox, measles, and mumps. As a result, these viruses are very contagious; they are easily spread from person to person.

Some viruses, such as the poliomyelitis (polio) virus, can be transmitted in contaminated food or water. The virus gains entry to the host through the mouth and digestive system. Other viruses will also gain entry after contact, which may be direct (person to person) or indirect (via an inanimate object). Viruses will also enter a host if they are directly introduced into the bloodstream, which can occur via a cut or wound or through use of a contaminated needle. Hepatitis B virus and the human immunodeficiency virus (HIV), which causes acquired immunodeficiency syndrome (AIDS), can infect individuals in this manner. Transmission of these viruses occurs

Information on Viral Infections

Causes: Exposure to viruses, usually through contact with infected humans, animals, or vectors
Symptoms: Wide ranging; may include rash, fever, muscle aches, headaches, pain, sore throat
Duration: Acute to chronic
Treatments: Antiviral agents, supportive therapy

at a high rate among intravenous drug users who share needles. In addition to the above methods of transmission, mosquitoes may transmit viruses such as the encephalitis virus and the yellow fever virus.

All viruses must first attach themselves to their respective host cells. This phase of viral infection is sometimes referred to as adsorption. The attachment process is very specific and is controlled (mediated) by receptors present on the host cell, most of which are glycoproteins. It is the specific nature of this attachment process that accounts for the fact that a virus will infect host cells of only one species. Some viruses are also specific for the type of host cell to which they will adsorb. For example, poliovirus adsorbs only to cells of the central nervous system and gastrointestinal tract.

Following adsorption, the virus penetrates the host cell. In the case of bacteriophages, only the viral genome reaches the interior of the host cell; the protein coat of the virus remains outside. In contrast, the entire animal virus penetrates its host cell. Once inside, the viral genome is separated from the protein coat and envelope. During this stage of viral infection, the virus cannot be visualized by electron microscopy.

The viral genome is responsible for the next stages of viral infection. Many viruses begin a process that will eventually result in the replication of the viral genome and the production of progeny viruses. These viruses are referred to as lytic viruses because the death and lysis of the host cell accompany infection. The infecting lytic virus uses many of the host cell's biochemical processes to replicate its DNA or RNA. It also causes the host to make proteins that will constitute the capsids of the newly made viruses. New viral particles assemble spontaneously. In many cases, hundreds of these progeny will be released as the host cell disintegrates. These newly produced viruses are then available to infect other cells. This type of virus causes diseases such as chickenpox and polio. In some cases, progeny viruses are continuously shed from host cells. The host cell remains viable for long periods of time and releases large numbers of viruses.

Some viruses do not produce progeny after they penetrate host cells. Instead of being used to produce new viruses, the genetic material of these viruses becomes part of the host cell genome in a process called integration. These viruses are referred to as lysogenic or temperate viruses. In order for these viruses to integrate into the host cell genome, they must either consist of double-stranded DNA or be capable of forming double-stranded DNA within the host cell. RNA viruses that are capable of lysogeny contain an enzyme known as reverse transcriptase that enables the virus to produce a DNA copy of the viral RNA. These viruses are known as retroviruses. Several medically important viruses, such as some tumor viruses and HIV, belong to this category.

Although integrated into the viral genome, lysogenic viruses do not multiply to produce new viral particles. They remain in an apparently latent state. There is evidence, however, that these viruses can make some types of protein and, in some cases, can alter the properties of their host cells. For example, when a virus called SV40 integrates into the genome of certain host cells, it will cause these cells to divide rapidly and grow in a manner that resembles tumor cells. Not all lysogenic viruses remain latent. Ultraviolet light is known to cause latent herpesvirus to switch to a lytic mode of infection, an effect known as induction. Other factors, such as stress, may also be responsible for viral induction.

Diagnosis and Treatment

The extent of a viral disease can usually be explained by the biological properties of the particular virus involved. Some viral infections may be mild, such as the common cold, or entirely unnoticed. Other viral infections can be more serious, debilitating, or even fatal, such as polio, influenza, and AIDS. In some cases, viral infection is acute; an individual is sick for a short period of time and then fully recovers. Other viral infections are chronic; the virus persists for long periods of time. The disease that it causes periodically erupts and then subsides.

Diagnosis of viral diseases often relies on an analysis of the symptoms associated with each type of viral infection. Some viral illnesses cause typical rashes such as those seen in chickenpox, measles, and rubella. Influenza virus infection results in typical flulike symptoms, including throat pain, fever, and muscle aches. It is much more difficult to diagnose viral infections when the virus is latent or not actively causing damage to the host. Sometimes it is important to detect individuals who are infected with a latent virus or who are not symptomatic. Such individuals may be carriers of the virus and thus have the potential to transmit the disease to others. It is possible to identify such individuals by testing for the presence of viral proteins or by examining their immune response to the virus.

The major host defense against viral infections in higher organisms is the immune system. Cells of the immune system recognize many disease-causing viruses, either as virions circulating within the host or by the presence of virus-specific proteins on infected host cells. In either case, the virus is eliminated, although damage to host cells is sometimes a natural consequence of this type of protection. This active immune response against the virus will often result in lifelong protection from subsequent infections by the same virus. It is extremely rare for a person who has recovered from measles or mumps to have another occurrence of that particular disease.

Some viruses are not completely eliminated when recovery occurs. Varicella zoster virus is the cause of chickenpox, a common childhood disease. Chickenpox usually runs its course in about two weeks, and complete clinical recovery is observed. Yet, the virus is not necessarily eliminated. It has been tracked to the nervous system, where it can remain dormant for decades. The virus can be reactivated, usually in older adults or in those individuals whose immune systems are compromised. It will travel via the nerves and cause shingles (herpes zoster). Shingles is a condition characterized by a burning rash, itching, tingling, and pain that may be quite severe.

Vaccines. Vaccines protect against viral infections by utilizing the host's own immune system. For use in vaccines, the virus is either inactivated, and thus is no longer capable of

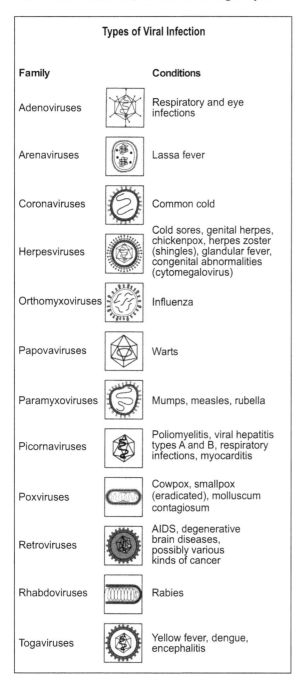

Types of Viral Infection

Family		Conditions
Adenoviruses		Respiratory and eye infections
Arenaviruses		Lassa fever
Coronaviruses		Common cold
Herpesviruses		Cold sores, genital herpes, chickenpox, herpes zoster (shingles), glandular fever, congenital abnormalities (cytomegalovirus)
Orthomyxoviruses		Influenza
Papovaviruses		Warts
Paramyxoviruses		Mumps, measles, rubella
Picornaviruses		Poliomyelitis, viral hepatitis types A and B, respiratory infections, myocarditis
Poxviruses		Cowpox, smallpox (eradicated), molluscum contagiosum
Retroviruses		AIDS, degenerative brain diseases, possibly various kinds of cancer
Rhabdoviruses		Rabies
Togaviruses		Yellow fever, dengue, encephalitis

causing an infection, or infectious but of a much milder strain. Viruses are commonly inactivated for vaccine preparation by chemical treatments that essentially kill the virus. The virus is then no longer able to infect and multiply within host cells. These types of vaccines must be administered at repeated time intervals (months or years, depending on the vaccine) to ensure a sufficient level of immunity.

Live viruses are used in some vaccines, but the harmful or pathogenic form of the virus is never employed. Instead, a weaker version of the virus is selected. These weaker variants, called attenuated strains, can sometimes be found when the virus is grown under laboratory conditions. The advantage of live viral vaccines is that the virus can multiply within the host and cause a significantly higher stimulation of the host's immune system than is usually seen with inactivated viral vaccines. Attenuated strains of the poliovirus are used to produce the oral polio vaccine that is commonly administered to infants. In rare cases, serious problems do occur with live vaccines. A few individuals among the millions who have been vaccinated, or their family contacts, have been known to develop polio as a result of exposure to the live polio vaccine.

Another method of vaccine preparation involves the use of parts of the viral envelope, particularly the viral-coded proteins. These proteins can be mass-produced using modern genetic engineering technology and then incorporated into various vaccine preparations. This method has the advantage of reducing the risks involved with live vaccines.

The important result of vaccination is that the immune system is stimulated to recognize the virus and thus eliminate its harmful form when the virus is next encountered. Vaccination programs have been highly effective in decreasing the incidence of viral diseases in countries where they are administered. The most striking success of a major vaccination program was the virtual global elimination of naturally occurring smallpox, declared official by the World Health Organization in 1980.

For some viral infections, the immune system does not offer adequate protection from the harmful effects of the virus. In still other cases, effective vaccines that offer long-term protection against viral infection have not been developed. With some viral infections, an encounter with the virus does not guarantee immunity from future infections: the virus is able to alter its envelope proteins and thus appears different to the immune system when it is encountered again. This is the case with influenza viruses.

Chemical agents. Chemical antiviral agents have also been developed. These chemical agents have been useful because they limit or inhibit important steps in the viral reproductive cycle. For example, acyclovir inhibits the replication of viral DNA in herpesviruses. Among the problems encountered with the use of these chemical agents, however, are their restricted action (they work only for certain viruses) and their toxic effects on the host.

A naturally produced agent with antiviral activity is interferon. Interferon is actually a group of proteins produced by the host during a viral infection. These proteins are active only in the host species in which they are produced. They have the ability to interfere with viral multiplication and are therefore potentially useful agents in the treatment of viral infection and certain human cancers.

Cancer and viruses. The link between viruses and cancer, induced in experimental animals, was established in the early part of the twentieth century. The role of viruses as causative agents of human cancers has been less conclusive. Many viruses are associated with human cancers. They are often integrated into the genomes of cancer cells. Yet, the presence of a virus and its association with a certain type of cancer do not constitute proof that the virus is actually responsible for the cancerous condition. There is evidence that a type of liver cancer, hepatocellular carcinoma, may be caused by hepatitis B or C virus. A specific form of leukemia has been linked to human T-cell leukemia viruses. The Epstein-Barr virus is associated with a rare type of cancer, Burkitt's lymphoma. Viruses may be involved in many other types of human cancer, along with other genetic and environmental factors.

The growing evidence for the involvement of viruses in human cancers, either directly or indirectly, provides further impetus for developing an understanding of the biology of these viruses, as well as methods to protect individuals from infection. Molecular biologists continue to elucidate the strategies by which cancer viruses gain entry into host cells and alter the properties and functions of these cells. Understanding such events will provide important clues that could be utilized to interrupt the processes that cause normal cells to become cancer cells.

Prevention. Very few antiviral agents have proven effective in combating viral illnesses. One of the best approaches in dealing with viral infection is prevention. This can be accomplished by identifying the mode of transmission of the virus and developing measures to block the transmission whenever possible. The most powerful method of preventing viral diseases, however, is through the use of vaccines to immunize individuals against viral infection. Vaccine programs have been tremendously successful in eliminating smallpox worldwide and in greatly reducing the number of new cases of polio and chickenpox throughout the Western Hemisphere and Europe. Continued efforts are needed to produce safe and effective vaccines. These vaccines must also be stable and easily administered so that they can be used in parts of the world where populations need protection from serious viral diseases.

Preventive measures cannot be used in all cases. For example, it is extremely difficult to block the transmission of viruses that are carried in the air. There are also many viral diseases for which safe vaccines may not be available. Furthermore, some viruses are able to evade the immune defenses of the host, thus greatly reducing the usefulness of a vaccine. The influenza virus has a strategy for escaping detection by the host's immune system. This virus is able to alter its envelope proteins so that the newer forms are no longer recognized by the immune system of an individual who has recovered from a previous bout with the flu. Thus, an individual who has had one strain of flu is susceptible to another occurrence of the illness caused by a different strain. Although flu vaccines have been developed, their usefulness is limited by the changing nature of the virus.

Perspective and Prospects

From their discovery as the causative agent of tobacco mosaic disease in the late 1890s by the Dutch microbiologist Martinus Beijernick, viruses have been implicated in numerous plant and animal diseases. Human diseases caused by viruses range from very mild to fatal and are often difficult to treat. Epidemics caused by viruses have plagued humankind for centuries. Outbreaks of smallpox, polio, yellow fever, and other viral diseases were once quite commonplace. Viral illnesses such as influenza still appear yearly in epidemic proportions. A severe worldwide outbreak of influenza was responsible for the deaths of twenty million people between 1918 and 1919.

The virus that causes AIDS, the human immunodeficiency virus (HIV), has the potential to cause millions of deaths worldwide. It is spread relatively easily, and the time between exposure and apparent disease can be a decade or longer. Many experts are working to create a vaccine for HIV/AIDS.

—*Barbara Brennessel, Ph.D.; updated by L. Fleming Fallon, Jr., M.D., Ph.D., M.P.H.*

See also Acquired immunodeficiency syndrome (AIDS); Adenoviruses; Avian influenza; Cancer; Canker sores; Chickenpox; Childhood infectious diseases; Chlamydia; Chronic fatigue syndrome; Cold sores; Common cold; Coronaviruses; Cytomegalovirus (CMV); Diarrhea and dysentery; Disease; Ebola virus; Emerging infectious diseases; Encephalitis; Enteroviruses; Epidemics and pandemics; Epidemiology; Epstein-Barr virus; Fever; Fifth disease; Hand-foot-and-mouth disease; Hanta virus; Hepatitis; Herpes; H1N1 influenza; Human immunodeficiency virus (HIV); Human papillomavirus (HPV); Infection; Influenza; Insect-borne diseases; Keratitis; Marburg virus; Measles; Microbiology; Monkeypox; Mononucleosis; Mumps; Nausea and vomiting; Noroviruses; Parasitic diseases; Pelvic inflammatory disease (PID); Pityriasis rosea; Poliomyelitis; Pulmonary diseases; Rabies; Retroviruses; Rheumatic fever; Rhinoviruses; Roseola; Rotavirus; Rubella; Severe acute respiratory syndrome (SARS); Sexually transmitted diseases (STDs); Shingles; Smallpox; Tonsillitis; Viral hemorrhagic fevers; Warts; West Nile virus; Yellow fever; Zoonoses.

For Further Information:
Biddle, Wayne. *A Field Guide to Germs.* 3d ed. New York: Anchor Books, 2010.
Centers for Disease Control and Prevention, May 2013.
Collier, Leslie, John Oxford, and Paul Kellam. *Human Virology.* 4th ed. New York: Oxford University Press, 2011.
Fettner, Ann Giudici. *The Science of Viruses: What They Are, Why They Make Us Sick, How They Will Change the Future.* New York: Quill/William Morrow, 1993.
Garrett, Laurie. *The Coming Plague: Newly Emerging Diseases in a World out of Balance.* New York: Penguin, 1995.
Henig, Robin Marantz. *A Dancing Matrix: Voyages Along the Viral Frontier.* New York: Vintage Books, 1994.
Knipe, David M., and Peter M. Howley, et al, eds. *Fields" Virology.* 5th ed. Philadelphia: Wolters Kluwer Health/Lippincott Williams & Wilkins, 2007.
Montagnier, Luc, and Stephen Sartarelli. *Virus: The Co-Discoverer of HIV Tracks Its Rampage and Charts the Future.* New York: W. W. Norton, 2000.
"Overview of Viral Infections." *Merck Manual Home Health Handbook*, Nov. 2009.

Radetsky, Peter. *The Invisible Invaders: Viruses and the Scientists Who Pursue Them.* Rev. ed. Boston: Little, Brown, 1994.

Regush, Nicholas. *The Virus Within: A Coming Epidemic.* New York: Plume, 2001.

Robertson, Erle S., ed. *Cancer Associated Viruses.* New York: Springer, 2012.

Ryan, Frank. *Virus X: Tracking the New Killer Plagues out of the Present and into the Future.* New York: Little, Brown, 1998.

Sompayrac, Lauren. *How Pathogenic Viruses Work.* Boston: Jones and Bartlett, 2002.

Strauss, James, and Ellen Strauss. *Viruses and Human Disease.* 2d ed. Boston: Academic Press/Elsevier, 2008.

"Viral Infections." *MedlinePlus*, May 23, 2013.

"Viruses." *Microbe World.* American Society for Microbiology, 2012.

Wagner, Edward K., and Martinez J. Hewlett. *Basic Virology.* 3d ed. Malden, Mass.: Blackwell Science, 2008.

VISION

Biology

Also known as: Eyesight, sight

Anatomy or system affected: Eyes, nervous system

Specialties and related fields: Neurology, ophthalmology, plastic surgery

Definition: One of five special senses. Light enters the eye and is then focused through specialized structures onto the retina, which responds with chemical reactions translating light into nerve impulses that travel to the brain to be interpreted as images.

Key terms:

anterior chamber: the space between the cornea and lens; filled with aqueous

aqueous: watery fluid in the anterior chamber

blindness: legally in the United States, vision less than 20/200 or peripheral vision less than 20 degrees

cones: specialized photoreceptors that sense color and detailed vision in bright light

cornea: the clear central structure on the front of the eye analogous to a vehicle windshield

diplopia: double vision

iris: the colored part of the eye; acts like a shutter to let in more or less light

low vision: impairment of vision requiring visual aids

optic nerve: the largest nerve in the body; takes information from retina to brain

photoreceptors: specialized cells that translate light into electrical information, which is transferred via nerves to the brain

refractive error: a condition requiring corrective lenses

retina: the multilayered structure lining the back of the eye; functions like camera film to sense light and transfer images to the brain

rhodopsin: a chemical within photoreceptors that translates light into electrical impulses

rods: specialized photoreceptors that provide peripheral vision and vision in dim light

strabismus: muscle imbalance between eyes

vitreous: a clear gel that fills the back of the eye between the lens and the retina

Structure and Functions

Vision is one of five special senses. Vision provides information about the environment and is important in balance. Loss of vision limits activities but is not life-threatening. "Low vision" is a term to describe partial vision loss that can be treated with visual aids such as magnifiers. The word "blind" is often used incorrectly. Criteria for legal blindness varies from country to country and is less than 20/200 in the United States. No light perception means that there is no vision at all.

The most common method to measure vision is the standard eye chart. A vision of 20/20 is considered normal vision. This means that at a standard distance of twenty feet, a person can read a specific line on a standardized eye chart. Vision of 20/40 means that the individual has to be at a distance of twenty feet to see what normally can be seen at forty feet. When the second number is less than twenty—for example, 20/15—then the vision is better than 20/20.

Other vision functions can also be measured. Color vision measures the ability to distinguish colors. Red-green color blindness is the most common color deficit. Contrast sensitivity measures the ability to distinguish shades of gray. It is possible to read 20/20 but to have reduced visual function, such as reduced contrast sensitivity, which would make it difficult to do activities in low light. Stereo vision is made possible by the two eyes working together. Stereo vision is important for tasks such as threading a needle. If vision is impaired in one eye, then stereo vision is reduced. If vision is similar in the two eyes but they are not aligned properly, then double vision (diplopia) results. Peripheral vision is the ability to see to the sides and is measured by visual field testing. Finally, the lens in the eye can focus but becomes weak with age. Focus ability allows the vision to transition between near and far. By forty years or older, the focus ability is usually weak enough that bifocal or reading glasses are needed.

The process of vision begins when light enters the eye. Light travels first through the clear central cornea, which is analogous to a car windshield. The cornea is approximately 550 microns thick at its thinnest central point. Corneal structure includes collagen connective tissue molecules that are aligned to allow for the cornea to be clear. Light rays entering the eye are parallel and must be focused to allow for vision to be possible. The corneal curvature begins the process of bending the light rays to bring them into focus on the retina at the back of the eye. The cornea provides the majority of focusing power for the eye.

After the cornea, light traverses the anterior chamber, which is filled with a watery substance called aqueous. The anterior chamber is the space between the iris (the colored part of the eye) and the cornea. Light will then travel through the pupil, the space in the center of the iris. The iris is similar to the shutter in a camera and will expand and constrict to let more or less light into the eye. The pupil usually looks dark because the light enters this space but does not exit. The exception is when light bounces off the retina and exits through the pupil, such as happens with red-eye effect from a camera flash.

Behind the iris is the lens. The lens focuses light onto the

Anatomy of the Eye

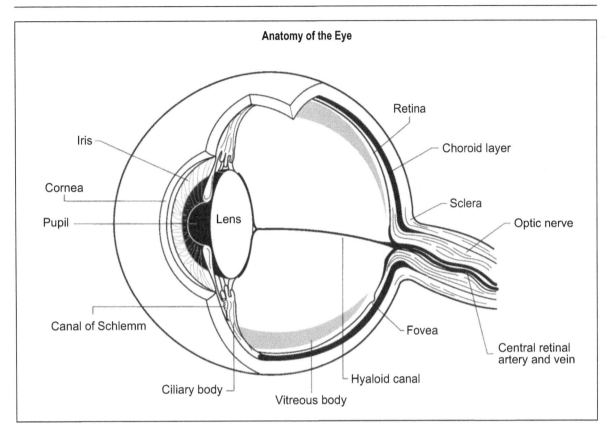

retina and allows for the transition of vision between far and near. The change in focus, called accommodation, decreases with age. After passing through the lens of the eye, the light enters the posterior chamber, which is filled with a clear gel called vitreous. The posterior chamber is the space between the lens and the retina.

The retina lines the back of the eye and contains approximately 120 million specialized cells called photoreceptors. Photoreceptors around the peripheral retina are called rods and are important for peripheral vision and night vision. The central part of the retina is called the macula, and at the center of the macula is the fovea, which is the most sensitive to color and provides sharp central acuity. The fovea contains approximately 35,000 photoreceptors called cones and no rods. There are about twenty rods for each cone.

The layers of the retina include the pigment epithelium, outer segments of the photoreceptor cells, outer nuclear layer, outer plexiform layer, inner nuclear layer, inner plexiform layer, ganglion cell layer, and axon layer. Underneath the retina is the choroid vascular, which provides blood flow to the retina. Retinal veins and arteries also nourish the retina. There are no blood vessels in the fovea.

When light strikes the retina, a molecule within the photoreceptors called rhodopsin undergoes a chemical structural change from a *cis* to a *trans* configuration. This hyperpolarizes the cell, causing an increase in negative charge. The cells within the retina have a hierarchy of on-cen-

ter and off-center receptive fields that interact to distinguish gradations of light intensity and color. These electrical messages are passed from the photoreceptor cells to bipolar cells and then to ganglion cells. The ganglion cells then communicate with the visual areas of the brain via the optic nerve.

After light is translated into neural information by retinal cells, information from each eye travels through the optic nerve to the optic chiasm. At the chiasm, the two nerves meet and the central half of each set of nerve fibers crosses and joins with fibers from the fellow eye. The neural pathways continue in parallel to the right and left brain, along the optic tract to the lateral geniculate nucleus and to the primary visual cortex. The visual cortex provides an interpretation of the visual images from each eye and fuses them into a single image. A stroke to these areas of the brain will cause an identical defect to the opposite side of the vision in each eye. For example, a right stroke will cause a left field defect that will affect both eyes.

Each eye, also called the globe, is about twenty-four millimeters long and can distinguish light from three hundred nanometers (near ultraviolet) to two thousand nanometers (near infrared). The globes are positioned within the bony space within the skull called the orbit. Orbital bones are particularly strong around the orbital rim but very thin and weaker toward the back of the orbital roof and orbital floor. This feature protects the eye from trauma, as the orbital bones will fracture before the eye is ruptured. This is called a blowout fracture.

The orbit contains fatty tissue, connective tissue, the lacrimal gland (important for tearing), and the extraocular muscles. Six extraocular muscles are attached to each eye to provide the ability of the eyes to move synchronously. The inferior oblique, inferior rectus, medial rectus, superior rectus, iris, and lid are supplied by the third nerve. Injury to the third nerve can lead to diplopia, ptosis (droopy lid), and pupil abnormalities. The lateral rectus is supplied by the sixth cranial nerve, and the superior oblique is supplied by the fourth cranial nerve. The oblique muscles provide rotational movement. The extraocular muscles coordinate the eyes to provide a single image. An imbalance of muscles can cause diplopia.

The orbit is covered by the eyelids. To maintain clear vision, the cornea must be covered with a film of tears. If the cornea becomes too dry or swollen, then it will lose clarity. Disorders of the lacrimal gland and lid disorders can lead to dry eyes, which will impair vision. The lids, lacrimal gland, extraocular muscles, structures within the eye, optic nerve, and brain must all be working properly to provide normal vision.

Disorders and Diseases

Numerous diseases and disorders can affect vision. The most common disorders are nearsightedness (myopia), farsightedness (hyperopia), and astigmatism, which can be corrected by glasses and contact lenses.

A nearsighted eye is too long or the cornea is too steep, which results in the light from a distance coming to a focal point in front of the retina. The farsighted eye is too short or the cornea is too flat, and light from a distance will come to a focal point past the retina. Astigmatism usually means the cornea is not spherical but is shaped more like a football, with two different radii of curvature. In the astigmatic eye, light from a distance will have two focal points, which results in a tilted image. Refractive errors can be treated with glasses, contact lenses, or laser vision correction.

Uncorrected refractive error or other childhood conditions can lead to amblyopia, also known as a lazy eye. If these problems are not corrected before age seven, then the eye will not develop the proper neural connections and vision is permanently reduced. Treatment with surgery, glasses, or patching can help many patients with amblyopia.

Strabismus is also called a wandering eye or squint. Strabismus commonly develops in childhood and causes an eye turn. Adult causes of strabismus include stroke, thyroid orbitopathy, or trauma. Strabismus can lead to amblyopia in a child or diplopia. Prism glasses, patching, or surgery may be recommended.

The focus ability of the lens, accommodation, decreases with age, resulting in the need for reading glasses or a bifocal eyeglass for reading sometime after the age of forty. Other common eye diseases include cataract, glaucoma, and macular degeneration. Cataract is clouding of the lens and is treated by cataract removal (removal of the lens of the eye) and replacement with a clear lens implant. Glaucoma can be hereditary and involves the loss of peripheral vision due to damage to the optic nerve as a result of high eye pressure.

Glaucoma can also occur with a normal pressure and, if not treated, will result in tunnel vision. Macular degeneration may be hereditary and can lead to the loss of central vision. Vitamins, injections, and laser treatment may sometimes be helpful in the treatment of macular degeneration.

Numerous other eye disorders and diseases can lead to a partial or complete loss of vision. Healthy lifestyle choices such as not smoking, eating a healthy diet, and exercising may help prevent many eye disorders. Eye examination by a qualified optometrist or ophthalmologist in childhood and routinely throughout life can aid in the early detection of eye disorders. Eye disorders can often be prevented or treated if detected early.

Perspective and Prospects

Millions of people are affected by eye disorders and injury, and billions of dollars are spent each year on such things as contact lenses and cataract surgery to correct these issues. Many eye injuries can be prevented with the proper protective eyewear for sports and other activities, such as using power tools.

Vision has fascinated scientists and writers since classical Greek writers theorized that vision was made possible by light rays emanating from the eyes. Other theories included a process by which images send copies of themselves to the eye. It was the work of Johannes Kepler, Galileo Galilei, Christoph Scheiner, and Willibrord Snellius (Snell) in the seventeenth century that began the true understanding of the vision process.

Some research suggests that many people are more afraid of going blind than of dying, and those with eye disorders such as an eye turn have lower socioeconomic success. However, there are many examples of success in spite of vision loss, including musician Stevie Wonder, artist Claude Monet, and activist Helen Keller. Fortunately, vision loss can often be avoided by proper eye protection and regular eye examinations.

—*E. E. Anderson Penno, M.D., M.S., FRCSC*

See also Albinos; Astigmatism; Behçet's disease; Blindness; Blurred vision; Cataract surgery; Cataracts; Chlamydia; Color blindness; Conjunctivitis; Corneal transplantation; Diabetes mellitus; Eye infections and disorders; Eye surgery; Eyes; Glaucoma; Gonorrhea; Keratitis; Laser use in surgery; Macular degeneration; Microscopy, slitlamp; Myopia; Ophthalmology; Optometry; Optometry, pediatric; Refractive eye surgery; Sense organs; Strabismus; Toxoplasmosis; Transplantation; Vision disorders.

For Further Information:

Badash, Michelle, and Eric L. Berman. "Nearsightedness and Farsightedness." *Health Library*, September 1, 2011.

"The Eye and How We See." *Prevent Blindness America*, 2011.

"Eyes and Vision." *MedlinePlus*, June 26, 2013.

Ferkat, Sharon, and Jennifer S. Weizer. *All About Your Eyes: A Practical Guide in Plain English from the Physicians at the Duke University Eye Center.* Durham, N.C.: Duke University Press, 2006.

"Living EyeSmart." *EyeSmart.* American Academy of Ophthalmology, 2013

Tortora, Gerard J., and Bryan Derrickson. *Principles of Anatomy and Physiology.* 14th ed. Hoboken, N.J.: John Wiley & Sons, 2013.

Vorvick, Linda J., Franklin W. Lusby, and David Zieve. "Standard Ophthalmic Exam." *MedlinePlus*, February 10, 2011.

West, John B., ed. *Best and Taylor's Physiologic Basis of Medical Practice.* 11th ed. Baltimore: Williams & Wilkins, 1985.

VISION CORRECTION. *See* REFRACTIVE EYE SURGERY.

VISION DISORDERS

Disease/Disorder

Anatomy or system affected: Eyes

Specialties and related fields: Geriatrics and gerontology, ophthalmology, optometry

Definition: Poor vision caused by diseases or abnormalities of the eyes.

Key terms:

aqueous fluid: a clear, watery liquid that fills the region inside the front of the eyeball between the lens and cornea

cataract: a loss of transparency in the lens of the eye, commonly associated with aging

cornea: the transparent, curved front surface of the eyeball, which provides protection and focuses light

glaucoma: an increase in the eye's internal pressure that can damage the optic nerve and eventually lead to blindness

laser: a very intense beam of light; used in eye surgery for glaucoma, a detached retina, or hemorrhaging blood vessels

macular degeneration: a deterioration of vision, primarily among the elderly, caused by small hemorrhages in the most sensitive central region of the retina

retina: a thin membrane, lining the inside back surface of the eyeball, where light is transformed into electrical signals that are transmitted to the brain

Causes and Symptoms

The most common defects in human vision are nearsightedness (myopia), farsightedness (hyperopia), and astigmatism. All three of these conditions are called refractive errors because the cornea-lens focusing system of the eye bends light rays either too much or too little, so that the image formed on the retina is blurred. Fortunately, refractive errors can be corrected by means of eyeglasses or contact lenses. Millions of people use some form of vision correction.

Myopia and hyperopia are caused by a mismatch between the focusing power of the cornea-lens combination and the length of the eyeball. For a nearsighted person, the incoming light comes to a focus in front of the retina; a diverging lens is needed to move the image farther back. For a farsighted person, the situation is reversed; a converging lens is prescribed to provide extra focusing power.

The problem of astigmatism is attributable to a difference in the focal length of the eye for two perpendicular directions, which can occur if the eyeball is slightly deformed (like a grape being squeezed between two fingers). The curvature of the corneal surface would be different in two perpendicular planes. An optometrist can correct for astigmatism by pre-scribing glasses with different focal lengths in the two planes. The prescription must specify the angle at which the deformation of the eyeball is maximized.

A vision problem that is common among older adults is the formation of cataracts, in which the lens of the eye becomes cloudy. Cataracts are a normal part of the aging process, like wrinkled skin or gray hair. In rare cases, however, children have them at birth or after an eye injury. Cataracts form on the inside of the lens capsule, not on the surface of the eye. Once started, their growth is irreversible. While vision can often helped through the use of eyeglasses and stronger lighting, the only entirely effective treatment is surgical removal of the defective eye lens, followed by implantation of an artificial (plastic) replacement. With developments in ophthalmology, such microsurgery has a success rate of better than 95 percent. What causes eye cataracts in the elderly is not yet well understood. One suggested explanation is the Maillard reaction, in which glucose and protein molecules combine when heated to form a brown product. This chemical reaction is responsible for the browning of bread or cookies during baking. The same process is thought to occur even at body temperature, but very slowly over a period of years. It has been suggested that the onset of cataract formation can be delayed by a good diet, regular exercise, and a generally healthy lifestyle.

Glaucoma is a vision problem that afflicts about 2 percent of the adult population, normally after the age of forty. Excessive fluid pressure develops inside the eye, causing damage to the optic nerve. Peripheral vision gradually decreases—a decrease that the patient may not even notice until it is detected by an optometrist during an eye examination. The usual treatments are medicated eyedrops to reduce pressure and laser surgery to improve fluid drainage. Glaucoma has nothing to do with red or watery eyes because these symptoms occur on the exterior of the eyeball.

The retina is a paper-thin membrane at the back of the eye, nourished by a network of tiny blood vessels. A frequent problem encountered by diabetics is the enlargement and possible hemorrhaging of these blood vessels. For older adults, macular degeneration is a condition associated with arteriosclerosis, sometimes leading to retinal bleeding. The most sensitive, central region of the retina deteriorates, causing an irreversible loss in reading ability that cannot be corrected with glasses.

Another retinal problem is its detachment from the back wall of the eye. This is an emergency situation requiring immediate medical attention. A detached retina can be caused by an accumulation of fluid behind the retina resulting from leakage through a small tear in the membrane. It can also come from a blow to the eye, as with a sports injury. Laser surgery has become an effective treatment for the various types of retinal damage.

Treatment and Therapy

During an eye examination, the optometrist tries to detect any deviations from normal vision. If the patient is nearsighted or farsighted or has astigmatism, appropriate corrective lenses can be prescribed. If cataracts, glaucoma, or a retinal problem

---

Information on Vision Disorders

Causes: Infection, disease, allergies, injury, cataracts, glaucoma, refractive errors (nearsightedness, farsightedness, astigmatism)
Symptoms: Vary; may include eye redness, itchiness, or inflammation; blurred or disrupted vision; bleeding or hemorrhaging from eyes
Duration: Acute to chronic
Treatments: Depend on cause; may include medicated eye drops, corrective lenses, laser surgery, antibiotics, corneal transplantation

---

exists, the patient will be referred to an ophthalmologist, who has received specialized medical training in eye surgery.

The history of eyeglasses has been traced back to the thirteenth century, when Roger Bacon, a Catholic scholar, wrote about using convex glass to make writing appear larger. Some medieval paintings show elderly noblemen wearing eyeglasses. No significant innovations were made until Benjamin Franklin invented bifocals in 1780, to aid people whose eyes did not focus properly at either near or far distances. Until the late 1940s, prescription eyeglasses were always made out of glass. Then plastic lenses were introduced; they had the advantages of lighter weight and greater resistance to breakage. The main problem with plastic is that it scratches more easily, but coatings have been developed to overcome this drawback.

An alternative to eyeglasses came in the 1950s with the development of contact lenses. They were made out of a hard plastic and covered the front of the cornea, floating on a thin layer of tears. They provided good vision but were uncomfortable to insert. Also, hard contacts cannot transmit oxygen and carbon dioxide to nourish the surface of the cornea, causing dryness and irritation for the wearer. Such lenses are now virtually obsolete. Daily-wear soft contact lenses became available in the 1970s. They were much more comfortable than the hard plastic material and were gas-permeable. The soft lenses had an affinity for infection-causing bacteria, however, requiring a tedious, nightly sterilizing procedure with heat or chemicals. The technology of contact lenses continues to evolve. More recent developments are soft contacts for extended wear (up to two weeks without removal), bifocal gas-permeable contacts, and inexpensive, disposable contacts (to be discarded after two or three weeks). Contact lens wearers are cautioned to have regular eye checkups to make sure that the cornea is not being damaged.

Starting in the 1970s, eye specialists began to investigate the possibility of reshaping the eyeball to do away with eyeglasses completely. The first attempt utilized a hard lens pressing directly against the cornea to flatten it, in much the same way that orthodontic braces are used to straighten teeth. The change induced in the shape of the eye generally was only temporary, so lenses still were needed afterward.

A Soviet physician, Svyatoslav Fyodorov, developed Radial Keratotomy (RK), a surgical procedure to flatten the cornea permanently. A series of shallow incisions is made in the outer part of the cornea in a radial pattern, like the spokes of a wheel. The center of the cornea is not touched. As the incisions heal, the cornea bulges slightly near the edges, thus reducing its curvature in the middle. In this way, a permanent cure for nearsightedness can be accomplished. While thousands of patients underwent RK surgery between 1980 and 1993, the procedure remained controversial. The main problem was that the number of incisions and their depth could overcorrect or undercorrect the original refractive error. Also, some ophthalmologists were concerned about possible long-term aftereffects of scars on the cornea. RK soon decreased in popularity.

Another technique to alter the shape of the cornea is called keratomileusis. The outer half of the patient's cornea is removed and frozen, and then reshaped with a computer-controlled lathe to a predetermined curvature. After thawing, the cornea is sewn back into place, where it acts as a permanent contact lens. Keratomileusis can correct both myopia and hyperopia.

The laser, invented by physicists in the 1960s, is a very intense beam of light that can be adapted particularly well for surgery on the retina of the eye. The light beam passes successively through the transparent cornea, aqueous fluid, and lens without being absorbed. Its energy is then concentrated into a tiny spot on the retina, causing localized vaporization, or "welding," to occur. Laser-assisted in situ keratomileusis (LASIK) became quite popular at the end of the twentieth century. In LASIK surgery, the cornea is reshaped to help patients overcome myopia, hyperopia, or astigmatism. The procedure is done with a cool beam laser that removes thin layers of tissue from selected sites on the cornea to change its curvature. Success rates are high: 90 to 95 percent of the patients get 20/40 vision, and 65 to 75 percent of the patients get 20/20 vision or better. Lasers can also be used to excise leaking blood vessels and to repair or reattach a damaged retina.

Another surgical technique is to use a corneal transplant from an organ donor. The new cornea is shaped to the proper curvature with a lathe and is sewn on top of the patient's own cornea.

The standard treatment for cataracts is surgical removal of the defective lens, followed by implantation of an artificial, plastic lens. Ophthalmologists routinely perform cataract surgery using only local anesthetic, so that the patient can go home without an overnight hospital stay.

Glaucoma, a condition of excess pressure in the eye, affects millions of people and has caused thousands of cases of blindness. The first line of treatment is the use of daily medication in the form of eyedrops to reduce the fluid pressure. Eventually, surgery may be necessary. The procedure used enlarges an opening at the edge of the iris to allow for better drainage of the aqueous fluid between the lens and cornea. The incision can be made with either a miniature scalpel or a laser. Glaucoma damage to the optic nerve cannot be repaired, but prompt treatment can prevent further deterioration of vision.

Perspective and Prospects

The human eye is the most important sense organ for individuals to gather information about their environment. An amazingly high 40 percent of all nerve fibers going to the brain come from the retina of the eye. Any defect or deterioration from normal vision is a serious limitation. During the Middle Ages, few people learned to read and write, so the need for seeing at close range was not important. In modern society, however, people with poor eyesight are greatly handicapped. For example, students, computer operators, airplane pilots, and athletes cannot function without good vision.

Society is gradually becoming more sympathetic to people with handicaps, including blindness. Braille printing, guide dogs, and books recorded on audiotape are helpful developments for the blind. The U.S. Congress in 1992 passed the Americans with Disabilities Act, which mandates improved access for the visually impaired in facilities that serve the general public. Nevertheless, retaining good vision and preventing further deterioration will continue to be a vital part of overall health care.

—Hans G. Graetzer, Ph.D.

See also Albinos; Astigmatism; Behçet's disease; Blindness; Blurred vision; Cataract surgery; Cataracts; Chlamydia; Color blindness; Conjunctivitis; Corneal transplantation; Diabetes mellitus; Eye infections and disorders; Eye surgery; Eyes; Glaucoma; Gonorrhea; Keratitis; Laser use in surgery; Macular degeneration; Microscopy, slitlamp; Myopia; Ophthalmology; Optometry; Optometry, pediatric; Refractive eye surgery; Sense organs; Strabismus; Toxoplasmosis; Transplantation; Vision.

For Further Information:

Anshel, Jeffrey. *Healthy Eyes, Better Vision: Everyday Eye Care for the Whole Family.* Los Angeles: Body Press, 1990.
Berns, Michael W. "Laser Surgery." *Scientific American* 264 (June, 1991): 84–90.
Buettner, Helmut, ed. *Mayo Clinic on Vision and Eye Health: Practical Answers on Glaucoma, Cataracts, Macular Degeneration, and Other Conditions.* Rochester, Minn.: Mayo Foundation for Medical Education and Research, 2002.
Cassel, Gary H., Michael D. Billig, and Harry G. Randall. *The Eye Book: A Complete Guide to Eye Disorders and Health.* Baltimore: Johns Hopkins University Press, 2001.
"Eye Health and Safety." *Prevent Blindness America,* 2011.
"Healthy Eyes." *National Eye Institute,* 2013.
Parker, James N., and Philip M. Parker, eds. *The Official Patient's Sourcebook on Myopia.* San Diego, Calif.: Icon Health, 2004.
"Refractive Errors." *MedlinePlus,* May 20, 2013.
Sardegna, Jill, et al. *The Encyclopedia of Blindness and Vision Impairment.* 2d ed. New York: Facts On File, 2002.
Sutton, Amy L. *Ophthalmic Disorders Sourcebook.* 3d ed. Detroit, Mich.: Omnigraphics, 2008.
Sutton, Amy L., ed. *Eye Care Sourcebook: Basic Consumer Health Information About Eye Care and Eye Disorders.* 3d ed. Detroit, Mich.: Omnigraphics, 2008.
"Vision Impairment and Blindness." *MedlinePlus,* May 28, 2013.
"What Is Low Vision?" *EyeSmart.* American Academy of Ophthalmology, 2013.

VITAMIN D DEFICIENCY

Disease/Disorder

Anatomy or system affected: All

Specialties and related fields: Nutrition, preventive medicine

Definition: An illness that results from a deficiency of vitamin D in the diet.

Vitamin D has become a popular topic in the general public due to its attention in the media and supposed role in prevention and treatment of many chronic diseases. In recent years, vitamin D deficiency has especially been recognized as a pandemic with prevalence between 25-54 percent in adults older than 60 years of age. Older adults are the most vulnerable population to a vitamin D deficiency due to their decreased exposure to natural sunlight, increased prevalence of malnutrition and intestinal malabsorption.

Vitamin D is considered a prohormone, which is an inactive substance that can be converted to a hormone. Vitamin D is a fat-soluble vitamin synthesized in the skin through ultraviolet light and obtained in foods such as oily fish, eggs and fortified foods (milk, eggs, cereals). It can be produced by phytoplankton, zooplankton and most animals exposed to sunlight. Vitamin D exists in supplemental, pharmaceutical and metabolite forms as vitamin D_2 (ergocalciferol) and vitamin D_3 (cholecalciferol). Vitamin D_2 is synthesized "from yeast and used for food fortification" in comparison to Vitamin D_3, which is made in the skin when exposed to ultraviolet rays emitted from sunlight. Vitamin D_2 can be ingested through plant sources, while Vitamin D_3 is obtained through animal sources.

Vitamin D status is generally defined by the following reference ranges of serum 25 hydroxyvitamin D: deficiency equals less than 20 ng/mL (50 nmol/L); insufficiency equals 21-29 ng/mL (52-72 nmol/L); sufficiency equals 30 ng/mL (75 nmol/L); and toxicity equals greater than 150 ng/mL (374 nmol/L). In 2010, the Institute of Medicine (IOM) updated the Dietary Reference Intake (DRIs) for calcium and vitamin D. Assuming minimal sun exposure, the recommended DRIs for vitamin D is 600 IUs per day for most everyone in the United States and Canada and 800 IUs for those age 71 and older.

The most efficient and plentiful source of vitamin D is direct sunlight. It is important to note that sunscreens SPF 8 and above not only reduce but also prevent vitamin D production. The amount of unprotected sun exposure is dependent upon latitude/climatic locations and skin type. Vitamin D produced in the skin lasts at least twice as long in the blood as vitamin D ingested from the diet.

Vitamin D is naturally present in mushrooms and oily fish (i.e. swordfish, tuna fish, salmon, sardines) and available in fortified foods such as milk, yogurt, cheese, margarine, orange juice, and breakfast cereals. Using the National Health and Nutrition Examination Survey (NHANES) data, Bailey et al. determined that 53 percent of the U.S. population reported using any dietary supplement (2003-2006) and 37 percent used vitamin D (2005-2006). However, supplements only increase serum vitamin D levels by 30 ng/ml.

Once vitamin D is obtained through endogenous production in the skin through UV rays or consumed through a dietary source, it enters the bloodstream via vitamin D receptors (VDRs). These receptors exist everywhere throughout the body on cells of the target organs such as the kidneys, bone, intestinal tissues and brain. Vitamin D then travels to the liver as a metabolite (25-hydroxyvitamin D) in its major circulating form and to the kidneys where it is converted to its active form (1-25-hydroxyvitamin D). The main function of vitamin D is in the regulation of calcium and phosphorus levels found in the body. This regulation is done in conjunction with parathyroid hormone (PTH). PTH stimulates 1-25-hydroxyvitamin D, the active form of vitamin D, which increases the production of calcium from the intestinal lumen and bone. Likewise, an increase in 1-25-hydroxyvitamin D increases phosphate absorption from the intestine and decreases phosphate urinary excretion while also slightly increasing intestinal calcium absorption.

Vitamin D promotes skeletal health and bone mineralization. The most established data on the benefits of vitamin D are related to the skeletal system. There is an increasing amount of evidence on the neurological effects of vitamin D. Additionally, vitamin D improves coronary artery disease through lipid lowering effects, promotes immunomodulation, and aids in the response to viral infections. Recent evidence shows that it may also inhibit airway remodeling in COPD, increase peripheral insulin sensitivity and improve islet beta cell function. Vitamin D has also been shown to have oncologic benefits by altering gene expression and possible lowering the incidence of colorectal and breast cancer.

According to Chu, vitamin D_3 has skeletal benefits such as fall and fracture risk prevention, as well as for osteoporosis in the elderly. Although many findings have been made in regard to the skeletal effects of vitamin D, there are still mixed and inconclusive results from numerous studies and testing related to non-skeletal effects. Non-skeletal effects of vitamin D insufficiency are not as widely studied but are currently being explored, particularly in relation to cardiovascular disease, diabetes mellitus, cancer, and immune dysfunction. Increasing evidence has shown that vitamin D has beneficial neurological effects on cognition, memory, and mood.

Depression is one of the most prevalent mental health disorders in older adults, affecting approximately 15 out of every 100 adults over age 65 in the United States. Some also falsely attribute depression as a normal disorder of aging, so it often goes underreported and undertreated. There are many risk factors that predispose older adults to depression. These include stressful life events, lack of social support, socioeconomic factors, medication side effects, pain, decreased sleep, and anxiety disorders. The increase and worsening of medical conditions and physical decline in diabetes, dementia, Parkinson's disease, and stroke also increase the risk of depression.

By detecting a vitamin D deficiency, primary care providers may be able to prevent conditions in late life, such as depression, and improve quality of life in older adult patients. Preventing and treating vitamin D deficiency may potentially improve the morbidity and mortality associated with depression and other health outcomes in older adults. This can have a significant impact on medical practice as primary care providers are at the forefront of health promotion, health maintenance and patient education.

—Elizabeth Farrington, AGPCNP-BC

For Further Information:
Aloia, J. F. "Clinical Review: The 2011 Report on Dietary Reference Intake for Vitamin D: Where Do We Go from Here?" Journal of Clinical Endocrinology & Metabolism, 96 (2011): 2987-2996.

Bailey, R., K. Dodd, J. Goldman, J. Gahche, J. Dwyer, A. Moshfegh, C. Sempos, and M. Picciano. "Estimation of Total Usual Calcium and Vitamin D Intakes in the United States." The Journal of Nutrition, 140 (2010): 817-822.

Chu, M. P., K. Alagiakrishnan, and C. Sadowski. "The Cure of Ageing: Vitamin D-Magic or Myth?" Postgraduate Medical Journal, 86 (2010): 608-616.

DeLuca, H. "Overview of General Physiologic Features and Functions of Vitamin D." American Journal of Clinical Nutrition, 80:6 (2004):1689S-1696S.

Fiske, A., J. Wetherell, and M. Gatz. "Depression in Older Adults." Annual Reviews of Clinical Psychology, 5 (2009): 363-389.

Geriatric Mental Health Foundation. "Depression in Late Life: Not a Natural Part of Aging." Retrieved from Geriatric Mental Health Foundation website: http://www.gmhfonline.org/gmhf/consumer/factsheets/depression_latelife.html

Hankey, C., and W. Leslie. (2011). "Nutritional Issues and Potential Interventions in Older People." Reviews in Clinical Gerontology, 21 (2011): 286-296.

Holick, Michael F. The Vitamin D Solution: A 3-Step Strategy to Cure Our Most Common Health Problem. New York: Hudson Street Press, 2010.

Institute of Medicine, Food and Nutrition Board. "Dietary Reference Intakes for Calcium and Vitamin D." National Academy Press, 2010. Retrieved from http://www.iom.edu/Reports/2010/Dietary-Reference-Intakes-for-Calcium-and-Vitamin-D/Report-Brief.aspx

Nguyen, H. C. T., and A. Chernoff, A. (2012, April 20). "Vitamin D3 25-hydroxyvitamin D." Medscape Reference: Drugs, Diseases & Procedures. Retrieved from http://emedicine.medscape.com/article/2088694-overview

Peacock, M. "Calcium Metabolism in Health and Disease." Clinical Journal of the American Society of Nephrology, 5 (2010): S23-S30.

Phinney, K., M. Bedner, S. Tai, W. Vamathevan, L. Sander, K. Sharpless, S. Wise, J. Yen, R. Schleicher, M. Chaudhary-Webb, C. Pfeiffer, J. Betz, P. Coates, and M. Piacciano. "Development and Certification of a Standard Reference Material for Vitamin D Metabolites in Human Serum." Analytical Chemistry, 84 (2012): 956-962.

Rosen, C. "Vitamin D Insufficiency." New England Journal of Medicine. 364 (2011):248-254.

Tuohimaa, P. "Vitamin D and Aging." Journal of Steroid Biochemistry and Molecular Biology, 114, no. 1-2 (2009): 78-84.

Vitamin D Council. "About Vitamin D." Retrieved from http://www.vitamindcouncil.org/about-vitamin-d/

Wilkins, C., Y. Sheline, C. Roe, S. Birge, and J. Morris. "Vitamin D Deficiency Is Associated with Low Mood and Worse Cognitive Performance in Older Adults." American Journal of Geriatric Psychiatry, 14, no. 12 (2009): 1032-1040.

VITAMINS AND MINERALS

Biology

Anatomy or system affected: All

Specialties and related fields: Endocrinology, family medicine, internal medicine, nutrition

Definition: Chemicals that supply the body with the means of metabolizing (extracting and using the energy from) the macronutrients (fats, carbohydrates, and proteins) it ingests; essential ingredients of the diet.

Key terms:

fat-soluble vitamins: vitamins that, because of their structure and solubility, migrate to fatty tissues in the body, where they are stored

macronutrients: materials ingested in large amounts to supply the energy and materials for physical bodies

megadose: ten or more times the recommended daily allowance of a nutrient

micronutrients: substances of which only milligrams are needed in the daily diet, such as vitamins and minerals

mineral: an inorganic salt of particular metals or elements needed for good health

recommended daily (or dietary) allowance (RDA): the intake levels of the essential nutrients that are considered adequate to meet the known nutritional needs of most healthy persons

trace elements: elements needed in the diet at levels of less than 100 milligrams per day

vitamin: an organic compound constituent of food that is consumed in relatively small amounts (less than 0.1 gram per kilogram of body weight per day) and that is essential to the maintenance of life

water-soluble vitamins: vitamins that, because of their structure, show strong solubility in water; they normally pass through the body in a relatively short time

Structure and Functions

Vitamins are organic compounds (that is, compounds made up of carbon, oxygen, nitrogen, sulfur, or hydrogen) that are constituents of food and that are crucial to the maintenance of life and good health. They make possible the production of energy and the formation of coherent body tissues from the macronutrients normally consumed in a regular diet. They are, among other things, coenzymes that serve as oxidizing, reducing, and transfer chemicals at the active sites of enzymes. Vitamins are part of the one hundred or so organic compounds that are of the proper size and stability to be absorbed from the digestive tract into the bloodstream without digestion or breakdown. Nevertheless, they are not produced in the body in amounts large enough to keep a person healthy—because they have always been available in food, there was probably no need for the human metabolism to produce them. Vitamins are synthesized by plants, and therefore plants constitute the principal natural source of these compounds.

Vitamins are divided into two main groups: the water-soluble and the fat-soluble vitamins. Structural differences account for the two types of solubility. Fat-soluble vitamins (such as vitamins A, D, E, and K) consist mainly of hydrocarbon groupings (nonpolar hydrocarbon chains and rings compatible with nonpolar oil and fat) and are structurally similar to fats, whereas water-soluble vitamins have polar hydroxyl (-OH) and carboxyl (-COOH) groups that are attracted to and form hydrogen bonds with water. One of the most important differences between vitamins is the result of their solubility: Fat-soluble vitamins are stored in the body tissues and organs for relatively long periods of time, while water-soluble vita-

mins are eliminated from the body in a relatively fast manner, sometimes in a matter of hours.

Vitamin A (retinol) maintains the health of eyes, skin, and mucous membranes and is particularly important for good vision in dim light. There are various physiological equivalents to vitamin A, that is, compounds with closely related structures that can be used as the vitamin itself. Beta carotene is a provitamin (a substance that can be easily converted to a vitamin) of vitamin A found in carrots. The vitamin can also be found in liver and liver oils. Lack of vitamin A can cause night or total blindness.

The B vitamins are often considered as a group, called the B complex, because they work together as coenzymes in biochemical reactions leading to growth and energy production. They are water soluble and easily eliminated from food in the cooking process. Members of this group include pyridoxine (B_6), involved in at least sixty enzyme reactions (mostly in the metabolism and synthesis of proteins); thiamine (B_1), a coenzyme in carbohydrate metabolism and involved in energy production, digestion, and nerve activity; riboflavin (B_2), used in obtaining energy from foods; pantothenic acid (B_3), needed for proper growth; niacin (B_4), needed for the production of healthy tissues; cobalamin (B_{12}), involved in the production and growth of red blood cells; and folic acid (B_9), also involved in the production of red blood cells and in metabolism. They are present in various foods, especially meat and dairy products. Deficiency symptoms include anemia, skin disorders, and nervous system disorders.

Vitamin C, or ascorbic acid, is involved in the destruction of invading bacteria, in the synthesis and activity of interferon (which prevents entry of viruses into cells), in decreasing the effect of toxic substances (such as drugs and pollutants), and in the formation of connective tissue. Humans are one of the few species of animals for which ascorbic acid is actually a vitamin, since other species produce it in their metabolic processes. Deficiency symptoms include the degeneration of tissue and scurvy. Vitamin C is found mostly in citrus fruits.

Vitamin D (calciferol) promotes the absorption of calcium and phosphorus through the intestinal wall and into the bloodstream. Its deficiency induces the disease rickets and, in adults, the malformation of bones. Unlike other vitamins, it forms in the body through the action of the sun's ultraviolet light. As with the vitamin B complex, vitamin D has a set of closely related molecular structures, called D_1, D_2, D_3, and so on. All these structures have the same physiological function. Because of limited sun exposure, copious clothing, and indoor living and working conditions, humans need to add vitamin D to their diet, as in fortified milk, cod liver oil, or vitamin supplements.

Vitamin E (alpha tocopherol) is an antioxidant of polyunsaturated fatty acids (fatty acids with numerous double bonds). These fatty acids readily form peroxides, which are particularly damaging because they can lead to runaway oxidation in cells. Vitamin E protects the integrity of cell membranes, which contain considerable amounts of fat. It also helps maintain the integrity of the circulatory and central nervous systems; is involved in the functioning of the kidneys, lungs, liver, and genitalia; and detoxifies poisonous materials absorbed by the body. Since aging, in some theories, is considered to be the cumulative effect of free radicals (reactive atoms) running wild in the body, the antioxidant properties of vitamin E may make it a good candidate for inhibiting aging, or at least preventing premature aging. Its deficiency symptoms in humans are unknown. Vitamin E is present in various foods, especially in grain oils.

Biotin (also called vitamin H) participates in metabolism by acting as a carboxyl carrier for a number of enzymes. Its sources are liver, cereals, and egg yolks. Symptoms of deficiency include alopecia (the loss or absence of hair) and skin rashes.

Vitamin K completes the list of vitamins. It participates in the clotting of blood, and its deficiency can cause hemorrhage and liver damage. This vitamin is commonly found in plants and vegetables.

The term "minerals," when used in a nutritional context, includes all the nutritional chemical elements of foods obtained from macronutrients, except for carbon, hydrogen, nitrogen, oxygen, and sulfur. This term also refers to metal elements combined with others in compounds such as soluble inorganic salts. It is in this combined form that they serve indispensable functions in the body.

Minerals pass slowly through the body and are excreted in the feces, urine, and sweat. Therefore, they must be replaced and an appropriate balance continuously maintained. Because living beings cannot generate minerals in their own bodies, they must obtain them from foods or food supplements. Plants pick up minerals directly from the soil, and animals get them from the plants that they ingest. As opposed to vitamins, which are synthesized by plants, minerals cannot be generated if they are not in the soil. Among their many functions, minerals are components of enzymes, are structural components of body parts such as bones, are involved in maintaining the electrolyte balance in body fluids, and transport materials, as hemoglobin does in blood.

There are seventeen known minerals, although many others may exist. Since most of them are present in the body in relatively small amounts, their functions have been determined through the symptoms of various dietary deficiencies. Minerals can be grouped into two classes. The major elements—calcium, phosphorus, and magnesium—are required in amounts of 1 gram or more per day. The trace elements, such as chlorine, chromium, cobalt, copper, fluorine, iodine, iron, manganese, molybdenum, nickel, selenium, sulfur, vanadium, and zinc, are needed in milligram or microgram quantities each day.

Calcium, probably the best-known mineral, is present in the body in a greater amount than any other mineral: up to 1.5 or 2.0 percent of total body weight, with 99 percent of it in bones and teeth. In the nervous system, it is used to slow down the heartbeat, and it is metabolized in the body by a hormone synthesized from calciferol (vitamin D). Excess calcium can give rise to kidney stones. Its deficiency is common in postmenopausal women, who produce less estrogen. This decrease encourages bone dissolution, and when bones are dissolved, calcium is lost. Calcium is found in milk and dairy products, fish, and green vegetables. Phosphorus, the second most common mineral, is a structural component of bones and soft tissue. It is found in nearly all foods.

Sodium and potassium cations (positively charged atoms) are components of many minerals. They work in the conservation of electrolytic balance in cell fluids. Potassium governs the activity of many cellular enzymes, while sodium keeps the water content of cellular fluids in a healthy balance. For the body to work properly, it needs the appropriate ratio of sodium to potassium. Potassium ions concentrate inside the cell, while sodium ions concentrate outside the cell. Natural unprocessed foods have high sodium-to-potassium ratios. Because sodium and potassium compounds are very soluble in water, however, they dissolve during processing and cooking and are discarded. Sodium is replenished by adding salt to food, but this is not the case with potassium, which is not added to food. Care must be taken in this matter, either by eating more fresh foods or by using a specialized table salt that contains a mixture of sodium chloride and potassium chloride. The retention of sodium leads to water retention and edema (swollen legs and ankles) and to high blood pressure in some individuals. Sodium is mostly found in table salt, and potassium is found in meat, dairy products, and fruit.

Magnesium and chloride ions are the most common minerals in cell fluids, as they regulate fluid balances and electrical charges. Magnesium controls the formation of proteins inside the cell and the transmission of electrical signals from cell to cell. Chloride is present in the stomach as hydrochloric acid, or stomach acid. Magnesium is found in whole-grain cereals, dried fruits, and leafy green vegetables, and chloride is found in table salt.

Trace elements work in various ways, with most of them incorporated into the structure of enzymes, hormones, and related molecules or acting in conjunction with vitamins. Among the trace elements, one of the more important ones is iron, which is a critical part of the hemoglobin molecule of red blood cells and is involved in oxygen transport. Fluoride, another trace element, helps harden the enamel of teeth to make them resistant to decay; zinc plays an important role in growth, the healing of wounds, and the development of male sex glands; and manganese is needed for healthy bones and a well-functioning nervous system. Iodine is involved in the proper operation of the thyroid gland, chromium is important in the metabolism of glucose, and cobalt aids in cell function. Copper and selenium are other trace elements needed by the body. Most trace elements are found in fish, meat, fruits, and vegetables.

Related Diseases

Vitamin deficiencies are not common in the United States and other Western countries. A well-balanced diet provides ample vitamins of all kinds. Megadoses of vitamins can create harmful effects, however, as a toxic dose exists for many vitamins. For example, vitamin A, when taken in excess, can cause headache, nausea, vomiting, fatigue, swelling, hemorrhage, pain in the arms and legs, and birth defects. An acute deficiency of the vitamin, however, can impair vision and eventually cause blindness. Consequently, there must be a balance in vitamin intake. This balance can be achieved by following the recommended daily (or dietary) allowances (RDAs).

In the United States, the Food and Nutrition Board of the National Academy of Sciences and the National Research Council determined the daily needs for some vitamins and minerals. The Food and Drug Administration (FDA) made these findings the basis for its list of RDAs. These allowances are presented in units of grams or milligrams, and these amounts are determined using international units of biological activity. (Some vitamins come in several forms, all of which are physiologically equivalent.) RDAs do not cover every single vitamin and mineral needed for good health, nor do they cover the more extreme nutritional requirements that result from illness or unusual genetic makeup. They just serve as general guidelines for healthy individuals. For some substances lacking specific RDAs, such as chromium and a handful of other elements, the FDA lists the daily ranges of these micronutrients that it considers to be safe and effective. RDAs depend on gender, age, weight, and other conditions and are normally presented in food labels as percentages of the daily dietary requirement.

In 2005, the U.S. Department of Agriculture (USDA) updated the Food Guide Pyramid. The new pyramid emphasizes the need for physical activity (thirty minutes of moderate or vigorous exercise per day) and the importance of variety in diet. Consumers can get personalized recommendations, based on their age and gender, at MyPyramid.gov. Unlike the older food pyramids, the 2005 version suggests food quantities in cups and ounces, rather than as servings, which was ambiguous and confusing to consumers. For example, for a 2,000 calorie per day diet, the recommendations are six ounces of whole grains, two and a half cups of vegetables, two cups of fruit, three cups of dairy, and five and a half ounces from the meat and bean subgroup.

The main criticisms of the 2005 food recommendations are that they do not mention any specific foods from which to abstain, that people who do not have Web access cannot obtain personalized recommendations, and that the beef and dairy industry lobbies play a role in the USDA's decisions about these matters. Consumers should keep in mind that the primary role of the USDA is to promote agriculture in the United States. Politics are embedded in decisions made about diets, and recommending that people eat less is not good for business. Some nutritionists and scientists believe that diet matters should be under the auspices of a more neutral party, such as the National Institutes of Health (NIH).

The activity of a vitamin or mineral depends only on its molecular structure, not on its source. Therefore, the synthetic vitamins found in food supplements provide the same nutrients as naturally occurring ones. It is crucial to remember, however, that other substances or nutrients are present in the food that is being consumed to obtain the necessary vitamin and mineral requirements. Authentic food often contains additional substances that enhance the absorption and utilization of its nutrients. For example, the calcium that is naturally present in food is more likely to carry with it any vitamin D or phosphorus that the body might need for its optimum use than is the calcium found in an antacid tablet or a food supplement. A balanced diet provides a diversity of nutrients that no pills can match.

The major medical use of the vitamins is in curing the deficiency diseases—that is, those caused by their absence from the diet. Nine vitamins have been judged by an FDA panel to be safe and effective as over-the-counter drugs. Supplementation is commonly thought of as a means of maintaining nutritional equilibrium in the body.

Many different analytical methods—such as ultraviolet-visible and infrared spectroscopy; paper, thin-layer, and gas-liquid chromatography; and mass spectroscopy—as well as biological assays have been used for the detection and identification of vitamins. They have greatly helped to explain the complex structures of these compounds. These methods are also used in the determination of the vitamin content of a particular food item, providing the consumer with valuable nutritional information.

Perspective and Prospects

Vitamin deficiency diseases such as scurvy, beriberi, and pellagra have plagued the world at least since the existence of written records. The concept of a vitamin or "accessory growth factor" was developed in the early part of the twentieth century. In 1912, Casimir Funk, a Polish biochemist, isolated a dietary growth factor from the outer covering of rice grains and found that, when added to the food of those who had beriberi, it cured the disease. The factor was an organic compound called an amine (that is, a compound containing nitrogen combined with carbon and hydrogen). Funk coined the term "vitamine" (meaning "life-giving amine") for the compound, which is now called thiamin or vitamin B_1. In the next five decades, there was an exciting era of the isolation, identification, and synthesis of vitamins. It was soon found that these compounds were not all amines, and the term was changed to "vitamins." As more information on the structure of vitamins was obtained, names changed from general ones (such as vitamin C) to more specific ones (such as ascorbic acid). These discoveries led to the availability of inexpensive synthetic vitamins and to a dramatic reduction in overt vitamin deficiency disease.

Small amounts of vitamins are essential for good health, but the benefits of taking megadoses of certain vitamins to prevent or cure certain ailments are often debated. Even so, there is evidence that the use of high levels of vitamins can prevent or alleviate a number of diseases. Improvements in the analytical methods used in the detection and identification of vitamins have led to better and more sensitive detection limits for these compounds. The result has been increased knowledge of vitamins and minerals and their function.

In 2002, the American Medical Association endorsed the notion that adults should take a multivitamin daily. This reversed the organization's long-standing antivitamin stance that vitamins were a waste of time and money for all people except pregnant women and for some people with chronic illnesses. The current recommendation, published in the *Journal of the American Medical Association*, acknowledges that vitamins may prevent some kinds of chronic diseases, such as heart disease, cancer, and osteoporosis. Nevertheless, the efficacy and safety of regular intake of multivitamins remains a subject of debate in the medical community. In a 2013 book entitled *Do You Believe in Magic?: The Sense and Nonsense of Alternative Medicine*, Dr. Paul Offit of the University of Pennsylvania cites several studies suggesting that regular intake of vitamin supplements increases risk of disease. However, critics like Dr. Dallas Clouatre of the American College of Nutrition argue that many vitamin studies rely on unscientific data—such as self-reporting through questionnaires.

—*Maria Pacheco, Ph.D.;*
Lisa Levin Sobczak, R.N.C.;
updated by LeAnna DeAngelo, Ph.D.

See also Anorexia nervosa; Antioxidants; Beriberi; Bulimia; Cholesterol; Dietary reference intakes (DRIs); Digestion; Eating disorders; Ergogenic aids; Food biochemistry; Food Guide Pyramid; Food poisoning; Hyperlipidemia; Kwashiorkor; Lactose intolerance; Lead poisoning; Macronutrients; Malnutrition; Nutrition; Obesity; Osteoporosis; Phenylketonuria (PKU); Poisoning; Rickets; Scurvy; Self-medication; Supplements; Wilson's disease.

For Further Information:

Balch, James F., and Phyllis A. Balch. *Prescription for Nutritional Healing: A Practical A to Z Reference to Drug-Free Remedies Using Vitamins, Minerals, Herbs, and Food Supplements*. 4th rev. ed. Garden City Park, N.Y.: Avery, 2008.
Duyff, Roberta Larson. *American Dietetic Association Complete Food and Nutrition Guide*. 3d ed. Hoboken, N.J.: John Wiley & Sons, 2007.
Lieberman, Shari, and Nancy Bruning. *Real Vitamin and Mineral Book*. 4th ed. New York: Avery, 2007.
Murray, Michael. *The Pill Book Guide to Natural Medicines: Vitamins, Minerals, Nutritional Supplements, Herbs, and Other Natural Products*. New York: Bantam, 2002.
Offit, Paul A. Do You Believe in Magic?: The Sense and Nonsense of Alternative Medicine. New York: Harper, 2012.
Preidt, Robert. "Too Little Vitamin D May Hasten Disability as You Age." *MedlinePlus*. July 17, 2013.
Shelton, C.D. *Vitamins, Minerals & Supplements: Essential or Over-Hyped?* Seattle: Amazon Digital Services Inc., 2013.
Weil, Andrew. *Eight Weeks to Optimum Health: A Proven Program for Taking Full Advantage of Your Body's Natural Healing Power*. Rev. ed. New York: Ballantine Books, 2007.

VITILIGO

Disease/Disorder

Anatomy or system affected: Immune system, skin
Specialties and related fields: Dermatology, endocrinology
Definition: A disorder that occurs when cells that make pigment (color) in the skin are destroyed, leading to white patches on the body. It may also affect the eyes and the mucous membranes of the mouth and nose, and it may cause hair to gray.

Key terms:

autoimmune disorders: conditions in which the body attacks its own cells and tissues
immune system: a body system in which blood cells, proteins, and organs fight infection and other cellular issues such as cancer through antibody development
melanin: the substance in the skin responsible for color (pigment); tanning from sun exposure is caused by melanin

Causes and Symptoms

There is no known cause for vitiligo, but it may be an autoimmune disease or a disorder in which one or more genes contribute to its development. The white patches that develop on the skin are caused when melanocytes in the skin, cells that produce melanin, are destroyed. The color of the skin is determined by the amount of melanin that the body produces. Contributing factors to the development of vitiligo may include emotional distress, sunburn, or preexisting autoimmune diseases such as hyperthyroidism, but they are not considered causative.

Vitiligo usually develops before the age of forty and affects all races and sexes equally, with up to 2 percent of the population affected. The disorder may run in families; those with a family history of vitiligo or premature graying of the hair are at an increased risk.

The primary symptom of vitiligo is the loss of pigment in the skin leading to the development of widespread, irregularly shaped white patches on the body. The white patches are more evident in dark-skinned individuals and are much less noticeable in fair-skinned individuals. The patches may develop rapidly. Cycles of depigmentation followed by stable periods may occur throughout the lifetime of the affected individual. The areas commonly affected are the areas exposed to the sun, body folds such as the armpit and groin area, body openings, the area around moles, and areas of previous injury to the skin. Premature graying of the hair, including eyelashes, eyebrows, and beards, may also be symptomatic of vitiligo. The course of the disease is difficult to predict, and the spread of the white patches may spontaneously stop, but in most cases, the entire surface of the body is ultimately affected.

Treatment and Therapy

If an individual notices areas of skin that are losing color, early graying of hair, or loss of eye color, then a doctor should be consulted. A dermatologist, a doctor who specializes in disease of the skin, is usually the physician of choice to treat vitiligo, but other specialists may be involved. There is no cure for vitiligo. The goal of treatment is to restore color to the skin and stop future depigmentation, if possible.

The diagnosis of vitiligo begins with a thorough patient examination and history, including any family history of vitiligo or autoimmune disease, unusual sun exposure, sunburn or other skin condition in the period of time just prior to onset of the white patches, and recent stress or physical illness. Blood may be drawn to determine if there are thyroid or other blood-related dysfunctions. A referral to an ophthalmologist (a doctor who specializes in the eye) for a comprehensive eye examination for inflammation may be indicated.

Treatment depends on the site and extent of the discolored areas. Therapeutic cosmetics may be used to camouflage white patches and are readily available in most department stores. The use of sunscreen is important to prevent normal skin from becoming increasingly darker than the vitiligo patches, especially in fair-skinned individuals. Sunless tanning preparations may also be used to tint areas of skin.

Topical corticosteroids may be useful in the early stages of the disease. Vitamin D derivatives may be used in conjunction with corticosteroids or with ultraviolet light. Other topical ointments may be used in small areas of vitiligo, although studies are small and side effects including an increased risk of lymphoma and skin cancer are possible. Topical psoralen with ultraviolet A (PUVA therapy), or photochemotherapy, may be effective, although severe sunburn, blistering, and other complications may occur. If more than 20 percent of the body is involved, oral PUVA may be used. Regardless of medical treatment, frequent visits to the doctor's office and careful monitoring are needed.

Narrowband ultraviolet B (UVB) therapy is a newer approach to treating vitiligo. No medicine is needed prior to application of the ultraviolet light. More research is needed, although small clinical trials have shown promise. Depigmentation therapy using monobenzyl ether of hydroquinone twice a day lightens all areas of the skin to match the areas of vitiligo in individuals with depigmentation that affects more than half the body. Autologous skin grafts and tattooing are options that may restore pigmentation or provide color to affected areas.

Perspective and Prospects

Support for the individual experiencing vitiligo is important, as the altered appearance caused by visible white patches may cause emotional distress. The extent of treatment may be determined by the psychological impact of the disease on the individual. Younger people and dark-skinned individuals may find the discoloration more disruptive in their daily lives and seek more aggressive therapies. Support groups are also available in many areas or online through organizations related to vitiligo therapy.

Research is being done to grow melanocytes in the laboratory from the patient's own skin that can be transplanted into the areas of depigmentation. Studies are also being conducted with other medicines, and piperine found in black pepper has been found to be effective at repigmentation of skin in mice. While there are no significant clinical trials, alternative medi-

cines have been tried in individuals with slow-spreading vitiligo. Patients should talk to their doctors before trying any over-the-counter treatments.

—*Patricia Stanfill Edens, Ph.D., R.N., FACHE*

See also Age spots; Albinos; Birthmarks; Dermatology; Dermatology, pediatric; Dermatopathology; Eye infections and disorders; Eyes; Grafts and grafting; Hair; Pigmentation; Plastic surgery; Skin; Skin disorders; Skin lesion removal; Sunburn; Tattoos and body piercing.

For Further Information:

American Academy of Dermatology. "Vitiligo."
Halder, Rebat M., and Jonathan Chappell. "Vitiligo Update." *Seminars in Cutaneous Medicine and Surgery* 28, no. 2 (June, 2009): 86–92.
Isenstein, Arin, Dean Morrell, and Craig Burkhart. "Vitiligo: Treatment Approach in Children." *Pediatric Annals* 38, no. 6 (June, 2009): 339–44.
National Library of Medicine and National Institutes of Health. "Vitiligo."
National Vitiligo Foundation.
Rosenblum, Laurie B. "Vitiligo." *Health Library*, September 12, 2012.
TaÃ⁻eb, Alan, and Mauro Picardo. "Clinical Practice: Vitiligo." *New England Journal of Medicine* 360, no. 2 (January 8, 2009): 160–69.
"Vitiligo." *Mayo Clinic*, April 21, 2011.
"Vitiligo." *MedlinePlus*, July 11, 2012.

VOICE AND VOCAL CORD DISORDERS
Disease/Disorder
Anatomy or system affected: Respiratory system, throat
Specialties and related fields: Otorhinolaryngology, speech pathology
Definition: Physical disorders of the vocal system in the larynx, pharynx, or oral cavity.

Causes and Symptoms

The human vocal apparatus consists of the larynx (voice box), the vocal tract (the pharynx and the nasal and oral cavities), and the nose and mouth (sound radiators). The main sound source is the larynx, containing the vocal cords; the thyroid, forming the projection on the front of the neck known as the Adam's apple; and the arytenoids, which control the size of the glottis (the opening between the vocal cords). The arytenoids are usually well separated to permit breathing; however, they pull together and vibrate during vocalization. Disorders of the vocal system may occur at the larynx or the palate (the roof of the mouth). Such disorders are sometimes caused by nonorganic emotional disturbances.

Laryngitis, or inflammation of the larynx, may be acute or chronic. The acute form may be caused by bacterial infection, chemical agents (such as chlorine), overuse of the vocal cords, or trauma. During acute laryngitis, the membrane lining the larynx swells and secretes a thick mucous substance that obstructs the vocal cords. Vocal strain following prolonged talking or singing may cause chronic hoarseness or roughening of the voice. Abuse of the voice consists of yelling or screaming, being forced to talk loudly in noisy surroundings, or having a faulty vocal technique.

Chronic laryngitis, produced by excessive smoking, alcoholism, or constant abuse of the vocal cords, dries the mucous membrane and often results in nodular growths on the vocal cords. These growths obstruct the normal functioning of the cords or cause erratic vibration. Hoarseness is symptomatic of a vocal cord problem. Sinusitis or any pulmonary disease that results in a chronic cough is particularly damaging to the voice. Chronic bronchitis may permanently injure the vocal apparatus because coughing is particularly traumatic to the vocal folds, which close tightly just prior to the cough and then open abruptly to permit the explosive air blast.

When the palate is not fused, a congenital deformity termed cleft palate, sound in the mouth cavity leaks into the nasal cavity. The resulting speech sounds have a nasal quality. (For normal speech, nasal sounds are produced when the soft palate at the back of the throat opens to allow sound into the nasal cavity.) The speaker with cleft palate may not be able to develop sufficient pressure in the mouth cavity to enunciate stops and fricatives.

Laryngeal granuloma, or contact ulcer, is a vocal cord lesion resulting from the insertion of a tube into the trachea (as with general anesthesia) or from an inappropriate configuration of the vocal cords during speech. This condition is suspected when a patient complains of pain or hoarseness after prolonged talking. Symptoms are slight hoarseness and a peculiar feeling in the throat.

A papilloma, or vocal nodule, is a small, benign, wartlike growth (polyp) attached to the vocal cords. It most often occurs in singers, announcers, and people who frequently use their voices strenuously. A patient with a vocal nodule may complain of chronic hoarseness or some ill-defined difficulty in speaking.

Laryngeal carcinoma is a malignant tumor caused by chronic irritation or by alcohol and tobacco abuse. Both types of laryngeal carcinoma—intrinsic, which attacks the vocal cords, and extrinsic, which grows in the area above the vocal cords—produce immediate symptoms of hoarseness, discomfort, and coughing. In the intrinsic form, if the symptoms are diagnosed correctly in the early stages of tumor growth, the patient has a good chance of recovery after the tumor is removed.

Treatment and Therapy

There are two treatments for chronic laryngitis. Surgery, followed by vocal exercises to correct the cause, will restore the contours of a larynx that has developed polyps or become thickened. In some cases, however, the larynx appears entirely normal but the voice tires or roughens with prolonged use. The problem is repeated vocal cord strain from excessive subglottal pressure or the inappropriate application of breath during phonation. Relief must come from a voice teacher or speech therapist.

A cleft palate is surgically corrected by closing the hole in the palate. When the original palate is inadequate for simple closure, plastic surgery may restore it to its intended purpose, or a prosthesis may be fitted to effect an artificial closure.

Laryngeal granuloma is readily corrected by surgically removing the lesion. When the ulcer occurs as a result of prolonged talking, speech therapy or vocal training will prevent a recurrence. After careful diagnosis, a vocal nodule (polyp) is also removed by means of surgical forceps. The patient is ordinarily restored to normal talking or singing within two to six weeks. Since nodules usually result from vocal abuse, the cause must also be identified and corrected.

Carcinoma of the larynx can be successfully removed surgically, or treated by radiotherapy, when detected early. The extent of surgical intervention is directly dependent on the site and extent of the tumor. If the tumor is restricted to the surface of the vocal folds, a laryngofissure may be performed, but more extensive penetration requires a laryngectomy. When the tumor is known to be of low malignancy, a hemilaryngectomy and immediate skin graft preserve the natural airway and leave a functional, although inefficient, voice.

—*George R. Plitnik, Ph.D.*

See also Aphasia and dysphasia; Bronchitis; Cleft lip and palate; Cleft lip and palate repair; Hearing loss; Laryngectomy; Laryngitis; Mouth and throat cancer; Nasopharyngeal disorders; Otorhinolaryngology; Pharyngitis; Pharynx; Sinusitis; Sore throat; Speech disorders; Stuttering; Tumor removal; Tumors.

For Further Information:

Colton, Raymond H., Janina K. Casper, and Rebecca Leonard. *Understanding Voice Problems: A Physiological Perspective for Diagnosis and Treatment.* 3d ed. Philadelphia: Lippincott Williams & Wilkins, 2006.

LaRusso, Laurie, and Brian Randall. "Laryngitis." *Health Library*, Jan. 9, 2013.

Mathieson, Lesley. *Greene and Mathieson's The Voice and Its Disorders.* 6th ed. Philadelphia: Whurr, 2006.

Ramig, Lorraine Olson, and Katherine Verdolini. "Treatment Efficacy: Voice Disorders." *Journal of Speech, Language, and Hearing Research* 41, no. 1 (February, 1998): S101–S116.

Rammage, Linda, Murray Morrison, and Hamish Nichol. *Management of the Voice and Its Disorders.* 2d ed. San Diego, Calif.: Singular, 2001.

Rubin, John S., Robert T. Sataloff, and Gwen S. Korovin, eds. *Diagnosis and Treatment of Voice Disorders.* 3d ed. San Diego, Calif.: Plural, 2006.

Strong, W. J., and G. R. Plitnik. *Music, Speech, Audio.* Provo, Utah: Soundprint, 1992.

"Throat Cancer." *MedlinePlus*, May 24, 2013.

Tucker, Harvey M. *The Larynx.* 2d ed. New York: Thieme Medical, 1993.

"Voice Disorders." *MedlinePlus*, May 26, 2013.

VOMITING. *See* NAUSEA AND VOMITING.

VON WILLEBRAND'S DISEASE
Disease/Disorder

Also known as: Pseudohemophilia, angiohemophilia, vascular hemophilia

Anatomy or system affected: Blood, blood vessels, joints, reproductive system, skin

Specialties and related fields: Dentistry, dermatology, family medicine, gastroenterology, gynecology, hematology, vascular medicine

Definition: A genetic disorder characterized by the lack of a clotting factor and manifested by excessive bleeding.

Causes and Symptoms

Von Willebrand disease (vWD) is a genetic disorder affecting the normal clotting function of platelets in the blood. There are three types of vWD that run in families, all due to inheriting a gene mutation. The pattern of inheritance may be autosomal dominant or autosomal recessive, although with either, both males and females are affected equally; some persons could be carriers of the defective gene without exhibiting any symptoms. There is another form of vWD called acquired von Willebrand syndrome. This disease is not caused by inheriting a gene mutation, and thus does not run in families. This disease is characterized by the qualitative or quantitative deficiency of von Willebrand factor (vWF). This glycoprotein, present in platelets and the endothelium of blood vessels, facilitates the adhesion of platelets to one another to form a stable clot when there has been injury to a blood vessel. Therefore, patients with vWD exhibit the signs and symptoms of blood clotting abnormality.

Three types of vWD are recognized: type I vWD, with decreased levels of the protein vWF; type II vWD, with normal levels but decreased activity of vWF; and type III vWD, the most severe form of the disease, with a nearly complete deficiency of vWF.

Patients with mild or moderate vWD (type I or type II) can become symptomatic at any age and usually exhibit one or more of the following symptoms: easy bruisability, bleeding gums, frequent nosebleeds, bleeding points under the skin (subcutaneous hemorrhages), prolonged bleeding after injury or surgery of any kind, and, in women, menorrhagia, or excessive bleeding during menstrual periods. Patients with severe type III vWD become symptomatic at an early age and exhibit symptoms similar to hemophilia, with bleeding into and pain in the joints (hemathrosis), spontaneous bleeding into the gastrointestinal tract and from the mucous membranes that is potentially life-threatening, and painful bleeding into the muscles (hematomas). Some patients with type III disease also have multiple episodes of acute gastrointestinal bleeding and are often misdiagnosed. Some patients also have decreased factor VIII, which is deficient in hemophilia. The symptoms of vWD appear to decrease with advancing age, and they are milder in pregnancy, when factor VIII levels are high. Typically, bleeding time is prolonged in all patients with vWD.

The disease is diagnosed in the laboratory using specialized blood tests, such as the von Willebrand factor antigen (which measures the amount of vWF in blood), Ristocetin cofactor (which measures the function of vWF in blood), vWF multimers, and factor VIII levels. A careful family history of the disease should help distinguish it from the rarer hemophilia. A correlation of family history, laboratory findings, and clinical findings may be needed in order to diagnose the condition in mild cases of vWD, in which diagnosis is difficult.

A few cases of acquired vWD have been identified, with antibodies against vWF being present. Such persons may be otherwise healthy or may also exhibit other immune-mediated diseases.

Treatment and Therapy

The aim of therapy for vWD is to stop the bleeding and to prevent further episodes. Both goals can be met by increasing vWF and/or factor VIII levels in the blood. This result can be achieved by many methods, the most common being the administration of the drug DDAVP (desmopressin acetate) by a nasal or intravenous route. This drug does not seem to have a beneficial effect in type III disease, and these patients may need intravenous infusions of concentrates of factor VIII and vWF. For women with heavy menstrual bleeding, estrogen therapy in the form of oral contraceptive (birth control) pills is a good alternative, as it has been observed that estrogen increases the levels of vWF in the blood. Local antifibrinolytic drugs, which delay the dissolution of the clot, are useful in milder presentations of the disease (such as nosebleeds) or following dental procedures.

Preventive care should be taken by all persons suspected of having vWD. Adequate care and treatment taken prior to any dental procedure or surgical intervention should prevent the excessive loss of blood. Children with the disease are advised against engaging in rough and vigorous sports activities with a high potential for injury. Patients should also be cautioned against the excessive intake of aspirin and other nonsteroidal anti-inflammatory drugs (NSAIDs), as they worsen the symptoms of vWD.

Perspective and Prospects

In 1925, Finnish physician Erik von Willebrand identified a bleeding disorder in the natives of the Aland Islands and named it after himself. Later, it was found that the disease was

---

Information on Von Willebrand's Disease

Causes: Genetic disorder

Symptoms: Depend on type; may include easy bruising, bleeding gums, frequent nosebleeds, subcutaneous hemorrhages, prolonged bleeding after injury or surgery, menorrhagia in women, spontaneous bleeding, hematomas

Duration: Chronic

Treatments: DDAVP (desmopressin acetate) nasally or intravenously, intravenous factor VIII and vWF, oral contraceptives, antifibrinolytic drugs, care prior to dental or surgical procedures

2372 • Von Willebrand's disease

caused by a defect in one of the clotting factors, and the factor was also named after the brilliant physician. Today, vWD is recognized as the most common inherited bleeding disorder; it is thought to affect 1 to 3 percent of the population, with an equal distribution between the two sexes. It is important to distinguish this condition from the better-known hemophilia. The diagnosis of vWD in women is significant, as it is a popular misconception that bleeding disorders occur only in men.

The present drug therapy available to combat the disease is quite effective in reducing the bleeding that occurs. Modern-day medicine has reduced the problems of blood infections associated with the administration of cryoprecipitates. Further research is being conducted to develop an effective recombinant vWF.

—*Rashmi Ramasubbaiah, M.D.,*
and Venkat Raghavan Tirumala, M.D., M.H.A.

See also Bleeding; Blood and blood disorders; Circulation; Genetic diseases; Hematology; Hematology, pediatric; Hemophilia; Nosebleeds; Transfusion; Vascular medicine; Vascular system.

For Further Information:

Fauci, Anthony S., et al, eds. *Harrison's Principles of Internal Medicine.* 18th ed. New York: McGraw-Hill, 2012.

Gersten, Todd, Linda J. Vorvick, and David Zieve. "Von Willebrand Disease." *MedlinePlus*, Feb. 16, 2012.

Greer, John, et al., eds. *Wintrobe's Clinical Hematology.* 12th ed. Philadelphia: Wolters Kluwer/Lippincott Williams & Wilkins Health, 2009.

Judd, Sandra J., ed. *Genetic Disorders Sourcebook: Basic Consumer Information About Hereditable Disorders.* 4th ed. Detroit, Mich.: Omnigraphics, 2010.

"Platelet Disorders." *MedlinePlus*, May 22, 2013.

Rosenblum, Laurie, and Michael Woods. "Von Willebrand Disease." *Health Library*, Nov. 26, 2012.

Ruggeri, Zaverio M., ed. *Von Willebrand Factor and the Mechanisms of Platelet Function.* New York: Springer, 1998.

Westphal, Robert G., and Dennis M. Smith, Jr., eds. *Treatment of Hemophilia and Von Willebrand's Disease: New Developments.* Arlington, Va.: American Association of Blood Banks, 1990.

"What Is von Willebrand Disease?" *National Heart, Lung, and Blood Institute*, June 1, 2011.

WEANING

Procedure

Anatomy or system affected: Gastrointestinal system, stomach

Specialties and related fields: Family medicine, nutrition, pediatrics

Definition: The training of an infant to accept food other than breast milk.

Key terms:

engorgement: an uncomfortable, often painful condition in which the breasts are overly full with milk

overfeeding: the provision of more milk or formula for an infant than is necessary; may result in regurgitation

Indications and Procedures

For a woman who is well-informed about breast-feeding, the appropriate time to wean her infant will become clear if she is sensitive to the child's cues. Other factors affecting a mother's decision to wean her child include family or cultural pressures, pressure from the partner, and personal beliefs about when weaning should occur. Often, weaning takes place between periods of great developmental activity for the child: between eight to nine months, twelve to fourteen months, eighteen months, two years, or three years of age. Most babies are weaned before nine months of age.

Mothers who want to wean their children from breast milk to a bottle before nine months of age need to prepare the child for the process by introducing a bottle when the infant is about six to eight weeks old. They can do so without compromising the nutrition of breast milk by pumping and offering breast milk occasionally through a bottle. Infants who are not used to the bottle after that age are more reluctant to accept it later. If the mother decides to wean the baby before one year of age, a commercial formula should be used for supplementation. Cow's milk is not appropriate for infants under one year of age. Honey should never be used to sweeten the formula because of the danger of infant botulism.

When a mother decides to wean her child from breast milk, she should supplement one bottle (or cup) of formula for the least important breast-feeding session of the day. This should be done over a period of two days to a week. If weaning is conducted abruptly, the mother's breasts may become painfully engorged with milk. Breast-feeding sessions associated with meals can be easily forgone, as the child has less desire for milk during those times. Gradually, the mother can substitute more breast-feeding sessions with bottle-feeding. Many mothers continue to breast-feed their infants in the morning and/or in the evenings for many months before weaning is completed. This has many advantages, in that both the baby and the mother will have time to adjust to their new feeding schedule. Weaning mothers should continue to drink plenty of fluids, as restricting fluid intake will not prevent engorgement. Typically, this late form of engorgement passes in one or two days after the weaning process begins.

When bottle-feeding babies, mothers should assume the same position with their infants as they did when breast-feed-

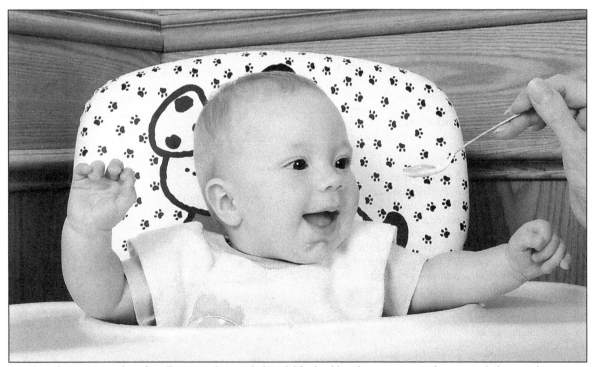

An infant who can sit upright and swallow properly is ready for solid foods, although many more months may pass before complete weaning takes place. (PhotoDisc)

ing. Most women cradle their infants in the crook of their arm for comfort and intimacy. The bottle's nipple should have a hole big enough to allow milk to flow in drops when turned upside down. Too big a hole, however, can lead to overfeeding and regurgitation by the baby. Cleanliness is important when bottle-feeding; appropriate methods of formula preparation and the sterilization of bottles must be followed.

Related to weaning is getting an infant to discontinue the use of a pacifier. Just as in weaning a baby from breast milk, this process has to be gradual and gentle. The best time to wean a baby from a pacifier is when he or she becomes more mobile, in order to prevent the pacifier from becoming a habit. The parent can remove the pacifier after the baby is asleep. Gradually, pacifier use can be restricted to nap time and bedtime. Parents should encourage the baby to stop using the pacifier by offering praise and being patient.

Once a baby starts to use a cup, it is important to make sure that the cup is heavy enough to be stable on a flat surface such as a table or high chair tray. The cup needs to be small enough for the baby to hold properly. Special training cups with spill-proof tops are widely available. Using a floor mat often saves the parent time in cleaning up after a spill.

Uses and Complications

If both the mother and the child are comfortable with the timing of the weaning, it can be accomplished with minimal difficulty. Nevertheless, weaning is a time of emotional separation for mother and child, and they may be unwilling to give up the closeness that nursing offers. Hence, it is important to plan comforting, consoling, and play activities to replace breast-feeding. Weaning is best conducted in a gradual manner.

One worry that mothers often express when switching from breast to bottle is uncertainty as to how much milk an infant needs. Parents should avoid overfeeding or feeding infants every time they cry. They should also avoid setting artificial goals such as "the baby must consume 8 ounces," feeding the infant until the goal is reached even though the baby may no longer be hungry. Overfeeding results in obesity.

Perspective and Prospects

In recent years, the American Pediatrics Association has emphasized the importance of breast-feeding through a baby's first year. Physiologically, breast milk helps the infant fight infections by supplying antibodies and by coating the intestines with bacteria-fighting liquids. Developmentally, it has been found that breast-feeding mothers are more likely to engage in frequent interactive behavior with their infants, report that their infants have "easy temperaments," and engage in more flexible caregiving. It has been found that infants who are breast-fed retain an advantage in cognitive ability as measured by intelligence quotient (IQ) tests well into their third year of life.

For a majority of women who end breast-feeding prior to one year, inadequate milk supply and employment are the major reasons cited. Whether the result of choice or necessity, weaning is a natural process and a milestone for both mother and child.

—Gowri Parameswaran

See also Bonding; Breast-feeding; Developmental stages; Food poisoning; Malnutrition; Nutrition; Obesity, childhood; Pediatrics; Teething; Thumb sucking.

For Further Information:

Arvedson, Joan. "Weaning Preparation for Children Fed by G-Tube." *The Oley Foundation*, June 26, 2013.

Bengson, Diane. *How Weaning Happens*. Schaumburg, Ill.: La Leche League International, 1999.

"Breastfeeding." *womenshealth.gov*, August 1, 2010.

Bumgarner, Norma Jane. *Mothering Your Nursing Toddler*. Rev. ed. Schaumburg, Ill.: La Leche League International, 2000.

Hillis, Anne, and Penelope Stone. *Breast, Bottle, Bowl: The Best Fed Baby Book*. Rev. ed. Pymble, N.S.W.: HarperCollins, 2008.

Markel, Howard, and Frank A. Oski. *The Practical Pediatrician: The A to Z Guide to Your Child's Health, Behavior, and Safety*. New York: W. H. Freeman, 1996.

Meek, Joan Younger, and Sherill Tippins, eds. *American Academy of Pediatrics New Mother's Guide to Breastfeeding*. New York: Bantam Books, 2006.

Rolfes, Sharon Rady, Linda Kelly DeBruyne, and Eleanor Noss Whitney. *Life Span Nutrition: Conception Through Life*. 2d ed. St. Paul, Minn.: West, 1998.

"Solid foods: How to get your baby started." *Mayo Clinic*, June 6, 2013.

Spock, Benjamin, and Robert Needlman. *Dr. Spock's Baby and Child Care*. 8th ed. New York: Pocket Books, 2004.

WEIGHT LOSS AND GAIN
Biology

Anatomy or system affected: Gastrointestinal system, muscles, musculoskeletal system, psychic-emotional system, stomach

Specialties and related fields: Endocrinology, gastroenterology, nutrition, psychology

Definition: Weight loss occurs when more energy is expended than ingested, while weight gain occurs when more energy is ingested than expended; both conditions may exist as a consequence of changes in diet or physical activity or of physical or psychological disease.

Key terms:

basal metabolism: the energy used to fuel the involuntary activities necessary to sustain life (respiration, circulation, and hormonal activity)

energy balance: the state in which kilocalories from ingested food are equal to kilocalories expended

energy-yielding nutrient: nutrients that supply the body with energy (fat provides 9 kilocalories per gram, while carbohydrates and protein provide 4 kilocalories per gram)

kilocalorie: the amount of heat necessary to raise the temperature of a kilogram of water 1 degree Celsius; the unit of measure for the energy content of foods, also called a Calorie

nutrient density: the amount of nutrients provided per kilocalorie of food

wasting: severe weight loss characterized by the loss of muscle tissue and body fat deposits

Process and Effects

Whether a person gains or loses weight is dependent on the balance of energy expended versus energy ingested. Thus, weight is determined by how many kilocalories are in the foods eaten and how many kilocalories of energy are expended. Normal day-to-day fluctuations in weight are typically minor changes attributed to shifts in body fluid and are not related to energy balance (input versus output). Input kilocalories refer to those from fat, protein, carbohydrates, and alcohol. Although alcohol is not considered an energy-yielding nutrient, it provides 7 kilocalories per gram. Output kilocalories are used to maintain the body's basal metabolism; to chew, digest, and process food; to fuel muscular activity for physical exercise; and to help the body adapt to environmental changes. When energy intake exceeds output, a person gains weight. When energy output exceeds intake, a person loses weight.

Body weight is determined by the amounts of body fat, water, lean tissue (muscle), and bones. Ideally, what people want to lose when dieting is body fat, not lean tissue. It takes approximately 3,500 excess kilocalories to store a pound of body fat, whereas approximately 2,000 to 2,500 kilocalories are required to gain one pound of lean tissue. Any excess food kilocalories—whether from fat, carbohydrates, protein, or alcohol—can be converted into body fat. There is no limit to body fat stores.

During periods of caloric deficit (meaning that input is less than output), a person will lose weight. A deficit of 500 kilocalories per day translates into a loss of about one pound per week. Not all the body weight lost is fat. During a deficit or fasting, the body draws on stores to provide energy. During the first four to six hours without eating, either while sleeping during the night or while awake and active during the day, the body draws its energy primarily from liver carbohydrate stores called glycogen. If no food is consumed after these periods, the body begins to break down muscle (also called lean body tissue) as fuel. Although people lose weight under these circumstances, it is the result of muscle loss and fluid shifts, not fat loss. Body fat supplies fuel during fasting but cannot prevent muscle wasting unless a regular supply of carbohydrates is present. The fat used during fasting is not efficiently metabolized and can cause medical problems if the fast continues for more than a few days. Fat loss can be accomplished by eating balanced regular meals that contain fewer kilocalories than those typically eaten.

Caution should be used before an individual undergoes either a weight loss or a weight gain plan. Starvation diets or very low kilocalorie diets and meal skipping are not wise. These diets promote water and muscle loss, not a steady body fat loss. A reduction in kilocalories of about 500 per day will promote safe, effective fat loss without medical hazards. The central nervous system cannot use stored body fat as fuel, making prolonged fasting a dangerous practice. By consuming a balanced diet that contains all five food groups in moderate portions, exercising, and modifying poor dietary behaviors (such as snacking while watching television), an individual can achieve lasting weight loss. Nutrient-dense foods—those that are low in kilocalories and fat yet still contain ample amounts of vitamins and minerals—should be chosen. Understanding the kilocaloric content of foods is not always necessary if a person uses exchange lists (diabetic exchanges), which are portion-controlled groupings of foods with similar energy contents that can be used to form an adequate diet. Exercise is important because it not only tones the body but also allows for more energy expenditure. Research has shown that regular exercise speeds up the basal metabolic rate, which also helps control weight.

Usually individuals seeking weight gain want to gain muscle, not body fat. Weight gain of this type can be accomplished by physical conditioning and a high kilocalorie diet. The amount of muscle gained is under hormonal control. In healthy individuals, an excess of 700 to 1,000 kilocalories per day is sufficient to add 1 to 2 pounds per week. This excess must be accompanied by exercise training, however, or only body fat deposits will increase.

Healthy individuals desiring weight gain need to exercise and to ingest more kilocalories in order to increase muscle size. Consuming more kilocalories can be problematic, especially for athletes. These individuals must take time to eat perhaps five to six times per day. These individuals should eat more kilocalorically dense foods—the exact foods avoided during weight loss. Emphasis should still be placed on nutrient-wise choices, not simply empty kilocalories. If someone is underweight, increasing fat in the diet is not considered a major heart disease risk because the fat will prevent muscle wastage.

Complications and Disorders

Not all weight gain or loss is voluntary. Weight changes can be warning signs or consequences of disease. Several diseases are frequently accompanied by severe weight loss and wasting, such as acquired immunodeficiency syndrome (AIDS), cancer, colitis, chronic obstructive pulmonary diseases (such as emphysema), cystic fibrosis, and kidney diseases. Wasting is characterized by decreased muscle mass and depleted fat stores. This is a result of inadequacies in both kilocalories and nutrient intake. Lack of appetite, termed anorexia, could be a consequence of disease, drug therapy, or both, complicating a person's desire to eat. Severe weight loss is compounded by other nutrient losses caused by diarrhea, loss of blood, or drug interactions. Individuals with AIDS can experience extreme weight loss, perhaps losing up to 34 percent of ideal body weight.

Thus, with illness a vicious cycle occurs: A lack of adequate food energy promotes the risk of infection; infections require more food energy for healing, further depleting energy reserves; and patients lose more weight, placing them at greater risk for subsequent infections. Extreme weight loss makes AIDS patients prone to other infections, which subsequently compromise weight status because more kilocalories are needed to combat these infections. Similarly, patients with cancer, colitis, and chronic obstructive pulmonary disease who experience weight loss become nutritionally compromised, placing them at risk for infections and delayed wound healing. Extra kilocalories are required to support the

2376 • WEIGHT LOSS AND GAIN

labored breathing accompanying chronic obstructive pulmonary disease. People with emphysema, a type of this disease, are often too weak to ingest enough food to prevent weight loss. Diseases of the gastrointestinal tract magnify poor nutritional status because energy-yielding nutrients cannot be absorbed.

Weight loss is also a symptom of cystic fibrosis. Cystic fibrosis is a genetic disorder that affects the pancreas and lungs. Individuals with this disease become malnourished because the normal release of pancreatic digestive enzyme secretions is impaired and because of high nutritional needs to combat lung infections. In an effort to clear congested lungs, individuals with severe cystic fibrosis cough so forcefully that frequently they vomit any food substances that they were able to consume.

Treatment for illness-related weight loss is complex. Individuals do not always want to eat, for both physical and psychological reasons. More frequent meals, higher fat intakes, and even special nutritional supplements are required. In severe cases, intravenous solutions, tube feedings, and hyperalimentation (feeding higher-than-normal amounts of nutrients through tube feeding or veins) may be implemented.

Sudden, dramatic weight loss could be a sign of dehydration. Athletes exercising during hot weather must pay attention to weight loss after practice and replenish fluids immediately. Rapid weight loss in teenagers, especially girls, may be attributable to eating disorders such as anorexia nervosa (self-induced starvation) and bulimia (periods of binge eating followed by intentional vomiting, or purging). Being underweight increases the risk of infections and often causes infertility in women.

Patterns of weight gain or loss are important indicators of childhood growth. Rapid changes may signal illnesses or psychological problems that have manifested themselves as overeating or undereating. Tracking weight gain during pregnancy is also important. Gaining weight too rapidly may be a sign of fluid imbalance forewarning pregnancy complications. Weight gain may precipitate insulin-dependent (type 2) diabetes mellitus. Although people with this type of diabetes are overweight, they are hungry because the energy that they ingest cannot enter the body's cells; consequently they continue to overeat, fostering further weight gain. The location of excess weight on the body is also important. Individuals who gain excess weight in the waist area are considered to be at risk for hypertension, type 2 diabetes, and other disorders.

Perspective and Prospects

It is now well known that weight loss, the predominant goal of people with nonmedical weight-related concerns, cannot usually be achieved and sustained by dieting. It is estimated that one-fifth to one-third of the otherwise healthy adult population in the United States is "on a diet" at any given time. Going on a diet is not the way to get control of weight. Diets can produce weight loss; they rarely produce weight control over the long term. Repeated cycles of weight loss through deprivation of favorite high-calorie foods and weight gain

when the motivation to tolerate this deprivation wanes, so-called yo-yo dieting, are hazardous. The cycles usually reduce individual metabolic rates, reduce lean tissue, discourage the individual, and make subsequent weight loss extremely difficult.

Weight management is a long-term endeavor resulting from myriad short-term decisions. Success comes with setting and achieving realistic goals. Family or group support, positive and tolerant attitudes, regular meals representative of all food groups, and behavioral modification will sustain healthy weight. Twenty to thirty minutes of exercising the large muscle groups, every other day, can prove a modest, effective way to burn fat and increase one's metabolic rate. It also produces more lean muscle tissue, a goal for both dieters and gainers.

Whether weight gain or loss is the goal, healthful eating habits require one to make wise choices and understand that weight control is a lifestyle, not a quick fix. Individuals experiencing a weight gain or loss who are not voluntarily altering exercise or food intake should have a thorough physical examination to determine the root cause. In June 2013, the American Medical Association voted to classify obesity as a disease. The decision spurred a nationwide conversation about obesity treatment and prevention. In addition, it led some members of the United States Congress to consider expanding Medicare coverage to include weight-loss drugs and weight-reduction treatments.

—Wendy L. Stuhldreher, Ph.D., R.D.,
and Paul Moglia, Ph.D.;
updated by LeAnna DeAngelo, Ph.D.

See also Acquired immunodeficiency syndrome (AIDS); Alcoholism; Anorexia nervosa; Appetite loss; Bariatric surgery; Bulimia; Cancer; Cholesterol; Colitis; Cystic fibrosis; Diabetes mellitus; Dietary reference intakes (DRIs); Eating disorders; Emphysema; Food Guide Pyramid; Growth; Hyperadiposis; Hyperlipidemia; Malnutrition; Metabolic disorders; Metabolic syndrome; Metabolism; Nutrition; Obesity; Obesity, childhood; Pregnancy and gestation; Vitamins and minerals; Weight loss medications.

For Further Information:
Barasi, Mary E. *Human Nutrition: A Health Perspective.* 2d ed. New York: Oxford UP, 2003.
"Best Diets." *Consumer Reports* 70, no. 6 (June, 2005): 18-22.
Brownell, Kelly D. *The LEARN Program for Weight Management.* 10th ed. Dallas, Tex.: American Health, 2004.
Pollack, Andrew. "A.M.A. Recognizes Obesity as a Disease." *New York Times.* New York Times Co., Web. 18 June 2013.
Prescription Weight-Loss Drugs: Can They Help You?" *Mayo Clinic.* June 7, 2013.
Rolfes, Sharon Rady, Kathryn Pinna, and Eleanor Noss Whitney. *Understanding Normal and Clinical Nutrition.* 8th ed. Belmont, Calif.: Thomson/Wadsworth, 2009.
Stransky, Fred W., and R. Todd Haight. *The Good News About Nutrition, Exercise, and Weight Control.* Troy, Mich.: Momentum Books, 2001.
Summerfield, Liane. *Nutrition, Exercise, and Behavior: An Integrated Approach to Weight Management.* Pacific Grove, Calif.: Wadsworth/Thomson Learning, 2000.
Wardlaw, Gordon M., and Anne M. Smith. *Contemporary Nutrition.* 7th ed. New York: McGraw-Hill, 2008.

"Weight Loss: Gain Control of Emotional Eating." *Mayo Clinic*. December 1, 2012.

"Weight Loss: Choosing a Diet That's Right For You." *Mayo Clinic*. June 22, 2012.

WEIGHT LOSS MEDICATIONS

Treatment

Anatomy or system affected: Brain, endocrine system

Specialties and related fields: Endocrinology, family medicine, internal medicine, nutrition

Definition: The use of drugs to assist in weight loss.

Indications and Procedures

By the mid-1990s, several drugs had come onto the market showing promise in helping people achieve weight loss. The most widely sought and prescribed of these were Fen-Phen (combining serotonergic fenfluramine and amphetamine-like phentermine) and Redux (dexfenfluramine, with similar properties and actions to fenfluramine). Fen-Phen inhibited the brain's utilization of the neurochemical serotonin, which acts on the brain's appetite control center in the hypothalamus, and suppressed appetite directly, much as traditional over-the-counter diet pills do. Other drugs, less widely used, included phentermine, mazindol, and fluoxetine.

The hope and early evidence were that these medications would produce improved cardiac function, cholesterol and triglyceride profiles, blood sugar concentrations, and blood pressure; assist in the treatment of bulimia; and reduce weight in the obese and prevent weight gain in those at high risk for it, such as individuals who recently have quit smoking. The drugs were intended to assist those with morbid obesity, obese persons with serious medical conditions, and obese persons who had failed to manage their weight using more conservative nutritional and behavioral methods. At no point did researchers intend the medications as quick fixes for those unwilling to exercise or unwilling to change their eating habits. Nevertheless, many physicians prescribed them to patients who were not significantly obese or who were merely overweight.

Uses and Complications

Multiple studies across many different populations have tended to show the same results: Measurable weight loss in those taking the drugs was between 5 and 15 percent, with weight regained one year after patients had stopped taking the drug. The medications had few initial side effects—dry mouth, constipation, and drowsiness being the most common—and were unlikely to become physically addicting.

Health providers across all disciplines were particularly concerned, however, that some patients were coming to rely on these medications as alternatives to the sustained, hard work of developing lifestyle habits of healthy, proportional eating and exercise. In addition, concerns grew over the drugs" potential to cause neurotoxicity and primary pulmonary hypertension. Fen-Phen, in particular, was responsible for numerous reports of valvular heart disease and pulmonary hypertension.

Perspective and Prospects

In 1997, the Food and Drug Administration (FDA) withdrew approval of Fen-Phen and Redux for treating obesity, and their marketing and distribution were discontinued. Class-action lawsuits were filed—former Fen-Phen users alone have filed approximately fifty thousand lawsuits against the makers of the drug—and large settlements were reached for those who had used Fen-Phen and other such drugs.

The government then set its sights on dietary products containing ephedra. Manufacturers claimed that ephedra, a botanical source of ephedrine, is a "fat-burning" supplement that could boost energy and enhance athletic performance, but reports began to surface about seizures, strokes, heart attacks, and even deaths in otherwise healthy users. In 2003, the FDA banned the use of ephedra.

—Paul Moglia, Ph.D.;
updated by LeAnna DeAngelo, Ph.D.

See also Addiction; Anorexia nervosa; Appetite loss; Bariatric surgery; Bulimia; Caffeine; Eating disorders; Malnutrition; Nutrition; Obesity; Obesity, childhood; Weight loss and gain.

For Further Information:

Berke, Ethan M., and Nancy E. Morden. "Medical Management of Obesity." *American Family Physician* 62, no. 2 (July 15, 2000): 419-427.

Finn, R. "Pharmacotherapy May Help Some Obese Teens." *Internal Medicine News* 38, no. 19 (June, 2005): 45.

Marcovitz, Hal. *Diet Drugs*. Farmington Hills, Mich.: Lucent Books, 2007.

Mitchell, Deborah R., and David Dodson. *The Diet Pill Guide: A Consumer's Book to Prescription and Over-the-Counter Weight-Loss Pills and Supplements*. New York: St. Martin's Griffin, 2002.

Peikin, Steven R. *The Complete Book of Diet Drugs: Everything You Need to Know About Today's Prescription and Over-the-Counter Weight Loss Products*. New York: Kensington Books, 2002.

Whelan, S., and T. A. Wadden. "Combining Behavioral and Pharmacological Treatments for Obesity." *Obesity Research* 10, no. 6 (June, 2002): 560-574.

WELL-BABY EXAMINATIONS

Procedure

Anatomy or system affected: All

Specialties and related fields: Neonatology, nursing, pediatrics, perinatology

Definition: The art and scientific procedure of the pediatric physical examination.

Key terms:

alopecia: hair loss

dehydration: excessive loss of the body's water content; in infants, manifests as increased pulse, sunken fontanelle, decreased blood pressure, dry mucous membranes, and decreased skin turgor

periodic breathing: rapid breathing followed by several seconds of no breathing; more than ten-second pauses are abnormal

trichotillomania: excessive hair pulling

Indications and Procedures

A pediatrician or nurse practitioner usually performs the

routine physical examination of an infant. Because the child may be frightened, some steps in the examination may be performed while the baby is being held in the parent's lap. If the baby or child is ill, the health care provider will look for signs of dehydration and possible lethargic mental status. Dehydration is always checked in cases where fever is present. A child's normal oral temperature is similar to an adult's (98.6 degrees Fahrenheit). A rectal temperature will typically be 1 degree higher. It is not uncommon for a young child to have a temperature of 105 degrees with even a minor infection.

Respiration and pulse are measured. Young children and infants breathe with their diaphragm; therefore, the movements of the abdomen can be counted. Periodic breathing is common in infants. Respiratory rates for newborns are 30 to 50 respirations per minute. Toddlers average rates of 20 to 40 respirations per minute. The pulse of a newborn baby is detected best over the brachial artery. The rate is usually in the range of 120 to 160 beats per minute; this figure declines as the child grows older.

Blood pressure, length, weight, and head circumference are measured and checked against charts showing norms. Infants are weighed without clothing and are measured on a firm table. The head is measured at the maximum point of the occipital protuberance posteriorly and at the mid forehead anteriorly. The shape of the child's head, such as flatness or swelling, is observed. Hair is checked for quantity, color, texture, and infestations. The presence of a fungus can be indi-

cated by alopecia (hair loss), but this cause must be distinguished from trichotillomania. Hypothyroidism can be indicated by dry, coarse hair.

An eye examination can give information about systemic problems and about the eyes themselves. The eyes are observed working together; reaction to light, pupil size, cornea haziness, excess tearing, vision, visual fields, and the distance between the eyes are checked. Observations for nystagmus (involuntary movement of the eyes) and for the abnormal upward outward eye slant and epicanthal folds associated with Down syndrome are also made. Newborns have about 20/400 vision, which improves to 20/40 by six months of age.

During an ear examination, the tympanic membrane is checked for perforations, color, lucency, and bulging (indicating pus and/or fluid) in the middle ear. A rough hearing acuity may be determined by eliciting from the child a startle reflex to sound.

The nose is checked interiorly, and the nasal mucus is checked for watery discharge (indicating allergy) and mucopurulent discharge (indicating infection). The nasal septum and passages are also checked, and any foreign bodies are removed.

The oral cavity examination consists of checking the lips for asymmetry, fissures, clefts, lesions, and color. The tongue is examined for color, size, coating, and dryness. The tonsils are observed for signs of infection and color, while the palate is observed for arch and possible lesions. The throat is exam-

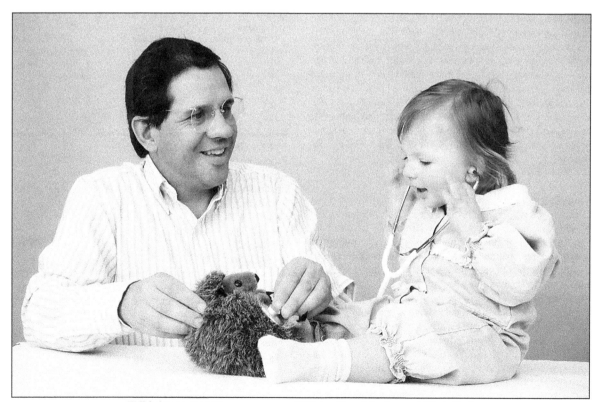

Well-baby examinations assess a young child's health and development. (PhotoDisc)

ined for signs of inflammation and other problems. The neck is checked for tilt and range of motion. The thyroid gland is palpitated and evaluated for symmetry, consistency, and surface characteristics. Any other swellings are noted and their causes determined.

The neurologic examination is extensive and begins with an assessment of a child's milestones. An infant's primitive reflexes—Moro, asymmetric tonic neck, Babinski, palmar grasp, rooting, and parachute reflexes—are checked. Cranial nerves that can be assessed at the child's stage of development may be assessed. General sensation and response to touch and muscle tone and movement are checked for unusual responses. The musculoskeletal system and extremities are checked for gross deformities and congenital anomalies. Gait and stance are observed, as well as muscle tone and range of motion. Posture in older children may be observed for spinal curvatures.

The lungs are checked to evaluate air movement, to identify breath sounds and chest sounds, and to inspect the shape of the chest. The physician will note any physical deformities and listen to rhythms that could indicate abnormal blood circulation. Indications of circulatory system problems in infants are cyanosis, clubbing of fingers or toes, tachycardia (rapid heart rate), peripheral edema, and tachypnea (rapid breathing). Examination of the abdominal contour and auscultation and palpation of the abdomen are done. In newborns, the genitals are checked for ambiguity, and the rectal area is checked for fissures or anal prolapse. Skin is checked for color, pigmentation, rashes, or burns.

Vaccinations—either oral or by injection—and boosters are a part of some well-baby visits. Occasionally, blood or urine samples are taken for analysis.

Uses and Complications

The challenge of keeping the child calm enough for the clinician to perform a valid exam is important in the diagnostic process. Although an older child can usually be examined easily in standard adult order, this does not work well for pediatric patients. The younger the patient, the more important it is that crucially affected areas be examined first, before the child becomes upset or cries. Clinicians and parents should work together to minimize a child's fears during the examination.

—*Patricia A. Ainsa, M.P.H., Ph.D.*

See also Bones and the skeleton; Cardiology, pediatric; Childhood infectious diseases; Cognitive development; Colic; Cradle cap; Dermatology, pediatric; Developmental disorders; Developmental stages; Diagnosis; Diaper rash; Endocrine system; Endocrinology, pediatric; Failure to thrive; Gastroenterology, pediatric; Gastrointestinal system; Growth; Immune system; Immunization and vaccination; Motor skill development; Neonatology; Nervous system; Neurology, pediatric; Obesity, childhood; Physical examination; Pulmonary medicine, pediatric; Reflexes, primitive; Reproductive system; Respiration; Screening; Signs and symptoms; Umbilical cord; Urinary system; Urology, pediatric; Weight loss and gain.

For Further Information:
Albright, Elizabeth K. *Pediatric History and Physical Examination.* Updated and revised ed. Laguna Hills, Calif.: Current Clinical Strategies, 2003.

Barness, Lewis A. *Manual of Pediatric Physical Diagnosis.* 6th ed. St. Louis, Mo.: Mosby Medical, 1991.

"Children's Health." *MedlinePlus*, June 26, 2013.

Hay, William W., Jr., et al., eds. *Current Diagnosis and Treatment in Pediatrics.* 19th ed. New York: Lange Medical Books/McGraw-Hill, 2009.

"Middle Childhood (9-11 years of age)." *cdc.gov*, August 15, 2012.

"Preschoolers (3-5 years of age)." *cdc.gov*, August 12, 2012.

Sanghavi, Darshak. *A Map of the Child: A Pediatrician's Tour of the Body.* New York: Henry Holt, 2003.

Schwartz, M. William, ed. *Schwartz's Clinical Handbook of Pediatrics.* 4th ed. Philadelphia: Wolters Kluwer/Lippincott Williams & Wilkins, 2009.

Zitelli, Basil J., and Holly W. Davis, eds. *Atlas of Pediatric Physical Diagnosis.* 5th ed. St. Louis, Mo.: Mosby/Elsevier, 2007.

WERNICKE'S APHASIA
Disease/Disorder

Also known as: Sensory aphasia or fluent aphasia

Anatomy or system affected: Brain

Specialties and related fields: Neurology, neuropsychology, neuroscience, neurosurgery, psychology, speech pathology

Definition: An acquired language disorder that mostly causes difficulties in comprehension of oral language.

Key terms:

Broadmann's areas: areas of the brain that are differentiated based on the cellular structure of the cerebral cortex

paragrammatism: confused or incomplete use of grammatical structures, as in case of substitution of function words and grammatical morphemes (the man are singing instead of the man is singing)

paraphasias: a type of partial aphasia that is characterized by a person who uses words incorrectly

phonological/phonemic error: a phoneme substitution/omission of the target word (boat or oat instead of goat); this type of error is also called phonological paraphasia

semantic error: the use of a word that resembles in meaning the target word (cat instead of dog); this type of error is also called semantic paraphasia

Causes and Symptoms

Wernicke's aphasia is generally caused by a focal brain damage due to strokes, head trauma, brain tumors, or brain infections. People suffering from Wernicke's aphasia showed a lesion in the middle-posterior tract of the first left temporal circonvolution, the so called Wernicke's area or Broadmann's area 22, and in the adjacent cortico-subcortical areas.

The classical definition of aphasic syndromes consists of various categorization systems. Some authors categorize according to the type of language errors. Others take into consideration language production and related impairments in spontaneous speech. However, in past decades a classification has been suggested on the basis of specific clusters of aphasic disorders. In particular, aphasia syndromes are differentiated in two groups: fluent and nonfluent. Wernicke's aphasia, as well as anomic aphasia, transcortical sensory aphasia and conduction aphasia, are considered fluent aphasias, while Broca's aphasia, global aphasia and transcortical motor aphasia are forms of the nonfluent type. Fluent types are characterized by fluent speech, no articulation disorders, but difficulties in auditory comprehension and/or repetition and the presence of paraphasias. Nonfluent types are characterized by difficulties in articulation and spoken language with relatively preserved auditory comprehension.

Here are the main symptoms of Wernicke's aphasia: Auditory comprehension is impaired, generally both at the level of sentences and discourse and at the level of single words. Repetition is also compromised as well as naming that is affected by semantic and phonological omissions and substitutions due to word finding retrieval problems. Spontaneous speech is well articulated and connected and produced effortlessly, but phonemic errors as well as semantically and nonsemantically related substitutions are frequent.

Treatment and Therapy

People who became aphasic after a stroke or a traumatic brain injury generally undergo a variable degree of recuperation in the period following injury referred to as "spontaneous recovery." This effect is maximal in the first 6 months, even if there is evidence that improvement can be observed up to 2 years post onset. While all studies indicate that the initial severity, defined with global impairment measures, is the strongest predictor of recovery, the type of aphasic syndrome (e.g., Broca's aphasia, Wernicke's aphasia) is not a good independent predictor. Many other factors influence spontaneous recovery like etiology, handedness, age, multilingualism, and hemispheric asymmetries as well as social support and mood. The presence of spontaneous recovery suggests that neuroplasticity could be allowing the damaged brain to regain previously lost functionality. Despite the importance of spontaneous recovery, treating language deficits is essential. When planning and setting the therapeutic goals for aphasia therapy, it is important to use diagnostic tools that provide an overview of an aphasic person's abilities and disabilities in both the language and associated cognitive domains, in order to guarantee an impairment-specific training. Generally, in the case of Wernicke's aphasia, it is important to first treat auditory comprehension deficits through different tasks, like matching photos or pictures with words and sentences. Concerning pharmacological treatments, in the subacute to chronic phase, drugs may provide useful adjuvant therapy, but only in the presence of specific language and speech therapies.

Perspective and Prospects

Even if a diagnostic label like "Wernicke's aphasia" can be useful to communicate information among different clinicians, recently the limits of the classic approach have been emphasized. Only roughly defined linguistic parameters and tasks are employed. An enormous variability is seen in the relative severity of each of the constituting symptoms in each syndrome. Many observed cases would not unambiguously fit one classic aphasia type. As a result, what is considered in one hospital as an instance of one type of aphasia may be occasionally classified otherwise in another hospital. The new approach to the study of language disorders has been influenced by theoretical linguistics and by cognitive neuropsychology. Each clinical condition should be described in terms of damage to representation and processes involved in a given task. The content and the format of concerned representations should be specified. Thus, the description of aphasic disorders would overcome the traditional classification of Wernicke's aphasia, global aphasia and so on, in order to take into consideration the different levels of grammar: the phonological, the morpho-syntactic and the lexicosemantic level. Moreover, for each of these levels, a distinction between production impairments and comprehension deficits is necessary. Only this description and analysis of deficits helps clinical neuropsychologists or speech therapists to construct specific rehabilitation protocols for each patient. Then, impairment-specific training will aim primarily at relearning degraded linguistic knowledge, reactivating impaired linguistic modalities such as oral and written comprehension, and learning explicit compensatory linguistic strategies.

—Valentina Chiarelli, Ph.D.

See also Aphasia and dysphasia

For Further Information:

Berthier, M.L. "Poststroke Aphasia: Epidemiology, Pathophysiology and Treatment." *Drugs Ageing* 22, no. 2 (2005): 163-182.

Denes, G., and L. Pizzamiglio. *Handbook of Neuropsychology.* London: Erlbaum, 1999.

Hillis, A.E. *The Handbook of Adult Language Disorders: Integrating Cognitive Neuropsychology, Neurology and Rehabilitation.* New York: Psychology Press, 2002.

Whitworth, A., J. Webster, and D. Howard. *A Cognitive Neuropsychological Approach to Assessment and Intervention in Aphasia: A Clinician's Guide.* New York: Psychology Press, 2005.

WEST NILE VIRUS

Disease/Disorder

Also known as: West Nile encephalitis, West Nile meningitis

Anatomy or system affected: Brain, nervous system, psychic-emotional system

Specialties and related fields: Environmental health, epidemiology, neurology, pathology, public health, virology

Definition: A mosquito-borne virus affecting humans, birds, and possibly other warm-blooded animals.

Key terms:

arbovirus: any virus transmitted by an arthropod such as a mosquito or fly; the term is an abbreviation of "arthropod-borne virus"

emerging disease: a disease whose incidence in target organisms such as humans has suddenly increased

encephalitis: any disease that manifests symptoms of swelling of the meninges, or linings of the brain

meninges: the three protective layers or linings of the brain, called the pia mater, dura mater, and subarachnoid

Causes and Symptoms

For most of the twentieth century following its discovery in Uganda, West Nile virus, an organism that can cause severe inflammation of the spinal cord and brain, was known only in Africa, southeast Europe, and southwest Asia. As the century came to a close, however, the potentially fatal disease emerged in the Western Hemisphere, in the New York City metropolitan area. Since then, it has spread across the continental United States, seven Canadian provinces, Mexico, the Caribbean, and parts of Central America. One of the hallmarks of the disease is dead birds, such as crows, who are also susceptible to the virus.

The first North American cases of the mosquito-borne West Nile virus were found in patients from New York in 1999, and its resurgence in following summers indicates that this disease has become established. The virus is a member of the Japanese encephalitis complex most closely related to St. Louis encephalitis, which also occurs in North America. This group of encephalitis viruses includes the Japanese, Murray Valley, and Stratford complex of viruses. The West Nile virus is also called West Nile encephalitis or West Nile meningitis.

The West Nile virus is called an arbovirus, which is an abbreviation for "arthropod-borne virus." Mosquitoes are the only known agents of transmission of the virus. Other blood-feeding animals, such as ticks and flies, may carry the virus, but so far none of them has been shown to transmit the viral disease to humans. The disease cannot be transmitted from one person to another or between animals and humans other than through a vector mosquito.

A potential transmission cycle begins when a mosquito becomes infected with the disease by feeding on an infected animal, usually a bird or mammal. The virus enters the mosquito's bloodstream and is eventually carried to its salivary glands. The virus incubates within the salivary glands for an unknown period of time. During the mosquito's next blood meal, some of the saliva containing the virus may be injected. Once inside the individual, the virus multiplies and is carried via the bloodstream to all the tissues of the body. In about 1 in 150 individuals, some of the virus makes its way past the blood-brain barrier and into the brain. In humans, the pathology of the West Nile virus disease manifests as a type of encephalitis, a swelling of the meninges, or tissue linings, of the brain.

The first symptoms of infection usually appear within three to fifteen days following exposure, and they may include fever, headache, general body aches, swollen lymph glands, and sometimes a skin rash. In more serious cases, symptoms such as high fever, stiffness, disorientation, stupor, coma, tremors, convulsions, and muscle weakness and paralysis may progressively occur.

Treatment and Therapy

Severely infected individuals are hospitalized and treated with a battery of life-support therapies, including intravenous fluids, ventilation to aid breathing, and inoculations to prevent the occurrence of pneumonia and other secondary infections. In many cases, the symptoms may last several weeks. In severe cases, brain damage and other neurological disorders may be permanent. Fatalities result from swelling of the brain and associated neurological pathologies. At present, there is no treatment for the disease.

Perspective and Prospects

West Nile virus is a classic emerging disease. It was first isolated in 1937 in the West Nile Valley of Uganda in humans and animals, notably horses and birds. The virus quickly spread throughout much of interior Africa, following the course of the Nile River southward into Uganda and neighboring countries, then westward into the Republic of the Congo, then still farther south into Botswana and Zimbabwe. Spreading northward along the Nile River, the virus reached Egypt in 1950, then spread across the Middle East, Eurasia, and Oceania. By 1997, the virus was documented in Italy, France, and Romania. The first cases of West Nile virus in North America were reported in the early summer of 1999 in New York. Twelve states reported cases in 2001, and all states but Alaska and Hawaii had reported the disease by 2005. The numbers of both infections and fatalities in the United States decreased between 2008 and 2011. However, in 2012, there were over 5,600 reported cases of West Nile in the United States, including over 280 deaths. The number of reported cases in Canada in 2003 reached about 1,400; by 2005, only 200 persons were diagnosed. In 2012, approximately 450 cases of West Nile were reported in Canada.

The transmission and fatality rates in humans are actually very low, for several reasons. First, the incidence of infected mosquitoes in an area is typically small, generally on the order of about 1 percent or less, even in regions that have had a long history of West Nile virus. Second, acquiring the virus from the bite of an infected mosquito is not certain, as particles of the virus may or may not be transmitted into the human bloodstream during the blood meal. Finally, small amounts of virus may not produce the "full-blown" disease in humans. The Centers for Disease Control and Prevention (CDC) suggest that about 1 in 150 people bitten by an infected mosquito becomes severely ill with the disease. Healthy people may simply fight off the viral infection without manifesting any symptoms at all. Others experience a variety of generally mild, flulike symptoms, which may include malaise, aching

---

Information on West Nile Virus

Causes: Viral infection transmitted by mosquitoes
Symptoms: Fever, headache, body aches, swollen lymph glands, sometimes rash; in severe cases, high fever, stiffness, tremors, convulsions, muscle weakness and paralysis, disorientation, stupor, brain swelling, coma, sometimes death
Duration: Several weeks
Treatments: In severe cases, hospitalization and life-support therapies (intravenous fluids, ventilation, inoculations against secondary infections)

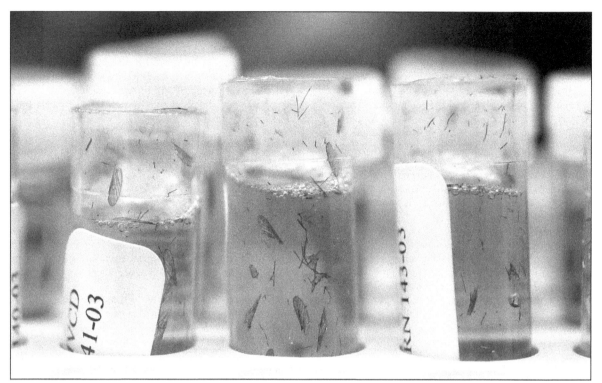

Vials are filled with mosquitoes to be tested for the presence of West Nile virus in California in August, 2003. (AP/Wide World Photos)

bones, and headaches.

CDC estimates of fatality rates are uncertain but suggest that one in one thousand infected people actually dies from the disease, but some estimates place the fatality rate at 3 to 15 percent. As with many viral diseases, the effect of West Nile virus increases with age; the young and healthy seem to develop very few symptoms and almost no residual traces of the disease, but people fifty and older or individuals with compromised immune systems are most at risk. Individuals who survive exposure apparently develop a long-term immunity to the virus.

At present, the only way to prevent becoming infected with West Nile virus is to avoid being outdoors in areas where mosquitoes are plentiful or, alternately, to confine outdoor activities to midday hours, when mosquitoes are least active. When outdoors, one should use a recommended mosquito repellant and wear long pants and a long-sleeved shirt.

Among mammals, horses seem most susceptible to the West Nile virus, but the virus has also been documented in dogs, cats, rabbits, skunks, bats, chipmunks, mice, and squirrels. At least seventy species of birds have been found with the disease, of which sparrows, ducks, pigeons, starlings, and crows are the best-known examples. Of these animals, crows seem most at risk, or at least seem to show the highest incidence of infection and mortality, but this may reflect their size and coloration, both factors making them easily seen. Despite public concern over the incidence of West Nile virus in birds and other mammals, tests have shown that the virus cannot be transmitted simply by handling dead birds. There are no records of animal-to-animal or animal-to-human transmission of West Nile virus. However, it is always advisable to wear gloves and avoid the animal's body fluids when handling animals found dead or known to be infected with West Nile virus.

—Dwight G. Smith, Ph.D.;
updated by David M. Lawrence

See also Brain; Brain disorders; Emerging infectious diseases; Encephalitis; Epidemics and pandemics; Insect-borne diseases; Meningitis; Nervous system; Neurology; Neurology, pediatric; Viral infections; Zoonoses.

For Further Information:
Despommier, Dickson D. *West Nile Story.* New York: Apple Tree, 2001.
Emerging Infectious Diseases Journal 7, no. 4 (August, 2001).
Giesecke, Johan. *Modern Infectious Disease Epidemiology.* 2d ed. New York: Oxford University Press, 2002.
Lashley, Felissa R. "West Nile Virus." In *Emerging Infectious Diseases: Trends and Issues*, edited by Lashley and Jerry D. Durham. New York: Springer, 2002.
Neale, Todd. "West Nile Virus 'Stumps' CDC." *medpagetoday.com* . 27 Sept. 2012:Web. 4 Jun. 2013.
Sfakianos, Jeffrey N. *West Nile Virus.* Rev. ed. Philadelphia: Chelsea House, 2005.
White, Dennis J., and Dale L. Morse, eds. *West Nile Virus: Detection, Surveillance, and Control.* New York: New York Academy of Sciences, 2003.

WHIPLASH
Disease/Disorder
Anatomy or system affected: Head, ligaments, neck, spine
Specialties and related fields: Orthopedics, physical therapy
Definition: An injury to the muscles and ligaments in the neck that is usually the result of riding inside a motor vehicle that is hit from behind.

Causes and Symptoms

When a moving car collides with an obstacle, the driver and passengers suddenly feel themselves thrown forward. If an occupant's head hits the dashboard or windshield, then serious injury can result. Seat belts, a padded dashboard, and air bags can reduce the severity of the impact. Conversely, when a car is hit by another vehicle from behind, the occupants will feel an extra forward push against the trunk of their body while the head snaps backward. This so-called whiplash effect is like the crack of a whip made by the driver of a team of horses, in which the whip handle is rapidly moved forward while the end of the rope snaps backward. In a rear-end automobile collision, if a person's head flies backward beyond its normal range of motion, then the muscles and ligaments of the neck can be damaged. The person may not feel pain right away, but it can show up after a delay of some days. In severe cases, vertebrae of the spine can be knocked out of alignment or fractured. Most commonly, injury occurs at the junction of the fourth and fifth vertebrae. The upper four vertebrae are flexible and act as the lash, while the lower ones act as the handle of the whip.

Information on Whiplash

Causes: Usually an automobile collision
Symptoms: Neck pain (sometimes delayed), muscle spasms; in severe cases, fracture or misalignment of vertebrae
Duration: Acute
Treatments: Initial avoidance of activity, aspirin or other anti-inflammatory drugs, neck collar to limit motion, physical therapy (heat treatment, massage, stretching exercises)

Treatment and Therapy

Various treatments for whiplash are available, depending on the severity of the injury. Physically demanding activities such as sports or heavy lifting should be avoided. For pain control, aspirin or other anti-inflammatory drugs can be taken. If muscle spasms occur, then a physician may prescribe physical therapy, which includes heat treatment, massage, and stretching exercises. Wearing a neck collar can be useful to limit the motion of the head so that the muscles and ligaments can heal.

Perspective and Prospects

Most automobiles have a headrest attached to the top of each seatback. Its purpose is to prevent an occupant's head from snapping backward in a rear-end collision. Whiplash injuries happen frequently in cases such as a multiple-car pileup on an interstate highway. Slower speeds and a greater distance

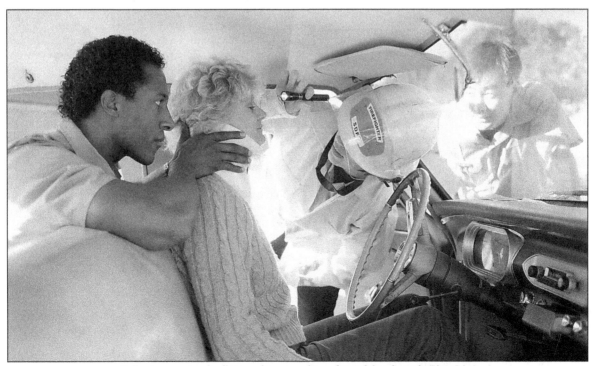

Following a rear-end collision, a brace may be used to stabilize the neck. (PhotoDisc)

between cars are especially important during foggy driving conditions or on an icy road.

Whiplash injury is not limited to car accidents. In football, a quarterback sometimes is tackled from behind, causing the same effect as a car collision from the rear. On the ski slope, a skier may lose control and crash into someone who has stopped to rest. During the snow season, some mountain towns have a tubing hill where people can slide down on inflated inner tubes, with frequent collisions resulting. Any activity that causes excessive flexion of the neck muscles and ligaments can result in whiplash injury.

—*Hans G. Graetzer, Ph.D.*

See also Accidents; Head and neck disorders; Headaches; Ligaments; Muscle sprains, spasms, and disorders; Muscles; Physical rehabilitation; Spine, vertebrae, and disks; Sports medicine.

For Further Information:

American Medical Association. *American Medical Association Family Medical Guide*. 4th rev. ed. Hoboken, N.J.: John Wiley & Sons, 2004.

Carson-DeWitt, Rosalyn. "Whiplash." *Health Library*, June 24, 2013.

Foreman, Stephen M., and Arthur C. Croft. *Whiplash Injuries: The Cervical Acceleration/Deceleration Syndrome*. 3d ed. Philadelphia: Lippincott Williams & Wilkins, 2002.

Kasper, Dennis L., et al., eds. *Harrison's Principles of Internal Medicine*. 16th ed. New York: McGraw-Hill, 2005.

Komaroff, Anthony, ed. *Harvard Medical School Family Health Guide*. New York: Free Press, 2005.

"Neck Pain." *American Academy of Orthopaedic Surgeons*, November 2009.

Rook, Jack L. *Whiplash Injuries*. Philadelphia: Butterworth-Heinemann, 2003.

"Whiplash." *MedlinePlus*, June 4, 2011.

WHOOPING COUGH

Disease/Disorder

Also known as: Pertussis

Anatomy or system affected: Chest, heart, neck, respiratory system, throat

Specialties and related fields: Bacteriology, critical care, family medicine, otorhinolaryngology, pediatrics

Definition: A highly contagious respiratory disease characterized by uncontrollable coughing that ends in a loud whoop as the patient attempts to inhale.

Key terms:

catarrhal stage: the early stage of pertussis, characterized by sneezing and dry cough

DPT vaccine: a trivalent vaccine that provides immunization against diphtheria, pertussis, and tetanus

dyspnea: difficulty in breathing

epiglottis: tissue that lies over the larynx to prevent food from entering the windpipe

paroxysmal stage: the second stage of pertussis, characterized by deep, rapid coughing accompanied by sharp intakes of breath with sound of "whooping"

Causes and Symptoms

The etiological agent of whooping cough is *Bordetella pertussis*, a small, gram-negative, rod-shaped bacterium. A similar organism, *Bordetella parapertussis*, causes a less severe form of the disease. Symptoms and tissue damage are the result of a toxin secreted by the organism.

The diagnosis of pertussis is primarily clinical, based on the characteristic whoop that accompanies the paroxysmal stage. The most definitive diagnosis involves the actual isolation of the organism. Most pathogenic strains of *Bordetella* are fastidious in their requirements. Nasal swabs from the patient are obtained, with the organism grown on a special Bordet-Gengou medium.

The clinical manifestation of whooping cough is arbitrarily divided into the catarrhal, paroxysmal, and convalescent stages. The average incubation period following exposure is about seven days. During this period, the patient develops a dry cough, often accompanied by sneezing. A mild fever may be present. Early symptoms resemble those of bronchitis or influenza.

The severity of the cough gradually increases over the next ten to fourteen days; it may be triggered by exercise or even eating. As the patient enters the paroxysmal stage, the cough becomes deeper and more pronounced. It is often characterized as a series of short bursts, followed by a whooping sound as the patient attempts to inhale; the sound itself is caused by possible spasm of the epiglottis.

Large quantities of mucus may be expelled during the coughing spells, which in severe cases may occur forty to fifty times a day. The patient may exhibit dyspnea and become cyanotic from lack of air. In infants, choking is common during this stage and can prove fatal. The severity of the cough has also been known to result in hemorrhaging from the throat.

The paroxysmal stage of the disease lasts from four to six weeks. Gradually, the cough disappears as the patient enters the convalescent stage. The entire period of illness may last ten weeks, with the cough persisting for months afterward; coughing may recur during another respiratory illness.

The disease is highly contagious, with the agent passing from person to person by means of respiratory droplets. The patient is most infectious during both the catarrhal stage and the early portion of the paroxysmal stage, a period lasting two to three weeks.

Treatment and Therapy

Routine treatment of whooping cough consists of bed rest and the provision of adequate food and water. Infants are most at risk and are generally hospitalized. The administration of oxygen may be helpful in the relief of dyspnea and cyanosis. If

---

Information on Whooping Cough

Causes: Bacterial infection

Symptoms: Dry, hacking cough that becomes deep and uncontrollable, followed by whooping sound upon inhalation; fever; excess mucus production

Duration: Six to eight weeks

Treatments: Antibiotics (erythromycin), supportive therapy

there is prolonged vomiting, intravenous therapy may be necessary. Administration of corticosteroids has also been shown to ameliorate the severity of the cough.

Because paroxysmal symptoms are associated with production of a toxin secondary to the initial infection, antibiotics are of little help. An antibiotic such as erythromycin, however, may be administered to reduce secondary infections or to limit transmission to other persons. If erythromycin is administered early during the development of the disease, during the incubation period, or even during the first week of the catarrhal stage, it may prevent the disease or limit its severity. Persons coming into contact with the patient should also receive a course of antibiotic treatment.

Immunoglobulin is available, but its effectiveness is in dispute. Active immunization with pertussis vaccine is recommended to protect against the initial infection. Usually, this is a portion of the DTaP vaccine administered in a series of injections beginning at about two months of age.

Perspective and Prospects

The earliest known description of whooping cough was that by G. Baillou in 1578. It was Robert Watt, an English physician, who in 1813 provided the first complete clinical description of the disease. Watt also described the results of autopsies that he had performed on children who had died of the disease during his thirty years of observations; two of these children were his own. Watt also noted the highly contagious nature of whooping cough.

In 1906, Jules Bordet and his brother-in-law, Octave Gengou, isolated the infectious agent from the sputum of Bordet's son, who had contracted the disease. Known initially as *Haemophilus pertussis*, the organism was eventually renamed *Bordetella pertussis* after its discoverer. Bordet also determined that the virulent nature of the disease resulted from the production of a toxin. The special substance needed to grow the organism in the laboratory became known as Bordet-Gengou medium.

Initial attempts to develop a pertussis vaccine by Bordet and Gengou using inactivated toxin were largely unsuccessful. In the 1940s, however, an inactivated whole cell suspension was introduced and proved effective in immunizing children against the disease. In the United States, the pertussis vaccine was combined with inactivated diphtheria and tetanus preparations into a trivalent vaccine, DPT, that proved effective in immunizing children against all three diseases simultaneously.

Because of side effects in some children receiving the pertussis preparation, such as fever, vomiting, and mild seizures, questions developed as to the safety of the vaccine. In 1997, a new vaccine, DTaP, was introduced after researchers learned it was much less likely to cause the adverse reactions found with the DPT vaccine. The *a* in DTaP stands for "acellular," which means there are no whole bacteria in the vaccine. While the DPT vaccine uses whole, inactivate pertussis bacteria, the DTaP uses only the parts of the bacteria that help children develop immunity to it. Since human beings represent the only reservoir of whooping cough, the disease may eventually face eradication.

—*Richard Adler, Ph.D.*

See also Antibiotics; Bacterial infections; Childhood infectious diseases; Coughing; Immunization and vaccination; Lungs; Pulmonary diseases; Pulmonary medicine; Pulmonary medicine, pediatric; Respiration; Wheezing.

For Further Information:

Alan, Rick, and Brian Randall. "Whooping Cough." *Health Library*, Nov. 26, 2012.

Cohen, Jonathan, et al, eds. *Infectious Diseases*. 3d ed. St. Louis, Mo.: Mosby, 2010.

Kliegman, Robert M., et al, eds. *Nelson Textbook of Pediatrics*. 19th ed. Philadelphia: Saunders/Elsevier, 2011.

Larsen, Laura. *Childhood Diseases and Disorders Sourcebook: Basic Consumer Health Information About Medical Problems Often Encountered in Pre-adolescent Children*. 3d ed. Detroit, Mich.: Omnigraphics, 2012.

"Pertussis (Whooping Cough)." *Centers for Disease Control and Prevention*, May 7, 2013.

"Pertussis (Whooping Cough) " What You Need to Know." *Centers for Disease Control and Prevention*, May 8, 2013.

Ryan, Kenneth J., and C. George Ray, eds. *Sherris Medical Microbiology: An Introduction to Infectious Diseases*. 4th ed. New York: McGraw-Hill, 2004.

"Whooping Cough." *MedlinePlus*, May 21, 2013.

Woolf, Alan D., et al., eds. *The Children's Hospital Guide to Your Child's Health and Development*. Cambridge, Mass.: Perseus, 2002.

WILLIAMS SYNDROME
Disease/Disorder

Anatomy or system affected: face, heart, kidneys, bladder, bowels, ears, eyes, muscles, skin, brain, spine, endocrine system

Specialties and related fields: genetics, cardiology, nephrology, audiology, optometry/ophthalmology, physical therapy, occupational therapy, neurology, endocrinology, neuropsychology, psychology/psychiatry, orthodontics

Definition: A rare neurodevelopmental disorder caused by a microdeletion within a specific region of chromosome 7 (7q11.23), typically encompassing approximately 25 to 28 adjacent genes; this chromosomal region has been named "Williams Beuren Syndrome chromosome region 1" (WBSCR1).

Key terms:

arteriopathy: any disease of the artery

autosomal dominant: a disease in which a person only needs to receive the abnormal gene from one parent in order to inherit the disease

hypertension: high blood pressure

hypercalcemia: abnormally high level of calcium in the blood

malocclusion: a misalignment of teeth or incorrect relation between the teeth of the two dental arches

microdeletion: a genetic mutation resulting from the deletion of a small part of a chromosome, usually involving many genes

supravalvular aortic stenosis: a narrowing of the aorta (the large blood vessel that carries blood from the heart to the rest of the body)

Causes and Symptoms

Williams syndrome is caused by the deletion of genetic material on one copy of chromosome 7. The condition affects males and females equally. The prevalence of this condition is estimated to be approximately one in 10,000 worldwide. Most cases are sporadic and occur in a single family member only, but occasionally, parent-to-child transmission is observed. In familial cases, Williams syndrome is inherited as an autosomal dominant trait. Diagnosis is typically confirmed by genetic testing known as a FISH (fluorescent in situ hybridization) test that detects a deletion of one of the critical genes, the Elastin (ELN) gene, which lies in the middle of the deleted region. The ELN gene encodes the protein elastin. According to investigators, many genes within the 7q11.23 chromosomal region may play a causative role in Williams syndrome, including those known as the ELN (elastin) gene, the LIMK1 (or LIM kinase-1) gene, and the RFC2 (replication factor C, subunit 2) gene. The LIMK1 gene is believed to be involved with the visual-spatial problems associated with Williams syndrome.

Williams syndrome is characterized by a wide spectrum of symptoms that may change, persist, resolve, improve, or increase with age. Babies with Williams syndrome usually experience growth delays before and after birth, and developmental delays are common. As time goes on, the following features may also become apparent: short stature, a varying degree of intellectual disability, distinctive facial features that typically become more pronounced with age (small upturned nose, flattened nasal bridge, flat cheek bones, full cheeks, puffiness around the eyes, full lips, and small irregular teeth). A star-like (stellate) pattern in the iris of the eye may be apparent in about 50 percent of children with this disorder.

Children with Williams syndrome may feed poorly, and fail to gain weight and grow at the expected rate. Symptoms such as vomiting, gagging, diarrhea, and constipation are common during infancy. Some infants may have elevated levels of calcium in their blood (hypercalcemia), leading to loss of appetite, irritability, confusion, weakness, fatigue, and/or abdominal and muscle pain. Calcium levels usually return to normal around the age of 12 months. However, in some cases, hypercalcemia may last into adulthood. Growth may be delayed during the first four years of life. However, growth spurts usually occur between the age of five and 10 years.

Other defining features include: abnormal brain development (such as smaller brain size and unusual brain shape); extreme cognitive impairments in visual-motor and visual-spatial functions (regardless of level of intellect); a distinctive outgoing, friendly, and empathetic personality; a short attention span and distractibility. Learning difficulties may also be present (particularly in nonverbal domains, such as mathematics, but literacy can also be affected). Language is impaired, but of note, superficially fluent social language, eagerness to please and some relative language strengths (e.g., vocabulary, rote social phrases) can be misleading and mask underlying areas of language and cognitive deficit.

Williams syndrome is also associated with high levels of anxiety (generalized anxiety disorder, specific phobias), and Attention Deficit Hyperactivity Disorder (ADHD) is more prevalent here than in the general population. Depression is also of concern, especially in adolescents and adults.

Because they lack the elastin protein, people with Williams syndrome may have disorders of the circulatory system and heart defects (elastin arteriopathy, most commonly supravalvular aortic stenosis). Williams syndrome may also be associated with connective tissue abnormalities (hoarse voice, hernias, bowel/bladder diverticulae, rectal prolapse, constipation, joint limitation or laxity, and soft, lax skin, premature skin aging), endocrine abnormalities (idiopathic hypercalcemia, hypercalciuria, hypothyroidism, early puberty); hypotonia, and hyperextensible and stiff joints are also common. Abnormal curvature of the spine (scoliosis or kyphosis) and awkward gait may be present.

Affected individuals may also experience auditory/hearing difficulties (e.g., chronic middle ear infections, hypersensitivity to sound known as hyperacusis; hearing loss can occur, especially with age). Visual problems (e.g., inward deviation of the eyes, squint, farsightedness, poor depth perception, cataracts) and dental abnormalities (e.g., malocclusion, small and underdeveloped teeth) can occur.

Treatment and Therapy

There is no cure for Williams syndrome, but with regular monitoring and appropriate intervention, most affected individuals can lead active and full lives. Patients must be continually monitored and treated for symptoms throughout their lives. Treatment of most symptoms does not differ from that in the general population. It can help to have treatment coordinated by a geneticist who has experience with the disorder.

Early intervention programs, special education programs, psychometric assessments and vocational training address developmental, intellectual and learning disabilities. Programs may include speech/language, physical, occupational, feeding, and sensory integration therapies. Psychological and psychiatric evaluation and treatment provide individualised behavioural counseling, cognitive and behavioural interventions and medications may be required, especially for anxiety and ADHD. Surgery may be required for cardiac, renal, or other medical defects. Treatment of hypercalcemia may include diet modification, avoidance of dietary supplements, and/or medication. Other symptoms would be treated according to standard protocols.

Guidelines typically suggest cardiology evaluations annually in early childhood and every 2 to 3 years thereafter throughout adulthood. Additional periodic evaluations include: serum calcium studies every four to six months before the age of two years and every two years thereafter; assessment of thyroid function and oral glucose tolerance every three years; and renal and bladder ultrasound examination every ten years. Regular vision and hearing assessments are recommended and should continue into adulthood. Reviews may be more frequent or may include monitoring of other symptoms, depending on an individual's clinical history.

The risk of hypertension increases with age and should be monitored regularly (blood pressure must be taken from both arms). Continued monitoring of gastrointestinal, musculoskeletal, weight gain/loss, dental problems, mental health are important throughout childhood, adolescence, and into adulthood.

Perspective and Prospects

The first reported case of Williams syndrome was published in the early 1960s. In the 1970s and even 1980s, it was not uncommon for affected children to go undiagnosed until late childhood or even into adulthood. With the aging population, there are also likely to be many older adults with the disorder who have not been diagnosed. The increased awareness of Williams syndrome within the general medical field and the opportunity for genetic testing since the 1990s has led to much earlier and more accurate diagnoses, with the syndrome now typically diagnosed in the first year of life.

Of note, despite the social phenotype of Williams syndrome, many individuals experience difficulties with forming and maintaining friendships; social isolation, loneliness, and depression are common, particularly in adults. There is an ongoing need for structure and routine and vocational and vacational activities to provide opportunity for regular social interactions and to promote daily independence.

There has been an exponential growth in research on Williams syndrome, particularly in the last decade; more research is needed into intervention approaches to bridge the gap between research and clinical practice. Remediation techniques that utilize cognitive strengths to help compensate for other weaknesses are proving beneficial for some individuals with Williams syndrome, such as verbal mediation to assist with spatial navigation, drawing, and handwriting.

Of note, clinical and cognitive variability within the disorder indicates that individually tailored management and interventions are required and should be informed by the detailed evaluation of a particular individual's needs and their individual profile cognitive of strengths and weaknesses.

—*Melanie Porter, Ph.D.*

See also Genetic diseases; Genetics and inheritance

For Further Information:

Canadian Association for Williams Syndrome: http://www.williams-syndrome.org

Genetic and Rare Diseases (GARD) Information Center: http://rarediseases.info.nih.gov/GARD/AboutGARD.aspx.

NIH/National Institute of Child Health and Human Development: http://www.nichd.nih.gov/.

Williams Syndrome Association: http://www.williams-syndrome.org.

Williams Syndrome Association of Australia: http:// www.agsa-geneticsupport.org.au

The Williams Syndrome Foundation (UK): http://www.williams-syndrome.org.uk

WILSON'S DISEASE
Disease/Disorder

Also known as: Hepatolenticular degeneration

Anatomy or system affected: Brain, liver, nervous system, psychic-emotional system

Specialties and related fields: Biochemistry, gastroenterology, internal medicine, neurology

Definition: An inherited disease of abnormal copper metabolism, leading to copper accumulation and toxicity in the liver and brain.

Causes and Symptoms

Wilson disease is an autosomal recessive disorder of copper metabolism, resulting in excess copper accumulation and toxicity in the body. The gene in Wilson disease is located on chromosome 13 and codes for a copper-transporting protein. The normal mechanism of elimination of excess copper in humans is excretion of extra copper in the bile for loss in the stool. The genetic mutation in this disease causes defective, reduced excretion of copper into the bile by the liver. The resultant excessive copper accumulation in the liver and brain causes liver damage and neurologic as well as psychiatric abnormalities.

Wilson disease typically manifests itself between the ages of ten and forty, although it may also appear in earlier childhood as well as later in life. Typical signs and symptoms are related to damage to the liver and brain. Liver involvement in Wilson disease may vary from hepatitis or chronic cirrhosis to acute liver failure. Neurologic symptoms and signs often involve areas of brain that control movement. Patients may have slurred speech, tremor and rigidity in the extremities, and dystonia, a syndrome of sustained muscle contractions causing abnormal postures or movements. Other symptoms include seizures, mental changes, and transient periods of coma. Psychiatric abnormalities may also be prominent and may be the initial presentation. Behavioral changes include impaired school performance, labile moods, depression, and psychosis.

Useful screening tests for Wilson disease include serum ceruloplasmin, twenty-four-hour urine copper, and slitlamp examination for Kayser-Fleischer rings. Blood ceruloplasmin is usually low in Wilson disease, although approximately 10 to 25 percent of patients will have a normal value. Urinary copper values are typically elevated in symptomatic patients. Kayser-Fleisher rings, which are caused by copper deposits in the cornea of the eye, can be detected reliably only by slitlamp microscopy examination. They are almost always seen in patients with neurologic or psychiatric symptoms but may not be present in patients with symptoms related to liver damage. The gold standard for diagnosis in Wilson disease is liver biopsy, which reveals an elevated amount of copper in the liver.

Treatment and Therapy

Given the diverse initial presentations of Wilson disease, early diagnosis is often difficult. It is important, however, because effective treatments exist. Treatment is aimed toward the prevention of copper accumulation, the reduction of copper absorption through the promotion of its excretion in the urine or bile, or a combination of these mechanisms. Pharmacologic treatments include penicillamine and trientine, two drugs that act by removing copper (chelating agents); zinc,

Information on Wilson's Disease

Causes: Genetic defect in copper metabolism
Symptoms: Liver damage (hepatitis, cirrhosis, liver failure); neurologic problems (slurred speech, tremor, rigidity in extremities, dystonia, seizures, mental changes, transient periods of coma); psychiatric abnormalities (behavioral changes, moodiness, depression, psychosis)
Duration: Chronic
Treatments: Chelating agents (penicillamine, trientine), zinc, tetrathiomolybdate, liver transplantation

which blocks copper absorption; and tetrathiomolybdate, which is experimental. Liver transplantation can be helpful in the patient with end-stage liver disease.

—*Winona Tse, M.D.*

See also Genetic diseases; Liver disorders; Liver transplantation; Metabolic disorders; Metabolism; Nervous system; Neurology; Neurology, pediatric; Vitamins and minerals.

For Further Information:

Brewer, George J. *Wilson's Disease: A Clinician's Guide to Recognition, Diagnosis, and Management*. Boston: Kluwer Academic, 2001.
Hoogenraad, Tjaard U. *Wilson's Disease*. Philadelphia: W. B. Saunders, 1996.
"NINDS Wilson Disease Information Page." *National Institute of Neurological Disorders and Stroke*, June 14, 2012.
Parker, James N., and Philip M. Parker, eds. *The 2002 Official Patient's Sourcebook on Wilson's Disease*. San Diego, Calif.: Icon Health, 2002.
Rosenblum, Laurie, and Michael Woods. "Wilson Disease." *Health Library*, Apr. 26, 2013.
Rowland, Lewis P., Timothy A. Pedly, and H. Houston Merritt, ed. *Merritt's Neurology*. 12th ed. Philadelphia: Lippincott Williams & Wilkins, 2010.
Schilsky, M. L. "Diagnosis and Treatment of Wilson's Disease." *Pediatric Transplantation* 6 (2002): 15–19.
"Wilson Disease." *MedlinePlus*, May 20, 2013.
"Wilson Disease." *National Digestive Diseases Information Clearinghouse (NDDIC)*, Apr. 30, 2012.

WISDOM TEETH

Anatomy
Also known as: Third molars
Anatomy or system affected: Gums, mouth, teeth
Specialties and related fields: Dentistry
Definition: The common term for the permanent third molars, which usually appear between the ages of seventeen and twenty-four.

Structure and Functions

The third molars are called wisdom teeth because they appear much later than the other permanent teeth, at an age when people are supposedly wiser than they were as children. The average number of wisdom teeth is four, but it is possible to have more or less. They come in behind the second molars on the upper left, upper right, lower left, and lower right. Wisdom teeth are no longer considered necessary. People now eat soft diets and have better dental care, which prevents decay and molar loss. Thus, the second molars are sufficient.

Wisdom teeth become impacted if the tooth cannot erupt because of gum or bone hardness and/or lack of space. Impacted wisdom teeth fall into four categories: Mesioangular refers to a tooth that is angled forward toward the front of the mouth; vertical refers to a tooth that does not fully erupt through the gum line; horizontal refers to a tooth that angles forward, growing into the roots of the second molar; and distoangular refers to a tooth that is angled backward.

Disorders and Diseases

Wisdom teeth may become infected when saliva, bacteria, or food particles collect around them, causing pain, decay, swelling, and, in severe cases, trismus (inability to open the mouth fully). The infection can spread to the cheek and neck. In rare cases, the infection has been linked to heart disease. Infected wisdom teeth are usually extracted.

Wisdom teeth may also be removed even if no infection is present, such as when a younger patient is having lengthy orthodontic treatment to straighten teeth, as unremoved wisdom teeth may erupt and damage the straightened teeth. Also, older patients who need dentures should have any latent wisdom teeth removed. Should wisdom teeth erupt beneath a denture, it could cause severe irritation. The patient could suffer considerable pain and must replace the dentures, as the shape of the jaw will have changed.

There is a possibility of nerve damage during tooth extraction. Two nerves are close to the lower wisdom teeth. One of them, the inferior alveolar nerve, supplies sensation to the lower teeth on the right and the left side of the mouth, and a sense of touch to the right and left half of the chin and lower lip. The second nerve, the lengual, supplies a sense of touch and taste to the tongue and the gums. Injury can occur as a result of a faulty extraction or by a dental drill. Such injuries are rare, but damage can be prolonged or permanent.

Treatment after extraction usually consists of packing gauze pads in the hole for half an hour to control bleeding. Swelling is controlled by the use of cold packs. After twenty-four hours, rinsing with warm saltwater every two hours will help healing. For minor discomfort, aspirin or ibuprofen can be taken.

Perspective and Prospects

Researchers from the United States and Australia have made stem cell studies on the dental pulp found in extracted wisdom teeth. These stem cells have the potential to save injured teeth and grow jawbone. As research progresses, it may be possible to use these stem cells to restore cells damaged by conditions such as Parkinson's disease.

—*Billie M. Taylor, M.S.E., M.L.S.*

See also Dental diseases; Dentistry; Dentistry, pediatric; Dentures; Orthodontics; Teeth; Tooth extraction; Toothache.

For Further Information:

Fields, Helen, and Margaret Mannix. "Not so Wise Wisdom Teeth." *U.S. News and World Report* 139, no. 12 (October 13, 2005): 53.

Goldie, Maria Perno. "Stem Cell Research: A New Era." *Access* 19, no. 9 (November 2005): 28-30.

"Hold On to Your Wisdom Teeth." *Consumer Reports on Health* 5, no. 8 (August 1993): 84-85.

"Impacted tooth." *MedlinePlus*. April 5, 2012.

"Just Ask Us." *Current Health* 27, no. 2 (October 2000): 94.

Roeder, Felix. "Necessity of 3D Visualization for the Removal of Lower Wisdom Teeth: Required Sample Size to Prove Non-Inferiority of Panoramic Radiography Compared to CBCT." Clinical Oral Investigation. 16.3 (2012): 699–706.

Steinmeh, Eric. "Yanking Those Wisdom Isn't Always Necessary." *Health* 19, no. 8 (October 2005): 91.

"Wisdom Teeth." *American Association of Oral and Maxillofacial Surgeons*. July 25, 2013.

WISKOTT-ALDRICH SYNDROME

Disease/Disorder

Also known as: Aldrich syndrome, eczema-thrombocytopenia-immunodeficiency syndrome

Anatomy or system affected: Blood, ears, immune system, lungs, skin

Specialties and related fields: Dermatology, genetics, immunology, oncology, pediatrics

Definition: An X-linked genetic disorder characterized by thrombocytopenia, infections, and eczema in childhood.

Causes and Symptoms

Wiskott-Aldrich syndrome is a rare primary inherited immunodeficiency disorder, involving both T and Bdf lymphocytes. Also, the disease is characterized by the deficiency of platelets, which are integral cells required for blood clotting. In the classical form, it is manifested soon after birth and through the first year of life, with the symptoms of recurrent sinopulmonary infections (from a decreased immune system); bleeding into the skin, bowels, gums, or joints (from defective platelets); and eczematous scaly skin rash. Autoimmune manifestations in the form of anemia and or malignancies such as lymphoma or leukemia later in adolescence or young adulthood are also reported.

The disease is seen in its classical form as a result of the ineffective production of Wiskott-Aldrich syndrome protein (WASP), which determines the severity of the disease—the greater the deficiency of the WASP, the more severe the disease. Defective production of WASP is caused by a mutation or error in the WASP gene, located on the short arm of the X chromosome. This mutation is inherited in an X-linked recessive fashion, and therefore, primarily boys are affected by the disease. In extremely rare cases involving girls, similar genetic mutations have not been noted.

Wiskott-Aldrich syndrome is suspected in any male child who has bleeding, typically bloody diarrhea in infancy. Older children may even have a low platelet count and abnormally small platelets when a routine blood smear is done during an infection. Otitis media, sinusitis, and pneumonia are quite common infections for these children, and viral infections are also seen as a result of the abnormal immune response.

The clinical presentation depends on the severity of the WASP deficiency and may differ from patient to patient. It may range from just thrombocytopenia (low platelet count) to all three classic symptoms of eczema, recurrent infections (because of immunodeficiency), and bleeding (because of low platelets). The disease X-linked thrombocytopenia is considered a different form of Wiskott-Aldrich syndrome. The first presentation of the disease is usually within the first year of life, soon after birth, and most often is as a result of immunodeficiency or thrombocytopenia. The most characteristic feature of Wiskott-Aldrich syndrome is reduced platelets. Also, a defect in the function of platelets is noticed in some forms of the disease, manifested as bleeding gums, prolonged epistaxis (nosebleeds), or bleeding into joints or bowels.

Eczema is a common symptom of Wiskott-Aldrich syndrome. It may be localized or generalized, with itchy rashes all over the body. Scratching of such rashes might lead to bleeding and infections. Recurrent infections are common in the syndrome because of the deficiency of T and B lymphocytes (white blood cells). As both T and B cells are affected, the infections may be attributable to bacteria, fungi, or viruses. Other manifestations of the disease are autoimmune anemia, leukemia, and lymphoma, which are seen more often in older boys and adults.

A diagnosis of Wiskott-Aldrich syndrome must be considered in any boy with unusual bleeding, recurrent infections, and eczema. The characteristic platelet features of low count and abnormally small size are also evident in the cord blood of a newborn. The blood test for platelet count and size is, therefore, the most useful one. In older children, other tests such as serum immunological studies for antibodies and negative skin tests for T cell function are done. Confirmation of the diagnosis is by measuring the levels of WASP in the blood or by detecting WASP gene mutation through genetic studies.

In families with a boy diagnosed with Wiskott-Aldrich syndrome, prenatal testing of the mother before subsequent pregnancies should be performed by amniocentesis or chorionic villus sampling, as there is a 50 percent chance of a mother transferring the abnormal gene to her baby.

Treatment and Therapy

The treatment of Wiskott-Aldrich syndrome is prolonged and involves multiple approaches. Family support is of vital importance in the treatment of chronic illnesses. Bleeding often results in anemia that requires blood transfusions for correction. To counter recurrent infections, these boys require appropriate antibiotics, which must be determined after careful culture and sensitivity tests. As a result of the abnormality of the immune system, vaccinations might not prove very effective. In fact, live virus vaccines are contraindicated in these patients and must be avoided. Instead, patients are given intravenous immunoglobulins (IVIGs), or preformed antibodies, to decrease the chances of bacterial infections. The treatment of eczema involves avoiding frequent bathing and applying bath oils and moisturizing creams after a bath;

Information on Wiskott-Aldrich Syndrome

Causes: Genetic protein deficiency affecting lymphocytes and platelets

Symptoms: Thrombocytopenia; eczema; recurrent sinus and pulmonary infections; bleeding into skin, bowels, gums, or joints

Duration: Chronic

Treatments: Blood and platelet transfusions, antibiotics, intravenous immunoglobulins, removal of spleen, bone marrow transplantation, cord blood stem cell transplantation

topical steroids are often helpful. Systemic antibiotics are of help in some cases of eczema. Platelet deficiency is corrected by transfusing platelets into the bloodstream. Surgical removal of the spleen is of some beneficial effect in checking the thrombocytopenia. Avoiding allergens is an important way to prevent the exacerbation of eczema. Bone marrow transplantation and cord blood stem cell transplantation are the only methods of curing the disease permanently.

Perspective and Prospects

In 1937, Alfred Wiskott first discovered this disease in three brothers with low platelet counts. In 1954, Robert Anderson Aldrich identified it as an X-linked recessive disease. When the disease was first identified, the prognosis was dismal, with a life expectancy of just two to three years. The discovery of and advances in antibiotics, immunoglobulins, bone marrow transplantations, and cord blood stem cell transplantation have improved the prognosis greatly. Today, it is not unusual to see patients with Wiskott-Aldrich syndrome lead productive lives as adults without developing the complications of the disease.

—*Rashmi Ramasubbaiah, M.D.*

See also Autoimmune disorders; Bleeding; Blood and blood disorders; Bone marrow transplantation; Eczema; Genetic diseases; Hematology; Hematology, pediatric; Immune system; Immunodeficiency disorders; Immunology; Immunopathology; Stem cells; Thrombocytopenia.

For Further Information:

"Bleeding Disorders." *MedlinePlus*, May 24, 2013.

Dugdale, David C. III, Yi-Bin Chen, and David Zieve. "Thrombocytopenia." *MedlinePlus*, Mar. 14, 2012.

Fauci, Anthony S., et al, eds. *Harrison's Principles of Internal Medicine*. 18th ed. New York: McGraw-Hill, 2012.

Frazier, Margeret Schell, and Jeanette Wist Drzymkowski. *Essentials of Human Diseases and Conditions*. 5th ed. St. Louis, Mo.: Saunders/Elsevier, 2013.

Greer, John, et al, eds. *Wintrobe's Clinical Hematology*. 12th ed. Philadelphia: Wolters Kluwer/Lippincott Williams & Wilkins Health, 2009.

Porter, Robert S., et al., eds. *The Merck Manual Home Health Handbook*. Whitehouse Station, N.J.: Merck Research Laboratories, 2009.

"Wiskott-Aldrich Syndrome." *Genetics Home Reference*, May 20, 2013.

WORLD HEALTH ORGANIZATION

Organization

Definition: A specialized agency of the United Nations that fights illness and disease all over the globe.

Key terms:

ecology: a branch of science concerned with the relationships among organisms and their environments

ecosystem: an ecological community considered together with the nonliving factors of its environment

epidemic: an unarrested spread of something, as of a disease

epidemiology: a science that deals with the incidence, distribution, and control of disease in a population

etiology: the investigation of the causes of any disease

meningitis: inflammation of a membrane that envelops the brain or spine, often caused by bacteria

pandemic: pertaining to a high proportion of a population

vaccine: any substance for preventive inoculation to build immunity

Functions and Responsibilities

The World Health Organization (WHO) is a specialized agency of the United Nations. With its headquarters in Geneva, Switzerland, the organization has grown from twenty-six member countries in 1948 to 194 by 2013, improving health conditions on every continent of the earth. It functions under the aegis of the United Nations" Economic and Social Council. The governing body of WHO is the World Health Assembly, which is composed of delegations from all member states. The assembly decides the policies, programs, and budget of the organization. Every three years, the assembly elects members of its thirty-four-member executive board, which oversees the programs and budget for the coming year. These plans are presented for approval by the director general, appointed every five years, who, with a staff of approximately two thousand, is responsible for conducting investigations and surveys.

The World Health Organization is divided into six regional subdivisions working in Europe, the Americas, Africa, the eastern Mediterranean, southeastern Asia, and the western Pacific. These regional organizations have headquarters in Copenhagen, Denmark; Washington, DC; Brazzaville, Congo; Cairo, Egypt; New Delhi, India; and Manila, Philippines; respectively.

The regular budget is contributed directly to WHO by its member states. The United Nations also devotes many resources to funding for technical assistance to underdeveloped countries, of which a substantial part is for health work. Other financial sources are individual donations for promoting good health practices and eradicating malaria. Despite these incomes, there is a continual drain on funds because many underdeveloped countries cannot afford to pay for the drugs, vaccines, or technical medical assistance that they receive.

One of WHO's enduring achievements has been to communicate to the world an understanding and acceptance of the idea of a common, basic list of drugs. The Model Lists of Essential Medicines—the editions of which are broken down into separate lists for adults and children, each separated into lists of core and complemetary drugs—have been a powerful tool in providing scientific justification for the improvement of health standards and practices through publicity, workshops, and training in the developing world. The first list of essential drugs was published in 1977 and included 205 drugs; the list published in 2002 contained 320 preparations; and the list published in 2013 contained more than 350 medicines. The growing lists of drugs are included based on recommendations of expert committees from both developing and developed countries. The committees consist of clinical pharmacologists, health officials, and university professors. The drugs are chosen for efficacy, safety, quality, and stability. By emphasizing generic agents, the list has stimulated international competition among drug suppliers and has brought down prices—an important consideration since some countries spend 40 percent of their slim health budgets on drugs.

WHO concerns itself with the needs of those billions of people in the world who are still without regular access to the most basic drugs at the primary health care level. It seeks to establish equitable access to essential drugs for people. The organization has helped more than 90 percent of its member nations to develop a partly or fully developed essential drugs policy. The Model Lists of Essential Medicines are a valuable resource for countries trying to develop their own national lists. Changes have been made in the lists for several reasons, including oversight or omission, accumulation of more conclusive evidence of the therapeutic advantages of various drugs, and changes in the perceived role of the overall list itself.

WHO attacks communicable diseases in every country through prevention, control, and treatment. The cornerstone of prevention and control is education. Public information is of crucial importance in controlling epidemics. Also vital to many populations is information on nutrition, breast-feeding, personal hygiene, cleanliness, and the use of safe water. Stress is placed on the public's ability to play an important role in prevention and early detection. With full and accurate information, symptoms may be correctly interpreted and conditions correctly diagnosed, thus preventing the spread of disease.

Various WHO commissions continue working on projects to improve health standards. Efforts continue for increasing the number of trained medical personnel in many countries. Systems for selecting, procuring, storing, and distributing drugs and supplies more efficiently are continually being refined. WHO is cognizant of a global range of concerns, from promoting a healthy environment to revising guidelines for ethical conduct in research on an international level.

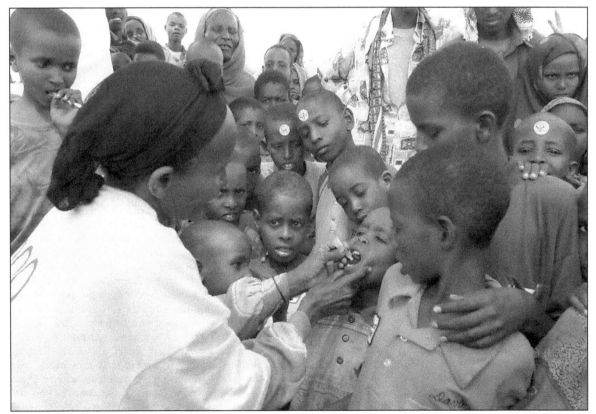

A World Health Organization (WHO) official gives a dose of polio vaccine to Somali children in Somalia in 2000. (AP/Wide World Photos)

Efforts around the World

The World Health Organization monitors the spread or decline of disease all over the world. An example of how beneficial such knowledge can be when applied internationally is the organization's work on inoculation in Egypt and Brazil. Public information services led to its success. In 1973, a study supported by WHO to test the effectiveness of a newly perfected meningitis vaccine was conducted in Egypt, with 250,000 schoolchildren participating. After the first year, it was clear that the vaccine was extremely effective.

Then a major meningitis epidemic broke out in Brazil. King Faisal of Saudi Arabia, aware of the successful results in Alexandria, Egypt, donated four million US dollars to send the vaccine to Brazil in order to reduce international concern. Immunization against meningitis was later carried out in Sudan, with the population of Khartoum and surrounding areas receiving vaccinations in 1987 when the disease began to break out across the country.

In Saudi Arabia, vaccination against meningitis is particularly important in preventing disease at the time of the annual pilgrimage to the holy city of Mecca. The health authorities ask that all pilgrims be vaccinated against meningitis before they arrive in Saudi Arabia, and, if they have not done so, then they are offered vaccination on arrival. People living in the pilgrimage area—in the cities of Jeddah, Mecca, and Medina—who come into contact with the pilgrims are also vaccinated against meningitis regularly; thus, no cases are expected among them.

The exchange of information has also led to spectacular success in Egypt in the control of diarrheal diseases. Authorities have used a proven method: after recognizing the seriousness of the problem, they have developed a simple preventive message and have used public personalities to deliver it. Egypt has also made effective use of all information channels, employing various methods to give the same message. Egypt's national program to control diarrheal diseases is recognized as one of the best in the world. It has demonstrated the value of using the media for advocating health. The country is no longer concentrating only on curing these diseases but instead is giving equal emphasis to prevention. These practices are also used to educate mothers about nutrition, breast-feeding, personal hygiene, cleanliness, and the use of safe water for drinking, cooking, and bathing.

Vaccinating newborns against the hepatitis B virus, a contagious infection of the liver, is another successful campaign by WHO. Immunizing poor children is an ongoing, worldwide program. Medical experts are also looking ahead at trying to take care of the orphaned children of the victims of acquired immunodeficiency syndrome (AIDS).

Prenatal care and safe childbirth practices are also global concerns of WHO, which contends that there is no need to die in giving birth. Every time a woman in Africa becomes pregnant, her risk of dying as a result is more than one hundred times greater than for a woman in the industrialized world. Conferences are held regularly in order to try to stop this waste of life. Involved in the exchanges and preparations are public health officials, midwives, doctors, and the representatives of nongovernmental agencies.

Epidemiological studies have brought together twenty-two French-speaking governments in Africa to act to reduce maternal mortality. Apart from such specific causes as excessive blood clots, difficult confinements, infections, and other complications, factors in maternal mortality include anemia, malnutrition, malaria, or simply overwork—many African women toil twelve to fourteen hours a day.

WHO contends that the heavy price that African women pay for maternity is not inevitable. There are inexpensive methods that can put a stop to such tragedy. Some of the most important are family planning, prenatal and postnatal care, supervision of the confinement, and recourse to well-equipped and well-staffed primary health care centers. To achieve these goals, WHO coordinates the mobilization of resources with the help of both national commitment and international cooperation.

Heavy publicity efforts are part of the multifaceted WHO campaign to cope with the global AIDS toll. Statistics show that human immunodeficiency virus (HIV) infection has spread rapidly among women and children in sub-Saharan Africa and in Asia. In 2011, an estimated thirty-four million people were living with HIV; more than two-thirds of the 2.5 million people newly infected that year were living in sub-Saharan Africa. Millions of HIV-infected babies are born to infected women. AIDS is the sixth leading cause of death worldwide, and it has been the number one cause cause of death among women aged twenty to forty in some central African cities. AIDS has also eroded many of the gains developing countries made in decreasing infant mortality rates during the 1980s and 1990s. Globally, by the end of 2001, there were approximately 14 million children orphaned after one or both parents died of AIDS. By 2011, 230,000 children were living with HIV.

Experts working in the field of AIDS have noted that one of the greatest obstacles to prevention is the general lack of basic health care in the developing world, as well as among the poor in urban cities. A lack of resources and medicine compounds the seriousness of AIDS in sub-Saharan African countries. At times, there is no money to buy medicine, even if the supply of medicine exists. Experts also note that women's status and their typical lack of control over their own sexuality have had dire consequences for the AIDS epidemic in developing countries.

While scientists work toward a cure for curing HIV/AIDS, WHO recommends treating and suppressing the progression of HIV with a combination of at least three antiretroviral (ARV) drugs. Unfortunately, access to these medications is often severely limited for people with the disease in Africa and Asia. WHO continues to promote better distribution and use of drugs in the developing world, and it is also financing drug development studies for promising agents in these countries. In 2003, WHO announced its ambitious "3 by 5" program—getting three million people on critically important antiretroviral (ARV) therapy by the end of 2005. Only 300,000 people globally had access to ARV, but experts estimated that five to six million people infected with HIV in the developing world needed it. The initiative fell short of its goal, but the number of people receiving ARV tripled.

The fight against communicable diseases continues to be fought and won on various fronts. Oral rehydration tablets to cope with diarrhea among children, for example, have proven effective, reducing infant mortality in many countries by 50 percent. Early in the 1950s, Professor Samir Najjar of Lebanon produced a formula for oral rehydration that differed only slightly from the present oral rehydration formula. Then in 1962, a hospital training course in oral rehydration was organized in Alexandria, Egypt, another pioneering effort. Eventually, oral rehydration salts became the standard worldwide treatment of diarrhea in the 1970s.

Perspective and Prospects

The World Health Organization's efforts to fight diseases of all kinds and to improve health are so impressive that international successes in all fields seem almost inevitable. Yet the world's health problems also have a larger cause, one that is more difficult to solve. It is now increasingly evident that many diseases stem from the degradation to the environment caused by humans. The harmful effects of industrial development on the global ecosystem are now better known. Some of these ecological wounds are depletion of the ozone layer, acid rain, changes in climate, deforestation, and chemical pollution.

In Europe in 1984, thirty-two member nations of WHO agreed to a single health policy, including environmental issues. It contains measurable objectives to which each nation has agreed to be publicly accountable on an annual basis. The program is called Health for All, and it is based on four sweeping policy goals. The goals have thirty-eight targets supported by more than one hundred measurable indicators, all of which are aimed at achieving a symbolic health standard and improving the environment of Europe.

Communicable diseases are a continual problem. Susceptible populations have to be monitored for their appearance, and the latest medical information and practices need to be made accessible. Like environmental problems, the spread of diseases must be prevented, controlled, treated, and, wherever possible, eradicated completely.

In 1988, WHO undertook a program to eradicate polio on a global scale, using the polio vaccine. The polio vaccine confers long-lasting immunity and is easy to administer. It is routinely used to immunize children and adults against polio throughout the world. By 2013, WHO's highly successful program had eliminated polio in all but three countries worldwide—Nigeria, Afghanistan, and Pakistan—down from more than 125 countries when the Global Polio Eradication Initiative was first launched.

Millions more children have also been immunized against diphtheria, pertussis (whooping cough), measles, and tetanus. Using advanced biotechnology, scientists are working on keeping vaccines cool in transit to recipients in the tropics.

Still other endeavors by WHO are "no tobacco" days, vaccination programs against hepatitis B virus, laws to facilitate the distribution of drugs and medical supplies, the reduction of prices charged by manufacturers, the provision of more X-ray machines, the elimination of iron deficiency among the destitute, and advanced research on amino acids.

In the area of nutrition, WHO has helped publicize that requirements for each amino acid may be higher than previously recommended. Amino acids are the molecular units that combine to make proteins. Adult humans need eight amino acids in the diet. Other amino acids required for protein synthesis are manufactured in the body and do not need to be consumed in food. With these higher levels accepted, as WHO recommends, better protein nutrition can be achieved and food aid programs can be improved.

—Walter Appleton

See also Acquired immunodeficiency syndrome (AIDS); Centers for Disease Control and Prevention (CDC); Childbirth; Childbirth complications; Childhood infectious diseases; Diarrhea and dysentery; Environmental diseases; Environmental health; Epidemiology; Ethics; Hepatitis; Immunization and vaccination; Malnutrition; Meningitis; National Institutes of Health (NIH); Nutrition; Poliomyelitis; Preventive medicine; Tropical medicine; Tuberculosis.

For Further Information:

Beigbeder, Yves. *The World Health Organization.* Boston: M. Nijhoff, 1998.

Burci, Gian Luca, and Claude-Henri Vignes. *World Health Organization.* Frederick, Md.: Aspen, 2004.

"European Health for All Database." *World Health Organization,* Aug. 2012.

Grahame, Deborah A. *World Health Organization.* Milwaukee: Gareth Stevens, 2003.

"HIV/AIDS." *World Health Organization,* 25 July 2013.

Lee, Kelley, and Jennifer Fang. *Historical Dictionary of the World Health Organization.* 2d ed. Lanham, Md.: Scarecrow Press, 2013.

"Poliomyelitis." *World Health Organization,* Apr. 2013.

"The Top Ten Causes of Death." *World Health Organization,* July 2013.

"WHO Model Lists of Essential Medicines." *World Health Organization,* Apr. 2013.

World Health Organization. *The Fourth Ten Years of the World Health Organization: 1978–1987.* Geneva, Switzerland: World Health Organization, 2011.

World Health Organization. *World Health Statistics 2012.* Geneva, Switzerland: World Health Organization, 2012.

WOUNDS

Disease/Disorder

Anatomy or system affected: All

Specialties and related fields: Critical care, emergency medicine, family medicine, internal medicine

Definition: Breakdown in the protective function of the skin; resulting in disruptions or breaks in the continuity of any body tissue.

Wounds might arise because of violence, accident, or intentional procedure, such as surgery. They may be classified according to the instrument responsible, such as a knife, bullet, or shrapnel, or according to the way in which they occurred, such as a burn or a crushing wound.

Surgeons describe wounds according to their general appearance. A wound may be described as incised, when a sharp cutting instrument is involved; lacerated, when the tissue is damaged, cut, or torn; abrasion, when a superficial layer of skin is removed; contused, when a forceful blow to the tissue leaves the skin intact, causing bluish/blackish discoloration; avulsed, when part of the tissue is torn apart; punctured, when the outer opening is rather small; penetrating; and nonpenetrating, when the external tissue remains intact. Fractures are also classified in several terms, such as incomplete, complete, closed, or open. The depth of the tissue injury classifies burns as first, second, or third degree.

Generally, wounds may be classified as open or closed. Closed wounds involve no external hemorrhage, and their degree of seriousness is related to the force of the blow and its direction, the age of the victim, and other physiological and anatomical factors. Normally, internal hemorrhage stops abruptly or by applying direct pressure, with the blood and fluid absorbed within a few days. More bleeding occurs when larger internal vessels are damaged, with subsequent collection of the blood in tissues, forming a hematoma that may take several weeks to be absorbed. The impact on a body part may result in damage to a part that is not directly involved at the time of impact. Thus, a fall on an outstretched hand may injure not only the flesh and bones of the hand itself but also the scaphoid part of the wrist, or even the elbow or shoulder. During a car accident, a stationary body part may be heavily affected by the transmission of impact from a relatively mobile part; when occurring in the neck, this type of injury is commonly known as whiplash. First aid procedures for fractures, sprains, and strains include ice packs, crutches, elevation, and splinting.

Infections resulting from wounds. Open wounds take place when the skin and/or mucous membranes are broken, thus allowing the invasion of hazardous foreign material, such as bacteria or dirt, into the tissues. This invasion may lead to infection, which is particularly serious when the disruption of the skin is considerable. Generally, injuries from sharp instruments (such as a needle, knife, or bullet) cause little tissue damage, except to the part that they penetrate. The great danger lies in the injury of a vital organ and from the foreign objects that are on the surface of the instrument. Injuries from irregular objects (such as bomb fragments or a jagged knife) create much more damage, which leads to longer recuperation periods. Skin is elastic and well supplied with blood, which means that superficial cuts heal easily. The subcutaneous fatty tissues and muscles are not as rich in blood supply, and their damage is more serious and long-lasting, especially because it is easier for infection to occur. Fragmentation of bone in an open wound is particularly troublesome, since the fragments cannot survive without blood and will act as foreign substances, thus creating a serious infection. Injuries to joints, nerves, or major capillaries (such as arteries) will complicate the state of the open wound.

The contamination of the wound may start immediately after the causative incident. Nonbacterial contamination is more serious when organic substances are involved. In bacte-

Information on Wounds

Causes: Violence, accidents, surgery
Symptoms: May include bruising, bleeding, swelling, pain
Duration: Acute
Treatments: Disinfecting, bandaging, antibiotics, surgery if needed

rial contamination, the most serious results are seen with virulent bacteria that are nourished by dead tissue and organic foreign material, sometimes leading to gas gangrene. Such infection generally spreads unchecked and can be stopped only by surgical removal or amputation, in order to avoid death. Other infections are caused by streptococcal and staphylococcal bacteria and are characterized by the local production of swelling, redness, and pus. Finally, tetanus is another type of wound infection. It starts with serious muscle spasms a few days after the injury and, left untreated, often leads to death.

The healing process. When an open wound occurs, the tissues are cut and the edges of the wound separate, pulled apart by the elasticity of the skin. Blood flowing from the wound fills the resulting cavity, fibrin is produced, and the blood clots, creating a scab. During the first twenty-four hours after the injury, the scab shrinks, drawing the edges of the skin together. Special cells called histiocytes and macrophages digest the debris in the wound, such as blood seepage, dead cells, and other foreign bodies, 2-3 days after the injury. Connective tissue cells called fibroblasts grow inward from the margins of the wound to close the cavity 3-5 days after injury. The fibroblasts produce a protein called collagen that provides strength to the new skin.

The red-colored capillaries slowly disappear and are replaced by white collagen. Thus, upon removal of the scab, a layer of reddish granulation tissue appears, which covers the subcutaneous tissue. A thin, gray membrane extends outward from the skin edges and covers the whole surface. Contraction brings the epithelial sheets from the two sides together, and eventually the skin around the wound is reproduced. Wounds that cross normal skin creases become depressed below the level of the surrounding skin. The resulting scars, which are very low in capillaries, do not become tanned with sunlight exposure, and they produce neither hair nor sweat, which is indicative of skin that is less than fully functional. They are much whiter than the surrounding skin.

Treatment. Medical treatment of wounds requires first the control of bleeding by direct pressure or bandaging. In the case of small cuts, local irrigation and the use of disinfection include the external use of oxidizing agents (such as hydrogen peroxide) and of nonpolar ointments (such as petroleum jelly) to combat invading polar bacteria. A large area of injury or dead tissue is managed surgically, either by debridement or through amputation. Sutured wounds heal faster because stitches bring the skin edges together. Foreign surgical material introduced in a wound may be absorbed by the tissues, which is exactly what happens when catgut is used to close the wounded tissue. Body factors are also crucial in the overall healing; these include age, the concurrent presence of diseases such as uncontrolled hypertension and diabetes, and nutrition that includes adequate quantities of protein and antioxidants, such as vitamin C. Hospitals take elaborate precautions to prevent infections through sterilization, hand sanitation, good air filtration, the use of ultraviolet light to kill bacteria in the operating room, and the administration of antibiotics. The skin in the area of any surgery is treated with antiseptics and is carefully protected with sterilized cloth.

—Soraya Ghayourmanesh;
updated by Anubhav Agarwal, M.D.

See also Amputation; Bites and stings; Bleeding; Bruises; Burns and scalds; Concussion; First aid; Fracture and dislocation; Fracture repair; Frostbite; Gangrene; Grafts and grafting; Healing; Infection; Laceration repair; Lesions; Necrotizing fasciitis; Plastic surgery; Shock; Skin; Tetanus; Toxic shock syndrome; Transfusion

For Further Information:

Collier, Mark. "Understanding Wound Inflammation." *Nursing Times* 99, no. 25 (2003): 63-64. Recognizes and manages the signs and consequences of clinically infected wounds.

Cutting, K.F., and K.G. Harding. "Criteria for Identifying Wound Infection." *Journal of Wound Care* 3, no. 4 (1994): 198-201. Explains how to recognize signs of inflammation/increasing bacterial burden/clinical infection and to reduce risk of complications

Gulli, Benjamin, Les Chatelain, and Chris Stratford, eds. *American Academy of Orthopaedic Surgeons. Emergency Care and Transportation of the Sick and Injured.* 9th ed. Sudbury, MA: Jones and Bartlett, 2005. Includes new and expanded coverage of patient assessment, anatomy and physiology, stroke and seizure, trauma injuries, and special chapters on pediatrics and geriatrics.

Handal, Kathleen A. *The American Red Cross First Aid and Safety Handbook.* Boston: Little, Brown, 1992. A comprehensive, fully illustrated guide outlining basic first aid and emergency care steps to be taken until medical assistance can be obtained. Updated materials can also be obtained directly from local Red Cross Association chapters listed in telephone books.

Krohmer, Jon R., ed. *American College of Emergency Physicians First Aid Manual.* 2nd ed. New York: DK, 2004. An excellent reference guide illustrated with photographs and written in a clear, step-by-step format. Covers many first aid methods, from resuscitation of conscious and unconscious choking victims, to how to deal with bleeding, shock, spinal injuries, poisoning, seizures, fractures, and bandages.

Marsh, J.L., et al. "Fracture and Dislocation Classification Compendium-2007: Orthopaedic Trauma Association Classification, Database and Outcomes Committee." *Journal of Orthopedic Trauma* 21 (November/December 2007): 1-133. This new classification compendium republishes the Orthopaedic Trauma Association's (OTA) classification.

Subbarao, Italo, et al., eds. *American Medical Association Handbook of First Aid and Emergency Care.* Rev. ed. New York: Random House Reference, 2009. Covering urgent emergency situations as well as the common injuries and ailments that occur in every family, this AMA guide takes the reader step by step through basic first aid techniques.

Thygerson, Alton L. *First Aid and Emergency Care Workbook.* Boston: Jones and Bartlett, 1987. Concise information packed into a workbook format, produced in cooperation with the National Safety Council. Charts, drawings, photographs, and tables outline common emergency care, covering a wide range of topics for the general public.

Youngson, R.M. *First Aid.* New York: HarperCollins, 2003. Gives clear, step-by-step instructions for the handling of accidents or illness of all types and degrees of severity.

X RAYS. *See* IMAGING AND RADIOLOGY.

XENOTRANSPLANTATION
Procedure
Anatomy or system affected: All
Specialties and related fields: Biotechnology, ethics, general surgery, immunology
Definition: The transfer of cells, tissues, or organs from non-human animal donors to human recipients for therapeutic purposes.
Key terms:
gene: a piece of deoxyribonucleic acid (DNA), or sometimes ribonucleic acid (RNA), that directs a specific activity within a cell, such as the production of a protein
genetic engineering: the transfer of genes, often from one species to another
rejection: the destruction of transplanted organs by the immune system

Indications and Procedures

The transplantation of organs from human donors to human recipients has been established practice in medicine since the first successful kidney transplant was performed in 1954. Its applications have been limited, however, for two major reasons. First, the demand for human-donated organs always exceeds the supply. Second, the human body naturally rejects transplants. When the immune system recognizes compounds on the surfaces of cells from any source that is "not self," a chain reaction begins. Antibodies attack foreign proteins and mark them for destruction by white blood cells. Enzymes attack the walls of blood vessels in a transplanted organ, destroying it within hours. To prevent rejection, transplant recipients must take immunosuppressive drugs for months or years. Blocking their immune response, however, makes transplant patients susceptible to infections, some of which can be deadly.

Xenotransplantation—the transfer of cells, tissues, or organs from nonhuman animal donors to human recipients for therapeutic purposes—might solve both of these problems. A large supply of organs can, in theory, be farmed in animals such as pigs. Also, theoretically, organs can be tailor-made to prevent rejection. Genetic engineering techniques should be able to replace animal proteins and sugars on the surfaces of cells with human ones, thus creating an organ that the recipient's immune system is tricked into accepting as "self."

This genetic engineering is accomplished by transferring genes from humans to animals specially bred and farmed to serve as organ donors. To achieve this, a fertilized egg is removed from the uterus of a female donor animal. Next, human protein-coding genes are inserted into the nucleus of the fertilized egg. Finally, the egg is returned to the animal's uterus and allowed to develop normally. If the human genetic material is preserved and activated, then the cells of the animal that develops from the egg will manufacture human proteins on the surfaces of its cells.

Uses and Complications

One concern about xenotransplantation is that new diseases might be introduced into humans from other animals. All animals carry endogenous viruses that are part of their genetic makeup. Endogenous viruses are harmless in their natural hosts, but they can prove deadly when they cross from one species to another. For example, the Hong Kong flu virus lay harmlessly in waterbirds for many years. It then struck chickens and caused massive deaths on poultry farms, and now it infects and sometimes kills people. How the virus migrated to humans remains unknown. Also, diseases can be minor in some animals but major in humans. The herpesvirus B is one example. It gives monkeys mild cold sores but causes fatal encephalitis in people. The concern is that a virus imported into the human population through xenotransplantation might subsequently spread through other means, such as blood, air, water, or food.

Issues of morality, ethics, and religion also arise. Although the genetic makeup of other primates most closely matches that of humans, many people believe that using apes and monkeys as organ donors would be morally unacceptable. One answer to such objections is to use animals that are routinely raised and slaughtered for food. Pigs are easy to breed and care for, and they produce large litters. Their size and weight are similar to humans. Few people object to killing pigs. Much xenotransplantation research involves the development of pigs as potential organ donors. If pig cells can be induced to display human proteins on their surfaces, then the human body will, in theory, accept organs donated from them.

Animals used as transplant donors could not come from ordinary farms because the possibility of transferring infections would be too great. The animals would need to be raised in germ-free medical facilities. Animal rights advocates condemn organ farms as cruel. Despite such objections, public opinion supports further research on xenotransplantation. In a 1998 survey sponsored by the National Kidney Foundation, nearly two-thirds of respondents judged xenotransplantation an acceptable alternative to human donor transplants.

Perspective and Prospects

Xenotransplantation is not a new idea. In 1906, with no knowledge of the immune system, French surgeon Mathieu Jaboulay transplanted a kidney from a pig and a liver from a goat to human patients, both of whom died. In 1964, Thomas Starzl at the University of Pittsburgh transplanted baboon kidneys into two humans. Both patients died from infections accompanied by kidney failure. That same year, a chimpanzee-to-human transplant fared a little better. The patient lived for nine months before the kidney failed.

In 1984, a child the press called "Baby Fae" was born prematurely with a severely malformed heart. She could not live long without a transplant. No human heart small enough was available, so surgeons at Loma Linda University in California gave Baby Fae the heart of a baboon. The operation went well, but Fae died of organ rejection and infection after the surgery.

In 1992, two liver transplants from baboons were attempted. The livers functioned well, but the patients died from infections. That same year, two women received livers from pigs. The transplants were not meant to be permanent but were intended as "bridges" until human donors could be found. In both women, the livers functioned well, but one woman died before a human organ could be located.

In 1995, British scientists succeeded in transplanting pig hearts into monkeys. Half the monkeys survived for forty days, but long-term survival was not achieved, and attempts to transplant whole organs declined after that. Instead, researchers turned to cell transplants. Since 1995, brain cells from pigs have been used with some success in the experimental treatment of people with Parkinson's disease. In 2002, researchers in Virginia announced that they had successfully bred pigs lacking a specific sugar molecule on their cell surfaces known to trigger the rejection response in humans. Xenotransplantation advocates hope that this and similar developments will spur further progress in the field.

—Faith Hickman Brynie, Ph.D.

See also Animal rights vs. research; Cloning; Ethics; Genetic engineering; Grafts and grafting; Heart transplantation; Immune system; Immunology; Kidney transplantation; Liver transplantation; Systems and organs; Transplantation; Zoonoses.

For Further Information:

Brynie, Faith Hickman. *101 Questions About Your Immune System You Felt Defenseless to Answer . . . Until Now.* Brookfield, Conn.: Twenty-first Century Books, 2000.

Cooper, David K. C., and Robert P. Lanza. *Xeno: The Promise of Transplanting Animal Organs into Humans.* New York: Oxford University Press, 2003.

Fovargue, Sara. *Xenotransplantation and Risk: Regulating a Developing Biotechnology.* New York: Cambridge University Press, 2012.

Munson, Ronald. *Raising the Dead: Organ Transplants, Ethics, and Society.* New York: Oxford University Press, 2004.

"Organ Transplantation." *MedlinePlus*, May 23, 2013.

Schicktanz, Silke, et al. *Teaching Ethics in Organ Transplantation and Tissue Donation.* Akron, Ohio: University of Akron Press, 2011.

Tramper, Johannes, and Yang Zhu. *Modern Biotechnology: Panacea or New Pandora's Box?* Wageningen, the Netherlands: Wageningen Academic Publishers, 2011.

"Xenotransplantation." *US Food and Drug Administration*, Feb. 4, 2010.

YEAST INFECTIONS. *See* CANDIDIASIS.

YELLOW FEVER
Disease/Disorder

Anatomy or system affected: Blood, circulatory system, liver

Specialties and related fields: Environmental health, epidemiology, public health, virology

Definition: An acute tropical and subtropical disease spread by infected mosquitoes from human to human or from infected monkeys to humans.

Key terms:

endemic: referring to a disease that has a reservoir in a particular area and that can be expected to occur at some time and level of intensity

epidemic: an incidence of a disease well in excess of the constant rate expected in an area where it is endemic

flaviviruses: a family of ribonucleic acid (RNA) viruses that are transmitted by an arthropod vector; examples include yellow fever, dengue, and St. Louis and Japanese tick-borne encephalitis

hemorrhage: excessive or heavy and uncontrollable bleeding from blood vessels

jaundice: a yellowish skin discoloration symptomatic of yellow fever and other diseases that affect the production and processing of bile

zoonosis: a disease that can be transmitted by animals such as vertebrates to humans; sylvan yellow fever is transmitted from vertebrate reservoirs such as monkeys to humans via mosquitoes

Causes and Symptoms

Yellow fever is a viral disease of humans spread by infected mosquitoes. The infectious agent is a flavivirus. Yellow fever is primarily a disease of tropical and pantropical areas of South America and sub-Saharan Africa. The absence of yellow fever from Asia is curious but may be explained by the lack of suitable reservoirs. Three types of yellow fever are recognized, sylvan yellow fever, intermediate yellow fever, and urban yellow fever.

All three types are highly communicable, but none are directly transmitted via personal contact between humans. A human contracts the disease through the bite of an infected mosquito that, in turn, has taken a blood meal from an infected monkey or other human. The viral incubation period within the mosquito is nine to twelve days. The virus then appears in the saliva and can be transmitted during the mosquito's next blood meal. Thereafter, the mosquito carries the virus throughout its life.

Sylvan yellow fever is also known as jungle yellow fever. Forest monkeys are its primary reservoir, but marmosets and marsupials may also harbor the disease. Sylvan yellow fever is spread from monkey to monkey by the bite of infected *Sabethes* or *Haemagogus* mosquitoes, which breed in water-filled tree holes.

People who visit or work in rain forest environs, such as miners, engineers, wildlife biologists, and foresters, are at risk of contracting the disease. Sylvan yellow fever is rare or nonexistent outside tropical rain forests, but cases are reported every year in areas where it is endemic. The intermediate, or savannah, cycle of yellow fever is trasmitted from an infected mosquito to a human living or working near an area that borders the rain forest. This cycle of the virus can also be trasmitted from monkey to human, or from human to human, via the infected mosquito.

Urban yellow fever is spread by the *Aedes aegypti* mosquito, which is the main reservoir of the disease, along with humans. *Aedes* commonly lives and breeds in trash dumps and waste places around human habitations. Urban yellow fever often results in thousands of cases and high fatality rates.

In humans, the first symptoms of yellow fever typically appear from three to six days following the bite of an infected mosquito. Symptoms vary widely; the mildest cases may pass unnoticed, but in more severe cases the patient shows a number of flulike symptoms, such as muscle aches, backaches, headache, high fever, chills, nausea, and vomiting. Liver damage may occur as early as the fourth or fifth day of the illness, leading to progressive and extensive jaundice. In the most severe cases, periods of nausea, vomiting, renal failure, and extensive bleeding (hemorrhage) may prove fatal. The fatality rate may range from as low as 5 percent in indigenous populations to 50 percent or more during epidemics. Higher fatality rates are typically seen in nonindigenous people.

Clinical diagnosis of yellow fever is aided by isolation of the virus in mice, by microscopic examination of liver tissue for necrotic lesions that characterize this disease, by detection of the yellow fever viral antigen in blood or liver tissue fluid of the infected patient, or by detection of the viral genome in liver tissue. Diagnosis can also be determined serologically through the detection of specific antibodies.

Treatment and Therapy

There is no specific antiviral drug for yellow fever, so treatment goals include providing symptom relief, such as oxygen support, medications to reduce fever and pain, and the administration of vitamin K and replacement fluids. Dialysis may be required for patients suffering from kidney failure. Complete recovery may take several weeks, after which the individual has a lifelong immunity to yellow fever.

Perspective and Prospects

Yellow fever has long been a dreaded tropical and subtropical disease of humans. Throughout the centuries of exploration, yellow fever epidemics occurred with alarming regularity, and high fatality rates were seen among nonindigenous visitors and settlers in regions where the disease is endemic. The presence of yellow fever on a ship was indicated by flying the fever flag or yellow jack.

Despite modern medical advances, yellow fever remains a problem in many areas—the disease is endemic to forty-four countries in Africa and South America. Small numbers of cases of sylvan yellow fever occur every year in certain areas of Amazonia and northern South American countries, includ-

Information on Yellow Fever

Causes: Viral infection transmitted by mosquitoes
Symptoms: Vary widely; may include muscle aches, backaches, headache, high fever, chills, nausea, vomiting, liver damage leading to jaundice, kidney failure
Duration: Several weeks, sometimes fatal
Treatments: Alleviation of symptoms through oxygen support, medications for fever and pain, vitamin K supplements, replacement fluids, dialysis for kidney failure

ing Peru and Bolivia. In central Africa, the yellow fever belt extends from Ethiopia westward through Senegal, Sudan, and Ghana. Both occasional cases and epidemics occur irregularly. Between 1986 and 1988, for example, thirty thousand cases of yellow fever were reported in Nigeria, and ten thousand people died. The World Health Organization (WHO) estimates that there are 200,000 cases of yellow fever worldwide each year, which cause approximately 30,000 deaths.

Walter Reed was the first to describe the epidemiology of yellow fever and to recognize the importance of the mosquito vector in its spread. His research elucidated control and eradication measures that provide containment during epidemics. It was largely through his insights that yellow fever was eliminated from urban areas and was one of the main reasons that the Panama Canal could be completed by the United States after the failure of the French effort led by Ferdinand de Lesseps, the architect of the Suez Canal.

The traditional and still most effective method of preventing urban yellow fever is the eradication of the *Aedes aegypti* mosquito vector. Control measures involve a combination of insecticide spraying and the cleanup or removal of potential breeding sites. The prevention of yellow fever can also be achieved through the vaccination of all people within the endemic regions. A single vaccination with an attenuated strain of virus grown in chick embryos has been shown to be effective for thirty or more years, but revaccination is recommended every ten years.

The elimination of sylvan yellow fever is probably impossible because of the difficulty of eradicating jungle populations of *Sabethes* and *Haemagogus* mosquitoes. Prevention must therefore be achieved through defensive measures for people who work in or visit jungle areas, including immunization and the use of protective clothing, netting, and mosquito repellents.

—Dwight G. Smith, Ph.D.

See also Bites and stings; Epidemiology; Insect-borne diseases; Jaundice; Tropical medicine; Viral infections; Zoonoses.

For Further Information:

Delaporte, François. *The History of Yellow Fever: An Essay on the Birth of Tropical Medicine.* Translated by Arthur Goldhammer. Cambridge, Mass.: MIT Press, 1991.
"Hemorrhagic Fevers." *MedlinePlus*, May 20, 2013.
Heymann, David L., ed. *Control of Communicable Diseases Manual.* 19th ed. Washington, D.C.: American Public Health Association, 2008.
Kettle, D. S., ed. *Medical and Veterinary Entomology.* 2d ed. Wallingford, England: CAB International, 1995.
Murphy, Jim. *An American Plague: The True and Terrifying Story of the Yellow Fever Epidemic of 1793.* New York: Clarion Books, 2003.
Rymaruk, Jen, and Lawrence Frisch. "Yellow Fever." *Health Library*, June 20, 2012.
Wills, Christopher. *Yellow Fever, Black Goddess: The Coevolution of People and Plagues.* Reading, Mass.: Addison-Wesley, 1996.
"Yellow Fever." *Centers for Disease Control and Prevention*, Dec. 13, 2011.
"Yellow Fever." *World Health Organization*, May 2013.

YOGA

Treatment

Anatomy or system affected: Muscles, nervous system, psychic-emotional system

Specialties and related fields: Alternative medicine, preventive medicine

Definition: An ancient Indian system of physical exercises, breath control, and meditation aimed at attaining bodily and mental control and well-being.

Introduction

The word "yoga" comes from the Sanskrit word *Yuj*, meaning to "yoke," "join," or "unite." The word implies joining or integrating all aspects of the body with the mind to achieve a healthy and balanced life. The true purpose of the ancient practices of yoga is to bring a proper balance between the physical and mental aspects of a person and to awaken the subtle energies of the body. Yoga cultivates muscular strength, endurance, and flexibility and enhances the practitioner's mental acuity. Meditative breathing calms a person's nerves and sharpens a person's focus. With regular yoga practice, individuals are known to gain physical health, mental relaxation, and inner tranquillity.

Yoga has been practiced in India, in one form or another, for more than four thousand years. More than two thousand years ago, the Indian scholar Patanjali codified the various yoga practices into a written collection called the *Yoga Sutras*. According to Patanjali, there are three critical components of yoga: physical postures (*asanas*), breath control (*pranayama*), and meditation. The main purpose of *asanas* and *pranayam* is to cleanse the body, unlock energy paths, and raise the level of consciousness. Yoga styles have come to include a strong component of meditation to enhance the union of mind, body, and soul. Patanjali showed how, through the practice of yoga, one can gain mastery over mind and emotion. Advanced yoga practitioners are known to have incredible control over several autonomic functions such as respiration, heart rate, and blood flow.

Many of the bodily functions previously thought to be involuntary can be controlled in a relaxed state achieved through the regular practice of yoga.

Yoga *asanas* offer a simple yet profound technique for promoting muscle flexibility and deep relaxation. Practicing a variety of *asanas*, in combination with *pranayam*, is believed to clear the nervous system, causing energy to flow without obstruction and ensuring its even distribution through the body during *pranayam*. Advanced practitioners of yoga claim to experience a pure state of joy while practicing the various yoga *asanas*. Yoga *asanas* are designed to switch constantly from one posture to another. Holding the most intense *asanas* builds strength and endurance, while flexing postures are known to provide muscles with a greater range of motion in the hip and shoulder joints.

There are many forms and schools of yoga. The form most commonly practiced in Western countries is hatha yoga. It places special emphasis on physical postures, which are integrated with breath control and meditation. Hatha yoga thus emphasizes a balance of mind, body, and spirit.

Health Benefits

Research, mostly performed in India, suggests a wide variety of positive health effects from the daily practice of yoga, including, but not limited to, pain reduction in arthritis and carpal tunnel syndrome, reduction of coronary artery disease, and relief from asthma and other respiratory ailments. Situated in Bangalore, India, the Swami Vivekananda Yoga

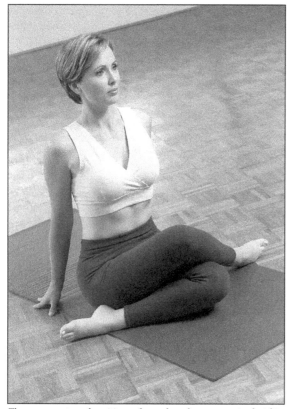

The movements and positions of yoga have been recognized within medicine for their promotion of flexibility and strength. (© Bruce Shippee/Dreamstime.com)

Anusandhana Samsthana (SVYASA) University treats people with such ailments as asthma, arthritis, heart disease, high blood pressure, psychiatric ailments, and eating disorders. The center uses an integrated approach of yoga therapies that includes *asanas*, chanting, *kriya* (yoga cleansing techniques), meditation, *pranayam*, and lectures on yoga philosophy. The system has been shown to benefit people with asthma, intellectual disabilities, rheumatoid arthritis, and type 1 diabetes mellitus. It is believed to improve visual perception, manual dexterity, and spatial memory.

With support from other organizations, SVYASA has been engaged in a vast variety of research, including studies regarding the use of yoga to treat obsessive-compulsive disorder; the effects of yoga on people with multiple sclerosis; and the use of yoga for assessing alertness, ability to focus, flexibility, balance, quality of life, and fatigue in healthy elderly people. *Pranayam* has been shown to lower blood pressure in people with hypertension, to alleviate discomfort from gastritis, and to reduce stress and anxiety.

One difficulty with the work in India, however, has been a lack of rigor in research design and protocol. For example, the yoga practices are traditionally combined with chanting, discourse, and other activities, and it is difficult to determine the effects of such extra variables when comparing the results of one study with another.

Perspective and Prospects

With growing interest in alternative therapies, several individuals and institutions have initiated extensive studies on the effects of yoga. For example, researchers at Ball State University found that fifteen weeks of yoga training brought a 10 percent improvement in lung capacity. Yoga has been found to help fight cardiovascular disease when used in conjunction with other lifestyle changes, such as a low-fat diet. The National Institutes of Health (NIH) is supporting research on yoga, including its use for treating insomnia and chronic lower back pain.

In a study at the University of Iowa, some patients with chronic fatigue syndrome were shown to benefit from yoga. Yoga prevailed among numerous conventional and alternative therapies as an effective fatigue fighter. At the end of the two-year study, yoga was the only therapy linked to a statistically significant positive outcome by linear regression analysis.

Marian Garfinkel, a yoga teacher turned researcher, has demonstrated that practicing certain yoga postures can relieve the symptoms of carpal tunnel syndrome, the common ailment resulting from repetitive hand activities such as typing. Patients practicing prescribed yoga postures showed significant improvement in grip strength and suffered less pain. There was also improvement on a nerve test used to measure the severity of carpal tunnel syndrome. Studies are in progress to observe the effect of yoga on osteoarthritis of the knee and on repetitive strain injuries.

Because each patient is unique, with different abilities and weaknesses, a yoga approach should be tailored to specific problems as well as specific potentials. It is also important to look at the studies in which yoga did not prove effective and to determine which variables led to these failures.

—*Tulsi B. Saral, Ph.D.*

See also Alternative medicine; Carpal tunnel syndrome; Chronic fatigue syndrome; Hypertension; Meditation; Stress; Stress reduction.

For Further Information:

Birkel, Dee Ann. *Hatha Yoga: Developing the Body, Mind, and Inner Self.* 3d ed. Dubuque, Iowa: Eddie Bowers, 2000.

Garfinkel, M. S., et al. "Yoga-Based Intervention for Carpal Tunnel Syndrome." *Journal of the American Medical Association* 280 (1998): 1601–3.

Iyengar, B. K. S. *Light on Yoga.* Rev. ed. New York: HarperCollins, 2001.

Mayo Clinic. "Yoga: Fight Stress and Find Serenity." *Mayo Foundation for Medical Education and Research,* January 15, 2013.

Mishra, Rammurti S. *Fundamentals of Yoga: A Handbook of Theory, Practice, and Application.* Reprint. New York: Julian Press, 1987.

National Center for Complementary and Alternative Medicine. "Yoga for Health." *National Institutes of Health,* May 2012.

Wren, A. A., et al. "Yoga for Persistent Pain: New Findings and Directions for an Ancient Practice." *Pain* 152 (2011): 477–80.

ZOONOSES

Disease/Disorder

Anatomy or system affected: All

Specialties and related fields: Bacteriology, epidemiology, public health, virology

Definition: Diseases that can be transferred to humans from their primary animal hosts, including farm animals, laboratory research animals, tropical insects and animals, and common house pets, and including poliomyelitis, malaria, rabies, and toxoplasmosis.

Key terms:

inoculate: to introduce immunologically active material in order to treat or prevent a disease

malaise: a feeling of lack of health or debility, often indicating or accompanying the onset of illness

mycobacterium: any of a genus of nonmotile aerobic bacteria that are difficult to stain and include numerous saprophytes and the organisms causing tuberculosis and leprosy

organism: a complex structure of interdependent and subordinate elements whose relations and properties are largely determined by their function as a whole

pathogen: a specific causative agent (as a bacterium or virus) of disease

rabies: an acute virus disease of the nervous system of warm-blooded animals, usually transmitted through the bite of a rabid animal

toxoplasma: any of a genus of parasitic microorganisms that are typically serious pathogens of vertebrates

toxoplasmosis: the infection of humans, other mammals, or birds with disease caused by toxoplasmas that invade the tissues and may seriously damage the central nervous system, especially that of an infant

tuberculosis: a highly variable, communicable disease of humans and some other vertebrates caused by the tubercle bacillus; characterized by toxic symptoms of allergic manifestations that in humans primarily affect the lungs

vaccinate: to administer a vaccine, usually by injection

vaccine: a preparation of killed microorganisms or living, virulent organisms that is administered to produce or increase immunity to a particular disease

Causes and Symptoms

There are many types of contact between humans and animals. Some produce pleasure, such as stroking a kitten's fur; some have strictly utilitarian considerations, such as farming or meat processing; and some are to help animals themselves, such as the veterinary sciences. Unfortunately, some also result in the transmission of infectious diseases to humans, which are called zoonoses. The most common symptoms of zoonoses are headache, fevers, general malaise, diarrhea or bloody stool, and sometimes skin rashes, eruptions, or inflammation (in the event of a bite or sting).

Approximately 150 types of zoonoses can be transmitted either directly or indirectly to human beings. Direct exposure results from coming in contact with an infected animal or its excrement, blood, or saliva. Indirect exposure results from being bitten by an insect carrying an infected animal's blood. In either case, a disease may or may not develop.

Although many diseases transmissible to humans from animals now can be cured, it is important to avoid the methods of transmittal, especially the handling of infected animals. Humans must wash their hands after handling animals, especially after cleaning cages or litter boxes. Small children should be discouraged from kissing and cuddling pets. In rural or mountainous areas, humans should be discouraged from handling wild animals. In some communities, especially rural areas, keeping wild animals such as wolves or raccoons as pets is popular. Unfortunately, wild animals can carry many serious diseases that can be passed to humans, notably rabies.

Incubation periods for zoonoses can range from a few days to several years. If it is suspected that a human has contracted a disease from an animal, it is important to seek medical attention. Most zoonoses can be diagnosed and treated. In most cases, treatment will clear up the disease with no lasting aftereffects. If the infected person waits too long for treatment, however, therapy may take longer, and problems may persist. In rare cases, surgery is necessary, and in even rarer cases, death can occur.

Zoonoses vary greatly in their sources and symptoms. Among the most important of these diseases are anthrax, brucellosis, cat-scratch fever, encephalitis, Lyme disease, malaria, cattle tuberculosis, plague, rabies, ringworm, Rocky Mountain spotted fever, roundworm, salmonella poisoning, sporotrichosis, and toxoplasmosis.

Anthrax is an infectious disease of warm-blooded animals such as cattle or sheep, caused by the bacterium *Bacillus anthracis*. The disease can be transmitted to humans by the handling of infected products, such as the animals" hair. The disease is characterized by lesions in the lungs and by external ulcerating nodules.

Brucellosis is characterized by repeated fevers accompanied by weakness and joint pain. It is contracted from the amniotic and fetal membranes of pregnant and newborn animals. More typical in farm animals, it can also be present in dogs that are bred. While it is not fatal, it does cause severe flulike symptoms. It can be difficult to treat and cure completely.

Not as serious as toxoplasmosis, which can also be transmitted through a bite or scratch from a cat, cat-scratch fever is a bacterial infection that can result when a human is bitten, nipped, or scratched by a feline. Symptoms include a blistery inflammation at the site of the infection, fever, malaise, and sometimes swelling of the lymph nodes. Such symptoms appear two to ten days after the skin is broken and generally last about a month. The infection will generally clear up on its own, but, after washing the affected area with soap and water, a consultation with a physician is recommended. Approximately twenty thousand people are infected annually with cat-scratch fever, mostly children. It is important for parents to instruct children not to play roughly with cats.

The bite of mosquitoes infected with encephalitis can

cause this disease in humans. The illness is an infection of the lining of the brain; symptoms include a high fever, general malaise, and usually a very strong headache. Another disease transmitted by the bite of mosquitoes is malaria, which is caused by sporozoan parasites. Symptoms include intermittent chills and fever. Malaria may persist for years, and once the disease has been contracted, those affected are discouraged from donating blood, to avoid passing it on to others.

Lyme disease is an insect-related disease that is usually caused by the bite of a deerfly or tick. The disease was named for an area of Connecticut where it was first discovered. A doctor treating patients with flulike symptoms and skin inflammations realized that patients complaining of the symptoms had all been walking in woody areas and had been in contact with brush, weeds, and flowers where the tiny ticks and deerflies could have been harbored. The insects preyed on deer and other animals in the area, then probably jumped off or were brushed off the host animal into the grass. (Bitten animals may become infected with the disease as well.) Cases of Lyme disease have been found across the United States, with the highest percentage being reported in the Midwest and on the East Coast. Although humans can develop the disease from a tick or deerfly bite, there is no evidence yet that a bite or scratch from an infected animal can transmit the disease.

The bacterium *Borrelia burgdorferi* is responsible for Lyme disease. Its symptoms include inflammation, skin lesions and redness, joint inflammation, fever, fatigue, general malaise, and headaches or a stiff neck. These symptoms may last for weeks after the bite. Nerve-related disorders and heart ailments may follow the preliminary symptoms. Early treatment is a fourteen-day regimen of antibiotics, which can then be followed by treatment with antimicrobial agents until symptoms cease. Later stages of Lyme disease, such as arthritis and heart disorders, can be treated with penicillin-type antibiotics. Nevertheless, joint and muscle pain may persist for several weeks.

Rocky Mountain spotted fever is another disease caused by tick bites. The disease is found in all areas of the United States, not only in the Rocky Mountains. Symptoms include headache, fever, and skin rash. Early diagnosis and antibiotic treatment are very important in order to prevent more serious complications.

An infection that often strikes herded animals such as cows, deer, or elk is a subspecies of tuberculosis caused by *Mycobacterium bovis*. Individuals who come in contact with such animals, such as veterinarians, farmers, and slaughterhouse workers, are most susceptible to this disease because they breathe in the tiny droplets of bacteria. In addition to lung infections, other diseases are reported to be associated with the *M. bovis* bacterium. Treatment for infected individuals is with antibiotics.

Plague is an infectious disease transmitted by the bite of a rodent flea infected with the bacillus *Yersinia pestis*. Two forms of plague affected millions of humans in Asia and Europe during the Middle Ages and continue to occur today, although not in epidemic form. Bubonic plague results in the formation of buboes, or swellings of the lymph glands. The

---

Information on Zoonoses

Causes: Diseases transferred to humans from animal hosts

Symptoms: Headache; fever; general malaise; diarrhea or bloody stool; rashes, eruptions, or inflammation (from bite or sting)

Duration: Acute to chronic

Treatments: Depend on cause; may include supportive therapy, antibiotics, antiviral drugs, antifungal agents

---

Black Death was caused by the same bacterium and was probably pneumonic plague; this form is transmissible between people and is characterized by black patches appearing on the skin of its victims. Both types cause fevers and heavy coughing. Before the discovery of antibiotics, most victims died from this very contagious disease.

Rabies is an acute viral disease of the nervous system of warm-blooded animals, usually transmitted through the bite of the infected animal. Rabies can be found in a small number of animal species across the world. There are two main types: urban rabies, carried mainly by domesticated animals such as dogs; and sylvatic rabies, carried by wild animals such as bats. Symptoms of the disease include fever, nausea, vomiting, shortness of breath, abdominal pain, and a cough. If left untreated, the muscles become paralyzed and breathing and heartbeats stop, causing death. There are three methods of treating the disease: vaccination of people at risk of exposure before any exposure has occurred; animal control and immunization, especially preexposure immunization; and postinfection treatment, usually a series of expensive, painful shots.

Generally, the incubation period for rabies in humans is three weeks to three months. There have been cases, however, in which the victim was bitten by a rabid animal a year before the onset of the disease. Two documented cases showed that the victims were bitten by infected dogs while traveling in Asia six or seven years prior to the onset of the illness. The World Health Organization (WHO) estimates that approximately 55,000 people die of rabies every year. While domesticated animals, such as dogs and cats, can be treated against the development of rabies, it is difficult to inoculate wild animals, mostly because vaccines are not licensed for use on them. One method to attempt to control rabies in wild animals is the use of edible bait laced with vaccine.

Ringworm is a skin disease caused by a fungus, not a worm. The fungus usually occurs on exposed skin, especially the scalp, and looks inflamed and scaly. Diagnosis in animals is made by exposing the hair or fur to an ultraviolet lamp (the infected area will appear greenish in color). In humans, antifungal soaps or drugs will cure the disease.

Salmonella bacteria in food cause gastroenteritis, inflammation of the mucous membrane of the stomach and intestine. Symptoms of the disease are severe, bloody diarrhea and sometimes dehydration. The illness is very contagious and often spread rapidly in daycare or home settings. Although salmonella bacteria are usually found in uncooked meat, they can also be present in pet turtles raised on farms—as many as 20 percent of turtle eggs may carry the bacteria. Thus parents buying pet turtles for their children may unknowingly bring the disease into their homes. Many of these strains of salmonella are quite resistant to commonly used antibiotics, thus making treatment difficult and allowing the disease to spread.

Most spider bites result in redness and itchiness or soreness at the site. They usually heal by themselves in a few days. The bites of some venomous spiders, however, such as the brown recluse, or violin, spider (*Loxosceles reclusa*), can cause serious complications in humans. Symptoms of the bite of a brown recluse spider include an eruption that turns black in the center, surrounded with a characteristic bull's-eye pattern of red, white, and blue circles. The sore is accompanied by flulike symptoms, weight loss, and extreme fatigue. If treatment is not sought, the flesh at the site becomes gangrenous, and surgery is necessary.

Almost all newborn puppies carry roundworms, and because children love to cuddle puppies, the children often pick up the worms without knowing it. Symptoms in humans are a cough, fever, headache, and poor appetite. Treatment for both humans and puppies is with anthelminthic (worm-destroying) drugs. It is important that all puppies be seen by a veterinarian when very young.

Sporotrichosis is a fungal infection transmitted by cats. The fungus is found as mold on decaying vegetation, soil, and timber, usually found along southern US waterways and in places with similar climates. Left untreated, the fungus can spread throughout the human body. The organism enters the body through a cut or abrasion in the skin or through inhalation of the fungus. Therefore, it is a good idea to wash one's hands after handling cats.

Protozoan toxoplasmas are found in undercooked meat, on unwashed raw fruits, and in the feces of cats, and cause a condition called toxoplasmosis. The toxoplasmas may enter the human body through the skin or by respiration. Extreme care should be taken, especially by pregnant women, when disposing of used cat litter. In pregnant women, the disease invades fetal tissues, causing damage to the baby's central nervous system. The antibiotic spiramycin is effective in combating the disease's effects. Toxoplasmosis also poses a threat to AIDS patients as a major cause of encephalitis (inflammation of the brain or brain's lining). Experiments have been conducted with the drug clindamycin in treating toxoplasmic encephalitis in AIDS or HIV-positive patients; however, such side effects as diarrhea and rashes have resulted.

Treatment and Therapy

Zoonoses are transmitted either directly from an animal (by handling it or coming in contact with its feces or saliva) or indirectly (by being bitten or stung by an insect that is carrying tainted blood from an infected animal). Symptoms of infection in humans usually consist of headache, fevers, general malaise, nausea, diarrhea, and skin eruptions or inflammation. If any of these symptoms is present after receiving an animal bite or scratch, or even after handling an animal, a visit to medical personnel is necessary.

Prevention plays the largest part in avoiding transmission of these diseases. People should wash their hands after touching or being in contact with animals, even if they do not appear to be sick or infected. Parents should instruct children to be careful when playing with pets. Humans should not care for wild animals as house pets. Hunters and hikers should take care when traveling through wooded areas so as not to pick up ticks or other insects; wearing clothing that covers the body, with socks rolled over pant legs and gloves fitting over long sleeves, can help in these instances. Finally, pregnant women should avoid contact with animal feces (someone else, for example, should change the cat's litterbox) in order to avoid contracting toxoplasmosis.

Perspective and Prospects

Zoonoses have been in existence ever since humans and other animals have been together. There is probably no way to completely eliminate such diseases from the human world. Since zoonoses can be transmitted in any environment in which animals and humans live, work, or play together, such eradication would be impossible. It is, therefore, extremely important for people to take precautions when handling animals or animal by-products (such as meat).

Although there are approximately 150 known zoonoses, new diseases that are transmissible between humans and animals are being identified. Most zoonoses are relatively rare and can be treated once a proper diagnosis is made by medical personnel. With common sense and precautionary measures, the contraction of such diseases can be controlled.

—*Carol A. Holloway*

See also Anthrax; Babesiosis; Bacterial infections; Bites and stings; Chagas' disease; Chronic wasting disease (CWD); Creutzfeldt-Jakob disease (CJD); Ebola virus; Ehrlichiosis; Emerging infectious diseases; Encephalitis; Food poisoning; Fungal infections; Influenza; Insect-borne diseases; Leishmaniasis; Lice, mites, and ticks; Lyme disease; Malaria; Monkeypox; Parasitic diseases; Pinworms; Plague; Poliomyelitis; Prion diseases; Protozoan diseases; Rabies; Rocky Mountain spotted fever; Roundworms; Salmonella infection; Schistosomiasis; Severe acute respiratory syndrome (SARS); Tapeworms; Toxoplasmosis; Tuberculosis; Typhus; Viral infections; West Nile virus; Worms; Xenotransplantation; Yellow fever.

For Further Information:

"Animal Diseases and Your Health." *MedlinePlus*, May 23, 2013.

Biddle, Wayne. *A Field Guide to Germs*. 3d ed. New York: Anchor Books, 2010.

"Disease Risks for People." *American Veterinary Medical Association*, May 7, 2012.

"Diseases from Wildlife." *Centers for Disease Control and Prevention*, Nov. 4, 2009.

Durani, Yamini. "Pets and Your Health." *TeensHealth*. Nemours Foundation, Mar. 2012.

Folkenberg, Judy. "Pet Ownership: Risky Business?" *FDA Consumer* 24 (April, 1990): 28–30.

Hugh-Jones, Martin E., et al. *Zoonoses: Recognition, Control, and Prevention*. Malden, Mass.: Blackwell, 2008.

"Healthy Pets Healthy People." *Centers for Disease Control and Prevention*, Sept. 28, 2012.

"Human Rabies: Strain Identification Reveals Lengthy Incubation." *The Lancet* 337, no. 8745 (April 6, 1991): 822.

Krauss, Hartmut, et al. *Zoonoses: Infectious Diseases Transmissible from Animals to Humans*. 3d ed. Washington, D.C.: ASM Press, 2003.

Palmer, S. R., Lord Soulsby, and D. I. H. Simpson, eds. *Zoonoses: Biology, Clinical Practice, and Public Health Control*. New York: Oxford University Press, 2003.

"Rabies." *World Health Organization*, Mar. 2013.

"Salmonella and Pet Turtles." *Child Health Newsletter* 8 (April, 1991): 21.

Schlossberg, David, ed. *Infections of Leisure*. 4th ed. Washington, D.C.: ASM Press, 2009.

Swabe, Joanna. *Animals, Disease, and Human Society: Human-Animal Relations and the Rise of Veterinary Medicine*. New York: Routledge, 1999.

Woodruff, Bradley A., Thomas R. Eng, and Jeffrey L. Jones. "Human Exposure to Rabies from Pet Wild Raccoons in South Carolina and West Virginia, 1987 Through 1988." *American Journal of Public Health* 81, no. 10 (October, 1991): 1328.

"Zoonoses: Unseen Dangers." *Current Health* 17 (March 2, 1991): 11–13.

GLOSSARY

Abandonment. The failure of a health care provider to continue emergency medical treatment.

Abdomen. The part of the body between the thorax (chest) and the pelvis.

Abortion. Termination of a pregnancy before the stage of viability (about twenty weeks); may occur from natural causes (spontaneous abortion) or may be induced by medical intervention.

Absorption. A process transporting digested food from the small intestine into blood vessels, blood, and body cells.

Acetylcholine. A chemical released by motor neuron terminals that causes muscle contraction.

Acid reflux disease. A chronic digestive disorder in which the lower esophageal sphincter (LES), designed to keep digestive juices in the stomach, relaxes and permits gastric acid to rise into the esophagus, causing a burning sensation.

Acidosis. A state of excess acidity in the body's fluids; metabolic acidosis involves the kidneys, while respiratory acidosis involves the lungs.

Acne. A group of skin disorders; acne vulgaris usually affects teenagers, while acne rosacea usually afflicts older people.

Acquired immunodeficiency syndrome (AIDS). A progressive loss of immune function and susceptibility to secondary infections that arises from chronic infection with the human immunodeficiency virus (HIV).

ACTH. *See* Adrenocorticotropin (ACTH).

Action potential. An electrochemical event in which nerve cells send signals along their cellular extensions in the nervous system.

Active euthanasia. The administration of a drug or some other means that directly causes death.

Active immunity. Immunity resulting from antibody production following exposure to an antigen.

Activities of daily living. General personal care activities such as eating, dressing, and bathing.

Acupressure. An ancient Chinese mode of therapy performed by applying pressure to specific points on the body.

Acupuncture. Insertion of long, fine needles at particular points on the body located along one of fourteen major meridian lines, thought to be the major channels of life force. Developed by the Chinese.

Acute. Referring to a disease process of sudden onset and short duration.

Acute confusion. A transient condition caused by social and/or biological stressors, which may include inattention, disorganized thinking, other mental impairments, and emotional problems.

Acute rejection. The rejection of a transplanted organ by cells of the immune system; acute rejection is common days to weeks after cadaveric organ transplants and can usually be treated successfully with antilymphocytic drugs.

Acute respiratory distress syndrome (ARDS). Respiratory failure caused by filling of the lungs with fluid from the capillaries, leading to a shortage of oxygen in the body that can eventually lead to death if not treated.

Adaptation. A decreased sensitivity to a stimulus, even though the stimulus may still be present, resulting in slowing of nerve impulses until the impulses stabilize or stop entirely.

Addiction. A psychological and sometimes physiological process whereby an organism comes to depend on a substance; characterized by a persistent need to use the substance, increases in the dosage used in order to counteract tolerance, and withdrawal symptoms when the substance is withheld or the dosage is reduced.

Addison's disease. A chronic condition in which the adrenal glands do not produce adequate amounts of corticosteroid hormones.

Adenohypophysis. Another name for the anterior lobe of the pituitary gland.

Adenoids. A group of lymph nodes located above the tonsils, at the back of the nasal passage; usually disappear after childhood but are sometimes surgically removed (adenoidectomy) if they become swollen and cause blockage or infection.

Adenosine triphosphate (ATP). A high-energy compound found in the cell that provides energy for all bodily functions.

Adenoviruses. Medium-sized viruses that can cause respiratory infections and diarrhea by infecting the tissue linings of the respiratory and urinary tracts, the intestines, and the eyes.

Adhesion. The "gluing" together by scar tissue of internal organs and tissues, often caused by endometriosis or infections; a common cause of pelvic pain.

Adipose tissue. Fat; a soft tissue of the body composed of cells (adipocytes) that contain triglyceride, a compound consisting of glycerol and fatty acids.

Adjustment (chiropractic). A thrust delivered into the spine or its articulations in order to reestablish normal joint and nerve function.

Adjuvant therapy. Therapy used in addition to surgery in order to control the growth of remaining cancer cells.

Adrenal glands. Small organs near the kidneys that are responsible for the production of certain sex hormones, including testosterone and small amounts of estrogen, and of hormones involved in metabolism and stress responses.

Adrenalectomy. Surgical removal of one or both of the adrenal glands.

Adrenocorticotropin (ACTH). A hormone made in the pituitary gland in the brain that stimulates the adrenal cortex to make steroid hormones.

Adrenoleukodystrophy. A variable X-linked genetic disorder with symptoms ranging from adrenal insufficiency to progressive neurological deterioration.

Advanced life support (ALS). Procedures to sustain life such as intravenous therapy, pharmacology, cardiac monitoring, and electrical defibrillation.

Adverse reaction. An undesirable event caused by the taking of a drug; onset could be immediate or develop over time.

Aerobic exercise. Exercise that requires oxygen for energy production and that can be sustained for prolonged periods of time; involves large muscle groups, increases the heart rate and/or breathing rate, and is rhythmic and continuous.

Aerobic respiration. The chemical reactions that use oxygen to produce energy.

Aerospace medicine. The medical specialty concerned for the health of the operating crews and passengers of air and space vehicles.

Affective disorders. Mental conditions characterized by a primary disturbance of mood as distinct from thinking or behavior.

Ageism. Discrimination against individuals based on their age; the overlooking of individuals' abilities to make positive contributions to society because of their age.

Agglutination. A clumping of blood cells caused by antibodies joining with antigens on the cell surfaces.

Aging. The process of growing older, which begins at conception and eventually leads to death; the gradual effects of aging include changes in every organ and body system.

Agonist. A drug that acts in a similar fashion to a hormone or neurotransmitter normally found in the body.

AIDS. *See* Acquired immunodeficiency syndrome (AIDS).

Akathisia. An unpleasant sensation of "inner" restlessness that compels the patient to move or walk.

Alcohol. An organic compound containing a hydroxyl group attached to a carbon atom; ethyl alcohol is the compound found in alcoholic beverages.

Alcoholism. The compulsive drinking of and dependency on alcoholic beverages; viewed as psychological in origin, it can be arrested but not cured.

Aldosterone. A hormone produced by the adrenal gland that helps regulate the salt (sodium) and water balance in the body by increasing both sodium and water retention.

Alkalosis. A condition of abnormally low carbon dioxide levels that results from hyperventilation (rapid breathing).

Alkylating agents. Drugs that introduce alkyl groups to biologically important cell constituents, whose function is then impaired.

Alleles. Alternate forms of a gene; an individual has two alleles of each gene (one from each parent), which may be the same or different.

Allergen. A substance (such as pollen, dust, or animal dander) that causes an allergic reaction.

Allergic rhinitis. Acute or seasonal nasal stuffiness and sneezing that follows the exposure to allergens like pollen or animal dander; hay fever is one form of allergic rhinitis.

Allergies. Exaggerated immune reactions to materials that are intrinsically harmless; the body's release of pharmacologically active chemicals during allergic reactions may result in discomfort, tissue damage, or, in severe responses, death.

Allied health. A designation used to describe the services and personnel that support the providers of direct patient care within the larger health care system.

Allogeneic. Of the same species.

Allograft. A graft of tissue from one individual to another individual, usually between close relatives.

Alloimmunization. Immunization by means of antibodies from another person.

Allopathic medicine. The traditional course of study leading to a doctorate in medicine; most practicing physicians are allopathic physicians.

Alopecia. Hair loss, especially if noticeable or significant.

ALS. *See* Advanced life support; Amyotrophic lateral sclerosis.

Alternative medicine. Any of a variety of nontraditional therapies and treatments (such as acupuncture, herbal medicine, and homeopathy) that are not practiced by the established medical community. These alternative treatments range in the degree to which their efficacy and legitimacy have been accepted, from highly experimental and non-science-based to well established.

Alveolar cell. Also known as an acinar cell; the fundamental secretory unit of the mammary glandular tissue.

Alveoli. Tiny air sacs deep within the lungs.

Alzheimer's disease. A progressive disease characterized by a loss of brain cells; it causes increasing memory impairment and cognitive deficits.

AMA. *See* American Medical Association (AMA).

Ambulatory care. Health care provided outside the hospital, usually in a clinic, office, or home.

Amenorrhea. A lack of menstruation in girls by the age of eighteen or its suppression, often as a result of overly strenuous exercise, rapid weight loss or gain, or emotional trauma.

American Board of Emergency Medicine. The agency certifying medical doctors as emergency medicine specialists; sets criteria for training and knowledge to become board certified in emergency medicine.

American College of Emergency Physicians. Supports quality emergency care and promotes the interests of emergency physicians.

American Medical Association (AMA). The largest voluntary association of physicians in the United States, with most of its members engaging directly in the practice of medicine.

Amino acid. The fundamental building block of proteins; there are twenty amino acids.

Amnesia. An impairment of memory, which may be total or limited, sudden or gradual.

Amniocentesis. A procedure in which a small amount of fluid is removed from the amniotic sac of a pregnant woman to detect abnormalities that may be present in the fetus.

Amniotic fluid. Fluid within the amniotic cavity produced by the amniotic sac during the early embryonic period (two to eight weeks) and later by the fetus' lungs and kidneys; it protects the fetus from injury and helps to maintain a stable temperature.

Amniotic sac. A thin, tough, membranous sac that contains amniotic fluid and the embryo or fetus of mammals, birds, and reptiles.

Amputation. Surgical removal of all or part of a limb or digit (finger or toe), often as a last resort to prevent fatal infection from gangrene.

Amygdala. Front portion of the temporal lobe of the brain.

Amylase. The enzyme responsible for breaking down carbohydrates in the small intestine; amylase enters the intestinal tract from the salivary glands and the pancreas.

Amyloidosis. A condition characterized by the deposit of waxy substances in animal organs.

Amyotrophic lateral sclerosis (ALS). Also called Lou Gehrig's disease; the most common form of motor neuron disease, in which the nerves that control muscle movement degenerate in the brain and spinal cord.

Anabolic steroids. A class of steroids that stimulate body reactions to build up more complex molecules and structures from simpler molecules; most are synthetic derivatives of testosterone.

Anaerobic. Occurring in the absence of oxygen.

Anal incontinence. The inability to control defecation.

Anal intraepithelial neoplasia. Precursor lesions to the development of anal cancer.

Analgesic. A medication (such as aspirin) that reduces or eliminates pain.

Analyte. Any chemical substance undergoing measurement; includes charged electrolytes found in the blood, such as sodium or potassium.

Anaphylaxis. Severe allergic reaction involving the circulatory and respiratory systems; often fatal without immediate treatment.

Anastomosis. The surgical connection of one tubular organ to another.

Anatomy. The structure of the human body-its parts, systems, and organs.

Androgens. Hormones that regulate sexual differentiation and the development and maintenance of male sex characteristics.

Andrology. The study of the physiological functions relating to male reproductive capacity.

Anemia. A condition characterized by a deficiency of red blood cells or hemoglobin; anemia is sometimes caused by a decrease in hemoglobin production, an increase in cell destruction, or blood loss.

Anesthesia. A state characterized by the loss of sensation, caused by or resulting from drugs that induce pharmacological depression of normal nerve function.

Anesthesiology. The branch of medicine specializing in the application of anesthetics.

Anesthetic. A pharmacologic agent used to block nerve conduction and reduce sensations.

Anesthetist. A health care specialist who administers anesthetics.

Aneuploidy. An abnormal number of chromosomes.

Aneurysm. A localized enlargement of a vessel, usually an artery, caused by the stretching of a weak place in the vessel wall.

Aneurysmectomy. Surgical removal of an aneurysm.

Angina. Pain in the chest caused by insufficient blood flow to the heart muscle.

Angiography. A radiological technique for visualizing the interior of the arteries; involves the placement of a catheter in an artery and the injection of dye.

Angioplasty. Compression of arterial plaque by insertion of a catheter into the artery and inflation of a balloon at the end of the catheter.

Anomia. An inability to remember the names of persons or objects even though the patient sees and recognizes the persons or objects.

Anorectal. Associated with the anal portion of the large intestine.

Anorexia nervosa. An eating disorder characterized by a compulsive aversion to food, caused by a fear of obesity and a distorted body image, that may result in severe malnutrition.

Anoscopy. Examination of the anal canal via a small tubal instrument inserted a few inches into the anus.

Anoxia. Oxygen deprivation.

Antagonist. A drug that acts to block the effects of a hormone or neurotransmitter normally found in the body.

Anterior. Toward the front of the body.

Anterior chamber. Space between the cornea and lens; filled with aqueous humor.

Antibiotic. Any substance that destroys or inhibits the growth of microorganisms, such as bacteria.

Antibody. A protein produced in the body by the immune system that recognizes and binds selectively to foreign material (antigens) to facilitate their elimination; antibodies combat bacterial, viral, chemical, and other invasive agents in the body.

Anticholinergic. Referring to drugs that oppose the action of acetylcholine in nerve-impulse transmission.

Anticoagulant. A drug that reduces the clotting of the blood.

Anticonvulsant. An agent that prevents or relieves seizures.

Antidepressants. A group of drugs used for the treatment of clinical depression.

Antidote. Anything that counteracts the effect of a substance.

Antiemetic. A drug that prevents or relieves the symptoms of nausea and/or vomiting.

Antifungal agent. A drug that kills or inhibits the growth of fungi.

Antigen. A molecule that induces the production of antibodies; antigens are generally proteins.

Antihistamines. Over-the-counter and prescription drugs that reduce the effects of histamines, thus treating allergy symptoms.

Antihypertensive drugs. Medicines designed to reduce and control elevated blood pressure.

Anti-inflammatory drugs. Drugs that counter the effects of inflammation, either locally or throughout the body; the three classes of these drugs are steroidal, immunosuppressant, and nonsteroidal.

Antimetabolites. Chemotherapeutic agents that act by inhibiting enzymes in the DNA synthetic pathway or by incorporating in DNA itself.

Antioxidants. Chemicals that destroy free radicals or neutralize them before they can do damage to a cell's mechanism; they are produced as a by-product of a normal process of metabolism.

Antiserum. The fluid portion of blood that contains specific antibodies.

Anxiety. A condition characterized by nervousness or agitation.

Anxiety disorders. Problems in which physical and emotional uneasiness, apprehension, and fear are the dominant symptoms.

Aorta. A large artery from the left ventricle of the heart that supplies oxygenated blood to the body.

Aphasia. The total absence of such language skills as speaking, reading, writing, and comprehension.

Apheresis. The removal of whole blood from a donor, followed by its separation into components, the retention of the desired component, and the return of the recombined remaining elements.

Aphrodisiacs. Substances thought to induce sexual desire or lust or to enhance sexual performance.

Apnea. Lack of airflow for more than ten seconds.

Apothecary. A pharmacist or druggist.

Appendectomy. The surgical removal of the vermiform appendix.

Appendicitis. Inflammation of the vermiform appendix, which may require its removal.

Aqueous humor. A clear, watery liquid that fills the region inside the front of the eyeball between the lens and cornea; also called the vitreous humor.

Areola. The pigmented tissue immediately surrounding the nipple.

Aromatherapy. The use of scents to facilitate physical, mental, and emotional well-being.

Arrhythmia. A heart rhythm that is abnormal, either in speed or in force.

Arteries. Vessels that take blood away from the heart and toward the tissues.

Arteriosclerosis. Hardening and thickening of the walls of the arteries caused by a buildup of fatty deposits or plaques; also called atherosclerosis.

Arteriovenous malformation. A condition in which the capillary beds that connect the arteries and the veins are abnormal or defective, resulting in malnourishment of tissues, especially in the brain and spinal cord.

Arthritis. Joint inflammation.

Arthroplasty. Replacement or repair of a joint using metal or plastic parts.

Arthropods. Small animals including mites, ticks, insects, and related organisms that may be vectors to animal or human hosts.

Arthroscopy. The use of an endoscope to examine the interior of a joint.

Articulation. A joint between two bones of the skeleton; also called an arthrosis.

Artificial nutrition and hydration. The medical intervention of giving a patient nutrients and/or fluids through a tube placed in the stomach, the intestine, or a vein.

Aseptic techniques. Sterilization and other procedures that allow surgeons to operate in a germ-free environment.

Asphyxiation. An impaired exchange of oxygen and carbon dioxide in the lungs; if prolonged, this condition leads to death.

Aspiration. The breathing of material into the lungs (such as vomit or food particles); also, the removal of a substance using suction or a needle and syringe.

Assessment. The systematic process of collecting, validating, and communicating patient data; these data will include information gathered from the patient's history and the results of physical examination and laboratory tests.

Assisted reproductive technologies. A range of medical procedures that are used to assist couples in conception and prenatal care, with special focus on infertility and its cure.

Asthma. A disorder of the lungs, experienced as wheezing and mucus blockage of the bronchi.

Astigmatism. A visual disorder in which either the cornea of the eye or the lens is not symmetrical.

Asymptomatic. Lacking or without any symptoms.

Ataxia. An inability to coordinate the muscles in voluntary movement.

Atherosclerosis. A process in which plaque builds up on the walls of blood vessels.

Athlete's foot. A contagious fungal infection of the skin on the feet.

ATP. *See* Adenosine triphosphate (ATP).

Atrial fibrillation. Abnormal heart rhythm or muscle contractions in the atria as a result of disorganized electrical impulses.

Atrioventricular (A-V) node. A small region of specialized heart muscle cells that receives the electrical impulse from the atria and begins its transmission to the ventricles.

Atrium (*pl.* atria). One of the two upper chambers of the heart; the right atrium receives blood returning through the veins, while the left atrium receives oxygenated blood from the lungs.

Atrophy. The wasting of tissue, an organ, or an entire body as the result of a decrease in the size and/or number of the cells within that tissue, organ, or body.

Attenuation. The weakening or elimination of the pathogenic properties of a microorganism; ideally, the organism is rendered harmless.

Auditory nerve. The nerve that conducts impulses originating in hair cells of the cochlea to the brain for processing as the sensation of sound.

Auditory system. The human hearing mechanism, including the pinna, the external ear canal, the middle-ear structures, the cochlea, and the ascending neural pathway that terminates in the auditory cortex of the brain.

Aura. Sensory symptoms that may precede a seizure, a migraine or cluster headache, or a psychotic episode.

Auscultation. Active listening, usually with the aid of a stethoscope, to sounds generated by the body.

Autism. An emotional disturbance found in children in which communication, social interactions, and language skills are severely impaired.

Autoantibody. An antibody produced against tissue antigens within a host; self-antigens.

Autograft. A graft of tissue transferred from one part of an individual's body to another.

Autoimmune disorders. Disorders in which the immune system starts to attack the body's cells as foreign matter.

Autologous. Self-derived.

Automated external defibrillator (AED). A portable and automated device that can deliver lifesaving shocks to the heart.

Autonomic nervous system. The division of the nervous system that regulates involuntary actions, such as vital functions; comprises the sympathetic and parasympathetic systems.

Autopsy. Examination of a dead body to determine cause of death.

Autosomal dominant gene. A gene (other than the X or Y chromosome) that needs to be on only one chromosome in order to be expressed.

Autosomal recessive gene. A gene (other than the X or Y chromosome) that must be on both chromosomes in order to be expressed.

Autosomes. All chromosomes, except the X and Y chromosomes (sex chromosomes), that determine body traits.

Autotransplantation. The transplantation of tissue or organs in which the recipient serves as his or her own donor (such as a skin graft); may also refer to transplantation between genetically identical individuals (identical twins).

A-V node. *See* Atrioventricular (A-V) node.

Axon. The cellular extension of the neuron that conducts electrical information, transmitting it to the dendrite of the next neuron through the synaptic gap between them.

AZT. *See* Zidovudine.

B lymphocyte. A blood and lymphatic cell that plays a role in the secretion of antibodies.

Bacteremia. A condition in which bacteria enter the bloodstream and thus can be disseminated throughout the body.

Bacteria. Single-celled microorganisms that exist throughout the environment.

Bacterial endocarditis. Bacterial infection of the heart, which may scar or destroy a valve.

Bacteriology. The study of bacteria.

Balloon catheterization. The use of a balloonlike device on the tip of a catheter to widen blood vessels, as in angioplasty.

Bariatric surgery. Any surgical procedure changing the structure of the digestive system in order to achieve weight reduction.

Bariatrics. The medical management of obesity and related conditions.

Barium study. A medical procedure in which the patient drinks a liquid barium sulfate mixture prior to undergoing an X-ray examination of the chest and abdomen; used to identify problems in the upper gastrointestinal tract.

Barrier method. The use of a contraceptive that physically prevents sperm from meeting the ovum, including the male condom, female condom, diaphragm, cervical cap, and vaginal sponge.

Basal cell carcinoma. The most common type of skin cancer; it grows slowly and seldom spreads beneath the skin.

Basal cells. Cells at the base of the epidermis that migrate upward and become the principal source of epidermal tissue.

Basal ganglia. A group of interconnected deep brain nuclei that includes striatum, pallidum, subthalamic nucleus, and substantia nigra.

Basic life support (BLS). A variety of life-support procedures, including rescue breathing and chest compressions, often given to a heart attack victim by the first person responding to the patient; public training in such procedures is available from the Red Cross and the American Heart Association.

BCG. *See* Bacillus Calmette-Guérin (BCG).

Becquerel. The international unit of radioactivity, defined as a radioactive sample that is decaying at the rate of one nucleus disintegration per second.

Beneficence. A principle of medical ethics which requires that actions be taken for the patient's good.

Benign. Referring to a tumor made of a mass of cells that do not leave the site where they develop.

Benign senescent forgetfulness. A common source of frustration in old age, associated with memory impairment; unlike dementia, it does not interfere with the individual's social and professional activities.

Benzodiazepine. Any of a group of drugs with strong sedative and hypnotic action.

Bereavement. The general, overall process of mourning and grieving; considered to have progressive stages that include anticipation, grieving, mourning, postmourning, depression, loneliness, and reentry into society.

Beriberi. A serious vitamin deficiency caused by an inadequate intake of thiamine (B_1).

Bicarbonate. An incompletely neutralized carbonic acid lacking one hydrogen atom.

Biguanide. A medication to lower blood glucose by increasing sensitivity to insulin and possibly lowering the liver's glucose production.

Bile. Fluid produced by the liver and stored in the gallbladder to be secreted into the intestine; contains salts, bile pigments (bilirubin), cholesterol, and other waste products.

Biliary colic. A distinct pain syndrome characterized by severe intermittent waves of right-sided, upper abdominal pain, often brought on by the ingestion of fatty foods; pain occurs when a gallstone obstructs the outflow of bile and usually resolves when the gallstone moves away from the outflow area.

Bilirubin. A yellow-brown component of bile created when the liver breaks down old red blood cells.

Bioengineering. The combination of biological principles and engineering concepts and/or methodology to improve knowledge in both areas.

Biofeedback. Receiving information about involuntary

bodily responses in an effort to modify these responses to some extent, thus learning how to reduce stress and induce or maintain other positive behavior.

Bioflavonoids. Active flavonoids that work synergistically with vitamin C; they are not vitamins but are sometimes referred as vitamin P.

Bioinformatics. A computational discipline that provides the tools needed to study whole genomes and proteomes.

Biological sciences. Natural sciences that deal with the structure and behavior of living organisms; includes disciplines such as zoology, genetics, cell biology, biochemistry and molecular biology, and anatomy and physiology.

Biomechanics. The application of mechanical principles to the living body, specifically of forces used by muscles and gravity on the skeletal structure and how biomaterials such as collagen or elastin behave under those conditions.

Biomedicine. The branch of medical science concerned with the capacity of human beings to survive and function in abnormally stressful environments, as well as with the protective modification of such environments.

Biopsy. The removal of tissue from a suspected site of disease, such as cancer, in order to identify abnormal cells under microscopic examination.

Biopsychosocial model. A model that examines the effects of illness on all spheres in which the patient functions-the biological sphere, the psychological sphere, and the social sphere.

Biostatistics. The application of statistical analyses to the study of biological data.

Biotechnology. The medical application of biological and engineering knowledge at the molecular and genetic levels of natural systems in order to diagnose, treat, cure, or learn more about diseases.

Biphasic reaction. Delayed allergic reaction to an allergen, between one and four hours after the initial reaction.

Bipolar disorder. A syndrome characterized by alternating periods of mania and depression; formerly called manic-depressive disorder.

Birth defect. A genetic abnormality in the tissue development of a certain body part of the fetus; in some cases the defect is minor, but in others it may be medically dangerous to the fetus and/or the mother.

Blackout. Memory loss, usually as a result of taking substances known to disrupt memory, in which the affected person may function as if aware of what is happening, despite having no memory of activities.

Bladder. The organ that stores urine until it is discharged from the body.

Blastocyst. A small, hollow ball of cells that typifies one of the early embryonic stages in humans.

Blindness. Loss of sight; legal blindness in the United States means vision less than 20/200 or peripheral vision less than 20 degrees.

Blindsight. Refers to the ability of some people with damage to the occipital cortex to respond at above chance levels to stimuli presented in their blind visual field despite reporting that they could not see anything.

Blood. The fluid that circulates in the veins and arteries, carrying oxygen and nutrients through the body, transporting waste materials to excretory channels, and participating in the body's defense against infection.

Blood bank. A temporary storehouse of blood, kept at reduced temperatures, for transfusions into persons needing an additional supply; such transfers are vital in surgery and in unexpected emergency procedures.

Blood group system. A classification of individuals into groups on the basis of their possession or nonpossession of specific blood substances.

Blood pressure. A measure of how much the fluid in the blood vessels pushes against the walls of the vessels.

Blood testing. The withdrawal of blood from an individual and its analysis for one of many purposes, including blood typing and a search for acquired or genetic disease indicators.

Blood type. A blood classification group based on the presence or absence of certain antigens on red blood cells.

Blood typing. The identification of the blood-group substances of individuals so as to classify them in specific blood groups; individuals may have blood types A, B, AB, or O and be Rh negative or Rh positive.

BLS. *See* Basic life support (BLS).

Body dysmorphic disorder. A psychiatric somatoform disorder resulting in exaggerated preoccupation with an imagined or minor defect in physical appearance that causes significant impairment of social functioning.

Body mass index (BMI). Weight in kilograms divided by height in meters, squared (kg/m^2).

Bolus. Food that has been mixed with saliva and formed into a ball; the bolus passes from the mouth to the stomach through a process called swallowing, or deglutition.

Bone grafting. The transplantation of a section of bone from one part of the body to another, or from one individual to another.

Bone marrow. The soft substance that fills the cavities within bones and that is the site of blood cell production.

Bone marrow transplantation. The removal of bone marrow from an immunologically matched individual for infusion into a patient whose bone marrow has been destroyed.

Bone scan. A diagnostic technique using a radioactive tracer that is strongly absorbed by a tumor, whose location then can be detected by radiation counters.

Bones. Hard tissues that form the skeleton, providing support while allowing flexibility.

Botox. A neurotoxin produced by bacteria that causes botulism in very high doses and is also used as a therapeutic agent for a variety of conditions.

Botulism. Food poisoning caused by bacteria that produce a toxin that is absorbed by the digestive tract and spread to the central nervous system.

Bowman's capsule. The group of cells in the kidneys that forms the cup of a nephron; fluids that seep from glomerular capillaries into the hollow wall of the capsule will be transformed into urine during their passage through the renal tubule leading from the capsule.

Bradycardia. Slowness of the heartbeat.

Brain. The most complex organ in the body, which is used for thinking, learning, remembering, seeing, hearing, and many other conscious and subconscious functions.

Brain death. Irreversible brain damage so extensive that it is deemed there is no potential for recovery of emotional, cognitive, or executive functioning. In addition, the body's autonomic internal functions cannot support life.

Brain stem. The medulla oblongata, pons, and mesencephalon portions of the brain, which perform motor, sensory, and reflex functions (such as respiration) and which contain the corticospinal and reticulospinal tracts.

Breast. The mammary gland, along with the nipple in front of it and the surrounding fatty tissue.

Breast biopsy. The surgical removal of a lump or tissue from the breast to determine whether it is malignant.

Breast cancer. Malignancy occurring in breast tissue and possibly involving the associated lymph nodes.

Breech position. A commonly encountered abnormal fetal presentation in which the buttocks is delivered first, rather than the head; may require a cesarean section.

Bronchi. The right and left branches from the trachea that supply air into the lungs.

Bronchioles. Small conducting tubes in the lungs that carry air to the alveoli.

Bronchitis. An inflammation of the bronchial tree of the lungs.

Bronchoscopy. The visual examination of the respiratory system using a flexible tube composed of optic fibers.

Buffer. A solution that contains components that enable a solution to resist large changes in pH when small quantities of acids and bases are added.

Bulbourethral gland. The bulbous portion of the male urethra adjacent to the prostate gland.

Bulimia. A compulsive eating disorder characterized by food binges and purges (either through self-induced vomiting or the use of laxatives).

Bulla. A blister that develops on the surface of the lung; also called a bleb.

Burkitt's lymphoma. A highly aggressive lymphoma often presenting in extranodal sites or as an acute leukemia.

Bursa. A connective tissue sac filled with fluid that reduces friction at joints.

Bursitis. An inflammation of a bursa, one of the membranes that surround joints.

Bypass graft. A surgical procedure that reroutes blood around an obstruction, usually caused by atherosclerosis; the "new" artery can be either plastic or constructed from an expendable, healthy section of vein in another part of the patient's body.

Bypass surgery. Heart surgery to bypass a clogged artery by use of an unclogged vein, usually taken from the leg.

CABG. *See* Coronary artery bypass graft (CABG).

Caffeine. An addictive chemical substance found in foods such as coffee, tea, chocolate, and some soft drinks.

Calcification. The deposit of lime salts in organic tissue, leading to the buildup of calcium in the arterial wall.

Calcitonin. A hormone made and released by the thyroid gland that lowers the level of calcium in the blood by stimulating the formation of bone.

Calculi (*sing.* calculus). Any of a variety of stones formed by calcium deposits, cholesterol, and other materials that may accumulate in the kidneys, in the gallbladder, or elsewhere in the urinary or digestive tract.

Callus. An area of skin that has become thick and hard in response to repeated friction and pressure; also a bony deposit formed between and around the broken ends of a fractured bone during healing.

Calorie. The basic unit of energy; the amount of heat needed to raise the temperature of 1 kilogram of water by 1 degree Celsius.

Canaliculus. A small canal linking the upper and lower puncta (tear duct openings) to the lacrimal sac.

Cancer. Inappropriate and uncontrollable cell growth within specialized tissues, which threatens normal cell and organ function.

Cannula. A tube used to drain body fluids or to administer medications.

Capacitation. A change in sperm when in the female reproductive tract that causes them to swim more vigorously.

Capillaries. Minute blood vessels that connect the smallest arteries (arterioles) to the smallest veins (venules); they allow passage of oxygen and nutrients from the arteries into the tissues and passage of waste products from the tissues into the veins.

Capsid. The protein shell of a virus.

Carbohydrates. A group of organic compounds that includes the sugars and the starches; one of three classes of nutrients and a basic source of energy.

Carbon dioxide. The gas produced by the body from the use of oxygen; carbon dioxide and the hydrogen ions that it can create may become toxic if not excreted by the body.

Carcinogen. A chemical or radiation that causes changes in genes, leading to the cancerous state in a cell.

Carcinoma. A malignant neoplasm arising from the epithelial cells that make up the surface layers of skin or other membranes.

Cardiac. Related to the heart.

Cardiac arrest. The cessation of heart contractions or insufficient contractions to pump blood to the brain and other vital organs.

Cardiac catheterization. The guidance of a catheter into the heart or great blood vessels to measure function, assess problems, and identify treatment options.

Cardiac muscle. A type of muscle, found only in the heart, that makes up the major portion of the heart; involved in the movement of blood through the body.

Cardiac rehabilitation. The activities that ensure the physical, mental, and social conditions necessary for returning cardiac patients to good health.

Cardiology. The branch of medicine specializing in the diagnosis and treatment of heart disease.

Cardiomyopathy. A serious acute or chronic disease in which the heart becomes inflamed; it may result from multiple causes, including viral infection, and may involve obstructive damage.

Cardiopulmonary resuscitation (CPR). A method of restoring normal breathing to a patient in cardiac arrest using chest compressions and artificial ventilation.

Cardiovascular. Relating to or involving the heart and blood vessels.

Cardiovascular disease. Any of a group of diseases that affect the heart, including coronary artery disease, hypertension, congestive heart failure, congenital heart defects, and valvular heart disease.

Carotenoids. A group of fat-soluble pigments found in plants that have a strong antioxidant capability.

Carpal tunnel syndrome. Tingling and pain in the thumb, index, and middle fingers caused by pressure on a nerve that passes through an area in the hand called the carpal tunnel.

Carpus. The wrist.

Carrier. A person infected by an organism who can transmit that organism to other people but who is asymptomatic.

Cartilage. A strong, flexible connective tissue that lines the end of bones at a joint, providing a cushioning effect, and for other body structures supports the nose, ears, or bronchial tubes.

Case management. An interdisciplinary approach to medical care characterized by the inclusion of physical, psychological, social, emotional, familial, financial, and historical data in patient treatment.

Casuistry. A form of moral reasoning whereby specific cases about which there is moral uncertainty are compared to other cases about which there is moral certainty.

Catalysis. An increase in the speed of a chemical reaction.

Cataract. A dark region in the lens of the eye that causes gradual loss of vision.

Cataract surgery. The removal of an eye lens with cataracts and the implantation of a plastic replacement using microsurgery.

Catheter. A flexible tube that is inserted into a small opening or incision in the body.

Catheterization. The insertion of a tube into a cavity of the body to withdraw fluids from or introduce fluids into that cavity.

Cathode-ray tube (CRT). A display device used for the presentation of nuclear medicine data; it displays images in real time.

Cauterization. A means of sealing blood vessels with heat, used to prevent bleeding.

Cavities. Disintegrations in tooth enamel; also called tooth decay or dental caries.

CDC. *See* Centers for Disease Control and Prevention (CDC).

Cecum. The dividing passageway between the small intestine and the large intestine (or colon).

Cell. The basic functional unit of the body, which contains a set of genes and all the other materials necessary for carrying out the processes of life.

Cellular biology. The study of the processes that take place within a cell.

Cellular respiration. The chemical reactions that produce energy in the cell; these reactions can be aerobic or anaerobic.

Cellular transformation. The process in which a cell becomes cancerous, which begins with abnormal changes in gene expression and cell differentiation.

Cellulitis. Infection of the skin and underlying tissue.

Cementum. The outer covering of the root of a tooth.

Centers for Disease Control and Prevention (CDC). The government agency charged with monitoring the spread of infectious diseases in the United States.

Central nervous system. The brain and spinal cord.

Centrifugation. The spinning of blood or another fluid to separate out certain components for laboratory analysis.

Cerebellum. The part of the brain in the lower rear of the head located just above the brain stem; controls balance, coordination, and motion.

Cerebral palsy. A group of nonprogressive disorders of the upper neurologic system resulting in abnormal muscle tone and lack of muscular control.

Cerebrospinal fluid (CSF). The extracellular fluid of the central nervous system; it flows through the ventricles of the brain and the central canal of the spinal cord, circulating nutrients and providing a cushion for the brain.

Cerebrum. The largest and uppermost section of the brain, which integrates memory, speech, writing, and emotional responses.

Certification. The formal notice of certain privileges and abilities after completion of certain training and testing.

Cervical vertebrae. The first seven bones of the spinal column, located in the neck.

Cervix. The entrance to the uterus from the vagina; it secretes mucus, which appears as vaginal discharge.

Cesarean section. Delivery of a baby through the lower abdomen by means of surgery.

Chemical weapons. Synthetic chemical agents used as weapons, or devices used to disseminate them.

Chemoreception. Sensitivity to chemical stimuli.

Chemoreceptors. Specific structures that respond to chemical stimuli, producing such sensations as taste and odor.

Chemotherapeutic index. For antibiotics, the ratio of the maximum dose that can be administered without causing serious damage to a person to the minimum dose that will cause serious damage to the infecting microorganism; a measure of selective toxicity.

Chemotherapy. The use of chemicals to kill or inhibit the growth of cancer cells.

Chest. The region of the body from the diaphragm to the neck, both within the rib cage (heart and lungs) and in front of it (breasts and muscles).

Chest compression. Pressure applied to the bottom half of the breastbone to pump blood from a heart in cardiac arrest.

Chiari malformations. A group of disorders where the cerebellum, the part of the brain in the lower rear of the head that controls motion, extends below the opening of the spinal canal (the foramen magnum).

Chickenpox. A very contagious but mild disease caused by the herpes zoster virus whose symptoms include fever, abdominal pain, and skin eruptions.

Chiropractic. Manipulation of the musculoskeletal and nervous structures (often the spine) to allow the body to use its natural recuperative systems to restore or maintain health.

Chlamydia. A sexually transmitted disease characterized by discharge, pain, and swelling of the genitals; if a pregnant woman is infected, the disease can infect her infant's eyes during childbirth.

Choking. A condition in which the breathing passage (windpipe) is obstructed.

Cholecystectomy. The surgical procedure that results in the removal of the gallbladder in its entirety. The two main techniques are the traditional open method and the laparoscopically aided method.

Cholecystitis. Inflammation or bacterial infection of the gallbladder, usually caused by the presence of gallstones.

Cholelithiasis. The formation of gallstones in the gallbladder or the ducts that connect the gallbladder to the liver or small intestine.

Cholera. An infection of the small intestine caused by *Vibrio cholerae*, a comma-shaped bacterium.

Cholesterol. A waxy essential substance present in all cells and transported in the blood.

Chondrocyte. A cell found disseminated at different locations throughout cartilage.

Chorionic villi. The fingerlike projections of the placenta that function in oxygen, nutrient, and waste transportation between a fetus and its mother.

Chorionic villus sampling. Removal of a small portion of chorionic villi for genetic analysis.

Chromosomal abnormality. Any change to the number, shape, or appearance of the forty-six chromosomes in each human cell; the presence of many such abnormalities will prevent the normal development of an individual and lead to miscarriage.

Chromosomes. The parts of a cell's nucleus that contain genetic information, made of DNA covered with protein; each human cell has twenty-three pairs of chromosomes.

Chronic. Referring to a lingering or long-term disease process.

Chronic fatigue syndrome. A multifaceted disease state characterized by debilitating fatigue.

Chronic obstructive pulmonary disease (COPD). A progressive, irreversible disease of the lungs that causes expiratory airflow obstruction; the most common form is a combination of chronic bronchitis and emphysema.

Chronic rejection. The rejection of a transplanted organ months or years after transplantation.

Chronic wasting disease (CWD). A neurological disease of deer and elk caused by an infectious protein particle called a prion.

Chyle. The product that results from the emulsification of fat by pancreatic juice during the digestive process.

Chyme. The semiliquid state of food as it is found in the stomach and first part of the small intestine.

Cilia. Hairlike structures on cells that sweep mucus, containing bacteria and foreign particles, out of the airways.

Ciliary body. A ring of tissue that surrounds the eye; the uveal portion of this tissue contains the ciliary muscle that adjusts the degree of curvature of the lens.

Circadian rhythm. A cyclical variation in a biological process or behavior that has a duration of slightly greater than twenty-four hours.

Circulation. The flow of blood throughout the body; the circulatory system consists of the heart, lungs, arteries, and veins.

Circulator. The worker in the operating room whose responsibility is to keep records and to open sterile supplies for the team members wearing gowns and gloves.

Cirrhosis. A condition of the liver in which injured or dead cells are replaced with scar tissue.

Claudication. Muscle cramps that occur when arterial blood flow does not meet the muscles' demand for oxygen.

Cleavage. The process by which the fertilized egg undergoes a series of rapid cell divisions, which results in the formation of a blastocyst.

Cleft lip. Incomplete fusion of the two sides of the lips during embryonic development; often associated with cleft palate.

Cleft palate. Incomplete fusion of the two sides of the palate in the mouth during embryonic development.

Clinic. A site for outpatient care.

Clinical examination. The physical examination of a patient, including medical history and an evaluation of environment.

Clinical laboratory. A general term for those areas of a medical facility where analyses of body fluids are performed.

Clinical trial. A research study to compare standard treatment against potentially better treatment.

Cloning. The making of identical copies; the techniques that genetic engineers use to recombine DNA from different sources and to reproduce those fragments in bacteria or other organisms.

Clot. A clumping of platelets, blood, fibrin, and clotting factors that normally accumulates in damaged tissue as part of the body's healing process; also called a thrombus.

Clotting factors. Chemicals circulating in the blood that are necessary for the process of blood clotting.

Cluster headaches. Headaches characterized by intense pain behind one eye.

CME. *See* Continuing medical education (CME).

Coagulation. The process of blood clotting.

Cochlea. A structure in the inner ear that receives sound vibrations from the ossicles and transmits them to the auditory nerve.

Cognitive. Relating to the mental process by which knowledge is acquired.

Cognitive functioning. A general term describing mental processes such as awareness, knowing, reasoning, problem-solving, judging, and imagining.

Cold sores. Thin-walled vesicles around the mouth that are infectious.

Colitis. Inflammation of the large intestine (colon), which usually is associated with bloody diarrhea and fever.

Collagen. A protein found in bone and other connective tissues; collagen fibers are well suited for support and protection because they are sturdy, are flexible, and resist stretch.

Collaterals. Small vessels that enlarge to compensate for the obstruction or narrowing of another vessel.

Collecting duct. Tubular canal that transports milk from the milk duct to the nipple.

Collimator. A device used for restricting and directing gamma rays by passing them through a grid made of metal, which absorbs the rays.

Colon. The large intestine, divided from the small intestine by the cecum (a controlled passageway) and ending at the sigmoid, which leads food waste into the rectum.

Colon therapy. The irrigation of the colon with water in order to detoxify it.

Colonoscopy. An endoscopic procedure used for visualization of the large intestine.

Color blindness. A genetic condition of the eye in which the patient is unable to distinguish between some colors.

Colostomy. The surgical creation of an artificial opening for the colon.

Colostrum. Thin, yellow milky secretions of the mammary gland just a few days before and after childbirth; it contains more proteins and less fat and carbohydrates than does milk.

Coma. A loss of consciousness from which a person cannot be aroused; a symptom signifying a variety of possible causes.

Commissurotomy. The severing of the corpus callosum, the fiber tract joining the two cerebral hemispheres.

Common cold. An acute respiratory tract infection including stuffy or running nose, sore throat, sneezing, fever, wheezing, and nasal pressure headache.

Communicative skills. Those skills required to express thoughts, desires, and feelings effectively through verbal and nonverbal communication.

Complement. A series of about twenty serum proteins that, when sequentially activated by immune complexes, may trigger cell damage.

Complication. A secondary medical problem that develops from an existing problem.

Compound. To mix or combine; to make by combining parts or elements.

Compulsion. A persistent, irresistible urge to perform a stereotyped behavior or irrational act, often accompanied by repetitious thoughts (obsessions) about the behavior.

Computed tomography (CT) scanning. A method of displaying the outline of a tumor or other structure, utilizing a computer to combine information from multiple X-ray beams.

Conception. A process encompassing all the events from fertilization of an egg to its first cell divisions.

Concordance. The inheritance of the same trait by both twins.

Concussion. Temporary neural dysfunction, causing confusion, dizziness, nausea, headache, lethargy, and short-term amnesia; often results when the head is struck by a hard blow or shaken violently.

Conductive loss. A hearing loss caused by an outer-ear or middle-ear problem that results in reduced transmission of sound.

Cones. Specialized photoreceptors that sense color and detailed vision in bright light.

Confidential. Referring to a situation distinguished by the willing disclosure of intimate, potentially damaging information because of assurances that the information will be protected from general distribution or unauthorized disclosure.

Congenital. Referring to a condition present at birth.

Congenital adrenal hyperplasia. A family of genetic conditions that affect hormone production by the adrenal glands.

Congenital disorders. Abnormalities present at birth that occurred during fetal development as a result of genetic errors, exposure to toxins and microorganisms, illness, or unknown causes.

Congenital heart disease. Conditions resulting from malformations of the heart that occur during embryonic and fetal development.

Congestive heart failure. Abnormal heart function characterized by circulatory congestion caused by cardiac disorders, especially myocardial infarction of the ventricles.

Conjunctivitis. An inflammation of the white part of the eye, the conjunctiva.

Connective tissue. The tissue in the body that binds and supports body parts, such as tendons and ligaments.

Conscious. Having an awareness of one's existence, behavior, and surroundings.

Constipation. The slow passage of feces through the bowels or the presence of hard feces.

Contact dermatitis. A common skin allergy characterized by inflamed skin; it occurs when skin comes in contact with substances such as poison ivy or allergenic cosmetics.

Contact lens. A small, shell-like glass or plastic lens that rests directly on the external surface of the eye; used to correct refractive error as an alternative to spectacles, to protect the eye, or to serve as a prosthetic device promoting a more normal appearance of a disfigured eye.

Continuing medical education (CME). Medical coursework given by hospitals, medical societies, and conferences.

Continuous care. Services provided for extended periods of time, such as shifts of eight, ten, twelve, or twenty-four hours.

Contraception. Avoidance of conception by either natural means (such as abstinence) or artificial means (use of condoms, spermicides, diaphragms, intrauterine devices, or chemical hormone regulators such as birth control pills).

Contraction. A squeezing action of the muscles, such as the squeezing of the uterus that results in birth.

Contraindication. A condition that makes a particular treatment not advisable; contraindications may be absolute (should never be used) or relative (should be used only with caution when the benefits outweigh the potential problems).

Control group. A group of patients receiving either a standard treatment or a placebo, allowing comparison with the experimental treatment.

Contusion. A bruise; injury to tissue without breaking the skin.

Convulsion. An instance of amplitude-random and high-frequency electrical activity in the brain.

Cooper's ligament. Projections of breast parenchyma covered by fibrous connective tissue that extend from the skin to the deep layer of superficial fascia.

COPD. *See* Chronic obstructive pulmonary disease (COPD).

Cornea. The curved, transparent front surface of the eyeball, which provides protection and partial light focusing.

Coronary arteries. The arteries that supply blood to the heart muscle.

Coronary artery bypass graft (CABG). A surgical procedure in which a blocked coronary artery is bypassed using a vein or artery; this intervention provides a blood supply to areas beyond the distal attachment of the graft.

Coronary artery disease. Formation of fatty deposits or plaque on the blood vessel walls; results in a narrowing of the coronary arteries and a concomitant reduction of oxygen supply to the heart muscle.

Coroner. An officer, often a layperson, who holds inquests in regard to violent, sudden, or unexplained deaths.

Corpus luteum. A yellow cell mass produced from a graafian follicle after the release of an egg.

Corpuscle. A minute particle; a protoplasmic cell floating free in the blood.

Correlation. A number between −1 and +1 that describes the strength and direction of the relationship between two variables.

Corrosives. Having a burning (caustic) and locally destructive effect.

Cortex. The outer layer of the adrenal gland; the area that produces steroid hormones.

Corticosteroid. A fatlike molecule (or steroid), produced by the adrenal gland or made synthetically, that can be used to treat inflammation.

Cortisol. A glucocorticoid that raises blood sugar levels, elevated in response to physical or psychological stress.

Cosmetic surgery. The application of plastic surgical techniques to alter the patient's appearance.

CPR. *See* Cardiopulmonary resuscitation (CPR).

Craniotomy. Any surgical incision into the cranium.

Creatine phosphate. An energy-containing molecule present in significant quantities in muscle tissue; energy is stored in a high-energy bond similar to that of ATP.

Creatinine. A nitrogen-containing by-product of metabolism; levels of creatinine may be indicative of kidney function.

Critical care. A multiprofessional health care specialty that cares for patients with severe, life-threatening illness and injury.

Crohn's disease. A chronic inflammation of the bowel, often

as a result of an autoimmune disease.

Croup. A respiratory disease that causes a severe, barking cough.

Crown. That portion of the tooth, normally covered with enamel, which is exposed in the oral cavity above the gingiva (gum).

CRT. *See* Cathode-ray tube (CRT).

Cryogenic agent. One of various mediums used to achieve the low temperatures needed to produce therapeutic effects.

Cryoprobe. An instrument used by physicians to apply cryogenic agents to diseased tissue; cryoprobes have differently shaped tips that affect the size and depth of the freezing.

Cryosurgery. The destruction of tissue by the application of extreme cold.

Cryotherapy. Use of cold temperatures to treat disease.

Crypt. A pit or cavity in the surface of a body organ (such as a tonsil).

CSF. *See* Cerebrospinal fluid (CSF).

CT scanning. *See* Computed tomography (CT) scanning.

Culdocentesis. Retrieval of a small amount of fluid, by means of needle aspiration, from the rectovaginal pouch for diagnostic purposes.

Culture. A medium for growing bacteria in laboratory conditions.

Current. The flow of electrical charges through space or a material.

Cusp. The conical projection of the chewing surface of the tooth.

Cuspid. The longest anterior tooth; also called the canine tooth or the eyetooth.

Cutaneous. Pertaining to the skin.

Cuticle. Cutaneous or skin tissue that surrounds the nail plate on its proximal sides and provides a protective barrier to the nail bed; it is attached to the proximal nail fold and to the nail plate.

CWD. *See* Chronic wasting disease (CWD).

Cyanosis. A bluish skin color resulting from poor oxygenation of the blood.

Cyst. A swelling or nodule containing fluid or soft material, resulting from a blocked duct or abnormal growth in fluid-producing tissue.

Cystectomy. Surgical removal of the urinary bladder or the gallbladder; also, surgical removal of a cyst.

Cystic fibrosis. A genetic disease that affects the exocrine glands and most physical systems of the body, resulting in death usually between the ages of sixteen and thirty.

Cystitis. Inflammation of the bladder, primarily caused by bacterial infection and resulting in pain, urgency in urination, and sometimes hematuria (blood in the urine).

Cystoscopy. Use of an endoscope to examine the urinary bladder.

Cytokine. Small, regulatory protein of the immune system that mediate cell interactions.

Cytopathology. The study of disease states as they manifest themselves within cells.

Cytoskeleton. A network of filaments (including microtubules, microfilaments, and intermediate filaments) that supports the cytoplasm and extensions of the cell surface.

D & C. *See* Dilation and curettage (D & C).

Date rape. A forced sexual act during a date.

Debridement. The removal of all foreign material and contaminated and devitalized tissues from or adjacent to a traumatic or infected lesion until surrounding tissue is exposed.

Decompression surgery. Removal of tissue or bone pressing against the spinal cord or a nerve in order to make more space and relieve pressure.

Decongestants. Drugs that are taken in order to break up congested mucus, fluids commonly found in the sinuses during allergic reactions and colds, in order to reduce swelling in the sinuses.

Decubitus ulcer. Ulceration of the skin and subcutaneous tissues resulting from protein deficiency and prolonged, unrelieved pressure on bony prominences.

Deep tendon reflex. A brisk contraction of a muscle responding to a sudden stretch produced by a sharp tap of a rubber hammer on a tendon insertion of a muscle.

Deep vein thrombosis. The formation of a blood clot (thrombus) in a deep vein that prevents blood circulation.

Defibrillation. The application of electrical energy through the chest in order to correct abnormal heart function and restore a normal heart rhythm.

Delayed primary closure. A procedure in which the wound is left open four to six days and then sewn closed; used for infected or contaminated wounds.

Dementia. Impairment/loss of intellect and personality due to loss or damage of neurons in the brain.

Demyelination. A loss of the fatty, white substance that coats nerves.

Dendrite. The extension of the neuron that receives electrical information from neurotransmitters.

Dengue fever. A flulike viral illness, contracted by humans through the bite of an infected *Aedes* mosquito.

Dental arch. The arched bony part of the upper and lower jaws in which the teeth are found.

Dentin. The substance that constitutes the major portion of the tooth internally.

Dentistry. The study, diagnosis, treatment, and maintenance of the teeth, gums, and other parts of the oral anatomy; also known as odontology.

Deoxyribonucleic acid (DNA). A long, spiral-shaped molecule in chromosomes; the sequence of DNA subunits contains the genetic information of the cell and organism.

Department of Health and Human Services. A federal organization, headed by a member of the U.S. president's cabinet, concerned with the health of the nation's citizens.

Dependence. A condition related to maladaptive substance use and characterized by tolerance, withdrawal, and contrived use despite psychosocial or physical impairment because of use of the substance or efforts to acquire it.

Depression. A condition characterized by persistent feelings of despair, weight change, sleep problems, thoughts of death, thinking difficulties, diminished interest or pleasure in activities, and agitation or listlessness.

Dermatitis. A general term for nonspecific skin irritations that may be caused by bacteria, viruses, or fungi.

Dermatology. The study of the skin. its chemistry, physiology, histopathology, cutaneous lesions, and the relationships of these lesions to systemic disease.

Dermatopathology. The study of diseased skin tissue.

Dermatoses. Disorders of the skin.

Dermis. The second layer of skin, immediately below the epidermis; it contains blood and lymphatic vessels, nerves, glands, and (usually) hair follicles.

Detoxification. The process by which toxic substances are removed from the body, often as a function of the body's natural responses over time; in alternative medicine, such methods as juice therapy or colon therapy may be used to aid this process.

Development. The process of progressive change that takes place as one matures from birth to death; development can be gradual (as on a continuum) or ordered (as in distinctly different stages).

Developmental disorders. A group of conditions that indicate significant delays in or a lack of social skill development, with deficiencies in adaptive behaviors, poor language skills, and a limited capacity to communicate effectively.

Diabetes mellitus. A hormonal disorder in which the pancreas is unable to produce sufficient insulin to process and maintain a proper level of sugar in the blood; if left untreated, may lead to circulatory problems, heart disease, blindness, dementia, kidney failure, and death.

Diabetes insipidus. Less common than what most people mean when they refer to diabetes (see, diabetes mellitus), this is a condition arising from either an insufficient amount of "antidiuretic hormone' (ADH) being produced in the brain and thus unavailable to the kidneys, or from an impairment in the kidneys' response to ADH. The most salient symptoms of having diabetes insipidus are excessive thirst and excessive urination.

Diabetic nephropathy. Kidney disease associated with long-standing diabetes.

Diagnosis. The act of identifying a specific disease using signs and symptoms as evidence.

Diagnostic. Relating to the determination of the nature of a disease.

Dialysis. The filtration of crystalloid from colloid substances; most commonly used to refer to the medical procedure performed periodically on individuals whose kidneys have failed to remove waste products and other toxic substances that build up in the blood.

Diaphragm. The muscular partition that separates the abdominal and thoracic cavities; also, a contraceptive device that covers the cervix.

Diarrhea. Loose, watery, and copious bowel movements.

Diastole. The period of relaxation of the heart between beats.

Diastolic blood pressure. The pressure of the blood within the artery while the heart is at rest.

Diathermy. The heating of body tissues because of the resistance to the passage of high-frequency electromagnetic radiation, electric current, or ultrasonic waves; also known as electrocoagulation.

DIC. *See* Disseminated intravascular coagulation (DIC).

Dietary reference intake (DRI). The amount of nutrients needed daily by a healthy person to maintain health; age and gender affect the listed DRIs.

Differentiation. The process of gradual change of tissues in the embryo or fetus.

Diffusion. The process in which substances move from an area of high concentration to an area of low concentration; if given enough time, the concentration of the substance will be the same everywhere.

Digestion. The chemical breakdown of food materials in the stomach and small intestine and the absorption into the bloodstream of essential nutrients through the intestinal walls.

Digit. A finger or toe.

Dilation. The opening of the cervix to allow passage of the fetus through the birth canal.

Dilation and curettage (D & C). Dilation of the cervix to allow scraping of tissue from the endometrium (lining of the uterus); used to diagnose and treat disease and as an abortion method.

Diminished capacity. Partial insanity; a legal determination that a defendant does not have the ability to achieve the state of mind required to commit a crime.

Diopter. A unit of power of a lens equal to the reciprocal of the focal length of the lens in meters.

Diphtheria. A highly contagious bacterial infection that usually affects the respiratory system.

Diploid. Containing a double set of chromosomes.

Diplopia. Double vision.

Dipstick. A chemically treated paper strip used for the chemical analysis of urine or saliva.

Disarticulation. The amputation of a limb through a joint, without cutting the bone.

Disease. An abnormal condition of the body, with characteristic symptoms associated with it.

Disequilibrium. The sensation of being off-balance.

Disintegrative disorder. Deterioration in functioning following a period of normal development.

Disk. A soft, cushionlike structure that lies between bony vertebrae from the base of the skull to the sacrum of the pelvis; it has a soft liquid in the center and is surrounded by a thickened ligament.

Disk prolapse. The protrusion (herniation) of intervertebral disk material, which may press on spinal nerves.

Dislipidemia. Abnormal blood lipid levels, especially characterized by high serum triglycerides and very low-density lipoproteins (VLDLs) and depressed serum high-density lipoprotein (HDL) cholesterol.

Dislocation. The forceful separation of bones in a joint.

Disorder. An abnormal physical or mental condition.

Disseminated intravascular coagulation (DIC). A hemor-rhagic disorder that occurs as a complication of several different disease states and results from abnormally initiated and accelerated blood clotting.

Distal. Away from the point of origin.

Diuresis. Increased formation and excretion of urine.

Diuretic. A drug that stimulates the kidneys to eliminate more salt and water from the body.

Diverticulitis. The painful inflammation of diverticula.

Diverticulosis. A disease involving multiple outpouchings, or diverticuli, of the wall of the colon.

Diverticulum. A pouchlike, weakened region of the colon wall, which can cause pain and bleeding.

Dizygotes. Fraternal twins; born from two ova separately fertilized by two sperm.

Dizziness. A nonspecific term that includes vertigo, fainting, and disequilibrium.

DNA. *See* Deoxyribonucleic acid (DNA).

DNA testing. A technique for identifying a person based on matching unique gene-bearing proteins from an organic sample taken from that person (such as hair, blood, or tissue) with another organic sample.

Domestic violence. Assaultive behavior intended to punish, dominate, or control another in an intimate family relationship; physicians are often best able to identify situations of domestic violence and assist victims to implement preventive interventions.

Dominant allele. The version of a gene that produces a recognizable trait in offspring when present in only one of the two chromosomes of a pair.

Dominant genetic disease. A disease caused by a mutation in a gene that need be inherited from only one parent in order to exert its effect.

Dopaminergic. Related to the brain's neurotransmitter dopamine, which plays a role in such processes as mood, movement, and psychological functioning.

Doppler shift. The increase in frequency of sound waves as the source of the waves approaches the observer or instrument; Doppler techniques are often used to assess blood flow in body channels such as veins.

Down syndrome. An inherited disease caused by a defect in chromosome 21 that produces moderate to severe mental retardation.

DRI. *See* Dietary reference intake (DRI).

Drug. Any chemical substance that can be ingested into the body to modify bodily functions and responses.

Drug interactions. The chemical effects of taking drugs in combination, where the effects will reduce, magnify, or alter the desired effects of one or more of the drugs.

Duodenum. The initial part of the small intestine, where most of the digestion of food occurs.

Duplex scan. An ultrasound representation of echo images of tissues and blood vessels combined with a Doppler representation of blood-flow patterns.

Dura mater. Tissue layer between the brain and skull.

Durable power of attorney. Designation of a person who will have legal authority to make health care decisions if the patient becomes incapable of making decisions for himself or herself.

Dwarfism. Underdevelopment of the body, most often caused by a variety of genetic or endocrinological dysfunctions and resulting in either proportionate or disproportionate development, sometimes accompanied by other physical abnormalities and/or mental deficiencies.

Dys-. A prefix denoting wrong, painful, or difficult.

Dysfunction. The disordered or impaired function of a body system, organ, or tissue.

Dyskinesia. A neurologic disorder causing difficulty in the performance of voluntary movements.

Dyslexia. Severe reading disability in children with average to above-average intelligence.

Dysmenorrhea. Painful menstruation; primary dysmenorrhea is generally harmless and occurs in young women, while secondary dysmenorrhea may be caused by endometriosis, pelvic inflammatory disease, or tumors.

Dysmorphic. Abnormal in shape or appearance.

Dyspareunia. Painful sexual intercourse.

Dyspepsia. A general term applied to several forms of indigestion.

Dysphasia. A disturbance of such language skills as speaking, reading, writing, and comprehension.

Dysplasia. Any form of abnormal tissue development.

Dyspnea. Abnormal or uncomfortable breathing.

Dystrophy. A progressive condition that occurs when required nutrients do not reach tissues or organs, causing an inability of these structures to carry out their proper functions.

Dysuria. Painful or difficult urination, often the result of urinary tract infection or obstruction.

E. coli. See Escherichia coli.

Eardrum. The membrane separating the outer ear canal from the middle ear that changes sound waves into movements of ossicles; also called the tympanic membrane.

Ears. The organs responsible for both hearing and balance.

Eating disorder. An emotional disorder centering on body image that leads to a misuse of food, such as overeating, overeating and purging (bulimia), or undereating (anorexia nervosa).

Ecchymosis. Bleeding into the skin, subcutaneous tissue, or mucous membranes, resulting in bruising.

ECG waves. The repeated deflections of an electrocardiogram; one complete wave consists of a P wave, followed by a QRS complex, and then a T wave and represents one complete cardiac cycle, or heartbeat.

Echocardiogram. A graph of cardiac motion and heart valve closure produced by sending sound waves to the heart and recording their deflections.

Echocardiography. The use of sound waves to record activities within the heart and great arteries and to examine heart structures.

Eclampsia. Hypertension induced by pregnancy, in its convulsive form.

Ecology. A branch of science concerned with the relationships between organisms and their environments.

Ecosystem. An ecological community considered together with the nonliving factors of its environment.

-ectomy. A suffix denoting surgical removal; for example, an appendectomy is the removal of the appendix.

Ectopic pregnancy. The development of a fertilized egg in a Fallopian tube instead of the uterus; can be fatal to the mother unless it is corrected surgically.

Eczema. A skin disorder characterized by reddening, swelling, blistering, crusting, and scabbing; also called dermatitis.

Edema. The abnormal accumulation of fluid in tissues or cavities of the body, resulting in swelling.

EEG. *See* Electroencephalography (EEG).

Effector. A general term referring to skeletal, smooth, and cardiac muscles or glands that respond to impulses produced by the nervous system.

Efficacy. The extent to which a drug or procedure works as expected under ideal conditions, such as in the laboratory; efficacy must be proven before a drug or procedure may be applied in a clinical environment.

Ehrlichiosis. Infection by one of a group of intracellular bacteria transmitted to humans through tick bites.

Ejaculation. The release of sperm from the male's body during sexual activity.

Elastin. A protein that forms the main substance of yellow elastic fibers within connective tissue such as ligaments.

Elbow. The joint between the upper arm and the forearm.

Electric anesthesia. The use of pulses of electricity to deaden nerve cells or cause unconsciousness.

Electrical shock. The physical effect of an electrical current entering the body and the resulting damage.

Electrocardiography (ECG or EKG). The recording of heartbeat activity using electrodes attached to the chest.

Electrocauterization. The use of a high-frequency electrical current or electrically heated metal to sear tissue.

Electroconvulsive therapy. The use of electric shocks to induce seizure in depressed patients as a form of treatment.

Electrodermal response biofeedback. The monitoring and displaying of information about the conductivity of the skin; used for anxiety reduction, asthma treatment, and the treatment of sleep disorders.

Electroencephalography (EEG). The recording of brain-wave activity using electrodes attached to the scalp.

Electrolytes. Chemicals that, when dissolved in water, dissociate to form positive and negative ions so that the resulting solution is an electrical conductor.

Electromyograph. An instrument that is capable of monitoring and displaying information about electrochemical activity in a group of muscle fibers.

Electromyography (EMG). An electrodiagnostic technique for recording the extracellular activity (action and evoked potentials) of skeletal muscles at rest, during voluntary contractions, and during electrical stimulation.

Electron. A tiny particle with an electronic charge; a component of an atom.

Electron volt. A unit of energy defined as the energy acquired by an electron traveling through a potential difference of 1 volt.

Embolism. The blockage of an artery by matter (such as a blood clot) that has broken off from another area.

Embolus. Any particle in the arterial or venous system that travels with the flow of blood and eventually lodges in the lungs, brain, or other organ or blood vessel.

Embryo. In humans, the cells growing from conception until the eighth week of pregnancy.

Embryology. The study of the development of the (human) organism from conception to birth.

Emergency medical services. The complete chain of human and physical resources that provides patient care in cases of sudden illness or injury.

Emergency medicine. The branch of medicine that addresses conditions (such as cardiac arrest, severe wounds, poisoning, or seizures) requiring immediate medical treatment.

Emergency room (ER). A health care facility where rapid evaluation and treatment of sudden illnesses, accidents, and traumas occurs.

Emerging diseases. Those diseases that newly appear in a populace, or have been in existence for some time but are rapidly increasing in incidence, geographic range, or surface as new drug-resistant strains of viruses, bacteria, or parasitic species.

Emetic. Something that causes vomiting (emesis).

EMG. *See* Electromyography (EMG).

Emphysema. A disease characterized by an increase in the size of air spaces at the terminal ends of bronchioles in the lungs, which reduces the ability of the lungs to exchange oxygen and carbon dioxide.

Enamel. The tissue that covers the crown of the tooth; the hardest tissue in the body.

Encephalitis. Inflammation of the brain resulting in a variety of usually serious symptoms and sometimes death.

Encephalopathy. Any abnormality in the structure or function of the brain.

End-stage renal disease. The final phase of longstanding kidney disease, characterized by a nearly complete loss of kidney function.

Endarterectomy. A surgical technique for excising atherosclerotic plaque or the diseased endothelial lining of an artery.

Endemic disease. A disease that is usually present in a specific population such that the frequency of disease occurrence does not fluctuate greatly.

Endocarditis. Inflammation of the lining of the heart and its valves.

Endocrine. Referring to a process in which cells from an organ or gland secrete substances into the blood, which in turn act on cells elsewhere in the body.

Endocrine glands. Ductless glands that secrete hormones directly into the bloodstream.

Endocrine pancreas. Specialized secretory tissue dispersed within the pancreas called islets of Langerhans, which are responsible for the secretion of glucagon and insulin.

Endocrine system. The system of glands located throughout the body that produces hormones and secretes them directly into the blood for delivery by the circulatory system.

Endocrinology. The study of the endocrine system, the glands that produce hormones and the functioning of those hormones.

Endodontic disease. Diseases of the dental pulp found within teeth and diseases of the surrounding tissues, the gums.

Endodontics. The dental specialty that treats diseases of infected pulp tissue.

Endogenous. Something occurring or naturally found within the body.

Endolymph. Inner ear fluid.

Endometrial biopsy. A procedure designed to obtain a sample of the uterine lining (endometrium) for diagnostic analysis.

Endometriosis. A female reproductive disease in which cells from the uterine lining (the endometrium) grow outside the uterus, causing severe pain and sometimes infertility or the need for hysterectomy.

Endoplasmic reticulum. A system of cytoplasmic membrane-bound sacs that, with attached ribosomes, synthesize proteins destined to enter membranes or to be stored or secreted.

Endoscope. A lighted, flexible, hollow instrument used for examination and the placement of surgical instruments.

Endoscopic retrograde cholangiopancreatography (ERCP). An endoscopic procedure in which dye is injected into the common bile duct and pancreatic ducts for visualization with X rays.

Endoscopy. The process of passing a flexible fiber-optic instrument into an area of the body (such as the gastrointestinal tract) to allow visualization.

Endospore. A modified bacterial cell that is extraordinarily resistant to heat, desiccation, and other environmental extremes.

Endothelium. The inner surface of the cornea, which is separated from the rest of the eye by a layer of transparent fluid.

Endotracheal tube. A flexible tube inserted through the mouth or nose into the trachea (windpipe) to carry anesthetic gas and oxygen directly to the lungs.

Enema. Any one of a variety of procedures for cleaning out the lower colon or injecting food or diagnostic substances.

Energy. A measure of a system's capacity to do work.

Enteroviruses. A class of viruses capable of infecting multiple organ systems, such as the central nervous system, the skin, the eyes, and the heart.

Enuresis. *See* Bed-wetting.

Environment. The biological, physical, cultural, and mental factors that influence health; anything external to an individual.

Environmental diseases. Conditions and diseases resulting from largely human-mediated hazards in both the natural and artificial environments.

Environmental health. The control of all factors in the physical environment that exercise, or may exercise, a deleterious effect on human physical development, health, and survival.

Environmental medicine. The branch of medical science that addresses the impact of chemical and physical stressors and biological hazards on the individual or group in a community.

Environmental toxicology. The study of the impact of chemical pollutants on biological organisms; human health is the primary consideration, but the specialty also examines the effects of toxins on nonhuman organisms.

Enzyme. A protein secreted by a cell that acts as a catalyst to induce chemical changes in other substances, remaining apparently unchanged itself in the process.

Enzyme therapy. The administration of enzymes to aid digestive problems.

Epidemic. A widespread, rapid occurrence of an infectious disease in a community or region at a particular time.

Epidemiology. The study of the occurrence, frequency, causes, and distribution of diseases within a population.

Epidermis. The outer layer of the skin, consisting of a dead superficial layer and an underlying cellular section.

Epidural anesthesia. Anesthesia produced by injecting a local anesthetic between the vertebrae and beneath the ligamentum flavum into the extradural space; also known as extradural anesthesia.

Epilepsy. Uncontrollable excessive activity in either all or part of the central nervous system.

Epinephrine. A hormone that acts as a vasoconstrictor and cardiac stimulant.

Episiotomy. Surgical incision into the area between the anus and the vagina to enlarge the vaginal opening during childbirth.

Epi-Pen. A device that administers a prescribed dose of injectable epinephrine.

Epithelia. Tissues that originate in broad, flat surfaces, usually lining the surfaces of the body and organs.

ER. *See* Emergency room (ER).

ERCP. *See* Endoscopic retrograde cholangiopancreatography (ERCP).

Erectile dysfunction. A disorder whereby a male cannot achieve or maintain an erection suitable for sexual intercourse.

Erection. A complex phenomenon involving nerves, blood vessels, and the mind that leads to the entrapment of blood in the penis, making it rigid.

Ergonomics. The science of the relationship between the human form and its biomechanical environment.

Erythema multiforme. A skin disorder that produces multiple skin lesions and results from an allergic reaction or infection.

Erythema nodosum. Inflammation of the fatty layer of the skin resulting in red, painful bumps, usually located on the front of the legs.

Erythematous. Related to or marked by reddening.

Erythrocyte. The nonnucleated, disk-shaped blood cell that contains hemoglobin; also called a red blood cell.

Escherichia coli. A common bacterium that inhabits the human intestinal tract; used by genetic engineers to carry and propagate cloned DNA fragments and to produce pro-

teins from the cloned genes.

Esophagectomy. Surgical removal of all or part of the esophagus.

Esophagus. The muscular tube through which food passes from the throat to the stomach.

Essential nutrient. A substance that must be included in the diet because it cannot be synthesized by the body.

Ester. The relatively non-water-soluble compound formed when an alcohol reacts with a carboxylic acid.

Estrogen. The female sex hormone produced by the ovaries and the adrenal gland that is responsible for the development of female secondary sex characteristics; the three types naturally produced by the body are estradiol, estrone, and estriol.

Ether. A volatile liquid that causes unconsciousness when inhaled.

Ethics. A philosophical discipline that attempts to analyze systematically the way in which moral decisions are made; in medicine, ethics involves defining appropriate patient care, humane biological research, an equitable distribution of scarce medical resources, and a just health care delivery system.

Etiology. The investigation of the causes of any disease.

Eustachian tube. The tube connecting the middle ear to the back of the throat; air exchange through this tube equalizes air pressure in the middle ear with the outside air pressure.

Euthanasia. The medical inducement of death to relieve suffering; though performed routinely on non-human animals, euthanasia on humans is against the law in most, but not all, societies.

Evidence-based medicine. A method of basing clinical medical practice decisions on systematic reviews of published medical studies.

Evolution. A theory that explains the development of all organisms from simple ancestor organisms.

Excision. The surgical removal of an organ or tissue.

Excisional biopsy. Biopsy by incision to excise and completely remove an entire lesion, including adjacent portions of normal tissue.

Exercise. Physical movement that boosts metabolism and strengthens the body.

Exercise physiology. The science that studies the effects on the body of various intensities and types of physical activity, including cellular metabolism, cardiovascular responses, respiratory responses, neural and hormonal adaptations, and muscular adaptations to exercise.

Exocrine glands. Glands that excrete their products into tubes or ducts.

Exogenous. Originating outside the body.

Expiration. The act of breathing out, which partly collapses the lungs.

Extended care. Long-term, ongoing medical care for individuals with serious, chronic, or terminal conditions; may be performed in a medical or hospice facility or at the individual's home.

Extended care facility. A facility that can be found in several settings, outside the home, where specialized medical care can be rendered under a physician's orders.

Extension. Movement that increases the angle between the bones, causing them to move further apart; straightening or extension of the ankle occurs when the toes point away from the shin.

Exteroreceptors. Sensory receptors generally located on the skin or body surfaces that supply the brain with information about the external environment in which the body is located.

Extracellular fluid. The internal environment of the human body that surrounds the cells; the fluid contains ions, gases, and the nutrients needed by cells for proper functioning and is constantly circulated throughout the body by the blood and into tissues by diffusion.

Extracellular respiration. The process of oxygen transport from the lungs to the cells and carbon dioxide transport from cells back to the lungs.

Extracorporeal. Pertaining to something occurring outside the body, such as therapy.

Extubation. Removal of a breathing tube.

Eyes. The body structures that receive and transform information about objects into neural impulses that can be translated by the brain into visual images.

Face lift. The separation of the skin of the face from the underlying fascia and its tightening until the desired degree of wrinkle elimination is achieved; also called rhytidectomy.

Facial nerve. The seventh cranial nerve pair, which relays signals from the face and the front region of the tongue up to the pons of the brain stem; conducts impulses related to taste, salivation, and facial expression.

Fallopian tube. One of the two tubes through which egg cells travel from the ovaries, in which they originate, to the uterus.

Family medicine. The branch of medical practice concerned with treating individuals comprehensively on a long-term basis, often along with, or in the context of, all members of that person's immediate family.

Farsightedness. The inability of the eye to focus on close objects; also called hyperopia.

Fascia. Connective tissues such as tendons and ligaments.

Fasciculation. A brief, spontaneous contraction of muscle fibers associated with disorders of the lower motor neurons.

Fasciectomy. Surgical removal of any part of the fascia.

Fatigue. A general symptom of tiredness, malaise, depression, and sometimes anxiety associated with many diseases and disorders; in some cases, no specific cause can be found.

Fats. A group of organic compounds, also called lipids, that store energy; one of three classes of nutrients.

Fatty acid. An organic compound that is composed of a long hydrocarbon chain with a carboxyl group at one end.

Favorable. Indicating that a better outcome is more likely to occur.

FDG-PET. *See* Fluorodeoxyglucose-positron emission tomography (FDG-PET).

Fecalith. A hardened piece of fecal matter that often begins the events leading to appendectomy by blocking the appendix.

Fee-for-service. The traditional way of paying for medical care by billing patients when services are rendered (in contrast to a health maintenance organization).

Feedback. A system in which two parts of the body communicate and control each other, often through hormones; through such a system, hormones trigger other hormones' production (stimulatory feedback) or inhibition (inhibitory feedback).

Femur. The thigh bone.

Fenestration. The surgical opening of a passage in a closed or narrowing ear canal in order to allow sound to pass.

Fermentation. A chemical reaction that splits complex organic compounds into relatively simple substances.

Fertilization. The process in which the sperm head penetrates the ovum, resulting in the formation of an embryo.

Fetal alcohol syndrome. Growth retardation and mental or physical abnormalities in a child resulting from alcohol consumption by the mother during pregnancy.

Fetal surgery. Surgical intervention in utero, before birth, if the fetus has a life-threatening condition or congenital abnormality that can be alleviated.

Fetus. The unborn child from the eighth week after fertilization until birth.

Fever. A symptom associated with a variety of diseases and disorders, characterized by body temperature above normal.

Fiber. Food material derived from plant substances that retain the full structure of their cell walls despite the chemical effects of the digestive process.

Fiber optics. The transmission of light through thin, flexible tubes.

Fibrillation. Rapid and chaotic contractions of the heart muscle.

Fibrin. A fibrous insoluble protein formed from fibrinogen by the action of thrombin, especially in the clotting of blood.

Fibrinogen. A protein produced in the liver that is present in blood plasma and is converted to fibrin during the clotting of blood.

Fibrinolysis. The breakdown of fibrin, a major component of blood clots, that occurs after the broken vessel wall has healed; fibrinolytic agents are used to dissolve unwanted clots.

Fibroblast. A cell in connective tissue that gives rise to other cells that form binding and supportive tissue of the body.

Fibromyalgia. A connective, soft tissue disease involving chronic, spontaneous, and widespread musculoskeletal pain, as well as recurrent fatigue and sleep disturbance.

Fibrosis. Development of scar tissue consisting of excess fibrous connective tissue.

Fibula. The smaller of the two bones in the lower leg, on the lateral side.

Fight-or-flight response. A stressful biochemical reaction in animals, usually involving the adrenal hormone epinephrine, that prepares the animal for confrontation with predators or competitors.

Filtrate. Water and small solute molecules filtered from the blood by the glomerulus of the nephron.

Fistula. Any of a variety of abnormal openings from an internal organ to the body's surface.

Flagellum. A long, whiplike structure at the base of the sperm that propels it forward.

Flexion. A bending movement that decreases the angle of the joint and brings two bones closer together; for example, flexion of the ankle pulls the foot closer to the shin.

Flora. The microorganisms that are commonly found on or in the human body; also called microflora.

Fluid. An intracellular or extracellular solution of water and other substances, the concentrations of which must be regulated to achieve proper physiological functioning.

Fluorescein. A brightly colored dye used for diagnostic purposes.

Fluorodeoxyglucose-positron emission tomography (FDG-PET). A molecular imaging method in which radioactive sugar (FDG) is injected, accumulates in tissues with hypermetabolism, and is detected by its positron emission.

Fluoroscopy. Examination of the deep structures of the body by means of a fluoroscope, which renders visible X-ray shadows by projecting them on a screen.

fMRI. *See* Functional magnetic resonance imaging (fMRI).

Follicle. A small, saclike cavity for secretion or excretion, such as a hair follicle; also, spherical structures in the ovary that contain the maturing ova (eggs).

Food allergy. An abnormal response by the immune system to some foods, causing mild to severe symptoms that may become life-threatening.

Food group. Category of organic material from plants or animals that share similar characteristics.

Food poisoning. Food-borne illness caused by bacteria, viruses, or parasites consumed in food and resulting in acute gastrointestinal disturbance that may include diarrhea, nausea, vomiting, and abdominal discomfort.

Foramen magnum. An opening at the bottom of the skull where the nerves from the brain pass through and connect with the spinal cord.

Forearm. The region from the elbow joint to the wrist; also called the antebrachium.

Foremilk. The milk released early in a nursing session, which is low in fat and rich in nutrients.

Forensic. Having to do with a court of justice; forensic medicine and its various subspecialties apply medical science to the purposes of the law.

Forensic autopsy. A systematic investigation to determine the cause of death, providing the pathologist with information to state an informed opinion about the manner and mechanism of death in cases that are of public interest.

Forensic pathology. The branch of medicine that applies medical knowledge to legal situations, particularly crimes; forensic specialists, for example, gather data to determine the causes and circumstances surrounding a death that is believed to be a homicide.

Forensic toxicology. The branch of toxicology that interacts regularly with the legal community and law enforcement.

Fourier transform. A mathematical method that allows MRI to utilize one radio frequency pulse and thereby examine all wavelengths, as opposed to examining each wavelength individually with a continuous wave.

Fracture. A break in a bone, which may be partial or complete.

Free radical theory. The idea that aging may be brought about by the production within the body of very reactive chemicals (free radicals) that damage chromosomes and other cell parts.

Frequency. The number of complete events per period of time; for example, sound is measured in cycles per second, and one cycle per second is equal to 1 hertz.

Frontal lobe. The area of the brain in the front of the skull, responsible for executive functions; each cerebral hemisphere has one frontal lobe.

Frontotemporal dementia (FTD). A group of neurodegenerative disorders that affect the frontal and temporal lobes of the brain.

Frostbite. Localized freezing of tissue, usually of extremities exposed to low temperatures.

Frozen section. An extremely thin tissue section cut by a specially designed instrument called a microtome from tissue that has been rapidly frozen, for the purpose of microscopic evaluation and rendering a diagnosis.

Full-term. Referring to a gestation period of nine months.

Functional disease. A derangement in the way that normal anatomy operates; also, a disorder without any known organic basis (sometimes suggesting that the basis may be psychological).

Functional magnetic resonance imaging (fMRI). A radiologic technique that shows regional oxygen uptake, indicating brain activity.

Fungal infections. Infections caused by fungi, ranging from minor skin disease to serious, disseminated disease of the lungs and other organs.

Fungus (*pl.* fungi). A plantlike organism that does not produce its own food through photosynthesis, instead living as a heterotroph that absorbs complex carbon compounds from other living or dead organisms.

Gallstones. Particles of cholesterol and other substances that form in the gallbladder when the solubility of bile components is altered.

Gamete intrafallopian transfer (GIFT). A treatment for infertility in which sperm and eggs are introduced surgically into a Fallopian tube, where fertilization (and subsequent implantation in the uterus) are expected to occur naturally.

Gametes. The reproductive cells in either sex (the sperm and the ova).

Gamma camera. A type of radiation-detection instrument that detects gamma rays external to the body and makes an image of the radionuclide distribution in body organs; also known as a scintillation camera.

Gamma ray. A type of electromagnetic radiation that has the same physical properties as X rays but is emitted by unstable nuclei in their decay process; gamma rays are capable of penetrating soft tissue, thereby allowing their detection outside the body to produce images of organs.

Ganglion. A benign swelling or nodule surrounding a tendon, usually in the wrists, fingers, or feet.

Gangrene. Necrosis (tissue death) caused by obstruction of the blood supply; it may be localized to a small area or involve an entire extremity.

Gas exchange. The movement of oxygen and carbon dioxide across the membrane of the lungs and into the blood and tissues; other gases, such as nitrogen, may also cross the membrane.

Gastrectomy. Surgical removal of all or part of the stomach.

Gastric. Pertaining to the stomach.

Gastritis. Any inflammation of the stomach.

Gastroenteritis. An acute infectious process affecting the gastrointestinal system, usually leading to abdominal discomfort and diarrhea.

Gastroenterology. The medical specialty devoted to care of the digestive tract and related organs.

Gastrointestinal. Referring to the stomach and to the small and large intestines.

Gastrointestinal system. The gastrointestinal tract together with the salivary glands, pancreas, liver, and gallbladder.

Gastrointestinal tract. The digestive tract; a tubelike series of organs that includes the mouth, pharynx, esophagus, stomach, small intestine, large intestine, and anus.

Gastrostomy. Surgical incision into the stomach.

Gaucher's disease. A congenital disorder caused by a defect in lipid metabolism and characterized by cell hyperplasia in the liver, spleen, and bone marrow.

Gender. Strictly speaking, the behavioral and social aspects of being one sex versus the other; loosely used to refer to the biological and physical aspects of being male or female as well.

Gene. The basic unit of inheritance; at the molecular level, a gene consists of a segment of DNA that codes for a particular protein.

Gene regulation. The control of whether a gene is active (that is, encoding messenger RNA and protein) or inactive (that is, not encoding RNA or protein), a process often affected by hormones.

General anesthesia. Anesthesia that induces unconsciousness.

General practice. A primary care field in which health care is provided by physicians who usually have completed less than three years of residency training.

Generic drugs. Copycat versions of brand-name originals that are no longer protected by patents.

Genetic. Imparted at conception and incorporated into every cell of an organism.

Genetic counseling. Physician-provided advice to a couple who plan to have a child who might inherit a condition or disorder.

Genetic disease. A disease state that exists because of a decrease in or the absence of normal protein activity as the result of an alteration in the information carried in DNA.

Genetic engineering. A group of scientific techniques that allow scientists to alter genes; also called recombinant DNA research.

Genetic screening. A program designed to determine whether individuals are carriers of or are affected by a particular genetic disease.

Genetics. The study of the hereditary transmission of characteristics.

Genome. The total complement of genes inherited by an organism.

Genomics. The study of whole genomes.

Genotype. The genetic makeup of an individual; it is usually expressed as a list of alleles.

Genus. A category, below a family and above a species, used to classify living organisms and fossils.

Geriatrics. The branch of medicine that treats the conditions and diseases associated with aging and old age.

German measles. *See* Rubella.

Gerontology. The branch of medicine focused on the process of aging and the conditions and diseases that affect the elderly.

Gestation. The period from conception to birth in which the fetus reaches full development in order to survive outside the mother's body.

Gestational diabetes. A medical condition in which diabetes mellitus first occurs during pregnancy.

GIFT. *See* Gamete intrafallopian transfer (GIFT).

Gigantism. A rare endocrine disorder characterized by an overgrowth of all bones and body tissues.

Gingiva. The gum tissue surrounding the neck of the tooth.

Gingivitis. A superficial inflammation of the gums associated with the destructive buildup of dental plaque; if left untreated, it can result in periodontitis.

Gland. An organ or area of the body that produces, stores, and secretes fluids, exerting a profound effect on growth, energy production, chemical balance, reproduction, and health.

Glasses. A pair of ophthalmic lenses held together with a frame or mounting; also called spectacles.

Glaucoma. An eye disease characterized by increased intraocular pressure, which can lead to degeneration of the optic nerve and ultimately blindness if left untreated.

Glial cells. Nonexcitable cells of the nervous system; they include astrocytes, microglial cells, oligodendrocytes, and Schwann cells.

Glomerular filtration. The first step in urine formation; passive filtration in which fluids and solids dissolved in the fluid (solutes) are forced through a membrane, resulting in filtration of the blood.

Glomerulonephritis. Inflammation of the glomeruli, the clusters of blood vessels and nerves found throughout the kidney.

Glomerulus (*pl.* glomeruli). One of the very small units in the kidney, in which blood is filtered through a membrane.

Glossopharyngeal nerve. The ninth cranial nerve, which relays signals pertaining to or controlling salivation; it sends neurological information to and from the posterior region of the tongue to the medulla oblongata of the brain stem.

Glucagon. A pancreatic hormone that signals an elevated

concentration of glucose circulating in the blood.

Glucocorticoids. Steroid hormones that regulate the metabolism of glucose and other organic molecules.

Gluconeogenesis. The synthesis within the body of glucose from noncarbohydrate precursors.

Glucosuria. A condition in which the concentration of blood glucose exceeds the ability of the kidney to reabsorb it; as a result, glucose spills into the urine, taking with it body water and electrolytes.

Gluten. A protein found in wheat, barley, and rye grains.

Gluten intolerance. A chronic, immune-mediated condition of progressive, itchy skin lesions triggered by ingestion of gluten.

Glycerol. A three-carbon alcohol that has one hydroxyl compound on each carbon atom.

Glycogen. The form that glucose takes when it is stored in the muscles and liver.

Glycogen storage diseases. Inherited metabolic disorders that lead to the accumulation of an abnormal amount or type of glycogen in the liver, muscles, and heart.

Glycolysis. The chemical process of splitting a molecule of glucose in order to obtain energy for other cellular processes; at times of intense activity, glycolysis produces most of the energy used by muscles.

Glycoprotein. A protein to which is attached one or more sugar molecules.

Goiter. Enlargement of the thyroid gland in the neck.

Golgi complex. A system of membrane sacs in which proteins are chemically modified, sorted, and routed to various cellular destinations.

Gonad. The male or female organ (testis or ovary, respectively) in which the essential gametes are formed for reproduction.

Gonadotrophin. A hormone secreted by the pituitary gland; the primary gonadotrophins are luteinizing hormone (LH) and follicle-stimulating hormone (FSH).

Goniometry. The measurement of angles, particularly those for the range of motion of a joint.

Gonorrhea. An infection of the urogenital tract that is a common sexually transmitted disease.

Gout. Painful arthritis of the peripheral joints, often in the big toe, caused by uric acid buildup.

Graafian follicle. Any of the ovarian follicles that produce eggs.

Graft-versus-host disease. A genetic incompatibility between tissues in which immune system cells from the grafted tissue attack host tissue.

Grafting. A surgical graft of skin from one part of the body to another or from one individual to another.

Gram staining. The use of a stain to classify bacteria as either gram-positive (they retain the primary stain of crystal violet when subjected to treatment with a decolorizer) or gram-negative (no coloration).

Grand mal. A type of epileptic seizure characterized by severe convulsions, body stiffening, and loss of consciousness during which victims fall down.

Granulocyte. A white blood cell characterized by large numbers of cytoplasmic granules, including neutrophils, eosinophils, and basophils.

Granuloma. A nodular, inflammatory lesion that is usually small, firm, and persistent and contains proliferated macrophages.

Graves' disease. A common type of hyperthyroidism in which the thyroid gland produces an oversupply of hormone.

Gross pathology. The study of that which is visible to the naked eye (macroscopic) during inspection.

Growth. The development of the human body from conception to adulthood.

Guillain-Barré syndrome. An acute degeneration of peripheral motor and sensory nerves, known to physicians as acute inflammatory demyelinating polyneuropathy, a common cause of acute generalized paralysis.

Gum disease. Inflammation of the soft tissue that surrounds the teeth; in advanced disease, there is also loss of bone that holds the teeth in place.

Gynecology. The branch of medicine that focuses on the conditions and disorders affecting the female reproductive system.

Hair. Threadlike outgrowths of nonliving, mostly proteinaceous material that covers much of the body of humans and other mammals.

Hair transplantation. The surgical relocation of healthy hair follicles to a part of the scalp where shrunken follicles are producing short, thin hair or no hair.

Half-life. The time required for half of the nuclei in a radioactive sample to decay.

Hallucinations. The perception of sensations without relevant external stimuli.

Hammertoe. An abnormality of the tendon in a toe that causes the main joint to curve upward and can be painful as a result of shoe pressure.

Haploid. Containing only a single set of chromosomes; mature gametes are haploid.

Hard palate. The bony portion of the roof of the mouth, contiguous with the soft palate.

Harelip. *See* Cleft lip.

Hashimoto's thyroiditis. An inflammation of the thyroid gland caused when abnormal blood antibodies and white blood cells infiltrate and attack thyroidal cells.

HDLs. *See* High-density lipoproteins.

Headaches. Pain localized in the head or neck, often caused by tension but also the result of a range of disorders.

Healing. The process of mending damaged tissue by which an organism restores itself to health.

Health. A condition in which all functions of the body, mind, and spirit are normally active.

Health care system. The collection of services in a given country that provide hospital, emergency, preventative, and other outpatient care to citizens.

Health insurance. The promise by a company to pay specified costs related to the health care of an individual or group of individuals who pay premium fees.

Health maintenance. The practice of anticipating, finding, preventing, and/or dealing with potential or established medical problems at the earliest possible stage to minimize adverse effects on the patient.

Health maintenance organization (HMO). A group of general practitioners, specialists, and allied health professionals who provide medical services to subscribers who pay a regular maintenance fee.

Hearing loss. Loss of sensitivity to sound pressure changes as a result of congenital factors, disease, traumatic injury, noise exposure, or aging.

Heart. The muscle that pumps blood through the body by means of rhythmic contractions.

Heart attack. Sudden and permanent damage to a part of the heart muscle as a result of impaired blood flow through the coronary arteries; the common term for myocardial infarction.

Heart block. A delay or blockage of the electrical signal traveling through the heart muscle, which upsets the synchronization between contractions of the upper and lower chambers.

Heart failure. A condition in which the heart cannot pump enough blood to meet the body's needs.

Heart rate. The number of times the heart contracts, or beats, per minute.

Heart transplantation. The removal of a diseased heart and its replacement with a healthy donor heart.

Heart valve replacement. A surgical procedure involving the removal of a defective heart valve and its replacement with another tissue valve or with a mechanical valve.

Heat. The transfer of energy across a boundary because of a temperature difference.

Heat exhaustion. Mild shock caused by a decrease in the amount of fluid in the blood.

Heatstroke. A medical emergency in which high body temperatures result in organ damage.

Heel spur. A bony outgrowth on the heel of the foot.

Hematology. The study of the blood, including its normal constituents and such blood disorders as anemia, leukemia, and hemophilia.

Hematoma. A localized collection of clotted blood in an organ or tissue as a result of internal bleeding.

Hematopoiesis. The production of red and white cells and platelets, which occurs mainly in bone marrow; also called hematosis.

Hematuria. The abnormal presence of blood in the urine.

Hemiplegia. Paralysis or weakness on one side of the body.

Hemochromatosis. A multisystem disease characterized by increased iron absorption and storage.

Hemodialysis. The removal of toxins from blood through the process of dialysis.

Hemodynamics. The study of blood circulation.

Hemoglobin. The oxygen-carrying iron-containing pigment present in red blood cells that is responsible for oxygen exchange in cells and tissues.

Hemolysis. Breakdown of red blood cells and the release of hemoglobin.

Hemolytic anemia. Anemia resulting from hemolysis, the excessive destruction of red blood cells.

Hemophilia. A hereditary blood defect (occurring almost exclusively in males) characterized by delayed clotting of the blood and consequent difficulty in controlling bleeding even after minor injuries.

Hemorrhage. The loss of a large amount of blood in a short period of time.

Hemorrhagic fever. A disease in humans or other animals characterized by a high fever and a bleeding disorder, affecting multiple organ systems and, if severe, leading to death.

Hemorrhoids. Dilated blood vessels in the anus or rectum that are itchy and painful.

Hemostasis. The stopping of blood flow through the blood vessels, usually as a result of blood clotting.

Hepatic. Of or referring to the liver.

Hepatitis. Inflammation of the liver.

Hepatitis A virus. The virus associated with certain forms of hepatitis; generally contracted through fecal contamination of food and water.

Hepatitis B virus. The agent associated with severe forms of viral hepatitis; contracted through contaminated blood or hypodermic needles or through contaminated body fluids.

Hepatitis C virus. Formerly referred to as the etiological agent for non-A, non-B viral hepatitis; most often passed in contaminated blood.

Hepato-. A prefix denoting an association with the liver; for example, a hepatocyte is a liver cell.

Hepatocyte. The functional cell of the liver.

Herbal medicine. A nontraditional form of medicine that uses different types of herbs for therapy and health maintenance.

Hernia. A pouch of intestines and/or vital organs of the abdomen that protrudes through the abdominal wall.

Heterosexual. Being principally attracted to and aroused by opposite-gender persons.

Heterozygous. Having two different alleles for a particular gene.

Heuristics. Methods used to aid and guide in the discovery of a disease process when incomplete knowledge exists.

Hiatal hernia. A condition in which a portion of the stomach protrudes into the chest cavity through an opening in the diaphragm.

High-density lipoproteins (HDLs). A form of cholesterol in the blood that appears to be associated with a lower risk of arterial and heart disease.

Hindmilk. The milk released late in a nursing session, which is higher in fat content.

Hippocratic oath. A document written in the fifth century B.C.E. to offer guidelines for the emerging medical profession.

Hirsutism. Excessive hair growth.

Histamine. A compound released during allergic reactions that causes many of the symptoms of allergies.

Histamine II blockers. Various drugs that combat the chemical action of ulcers by reducing the secretion of gastric juices, or "stomach acids."

Histiocytosis. A group of relatively rare blood disorders characterized by the abnormal accumulation of white blood cells called histiocytes, leading to a wide range of adverse bodily responses.

Histocompatibility. Tissue compatibility, as determined by histocompatibility protein antigens present on the cell membranes of all tissue cells.

Histology. The branch of medicine that focuses on the study of cells and tissues as they relate to their function.

Histopathology. The histologic or microscopic description of abnormal pathologic tissue changes; these changes can be seen under the microscope.

HIV. *See* Human immunodeficiency virus (HIV).

HLAs. *See* Human leukocyte antigens (HLAs).

HMO. *See* Health maintenance organization (HMO).

Hodgkin's disease. A neoplastic disorder originating in the tissues of the lymphatic system, recognized by distinctive histologic changes and defined by the presence of Reed-Sternberg cells.

Holistic. The philosophy that individuals function as complete units or integrated systems and are not understood merely through their parts.

Holistic medicine. An approach to the practice of medicine based on the philosophy that treatment must occur taking into consideration the entire organism, both physiological and psychological.

Home care. The provision of outside services to a patient living in a home setting.

Homeopathy. A nontraditional approach to treatment based on a theory of Samuel Hahnemann, called the "law of similars," positing that substances which provoke disease may be used in small doses to treat the disease.

Homeostasis. The maintenance of a constant internal environment; the systems of the body work together to maintain constant temperature, pH, oxygen availability, water content, ion concentrations, and so on.

Homosexual. Being principally attracted to and aroused by persons of one's own gender; two synonymous terms are "gay," which can refer to all homosexuals or to homosexual males exclusively, and "lesbian," which refers only to homosexual females.

Homozygous. Having two identical alleles of a particular gene.

Hormone. A substance that creates a specific effect in an organ distant from its site of production.

Hormone receptor. A molecule contained in or on a cell that allows it to respond to a hormone; if receptors are not present, the hormone will have no effect.

Hormone therapy. The use of hormones as treatment, especially the use of estrogens, with or without progesterone, to treat menopausal symptoms.

Hospice. A program designed to ease the suffering and grief for terminally ill patients and their families; care can be rendered in the home or in a special hospice setting with special emphasis on the relief of pain.

Hospital. An institution focused on the management, prevention, and treatment of illness, utilizing a staff of medical and allied health professionals to provide medical, surgical, and psychiatric treatments, along with emergency care and evaluation.

Host. The body of the person or animal infected with a pathogen, especially a parasite.

Host-defense mechanisms. Immunological methods that the body uses to protect against external infectious agents and to maintain internal homeostasis, such as skin, sweat, urine, tears, phagocytes, and "helpful" bacteria.

Host-versus-graft disease. A tissue rejection in which the immune system cells of the graft recipient attack the grafted tissue from a donor individual.

Hot flashes. Temporary sensations of warmth experienced by perimenopausal and postmenopausal women in which the upper body feels hot, the skin turns red, and sweating occurs.

HPV. *See* Human papillomavirus (HPV).

Human immunodeficiency virus (HIV). The virus that causes acquired immunodeficiency syndrome (AIDS); it may be transmitted through blood or semen.

Human leukocyte antigens (HLAs). Structures located on the surface of each cell that are unique to an individual; also called transplantation antigens.

Humerus. The bone that forms the structural beam of the upper arm.

Huntington's disease. A genetic disease characterized by uncoordinated movements as a result of neuron degeneration.

Hydro-. A prefix denoting water or fluid.

Hydrocarbon. An organic compound composed of only hydrogen and carbon atoms that does not dissolve in water (water-insoluble).

Hydrocephalus. An excessive collection of cerebrospinal fluid in the brain.

Hydrocortisone. Pharmaceutical term for cortisol.

Hydrophilic. "Water-loving" or water-attracting; a term given to molecules or regions of molecules that interact favorably with water.

Hydrophobic. "Water-hating" or "water-repelling"; a term given to molecules or regions of molecules that do not interact favorably with water.

Hydrotherapy. A form of treatment that uses water, externally, to aid in recovery or ease pain.

Hygiene. The science of health and the prevention of disease.

Hyper-. A prefix denoting "high" or more than normal.

Hyperalimentation. Intravenous fluid providing nutrition.

Hyperandrogenism. Higher-than-normal levels of androgens in the blood.

Hyperglycemia. High blood glucose.

Hyperinsulinemia. Abnormally high serum insulin concentration.

Hyperlipidemia. The presence of abnormally large amounts of lipids in the blood.

Hypernatremia. A high salt concentration in the blood that can result in seizure and coma.

Hyperopia. The inability of the eye to focus on close objects; also called farsightedness.

Hyperparathyroidism. The excessive, uncontrolled secretion of parathyroid hormone.

Hyperplasia. A proliferation of cells in response to either normal or abnormal physiological processes.

Hypersensitivity. An overreaction by the immune system to the presence of certain antigens; this overreaction often results in some damage to the person as well as the antigen.

Hypertension. High blood pressure; a systolic pressure of at least 140 or a diastolic pressure of at least 90.

Hyperthermia. The elevation of the body core temperature of an organism above a normal range.

Hypertrophy. The growth of a tissue or organ as a result of an increase in the size of existing cells.

Hyperventilation. Breathing at a faster rate than what is needed for metabolism, resulting in the exhalation of carbon dioxide faster than it is produced.

Hyphae. The long, filamentous, often branching cells of many fungi.

Hypnosis. The induction of an altered state of consciousness.

Hypo-. A prefix denoting "low" or less than normal.

Hypocalcemia. Low blood levels of calcium.

Hypochondriasis. A condition in which patients believe strongly that they are suffering from one or more serious illnesses, even when this belief is unsupported by medical evidence.

Hypodermis. The layer of fat under the dermis that contains carotene.

Hypoglycemia. A condition in which the concentration of glucose in the blood is too low to meet the needs of key organs, especially the brain.

Hypoparathyroidism. The reduced secretion of parathyroid hormone.

Hypospadias. An abnormal urethral opening in the penis, either on the underside or on the perineum.

Hypotension. Decrease in blood pressure to the point that insufficient blood flow causes symptoms.

Hypothalamus. The region of the brain called the diencephalon, forming the floor of the third ventricle, including neighboring, associated nuclei.

Hypothermia. A subnormal body temperature; clinically, it is a sustained cooling of the body to lower-than-normal temperatures.

Hypothyroidism. A condition in which the thyroid gland produces an insufficient supply of hormone.

Hypoxia. A deficiency in the amount of oxygen reaching the body tissues.

Hysterectomy. The surgical removal of the uterus. In a total hysterectomy, the uterus, ovaries, and Fallopian tubes are removed.

Iatrogenic. Referring to a complication or negative reaction resulting from physician intervention or contracted as a result of actions taken in a clinical setting.

Idiopathic. Referring to a medical condition with no known cause.

IgE. *See* Immunoglobulin E (IgE).

Ileostomy. The surgical creation of a fistula through which the lower part of the small intestine (ileum) passes to create an artificial bowel.

Ileum. The lower third of the small intestine, which joins with the colon.

Illicit drugs. Drugs that are illegal to possess, have addiction potential, and lack approved medical uses.

Imaging. Any one of a wide variety of technologies for creating visual depictions of the internal structures of the body, including (among others) X radiation, MRI, CT scanning, PET scanning, ultrasonography, and radionuclide scanning.

Immune response. The reaction of an intricate system of cells, which identify, attack, immobilize, and remove foreign tissue from the body through chemical signals.

Immune system. A body system (including the thymus, bone marrow, and lymph tissues) and processes that protect the body from foreign substances by identifying and destroying them.

Immunity. Resistance to infection by a particular disease-causing microorganism, often acquired by vaccination.

Immunization. The process of creating an immunity to a disease through the introduction of vaccines or other agents designed to produce the immunity.

Immunoassay. The use of antibody-antigen recognition as the basis of a medically useful method of detecting and measuring a substance in body fluids.

Immunocompromised. Referring to a condition in which the immune system is impaired in some way, such as being not fully developed, deficient, or suppressed.

Immunodeficiency disorders. Genetic or acquired disorders in which the normal functioning of the immune system is disturbed.

Immunoglobulin. The globulin fraction of serum protein.

Immunoglobulin E (IgE). A type of antibody associated with the release of granules from basophils and mast cells; ordinarily, a relatively rare antibody, but in patients with atopic dermatitis, levels can be significantly higher than in the general population.

Immunology. The branch of medicine that studies the immune system. its function and processes and agents that affect its function either positively or negatively, including allergies.

Immunopathology. The study of conditions or diseases that impair the immune system.

Immunosuppression. A decrease in the effectiveness of the immune system; drugs are sometimes used to depress the immune system in order to lower the probability of rejection in organ transplantation.

Immunotherapy. Therapy using antibodies or other immune system components or using antigens designed to stimulate an immune response.

Implant. A section of endometrial tissue found outside the uterus; also, an artificial part or device inserted surgically in a part of the body (such as a breast).

Implantation. The process in which the embryo attaches to the uterine lining; also, the surgical process of adding an artificial body part, such as a pacemaker.

Impotence. The inability to achieve or maintain an erection.

In utero. A Latin term meaning "in the womb."

In vitro fertilization. Fertilization of an ovum outside the female body, in an artificial culture in a test tube or dish.

In vivo fertilization. Fertilization of an ovum naturally, within the female body.

Incidence. The number of new illnesses or events occurring over a specified period of time among a specific population.

Incision. A cut made with a scalpel.

Incisional biopsy. The biopsy of a selected sample of lesion.

Incisor. One of the front teeth, used primarily to cut or shear food with a scissoring motion.

Incontinence. The inability to control the expulsion of urine or feces.

Incubation period. The time between first exposure to an organism and onset of symptoms.

Incubator. In the nursery, a Plexiglas unit that encloses the premature or sick infant to allow strict temperature regulation.

Indigestion. A digestive disorder characterized by a burning sensation in the chest and throat, sometimes by abdominal pain, bloating, nausea, vomiting, and diarrhea; also called dyspepsia.

Infant. A young child from birth to twelve months of age.

Infarction. Damage resulting from insufficient blood supply to a tissue or organ.

Infection. The invasion of healthy tissue by a pathogenic microorganism, resulting in the production of toxins and subsequent injury of tissue.

Infectious disease. A disease that is capable of being transmitted; often caused by a microorganism.

Infectivity. The ability of an organism to enter and reproduce within a host.

Inferior. Situated below another part; for example, the ankle bones are inferior to the bones of the lower leg.

Infiltration. Movement of fluid into the tissue.

Inflammation. Irritation caused by such things as infection, injury, allergy, or toxins; symptoms include redness, swelling, warmth, pain, and drainage.

Influenza. Any one of a group of serious respiratory diseases caused by viruses; different strains of the "flu" have been responsible for worldwide epidemics.

Informed consent. The process of educating a patient fully about the purpose, benefits, and risks of a clinical trial or procedure and of obtaining authorization to perform it.

Inguinal hernia. The most common form of hernia, in which the hernial sac protrudes into the lower groin area.

Inhalant. Medication that is inhaled into the lungs.

Inheritance. The passage of traits from parents to offspring in discrete units called genes.

Injection. Administration into the skin, muscle, or blood vessels via needle.

Inner ear. An organ that includes the cochlea (for detection of sound) and the labyrinth (for detection of movement).

Inoculate. To introduce immunologically active material in order to treat or prevent a disease.

Inotropic agent. A drug that improves the ability of the heart muscle to contract.

Inpatient care. Evaluation and treatment services requiring an overnight stay in a medical facility.

Insane. In legal terms, a state wherein a person is said to be incapable of appreciating the wrongfulness of certain acts or of conforming to the requirements of the law.

Insemination. The placement of semen in the female reproductive tract, which may occur naturally as a result of sexual intercourse or artificially as a result of a medical procedure.

Insomnia. Disturbed sleep; insomnia can be caused by many factors, such as dysfunctional sleep cycle, breathing problems, leg jerking, underlying medical and psychiatric disorders, and the side effects of medication.

Inspiration. The act of breathing in, which expands the lungs.

Instinctual drives. Libido (the seeking of gratification of sexual impulses) and aggression (the seeking of gratification of destructive impulses).

Insulin. A hormone secreted by the pancreas that is essential in regulating blood glucose, as well as in assimilating carbohydrates for growth and energy.

Intensive care. Continuous medical treatment involving vigilant monitoring of the vital signs of patients with grave physical conditions.

Intermittent care. Services provided one or more times a week with each visit limited in time.

Internal medicine. The branch of medicine that focuses on the diagnosis and treatment of diseases, particularly of the internal organs, in adults; practitioners of internal medicine, called internists, often act as primary care physicians.

Internship. A synonym for the first year of residency training for a variety of master's- and doctoral-level practitioners in diverse fields.

Interstitial. Referring to the spaces within the tissues or other structures of the body, but not the large body cavities.

Interstitial pulmonary fibrosis (IPF). A disease characterized by scarring and thickening of lung tissue, which causes breathing difficulty.

Intervertebral disks. Flattened disks of fibrocartilage that separate the vertebrae and allow cushioned flexibility of the spinal column.

Intervertebral foramina. Openings between two adjacent vertebrae to permit the exit of nerve structures from the spinal cord.

Intestinal lumen. The inner cavity of the intestine, which represents the food (chyme) compartment.

Intestines. The section of the gut between the anus and the stomach, consisting of the rectum, colon, and small bowel (subdivided into the ileus, jejunum, and duodenum).

Intoxication. Poisoning of the body by toxins, such as drugs; also, alcohol intoxication (drunkenness).

Intracellular fluid. The fluid within cells.

Intraocular pressure. The degree of firmness of the eyeball, as controlled by the proper secretion and drainage of the aqueous humor.

Intravascular fluid. The fluid carried within the blood vessels; it is in a constant state of motion because of the pumping action of the heart.

Intravenous (IV) therapy. The introduction of medication into a vein with a special needle.

Intraventricular hemorrhage. Bleeding into or around the normal fluid spaces within the brain.

Intubation. The introduction of a tube into a body cavity, as into the larynx.

Invasive. Referring to any process (such as disease) that spreads throughout an area of the body or any procedure (such as diagnostic or therapeutic surgery) that requires entry into the body through the skin.

Involuntary muscle contractions. Muscle contractions that occur unconsciously, such as those of the intestines.

Ionization. A process in which a neutral atom loses one or more of its orbital electrons because of light, heat, or electrical collisions.

Ions. Small chemical substances that have a positive or negative charge; the most important ions with a positive charge are sodium, potassium, hydrogen, and calcium, while the most important negative ion is chloride.

IPF. *See* Interstitial pulmonary fibrosis (IPF).

Iris. The circular pigmented membrane behind the cornea, perforated by the pupil; the most anterior portion of the vascular tunic of the eye.

Iron-deficiency anemia. Anemia characterized by low serum iron concentration.

Ischemia. A local anemia or area of diminished or insufficient blood supply caused by mechanical obstruction of the blood supply (commonly, the narrowing of an artery).

Islets of Langerhans. Clusters of cells scattered throughout the pancreas; they produce three hormones involved in sugar metabolism. insulin, glucagon, and somatostatin.

Isokinetic. Referring to the resistance training that provides muscular overload at a constant preset speed.

Isotonic. A solution that causes no change in cell volume.

Isotypes. The different classes of antibodies.

Itching. An irritating skin sensation that provokes a desire to scratch the affected area; also called pruritus.

-itis. A suffix denoting inflammation; for example, laryngitis is an inflammation of the larynx.

IV therapy. *See* Intravenous (IV) therapy.

Jaundice. A yellowish coloration of the skin and mucous membranes caused by high levels of bilirubin in the blood; the result of liver malfunction.

Jejunum. A region of the small intestine located below the duodenum.

Jet lag. The malaise, headache, fatigue, gastrointestinal disorders, and other symptoms that may result from traveling across several time zones within a few hours.

Joint. The conjunction of two or more bones.

Joint replacement. *See* Arthroplasty.

Karyotype. An analysis of the chromosomes from the cells of an individual; it can be used to predict the chromosomal set of a fetus or the presence of a large chromosomal abnormality.

Keratin. An extremely tough protein that is the chief constituent of the epidermis, hair, nails, and tooth enamel.

Keratinocytes. Matrix basal epithelial cells that differentiate, fill with keratin, and form the dead horny substance making up the nail plate.

Keratitis. A state of inflammation of the cornea that may cause partial or total opacity, leading to loss of vision.

Keratoses. Wartlike growths caused by the excessive production of the skin protein keratin, usually occurring in elderly people.

Keratotomy. Surgical incision into the cornea of the eye to correct myopia (nearsightedness) or astigmatism.

Ketones. The by-products of fat metabolism; their presence may be indicative of diabetes mellitus.

Kidney transplantation. A surgical procedure that replaces the recipient's diseased, nonfunctioning kidney with a donated one.

Kidneys. The organs that control the amount and composition of body water by separating the blood into waste products (which leave the body as urine) and nutrients (which are returned to the blood).

Kilocalorie. The unit measurement of food energy, defined as the amount of heat needed to raise the temperature of 1 kilogram of water 1 degree Celsius; also known as a Calorie.

Kinase. An enzyme that catalyzes the transfer of phosphate from adenosine triphosphate (ATP) to another molecule.

Kinesiology. The study of the body's movement and the function of structures involved in that movement.

Knee. The joint between the thigh and the lower leg.

Knockout mouse. A mouse in which a specific gene has been inactivated or "knocked out."

Koch's postulates. Criteria for judging whether given bacteria cause a given disease, including that the bacteria must be present in every case, that they must be isolated from the host and grown in pure culture, that the disease must be reproduced when the culture is inoculated into a healthy susceptible host, and that the bacteria must be recoverable from the experimentally infected host.

Kupffer cells. Specialized cells in the liver that perform the function of removing bacterial debris from the blood that has circulated throughout the body.

Kwashiorkor. A protein-deficiency disease that may affect young children in developing countries.

Kyphoplasty. Considered a relatively minor invasive surgery for the relief of back pain, spinal fracture, or loss of vertebral height, it is performed usually in a hospital operating room under general anesthesia. A small incision is made in the back, a small tube is inserted, and a special balloon is inserted in the tube and slowly inflated. When the correct level is reached, a bone cement is infused to stabilize the new positioning of the vertebrae and surrounding area.

L-dopa (L-dihydroxyphenylalanine or levodopa). An amino acid that is the parent compound for dopamine; used to treat parkinsonism.

Labia. The folds of tissue along the external portion of a woman's vagina and urethra.

Labor. The physiological process by which the fetus and placenta are expelled from the uterus; labor involves strong uterine contractions.

Laboratory tests. The collection and analysis of body fluids such as blood and urine in order to establish a diagnosis or to monitor a treatment regimen.

Labyrinth. A structure consisting of three fluid-filled, semicircular canals at right angles to one another in the inner ear; they monitor the position and movement of the head.

Laceration. A torn, jagged wound, or an unintentional cut (as opposed to an incision).

Lacrimal. Pertaining to the secretion and conduction of tears.

Lacteals. Lymphatic capillaries in the villi of the small intestine that absorb fat, producing a milky substance called chyle.

Lactiferous duct. A single excretory duct from each lobe of mammary glandular tissue that converges yet opens separately at the tip of the nipple; the mammary gland has fifteen to twenty lactiferous ducts.

Lamellar keratoplasty. The partial removal or transplantation of a portion of the cornea; usually possible in younger patients or those with less advanced disorders.

Lamina (*pl.* laminae). An arch of the vertebral bones.

Laminaria. A type of seaweed that absorbs water and swells; it can be used to dilate the cervix.

Laminectomy. Surgical removal of part or all of a lamina to relieve pressure on the spinal cord; sometimes called fusion surgery.

Laparoscopy. A surgical procedure in which an instrument is inserted into the abdominal cavity through tiny incisions in the abdomen; usually performed without hospitalization.

Laparotomy. A surgical procedure, often exploratory in nature, carried out through the abdominal wall; it may be used to correct endometriosis.

Laryngectomy. Surgical removal of all or part of the larynx.

Laryngitis. Inflammation of the larynx, characterized by hoarseness in the voice and sometimes the inability to speak.

Larynx. The voice organ, lying between the pharynx and the trachea; commonly called the voice box.

Laser. An acronym for "light amplification by stimulated emission of radiation"; a laser produces a high-intensity light beam at a single wavelength.

Latent. Lying hidden or undeveloped within a person; unrevealed.

Lateral. On the outer side; for example, toward the little toe when in reference to the leg.

LDLs. *See* Low-density lipoproteins.

Lead poisoning. Poisoning as the result of ingestion or inhalation of abnormally high levels of lead, which disrupts kidney function and damages the nervous system.

Learning disabilities. A variety of disorders involving the failure to learn an academic skill despite normal levels of intelligence.

Leg. The lower extremity, excluding the foot; the upper leg runs from the hip to the knee, and the lower leg runs from the knee to the ankle.

Lens. A transparent, flexible structure, convex on both surfaces and lying directly behind the iris of the eye; it focuses light rays onto the retina.

Leprosy. A bacterial infection that affects the skin and nerves, causing symptoms ranging from numbness to disfigurement.

Lesion. A visible local tissue abnormality such as a wound, sore, rash, or boil, that can be benign, cancerous, gross, occult, or primary.

Leukemia. A condition characterized by the presence of an increased number of leukocytes in the blood, with the specific disorder classified according to the predominant proliferating cells, the clinical course, and the duration of the disease.

Leukocyte. A white or colorless blood corpuscle.

Leukodystrophy. A group of genetic disorders characterized by progressive deterioration of the white matter (myelin sheath) of the brain.

Leukopenia. An abnormal decrease in white blood cells.

Liability. Responsibility for wrongdoing.

Ligament. A tough, rubber band-like structure that connects one bone to another and prevents the abnormal motion of these bones in relationship to each other.

Light therapy. A nontraditional form of therapy that employs light to alleviate symptoms such as depression.

Lingual. Related to the tongue; in dentistry, the inner sides or faces of the teeth.

Lipases. Enzymes secreted by the pancreas into the small intestine that break down fatty materials (triglycerides) in the first intestinal stage of digestion.

Lipids. Any of a group of fatty substances including triglycerides, phospholipids, and sterols (such as cholesterol).

Lipopolysaccharide (LPS). A major component of the cell walls of gram-negative bacteria; the toxicity of LPS is associated with illnesses caused by gram-negative organisms.

Lipoproteins. Lipid aggregates that transport fat and cholesteryl esters in the circulation; associated apolipoproteins determine how rapidly they are taken up by the liver or other tissues.

Liposuction. A cosmetic method for removing body fat by a surgical vacuuming procedure.

Lithium. A drug used in the treatment of bipolar disorder.

Lithotripsy. Pulverization of stones (calculi) located in the kidneys, bladder, or urethra by means of high-frequency sound waves.

Liver. A vital organ that controls blood sugar levels; metabolizes carbohydrates, lipids, and proteins; stores blood, iron, and some vitamins; degrades steroid hormones; and inactivates and/or excretes certain drugs and toxins.

Liver transplantation. Surgery performed to replace a diseased, nonfunctional liver with one that is healthy and capable of carrying out normal liver functions.

Living will. A legally binding document instructing a physician whether or not to prolong life by externally administered life-support systems if the patient is unable to express his or her decision concerning physician-recommended forms of medical treatment.

Lobectomy. The removal of a lobe of the brain, or a major part of a lobe.

Lobotomy. The separation of either an entire lobe or a major part of a lobe from the rest of the brain.

Lobule. Small gland that, when sent appropriate hormonal cues, produces breast milk.

Local anesthesia. The injection of medication into the body that renders the immediate area free of pain, allowing surgery in that area to be performed.

Lockjaw. *See* Tetanus.

Long-term care. Health care or personal care performed for someone who is chronically unable to provide his or her own care; the cornerstone of assisted living.

Loss-of-control syndrome. A pattern of behavior characterized by violent and emotional outbursts, occasionally associated with temporal-lobe seizures.

Lou Gehrig's disease. *See* Amyotrophic lateral sclerosis (ALS).

Low-density lipoproteins (LDLs). A form of cholesterol in the blood that appears to be associated with a higher risk of arterial and heart disease.

Lower extremities. The legs (thighs, lower legs, and feet), which are attached to the pelvis at the hip joint and which consist of muscles, bones, blood vessels, lymph vessels, nerves, skin, and toenails.

LPS. *See* Lipopolysaccharide (LPS).

Lumbar puncture. A procedure to extract cerebrospinal fluid from the lumbar region of the spine (between the ribs and the pelvis), usually to diagnose disease (such as meningitis) or to administer therapeutic drugs (in leukemia treatment, for example).

Lumbar vertebrae. The five bones of the spinal column in the lower back, which experience the greatest stress in the spine.

Lumen. The space within an artery, vein, or other tube.

Lumpectomy. Surgical removal of a lump, often in the female breast.

Lungs. Vital organs that allow gas exchange between an organism and its environment.

Lupus. Systemic lupus erythematosus; a chronic inflammatory disease characterized by an arthritic condition and a rash.

Lyme disease. Lyme disease involves a mild-to-serious infection caused by the bacteria *Borrelia burgdorferi*, which is spread by the bite of infected ticks.

Lymph. The straw-colored fluid of the lymphatic system containing infection-fighting lymphocytes; as much as 1 to 2 liters is collected from tissue each day and returned to the bloodstream.

Lymph node. A small, oval structure that filters tissue fluids; lymph nodes are found in areas such as the armpits, groin, mouth, and neck, and serve as sites of immune response.

Lymphadenectomy. The removal of lymph nodes, one or more in a group.

Lymphadenopathy. Enlarged lymph nodes, which may be caused by any disorder related to the lymphatic vessels or lymph nodes.

Lymphatic system. A major part of the body's immune system, consisting of lymphatic vessels and lymph nodes, that transports lymph through tissues and organs and drains it back into the bloodstream.

Lymphocyte. A small white blood cell constituting about 25 percent of all blood cells; two basic types are B cells (antibody production) and T cells (cellular immunity).

Lymphoma. A group of cancers that affect lymphatic tissue.

Lysosome. An organelle inside cells that contains a variety of enzymes for breaking down cellular constituents.

Lysosyme. An enzyme found in body secretions that destroys bacteria by breaking down their walls.

Macrophage. A white blood cell that engulfs foreign substances and stimulates other immune cells.

Macular degeneration. The progressive breakdown of the macula, the part of the eye that allows for detailed sight in the center of the field of vision, with a dense concentration of rods and cones.

Magnetic field therapy. A practical and inexpensive modality that uses magnets to relieve chronic and acute pain incurred through overuse or trauma.

Magnetic resonance imaging (MRI). A type of scan that uses radio waves and a powerful magnet to produce detailed computer images.

Malabsorption. The abnormal utilization of nutrients from food.

Malaise. A feeling of lack of health or debility, often indicating or accompanying the onset of illness.

Malaria. A serious parasitic infection spread by mosquitoes and characterized by fever, chills, sweating, vomiting, and damage to the kidneys, brain, and liver.

Malignancy. Any condition that becomes progressively worse, especially the growth of a cancerous tumor.

Malignant melanoma. A fast-growing, highly dangerous form of skin cancer.

Malnutrition. A physical state characterized by an imbalance of dietary proteins, carbohydrates, fats, vitamins, and minerals, given an individual's physical activity and health needs.

Malocclusion. A condition in which the teeth of the upper and lower jaws do not fit together properly.

Malpractice. The failure to care for patients in accordance with professional standards, for which injured patients are allowed to sue for compensation.

Malpractice insurance. Insurance policies held by physicians in order to protect them financially in the event of a patient-initiated lawsuit alleging incidents of improper medical decisions or incompetence.

Mammary gland. Group of milk-producing cells consisting of lobules and ducts.

Mammography. The use of X rays to image the female breast, primarily in the detection and diagnosis of malignant breast tumors before they can be felt.

Mandible. The lower jaw, which is hinged to the skull.

Manic-depressive disorder. *See* Bipolar disorder.

MAOIs. *See* Monoamine oxidase inhibitors (MAOIs).

Marasmus. The condition that results from consuming a diet that is deficient in both energy and protein.

Marijuana. A plant containing a psychoactive substance with the potential for both recreational abuse and medical use.

Mass spectrometry. A very sensitive technique that accurately measures protein or peptide mass.

Mast cells. Cells in connective tissue capable of releasing chemicals that cause allergic reactions.

Mastectomy. Surgical removal of the female breast.

Mastication. The act of chewing food.

Mastitis. Infection of the breast, which results in inflammation, tenderness, swelling, and pain.

Mastoidectomy. The surgical removal of the temporal or mastoid bone, which is located behind the ear.

Materia Medica. The homeopathic pharmacopoeia, a list of remedies with their associated symptoms and uses.

Matrix. Organic or inorganic material occurring in connective tissues but located outside the cells.

Maxilla. The upper jaw, which is fixed to the skull.

Maxillofacial surgery. Surgery of the face and neck, a form of cosmetic and reconstructive surgery.

Maximal oxygen uptake. The maximum rate of oxygen consumption during exercise.

MCAT. *See* Medical College Admission Test (MCAT).

Measles. A childhood infectious disease, also known as rubeola, characterized by a rash and fever; it can be controlled through immunization.

Mechanoreceptors. Sensory receptors that, when mechanically deformed (such as being pressed on), send nerve impulses causing sensations of pressure and touch.

Medial. Closer to an imaginary midline dividing the body into equal right and left halves than another part.

Medicaid. A health care program in the United States made available to those with low-level income or who are disabled and unable to pay health insurance premiums.

Medical College Admission Test (MCAT). A test of problem-solving skills taken by all candidates to medical school in the United States; used to predict which students will be successful.

Medicare. A U.S. federal program that covers many of the hospital costs and doctor bills for elderly and disabled persons and those with end-stage renal (kidney) disease.

Medicine. The science and art of diagnosing, treating, curing, and preventing disease; relieving pain; and improving and preserving health. Also, any drug or other substance used in treating disease, healing, or relieving pain.

Meditation. A mental exercise to enhance personal understanding of the self and the universe.

Medulla. The central portion of the adrenal gland, the area that produces epinephrine (adrenaline).

Megadose. Ten or more times the recommended daily allowance of a nutrient, such as a vitamin.

Megaloblastic anemia. Anemia caused by the failure of red blood cells to mature; also known as pernicious anemia, Addisonian anemia, or maturation failure.

Meiosis. A special kind of cell division whereby four cells are produced; each cell has only half of the original number of chromosomes; meiosis produces the sex cells (eggs and sperm).

Meissner's corpuscles. Receptors at which the sense of a light touch or low-frequency vibrations are detected; also called corpuscles of touch.

Melanin. A polymer made up of several compounds (including the amino acid tyrosine) that causes pigmentation in the skin, hair, and eyes.

Melanoma. Cancer of the melanocytes, the cells that produce melanin.

Melatonin. A hormone produced by the pineal gland within the epithalamus of the forebrain; it is usually released into the blood during the night phase of the light-dark cycle.

Membrane. A thin layer of lipid and protein molecules that controls transport of molecules and ions between the cell and its exterior and between membrane-bound compartments within the cell.

Menarche. The first menstrual cycle.

Meningitis. The inflammation of the protective tissues surrounding the brain and the spinal cord.

Menopause. The permanent cessation of the menstrual cycle, signifying the conclusion of a woman's reproductive life.

Menorrhagia. Excessive or prolonged bleeding during menstruation.

Menstruation. The cyclic bleeding that normally occurs, usually in the absence of pregnancy, during the reproductive period of the human female; typically occurs at twenty-eight day intervals.

Mental retardation. A condition characterized by a below-average intelligence quotient (IQ) and deficits in adaptive functioning before the age of eighteen years; the degree of retardation ranges from mild to severe.

Meridians. Designated channels in the body that react to acupuncture or acupressure stimulation.

Merkel's disks. Sensory receptors in the skin located in deeper layers of the epidermis; also called tactile disks.

Mesothelioma. A malignancy originating from the mesothelial surfaces (the lining cells) of the pleural and peritoneal cavities, the pericardium, or the tunica vaginalis.

Messenger ribonucleic acid (mRNA). A single-stranded RNA that arises from and is complementary to double-stranded deoxyribonucleic acid (DNA); it passes from the nucleus to the cytoplasm, where its information is translated into proteins.

Metabolic equivalent (MET). A unit used to estimate the metabolic cost of physical activity; 1 MET is equal to 3.5 milliliters of oxygen consumed per kilogram of body weight per minute.

Metabolic rate. A measurement of the Calories (kilocalories) that are converted into heat energy in order to maintain body temperature and/or for physical exertion.

Metabolic syndrome. A constellation of metabolic changes that affect most major organ systems and may impinge on practically all systems of the body, beginning with excess weight or obesity.

Metabolism. The chemical and physical processes involved in the interconversion of foods and the maintenance of life.

Metabolites. The molecular breakdown products of a substance.

Metastasis. The transfer of disease-producing cells to other parts of the body.

Metastasize. To spread by means of the bloodstream to other parts of the body.

Methicillin-resistant *Staphylococcus aureus* (MRSA) infection. An infection caused by virulent and destructive bacteria that is resistant to common antibiotics and difficult to treat.

Methotrexate. A powerful drug, originally developed to treat cancer, that is used to treat patients with severe cases of psoriasis.

Microarrays. Miniature plastic or glass chips upon which tiny amounts of biological material are permanently spotted in a grid-like array.

Microbiology. The study of organisms too small to be seen by the unaided human eye, especially the identification, transmission, and control of microorganisms that cause disease.

Microcephaly. Abnormal smallness of the head.

Microorganism. An organism that is too small to be seen without a magnifying lens; also known as a microbe.

Microscopy. The use of a microscope to make extremely small objects appear larger.

Microsurgery. Surgery done with the aid of a microscope.

Micturition. The act of urinating.

Middle ear. The air-filled cavity in which vibrations are transmitted from the eardrum to the inner ear via the ossicles.

Migraine headaches. Severe, incapacitating headaches that may be preceded by nausea and vomiting or by visual, sensory, and motor disturbances.

Milk duct. Tubular canal that transports breast milk from the lobule to the collecting duct.

Milk line. A line that originates as a primitive milk streak on each front side of the fetus; it extends from axilla to vulva, where rudimentary breast tissues or nipples could be located.

Mineralocorticoids. Steroid hormones that regulate the body levels of sodium and potassium.

Minerals. Inorganic compounds that are essential for human life; seventeen are required in the diet.

Miscarriage. The expulsion of the embryo or fetus before it is viable outside the uterus; also called spontaneous abortion.

Mitochondrion. A membrane-bound cytoplasmic organelle that constitutes the primary location of oxidative reactions providing energy for cellular activities.

Mitosis. The type of cell division that occurs in nonsex cells, which conserves chromosome number by equal allocation to each of the newly formed cells.

Mitral valve. The valve between the heart's left auricle and ventricle.

Mitral valve prolapse. The inability of the mitral valve in the heart to close properly; also called mitral insufficiency.

Modality. The ability to distinguish one sensation from another; the ability to discriminate light or heavy touch, pain, pressure, vibratory, or hot and cold sensations from one another.

Molars. The back teeth, which are used to grind food into smaller portions prior to swallowing.

Molecular biology. The study of the interactions that occur among the molecules making up living organisms.

Molecule. A collection of atoms bonded together; normally neutral because it has an equal number of protons and electrons.

Momentum. The product of mass and velocity for a particle; inverse with wavelength (the distance between peaks of a wave).

Monkeypox. A rare disease, originating in the rain forests of Central and West Africa, that affects animals and humans and is caused by a virus.

Monoamine oxidase inhibitors (MAOIs). A class of drugs that relieve the symptoms of depression by inhibiting the enzyme that deactivates the brain chemical monoamine oxidase.

Monoclonal antibodies. Antibodies (proteins that protect the body against disease-causing foreign bodies such as bacteria and viruses) produced in large quantities from cloned cells.

Mononucleosis. An infectious respiratory illness caused by the Epstein-Barr virus.

Monozygotes. Identical twins; born of a single ovum that divides after a single sperm fertilizes it.

Morbid obesity. Excessive accumulation of fat (more than 100 pounds overweight or 100 percent overweight).

Morbidity. In medical statistics, the occurrence of clinical disease, in contrast to mortality (death) and occurrence (which includes subclinical infections).

Mordant. A chemical that acts to fix a stain within a physical structure; the role played by iodine in Gram staining.

Morgue. A place, usually cooled, where dead bodies are temporarily kept, pending proper identification, autopsy, or burial.

Mortality. Relating to death.

Motility. Spontaneous motion, such as of the gastrointestinal tract or of sperm.

Motion sickness. A feeling of nausea brought on by motion.

Motor. Referring to parts of the nervous system having to do with movement production.

Motor neuron. A nerve cell that functions either directly or indirectly to control movement in a target organ or body part.

Motor neuron diseases. Progressive, debilitating, and eventually fatal diseases affecting nerve cells in muscles.

Motor weakness. Muscle weakness resulting from the failure of motor nerves.

MRI. *See* Magnetic resonance imaging (MRI).

mRNA. *See* Messenger ribonucleic acid (mRNA).

MRSA infection. *See* Methicillin-resistant *Staphylococcus aureus* (MRSA) infection.

MSUD. *See* Maple syrup urine disease (MSUD).

Mucopolysaccharidosis (MPS). A genetic disorder characterized by accumulations of mucopolysaccharides in tissues.

Mucosa. The tissue lining the interior of the gastrointestinal tract, through which nutrients pass into the bloodstream.

Mucous membrane. The soft, pink layer of cells that produce mucus to keep body structures lubricated; found in the eyelids and in the respiratory and urinary tracts.

Mucus. A fluid excreted by many body membranes as a lubricant.

Müllerian ducts. The pair of tubes in the early embryo that will develop into the internal female organs (uterus, oviducts, and upper vagina).

Multiple sclerosis (MS). An incurable, debilitating disease of the nervous system.

Multipotent. Referring to stem cells derived from adults that may develop into one of several types of tissue.

Mumps. An infectious, viral childhood disease characterized by swelling of the salivary glands in front of and below the ears.

Murmur. The sound made by blood flowing backward through a heart valve.

Muscle. A bundle of contractile cells that is responsible for the movement of organs and body parts.

Muscle contraction. The shortening of a muscle that results in movement of a particular body part.

Muscle fibers. Elongated muscle cells that make up skeletal, cardiac, and smooth muscles.

Muscle relaxant. Any of a number of medications that can be used either to paralyze the muscles of the patient temporarily before a medical procedure or to alleviate neuromuscular pain and spasms.

Muscular dystrophy. A group of progressive genetic diseases that attack the muscles.

Musculature. The arrangement of skeletal muscles in the body.

Musculoskeletal. Pertaining to or comprising the skeleton and the muscles.

Mutagen. A chemical or an ionizing radiation that causes a change in the nucleotide sequence of the DNA of a gene, possibly affecting the gene's normal expression.

Mutation. Damage to a gene that changes how it works.

Myasthenia gravis. A disorder in which the nicotinic acetylcholine receptors located in junctions between nerve cells and muscles are attacked by the immune system, causing exhaustion of the muscles.

Mycetoma. A progressive and chronic fungal or bacterial infection that causes overgrowth of the infected tissue and the formation of sinuses filled with the infecting organism.

Myco-. A prefix denoting fungus.

Mycobacterium. Any of a genus of nonmotile aerobic bacteria that are difficult to stain and include numerous saprophytes and the organisms causing tuberculosis and leprosy.

Mycosis. Any disease of humans, plants, or animals caused by a fungus.

Myocardial infarction. *See* Heart attack.

Myocardium. The muscle tissue that forms the walls of the heart, varying in thickness in the upper and lower regions.

Myoclonus. Involuntary twitching or spasm of muscle.

Myomectomy. Surgical removal of a noncancerous muscle tumor (myoma).

Myopia. The inability of the eye to focus on distant objects; also called nearsightedness.

NAD. *See* Nicotinamide adenine dinucleotide (NAD).

Narcolepsy. A brain disorder characterized by brief, numerous, and overwhelming attacks of sleepiness throughout the day.

Narcotics. A group of potent painkilling drugs characterized by their ability to cause the user to develop tolerance and therefore dependency (physical addiction); such drugs include morphine, codeine, heroin, and other opium-like compounds.

Nasogastric tube. A tube fed through the nose to the stomach.

Nasopharyngeal. Referring to the nose and pharynx (the upper part of the throat that leads from the mouth to the esophagus).

Nausea. An unpleasant sensation followed by stomach and intestinal discomfort, which may lead to vomiting.

Nearsightedness. The inability of the eye to focus on distant objects; also called myopia.

Necropsy. A postmortem (after-death) examination of an animal's body, similar to an autopsy performed on a human corpse.

Necrosis. Tissue damage occurring as a result of cell death.

Needle biopsy. The obtaining of tissue fragments by the puncture of a tumor, through a large-caliber needle, syringe, and plunger; the tissue within the lumen of the needle is obtained through the rotation and withdrawal of the needle.

Negative feedback. A homeostatic control system designed to respond to a stress by returning body conditions to normal physiologic levels.

Negligence. Failure to perform an important or necessary medical technique, or the performance of such a technique in a careless or unskilled manner so as to cause further injury.

Neonatal intensive care unit. A hospital nursery with advanced equipment and specially trained staff to maintain the vital functions of sick newborns and to monitor their progress closely.

Neonatal period. The first month of life; derived from the Greek *neo* (meaning "new") and the Latin *natum* (meaning "birth").

Neonate. A newborn infant.

Neonatology. The study of diseases, conditions, and treatments of newborns (infants between the time of birth and approximately one month of age).

Neoplasm. An uncontrolled growth of cells, which can develop into a tumor; may be malignant (cancerous) or benign.

Nephrectomy. Kidney removal.

Nephritis. Any disease or pathology of the kidney that results in inflammation.

Nephrology. The study of kidney diseases.

Nephron. A tiny blood-processing unit located in the kidneys (composed of the renal corpuscle, the loop of Henle, and renal tubules) that carries out the processes that form urine; each kidney contains approximately one million nephrons.

Nephrotic syndrome. An abnormal condition of the kidneys characterized by a variety of conditions, including edema and proteinuria; often accompanies glomerular dysfunction and diabetes.

Nephroureterectomy. A procedure similar to a radical nephrectomy, with the additional removal of the ureter and a cuff of the bladder; performed to treat transitional cell carcinomas of the ureters and the pelvis of the kidneys.

Nerve. A bundle of sensory and motor neurons held together by layers of connective tissue.

Nerve compression. Excessive pressure causing a nerve to be pinched.

Nervous system. Comprising both the central and peripheral bodily systems that receive interpret, and regulate information from the brain and other organs.

Neural tube. The embryonic structure that gives rise to the central nervous system.

Neuralgia. Pain associated with a nerve, often caused by inflammation or injury.

Neuritis. An inflammatory or degenerative lesion of a nerve, marked by pain and the loss of normal reflexes.

Neurofibrillary tangles. A hallmark lesion of Alzheimer's disease and several other disorders consisting of intracellular aggregates of the structural protein tau.

Neuroglial cell. A supportive cell for neurons within the central nervous system of animals.

Neuroleptic. A pharmacological agent such as chlorpromazine that is used to treat psychotic symptomology.

Neurologic. Dealing with the nervous system and its disorders.

Neurology. The study of the central nervous system, which is composed of the brain and spinal cord.

Neuromuscular electrical stimulation (NMES). The application of electrical and current to elicit a muscle contraction.

Neuromusculoskeletal. Pertaining to the interrelationship between the body's nerves, muscles, and skeleton.

Neuron. The principal nervous system cell that conducts electrical information from its dendritic extensions, through its cell body, to its axonal extensions, and on to other cells and is capable of releasing neurotransmitters.

Neuropathy. Any disorder of the nerves.

Neuroscience. The scientific specialization that seeks to understand mental processes, occurrences, and disturbances in terms of underlying mechanisms in the brain and the nervous system.

Neurosis. A psychic disturbance and defect from childhood that develops into a particular pattern of emotional illness and dysfunctional behavior.

Neurosurgery. Surgery to correct disorders of the nervous system, including the brain.

Neurotoxicity. An excessive or unwanted effect of too much anesthetic drug on the nerves.

Neurotransmitter. A chemical substance released by one nerve cell to stimulate or inhibit the function of an adjacent nerve cell; a chemical message released by a neuron.

Neutrophil. A circulating white blood cell that serves as one of the principal phagocytes for the immune system.

Nicotinamide adenine dinucleotide (NAD). A molecule used to hold pairs of electrons when they have been removed from a molecule by some biological process; the empty molecule is denoted by NAD+, while it is denoted as NADH when it is carrying electrons.

Nicotine. A colorless, poisonous alkaloid derived from tobacco plants.

Night sweats. Hot flashes that occur at night, typically during sleep.

Nitrous oxide. A chemical compound that at room temperature forms a colorless gas (also known as laughing gas) used to produce anesthesia and analgesia during surgery.

NMES. *See* Neuromuscular electrical stimulation (NMES).

Nocturia. Involuntary nighttime urination.

Nondisjunction. A malfunction of mitosis, resulting in cells with an abnormal chromosome number.

Noninvasive. Referring to a procedure that does not require entering the body.

Nonmaleficence. A principle of medical ethics which requires that the actions taken not harm the patient.

Nonsteroidal anti-inflammatory drugs (NSAIDs). Drugs such as ibuprofen that are used to reduce swelling and pain.

Normal. A term of reference that can mean average (as in statistically normal), functional (as in adaptive), or socially appropriate (as in within cultural bounds of acceptability).

NSAIDs. *See* Nonsteroidal anti-inflammatory drugs (NSAIDs).

Nuclear medicine. The branch of medicine that employs radioactive substances to diagnose or treat disease.

Nucleic acids. Very large molecules, located on DNA molecules, that control the synthesis of proteins and carry basic information determining heredity.

Nucleolus. A nuclear structure formed through the activity of chromosome segments in the production of ribosomal RNA and the assembly of ribosomal subunits.

Nucleoprotein. A virally encoded protein that is directly associated with the viral nucleic acid.

Nucleotide. A chemical subunit of DNA; different sequences of linked nucleotides spell out instructions for the assembly of proteins.

Nucleus. A large spherical mass occupying up to one-third of the volume of a typical plant or animal cell; also, the dense, positively charged, central core of an atom, containing its massive protons and neutrons.

Null hypothesis. A statement about populations that can be tested statistically which presupposes that there are no differences in the terms of some numerical measure.

Nulliparity. Having never given birth to a viable infant.

Numbness. A reduction or loss of feeling in an area of skin.

Nursing. The profession of providing health care that assists a patient to recover from an illness, injury, or surgical or other procedure, performed in a variety of settings. Also, the act of breast-feeding.

Nursing home. A type of extended care facility that can be classified as either skilled or intermediate, depending on the type of care; physicians oversee medical care that is rendered around the clock by a nursing staff.

Nutrients. Substances needed by the body for maintenance, growth, and repair; the six classes of nutrients are carbohydrates, fats, proteins, vitamins, minerals, and water.

Nutrition. The study of those substances found in foods that are needed by the body for maintenance, growth, and repair, as well as those substances that increase the risk of disease.

Nystagmus. Rhythmic involuntary movements of the eyes.

Obesity. A medical condition defined as being in excess of 20 percent above ideal weight.

Obsession. A recurrent and persistent thought or impulse associated with continuous and involuntary preoccupation that cannot be expunged by logic or reasoning.

Obsessive-compulsive disorder. An anxiety disorder characterized by intrusive and unwanted thoughts and/or the need to perform ritualized behaviors.

Obstetrics. The branch of medicine specializing in the problems and needs of pregnant women and their fetuses from conception through delivery and postnatal care.

Obstruction. Partial or complete blockage of the gastrointestinal tract.

Obstructive sleep apnea. Periods of interrupted breathing during sleep due to airway obstruction in the nose or throat.

Occlusion. The fit of the upper and lower teeth when they are brought together; also, the blockage of any vessel in the body, which may be caused by a thrombus or other embolus.

Occult blood. Fecal blood, as detected by microscopic or chemical testing.

Occupational health. Those health disciplines collectively concerned with the conditions, diseases, and injuries that occur within or as a result of the work setting.

Occupational medicine. A medical specialty focused on providing all levels of preventive medical services to working men and women in order to preserve, maintain, or restore health and well-being.

Occupational toxicology. A subspecialty of environmental toxicology that focuses on the effects of chemicals on the health of a workplace population.

Odontology. The study of teeth.

Oedipus complex. The experience of having sexual feelings toward the parent of the opposite sex that can occur in young children.

Olfactory knobs. Unmyelinated, tiny, rounded nerve endings of the sensory cells found at the mucus-coated olfactory membrane; each knob has five to eight extensions, called olfactory hairs, that branch out into the nasal cavity and monitor the environment.

Oncogene. A gene or DNA segment that can cause cancer.

Oncology. The branch of medicine specializing in the study of tumors, especially malignant tumors, and their treatment.

Onychomycosis. Common nail disorder in which fungal organisms invade the nail bed, causing progressive changes in the color, texture, and structure of the nail.

Oocyte. A female germ cell that differentiates to become a mature ova.

Oophorectomy. Removal of the ovaries, which is often necessary in cases of severe endometriosis.

Oophoritis. Inflammation of the ovary.

Operating room. A room in which surgical procedures are performed.

Operator. A person who induces a hypnotic state; synonymous with "hypnotist" and "suggestor."

Ophthalmology. The branch of medicine concerned with the study of the eye and its structures, disorders, conditions, and treatments.

Opioids. Pain medications derived from opiates, such as morphine, oxycodone, codeine, and fentanyl, intended to control severe pain.

Opportunistic infections. Potentially life-threatening diseases occurring in persons with a weakened immune system, caused by microorganisms that typically do not cause severe illnesses in an otherwise healthy person.

Optic disc. The portion of the optic nerve at its point of entrance into the rear of the eye.

Optic nerve. The nerve that takes information from retina to brain; largest nerve in the body.

Optical fiber. A very thin thread made of high-purity glass, plastic, or quartz; used to transmit light from a laser into the body.

Optometry. The practice of diagnosing visual problems and diagnosing correctional devices such as eyeglasses and contact lenses.

Oral hygiene. Care of the teeth and mouth.

Oral surgery. The dental specialty that surgically removes diseased teeth and oral tissues and treats bone fractures of the jaws.

Organelles. Specialized parts of cells.

Organic. Pertaining to, arising from, or affecting a body organ.

Organic brain syndromes. Clusters of behavioral and psychological symptoms involving impaired brain function, where etiology is unknown; includes delirium, delusions, amnesia, intoxication, and dementias.

Organic disease. A disease caused or accompanied by an alteration in the structure of the tissues or organs.

Organic mental disorders. Mental and emotional disturbances from transient or permanent brain dysfunction, with known organic etiology; includes drug or alcohol ingestion, infection, trauma, and cardiovascular disease.

Organism. A complex structure of interdependent and subordinate elements whose relations and properties are largely determined by their function as a whole.

Organs. *See* Systems and organs.

Oroprioception. Ability to locate the body in space.

Orthodontics. The branch of dentistry that diagnoses and treats malformed teeth.

Orthognathic surgery. Jaw reconstruction.

Orthopedics. The branch of medicine that specializes in the surgical repair or correction of injured or malformed bones and joints and the structures (such as muscles) associated with them.

Orthotic device. A podiatric appliance or prosthesis that is used to correct a foot deformity.

Orthotopic. Referring to the placement of a transplanted organ in the position occupied by the original organ.

Oscillopsia. Sensation of bouncing vision.

Oscilloscope. An instrument that displays a visual representation of electrical variations on the fluorescent screen of a cathode-ray tube.

Osmosis. The diffusion of molecules through a semipermeable membrane until there is an equal concentration on either side of the membrane.

Ossification. The formation of bone tissue.

Osteoarthritis. A degenerative process in which components of the joints undergo thinning, resulting in loss of motion, pain, and often inflammation in the later stages.

Osteoblast. A bone cell that can produce and form bone matrix; osteoblasts are responsible for new bone formation.

Osteoclast. A large bone cell that can destroy bone matrix by dissolving the mineral crystals.

Osteocyte. The primary living cell of mature bone tissue.

Osteomyelitis. Infection of bone.

Osteopathic medicine. A form of medicine, founded by Andrew Taylor Still in 1874, that emphasizes the health of the musculoskeletal system as well as a holistic approach to the functioning of the body.

Osteoporosis. A loss of bone mass accompanied by increasing fragility and brittleness.

Ostomy. A popular term for any operation that results in a stoma.

Otitis. Any inflammation of the outer or middle ear.

Oto-. A combining form indicating "ear."

Otoliths. Granular bones of the inner ear.

Otologist. A medical doctor who specializes in diseases and disorders of the ear.

-otomy. A suffix meaning an opening or incision in an organ or structure; for example, a ureterotomy is an opening in the ureter.

Otorhinolaryngology. The branch of medicine concerned with the diseases, conditions, and treatment of the ear, nose, and throat.

Otosclerosis. A condition in which the stapes becomes progressively more rigid and hearing loss results.

Otoscope. An instrument for viewing the ear canal and the eardrum.

Outer ear. The visible, fleshy part of the ear and the ear canal; it transmits sound waves to the eardrum.

Outpatient care. Evaluation and treatment services not re-quiring an overnight stay in a medical facility.

Ovarian cysts. Benign growths in the ovaries, which may cause pain.

Ovariectomy. The removal of the ovaries.

Ovaries. The pair of structures in the female that produce ova (eggs) and hormones.

Over-the-counter drugs. Pharmaceutical products, vitamins, herbal remedies, and other medicines that can be purchased without a doctor's prescription.

Oviducts. The pair of tubes leading from the top of the uterus upward toward the ovaries; also called the Fallopian tubes.

Ovulation. The release of an ovum from its follicle in the ovary.

Ovum (*pl.* ova). The female gamete; a large round cell that carries the female's chromosomes and is released from the ovaries during ovulation.

Oxidation-reduction. The transfer of electron(s) from one now-positive substance (oxidation) to one now-negative (reduction).

Oxygen therapy. Application of pure or high-oxygen gas to assist in recovery from oxygen deprivation (as in respiratory diseases).

Oxygenation. The process of getting oxygen into the bloodstream.

Oxytocin. The maternal pituitary hormone that regulates milk production and uterine contraction.

Pacemaker. A device surgically implanted in a patient suffering from heart disease in order to maintain a healthy heartbeat; also, a region of the heart called the sinoatrial (S-A) node, which maintains the regular heartbeat.

Pacinian corpuscles. Receptors at which the sensations of heavy touch or deep pressure originate; also called lamellated corpuscles.

Pain. Physical distress that is often associated with disorder and injury.

Pain management. The alleviation of pain, either completely or to a point of tolerance, by means of a variety of therapies, both chemical (as with drugs) and physical (as with exercise therapy).

Palliative treatments. Therapies that reduce symptoms without completely eradicating a disorder.

Palpation. Application of the hands, or touching, to determine the size, texture, consistency, and location of body structures.

Palpitation. The sensation of being aware of one's own heartbeat, usually because the heart is beating rapidly or more forcefully than normal.

Palsy. Partial or complete paralysis of a nerve followed by muscle weakness and wasting.

Pancreas. A secretory organ, located behind the stomach and connected to the duodenum, that produces enzymes to digest food and insulin to metabolize sugar.

Pancreatitis. Inflammation of the pancreas.

Pandemic. An epidemic prevalent throughout a country, a continent, or the world.

Panic attack. A sudden feeling of intense apprehension, fear, doom, and/or terror that can cause shortness of breath, palpitations, chest pain, chills, nausea, and light-headedness.

Pap smear. A simple diagnostic test for the presence of cervical cancer involving the removal of cervical tissue cells and the subsequent biopsy of these cells.

Paralysis. The loss of muscle function or sensation as a result of trauma or disease.

Paramedic. A person who is not generally a physician but is trained to provide emergency treatment in critical situations, such as resuscitation after a heart attack or seizure, arrest of bleeding, dressing wounds, and setting broken bones.

Paramedical. Related to the science or practice of medicine.

Paranoia. Pervasive distrust and suspiciousness of others and a tendency to interpret others' motives as malevolent.

Paraplegia. Partial or complete paralysis of both legs caused by damage to the spinal cord.

Parasite. An organism whose principal food source is another living organism; in medicine, the term refers to both unicellular and multicellular animals.

Parasympathetic nervous system. The part of the autonomic nervous system that stimulates digestion, slows the heart, and dilates blood vessels, acting in opposition to sympathetic nerves.

Parathyroid gland. One of four small endocrine glands, situated underneath the thyroid gland, whose main product is parathyroid hormone; this hormone is responsible for the regulation of serum calcium levels.

Parathyroidectomy. Removal of part or all of one or both of the parathyroid glands.

Parenteral. Administered by injection or infusion.

Paroxysm. An uncontrolled spasm or convulsion that may be violent.

Parturition. The process or action of giving birth.

Passive euthanasia. Ending life by refusing or withdrawing life-sustaining medical treatment.

Passive immunity. Immunity resulting from the introduction of preformed antibodies.

Pathogen. An agent that is capable of causing a disease, including viruses, bacteria, protozoa, rickettsia, or parasitic worms.

Pathogenicity. The ability of an organism to cause disease.

Pathologic. Pertaining to the study of disease and the development of abnormal conditions.

Pathology. The study of the nature and consequences of disease.

Pathophysiology. An alteration in function as seen in disease.

Patient advocacy. The representation of the patient's interest in medical diagnosis and treatment decisions, in which the health care provider acts as an information source and counselor for the patient.

Patient assessment. The systematic gathering of information in order to determine the nature of a patient's illness.

Pediatric. Pertaining to neonates, infants, and children up to the age of twelve.

Pediatrics. The branch of medicine specializing in the conditions, diseases, and development of infants and children.

Pedodontics. The dental specialty that treats children.

Pelvic inflammatory disease (PID). An infection of the female reproductive organs that may be caused by a sexually transmitted disease.

Penis. The male genital organ containing the urethra, through which both urine and semen pass; sufficient erection of the penis is required for intercourse.

Pepsin. A substance in the stomach that breaks down most proteins.

Peptic ulcer. Open sores that develop in the lining of the stomach as a result of excessive secretion of gastric juices.

Peptidoglycans. Repeating units of sugar derivatives that make up a rigid layer of bacterial cell walls; found in both gram-positive and gram-negative cells.

Percussion. Gentle tapping by the medical examiner's finger, which has been positioned on the patient; a hollow sound is heard over air-filled structures, while a dull thud is heard over solid areas or liquid-filled structures.

Percutaneous transluminal coronary angioplasty (PTCA). A procedure undertaken to increase the internal diameter of a coronary artery by inflating a small balloonlike device at the site or sites where the artery has narrowed because of plaque buildup.

Perforation. An abnormal opening, such as a hole in the wall of the colon.

Perfusion. The flow of blood through the lungs or other vessels in the body.

Perfusionist. A health care specialist who operates extracorporeal circulation equipment when it is necessary to support or replace a patient's circulatory or respiratory function.

Peri-. A prefix denoting "around," either in a literal sense (as in "pericarditis") or in a figurative sense (as in "perinatal").

Pericarditis. A disease of the membrane that surrounds the heart, caused by an inflammation that can lead to constriction of the heart muscle.

Pericardium. A fluid-filled conical sac of fibrous tissue that surrounds the heart and the roots of the great blood vessels.

Perinatology. The branch of medicine that treats the mother and child during the late stages of pregnancy and the first month or so following birth.

Perineum. The short bridge of flesh between the anus and vagina in women and the anus and base of the penis in men.

Period. The length of one complete cycle of a rhythm; ultradian rhythms are about twenty-four hours (twenty to twenty-eight hours), and infradian rhythms are longer than twenty-eight hours.

Periodontics. The dental specialty that treats the diseases of the supporting tissues of the teeth.

Periodontitis. The inflammation and infection of the gums, which may cause loss of the supporting bone and eventually tooth loss.

Periodontium. Those tissues supporting the tooth in the jaws, including the gingiva, the jawbone, and the periodontal ligament that attaches the root of the tooth into the jaw.

Periosteum. The thick, fibrous membrane that covers the entire surface of a bone except for the cartilage within joints.

Peripheral. Referring to a part of the body away from the center.

Peripheral nervous system. A system consisting of the nerves not located in the central nervous system (brain and spinal cord); these nerves carry impulses from the central nervous system to the target muscles and relay sensory impulses from the rest of the body to the central nervous system.

Peripheral vision. Side vision, or the visual perception to all sides of the central object being viewed.

Peristalsis. The wavelike muscular contractions that move food and waste products through the intestines; problems with peristalsis are called motility disorders.

Peritoneal cavity. The abdominal cavity, which contains the visceral organs.

Peritoneal dialysis. The removal of toxins from blood by dialysis in the peritoneal cavity.

Peritoneum. The membrane lining the walls of the abdominal cavity and enclosing the viscera.

Peritonitis. Infection of the abdominal (peritoneal) cavity in which the visceral organs are found.

Peroxisome. A membrane-bound organelle that contains reaction systems linking biochemical pathways taking place elsewhere in the cell; also called a microbody.

Personality disorders. Pervasive, inflexible patterns of perceiving, thinking, and behaving that cause long-term distress or impairment, beginning in adolescence and persisting into adulthood.

Pertussis. A serious bacterial infection of the respiratory tract that usually strikes very young children; commonly known as whooping cough.

Pervasive developmental disorders. Disorders characterized by severe, impaired social interaction or communication skills, or stereotyped behavior, interests, and activities.

PET scanning. *See* Positron emission tomography (PET) scanning.

Petechiae (*sing.* petechia). Minute, pinhead-sized spots caused by hemorrhage or bleeding into the skin.

Petit mal. A mild type of epileptic seizure characterized by a very short lapse of consciousness, usually without convulsions or falling.

Peyer's patches. Lymphatic nodules in the ileum of the intestine; Peyer's patches are one kind of mucosal associated lymphoid tissue (MALT), which, unlike lymph nodes, is not enclosed by tissue capsules.

pH. A value that represents the relative acidity or alkalinity of a solution; values below pH 7.0 are acidic, while values above pH 7.0 are basic.

Phagocyte. Any cell capable of surrounding, ingesting, and digesting microbes or cell debris; in a certain sense, phagocytes function as scavengers.

Phagocytosis. The ingestion and destruction of a pathogen or abnormal tissue by specialized white blood cells known as phagocytes.

Pharmaceutical. Of or relating to pharmacy; a medicinal drug.

Pharmaceutical care. The responsible provision of drug therapy to improve a patient's quality of life.

Pharmacist. A person with a license to dispense or sell drugs prescribed by a medical practitioner, such as a dentist, physician, or veterinarian.

Pharmacodynamics. Changes in tissue sensitivity or physiologic systems in response to pharmacological substances.

Pharmacognosy. The preparation of medicinal agents from natural sources.

Pharmacokinetics. The action of pharmacological substances within a biological system; pharmacologic substance absorption, distribution, metabolism, and elimination by an organism.

Pharmacology. The science that deals with the chemistry, effects, and therapeutic use of drugs.

Pharmacy. The art or profession of preparing and dispensing drugs and medicine.

Pharyngitis. Inflammation of the pharynx.

Pharynx. The throat; the part of the respiratory-digestive passage that extends from the nasal cavity to the larynx (voice box).

Phenylketonuria (PKU). A genetic disease characterized by the absence of the enzyme that breaks down the amino acid phenylalanine; the resulting buildup can lead to brain damage.

Phlebitis. The inflammation of a vein, often in the legs; may be accompanied by blood clots.

Phlebotomy. The act or practice of opening a vein for letting blood.

Phobia. Any abnormal or exaggerated fear of a particular object or situation.

Photism. In synesthesia, a vivid light or color sensation induced by a different sensory stimulus.

Photocoagulation. The condensation of protein material by the controlled use of an intense beam of light (such as a xenon arc light or argon laser).

Photon. A particle of light whose energy depends on its wavelength (that is, its color); many billions of individual photons make up a light beam.

Photophobia. Dread or avoidance of light.

Photoreception. Sensitivity to light.

Photoreceptor. A light-responsive nerve cell or receptor that is located in the retina of the eye.

Phrenic. Of or relating to the diaphragm.

Phylogenetics. The building of evolutionary trees, such as to describe accurately the base-by-base changes in a particular protein from different species.

Physiatry. The branch of medicine dealing with the prevention, diagnosis, and treatment of disease or injury and the rehabilitation from resultant impairments and disabilities; it uses physical agents such as light, heat, cold, water, electricity, therapeutic exercise, mechanical apparatus, and pharmaceutical agents.

Physical deconditioning. A condition that results when a person who has previously been exercising (has become conditioned) stops exercising for a significant period of time.

Physical examination. A step in the diagnostic process in which the physician makes general observations about the patient and examines structures of the patient's body through touching (palpation), tapping (percussion), and listening, usually with the aid of a stethoscope (auscultation).

Physical modalities. The physical means of addressing a disease, which include heat, cold, electricity, exercises, braces, assistive devices, and biofeedback.

Physical rehabilitation. The discipline devoted to the restoration of normal bodily function, primarily of the muscles and skeleton.

Physical sciences. The branch of natural science that analyzes the nature and properties of energy and nonliving matter; includes disciplines such as physics, chemistry, astronomy, and geology.

Physician assistant. A health care provider who works under the supervision of a licensed physician and who is trained to perform physical examinations, diagnose illnesses, interpret laboratory tests, set fractures, and assist in surgeries.

Physiological. Characteristic of or appropriate to an organism's healthy or normal functioning.

Physiology. The study of how the body functions, both at the cellular level and at the anatomical level.

Phytochemicals. Nonnutritive chemicals produced by plants that provide health benefits to humans who eat foods derived from them.

PID. *See* Pelvic inflammatory disease (PID).

Pigmentation. The color of the skin, hair, and eyes, caused by the degree and distribution of melanin in the skin.

Piles. A common term for hemorrhoids.

Pilosebaceous. Referring to hair follicles and the sebaceous glands.

Pimple. The common term for a papule (a solid elevation in the skin) or a pustule (a papule containing pus).

Pituitary gland. A very small gland at the base of the brain that is referred to as the master gland; with the hypothalamus, it regulates most of the endocrine systems.

PKU. *See* Phenylketonuria (PKU).

Placebo. An inactive substance resembling the experimental drug that might be given to a control group, especially when no standard treatment exists.

Placenta. The oval, spongy tissue containing blood vessels that provides the fetus with nutrients and oxygen from the mother via the umbilicus.

Plague. A serious, and sometimes fatal, bacterial infection transmitted by fleas.

Plaintiff. A person or corporation that brings legal action against another person or corporation.

Plantar. Having to do with the sole of the foot.

Plantar warts. Warts that develop on the soles of the feet, usually at points of pressure; such a wart consists of a soft core surrounded by a calluslike ring.

Plaque. The fatty material composed of cholesterol, degenerating cells, and proteinaceous substances that can build up in the wall of any artery; also, an accumulation of decomposing matter on the teeth that promotes tooth decay.

Plasma. The fluid portion of blood, in which white and red blood cells are suspended and that contains water, proteins, minerals, nutrients, hormones, and wastes.

Plasma proteins. Any proteins found in the plasma of blood, which include those proteins necessary for blood clotting and some necessary for the transport of other molecules; most are produced by the liver.

Plasmin. An enzyme present in the blood that can dissolve clots; plasmin is normally found in its inactive form, plasminogen, until needed.

Plastic surgery. Surgery performed to repair defects of the skin and underlying tissues caused by injury or malformations.

Plasticity. A phenomenon of many animal nervous systems, particularly those in higher vertebrates, in which central nervous system neurons grow or alter themselves in response to input or injury.

Platelets. Specialized blood-clotting particles that travel in the blood and become sticky when they come in contact with a damaged blood vessel.

Pleura. A serous membrane that covers and protects the lungs.

Pleurisy. The inflammation and swelling of the pleurae, the membranes that enclose the lungs and line the chest cavity.

Pluripotent. Referring to stem cells that have the capacity to develop into most of the specialized tissues of the body, but not an entire individual.

PMS. *See* Premenstrual syndrome (PMS).

Pneumocystis pneumonia. A form of pneumonia caused by the single-celled parasite *Pneumocystis carinii*; dangerous mainly to persons with impaired immune systems, particularly patients with AIDS.

Pneumonia. An inflammation of the lungs or bronchial passageways caused by viral or bacterial infection.

Pneumothorax. The collapse of a lung or portion of a lung due to the introduction of air or another gas or of fluid into the pleural space surrounding the lungs.

Podiatry. The branch of medicine that treats diseases and conditions of the foot.

Poisoning. Exposure to any substance in a quantity sufficient to cause health problems.

Poisonous plants. Plants that cause gastrointestinal or dermatological reactions in humans.

Poliomyelitis. A viral illness that may cause meningitis and permanent paralysis; it can be prevented through immunization.

Polycystic kidney disease. A genetic disorder characterized by multiple, bilateral, grapelike clusters of fluid-filled cysts that slowly replace much of the mass of the kidney, reducing kidney function and leading to renal failure.

Polycystic ovary syndrome. A complex disorder related to dysfunctional ovulation, endocrine abnormalities, and multiple cysts on the ovary that result in fertility difficulties; related to obesity and diabetes and poses increased risk for cardiovascular disease.

Polycythemia. An abnormal increase in red blood cells.

Polydactyly. A congenital anomaly characterized by excess fingers or toes.

Polymerase chain reaction. A technique that multiplies small amounts of genetic material (DNA) into amounts that can be detected by specific genetic probes.

Polymethylmethacrylate. A material used in the fixation of bones.

Polypharmacy. The prescription of many drugs at one time, often resulting in excessive use of medications and adverse drug interactions.

Polyps. Abnormal growths arising from mucous membranes anywhere in the body.

Polyspermy. Entry of more than one sperm into an egg, resulting in too many sets of chromosomes.

Population. All the people, research animals, or other items of interest in a particular study.

Porphyria. One of several rare, genetic disorders caused by the accumulation of substances called porphyrins.

Portacaval. Referring to a type of shunt used to carry blood from the portal vein to the inferior vena cava, allowing blood to bypass the liver.

Portal system. A system of veins, unique to the liver, that carry nutrient-rich blood from the digestive organs to the liver.

Positive feedback. Physiological process in which a product feeds back to stimulate the process, resulting in additional production or the continuation of that process.

Positron emission tomography (PET) scanning. A technique for creating three-dimensional images of tissues in the body by tracking radioisotopes injected into the body, allowing for diagnosis of tumors or metabolic diseases and conditions, especially of the brain.

Positrons. A type of radiation, similar to electrons but with positive charge, emitted by radioactive atoms.

Posterior. Toward the back or rear of the body or any structure.

Postnasal drip. The discharge of nasal mucus into the back of the throat.

Postoperative. Referring to a the period of time following a surgical procedure.

Postpartum depression. Depression following childbirth brought on by hormonal changes and sometimes by underlying social or emotional problems.

Potency. The effectiveness of a drug.

Prader-Willi syndrome. A disorder caused by a deletion in chromosome 15, characterized by developmental and cognitive delays, overeating resulting in obesity, and behavioral difficulties.

Preeclampsia. Hypertension induced by pregnancy, in its nonconvulsive form.

Pregnancy. The development of an embryo or fetus within the uterus, which begins with conception.

Premature. Referring to a birth that is less than full term.

Premenstrual syndrome (PMS). A common condition involving tension, irritability, headaches, depression, and bloating in the week prior to menstruation.

Premolars. The teeth between the cuspids and the molars, used in crushing and grinding food; also called bicuspids.

Prep. A short form of the word "prepare"; to prep means to wash and shave the surgical area and to clean the skin surface immediately before a surgical procedure.

Prescription drugs. Medicines that can be obtained only with the prescription of a doctor.

Presenilins. Proteins linked to several forms of inherited Alzheimer's disease, which are believed to play a role in the production of Ab.

Pressure. The measure of how much a gas or a liquid pushes on the walls of its container.

Prevalence. The number of individuals at a particular time who have a disease or a given characteristic.

Preventive medicine. An approach to health care that emphasizes behaviors and therapies (such as exercise and proper diet) designed to minimize contraction of disease before it happens.

Prima facie. The concept that one ethical principle is morally binding unless the action it requires violates another equal or greater principle.

Primary care. General medical services provided in family practice, internal medicine, pediatrics, geriatrics, obstetrics, and emergency care (in contrast to specialties, such as urology or cardiac surgery).

Primary infection. A person's first infection with a particular agent such as a virus.

Privacy. The state of being free from unwanted or unauthorized observation, company, or other intrusion.

Probability. A number varying between 0 (for an impossible event) to 1 (for an absolutely certain event).

Procedure. Any medical treatment that involves physical manipulation or invasion of the body.

Proctology. The study and treatment of diseases of the rectum.

Prodromal. Sensation before an event occurs.

Progesterone or progestin. A hormone produced in the ovaries, adrenal gland, and placenta (of pregnant women) that prepares for and sustains pregnancy.

Prognosis. The predicted outcome of a disease.

Prolactin. A hormone secreted from the anterior pituitary gland that signals the breast to start and sustain milk production.

Prone. The position of the body when lying face downward, on the abdomen.

Prophylactic treatment. A treatment focusing on preventing disease, illness, or their symptoms from occurring.

Prostaglandins. Chemical messengers that are not carried in the blood and that function only locally; they cause pain, contractions, and a variety of other effects.

Prostate gland. An accessory reproductive gland whose main function is to secrete into semen vital additive components that increase the fertilizing potential of sperm.

Prosthesis. A fabricated, artificial substitute for a missing part of the body, such as a limb.

Prosthetist. An individual skilled in constructing and fitting prostheses.

Prosthodontics. The dental specialty that restores missing teeth with fixed or removable dentures.

Prostoglandular carcinoma. The general pathological nomenclature for cancers located in the prostate gland.

Protein. Large molecules made up of amino acids connected by peptide bonds; the sequence of amino acids in a protein determines its three-dimensional structure.

Protein kinase. An enzyme type that often is encoded by oncogenes; this enzyme attaches phosphate molecules to certain amino acids on specifically targeted proteins.

Proteinuria. The presence of protein (typically albumin) in the urine.

Proteome. The complete set of proteins in a particular cell type.

Proteomics. The study of proteomes.

Protozoan (*pl.* protozoa). A single-celled organism that is more closely related to animals than are bacteria and is often a vector of disease; only a few drugs are available that will kill protozoa without harming their animal hosts.

Provider. The medical practitioner within a clinic or hospital; providers may be physicians, nurses, dentists, or other licensed health care professionals.

Proving. The testing of a substance or remedy on healthy volunteers (provers), who take repeated doses and record in detail any symptoms produced by it.

Proximal. Toward the origin.

Psoriasis. A chronic skin disease characterized by red, scaly patches overlaid with thick, silvery gray scales.

Psyche. The human mind, which according to Sigmund Freud is divided into id, ego, and superego; the id contains instincts and repressed feelings, the ego directs everyday behavior, and the superego guides the ego.

Psychedelic drugs. Substances that cause alterations in perception and thinking, such as changes in awareness, sense of self, or hallucinations.

Psychiatry. The branch of medicine, practiced by physicians, that treats emotional and behavioral problems through both medication and non-drug therapies such as counseling.

Psychoanalysis. A form of treatment for mental illness that employs talk therapy designed to elicit information from the patient, which the analyst then interprets in the light of psychological theorizing.

Psychoanalyst. A person trained in psychoanalysis and in practice to diagnose and treat clients; psychoanalysts are often, but not always, licensed to practice in a particular state.

Psychogenic. Psychological (rather than physical) in origin; set off by psychologically stressful events.

Psychosis. A condition occurring where a person is severely out of touch with reality and unable to function in an adaptive manner.

Psychosomatic. Referring to physical symptoms caused or aggravated by psychological factors.

Psychosurgery. The surgical removal or destruction of part of the brain in order to treat a patient with a psychiatric disorder such as depression.

Psychotherapy. Treatment using the mind, body, and behavior to remedy problems related to disordered behavior or thinking, emotional problems, or disease.

Psychotic. Referred to a disabling mental state characterized by poor reality testing (inaccurate perceptions, confusion, disorientation) and disorganized speech, behavior, and emotional experience.

Psychotropic drugs. Substances primarily affecting behavior, perception, and other psychological functions.

PTCA. *See* Percutaneous transluminal coronary angioplasty (PTCA).

Puberty. The physiological sequence of events by which a child is transformed into an adult; the growth of secondary sexual characteristics occurs, reproductive functions begin, and the differences between males and females are accentuated.

Public health. Preventive measures intended to improve the health of all persons in a community.

Pulmonary. Related to the lungs and breathing.

Pulmonary edema. Accumulation of fluid in the lungs, which may lead to death.

Pulmonary hypertension. A rare disorder of the pulmonary circulation occurring mostly in young and middle-aged women.

Pulmonary medicine. The field of medicine concerned with all the diseases that may afflict the lungs or in which the lungs may be involved.

Pulmonary nodules. Small, round growths on the lung that contain either trapped microorganisms or cancer cells.

Pulp. The internal, living tissue of the tooth, consisting of nerves, blood vessels, and dental cells.

Pulse. The rhythmical dilation of an artery, produced by the increased volume of blood forced into the vessel by the contraction of the heart; the frequency of the pulse corresponds to the heart rate.

Pulsed laser. A laser technique used to deliver a light beam of high power for a very short time in order to localize the heating effect without damaging surrounding tissue.

Pupil. The opening at the center of the iris through which light passes.

Pyelonephritis. Inflammation of the kidney as the result of a bacterial infection in the bladder.

Pyloric stenosis. A narrowing of the passageway between the stomach and the duodenum.

Pyorrhea. The second stage of gingivitis.

Pyridostigmine bromide. A chemical that prevents damage from possible nerve gas exposure.

Pyrogens. Protein substances that appear at the outset of the process that leads to a fever reaction.

Qi gong. A Chinese meditative exercise that improves cardiovascular circulation, restores deep breathing, and relieves stress.

Quadriplegia. Partial or complete paralysis of the arms, legs, and trunk caused by damage to the spinal cord in the neck.

Quantum theory. The theory that energy, momentum, and other physical quantities appear in indivisible units of finite quantity.

Quickening. The stage during a pregnancy when the mother begins to feel the movements of the fetus, usually in the second trimester.

Rabies. A viral infection, usually transmitted through the bite of a rabid animal, that attacks the nervous system; it can be cured through immediate immunization but is nearly always fatal once symptoms occur.

Radial. Toward the edge of the forearm and hand containing the radius and thumb.

Radiation dose. The amount of radiation absorbed, depending on the intensity of the source and the time of exposure; measured in units of rads or grays.

Radiation sickness. Acute, sometimes fatal illness that occurs with exposure to a sudden, large dose of radiation.

Radiation therapy. The use of radiation to kill cancer cells or shrink cancerous growth; when high and full doses of radiation (measured in units called rads) are used, the patient is said to be given a "megavoltage."

Radical surgery. Any surgery that removes all of the organ or tissue affected by a disease, as well as tissue surrounding the area, in an attempt to eradicate the disease.

Radiculopathy. Pain distributed along a specific pathway resulting from irritation of a nerve root.

Radioimmunoassay. The quantitative measurement of a hormone using an unlabeled hormone to inhibit the binding of a radiolabeled hormone to an antibody.

Radioimmunotherapy. A cancer therapy using radionuclides; the radionuclides attach themselves to antibodies that tend to target cancer cells in the body, thus eradicating the cancer cells through selective irradiation.

Radioisotope. *See* Radionuclide.

Radiology. The branch of medicine that focuses on imaging technologies such as X rays, magnetic resonance imaging (MRI), scanning techniques, and ultrasonography.

Radionucleotide scanning. A technique that develops an image of an internal bodily structure by detecting radiation emitted from a substance injected into the body to see how the bodily structure reacts to it.

Radionuclide. An unstable atomic nucleus that, in the process of decay, emits radiation.

Radiopharmaceutical. A sterile, radioactively tagged compound that is administered to a patient for diagnostic or therapeutic purposes.

Radius. The shorter of the two forearm bones, on the thumb side.

Rash. A skin disorder, usually temporary, characterized by red, inflamed areas or spots; generally a symptom of an underlying condition, such as a skin disease, autoimmune disorder, infectious disease, or bleeding disorder.

RDA. *See* Recommended daily (or dietary) allowance (RDA).

Receptor. A molecular structure at the cell surface or inside the cell that is capable of combining with hormones or neurotransmitters and causing a change in cell metabolism.

Recessive allele. A version of a gene that must be present on both chromosomes of a pair in order to produce a recognizable trait in offspring.

Recessive genetic disease. A disease caused by a mutation in a gene that must be inherited from both parents in order for an individual to show the symptoms of the disease; such a disease may show up only occasionally in a family history, especially if the mutation is rare.

Recombinant DNA technology. Manipulation of genetic material or DNA whereby pieces of DNA are separated and interchanged in order to obtain a desired result.

Recombination. The reciprocal exchange of segments between the two chromosomes of a pair, producing new combinations of alleles.

Recommended daily (or dietary) allowance (RDA). Former term for dietary reference intake (DRI).

Reconstructive surgery. Surgery designed to rebuild or replace a body part malformed at birth, damaged as a result of injury, or surgically removed for therapeutic reasons.

Recovery room. The room where a patient returns to full consciousness after a surgical procedure; in an outpatient facility, patients can change clothes in the recovery room, which may serve double duty as the preoperative waiting room.

Rectal prolapse. The protrusion of the rectum through the anus.

Rectum. The intestinal storage area for feces between the colon and anus.

Recurrence. The appearance of an infection or disease after initial treatment has been completed.

Red blood cells. Blood cells that contain hemoglobin; their role is to transport oxygen.

Reduction. The restoration of a fractured bone to its normal position; also a decrease in the total volume or mass of breast tissue, usually to correct undesirable ptosis.

Reed-Sternberg cell. A large, atypical macrophage with multiple nuclei; found in patients with Hodgkin's disease.

Referred pain. Pain that is felt somewhere other than at the site of injury or disease, as a result of neural pathways.

Reflux. The abnormal backward flow of a fluid (such as bile or urine).

Refraction. The bending of light rays by the cornea and lens to form an image on the retina.

Regeneration. The renewal, regrowth, or restoration of destroyed or missing tissue; the production of new tissue.

Regional anesthesia. Insensibility caused by the interruption of nerve conduction in a region of the body.

Regression. Reverting to a pattern of behavior seen at an earlier age of development.

Regurgitation. The leakage of blood backward through a valve; also vomiting.

Rehabilitation. The restoration of normal form and function after injury or illness; the restoration of the ill or injured patient to optimal functional level in the home and community in relation to physical, psychosocial, vocational, and recreational activity.

Reiter's syndrome. An autoimmune disorder with associated symptoms of arthritis, urethritis, conjunctivitis, and ulcerations of the skin and mouth.

Rejection. A cellular and chemical attack by the immune system on transplanted tissues or organs, which are recognized as foreign to the body.

Reliability. The concept that repeated tests will produce the same result.

Renal. Referring to the kidneys.

Renal cell carcinoma. Cancer of the small tubules of the kidney; generally known as kidney cancer.

Renal failure. The inability of the kidneys to process waste products in the blood and excrete them through the urine.

Renal pelvis. The central pocket or sac of each kidney, which collects urine from all nephrons and channels it into the ureter.

Renal tubule. The tubular portion of a nephron that allows renal fluid to flow from the Bowman's capsule to the renal pelvis; these tubules, shaped like hairpins, are crucially important in the production of urine.

Repertory. In homeopathy, a published index of symptoms, with each heading listing the drugs known to cause the symptom.

Replication. The process by which the DNA of a cell is duplicated so that the information stored there can be passed on to new cells after cell division.

Reproductive system. The organs of the female (the vagina, uterus, Fallopian tubes, ovaries, and mammary glands) and the male (the penis, testes, vas deferens, and prostate gland) that are involved in the production or feeding of offspring.

Reservoir. An animal population that is infected with a disease that can be transmitted either to other animals or to humans; also called an alternate host.

Residency. A course of clinical medical education undertaken after receiving an M.D. or D.O. degree and leading to certification in a generalist or specialist branch of medicine.

Resorption. The process in which bones dissolve and return their components to the body fluids.

Respect for autonomy. A principle of medical ethics which requires that the autonomous decisions of patients be honored.

Respiration. A process that includes both air conduction (the act of breathing) and gas exchange (oxygen and carbon dioxide transfer between the air and blood).

Respirator. A machine that inflates and deflates the lungs, imitating normal breathing; connected to patient through a tube placed into the windpipe.

Respiratory diseases. Any of a wide variety of diseases that affect the lungs and/or the process of respiration, including emphysema, lung cancer, and pneumonia.

Respiratory distress syndrome. A life-threatening illness primarily of premature infants; immature lungs lack a vital substance that keeps the tiny air sacs (alveoli) from collapsing upon exhalation.

Rest pain. Pain noted in the most distal portion of the extremity at rest, relieved by analgesics.

Restless legs syndrome. A sensorimotor disorder characterized by uncomfortable and even painful sensations in the limbs, especially the legs, when at rest or trying to sleep.

Restoration. An item or material that is used to restore the structure and function of a compromised tooth.

Restriction endonuclease. An enzyme that responds to a specific, short sequence of nucleotides within a DNA molecule by binding to that sequence and breaking the DNA strands near the sequence.

Resuscitation. The return of a person to consciousness or the restoration of a person's vital signs after an injury, seizure, or heart attack by means of artificial respiration, cardiopulmonary resuscitation (CPR), electrical shock treatment, chemicals, or other means.

Retina. A thin membrane at the back of the eyeball where light is converted into nerve impulses that travel to the brain.

Retrocochlear hearing loss. Any disruption of neural information processing beyond the cochlea.

Retroviruses. RNA viruses that replicate by synthesizing a double-stranded DNA molecule that integrates into the host genome; they are known to infect virtually all animals and sometimes cause serious disease, including cancer.

Revascularization. Procedures to reestablish the circulation to a diseased portion of the body.

Reverse transcriptase. An enzyme that synthesizes double-stranded DNA from single-stranded RNA.

Reye's syndrome. A somewhat rare, noncontagious disease of the liver and central nervous system that strikes individuals under the age of eighteen.

Rh factor. Any one of several "factors," or elements present in the blood, according to one system of blood-type classification; the presence of the D factor can cause erythroblastosis fetalis, a type of hemolytic disease of the newborn.

Rh0(D) immune globulin (human). A type of gamma globulin protein injected into Rh-negative mothers who may have an Rh-positive fetus in order to protect the fetus from an immune reaction.

Rheumatic fever. A complication of untreated streptococcal infections characterized by swollen joints, rashes, fever, and sometimes heart disorders; evidence of heart valve damage may emerge later in life.

Rheumatoid arthritis. A disease affecting the muscles, cartilage, and joints characterized by stiffness, pain, and swelling.

Rheumatology. The study and treatment of rheumatoid arthritis and related diseases.

Rhinitis. Inflammation of the mucous membrane that lines the nose, resulting from an allergic reaction or a common cold virus.

Rhinoplasty. Surgical alteration of the structure of the nose, performed for both therapeutic and cosmetic reasons.

Rhinovirus. A microorganism causing respiratory illness; one of the most prevalent causes of the common cold.

Rhodopsin. A chemical within photoreceptors that translates light into electrical impulses.

Ribonucleic acid (RNA). The material contained in the core of many viruses that is responsible for directing the replication of the virus inside the host cell.

Ribosome. A cytoplasmic particle assembled from ribosomal RNA and ribosomal proteins that uses messenger RNA molecules as directions for synthesizing proteins.

Ribs. The bones that support the chest and define its outline.

Rickets. A deficiency in vitamin D, calcium, and phosphorus that results in soft bones.

Risk assessment. The process that establishes whether a health risk exists for a population exposed to a toxic substance.

Risk factors. The situations, circumstances, or conditions that increase the probability of the occurrence of disease or accident.

RNA. *See* Ribonucleic acid (RNA).

Rods. Specialized photoreceptors that provide peripheral vision and vision in dim light.

Root. That portion of the tooth which is below the crown and is embedded in a bony socket of the jaw.

Root canal treatment. Surgery to save a tooth whose pulp has become diseased or has died.

Root hair plexus. A network of sensory receptors located at hair roots that generates an impulse when hairs are moved.

Rosacea. The chronic inflammation of facial skin; also known as acne rosacea or adult acne.

Roseola. A common and contagious childhood disease characterized by high fever and a skin rash.

Rotator cuff surgery. The surgical correction of a muscle tear within the shoulder.

Rubella. A mild, contagious viral illness that is dangerous only when contracted by women during the early months of pregnancy, when it is likely to cause birth defects; also called German measles.

Rubeola. *See* Measles.

Ruffini endings. Sensory receptors that respond to heavy and continuous touch and pressure; also called type II cutaneous mechanoreceptors or the end organs of Ruffini.

Rule of nines. A system for designating areas of the body, represented by various body parts; used in determining the extent of a burn.

S-A node. *See* Sinoatrial (S-A) node.

Salicylates. A group of drugs that includes aspirin and related compounds used to relieve pain, reduce inflammation, and lower fever.

Salivary glands. The glands that produce saliva, a watery substance in the mouth that helps break down food.

Salmonella. Bacteria that cause a general infection of the gastrointestinal tract and lymphatic system when ingested.

Sample. The members of a population that are actually studied or whose characteristics are measured.

Sanatorium. An institution designed for the treatment of chronic illnesses, such as tuberculosis.

Sanitation. The application of measures designed to protect public health.

Saphenous vein. Vein from the upper leg that is often used to bypass a blocked coronary artery.

Saponification. A reaction in which a strong basic solution splits a molecule into a carboxylic acid unit and an alcohol

unit.

Sarcoidosis. An inflammatory disease, characterized by noncaseating granulomas, of unknown cause, affecting multiple systems, especially the lungs, lymph nodes, skin, and eyes.

Sarcoma. A malignant tumor originating in connective tissue, including bone and muscle.

Sarin. A nerve gas that can cause convulsions and death.

SARS. *See* Severe acute respiratory syndrome (SARS).

Scabies. Skin infestation by mites, causing a rash and severe itching.

Scarlet fever. An acute, contagious childhood disease caused by bacterial infection.

Schizophrenia. A mental disturbance characterized by psychotic features during the active phase and deteriorated functioning in occupational, social, or self-care abilities.

Schwann cell. A supportive cell for neurons in the peripheral nervous system of vertebrate animals that wraps around and insulates axons using the protein myelin.

Sciatica. Painful inflammation of one of the sciatic nerves.

SCID. *See* Severe combined immunodeficiency syndrome (SCID).

Scientific method. A method of scientific investigation involving observation, the formation of a hypothesis (a possible explanation), experimentation, and the reevaluation of data.

Scintillation. The production of flashes emitted by luminescent substances when excited by high-energy radiation.

Sclera. The opaque portion of the outer layer of the eye; commonly referred to as the "white of the eye."

Scleroderma. A rare autoimmune connective tissue disorder affecting various organs.

Scoliosis. Abnormal curvature of the spine, which is often progressive.

Screening. A strategy used by physicians and public health professionals to diagnose disease or the potential for disease at an early stage, when it may be treatable or preventable; may be a mandatory procedure for a specific population or a voluntary activity requested by individuals.

Scrotum. The genital skin sac that holds the testicles and related structures.

Scrub. To wash one's hands and forearms in preparation for donning gown and gloves, which protect the patient from the surgeon and staff and protect the surgeon and staff from the patient.

Scurvy. A disease caused by a prolonged inadequate intake of vitamin C.

Seasonal affective disorder. A depression that undergoes a seasonal fluctuation as a result of various factors, both unknown and known.

Sebaceous glands. Glands in the skin that usually open into the hair follicles.

Sebum. A semifluid, fatty substance secreted by the sebaceous glands into the hair follicles.

Secondary infection. A bacterial, viral, or other infection that results from or follows another disease.

Sedation. The use of medication to calm patients who are agitated or anxious, to relieve pain, or to relax patients experiencing discomfort from a device being used to support care (for example, a breathing tube inserted down the throat).

Seizure. A sudden, violent, and involuntary contraction of a group of muscles; may be paroxysmal and episodic, also called a convulsion.

Selective serotonin reuptake inhibitors (SSRIs). A class of antidepressant drugs that work by inhibiting the neurotransmitter serotonin, thus making more of it available to brain cells.

Semen. Fluid produced by a man's prostate gland that makes up 95 percent of the fluid that is ejaculated.

Seminoma. The most common cancer of the testes.

Semipermeable membrane. A barrier that allows some materials to pass but blocks others.

Semisynthetic. Referring to natural products, such as antibiotics, that have been chemically modified to be more useful for a particular application.

Senile plaques. A hallmark lesion of Alzheimer's disease, composed of Aβ amyloid.

Senility. An outmoded term for dementia often applied to the elderly.

Sense organs. Specialized structures anatomically suited to a particular sense-the eyes for vision, the nose for smell (olfaction), the taste buds for taste, the ears for hearing and balance, and the skin for such cutaneous sensations as warmth, cold, light touch, deep pressure, and pain.

Sensitivity. The ability of a screening technique to identify correctly people who have a disease.

Sensory. Referring to perception by the senses. touch, sight, hearing, smell, and other senses such as hunger.

Sepsis. An infection in the circulating blood.

Septic pyelophlebitis. Inflammation of the veins that carry blood away from the kidneys.

Septic shock. A dangerous condition in which there is tissue damage and a dramatic drop in blood pressure as a result of septicemia.

Septicemia. Serious, systemic infection of the blood with pathogens that have spread from an infection in a part of the body, characteristically causing fever, chills, prostration, pain, headache, nausea, and/or diarrhea.

Septum. A membrane that serves as a wall of separation; in the heart, the interatrial septum divides the two atria, and the interventricular septum divides the two ventricles.

Serology. The branch of medicine specializing in the clear portion of the blood called the serum, often focused on analysis of the serum as a means of diagnosing disease.

Seronegative. The test result seen when blood does not contain the specific antibody or antigen being sought and the particular antigen-antibody reaction is not present.

Seropositive. The test result seen when blood contains the specific antibody or antigen being sought and the particular antigen-antibody reaction is present.

Serotonin. An abundant chemical nerve signal in the brain that is involved in modulating aggression.

Serotype. A subgroup member within a larger species; simi-

lar, but not identical, to other members of the species.

Serum. The fluid part of blood, without red blood cells and clotting factors.

Set point. A mechanism, thought to be formed by a series of feedback systems, for maintaining such characteristics as temperature and body weight.

Severe acute respiratory syndrome (SARS). A recently recognized type of pneumonia caused by a novel coronavirus that may progress to respiratory failure and death.

Severe combined immunodeficiency syndrome (SCID). A syndrome in which the immune system is unable to produce T and B lymphocytes, resulting in catastrophic failure of the immune system.

Sex change surgery. A set of procedures designed to convert the secondary sexual characteristics of an anatomic male to those of a female or an anatomic female to those of a male.

Sex glands. The ovaries in the female and the testes in the male, which secrete hormones involved in reproduction.

Sex steroids. Steroid hormones such as androgens and estrogens that influence the activity of sexual organs and activity.

Sexual differentiation. The process by which an embryo becomes male or female under the influence of genetic and hormonal factors.

Sexually transmitted disease (STD). Any disease that can be acquired through sexual contact or passed from a pregnant woman to her fetus, including syphilis, gonorrhea, chlamydia, herpes, and AIDS.

Shigellosis. An intestinal infection caused by *Shigella* bacteria.

Shingles. A disease of the central nervous system characterized by painful red blisters that join together and rapidly rupture and become crusted.

Shock. A life-threatening condition in which the heart is unable to pump enough blood to the vital organs; symptoms include rapid and shallow breathing, clammy skin, low blood pressure, and dizziness.

Shock wave. A miniature explosion caused by intense local heating with a laser beam; used to fragment stones in the kidney or gallbladder.

Shunt. An opening established by surgery to maintain easy access to an internal area of the body for various purposes, such as application of medication or drainage of excess body fluids.

Sickle cell disease. An inherited blood disorder in which abnormally high amounts of hemoglobin cause red blood cells to become sickle-shaped and block capillaries.

Side effect. A secondary and usually adverse effect (as of a drug); also known as an adverse effect or reaction.

SIDS. *See* Sudden infant death syndrome (SIDS).

Sigmoidoscopy. Endoscopy performed on the lower section of the colon.

Sign. Objective evidence of disease; a finding noted by the physician during the course of the physical examination.

Signal-averaged electrocardiogram. A sophisticated ECG that detects subtle and potentially lethal cardiac conduction defects.

Silicone. A plastic made primarily of silicon polymer.

Sinoatrial (S-A) node. A cluster of cells above the right atrium that emit electrical signals that initiate contractions of the heart; also called natural pacemaker cells.

Sinusitis. The inflammation of the lining of the nasal sinuses.

Skeletal muscle. A type of muscle that attaches to bone and causes movement of body parts; the only type that is under conscious, voluntary control.

Skeleton. The bony framework of the body.

Skilled home care. Medically necessary care that requires a service by a professional such as a nurse or physical therapist.

Skin. The largest organ of the body, which is vital to the survival of an organism for its protection against dehydration and abrasion, regulation of body temperature, and sensory reception.

Skin biopsy. A removal of a piece of skin for the purpose of further microscopic examination.

Sleep apnea. A sleep disorder characterized by intermittent cessation of airflow through the upper airway.

Sleep disorder. Any abnormal pattern of sleep that threatens normal function, including conditions that cause too much as well as too little sleep, and that may be both organic and nonorganic in origin.

Sleeping sickness. An infectious protozoan disease transmitted through the bite of a tsetse fly.

Slipped disk. A supportive ligament surrounding a vertebra in the neck or back that has broken through the spinal column and into the spinal canal; also called a herniated disk or a ruptured disk.

Small intestine. The region of gut between the stomach and the colon that comprises the duodenum, jejunum, and ileum; also called the small bowel.

Smell. A special sense in which chemicals interact with receptor sites in specialized structures of the nasal cavity and the resulting nerve impulses are classified as certain kinds of odor.

Smooth muscle. Muscle that, when viewed under a microscope, does not have striations, which are stripes seen in skeletal muscle cells; smooth muscle contracts involuntarily and is related to the functioning of the stomach, intestines, and urinary bladder; involved in the movement of food through the digestive tract.

Sodium pentothal. A fast-acting anesthetic that is injected into the vein; first developed for military hospitals during World War II.

Soft palate. A structure of mucous membrane, muscle fibers, and mucous glands suspended from the posterior border of the hard palate in the mouth.

Soma. The body of a cell, where the cell's genetic material and other vital structures are located.

Somatoform disorder. A mental disorder whose symptoms focus on the physical body.

Sonography. The use of sound waves deflected from internal body organs to find growing masses (including fetuses) and abnormal lesions; also called ultrasound.

Spastic. Characterized by uncontrollable spasms.

Spasticity. A rigidity or resistance to passive limb movement, usually occuring in limbs that are weak, that respond in an impaired way to voluntary control, and whose weakness is thought to be due to observed lesions in the upper motor neurons.

Specific gravity. The density of a solution relative to that of water; abnormal values can be indicative of elevated sugar or protein levels in urine.

Specificity. The ability of a screening technique to identify correctly people who do not have a disease.

Spectrum of activity. The range of microbial species that can be inhibited by an antibiotic; broad-spectrum antibiotics can control more than one kind of infection, but narrow-spectrum antibiotics avoid unintentional damage to the normal microbiota.

Speech disorder. A dysfunction in the brain-coordinated use of speech organs, such as problems with language, vocal quality, articulation, fluency, and dementia.

Sperm. The male gamete; the mature sperm has an oval head that contains the male's chromosomes and a long tail that allows it to swim in fluid.

Spermicide. A chemical that kills sperm after they are ejaculated.

Sphincter. A ringlike muscle that acts as a one-way valve to control the flow of fluids and waste.

Sphincterectomy. Surgical removal of a sphincter.

Sphygmomanometer. A device that uses a column of mercury to measure blood pressure.

Spina bifida. A genetic abnormality in which the spine has failed to fuse, sometimes exposing the spinal cord and nerves.

Spinal anesthesia. The injection of an anesthetic at the base of the spine to produce loss of feeling in the lower part of the body and legs; also known as a subarachnoid block.

Spinal canal. A tube or tunnel that runs down the spine and contains the spinal cord, which carries the nerves from the brain to the body.

Spinal cord. A cord in the trunk containing nerve cells that transmit impulses to and from the brain.

Spinal nerves. Pairs of nerves connected to the spinal cord and numbered according to the level at which they emerge from the cord; each spinal nerve attaches to the spinal cord by an anterior and a posterior root.

Spinal stenosis. A condition in which the diameter of the spinal canal is decreased and thus compromises the spinal cord and spinal nerve roots.

Spinal tap. *See* Lumbar puncture.

Spine. The combined spinal cord and the vertebral (spinal) column.

Spinous processes. Bony projections from vertebrae (horizontally in the neck, tilting downward in the thoracic area, and horizontally in the lumbar area) that are connected to one another by the interspinous and supraspinous ligaments and that control extremes of trunk motion.

Spleen. A lymphatic organ, found between the stomach and the diaphragm, that destroys old blood cells and filters foreign material from the blood.

Splenectomy. Surgical removal of the spleen.

Spondylitis. Inflammation and stiffening of the joints between the vertebrae of the spine.

Spondylosis. A condition characterized by restriction of movement of the vertebral bones; occurs naturally as a child grows.

Spontaneously resolve. To get better without any treatment.

Sports medicine. A medical subspecialty concerned with the care and prevention of athletic injuries, primarily those related to the musculoskeletal system.

Sprain. An injury in which ligaments are stretched or torn.

Squamous cell carcinoma. A form of skin cancer starting as a small, painless lump and often resembling a wart; common in fair-skinned individuals, especially in later life.

Staging. A numerical classification system used by physicians to describe how far a cancerous growth has advanced.

Staining. The artificial coloring of tissue sections and cells to facilitate their microscopic study.

Stapes. A small bone within the middle ear; also called the stirrup because of its shape.

Staphylococcal infections. A variety of infections caused by staphylococcus bacteria, including boils, abscesses, pneumonia, bone infections, and toxic shock syndrome.

STD. *See* Sexually transmitted disease (STD).

Stem cell. A master cell from which other blood cells develop; these cells are located primarily in the bone marrow.

Stenosis. An abnormal narrowing or constriction of a canal or passageway in the body caused by the buildup of cholesterol, fats, or other substances (plaque); the swelling or overgrowth of cells, tissue, or an organ; or a deformity.

Stents. Wire mesh tubes permanently implanted to prop open arteries or veins.

Stereotaxic computed tomography. A method of imaging using a series of X rays that are compiled by a computer to give a three-dimensional image of internal structures.

Sterile field. An area in which only sterile supplies may be placed and which only those wearing sterile gowns and gloves may touch; includes the surgical wound, the surgical drapes, and the extra tables.

Sterilization. Any procedure that makes it impossible for a person to reproduce, whether chemical or surgical.

Sternum. The breastbone, which is found in the midline of the chest cavity and lying over the heart.

Steroids. A class of fat-soluble chemicals that are structurally related to one another and share the same chemical skeleton; includes hormones, drugs, and other molecules.

Sterol. A steroid that has long side chains of carbone compounds attached to it and contains at least one hydroxyl group; cholesterol is one type of sterol.

Stethoscope. An instrument for listening to sounds in the body, such as the heartbeat.

Stillbirth. A condition in which a fetus has died within the uterus and is born after the twenty-eighth week of pregnancy.

Stimulus. Anything capable of producing a response.

Stoma. A surgically created passage between the intestines and the outer skin.

Stone. A deposit of cholesterol and calcium that may form in the gallbladder, kidneys, ureters, bladder, or urethra; also called a calculus (*pl.* calculi).

Stool. The waste matter of digestion excreted from the body through the anus or a stoma.

Strain. An injury in which muscles or tendons are stretched or torn.

Stratum corneum. The outermost layer of the epidermis; its cells are normally dead, hard, and constantly removed by normal bathing.

Strep throat. A contagious bacterial infection by streptococcal bacteria that causes inflammation of the pharynx.

Streptococcal infections. A variety of infections caused by streptococcus bacteria, including tonsillitis, strep throat, pneumonia, endocarditis, urinary tract infections, and otitis media.

Stress. Physical, environmental, or psychological strain experienced by an individual that requires adjustment.

Stress reduction. A set of procedures with the goal of decreasing bodily and mental tension by increasing rest and coping skills.

Stricture. The narrowing of a passageway.

Stridor. The harsh, high-pitched sound produced by turbulent airflow through a partially obstructed airway.

Stroke. Permanent damage to part of the brain as a result of impaired blood flow.

Stroke volume. The blood volume leaving either the right or the left side of the heart with each beat; each side usually ejects the same volume per beat.

Stuttering. The repetition of sounds or syllables or the inability to formulate words in a spoken sentence.

Subclinical. Referring to a medical problem in which the patient has no symptoms of disease or symptoms so slight that the disease is not diagnosed.

Subcutaneous. Under the skin.

Subdural hematoma. Collection of blood (clotted and partially clotted) in the subdural space between brain tissue and the dura mater.

Subluxation. An incomplete or partial dislocation of a joint, which creates abnormal neurological and physiological symptoms in neuromusculoskeletal structures and/or other body systems via interference with nerve impulse transmission.

Substrates. Reactants that enzymes convert into products; every enzyme is specific for one specific substrate.

Succussion. Violent shaking at each stage of dilution in the preparation of a homeopathic remedy.

Sudden infant death syndrome (SIDS). The abrupt death of any infant or young child in which postmortem examination fails to demonstrate an adequate cause.

Suggestion. A communication that evokes a nonvoluntary response reflecting the ideational content of the communication.

Superinfection. An infection caused by destruction of the normal microbiota by antibiotic therapy, which allows for proliferation of a pathogen other than the one targeted by the antibiotic.

Superior. Above another part or closer to the head; the ankle bones are superior to the bones of the feet.

Supine. Lying face-upward.

Suppressor T cell. A type of T lymphocyte that is believed to modulate the immune response.

Surgery. The treatment of diseases or disorders by physical intervention, which usually involves cutting into the skin and other tissues.

Surgical pathology. The branch of pathology that deals with the interpretation of biopsies.

Surgical team. The people working together in the operating room during a surgical procedure, including the surgeon, first assistant, surgical technologist, anesthesiologist and/or anesthetist, and circulator.

Surgical technologist. A surgical team member whose primary functions are to prepare surgical instruments and hand them to the surgeon as needed and to prevent infection by maintaining a sterile field in the operating room.

Suspiciousness. A range of symptoms from increasing distrust of others to paranoid delusions of conspiracies.

Suture. A thread used to unite parts of the body.

Sympathectomy. The surgical process of removing or destroying nerves that may be afflicted by frostbite or other injury.

Sympathetic nervous system. The division of the autonomic nervous system concerned primarily with preparing the individual to expend energy.

Symptom. Subjective evidence of disease, provided by the patient.

Symptomatic disease. A disease or disorder that displays overt symptoms.

Symptomatic treatment. A treatment focusing on aborting disease, illness, or their symptoms once they have occurred.

Synapse. An area of close contact between nerve cells that is the functional junction where one cell communicates with another.

Syndactyly. A congenital anomaly characterized by the fusion of the fingers or toes.

Syndrome. A group or pattern of recognizable symptoms or conditions that occur together and indicate a specific disease, psychological disorder, or other abnormal condition.

Synergistic effects. The combined effects of drugs interacting with one another, such that the effects of the drugs together have a compounded effect, greater than that of any one alone.

Synesthete. A person who experiences synesthesia by virtue of having a second sensation evoked by a single stimulus.

Synovial. Referring to the lubricating fluid in the joints or the membrane surrounding the joints.

Synovium. The cellular lining of a joint, having a blood supply and a nerve supply; the synovium secretes fluid for lubrication and protects against injury and injurious agents.

Syphilis. A serious sexually transmitted disease that can be fatal if left untreated.

Systemic. Affecting the entire body.

Systems and organs. Groups of tissues and organs dedicated to particular functions, all of which must work together to perform efficiently.

Systole. The period of contraction of the heart when blood moves out of the heart chambers and into the arteries.

Systolic blood pressure. The pressure of the blood within the artery while the heart is contracting.

T lymphocyte. A type of immune cell that kills host cells infected by bacteria or viruses or produces a chemical compound that mediates the host cells' destruction.

Tachycardia. Rapid beating of the heart.

Tachypnea. Rapid breathing greater than twenty breaths per minute.

Target heart rate range. A heart rate range that is to be maintained during exercise training.

Tarsus. The ankle.

Taste. A special sense in which chemicals interact with receptor sites in specialized structures of the tongue, and the resulting nerve impulses are classified as certain kinds of taste.

Taste bud. A special sensing structure for taste found on taste-responsive papillae; taste buds are made of three cell types-gustatory or taste cells, supporting cells, and basal cells.

Taste cell. The cellular compartment of a taste bud that contains chemoreceptors; taste hairs, one type of chemoreceptor, are found at the taste pore (or entry point) of a taste cell.

Temporal lobes. Lateral portions of the brain cerebrum; responsible for language, memory, and emotion.

Temporomandibular joint (TMJ). The hinged joint that attaches the head of the mandible to the skull.

Tendinitis. Inflammation of a tendon or a tough band of tissue that connects muscle to the bone.

Tendon. A structure of tough connective tissue that attaches a muscle to a bone.

Tensile strength. The greatest stress that can be placed on a tissue without tearing it apart; it is relative to the strength of a tissue.

Teratogens. Substances that induce congenital malformations when embryonic tissues and organs are exposed to them.

Teratology. The study of congenital malformations.

Testes (*sing.* testis). The male reproductive organs, a pair of gonads that are suspended in the scrotum and produce sperm; also known as the testicles.

Testicular torsion. Twisting of the testicle in the scrotum, with compromise of the blood supply to the testicle, as a result of spermatic cord rotation.

Testosterone. The male sex hormone that gives rise to male fertility and secondary sexual characteristics, such as body hair and musculature.

Tetanus. An often fatal nervous system disease characterized by painful, sustained, and violent muscle spasms; it can be prevented through vaccination.

Thalassemia. An inherited form of anemia in which red

blood cells contain less hemoglobin than normal.

Thalidomide. A sedative and sleep-inducing drug that was found to produce phocomelia (a birth defect in which hands or feet are attached to the body by short, flipperlike stumps) in developing fetuses.

Thanatology. The study and investigation of life-threatening actions, terminal illness, suicide, homicide, death, dying, grief, and bereavement.

Therapeutics. The use of chemicals in the diagnosis, prevention, or treatment of disease.

Thermogenesis. The combustion of fuels to provide energy in excess of that required to perform biological work in order to maintain body temperature.

Thermoregulatory set point. The ultimate neural control that maintains the human internal body temperature at 37 degrees Celsius and can either raise or lower it as a defense mechanism against disease.

Thigh. The upper segment of the leg, from the hip joint to the knee.

Thoracic. Pertaining to the chest.

Thoracic duct. The largest lymphatic vessel, which collects lymphatic fluid and returns it to the bloodstream at the left subclavian vein in the region of the neck.

Thorax. The part of the trunk above the diaphragm, containing the ribs; also called the chest.

Thrombin. An enzyme that facilitates the clotting of blood by catalyzing a conversion of fibrinogen to fibrin.

Thrombocytes. Small, irregularly shaped cells in the blood that participate in blood clotting; also called platelets.

Thrombocytopenia. A bleeding disorder in which the blood contains an abnormally low count of functional platelets (thrombocytes).

Thromboembolism. The blockage of a blood vessel by a fragment that has broken off from a thrombus in another blood vessel.

Thrombolytic drugs. A group of drugs that dissolve blood clots by increasing the level of plasmin in the blood.

Thrombosis. The act of complete clotting of an artery or vein, through which no blood can then flow.

Thrombus. A blood clot that has formed inside an intact blood vessel; a thrombus can be life-threatening if it occludes a vessel that supplies the heart or brain.

Thymus. The lymphatic gland in which T lymphocytes mature; located in humans just below the thyroid.

Thyroid gland. A gland found in the neck that secretes the hormones responsible for the synthesis and breakdown of proteins and the metabolism of carbohydrates.

Thyroidectomy. Surgical removal of the thyroid gland.

Thyroxine. The chief hormone of the thyroid gland, an iodine-containing derivative of the amino acid tyrosine.

TIA. *See* Transient ischemic attack (TIA).

Tibia. The larger of the two bones in the lower leg, on the medial side.

Tincture. A homeopathic remedy in liquid form, normally with alcohol and water as a solvent; the most concentrated form is called the mother tincture, from which all dilutions are made.

Tinnitus. An auditory sensation originating in the head, without external stimulation; also called ringing in the ears.

Tissue. A specialized region of cells that forms organs within the body; the four principal types are epithelial, connective, nervous, and muscular; tissues have specific functions.

Tissue culture. A diagnostic method in which cells from plant or animal tissues bathed in sustaining liquid solution form a monolayer on a container that can be inoculated and observed for deterioration or destruction by replicating viruses.

Tissue plasminogen activator (TPA or tPA). A substance produced by the body to prevent abnormal blood clots by stimulating the formation of plasmin from plasminogen; can also be administered to dissolve blood clots.

Tissue typing. The process of identifying a person's transplantation antigens.

TMJ. *See* Temporomandibular joint (TMJ).

Tolerance. With repeated substance abuse, the need for increasing amounts of a substance to achieve the same effect.

Tomography. All types of body-section imaging techniques; that is, a visual representation restricted to a specified section or "cut" of tissue within an organ.

Tonsillectomy. Surgical removal of one or both tonsils.

Tonsillitis. Infection and inflammation of the tonsils; if severe or chronic, it may require removal of the tonsils.

Tonsils. Masses of lymphatic tissue lying on either side of the entrance to the throat near the back of the tongue.

Tooth decay. The common term for dental caries.

Tooth extraction. The surgical removal of a tooth because it is damaged by decay, disease, or trauma; threatening the health of other teeth; or near the site of significant disease.

Tooth pulp. The tissue at the center of teeth, surrounded by dentin.

Toothache. Pain in the teeth or gums ranging from a dull, throbbing sensation to intense, sharp pains.

Topical. Referring to treatments or procedures applied directly to the skin or mucous membranes that affect primarily the area in which they are applied.

Tort. A wrongful act for which civil courts, rather than criminal courts, are empowered to render justice.

Totipotence. The capacity for cells of a given tissue type to regenerate and replace killed or damaged cells within a given body region.

Touch. A special sense in which nerve endings and specialized structures in the skin and other tissues send the brain data about the organism's environment, both internal and external.

Toxemia. The presence of toxins in the blood produced by bacteria, which may be ingested or caused by an infection in the body; also called blood poisoning or septicemia.

Toxic shock syndrome. A potentially fatal infection causing failure of multiple organs of the body, most notably associated with tampon use.

Toxicokinetics. The study of the time course of chemical absorption, distribution, metabolism, and elimination of toxic chemicals in the body; when the chemicals considered are therapeutic drugs, the correct term is "pharmacokinetics."

Toxicology. The science devoted to the study of poisons.

Toxin. A poisonous substance that is a product of the chemical processes of a living organism.

Toxoid. A toxin that has been chemically treated to eliminate its toxic properties but that retains the same antigens as the original.

Toxoplasmosis. An infection caused by parasitic microorganisms that invade tissues and that may cause damage to the central nervous system, especially in fetuses.

TPA or tPA. *See* Tissue plasminogen activator.

Trace elements. Elements needed in the diet at levels of less than 100 milligrams per day.

Trace evidence. Minute, often microscopic, signs or indications of an event or a presence.

Tracer. A radioactive substance introduced into the body, the progress of which may be followed by means of an external radioactive detector; it must not affect the process that it is used to measure.

Trachea. The tube that leads from the throat to the lungs; commonly called the windpipe.

Tracheostomy. Surgical creation of an opening in the trachea.

Trachoma. A contagious eye infection, leading to blindness, that affects millions of people in developing countries.

Tract. A collection of nerve fibers (axons) in the brain or spinal cord that all have the same place of origin and the same place of termination.

Transcription. The process by which the information stored in DNA is copied into the structure of RNA for transport to the cytoplasm.

Transducer (probe). A device designed to transfer ultrasound waves into the body noninvasively, receive the returning echoes, and transform those echoes into electrical voltages.

Transference. The unconscious tendency of a person to re-create preexisting nonfunctional relationship patterns with others; psychoanalytic treatment depends on the development of transference between client and analyst.

Transfusion. Injection directly into the bloodstream of a large amount of blood or blood components, usually to correct loss of blood as a result of injury or during surgery.

Transgender. A general term for persons who deviate from masculine and feminine gender norms.

Transient ischemic attack (TIA). A brief loss of blood to the brain, accompanied by temporary impairment of vision and numbness.

Transitional cell carcinoma. Cancer arising from the lining of the urine collection system of the kidneys, ureters, and bladder.

Translation. The process by which the copied information in RNA is utilized in the production of a protein.

Transmission. The mode of acquiring a disease.

Transplantation. The movement of one part of the body (such as an organ) or one area of tissue to another, either within the same individual or from one individual to another.

Transsexuals. Individuals who genuinely believe that they exist in the body of the wrong sex, despite the fact that they are anatomically normal.

Transverse processes. Projections from the sides of vertebrae, to which are attached muscles and ligaments, that assist in motor function by enhancing leverage and limiting extremes of motion.

Transvestism. Also called cross-dressing; wearing clothing deemed appropriate for a person of the gender to which one is not socially and culturally identified.

Trauma. Physical injury to bodily tissue.

Trauma center. An emergency room (ER) that meets certain criteria for the delivery of care to those suffering severe injuries.

Treatment. Any specific procedure used for the cure or improvement of a disease or pathological condition.

Trephination. The opening of a hole in the skull.

Trephine. A specialized surgical instrument that is used to cut a perfectly vertical incision in bone or corneal tissue.

Triage. A process in which patient needs are evaluated and prioritized by a health care team and preliminary treatment plans are made.

Tricyclics. Medications used to relieve the symptoms of depression.

Trimester. An arbitrary division of a human pregnancy into three-month divisions based on development changes in the fetus over time.

Triple test. A blood test that screens for genetic defects.

Trisomy. The presence of an extra chromosome.

Tropical medicine. The area of medicine concerned particularly with diseases, often arthropod-borne (such as malaria, yellow fever, or schistosomiasis), that thrive in tropical latitudes.

Trunk. The central part of the body, to which the extremities are attached.

Tubal ligation. A procedure for rendering a woman sterile by cutting, constricting, or otherwise blocking the Fallopian tubes so that sperm cannot reach the ovum.

Tuberculosis. A chronic, highly infectious lung disease.

Tubular reabsorption. The process of returning important solutes that were filtered out of the blood back into the blood; these important solutes include glucose, amino acids, vitamins, and most ions.

Tubular secretion. The process of tubular reabsorption in reverse; important solutes moved from the filtrate to the urine include hydrogen and potassium ions, organic acids, ammonia, and creatine.

Tumor. An abnormal mass of tissue that may be malignant (growing larger) or benign (not spreading).

Turgor. Fullness and firmness; the quality of normal skin in a healthy young person.

Twins. The presence of two fetuses in the womb.

Tympanic membrane. The eardrum, which separates the external ear canal from the middle ear and ossicles and which transmits sound vibration to the ossicles.

Typhoid fever and typhus. Acute infectious diseases caused by bacteria or rickettsiae.

Ulcer. A lesion that destroys tissue.

Ulcerative colitis. An inflammatory disease that causes ulcers in the large intestine.

Ulna. The larger of the two forearm bones, forming the principal part of the elbow joint with the humerus.

Ulnar. Toward the edge of the forearm and hand containing the ulna and little finger.

Ultrasonic. Referring to any frequency of sound that is higher than the audible range-that is, higher than 20,000 cycles per second (20 kilohertz).

Ultrasonography. An imaging technique that employs sound waves to form an image, still or moving, of internal organs.

Ultraviolet radiation. Radiation that is potentially damaging to the skin; it is not visible to humans.

Umbilicus. The cord that contains the blood vessels connecting the fetus to the placenta.

Unconsciousness. A state in which an individual is unaware of either surroundings or self and lacks response to stimuli; includes sleep, fainting, and coma.

Universal coverage. Inclusion of all persons in health insurance, without exception.

Upper arm. The region from the shoulder joint to the elbow joint; also called the brachium.

Upper extremities. The arms (upper arms, forearms, and hands), which are attached to the shoulder blade at the shoulder joint and which consist of muscles, bones, blood vessels, lymph vessels, nerves, skin, and fingernails.

Urea. A waste product of protein metabolism, that represents the form in which nitrogen is eliminated from the body.

Uremia. The presence of excessive amounts of urea and other nitrogenous waste products in the blood.

Ureter. Either of the two tubes that carry urine from the kidneys to the bladder.

Ureterolithotomy. The surgical removal of a stone in the ureter.

Urethra. The tube that drains from the bladder to outside the body; in the male, the urethra passes through the penis and carries sperm during ejaculation, while in the female, the urethra opens in front of the vagina but does not have a reproductive function.

Urethritis. Inflammation or infection of the urethra as a result of bacterial infection.

Urethroplasty. Surgical repair of the urethra.

-uria. A suffix meaning the presence of a substance in urine; for example, hematuria refers to blood in the urine.

Urinalysis. Laboratory analysis of urine to determine presence, absence, or quantity of compounds that may point to disease.

Urinary bladder. A stretchable, muscular sac that functions to store urine.

Urinary system. A system, composed of the kidneys, ureters, urinary bladder, and urethra, that removes body waste, maintains the proper amount of body water, and regulates the acid-base balance of the blood.

Urinary tract infections (UTIs). Infections of the bladder, kidneys, urethra, and ureters (which connect the bladder to the kidneys); infection may be limited to one area of these organs or spread throughout the urinary tract.

Urine. Fluid collected in the kidneys that contains metabolic wastes, including urea and salts.

Urolithiasis. The formation of stones in the urinary tract.

Urology. The branch of medicine specializing in the urinary tracts of both sexes, and the genitourinary tract of the male.

Uterus. The organ that supports the embryo during its development.

UTIs. *See* Urinary tract infections (UTIs).

Uvea. The iris and ciliary body of the eye.

Uveitis. Inflammation of the uvea of the eye.

Vaccination. Induction of immunity in organisms by ingestion or injection of an etiological agent.

Vaccine. Any substance used for preventive inoculation to build immunity.

Vaccinia. A virus that causes a poxlike illness in cattle (cowpox); it serves as a smallpox vaccine in humans because of its similarity to the smallpox virus.

Vagina. The tube-shaped cavity of the female into which the male's penis is inserted during intercourse and through which a baby is delivered; the diaphragm, cervical cap, vaginal sponge, or spermicide can be inserted into the vagina as contraceptives.

Vaginitis. Inflammation and infection of the vagina.

Vagotomy. Surgical incision into the vagus nerve.

Vagus nerve. The tenth cranial nerve, which carries taste messages from the limited number of taste buds located in obscure sites such as the palate, epiglottis, uvula, and other structures at the entrance of the esophagus; also sends important information from the thoracic and abdominal viscera to the brain.

Valgus. A musculoskeletal deformity in which a limb is twisted outward from the body.

Validity, selective. A preliminary indication of a screening technique's capability to identify persons with preclinical disease as test-positive and those without preclinical disease as test-negative.

Valves. Structures that close periodically to allow the passage of blood, such as those that connect heart chambers to each other and to the great arteries.

Variable. Any quantity that varies, such as height or cholesterol level.

Varicocele. An enlarged vein surrounding the testicle as a result of incompetent venous valves; most commonly found surrounding the left testicle.

Varicosis. The distension of superficial veins, often in the legs; also known as varicose veins.

Varus. A musculoskeletal deformity in which a limb is twisted toward the body.

Vas deferens. The duct that carries the male seminal fluid.

Vascular. Relating to or containing blood vessels.

Vascular medicine. The diagnosis and management of diseases of the arteries, veins, and lymphatic system, exclusive of the heart and lungs.

Vascular system. The pipeline through which every cell of the body receives oxygen, vitamins, hormones, and the metabolic fuels necessary to sustain life.

Vascularized transplant. Transplanted tissue or organs that must have blood vessels reattached in the recipient in order to function (such as a kidney); corneal or bone marrow transplants are examples of nonvascularized transplants.

Vasculature. All the blood vessels, including the arteries (blood vessels carrying oxygenated blood away from the heart), the capillaries (the smallest blood vessels, where fluid and nutrients are exchanged between arteries and veins), and the veins (blood vessels that return deoxygenated blood to the heart).

Vasculitis. A number of conditions characterized by inflammation of blood vessels, both arteries and veins, that leads to decreased circulation in the affected tissue or organ, which can damage the tissue or organ.

Vasectomy. A surgical procedure to render a male sterile by cutting the two vas deferens, the ducts carrying sperm from the testes to the seminal vesicles.

Vasoconstriction. A decrease in the diameter of vessels transporting blood throughout the body, reducing blood flow and oxygen transport.

Vasodilation. An increase in the diameter of arteries, which decreases the amount of work required for the heart to move blood.

Vector. An organism, usually an insect or other arthropod, that transmits a disease from one host to another; the vector may itself be a host in which the pathogen multiplies, or it may merely transmit the pathogen mechanically.

Veins. Blood vessels that carry blood from the cells back to the heart.

Vena cava. A large vein that carries deoxygenated blood into the right atrium of the heart from the lower half of the body.

Venereal disease. Former term for sexually transmitted disease (STD).

Venipuncture. A method of obtaining blood from a vein using a tourniquet, needle, and syringe.

Venous insufficiency. An abnormality characterized by decreased blood return from the legs to the trunk that is caused by inefficient valves in the veins.

Venous thrombosis. The presence of blood clots in the veins, usually in the legs or arms.

Ventricles. Refers to the two lower chambers of the heart or the four fluid-filled cavities of the brain.

Ventriculoperitoneal. Referring to a type of shunt used to carry cerebrospinal fluid from the brain to the abdominal cavity.

Vertebra. A bony structure in the back with a central spinal canal surrounded by an arch; the back part of the arch (the lamina) and the front part of the arch (the pedicle) are joined together by muscles, ligaments, and cartilage for motion, stability, and posture.

Vertebroplasty. Considered a minor invasive surgery for back pain from osteoporosis, a back tumor, or back trauma, it is usually performed in an x-ray suite or hospital operating room under light sedation. A biopsy needle is inserted into the problem area and bone cement is injected under high pressure until the area is secured. The needle is then withdrawn.

Vertigo. A sensation of motion or spinning when not moving.

Vesicle. A fluid-filled blister.

Villi. Fingerlike projections on the intestinal lining that absorb essential body nutrients after enzymes break down chyme.

Virilization. The development of masculine sex characteristics in a female.

Virion. A single virus particle.

Virulence. Level of aggressiveness of an organism.

Virus. A subcellular particle that enters cells and causes cellular damage; it uses cellular mechanisms to reproduce itself.

Visual acuity. Clarity or clearness in vision.

Vital organs. Organs of the body essential to life, usually considered to be the brain, the heart, the lungs, the liver, and sometimes the kidneys.

Vitamins. Organic compounds, essential for life but required in very minute quantities, that participate in biochemical reactions and help to release energy from the three classes of nutrients.

Vitiligo. A disorder that occurs when cells that make pigment in the skin are destroyed, leading to white patches on the body; may also affect the eyes and the mucous membranes of the mouth and nose and cause hair to gray.

Vitrectomy. Surgical removal of the vitreous humor.

Vitreous humor. The clear, jellylike substance that fills the eyeball; also called the aqueous humor.

Voltage. Energy per unit charge; typical biological voltages range from hundredths to tenths of a volt.

Voluntary euthanasia. A patient's consent to a decision that results in the shortening of his or her life.

Vomiting. The regurgitation of the contents of the stomach.

Wasting. Severe weight loss characterized by the loss of both muscle tissue and body-fat deposits.

Wavelength. A property used to measure colors in the spectrum of light from infrared to ultraviolet; usually expressed in units of microns (1 micron is equal to one-millionth of a meter).

Wedge argument. A logically contrived argument supporting a morally acceptable action that subsequently leads to other actions that are considered morally unacceptable.

Whiplash. Injury to the ligaments, joints, and soft tissues of the neck region of the spine due to a sudden, violent jerking motion.

White blood cells. Colorless, large blood cells that work together to combat infections.

WHO. *See* World Health Organization (WHO).

Whole blood. Blood from which none of the elements has been removed.

Wilson's disease. An inherited disease of abnormal copper metabolism, leading to copper accumulation and toxicity in the liver and brain.

Withdrawal. A physical and mental condition following decreased intake of an abusable substance, with symptoms ranging from anxiety to convulsions.

Wolffian ducts. The pair of tubes in the early embryo that will develop into the internal male organs (the epididymis, the vas deferens, and the seminal vesicles).

World Health Organization (WHO). A specialized agency of the United Nations that fights illness and disease all over the globe.

Wounds. Injuries classified as open or closed depending on whether the skin is broken; types of open wounds include abrasions, lacerations, avulsions, punctures, and incisions.

X and Y chromosomes. The chromosomes that determine genetic sex; males carry an XY pair and females carry an XX pair.

X radiology. The use of ionizing radiation of short wavelength to detect abnormalities in primarily dense portions of the body.

X-ray tube. A high-voltage electronic device used to produce X rays; X-ray tubes are used in X-ray machines, fluoroscopes, and CT scanners.

X rays. Penetrating radiation produced by means of a high-voltage machine; useful for both the diagnosis and the treatment of cancerous tissue.

Xanthomatosis. A condition in which fatty deposits appear anywhere in the body, including various areas of the skin, internal organs, eyes, and tendons.

Xenobiotics. Drugs and chemical compounds foreign to the body; the terms "xenobiotic," "toxin," "drug," and "chemical" are used interchangeably when discussing toxicology, since all substances are poisonous at some concentration.

Xenotransplantation. The transplantation of tissue or organs between different species (such as baboon to human).

Yang. The Chinese concept of the positive, male element of the universe.

Yin. The Chinese concept of the negative, female element of the universe.

Yoga. A mental discipline, originating in India, designed to master consciousness, to offer spiritual insight, and to induce tranquillity.

Zeugmatography. A name applied to MRI characterizing the close relationship of nuclear magnetic forces and electromagnetic waves (from the Greek *zeugma*, meaning "to yoke together").

Zidovudine. A drug, formerly known as azidothymidine (AZT), used to treat HIV infection; it interferes with the functioning of the virus's reverse transcriptase enzyme.

Zona pellucida. A translucent layer surrounding the mammalian egg; it promotes fertilization by causing the acrosome reaction in the sperm and also prevents polyspermy.

Zoonoses. Diseases communicable between animals and humans.

Zygoma. The cheekbone.

Zygote. A fertilized ovum before multicelluar development begins.

SYMPTOMS AND WARNING SIGNS

WARNING SIGNS OF COMMON DISEASES

CANCER
Forms of cancer differ by age, race, and sex, but the most common cancers in industrialized countries are lung, reproductive organ (prostate gland, breast, uterus), and colon. Early detection is critical. Signs may include the following:
- Breast lump or nipple discharge
- Change in bowel habits (unexplained by diet or medications)
- Change in color, shape, size or texture of a skin mole
- Chronic cough
- Difficulty urinating
- Noninfectious swollen glands (lymph nodes)
- Vaginal bleeding between periods or in menopausal women

DIABETES
This disease has two forms. Type 1 begins in childhood or early adulthood, is usually detected quickly in pediatric visits, and requires insulin injections from the start, along with dietary restrictions. Type 2 presents itself in adulthood, usually without obvious symptoms at first. This form can be treated with diet and perhaps by medications; insulin is usually a last resort. It is important to recognize type 2 diabetes by these signs:
- Blurry vision
- Excessive thirst
- Excessive urination
- Frequent vaginal yeast infections
- Unexplained weight change

HYPERTENSION
High blood pressure is known as the "silent killer," as few symptoms present themselves. **Note:** This diagnosis depends on having several blood pressure readings higher than 140/90 on different occasions after rest. Risk factors include the following:
- Diabetes
- Family history of hypertension
- Increased age (although younger for African Americans)
- Kidney disease
- Medication side effect
- Obesity
- Poor diet (high sodium; low potassium, magnesium, calcium)
- Sleep apnea

STROKES AND MINISTROKES
Ministrokes are often overlooked but are warnings of possible vascular problems. Their symptoms are sudden and short-lived (lasting one to two hours):

- Disorders of equilibrium, movement, speech, vision
- Heaviness or weakness of limbs
- Numbness
- Continuation of symptoms beyond twenty-four hours implies that a stroke has occurred

SYMPTOMS AND POSSIBLE CONDITIONS

ABDOMINAL PAIN
Diffuse, nonlocalized
- Gastroenteritis (stomach or intestinal infection)

Lower left side
- Appendicitis (rarely)
- Diverticulitis
- Hernia
- Kidney stones
- Pelvic infection

Lower right side
- Appendicitis
- Kidney stones

Upper left side
- Kidney stones
- Ulcer

Upper right side
- Gallbladder inflammation or infection
- Kidney stones
- Liver disorder
- Ulcer

BACK PAIN (LOWER BACK)
- Arthritis
- Herniated disk
- Kidney stones
- Muscle injury
- Sciatica

BLOOD
In phlegm (coughing up blood)
- Blood clot in lung
- Bronchitis
- Lung cancer
- Pneumonia
- Tuberculosis

In stool
- Anal fissure
- Colorectal cancer
- Hemorrhoids
- Ulcer
- Ulcerative colitis or Crohn's disease

In urine
- Bladder infection
- Kidney stones

Breast Disorder
Discharge
- Breast cancer
- Contraceptive use
- Hormone therapy
- Medication side effect

Swelling and/or pain
- Benign tumors or cysts
- Cancer
- Trauma

Chest Pain
Deep, dull, poorly localized
- Angina
- Gallbladder inflammation or infection

Sharp, well localized
- Hernia
- Muscle injury
- Rib fracture
- Shingles
- Ulcer

Constipation
- Colorectal cancer (sudden onset of constipation)
- Dehydration
- Hemorrhoids
- Impaction
- Medication side effect

Cough
- Allergy
- Bronchitis
- Emphysema
- Pneumonia

Diarrhea
- Antibiotics and other drugs
- Appendicitis
- Colorectal cancer
- Diverticular disease
- Food intolerance
- Infections
- Ulcerative colitis or Crohn's disease

Dizziness
- Anemia
- Anxiety
- Heart-related problem
- Inner-ear problem
- Low blood pressure
- Low blood sugar
- Ministroke

Eye Discomfort
Burning
- Dryness

Discharge
- Allergic conjunctivitis
- Bacterial or viral conjunctivitis

Itching
- Allergy

Pain
- Foreign object
- Infection
- Inflammation
- Trauma

Redness
- Conjunctivitis
- Corneal disorder
- Glaucoma

Fainting
- Anxiety
- Blood pressure drop
- Heart-related problem
- Low blood sugar

Fatigue
- Anxiety
- Depression
- Malnutrition
- Obesity
- Poor physical conditioning
- Sleep disturbance

Fever
- Bacterial infection
- Fungal infection
- Viral infection

Gas (Flatulence)
- Food intolerance
- Peptic ulcer

Headache
- Eyestrain
- Migraine headache
- Sinusitis
- Tension headache

Heart Palpitations
- Anemia
- Anxiety
- Arrhythmias (abnormal heartbeat)
- Heart valve dysfunction
- Hyperthyroidism (overactive thyroid)

Heartburn
- Food intolerance
- Gallbladder inflammation or infection
- Gastric (acid) reflux
- Medication side effect
- Ulcer

JAUNDICE
- Excess vitamin A
- Gallbladder inflammation or infection
- Hepatitis
- Liver inflammation or infection
- Medication

NASAL DISCHARGE
Clear
- Allergies

Discolored
- Sinus infection

NAUSEA AND VOMITING
- Appendicitis
- Early pregnancy
- Food intolerance or poisoning
- Gallbladder inflammation or infection
- Gastric intestinal infection
- Hepatitis
- Ulcer

NOSEBLEED
- Aspirin or blood thinner
- Sinus infection
- Spontaneous small blood vessel rupture
- Trauma

PENILE DISCHARGE (PUS)
- Infection (bladder or prostate)
- Sexually transmitted disease (STD)

RECTAL BLEEDING
- Anal fissure
- Colitis
- Colorectal cancer
- Diverticulosis
- Hemorrhoids

SEIZURES
- Alcohol or drug withdrawal
- Epilepsy
- High fever
- Low blood sugar
- Low potassium

SHORTNESS OF BREATH
- Anemia
- Anxiety
- Asthma
- Blood clot in lungs
- Bronchitis
- Collapsed lung
- Congestive heart failure
- Heart attack
- Pneumonia

SINUS PAIN AND PRESSURE
- Allergy
- Infection

SWALLOWING DIFFICULTY
- Allergic reaction
- Infection (yeast)
- Neurological disease
- Strep throat
- Tonsillitis

SWOLLEN ANKLES
- Arthritis
- Congestive heart failure
- Excessive salt intake
- Kidney failure
- Malnutrition

SWOLLEN GLANDS
- Infection
- Leukemia
- Lymphoma

SWOLLEN JOINTS
Chronic
- Arthritis
- Trauma

Sudden
- Gout
- Infection
- Lyme disease
- Trauma

TREMOR
- Alcoholism
- Anxiety
- Benign old-age condition
- Dementia
- Medication
- Multiple sclerosis
- Parkinson's disease

URINATION DISORDER
Difficulty
- Enlarged prostate gland
- Infection and inflammation
- Sexually transmitted disease (STD)

Frequency (incontinence)
- Alcohol
- Bladder cancer
- Caffeine
- Diabetes
- Diuretic drugs
- Infection (bladder or prostate)
- Pregnancy

VAGINAL BLEEDING
Premenopause
- Cervical cancer
- Cervical polyps or warts
- Ectopic pregnancy
- Impending miscarriage
- Infection

Postmenopause
- Cervical cancer
- Infection
- Uterine cancer

VAGINAL DISCOMFORT
Discharge
- Infection

Itching
- Dryness
- Yeast infection

Pain
- Dryness
- Infection or inflammation
- Psychological muscular contractions

WEIGHT GAIN
- Diabetes
- Hypothyroidism (underactive thyroid)
- Medication

WEIGHT LOSS
- Alcoholism
- Anorexia
- Depression
- Hyperthyroidism (overactive thyroid)
- Loss of appetite (medication)

—Mel Siegel, M.A.; Connie Rizzo, M.D., Ph.D., consultant

Diseases and Other Medical Conditions

Abdominal disorders. Disorders affecting the wide range of organs found in the torso of the body, including diseases of the stomach, intestines, liver, and pancreas.

Abscesses. Any enclosed collection of pus, whether sterile or infected.

Accidents. An occurrence in a sequence of events that produces unintended injury, death, or property damage. Accident refers to the event, not the result of the event. Unintentional injury refers to the result of an accident and is the prefer red term in the health community for accidental injury.

Achalasia. A swallowing disorder that prevents the movement of food from the esophagus to the stomach.

Acid reflux disease. A chronic digestive disorder in which the lower esophageal sphincter (LES), which keeps digestive juices in the stomach, relaxes and permits gastric acid to rise into the esophagus, causing a burning sensation.

Acidosis. A state of excess acidity in the body's fluids; metabolic acidosis involves the kidneys, while respiratory acidosis involves the lungs.

Acne. A group of skin disorders, the most common of which, acne vulgaris, usually affects teenagers; another form, acne rosacea, usually afflicts older people.

Acquired immunodeficiency syndrome (AIDS). A disease state caused by infection with human immunodeficiency virus (HIV), leading to a progressive deterioration of the immune system and characterized by development of any of a large number of opportunistic infections.

Acute respiratory distress syndrome (ARDS). Respiratory failure caused by filling of the lungs with fluid from the capillaries, leading to a shortage of oxygen in the body that can eventually lead to death if not treated.

Addiction. A process whereby an organism comes to depend on a substance psychologically and/or physiologically. Physiological dependence is marked tolerance and/or withdrawal from the specific substance.

Addison's disease. A failure of adrenal cortex function in which production of any or all of the hormones synthesized by the cortex is decreased.

Adenoviruses. Medium-sized viruses that can cause respiratory infections and diarrhea by infecting the tissue linings of the respiratory and urinary tracts, the intestines, and the eyes.

Adrenoleukodystrophy. A variable X-linked genetic disorder with symptoms ranging from adrenal insufficiency to progressive neurological deterioration.

Agnosia. Inability to identify objects or persons using one or more of the senses, even though the basic sensory modalities are not defective.

AIDS. *See* Acquired immunodeficiency syndrome (AIDS).

Alcoholism. A condition in which dependence on alcohol harms a person's health, social functioning, or family life.

Allergies. Exaggerated immune reactions to materials that are intrinsically harmless; the body's release of pharmacologically active chemicals during allergic reactions may result in discomfort, tissue damage, or, in severe responses, death.

Alopecia. Temporary or permanent hair loss.

Altitude sickness. A condition resulting from altitude-related hypoxia (low oxygen levels).

Alzheimer's disease. A relentlessly progressive disease resulting in the loss of higher cognitive function; the most common form of dementia.

Amebiasis. Infection of the colon or associated organs by the parasite *Entamoeba histolytica*.

Amenorrhea. The absence of menstrual cycles.

Amnesia. The loss of memory due to physical and/or psychological conditions.

Amyotrophic lateral sclerosis. A progressive, degenerative neurological disorder that affects the cells in the brain and spinal cord.

Anal cancer. Cancer affecting the lower alimentary tract, including the interior anal canal from the anorectal ring to the anal verge with 5 centimeters of skin extending beyond, including the perianal skin.

Anemia. Anemia is defined as a decrease in the oxygen-carrying capacity of blood with a reduction in the red blood cell count and/or hemoglobin.

Aneurysms. A localized dilatation of a blood vessel, particularly an artery, that results from a focal weakness and distension of the arterial wall.

Angelman syndrome. A complex genetic disorder that causes developmental disabilities and neurological problems.

Angina. Chest pain ranging from mild indigestion to a severe crushing, squeezing, or choking sensation.

Ankylosing spondylitis. A chronic, progressive, inflammatory disease of the spine and other joints

Anorexia nervosa. Self-induced malnutrition resulting in a body weight 15 percent or more below normal for age and height, and, in women, characterized by the absence of three or more consecutive menstrual periods.

Anosmia. A complete loss in the ability to detect odors.

Anthrax. A bacterial infection of humans and other animals, especially herbivores, which occurs following entrance into the body of *Bacillus anthracis* spores through abrasions in the skin or by ingestion or inhalation.

Antibiotic resistance. The ability of micro-organisms to survive and reproduce in the presence of a drug that formerly killed or inhibited it.

Anxiety. Heightened fear or tension that causes psychological and physical distress; the American Psychiatric Association recognizes six types of anxiety disorders, which can be treated with medications or through counseling.

Aortic aneurysm. A dilation or ballooning of the arterial vessel wall to twice its original size, creating an area of weakness.

Aortic stenosis. Narrowing of the bicuspid or tricuspid valve, preventing blood flow from the left ventricle to the aorta.

Aphasia and dysphasia. Aphasia is loss of the comprehension or production of language, while dysphasia is impairment of comprehension or production of language.

Apnea. Cessation of breathing, from the Greek meaning without wind.

Appendicitis. Inflammation of the human vermiform appendix.

Arrhythmias. A disturbance of electrical conduction activity in the heart. Potential causes range from medications to diseases or conditions that delay or block an impulse in the conduction system.

Arteriosclerosis. Also called atherosclerotic disease or hardening of the arteries, a generalized disease that causes narrowing of the arteries because of deposits on the arterial walls and leads to a multitude of serious medical conditions, notably s troke and heart attack.

Arthritis. A group of more than one hundred inflammatory diseases that damage joints and their surrounding structures, resulting in symptomatic pain, disability, and systemwide inflammation.

Asbestos exposure. Asbestos is a naturally occurring fire-resistant mineral fiber historically used in a variety of applications ranging from lamp wicks to roofing shingles. Asbestos fibers consist of silica compounds that can irritate human tissue, resu lting in disorders such as asbestosis as well as cancers of the lung, larynx, and gastrointestinal system.

Asperger's syndrome. A pervasive developmental disorder involving clinically significant impairment in social interactions and repetitive or stereotyped patterns of behavior, but no particular problem with cognitive functioning.

Aspergillosis. Infection with fungi from the genus *Aspergillus,* which initially produce pulmonary hypersensitivity reactions or colonize the lung and then either grow within a pulmonary cavity or disseminate through the blood to other organs.

Asphyxiation. The state of unconsciousness or death resulting from oxygen deprivation

Asthma. A chronic inflammatory obstructive pulmonary disease that obstructs the airways to the lungs and makes it difficult or, in severe attacks, nearly impossible to breathe.

Astigmatism. A slight deformation of the eyeball that makes it impossible for a person to form a sharp image of two perpendicular lines simultaneously.

Ataxia. A lack of coordination while performing voluntary movements that may appear as clumsiness, inaccuracy, or instability.

Athlete's foot. A microscopic fungal infection that lives on the outer layers of skin, nails, or hair on the feet.

Atrial fibrillation. Abnormal heart rhythm or muscle contractions in the atria as a result of disorganized electrical impulses.

Atrophy. A wasting away or decrease in size and/or activity of a body part because of disease or other influences such as inactivity. Skeletal muscle can undergo atrophy because of disuse or neurological and musculoskeletal disease.

Attention-deficit disorder (ADD). A condition characterized by an inability to focus attention or to inhibit impulsive, hyperactive behavior; it is associated with poor academic performance and behavioral problems in children but also may be diagnosed in adults under c ertain conditions.

Auras. Warning sensations of varying kinds received by the patient prior to a seizure, migraine, or psychotic episode.

Autism. A neurodevelopmental disorder characterized by impairment in emotional expression and recognition, difficulty with social relationships, delayed and/or abnormal language and communication, and preoccupation with repetitive, stereotyped behaviors or interests.

Autoimmune disorders. Damage to the tissues or organs of the body caused by failure of the immune system to distinguish between self and nonself, producing autoantibodies or autoreactive T lymphocytes (T cells).

Avian influenza. Avian influenza is caused by several virus strains that attack birds; occasionally, a strain develops the ability to attack humans, sometimes triggering an epidemic. There is concern that the H5N1 strain could mutate into a form that i s highly contagious among humans and result in a pandemic.

Babesiosis. A parasitic disease that is transmitted to humans by the bite of an infected tick.

Back disorders. *See* Back pain; Spinal cord disorders.

Back pain. Acute or chronic and usually severe pain centered along the spine, usually in the lower back but also common in the neck and upper back.

Bacterial infections. Infectious diseases caused by bacteria, of which hundreds exist.

Balance disorders. Problems with balance that may be described by sufferers as dizziness or vertigo and usually are associated with the inner ear; balance disorders may result in falls and other accidents.

Baldness. *See* Hair loss and baldness.

Basal cell carcinoma. *See* Skin cancer.

Batten's disease. A progressive neurological disruption and deterioration of intellectual and physical development caused by mutated genes.

Bed-wetting. A condition characterized by an inability of the bladder to contain the urine during sleep, often a developmental condition in children.

Bedsores. Sores caused by sustained pressure with restricted blood flow to the skin.

Behçet's disease. A multisystem disease characterized by recurrent oral and genital ulcers.

Bell's palsy. A weakening or paralysis of facial muscles caused by damage to the seventh cranial nerve.

Benign prostatic hyperplasia. *See* Prostate enlargement.

Beriberi. A nutritional disease resulting from thiamine deficiency.

Bipolar disorders. Affective (mood-related) illness characterized by periods of depressed and elevated mood.

Birth defects. Congenital malformations or structural anomalies and their accompanying functional disorders that originate during embryonic development; they are involved in up to 6 percent of human live births.

Bites and stings. Injuries from animals or insects.

Bladder cancer. Cancer that forms in tissues of the bladder, including transitional cell carcinomas (cancers that form in cells in the innermost tissue layer of the bladder), which account for about 90 percent of all bladder cancer cases; squamous cel l carcinomas (cancers that begin in flat cells lining the bladder); and adenocarcinomas (cancers that begin in cells that release fluids). In 2002, 357,000 new cases and 145,000 deaths were attributed to the disease worldwide.

Bladder infections. *See* Urinary disorders.

Bladder stones. *See* Stone removal; Stones.

Blindness. The absence of vision, or its extreme impairment to the extent that activity is limited; about 95 percent of all blindness is caused by eye diseases, the rest by injuries.

Blindsight. The ability of some patients with occipital cortex damage to respond at above chance levels to stimuli presented in their blind visual field.

Blisters. A local swelling of the skin that contains watery fluid and is usually caused by burning or irritation.

Blood poisoning. *See* Septicemia.

Blue baby syndrome. A congenital heart disease consisting of four distinct defects that result in poorly oxygenated blood being delivered to the tissues, thereby causing a bluish discoloration of the skin and mucous membranes upon birth.

Blurred vision. A decrease in clarity of vision (visual acuity).

Body dysmorphic disorder. A psychiatric somatoform disorder resulting in exaggerated preoccupation with an imagined or minor defect in physical appearance that causes significant impairment of social functioning.

Bone cancer. Cancer of the bone, which may have originated there or have spread from another site in the body.

Bone disorders. The various traumatic events that can occur to the bones and the tissues surrounding them, such as fractures, dislocations, degenerative processes, infections, and cancer.

Bone fractures. *See* Fracture and dislocation.

Botulism. A paralytic illness caused by a powerful neurotoxin produced by the bacterium *Clostridium botulinum.*

Bowlegs. A deformity of the legs that can be temporary or persistent, depending on causation.

Brain damage. Mild, moderate, or traumatic brain injury, which occurs when cells that make up the brain die.

Brain disorders. Disorders of the brain can interfere with its role in the control of body functions, behavior, learning, and expression, while defects can also threaten life itself.

Brain tumors. An abnormal growth in or on the brain.

Breast cancer. A general term for a group of solid tumor malignancies arising in the tissues of the breast.

Breast disorders. A variety of benign breast conditions, including fibrocystic disease and mastitis, which cause discomfort and anxiety and can make self-examination and diagnosis of cancer difficult.

Breathing difficulty. *See* Pulmonary diseases; Respiration; Respiratory distress syndrome.

Bronchiolitis. An inflammation of the bronchioles that affects breathing and the transfer of oxygen to the bloodstream.

Bronchitis. An inflammation of the bronchial tree of the lungs.

Brucellosis. A bacterial infection transmitted to humans from infected livestock and wildlife that is usually acquired from unpasteurized dairy products.

Bruises. A bruise is an area of skin that has become discolored, usually as a result of trauma (a fall or hit to the affected area).

Bulimia. An eating disorder that is characterized by repeated, uncontrollable episodes of overeating followed by induced vomiting or laxative abuse to eliminate the undigested food.

Bunions. An enlargement that develops on the joint of the big toe, producing deformity, pain, and discomfort.

Burkitt's lymphoma. A highly aggressive lymphoma often presenting in extranodal sites or as an acute leukemia.

Burns and scalds. Injury to skin and other tissues caused by contact with dry heat (fire), moist heat (steam or hot liquid), chemicals, electricity, lightning, or radiation.

Bursitis. An inflammation of a bursa, one of the membranes that surround joints.

Calculi. *See* Stones.

Campylobacter infections. An acute disease, often spontaneously resolving, caused by bacterial infection; sometimes called food poisoning.

Cancer. Inappropriate and uncontrollable cell growth within one of the specialized tissues of the body, threatening normal cell and organ function and in serious cases traveling via the bloodstream to other areas of the body.

Candidiasis. An acute or chronic fungal infection of humans and animals that can be superficial or deep-seated, caused by a species of the fungus *Candida.*

Canker sores. Small, round ulcers of the mucous membranes that line the mouth.

Capgras syndrome. The delusional belief that at least one family member or friend or significant other has been replaced by an impostor

Carcinogens. A substance or agent that causes or precipitates cancer.

Carcinoma. A malignant neoplasm or tumor that arises in epithelial cells.

Cardiac arrest. A complete cessation of the mechanical and/or electrical activity of the heart.

Carpal tunnel syndrome. A common disorder that causes discomfort and decreased hand dexterity via excessive pressure on the median nerve at the wrist, often caused by repetitive wrist and hand movements.

Cataracts. Dark regions in the lens of the eye that cause gradual loss of vision.

2464 • DISEASES AND OTHER MEDICAL CONDITIONS

Cavities. Cavities are erosions of the surface of teeth that can excavate the tooth surface and damage tooth structure.

Celiac sprue. Inflammation of the small intestine resulting from an abnormal response to gluten in the diet.

Cerebral palsy. A motor disability evident early in life (often by one year of age and certainly by age two) that is caused by a brain abnormality present by the end of the newborn period (one month of age) and unchanged after that time.

Cervical, ovarian, and uterine cancers. Primary cancers of the female reproductive system.

Chagas' disease. An acute disease that is most common in children and caused by the protozoan *Trypanosoma cruzi.*

Charcot-Marie-Tooth Disease. A group of inherited neurological disorders that damage peripheral nerves.

Chest pain. *See* Angina; Heart attack; Pain.

Chiari malformations. A group of disorders where the cerebellum extends below the opening of the spinal canal (the foramen magnum). Chiari malformations are classified according to severity and how much of the brain extends into the spinal canal: Type I is the most common and may be asymptomatic, type II is considered the classic Chiari malformation, and types III and IV are rare and the most serious.

Chickenpox. A highly infectious viral disease occurring primarily in children. Chickenpox is characterized by weakness, fever, and a generalized body rash.

Childbirth complications. The difficulties that can occur during childbirth, either for the mother or for the baby.

Childhood infectious diseases. A group of diseases including diphtheria, tetanus, measles, polio, rubella (German measles), mumps, varicella (chickenpox), hepatitis, and pertussis (whooping cough).

Chlamydia. The most common sexually transmitted bacterial disease in the United States, which primarily infects the reproductive tract and is caused by the bacterium *Chlamydia trachomatis.*

Choking. A condition in which the breathing passage (windpipe) is obstructed.

Cholecystitis. An inflammation of the gallbladder.

Cholera. An acute bacterial disease transmitted by polluted water and contaminated food.

Chromosomal abnormalities. *See* Birth defects; Genetic diseases.

Chronic fatigue syndrome. Chronic fatigue syndrome is a multifaceted disease state characterized by debilitating fatigue.

Chronic granulomatous disease. An inherited immune system disorder that prevents particular white blood cells (phagocytes) from effectively killing micro-organisms and leads to recurrent infections.

Chronic obstructive pulmonary disease (COPD). A progressive, irreversible disease of the lungs that causes expiratory airflow obstruction. The most common form of COPD is a combination of chronic bronchitis and emphysema.

Chronic wasting disease (CWD). A neurological disease of deer and elk caused by an infectious protein particle called a prion.

Cirrhosis. The formation of scar tissue in the liver, which interferes with its normal function.

Claudication. Pain in the calf or thigh muscle brought on by walking and relieved by rest.

Cleft lip and palate. A fissure in the midline of the palate, resulting from the failure of the two sides to fuse during embryonic development; in some cases, the fissure may extend through both hard and soft palates into the nasal cavities.

Clostridium difficile infection. An acute, contagious gastrointestinal infection caused by the anaerobic, gram-positive, spore-forming bacillus, *Clostridium difficile.*

Club drugs. A slang term for a variety of substances of abuse that generally are used in social situations, have hallucinogenic properties, and may either excite or sedate the user.

Cluster headaches. The most severe headache syndrome, characterized by paroxysmal onset of one side of the head, short duration, and episodic occurrence. Cluster headaches are often confused with migraine headaches, which are a similar syndrome but with different causes, patterns, and treatments.

Coccidioidomycosis. A fungal infection acquired by inhaling the spores of particular soil-based fungi. It initially attacks the lungs and often resolves without causing symptoms, but it can cause pneumonia and disseminate throughout the body.

Cockayne Disease. A rare, inherited genetic disease characterized by short stature and premature aging.

Cold agglutinin disease. A disease characterized by the production of antibodies against red blood cells that destroy them and cause anemia.

Cold sores. An infectious disease characterized by thin-walled vesicles around the mouth.

Colic. As a general term, a paroxysm of acute abdominal pain caused by spasm, obstruction, or twisting of a hollow abdominal organ. As a specific entity, infantile colic is a group of behaviors displayed by young infants including crying, fac ial grimacing, drawing-up of the legs over the abdomen, and clenching of the fists.

Colitis. A potentially fatal but manageable disease of the colon that inflames and ulcerates the bowel lining, occurring in both acute and chronic forms.

Collodion baby. A baby is born encased in a tight, shiny membrane.

Color blindness. An inability to distinguish certain colors resulting from an inherited defect in the light receptor cells in the retina of the eye.

Colorectal cancer. Cancer occurring in the large intestine, which is the second deadliest type of this disease.

Common cold. A class of viral respiratory infections that form the world's most prevalent illnesses.

Concussion. Mild brain injury that briefly impairs neurological functions.

Congenital adrenal hyperplasia. A family of genetic conditions that affect hormone production by the adrenal glands.

Congenital disorders. An abnormality present at birth, which may be due to a genetic defect, exposure to a toxic or infectious agent in utero, or a deficiency or lack of a substance necessary for fetal development.

Congenital heart disease. Conditions resulting from malformations of the heart that occur during embryonic and fetal development, accounting for about 25 percent of all congenital defects.

Congenital hypothyroidism. Retardation of mental and physical growth arising from prenatal or neonatal hypothyroidism.

Congestive heart failure. *See* Heart failure.

Conjunctivitis. An acute inflammatory disease of the eye caused by infection or irritation.

Constipation. The slow passage of feces through the bowels or the presence of hard feces.

Cornelia de Lange syndrome. A disorder with distinctive physical abnormalities and mental retardation usually apparent at birth.

Corns and calluses. Areas of thickened skin that form as a result of constant pressure or friction over a bony prominence.

Coronaviruses. Viruses frequently infecting the upper respiratory system and capable of producing either the common cold or severe acute respiratory syndrome (SARS).

Coughing. A physiological act in which air is forcibly expelled from the lungs.

Craniosynostosis. The premature closing of the open areas between the bones in an infant's skull.

Cretinism. *See* Congenital hypothyroidism.

Creutzfeldt-Jakob disease (CJD). Creutzfeldt-Jakob disease (CJD) is a human central nervous system disorder that is characterized by distinctive lesions in the brain, progressive dementia, lack of coordination, and eventual death. Although uncommon, it is the most prevalent of the human spongiform encephalopathies, inherited or transmissible illnesses of uncertain etiology associated with proteinaceous molecules called prions. Mad cow disease is a spongiform encephalopathy that affects cattle but may be tra

Crohn's disease. A chronic disease process in which the bowel becomes inflamed, leading to scarring and narrowing of the intestines.

Crossed eyes. *See* Strabismus.

Croup. An inflammation of the larynx, throat, and upper bronchial tubes causing hoarseness, cough, and difficult breathing.

Cushing's syndrome. A hormonal disorder caused primarily by chronic exposure of body tissues to excessive levels of cortisol.

Cutis marmorata telangiectatica congenita. Congenital abnormalities of the small blood vessels in the skin that are also usually associated with other congenital abnormalities.

Cyanosis. Dark blue discoloration of the skin and nail beds resulting from decreases in the oxygenation of hemoglobin in the red blood cells in the arteries.

Cystic fibrosis. A disease that affects the exocrine glands and, secondarily, most physical systems, resulting in death usually between the ages of sixteen and thirty.

Cystitis. An inflammation of the bladder, primarily caused by bacteria and resulting in pain, a sense of urgency to urinate, and sometimes hematuria (blood in the urine).

Cysts. A walled-off sac that is not normally found in the tissue where it occurs. To be a true cyst, a lump must have a capsule around it. Cysts usually contain a liquid or semisolid core (center) and vary in size from microscopic to very large. They may occur in any tissue of the body in a person of any age.

Cytomegalovirus (CMV). A viral disease normally producing mild symptoms in healthy individuals but severe infections in the immunocompromised. Congenital infection may lead to malformations or fetal death.

Deafness. Deafness is either partial or complete loss of hearing. Hearing loss occurs most often in older adults, but people may be born deaf or become deaf at young ages.

Deep vein thrombosis. The formation of a blood clot (thrombus) in a deep vein that prevents blood circulation.

Dehydration. Excessive loss of body water, which is often accompanied by disturbances in electrolyte balance.

Delirium. A neurocognitive disorder characterized by a change in attention and awareness (i.e., reduced ability to direct, focus, sustain, and shift attention).

Dementias. A group of disorders involving pervasive, progressive, and irreversible decline in cognitive functioning resulting from a variety of causes; differs from mental retardation, in which the affected person never reaches an expected level of mental growth.

Dengue fever. A flulike viral illness, contracted by humans through the bite of an infected *Aedes* mosquito.

Dental diseases. Diseases that affect the teeth, such as dental caries, and the gums, such as gingivitis, pyorrhea, or cancer.

Depression. One of the most common psychiatric disorders to occur in most lifetimes, caused by biological, psychological, social, and/or environmental factors.

Dermatitis. A wide range of skin disorders, some the result of allergy, some caused by contact with a skin irritant, and some attributable to other causes.

Developmental disorders. A group of conditions that indicate significant delays in or a lack of social skill development with deficiencies in adaptive behaviors, poor language skills, and a limited capacity to communicate effectively.

Diabetes mellitus. A hormonal disorder in which proper blood sugar levels are not maintained; due either to insufficient production of insulin by the pancreas or to an inability of the body's cells to use insulin efficiently. If left untreated, diabetes mellitus leads to complications such as blindness, cardiovascular disease, dementia, kidney disease, and, eventually, death.

Diarrhea and dysentery. Intestinal disorders that may indicate minor emotional distress or a variety of diseases, some serious; diarrhea is loose, watery, copious bowel movements, whereas dysentery is a process, usually infectious and characterized by severe diarrhea, sometimes with passage of blood, mucus, and pus.

DiGeorge syndrome. A pediatric syndrome caused by a missing piece of chromosome 22 and characterized by congenital heart defects, the absence or hypoplasia of the thymus and parathyroid glands, cleft palate, and dysmorphic facial features.

Diphtheria. An acute, contagious disease found primarily in children, associated with toxin production by the bacterium *Corynebacterium diphtheriae*.

Disease. A morbid (pathological) process with a characteristic set of symptoms that may affect the entire body or any of its parts; the cause, pathology, and course of a disease may be known or unknown.

Dislocation. *See* Fracture and dislocation.

Disseminated intravascular coagulation (DIC). A hemorrhagic disorder that occurs as a complication of several different disease states and results from abnormally initiated and accelerated blood clotting.

Diverticulitis and diverticulosis. Diverticulosis is a disease involving multiple outpouchings, or diverticuli, of the wall of the colon; these diverticuli may become inflamed, leading to the painful condition called diverticulitis.

Dizziness and fainting. Dizziness is a feeling of light-headedness and unsteadiness, sometimes accompanied by a feeling of spinning or other spatial motion; fainting is a loss of consciousness as a result of insufficient amounts of blood reaching the brain. Both are symptoms of many conditions, which may be harmless or serious.

Down syndrome. A congenital abnormality characterized by moderate to severe mental retardation and a distinctive physical appearance caused by a chromosomal aberration, the result of either an error during embryonic cell division or the inheritance of defective chromosomal material.

Drowning. A drowning victim dies by suffocation from submersion in a liquid medium, usually water.

Drug addiction. *See* Addiction.

Dry eye. Dry eye syndrome (DES), or keratoconjuntivitis sicca, affects the outer layers of the eye, which must be continually moistened by the liquid content of the tears. The normal flow of tears may be reduced as a result of the aging process or various external causes, including wearing contact lenses. DES occurs more among women than among men.

Dwarfism. Underdevelopment of the body, most often caused by a variety of genetic or endocrinological dysfunctions and resulting in either proportionate or disproportionate development, sometimes accompanied by other physical abnormalities and/or mental deficiencies.

Dysentery. *See* Diarrhea and dysentery.

Dyskinesia. Abnormal involuntary movements with different causes and clinical presentations.

Dyslexia. Severe reading disability in children with average to above-average intelligence.

Dysmenorrhea. A common menstrual disorder characterized by painful menstrual flow that is more severe than the usual cramps experienced by women with menstruation.

Dysphasia. *See* Aphasia and dysphasia.

Dystonia. Dystonia is the term used to describe an array of movement disorders characterized by repetitive muscle spasms, tremor, or excessive muscle activation. Dystonia is generally intermittent in nature, often leading to twisting, abnormal contraction patterns in skeletal muscles. It affects men, women, and children of all ages, and is present in about 300,000 people in the United States alone. It is a chronic, nonfatal condition that in most cases does not affect longevity, cognition,

E. coli infection. Infection by a gram-negative bacillus that normally colonizes the gastrointestinal tract of humans and other mammals.

Ear infections and disorders. Infections or disorders of the outer, middle, or inner ear, which may result in hearing impairment or loss.

Eating disorders. A group of conditions characterized by disordered eating patterns, preoccupation with body size and weight, and distorted body image. Eating disorders can cause serious medical complications and even death. The causes of eating disorders are complex and involve biological, psychological, and societal factors.

Ebola virus. A virus responsible for a severe and often fatal hemorrhagic fever.

Eclampsia. *See* Preeclampsia and eclampsia.

Ectopic pregnancy. The implantation of an embryo outside the uterine endometrium, most commonly in the Fallopian tube.

Eczema. An inflammation of the skin.

Edema. Accumulation of fluid in body tissues that may indicate a variety of diseases, including cardiovascular, kidney, liver, and medication problems.

Ehrlichiosis. Infection by one of a group of intracellular bacteria transmitted to humans through tick bites.

Electrical shock. The physical effect of an electrical current entering the body and the resulting damage.

Elephantiasis. A grossly disfiguring disease caused by a roundworm parasite; it is the advanced stage of the disease Bancroft's filariasis, contracted through roundworms.

Embolism. A mass of undissolved matter traveling in the blood or lymphatic current.

Emerging infectious diseases. First introduced by Nobel laureate Joshua Lederberg, the phrase emerging infectious diseases applies to those diseases that newly appear in a populace or have been in existence for some time but are rapidly increasing in incidence, geographic range, or surface as new drug-resistant strains of viruses, bacteria, or parasitic species.

Emphysema. A disease of the lung characterized by enlargement of the small bronchioles or lung alveoli, the destruction of alveoli, decreased elastic recoil of these structures, and the trapping of air in the lungs, resulting in shortness of breath, reduced oxygen to the body, and a variety of serious and eventually fatal complications.

Encephalitis. A disease that involves inflammation of the brain.

End-stage renal disease. Stage 5 of chronic kidney disease, which causes irreversible damage to and near-complete failure of the kidneys.

Endocarditis. Inflammatory lesions of the endocardium, the lining of the heart.

Endocrine disorders. The endocrine system controls the metabolic processes of the body. Endocrine disorders occur when the normal function of the endocrine system is disrupted.

Endodontic disease. Disease of the dental pulp and sometimes also the soft tissues and bone around the tip of the root.

Endometriosis. Growth of cells of the uterine lining at sites outside the uterus, causing severe pain and infertility.

Enterocolitis. Inflammation of the small and large intestines, which may be caused by a severe bacterial infection.

Enteroviruses. A class of viruses capable of infecting multiple organ systems, such as the central nervous system, the skin, the eyes, and the heart.

Enuresis. *See* Bed-wetting.

Environmental diseases. Sicknesses caused or exacerbated by human exposure to physical, chemical, biological, or social environmental conditions, the duration and intensity of the exposure typically affecting the manifestation of symptoms and fatality-case ra tios. Acute environmental diseases may result in rapid decline of health status and warrant emergency response, while chronic conditions often result from long-term exposures to low levels of environmental risk factors.

Epidemics and pandemics. An epidemic is a widespread, rapid occurrence of an infectious disease in a community or region at a particular time. A pandemic is an epidemic prevalent throughout a country, a continent, or the world.

Epidermal nevus syndromes. A group of systemic diseases that have in common pigmented spots on the skin.

Epiglottitis. An acute, life-threatening inflammation of the epiglottis.

Epilepsy. A serious neurologic disease characterized by seizures, which may involve convulsions and loss of consciousness.

Epstein-Barr virus. An extensively occurring virus which infects almost all humans during their lifetime, often remaining latent in their systems but sometimes causing malignant tumors and various types of cancer.

Erectile dysfunction. A disorder whereby a male cannot achieve an erection suitable for sexual intercourse.

Esophageal cancer. *See* Mouth and throat cancer.

Ewing's sarcoma. A rare bone cancer involving any part of the skeleton but found commonly in the long bones (60 percent), the pelvis (18 percent), and the ribs (15 percent) of children and young adults.

Eye infections and disorders. Eye infections involve the invasion, multiplication, and colonization of microorganisms in the tissues of the eye. Eye disorders are derangement or abnormality of the functions of parts of the eye and the general impairment of function of the eye for precise and clear vision.

Facial palsy. *See* Bell's palsy.

Factitious disorders. Psychophysiological disorders in which individuals intentionally produce their symptoms in order to play the role of patient.

Failure to thrive. A disorder of early childhood growth that includes disturbances in psychosocial skills and development.

Fatigue. A general symptom of tiredness, malaise, depression, and sometimes anxiety associated with many diseases and disorders; in some cases, no specific cause can be found.

Fatty acid oxidation disorders. Inherited metabolic defects that prevent the breakdown of fatty acids in the liver, muscles, and heart.

Fetal alcohol syndrome. Prenatal alcohol exposure of the fetus, resulting in specific facial and central nervous system abnormalities, impairment of physical growth (especially linear growth), and other associated anomalies.

Fever. A symptom associated with a variety of diseases and disorders, characterized by body temperature above normal (98.6 degrees Fahrenheit, or 37 degrees centigrade or Celsius); considered very serious at 104 degrees Fahrenheit (40 degrees Celsius) and higher.

Fibrocystic breast condition. The most common type of noncancerous breast condition, affecting approximately 60 percent of all women, the majority of whom are premenopausal. Because of its widespread incidence, the condition is now considered to be a normal physiologic variant. It is characterized by stromal tissue and glandular (lobules and ducts) changes in the breast or breasts that result in lumpiness, thickening, and localized edema (swelling).

Fibromyalgia. A connective, soft tissue disease involving chronic, spontaneous, and widespread musculoskeletal pain, as well as recurrent fatigue and sleep disturbance.

Fifth disease. An infectious disease of children characterized by an erythematous (reddish) rash and low-grade fever.

Flat feet. A congenital or acquired flatness of the longitudinal arch of the foot.

Food allergies. An abnormal response by the immune system to some foods, causing mild to severe symptoms that may become life threatening.

Food poisoning. Food-borne illness caused by bacteria, viruses, or parasites consumed in food and resulting in acute gastrointestinal disturbance that may include diarrhea, nausea, vomiting, and abdominal discomfort.

Foot disorders. Disorders involving the muscles, bones, nerves, or skin of the feet.

Fracture and dislocation. A fracture is a break in a bone, which may be partial or complete; a dislocation is the forceful separation of bones in a joint.

Fragile X syndrome. A genetic disorder of variable expression, with mental retardation being the most common feature.

Frontal lobe syndrome. An organic disorder of the brain affecting cognitive ability, personality, and behavior.

Frontotemporal dementia (FTD). Frontotemporal dementia is a descriptive term for a group of neurodegenerative disorders that affect the frontal and temporal lobes of the brain.

Frostbite. Frostbite is localized freezing of tissue, usually of extremities exposed to low temperatures, that results in ice crystals forming within cells, thereby killing them.

Fructosemia. An inborn error of metabolism in which eating foods containing fructose or sucrose will result in high blood fructose levels.

Fungal infections. Infections caused by fungi-simple, plantlike organisms-that range from minor skin diseases to serious, disseminated diseases of the lungs and other organs; patients whose immune systems are impaired are at greater risk of serious funga l infections.

Galactosemia. An inherited disorder of carbohydrate metabolism in which an infant is unable to utilize galactose from food.

Gallbladder cancer. A rare type of cancer affecting the gallbladder (a muscular, membranous sac containing bile) and its surrounding organs.

Gallbladder diseases. A family of disorders affecting the gallbladder, usually causing abdominal pain but occasionally symptomless.

Gallstones. *See* Gallbladder diseases; Stone removal; Stones.

Ganglions. *See* Cysts; Ganglion removal.

Gangrene. Gas gangrene is an infectious disease usually caused by *Clostridium perfringens*, a spore-producing bacterium that is usually found in soil and the gastrointestinal tract of humans and other animals.

Gastritis. *See* Abdominal disorders; Gastroenteritis; Gastrointestinal disorders.

Gastroenteritis. An acute infectious process affecting the gastrointestinal system, usually leading to abdominal discomfort and diarrhea.

Gastrointestinal disorders. The many problems that can affect the gastrointestinal tract, such as infections, injuries, dysfunctions, tumors, congenital defects, and genetic abnormalities.

Gaucher's disease. A congenital disorder caused by a defect in lipid metabolism and characterized by cell hyperplasia in the liver, spleen, and bone marrow.

Gender identity disorder. A psychiatric classification describing persons experiencing a strong and persistent incongruity between their anatomy and the gender with which they identify. Gender identity disorder is not concurrent with either disorders of sexual development (intersex conditions) or with homosexuality.

Genetic diseases. A variety of disorders transmitted from parent to child through chromosomal material; most people experience disease related to genetics in some form, and research into this area is yielding greater understanding of the relationship be tween disease and hereditary proclivities toward disease, as well as new strategies for early detection and prevention or therapy.

Genital disorders, female. All maladies affecting the reproductive organs of women.

Genital disorders, male. Disorders and diseases of the male reproductive system, including sexual dysfunction, infertility, genital cancer, and sexually transmitted diseases.

Gestational diabetes. A medical condition in which diabetes, or unregulated blood glucose, first occurs during pregnancy.

Giardiasis. An acute or chronic parasitic infection of the gastrointestinal system.

Gigantism. A rare congenital disease that begins in children with pituitary gland tumors that make too much growth hormone, which yields pituitary giants who often die at relatively young ages. After adolescence, the disease is manifested as acro megaly, which is quite serious over the long term.

Gingivitis. A gum disease that begins when plaque and calculus cause gum inflammation and bleeding. It can lead to periodontitis, which is associated with tooth loss, cardiovascular disease, and diabetes.

Glaucoma. A group of eye diseases characterized by an increase in the eye's intraocular pressure; early diagnosis through regular eye examinations can manage the effects of the disease, while late diagnosis may result in impaired vision or blind ness.

Glomerulonephritis. *See* Nephritis.

Glioma. An excessive reproduction of glial cells that leads to tumor formation in the central nervous system that can cause damage to nervous tissue.

Gluten intolerance. A chronic, immune-mediated condition of progressive, itchy skin lesions triggered by the ingestion of gluten.

Glycogen storage diseases. Inherited metabolic disorders that lead to the accumulation of an abnormal amount or type of glycogen in the liver, muscles, and heart.

Goiter. An enlargement of the thyroid gland that is noncancerous and not caused by a temporary condition such as inflammation.

Gonorrhea. A common treatable sexually transmitted disease that primarily infects the reproductive tract and which is caused by the bacterium *Neisseria gonorrhea*.

Gout. A form of arthritis of the peripheral joints, often characterized by painful, recurrent acute attacks and resulting from deposits of uric acid in joint spaces.

Guillain-Barré syndrome. An acute degeneration of peripheral motor and sensory nerves, known to physicians as acute inflammatory demyelinating polyneuropathy, a common cause of acute generalized paralysis.

Gulf War syndrome. A popular term used to describe collectively a variety of symptoms, not a specific disease, suffered by veterans of the Gulf War.

Gum disease. Inflammation of the soft tissue that surrounds the teeth; in advanced disease, there is also loss of bone that holds the teeth in place.

Gynecomastia. An enlargement of the glandular part of the male breast that may affect one or both breasts and be painless or painful.

Hammertoes. Toes that are bent permanently at the joint nearest to the foot; the closely related term clawtoe denotes a toe that is bent at both joints.

Hand-foot-and-mouth disease. An enteroviral disease that usually affects children, causing vesicular eruptions on the hands, feet, oral mucosa, and tongue.

Hantavirus. An often-fatal viral infection carried by rodents that causes influenza-like symptoms and respiratory failure.

Harelip. *See* Cleft lip and palate.

Hashimoto's thyroiditis. An autoimmune disease that results in inflammation of the thyroid gland caused when abnormal blood antibodies and white blood cells infiltrate and attack thyroidal cells.

Hay fever. A damaging immune response to otherwise harmless foreign substances such as pollen grains and mold spores.

Head and neck disorders. Physical trauma or neurological problems affecting the head and neck, including the spinal cord.

Headaches. A general term referring to pain localized in the head and/or neck, which may signal mere tension or serious disorders.

Hearing loss. Loss of sensitivity to sound as a result of disease, infection, injury, noise, or aging.

Heart attack. Myocardial infarction; the sudden death of heart muscle characterized by intense chest pain, sweating, shortness of breath, or sometimes none of these symptoms.

Heart disease. One of the leading causes of death in many industrialized nations; heart diseases include atherosclerotic disease, coronary artery disease, cardiac arrhythmias, and stenosis.

Heart failure. A condition in which the heart cannot pump enough blood to meet the needs of the body because its ability to contract is impaired.

Heat exhaustion and heatstroke. Heat-related illnesses in which the body temperature rises to dangerous levels and cannot be controlled through normal mechanisms, such as sweating.

Hematomas. Localized, semisolid masses of pooled blood in tissue, caused by spontaneous or posttrauma blood leakage through the vessel walls of arteries, capillaries, or veins and subsequent clotting in surrounding tissue; they may occur in skin, soft tissue (muscles, mucosa), and organs or within the skull.

Hematuria. The presence of blood or red blood cells in the urine.

Hemiplegia. Paralysis of one side of the body, usually caused by brain damage.

Hemochromatosis. A multisystem disease characterized by increased iron absorption and storage.

Hemolytic disease of the newborn. The destruction of red blood cells in a fetus by antibodies transferred from the mother.

Hemolytic uremic syndrome. A predominantly childhood disorder produced primarily by a strain of *Escherichia coli* bacteria and characterized by acute kidney failure, hemolytic anemia, and a low platelet count.

Hemophilia. A genetic disorder characterized by the blood's inability to form clots as a result of the lack or alteration of certain trace plasma proteins.

Hemorrhage. *See* Bleeding.

Hemorrhoids. Blood-swollen enlargements of specialized tissues that help close the anus, as a result of intravenous pressure in the hemorrhoidal plexus; sometimes called piles.

Hepatitis. An inflammatory condition of the liver, characterized by discomfort, jaundice, and enlargement of the organ and bacterial, viral, or immunological in origin; may also result from use of alcohol and other toxic drugs.

Hermaphroditism and pseudohermaphroditism. Abnormal primary sexual characteristics caused by developmental defects.

Hernia. A pouchlike mass consisting of visceral material encased in properitoneal tissue (the hernial sac) protruding through an aperture in the abdomen-a result of a weakening in the abdominal wall.

Herniated disk. *See* Slipped disk.

Herpes. A family of viruses that cause such diseases as cold sores, genital herpes, chickenpox, shingles, and mononucleosis. The term herpes is also used to refer to an infection with herpes simplex, either type 1 or type 2.

Hiccups. Involuntary, spasmodic contractions of the diaphragm and the simultaneous closure of the glottis.

Hirschsprung's disease. A disease of the large intestine that makes bowel movements difficult or impossible.

Histiocytosis. A group of relatively rare blood disorders characterized by the abnormal accumulation of white blood cells called histiocytes, leading to a wide range of adverse bodily responses.

HIV. *See* Human immunodeficiency virus (HIV).

Hives. Pink swellings called wheals that may occur in groups on any part of the skin.

Hodgkin's disease. A neoplastic disorder originating in the tissues of the lymphatic system, recognized by distinctive histologic changes and defined by the presence of Reed-Sternberg cells.

H1N1 influenza. H1N1 influenza is an acute respiratory infection caused by the H1N1 subtype of the influenza A virus.

Human immunodeficiency virus (HIV). A retrovirus that attacks cells of the immune system, leading to a loss of immune function and the development of acquired immunodeficiency syndrome (AIDS).

Human papillomavirus (HPV). A group of viruses, some of which are sexually transmitted and associated with genital warts and genital cancer.

Huntington's disease. In this autosomal dominant genetic neurodegenerative disease, patients have uncoordinated movements as a result of neuron degeneration.

Hydroceles. A collection of fluid between the lining membranes protecting the testicles in the scrotum.

Hydrocephalus. A collection of excessive amounts of cerebrospinal fluid (CSF) within the cranial cavity, which can cause increased pressure within the brain and skull, leading to brain tissue damage and, in infants, enlargement of the skull.

Hyperadiposis. Having excess body fat; exceeding 200 percent of standard body weight as defined on a height-weight table.

Hypercholesterolemia. A high level of cholesterol in the bloodstream, which is considered a major risk factor for heart attack or stroke.

Hyperhidrosis. Excessive sweating, which may be generalized or limited to certain areas of the body, particularly the hands and feet. The paroxysmal form of this disorder affects approximately 1 percent of the population of the United States.

Hyperlipidemia. The presence of abnormally large quantities of lipids (fats) in the blood.

Hyperparathyroidism and hypoparathyroidism. Excessive, uncontrolled secretion (hyperpara- thyroidism) or reduced secretion (hypoparathyroidism) of parathyroid hormone.

Hyperplasia. A proliferation of cells in response to either normal or abnormal physiological processes.

Hypertension. An abnormally high blood pressure, an often silent cardiovascular condition that may lead to heart attack, stroke, and major organ failures.

Hyperthermia and hypothermia. Hyperthermia is the elevation of the body core temperature of an organism, while hypothermia is a decrease in that temperature; an extreme in either condition is a medical emergency. They both can be induced therapeutically in certain medical and surgical conditions.

Hyperventilation. Breathing at a faster rate than what is needed for metabolism, resulting in the exhalation of carbon dioxide faster than it is produced.

Hypochondriasis. Unwarranted belief about or anxiety over having a serious disease that is based on one's subjective interpretation of physical symptoms or sensations; the belief or anxiety is maintained in spite of appropriate medical assurances that there is no serious disease.

Hypoglycemia. The condition in which concentration of glucose in the blood is too low to meet the needs of key organs, especially the brain; this condition limits treatments for diabetes mellitus.

Hypoparathyroidism. *See* Hyperparathyroidism and hypoparathyroidism.

Hypotension. Blood pressure that not only is low but also causes symptoms such as dizziness in the affected individual. It has multiple causes, including blood loss, heart attack, trauma, reactions to medications, and overwhelming infection.

Hypothermia. *See* Hyperthermia and hypothermia.

Hypothyroidism. *See* Congenital hypothyroidism.

Hypoxia. An inadequate supply of oxygen to tissues caused by either oxygen delivery not being sufficient for tissue requirements or utilization of oxygen being ineffective.

Iatrogenic disorders. Health problems caused by medical treatments.

Immunodeficiency disorders. Genetic or acquired disorders that result from disturbances in the normal functioning of the immune system.

Impetigo. A superficial bacterial infection of the skin.

Impotence. *See* Sexual dysfunction.

Incontinence. Involuntary loss of urine or feces, primarily a social and hygienic problem that particularly affects the older population.

Infarction. A localized area of tissue damage or necrosis caused by absence of blood supply and oxygen to the part.

Infarction, myocardial. *See* Heart attack.

Infection. Invasion of the body by disease-causing organisms such as bacteria, viruses, fungi, and parasites; symptoms of infection may include pain, swelling, fever, and loss of normal function.

Infertility, female. The inability to achieve a desired pregnancy as a result of dysfunction of female reproductive organs.

Infertility, male. The inability to achieve a desired pregnancy as a result of dysfunction of male reproductive organs.

Inflammation. The reaction of blood-filled living tissue to injury.

Influenza. An acute respiratory infection caused by an influenza virus.

Insect-borne diseases. Diseases transmitted by insects, which have a significant health and economic impact worldwide, causing illness, disability, and death.

Insomnia. *See* Sleep disorders.

Interpartner violence. Psychological, physical, or sexual harm from a current or former partner, which can be actual or threatened within heterosexual or homosexual partnerships.

Interstitial pulmonary fibrosis (IPF). An inflammatory disease that results in the scarring and fibrosis of the lung alveolar tissue (air sacs).

Intestinal cancer. *See* Stomach, intestinal, and pancreatic cancers.

Intestinal disorders. Diseases or disorders of the small intestine, large intestine (or colon), liver, pancreas, and gallbladder.

Intraventricular hemorrhage. Bleeding into or around the normal fluid spaces within the brain.

Irritable bowel syndrome (IBS). A common intestinal disorder characterized by abdominal pain or discomfort and by altered bowel habits, consisting of diarrhea or constipation or alternating between diarrhea and constipation.

Ischemia. The interruption or temporary restriction of blood flow to a particular area of the body, such as an organ.

Jaundice. Yellow discoloration of skin resulting from increased levels of bilirubin in the blood.

Joint diseases. *See* Arthritis.

Juvenile rheumatoid arthritis. A usually chronic autoimmune disease of unknown cause, characterized by joint swelling, pain, and sometimes the destruction of joints.

Kaposi's sarcoma. A disease in which cancer cells are found in tissues, causing lesions on the skin and/or mucous membranes and spreading to other organs in the body.

Kawasaki disease. An inflammatory disease that affects numerous organs and systems in the body and typically occurs in children under the age of five.

Keratitis. An inflammation of the cornea caused most often by the herpes simplex virus.

Keratoses. *See* Warts.

Kidney cancer. A number of different malignant growths that occur in a kidney.

Kidney disorders. Disorders, from structural abnormalities to bacterial infections, that can affect the kidneys and may lead to renal failure.

Kidney stones. *See* Kidney disorders; Stone removal; Stones.

Klinefelter syndrome. A male chromosomal disorder causing infertility and significant femaleness.

Klippel-Trenaunay syndrome. A rare congenital syndrome characterized by hemangiomas of the vascular system that can affect bone or soft tissue throughout the body.

Kluver-Bucy syndrome. A behavioral disorder characterized by lack of emotional activity or responses similar to that often observed in patients with Alzheimer's disease.

Knock-knees. A deformity in which the knees are positioned close together or turn toward each other and the tibias and ankles are apart when the feet are placed in a normal standing position.

Korsakoff's syndrome. Korsakoff's syndrome is a neurological condition involving disturbances in the ability to form short-term memories, often resulting in confabulation and psychosis, and attributable to deficiencies in thiamine often associated with chro nic alcohol use.

Kwashiorkor. A form of malnutrition caused by inadequate protein intake.

Kyphosis. A marked increase of the normal curvature of the thoracic vertebrae or upper back, sometimes referred to as dowager's hump because of its prevalence in elderly women.

Lactose intolerance. Lactose intolerance is an inability to break down and absorb milk sugar, known as lactose, resulting in stomach pain, gas, and diarrhea if lactose is consumed.

Laryngitis. Inflammation of the larynx (voice box), often associated with common colds, bacterial infection, or straining the voice. The throat is dry, swallowing becomes difficult, and speech is a hoarse whisper.

Lead poisoning. A condition caused by high levels of lead in the blood. This major preventable environmental health problem is found in both children and adults, but more frequently in children.

Learning disabilities. A variety of disorders involving the failure to learn an academic skill despite normal levels of intelligence, maturation, and cultural and educational opportunity; estimates of the prevalence of learning disabilities in the general po pulation range between 2 and 20 percent.

Legionnaires' disease. A rapidly progressing bacterial pneumonia caused by infection with an organism of the genus *Legionella* and characterized by influenza-like illness, with high fever, chills, headache, and muscle aches.

Leishmaniasis. A complex of diseases caused by protozoan parasites of the genus *Leishmania*.

Leprosy. A bacterial infection that affects skin and nerves, causing symptoms ranging from mild numbness to gross disfiguration.

Leptospirosis. A bacterial infection acquired from domestic animals and wildlife. Humans become infected through contact with animal urine or water and soil contaminated with animal urine. Potentially fatal complications arise from infection of the k idneys, liver, lungs, brain, and heart.

Lesions. Any tissue damaged by injury or disease.

Leukemia. A family of cancers that affect the blood, characterized by an increase in the number of white blood cells.

Leukodystrophy. A group of genetic disorders characterized by progressive deterioration of the white matter (myelin sheath) of the brain.

Lice, mites, and ticks. Parasites that live on the human body, causing severe itching, skin rashes, and sometimes more serious diseases.

Lisping. The defective pronunciation of the sibilants s and z, usually substituted with a th sound.

Listeria infections. Infections caused by the bacterium *Listeria monocytogenes*.

Liver cancer. Malignancies of the liver, which may be primary (arising in the organ itself) but are more likely to be secondary (metastasizing from another site).

Liver disorders. As one of the most complex organs in the body, the liver is the target of a wide variety of toxins, infectious agents, and cancers that lead to hepatitis, cirrhosis, abscesses, and liver failure.

Lockjaw. *See* Tetanus.

Lou Gehrig's disease. *See* Amyotrophic lateral sclerosis.

Lumps, breast. *See* Breast cancer; Breast disorders; Breasts, female.

Lung cancer. The appearance of malignant tumors in the lungs, which is usually associated with cigarette smoking.

Lung diseases. *See* Pulmonary diseases.

Lupus. *See* Systemic lupus erythematosus (SLE).

Lyme disease. Lyme disease is caused by bacteria transmitted by ticks. Initial symptoms include a spreading rash at the site of the tick bite; later, the central nervous system, heart, or joints may be affected.

Lymphadenopathy and lymphoma. Lymphadenopathy, or enlarged lymph nodes, refers to any disorder related to the lymphatic vessels of lymph nodes; lymphoma is a group of cancers consisting of unchecked multiplication of lymphatic tissue cells.

Lymphatic disorders. *See* Lymphadenopathy and lymphoma.

Lymphoma. *See* Lymphadenopathy and lymphoma.

Macular degeneration. A degenerative disease of the central portion of the retina that results primarily in loss of central vision.

Malabsorption. The impaired absorption of nutrients from food into the bloodstream.

Malaria. One of the world's most serious and potentially fatal diseases, malaria is the result of a parasite transmitted into the bloodstream by mosquito bites. It is most common in subtropical zones, especially in Africa, Asia, and Latin America.

Malignancy and metastasis. Malignancy is the uncontrolled growth of tumor cells that invade and compress surrounding tissues and break through the skin or barriers within the body; metastasis describes the tendency of malignant cells to break loose from their tumor of origin to travel to other locations within the body.

Malnutrition. Impaired health caused by an imbalance, either through deficiency or excess, in nutrients.

Manic-depressive disorder. *See* Bipolar disorders.

Maple syrup urine disease (MSUD). A recessive autosomal genetic disease resulting in the absence, partial activity, or inactivity of a multisubunit enzyme responsible for metabolizing the branched-chain amino acids leucine, isoleucine, and valine.

Marburg virus. Marburg hemorrhagic fever is a rare, highly lethal disease caused by Marburg filovirus.

Marfan syndrome. A condition in which the connective tissue does not form correctly and tends to be too flexible. The abnormal chemical composition, especially of the skeleton and heart, leads to major medical characteristics that are sometimes in evidence only at puberty.

Marijuana. A plant containing a psychoactive substance with the potential for both recreational abuse and medical use.

Mastitis . A bacterial infection of the mammary gland.

Measles. A highly contagious disease contracted through a virus transmitted in respiratory secretions and characterized by a spreading skin rash.

Meckel's diverticulum. A pouch on the wall of the lower part of the intestine that persists from embryonic development.

Melanoma. A malignant disease which originates with the melanocytes in the skin. While there may be a variety of causes, the primary risk factor is extent of exposure to sunlight.

Memory loss. Total or limited impairment of memory that may be sudden or gradual.

Ménière's disease. A chronic inner ear disorder associated with endolymphatic hydrops causing sensorineural hearing loss, tinnitus, and vertigo.

Meningitis. An inflammation of the meninges of the brain and spinal cord.

Menorrhagia. Excessively heavy or prolonged menstrual flow.

Mental retardation. Significant subaverage intellectual development and deficient adaptive behavior often accompanied by physical abnormalities.

Mental illness. *See* Psychiatric disorders; *specific diseases*.

Mercury poisoning. Mercury is a naturally occurring element that can cause neurological damage in humans exposed to it.

Mesothelioma. A malignancy originating from the mesothelial surfaces (the lining cells) of the pleural and peritoneal cavities, the pericardium, or the tunica vaginalis. The distribution of mesothelioma may be unifocal or multifocal or may involve t he lining cells in a continuous manner. Approximately 80 to 90 percent of all cases have a pleural origin (malignant pleural mesothelioma).

Metabolic disorders. Disorders resulting from alterations in the pathways by which the body derives energy and synthesizes other molecules from carbohydrates, lipids, and proteins in food; usually caused by genetic defects that result in a missing or fault y enzyme.

Metabolic syndrome. A constellation of metabolic changes that affect most major organ systems and may impinge on practically all systems of the body, often beginning with excess weight or obesity.

Metastasis. *See* Cancer; Malignancy and metastasis.

Methicillin-resistant staphylococcus aureus (MRSA) infections. An infection caused by a virulent and destructive bacteria that is resistant to common antibiotics and difficult to treat. It may be localized to one area of the body or may become systemic (spread throughout the body).

Minimally conscious state. A condition of severely altered consciousness in which minimal, but definite, behavioral evidence of self or environmental awareness is demonstrated.

Miscarriage. A pregnancy that self-terminates within the first twenty weeks of gestation; the same condition occurring after twenty weeks is termed a stillbirth.

Mites. *See* Bites and stings; Lice, mites, and ticks; Parasitic diseases.

Mitral valve prolapse. The inability of the mitral valve in the heart to close properly.

Mold and mildew. Mold is a generalized term describing nonfruiting fungi, often microscopic and living in moist areas both outdoors and inside buildings, which consume nutrients and produce spores. Mold, which thrives in humid and closed spaces, has co ntributed to the development of effective pharmaceuticals but has also been blamed for various health problems and diseases.

Moles. Nonmalignant marks, pigmented spots, or growths on the skin.

Monkeypox. A rare disease, originating in the rain forests of Central and West Africa, that affects animals and humans and is caused by a virus.

Mononucleosis. An acute viral infectious disease that produces lymph node enlargement (hyperplasia).

Morgellons disease. A skin disorder characterized by a pattern of dermatologic symptoms described as insectlike sensations, with skin lesions varying from very minor to disfiguring, and associated with disabling fatigue, joint pain, and various neuropsych iatric symptoms. In the first decade of the twenty-first century, the cause, transmission, and treatment remained under investigation.

Mosquito bites. *See* Bites and stings; Insect-borne diseases

Motion sickness. A disorder characterized by nausea, vomiting, and vertigo and caused by a combination of repetitive back-and-forth and up-and-down movements.

Motor neuron diseases. Progressive, debilitating, and eventually fatal diseases affecting nerve cells in muscles.

Mouth and throat cancer. A malignancy of the lips, tongue, gums, salivary glands, or pharynx.

Mucopolysaccharidosis (MPS). A genetic disorder characterized by accumulations of mucopolysaccharides in tissues.

Multiple chemical sensitivity syndrome. An increasing intolerance to commonly encountered chemicals at concentrations well tolerated by other people.

Multiple sclerosis. A debilitating chronic inflammatory disease affecting the central nervous system.

Mumps. An acute, contagious childhood disease caused by a virus and characterized by swollen salivary glands.

Münchausen syndrome by proxy. A disorder in which a parent fabricates, simulates, or induces a medical condition in a child in order to receive attention and acknowledgment as the source of information about the child's health.

Muscle sprains, spasms, and disorders. Injuries, defects, or disorders of the muscles of the body.

Muscular dystrophy. A group of related diseases that attack different muscle groups, are progressive and genetically determined, and have no known cure.

Myasthenia gravis. A disorder characterized by selective muscle fatigue following repeated use; it is caused by an abnormal immune reaction to specific receptors on the muscle surface.

Myocardial infarction. *See* Heart attack.

Myopia. A visual defect that impairs the perception of distant objects.

Narcolepsy. An apparently inherited disorder of the nervous system characterized by brief, numerous, and overwhelming attacks of sleepiness throughout the day.

Nasopharyngeal disorders. Disorders of the nose, nasal passages (sinuses), and pharynx (mouth, throat, and esophagus).

Nausea and vomiting. Nausea is an unpleasant subjective sensation, accompanied by epigastric and duodenal discomfort, which often culminates in vomiting, the regurgitation of the contents of the stomach.

Neck injuries and disorders. *See* Head and neck disorders.

Necrosis. Tissue damage occurring as a result of cell death.

Necrotizing fasciitis. An invasive bacterial infection that occurs in the connective tissue between the skin and muscle known as the fascia, cutting off blood flow; it must be urgently treated surgically and, even in the best circumstances, has a high mortality rate.

Neonatal brachial plexus palsy. A motor disability evident early in life that manifests as weakness of the affected arm due to stretching or compression of the nerves of the brachial plexus during the perinatal period, with passive range of motion greater than active .

Nephritis. An inflammatory response of the kidneys, particularly of the glomeruli, to infectious agents or immunological challenges.

Neuralgia, neuritis, and neuropathy. Pathological conditions affecting the peripheral nerves of the body and interfering with the proper functioning of those nerves.

Neurofibromatosis. A genetic disease affecting the nervous system, skin, and bones that produces multiple nerve tumors (neurofibromas), deeply pigmented areas of skin (café-au-lait spots), and bone deformities.

Neurosis. A psychiatric disorder in which the patient continues to be rational and in touch with reality.

Niemann-Pick disease. This lipid disease group, resulting from inactive sphingomyelinase and cholesterol-modifying enzymes, causes lipid buildup in the brain and other organs, mental and physical debilitation, and a short life span.

Nonalcoholic steatohepatitis (NASH). Fatty inflammation of the liver that is not caused by alcohol.

Noroviruses. A family of viruses that cause acute gastroenteritis.

Numbness and tingling. Abnormalities of sensation that are attributable to nerve damage or disorders.

Obesity. A condition in which the body carries abnormal or unhealthy amounts of fat tissue, leading the individual to weigh in excess of 20 percent more than his or her ideal weight.

Obesity, childhood. Having a body mass index (BMI) at or above the 95th percentile for children of the same age and sex. Rapid changes from infancy through adolescence are part of normal and expected development, and the norm used to identify childhood obesity must be correct for that child's age and sex.

Obsessive-compulsive disorder. An anxiety disorder characterized by intrusive and unwanted but uncontrollable thoughts, by the need to perform ritualized behavior patterns, or both; the obsessions and/or compulsions cause severe stress, consume an excessive amount of time, and greatly interfere with a person's normal routine, activities, or relationships.

Opportunistic infections. Potentially life-threatening diseases occurring in people with weakened immune systems by microorganisms that typically do not cause severe illnesses in otherwise healthy people.

Orchitis. An inflammation of one or both testicles.

Osgood-Schlatter disease. Pain caused by the patellar (kneecap) tendon pulling away from the tibia (shin bone).

Osteoarthritis. A degenerative joint disease that results from the wearing away of the cartilage of bones, causing inflammation, swelling, and pain in affected joints and eventually causing joint stiffness and limitation of movement, misalignment, and knoblike bone growths in the hands.

Osteochondritis juvenilis. The disturbance of the blood supply to the tops of the thigh bones, resulting in their destruction.

Osteogenesis imperfecta. A genetic disorder of variable severity that results in frequent bone breaks.

Osteomyelitis. A secondary bacterial infection of the bone and bone marrow.

Osteonecrosis. A disorder that occurs when the blood supply to bone is cut off, causing the death of bone tissue and leading to the collapse of joints in the affected areas.

Osteoporosis. A condition resulting from reduced bone mass; fractures are the major complications and are associated with significantly increased risks of morbidity and mortality, especially in older women.

Ovarian cancer. *See* Cervical, ovarian, and uterine cancers.

Ovarian cysts. Benign growths that develop in the ovaries.

Overtraining syndrome. Perceptible and lasting decrease in athletic performance, often coupled with mood changes, which does not quickly resolve following a normal period of rest.

Paget's disease. A chronic disorder resulting in enlarged and deformed bones.

Pain. An unpleasant, subjective experience of physical or mental suffering, a symptom of a real or potential underlying cause, condition, or injury.

Palpitations. A perceived irregularity of the normal heartbeat.

Palsy. A paralysis or partial paralysis that is usually accompanied or followed by muscle weakness and muscle wasting over the affected area; in some cases, there may be residual electrical activity present, but the amount is usually small an d the activity cannot be controlled.

Pancreatic cancer. *See* Stomach, intestinal, and pancreatic cancers.

Pancreatitis. Inflammation of the pancreas, which may be acute or chronic.

Panic attacks. *See* Anxiety.

Paralysis. Pronounced weakness or the inability to produce movement in a part of the body resulting from a variety of causes.

Paranoia. Pervasive distrust and suspiciousness of others and a tendency to interpret others' motives as malevolent.

Paraplegia. A motor or sensory loss in the lower extremities, with or without involvement of the abdominal and back muscles.

Parasitic diseases. Diseases borne by parasites, or organisms that live within host organisms; parasites travel to their hosts via vectors that may include fleas, mosquitoes, rats, and other animals.

Parkinson's disease. A progressive neurological disease characterized by tremor, slow movement, and muscle rigidity and typically seen only in those over the age of forty.

Pelvic inflammatory disease (PID). A serious bacterial infection of the upper genital tract that is often sexually transmitted.

Peptic ulcers. *See* Ulcers.

Periodontitis. A disorder of the teeth resulting from advanced gingivitis, inflammation and infection of the bones and the ligaments supporting the teeth.

Peritonitis. An inflammation of the membrane lining the abdominal cavity (peritoneum), usually secondary to a bacterial infection.

Pertussis. *See* Whooping cough.

Pharyngitis. Inflammation of the mucous membranes of the pharynx or throat, often caused by a viral infection or bacteria.

Phenylketonuria (PKU). A genetic disorder caused by a deficiency of the liver enzyme phenylalanine hydroxylase.

Phlebitis. The inflammation of a vein, often seen in conjunction with blood clots within the deep and superficial veins outside the heart.

Phobias. Excessive fears of certain objects, people, places, or situations.

Pick's disease. A brain disease causing shrinkage of tissue in discrete areas (focal lesions) in the frontal and temporal anterior brain lobes, thus reducing verbal reasoning and speech production.

PID. *See* Pelvic inflammatory disease (PID).

Pigeon toes. Usually a temporary condition in which one or both feet point inward when the heels are placed in a normal standing position.

Pimples. *See* Acne.

Pinworms. A common parasitic nematode that resembles a white thread approximately 0.5 inch in length.

Pityriasis alba. A common skin disorder that causes light-colored, scaly patches of skin on the face, neck, and arms.

Pityriasis rosea. A skin disorder that manifests with a characteristic rash.

PKU. *See* Phenylketonuria (PKU)

Plague. An infection transmitted by fleas, which may prove fatal if left untreated.

Plaque, arterial. Fatty deposits within arterial walls.

Plaque, dental. Various kinds of bacteria that live in the mouth stick to each other and then to the tooth surface, both above and below the gums, causing tooth decay and gum disease.

Pleurisy. A syndrome of chest pain made worse by breathing.

Pneumocystis jirovecii. A small fungus that normally lives in the respiratory tract of most people, but causes pneumonia in those with dysfunctional immune systems.

Pneumonia. An inflammation of one of several possible areas of the respiratory system, mainly in the lungs or bronchial passageways, resulting from bacterial or viral infection.

Pneumothorax. The collapse of a lung or portion of a lung as a result of the introduction of air or another gas or of fluid into the pleural space surrounding the lungs.

Poisoning. Exposure to any substance in sufficient quantity to cause adverse health effects, from severe to fatal.

Poliomyelitis. A contagious viral illness capable of causing meningitis and permanent paralysis; in response to a dramatic increase in the frequency of cases in industrialized nations during the twentieth century, a vaccine was developed that has vir tually eliminated this disease in Europe and the Western Hemisphere.

Polycystic kidney disease. A genetic disorder characterized by multiple, bilateral, grapelike clusters of fluid-filled cysts that slowly replace much of the mass of the kidney, reducing kidney function and leading to renal failure.

Polycystic ovary syndrome. A complex disorder related to dysfunctional ovulation, endocrine abnormalities, and multiple cysts on the ovary that result in fertility difficulties. Polycystic ovary syndrome is related to obesity and diabetes and poses an increased risk for cardiovascular disease. In addition to these conditions, symptoms of hirsutism may be accompanied by depression or anxiety.

Polydactyly and syndactyly. Polydactyly is the presence of extra fingers or toes, while syndactyly describes two or more fingers or toes that are joined or fused together.

Polymyalgia rheumatica. An inflammatory disorder of the joints and connective tissues of the shoulders, neck, and hips.

Polyps. Abnormal growths arising from mucous membranes anywhere in the body. A polyp is considered pedunculated if it is attached to the mucous membrane by a narrow, long stalk of tissue; if no stalk is present, then the polyp is said to be se ssile.

Porphyria. One of several rare genetic disorders caused by the accumulation of substances called porphyrins.

Postherpetic neuralgia. A condition that can potentially produce severe pain in a specific nerve root/dermatome that was once previously exposed to the herpes zoster virus (chicken pox-shingles). Neuralgia is the pain that is produced from a nerve that is inf lamed or enduring destruction from a disease process. In the case of postherpetic neuralgia, the nerve damage is produced by the reactivation of the herpes zoster virus.

Postpartum depression. A physical and emotional condition that may be life-threatening, involving the symptoms of depression occurring from a month to a year following childbirth and thought to be caused in part to dramatic hormonal shifts occurring in conju nction with childbirth.

Post-traumatic stress disorder. A maladaptive condition resulting from exposure to events beyond the realm of normal human experience and characterized by persistent difficulties involving emotional numbing, intense fear, helplessness, horror, reexperiencing of traum a, avoidance, and arousal.

Prader-Willi syndrome. A disorder caused by a deletion in chromosome 15, characterized by developmental and cognitive delays, overeating resulting in obesity, and behavioral difficulties.

Precocious puberty. The early onset of puberty caused by the premature secretion of sex hormones, resulting in the commencement of sexual maturation prior to age eight in girls and age ten in boys.

Preeclampsia and eclampsia. Preeclampsia is a serious complication of pregnancy, occurring any time from the middle stages of pregnancy to just after birth, characterized by hypertension and proteinuria. Eclampsia is a potentially fatal condition, likewise occurr ing any time from the middle stages of pregnancy to just after birth, characterized by seizures or coma that has no other apparent cause.

Premature birth. Premature birth is childbirth occurring before the thirty-seventh week of pregnancy; premature infants are those babies born before this time.

Premenstrual syndrome (PMS). A disorder characterized by the cyclic recurrence of physical and behavioral symptoms during the days between ovulation and the first few days of menstruation.

Prion diseases. A variety of fatal neurological illnesses, inherited or transmissible, that are associated with abnormalities in proteins, called prions.

Progeria. Rare disorders characterized by many aspects of premature aging.

Prostate cancer. Malignancy occurring in the prostate gland, that is the most deadly cancer for men in the United States.

Prostate enlargement. A common condition in which the prostate gland enlarges as a man matures.

Proteinuria. Disorder involving the elimination of abnormally high amounts of protein in the urine. It is typically defined as the excretion of more than 150 milligrams of protein in the urine per day.

Protozoan diseases. Disease caused by protozoa, a diverse group of free-living, unicellular animals that function as parasites.

Pruritus. *See* Itching

Psoriasis. A chronic skin disease in which red, scaly patches develop, overlaid with thick, silvery-gray scales, causing physical discomfort as well as damage to self-esteem.

Psychiatric disorders. Clusters of psychological or behavioral symptoms that cause a person to experience serious emotional distress or significant mental impairment; these symptoms must be unusual or unexpected, or the patient must show evidence of more tha n one behavior that deviates from normal social expectations.

Psychosis. The most severe mental disorder, in which the individual loses contact with reality and suffers from such symptoms as delusions and hallucinations.

Psychosomatic disorders. Physical disorder influenced by psychological stressors, or disorders characterized by symptoms that result from unconscious psychological factors instead of an underlying medical condition.

Pterygium/Pinguecula. A thickening of conjunctiva of the eye that grows onto the cornea (pterygium) or degeneration of a portion of the conjunctiva (pinguecula).

Ptosis. Drooping of the upper eyelid, partially or completely covering the eye.

Pulmonary diseases. Diseases of the lungs, which may be serious or fatal; common pulmonary diseases include those caused by infection (bronchitis, pneumonia, tuberculosis), tobacco smoke (emphysema, lung cancer), and allergies (asthma).

Pulmonary edema. A lung ailment in which the pressure in the blood vessels in the lungs exceeds the pressure in the air sacs, resulting in fluid being pushed from the blood into the lungs. This makes it difficult to transfer gases between the blood and lungs.

Pulmonary hypertension. A rare disorder of the pulmonary circulation occurring mostly in young and middle-aged women.

Pyelonephritis. Inflammation of the kidney as the result of a bacterial infection in the bladder.

Pyloric stenosis. An obstruction of the stomach in infancy caused by muscular hypertrophy of the gastric outlet.

Quadriplegia. Devastating, permanent paralysis of all four extremities below the level of injury to the spinal cord.

Quinsy. An abscess usually forming in the peritonsillar space behind the tonsils.

Rabies. A virus that attacks the nerve cells and is most often transmitted by the bite of a rabid animal; control of the disease is accomplished through vaccination of pets and immediate immunization of humans if exposed to the disease; once s ymptoms occur in humans, the disease is nearly always fatal.

Radiation sickness. An acute illness that occurs when an individual is exposed to a sudden, large dose of nuclear radiation or X rays.

Radiculopathy. Pain distributed along a specific pathway resulting from irritation of a nerve root.

Rape and sexual assault. A crime of violence in which a person is forced to submit to sexual acts.

Raynaud's Phenomenon. The reduction of circulation in the extremities, inducing a cold- or stress-induced color change

Reiter's syndrome. An autoimmune disorder with associated symptoms of arthritis, urethritis, conjunctivitis, and ulcerations of the skin and mouth.

Renal failure. A breakdown of kidney function that prevents the removal of waste materials from the body.

Respiratory diseases. *See* Pulmonary diseases; Respiration; *specific diseases*.

Respiratory distress syndrome. A deficiency of surfactant in the neonatal lungs, causing generalized alveolar collapse leading to respiratory failure.

Restless legs syndrome. A sensorimotor disorder characterized by uncomfortable and even painful sensations in the limbs, especially the legs, when at rest or trying to sleep.

Retroviruses. Ribonucleic acid (RNA) viruses that replicate by synthesizing a double-stranded deoxyribonucleic acid (DNA) molecule that integrates into the host genome. They are known to infect virtually all animals and sometimes cause serious disea se, including cancer.

Reye's syndrome. A somewhat rare, noncontagious disease of the liver and central nervous system that strikes individuals under the age of eighteen.

Rheumatic fever. An inflammatory disease of the heart that may follow a streptococcal throat infection.

Rheumatoid arthritis. A chronic, systemic, and inflammatory autoimmune disease that affects the synovial membranes of joints and other organs in the body.

Rhinitis. A discharge from the nose caused by inflammation of the internal nasal structures.

Rhinoviruses. Disease-causing agents that are responsible for more common colds than any other respiratory virus.

Rickets. A disorder involving the softening and weakening of a child's bones, primarily caused by lack of vitamin D and/or lack of calcium or phosphate.

Ringworm. A group of fungal diseases caused by several species of dermatophytes and characterized by itching, scaling, and sometimes painful lesions.

Rocky Mountain spotted fever. An acute febrile illness caused by *Rickettsia rickettsii.*

Rosacea. A chronic inflammation and redness of the face that usually affects people between the ages of thirty and fifty; it is more common in women but is more severe in men.

Roseola . A disease characterized by a mild fever and a rash that mostly affects young children.

Rotavirus. A virus with a characteristic wheel-like appearance when viewed under an electronic microscope that causes viral gastroenteritis in children worldwide.

Roundworms. Worm-shaped animals that act as parasites of plants and animals.

Rubella. An acute, contagious childhood disease caused by a virus and characterized by a rash.

Rubinstein-Taybi syndrome. A syndrome typically characterized by small skeletal stature, mental retardation, and large thumbs and toes.

Salmonella infection. A broad spectrum of clinical diseases caused by many types of salmonella bacteria.

Sarcoidosis. An inflammatory disease of unknown cause characterized by noncaseating granulomas, that affect multiple systems, especially the lungs, lymph nodes, skin, and eyes. This disease is thought to be the result of a dysregulated immune respo nse to an infectious agent or environmental factor. If severe, sarcoidosis is treated with corticosteroids.

Sarcoma. A malignant tumor that develops in connective tissues of the body and can occur in children or adults.

SARS. *See* Severe acute respiratory syndrome (SARS).

Scabies. Skin infestation by mites, causing a rash and severe itching.

Scalds. *See* Burns and scalds.

Scarlet fever. An acute, contagious childhood disease caused by bacterial infection.

Schistosomiasis. A human disease caused by infection by one of several endoparasites of blood flukes.

Schizophrenia. A disorder characterized by disordered thinking and odd perceptions that cause dysfunction in major activities, sometimes including withdrawal from the world, delusions, and hallucinations.

Sciatica. Painful inflammation of one of the sciatic nerves.

SCID. *See* Severe combined immunodeficiency syndrome (SCID).

Scleroderma. A rare autoimmune connective tissue disorder affecting various organs.

Scoliosis. Abnormal curvature of the spine, often progressive, which can result in severe deformity and associated medical problems.

Scurvy. An illness that results from a deficiency of vitamin C (ascorbic acid) in the diet.

Seasonal affective disorder. A subtype of depression characterized by seasonal fluctuation.

Seizures. Asynchronous, paroxysmal discharges of neurons in the brain that result in body movements, unusual sensations, altered perceptions, and/or hallucinations that interfere with normal function and behavior.

Septicemia. Serious, systemic infection of the blood with pathogens that have spread from an infection in a part of the body, characteristically causing fever, chills, prostration, pain, headache, nausea, and/or diarrhea.

Severe acute respiratory syndrome (SARS). A newly recognized type of pneumonia, caused by a novel coronavirus, that may progress to respiratory failure and death.

Severe combined immunodeficiency syndrome (SCID). A syndrome in which the immune system is unable to produce T and B cells, resulting in catastrophic failure of the immune system. The underlying cause is a mutation in one of several key genes, and without specialized treatment, often with cells from a donor, death typically occurs before the age of one.

Sexual dysfunction. Impotence is the persistent inability of a man to achieve and maintain an erection adequate for penetration and sexual intercourse; frigidity is the disinterest in sex, usually applied to women, because of inadequate or unpleasurable s ensation during intercourse.

Sexually transmitted diseases (STDs). Diseases acquired through sexual contact or passed from a pregnant woman to her fetus, including diseases such as syphilis, gonorrhea, chlamydia, genital herpes, genital warts, viral hepatitis, and acquired immunodeficiency syndrome (A IDS).

Shaking. *See* Tremors.

Shigellosis. An intestinal infection caused by *Shigella* bacteria.

Shingles. Reactivation of a viral infection within a nerve cell that causes a characteristic skin rash.

Shock. Shock is a life-threatening condition that may occur in response to a variety of circumstances (allergic reaction, infection, injury, blood loss, heart attack, toxic substances in the blood) which causes the heart to be unable to pump enough blood to supply the vital organs, which are therefore deprived of oxygen and nutrients and lose normal function; symptoms include rapid and shallow breathing, clammy skin, low blood pressure, rapid and weak pulse, and dizziness and if untreate

Sickle cell disease. Genetic disorders of the hemoglobin molecule.

SIDS. *See* Sudden infant death syndrome (SIDS).

Sinusitis. Irritation and swelling of the sinuses.

Sjögren's syndrome. An autoimmune disorder resulting in the loss of tears and saliva.

Skeletal disorders and diseases. *See* Bone disorders.

Skin cancer. Malignancies of the skin (and sometimes spreading to the internal organs) caused by the ultraviolet radiation in sunlight.

Skin disorders. Diseases and conditions that affect the skin, ranging from harmless to life-threatening.

Sleep apnea. A sleep disorder characterized by intermittent cessation of airflow through the upper airway.

Sleep disorders. Any abnormal pattern of sleep which threatens normal function, including conditions that cause too much as well as too little sleep, and which may be both organic and nonorganic in origin.

Sleeping sickness. A parasitic disease caused by protozoa and transmitted to humans by the bites of infected tsetse flies.

Sleepwalking. Repeated episodes of arising from bed during sleep and walking about, without being conscious of the episodes or remembering them.

Slipped disk. A condition in which the soft, gelatinous center part of an intervertebral disk pushes out through a weakened portion of the disk, often placing pressure on a spinal nerve.

Smallpox. An acute, systemic, highly contagious disease caused by a viral infection; there are two forms, the more deadly and feared classic smallpox and a milder variety known as alastrim, which has a fatality rate of about 1 percent.

Smoking. The inhalation of tobacco in the form of cigarettes or cigars, which poses important health risks; those risks can be significantly decreased by smoking cessation, even in older age.

Snakebites. The penetration of skin or flesh by the fangs of a snake. Although a snakebite often involves a poisonous snake, not all bites include venom injection into the bloodstream.

Soiling. The passage of fecal material into inappropriate places, usually underclothes.

Sore throat. Discomfort and/or pain experienced in the throat, which sometimes indicates the presence of a more serious disorder.

Speech disorders. Dysfunction in the brain-coordinated use of speech organs, such as problems with language, vocal quality, articulation, fluency, and dementia.

Spider bites. *See* Bites and stings.

Spina bifida. A birth defect that results from a mistake early in the development of the spinal cord.

Spinal cord disorders. Conditions that adversely affect the spinal cord, which normally carries sensory information from the skin and muscles to the brain and returns with information to control movement.

Spinal fusion. *See* Laminectomy and spinal fusion.

Spinocerebellar ataxia. A group of inherited diseases that cause degeneration in the brain and spinal cord, resulting in progressive loss of coordination.

Split-brain. A condition that results from cutting the corpus callosum, which is the major connection between the two cerebral hemispheres of the brain.

Spondylitis. A form of arthritis that affects the spine.

Sprains. *See* Muscle sprains, spasms, and disorders.

Squamous cell carcinoma. *See* Skin cancer.

Staphylococcal infections. Infections caused by bacteria from the genus *Staphylococcus*.

Stenosis. An abnormal narrowing or constriction of a canal or passageway in the body that is caused by the buildup of cholesterol, fats, or other substances (called plaque); the swelling or overgrowth of cells, tissue, or an organ; or a deformit y.

Steroid abuse. The use of illegal anabolic steroids to increase athletic performance, with negative side effects on physical and psychological health.

Stevens-Johnson syndrome. A severe immune response-mediated hypersensitivity reaction to particular drugs or infections that causes a rash, sloughing of the skin, and the disruption of mucous membranes.

Stillbirth. Birth of a fetus or infant who has died prior to delivery.

Stings. *See* Bites and stings.

Stomach, intestinal, and pancreatic cancers. Malignant tumors of the small intestine, stomach, or pancreas, the latter two types being difficult to detect and treat.

Stones. Hard deposits of material in the body associated with urine and bile.

Strabismus. The improper alignment or crossing of the eyes.

Streptococcal infections. Infections caused by bacteria belonging to the genus *Streptococcus*, such as strep throat, scarlet fever, impetigo, cellulitis, rheumatic fever, and necrotizing fasciitis.

Stress. A psychophysiological response to perceived pressures in the environment, including danger; prolonged stress contributes to hormonal imbalances, immune system collapse, susceptibility to disease, cancer, and death.

Strokes. Stroke, or a cerebrovascular accident (CVA), is the severe reduction or cessation of blood flow to the brain, resulting in a variety of serious and often permanent impairments depending on the area of the brain affected. A transient is chemic attack (TIA) is a temporary, brief loss of blood to the brain, accompanied by temporary impairment of vision, numbness, or other symptoms; it may herald a stroke.

Sturge-Weber syndrome. A disorder associated with partial facial disfigurement which involves vascular accumulations that affect the central nervous system.

Stuttering. Breaks in the smooth flow of speech.

Styes. Inflammations of hair follicles or glands of the eyelids that become infected by bacteria, usually *Staphylococcus aureus*.

Subdural hematoma. Collection of blood (clotted and partially clotted) in the subdural space.

Substance abuse. A pattern of social, psychological, and/or biological problems caused by the way in which a person uses drugs such as alcohol, nicotine, and prescription or illegal drugs.

Sudden infant death syndrome (SIDS). The abrupt and inexplicable death of any infant or young child, and the most common cause of infant death between the ages of two weeks and one year; postmortem examination fails to demonstrate a definitive cause of death.

Suffocation. *See* Asphyxiation.

Suicide. The deliberate taking of one's own life, usually the result of a mental disorder although sometimes deliberated in the face of life-threatening physical illness, significant interpersonal stress, or when under the influence of one or m ore substances of abuse.

Syndrome. A group or pattern of recognizable symptoms or conditions that occur together and indicate a specific disease, psychological disorder, or other abnormal condition.

Synesthesia. A phenomenon wherein one sensory stimulus-a word or a musical note, for example-automatically induces a second, unstimulated sensory perception, typically a color.

Syphilis. A sexually transmitted disease caused by the spirochete bacterium *Treponema palladum* that can progress from a genital lesion to a systemic disorder involving multiple organs.

Systemic lupus erythematosus (SLE). A chronic, inflammatory autoimmune disease in which the immune system attacks the body's own structures. SLE can affect any organ or body system, especially the skin, joints, blood vessels, and kidneys. It is distinguished from two oth er forms of lupus: drug-induced lupus, which is caused by certain prescription medications, and discoid lupus, which primarily affects the skin.

Systemic sclerosis. A systemic disease characterized by extensive scarring in the skin, connective tissue, and internal organs.

Tapeworms. Flatworms of the phylum Platyhelminthes and class Cestoda that are parasitic in the digestive tract of humans and other animals.

Tardive dyskinesia. A medication-induced movement disorder characterized by involuntary movements.

Tay-Sachs disease. An inherited disorder in which products of fat metabolism (gangliosides) accumulate in and destroy the brain and spinal cord.

Temporal arteritis. Inflammation of the medium and large blood vessels that bring blood to the temporal area of the head; may also occur in vessels in other parts of the body.

Temporomandibular joint (TMJ) syndrome. A disorder that produces pain and stiffness in the joint between the lower jawbone (mandible) and the temporal bone of the skull.

Tendinitis. An inflammation of a tendon or tendon sheath.

Tendon disorders. Inflammation or tearing of the tendons.

Teratogens. Agents that alter normal fetal development during pregnancy and cause birth defects.

Testicles, undescended. Testicles that neither reside in nor can be manipulated into the scrotum.

Testicular cancer. A tumor that appears as a hard lump, often painless, on one or both testicles.

Testicular torsion. A twisting or rotation of the testicle (testis) or spermatic cord on its long axis, causing acute pain and swelling.

Tetanus. An often fatal disease of the nervous system characterized by painful, sustained, and violent muscle spasms; it is almost completely preventable through vaccination.

Thalassemia. A group of diverse genetic blood disorders affecting either β or α globin and resulting in decreased amounts of normal hemoglobin.

Throat, sore. *See* Sore throat.

Thrombocytopenia. A bleeding disorder in which the blood contains an abnormally low count of functional platelets (thrombocytes).

Thrombosis and thrombus. Thrombosis is an abnormal blood condition in which blood cells called thrombocytes (platelets) produce clots that move through the bloodstream and eventually clog blood vessels; a thrombus is such a clot.

Thyroid disorders. Underactivity (hypothyroidism) or overactivity (hyperthyroidism) of the thyroid gland.

TIAs. *See* Transient ischemic attacks (TIAs).

Ticks. *See* Lice, mites, and ticks.

Tics. Small, brief, recurrent, inappropriate, compulsive jerking movements or twitches, sometimes called habit spasms, often set off by stressful events and including tic douloureux, involving the trigeminal nerve, and Tourette's syndrome, a lifelong disorder associated with a large variety of tics.

Tingling. *See* Numbness and tingling.

Tinnitus. An auditory sensation originating in the head without external stimulation. This common disorder (often considered a symptom) affects up to 10 percent of the general population in the United States, with the highest prevalence in perso ns between forty and seventy years old.

Tiredness. *See* Fatigue.

Tonsillitis. Inflammation, infection, and enlargement of the palatine tonsils, two small masses of lymphoid tissue located on either side of the back of the throat, and frequently of the pharyngeal tonsils, or adenoids, which are located high in th e throat above the soft palate.

Tooth decay. *See* Cavities.

Torticollis. A form of dystonia (muscle rigidity) in which the neck muscles contract involuntarily, causing spasms, abnormal movements, and posture of the neck and head backward (retrocollis), forward (antercollis), or sideways (torticollis).

Tourette's syndrome. A disorder characterized by recurrent, multiple motor tics and one or more vocal tics that causes stress and impairs social functioning.

Toxemia. A common disorder of pregnancy characterized by hypertension and proteinuria (protein in the urine). When severe, toxemia can affect multiple organ systems and even lead to seizures.

Toxic shock syndrome. A potentially fatal infection causing failure of multiple organs of the body, most notably associated with tampon use.

Toxoplasmosis. A widespread, infectious disease caused by a protozoan parasite.

Trachoma. An infectious disease of the eyes that causes blindness.

Transient ischemic attacks (TIAs). Temporary interference with blood flow to the brain, resulting in transient strokelike symptoms.

Traumatic brain injury. Injury to the brain that usually results from an accident.

Tremors. Rhythmic, oscillating, and involuntary movements that vary with respect to frequency, amplitude, pattern, and anatomical site.

Trichinosis. A parasitic disease of humans caused by nematodes of the *Trichinella* genus and acquired by eating contaminated, undercooked meat.

Trichomoniasis. A sexually transmitted disease in which motile *Trichomonas vaginalis* protozoans become established in the genitourinary tract of men and women.

Tuberculosis. A chronic, highly infectious lung disease that can destroy tissue.

Tularemia. A highly infectious bacterial disease, caused by *Francisella tularensis*, that is of concern as a potential biological weapon.

Tumors. Abnormal growths of bodily tissues caused by genetic changes within normal cells; tumors may be benign (noninvasive) or malignant (invasive).

Turner syndrome. A genetic condition in which cells are missing all or part of an X chromosome.

Typhoid fever. An acute, systemic, febrile disease caused by bacteria that are transmitted through contaminated food or water.

Typhus. An acute, systemic, febrile disease caused by bacteria that are transmitted through the bite of a body louse.

Ulcerative colitis. An inflammatory bowel disease that causes open sores in the colon.

Ulcers. Ulcers, specifically those referred to as peptic ulcers, are open sores that develop on the mucous membranes that line the gastrointestinal tract and are caused by excessive secretion of gastric juices, particularly from the pancreas i nto the intestine.

Undescended testicles. *See* Testicles, undescended.

Uremia. A condition that occurs when an excess of urea and other waste elements accumulate in the blood as the result of reduced or inadequate kidney function, or both.

Urethritis. An infection or inflammation of the urethra, which may be caused by infective organisms, ingested irritants, or trauma.

Urinary disorders. Diseases or pathologies associated with any organs of urine production or secretion, such as the kidneys, ureters, urinary bladder, and urethra.

Uterine cancer. *See* Cervical, ovarian, and uterine cancers.

Varicose veins. The distension of superficial veins, usually affecting the legs and causing the appearance of twisted, swollen, blue veins, especially on the backs of the calves.

Vasculitis. A number of conditions characterized by inflammation of blood vessels, both arteries and veins, that leads to decreased circulation in the affected tissue or organ, which can damage the tissue or organ. Inflammation may be continuous o r spotty and can result in damage to the walls of the blood vessel, leading to destruction of the blood vessel or the formation of an aneurysm.

Venereal diseases. *See* Sexually transmitted diseases (STDs).

Venous insufficiency. An abnormality characterized by decreased blood return from the legs to the trunk that is caused by inefficient valves in the veins.

Vertigo. A sensation of motion or spinning when not moving.

Viral infections. A wide range of diseases, from mild (such as the common cold) to fatal (such as rabies, smallpox, and AIDS), caused by viruses, life-forms that function as intracellular parasites.

Vision correction. *See* Refractive eye surgery.

Vision disorders. Poor vision caused by diseases or abnormalities of the eyes.

Vitamin D deficiency. An illness that results from a deficiency of vitamin D in the diet.

Vitiligo. A disorder that occurs when cells that make pigment (color) in the skin are destroyed, leading to white patches on the body. It may also affect the eyes and the mucous membranes of the mouth and nose, and it may cause hair to gray.

Voice and vocal cord disorders. Physical disorders of the vocal system in the larynx, pharynx, or oral cavity.

Vomiting. *See* Nausea and vomiting.

Von Willebrand's disease. A genetic disorder characterized by the lack of a clotting factor and manifested by excessive bleeding.

Wernicke's aphasia. An acquired language disorder that mostly causes difficulties in comprehension of oral language.

West Nile virus. A mosquito-borne virus affecting humans, birds, and possibly other warm-blooded animals.

Whiplash. An injury to the muscles and ligaments in the neck that is usually the result of riding inside a motor vehicle that is hit from behind.

Whooping cough. A highly contagious respiratory disease characterized by uncontrollable coughing that ends in a loud whoop as the patient attempts to inhale.

Williams syndrome. A rare neurodevelopmental disorder caused by a microdeletion within a specific region of chromosome 7 (7q11.23), typically encompassing approximately 25 to 28 adjacent genes; this chromosomal region has been named Williams Beuren Synd rome chromosome region 1 (WBSCR1).

Wilson's disease. An inherited disease of abnormal copper metabolism, leading to copper accumulation and toxicity in the liver and brain.

Wiskott-Aldrich syndrome. An X-linked genetic disorder characterized by thrombocytopenia, infections, and eczema in childhood.

Wounds. Breakdown in the protective function of the skin; resulting in disruptions or breaks in the continuity of any body tissue.

Yeast infections. *See* Candidiasis.

Yellow fever. An acute tropical and subtropical disease spread by infected mosquitoes from human to human or from infected monkeys to humans.

Zoonoses. Diseases that can be transferred to humans from their primary animal hosts, including farm animals, laboratory research animals, tropical insects and animals, and common house pets, and including poliomyelitis, malaria, rabies, and tox oplasmosis.

Pharmaceutical List

Brand names are capitalized and generics are lowercased. The most common uses are presented here; other uses may apply when appropriate.

Abilify (aripiprazole)
- Bipolar disorders
- Mania
- Psychosis
- Schizophrenia

Abreva (docosonal)
- Facial herpes
- Oral herpes
- Skin infections

acarbose (Precose)
- Type 2 diabetes

Accupril (quinapril)
- Heart failure
- Hypertension

Accutane (isotretinoin)
- Severe acne

acetaminophen (Tylenol, Children's Tylenol, Tylenol with Codeine)
- Fever
- Pain

Actonel (risedronate)
- Osteoporosis
- Paget's disease (bone disease)

Actos (pioglitazone oral)
- Type 2 diabetes

Acuvail (ketorolac tromethamine)
- Postoperative ocular inflammation

acyclovir (Zovirax)
- Chickenpox
- Herpes

Adderall (amphetamine)
- Attention-deficit hyperactivity disorder (ADHD)

Advil (ibuprofen)
- Arthritis
- Menstrual cramps
- Minor aches and pains

albuterol (Combivent, Proventil, Ventolin)
- Bronchial asthma

Aldactone (spironolactone)
- Edema
- Hypertension

Aleve (naproxin sodium)
- Arthritis
- Menstrual cramps

Allegra (fexofenadine)
- Allergies

Alli† (orlistat)
- Obesity

alprazolam (Xanax)
- Anxiety
- Panic disorder

Altace (ramipril)
- Arrhythmia
- Heart failure
- Hypertension

Alupent (metaproterenol sulfate)
- Bronchial asthma

amantadine (Symmetrel)
- Influenza
- Parkinson's disease

Ambien CR (zolpidem tartrate)
- Insomnia

amoxicillin (Amoxil, Augmentin)
- Pneumonia
- Sinusitis

ampicillin (Unasyn)
- Abdominal infections
- Gynecological infections
- Skin infections

Anafranil (clomipramine)
- Obsessive-compulsive disorder (OCD)

Antivert (meclizine)
- Motion sickness
- Vertigo

Aricept (donepezil)
- Mild to moderate Alzheimer's dementia

aripiprazole (Abilify)
- Bipolar disorders
- Mania
- Psychosis
- Schizophrenia

aspirin salicylate (Bayer, Ecotrin)
- Arthritis
- Fever
- Pain
- Rheumatism

Atenolol (tenormin)
- Angina
- Hypertension

Atripla (efavirenz, emtricitabine, and tenofovir)
- Human immunodeficiency virus (HIV) infections

Augmentin (amoxicillin)
- Pneumonia
- Sinusitis

Axid (nizatidine)
- Acid reflux
- Ulcers

azithromycin (Zithromax, Zmax)
- Pneumonia
- Sinusitis

Azmacort (triamcinolone acetonide)
- Asthma

Azulfidine (sulfasalazine)
- Arthritis
- Colitis

bacitracin/polymixin b (Polysporin)
- Minor cuts, scrapes, and burns

Bactrim (sulfamethoxazole)
- Infections

Bayer (aspirin salicylate)
- Fever
- Pain

belladonna alkaloids/phenobarbital (Donnatal)
- Intestinal inflammation
- Irritable bowel syndrome

Benadryl Allergy (diphenhydramine)
- Allergies
- Colds

Bentyl (dicyclomine)
- Irritable bowel syndrome

benzoyl peroxide (Benzac)
- Acne

betamethasone (Diprolene, Lotrisone, Luxiq, Taclonex)
- Dermatosis
- Fungal skin infections
- Psoriasis

bismuth subsalicylate (Pepto-Bismol)
- Diarrhea

Boniva (ibandronate)
- Osteoporosis

Brethine (terbutaline sulfate)
- Asthma
- Chronic bronchitis
- Emphysema

bromocriptine (Parlodel)
- Parkinson's disease

buproprion (Wellbutrin)
- Depression

Buspar (buspirone)
- Depression

calcium polycabophil (Fibercon)
- Constipation
- Diarrhea

Cambia (diclofenac potassium)
- Migraine headaches

carbamazepine (Tegretol)
- Neuralgia
- Seizures

carbidopa (Sinemet)
- Parkinson's disease

Cardizem LA (diltiazem)
- Angina
- Hypertension

Cardura (doxazosine)
- Hypertension
- Urinary retention

cefaclor (Ceclor CD)
- Bronchitis
- Pharyngitis
- Skin infections
- Tonsillitis

Cefprozil (cefzil)
- Infections

Ceftin (cefuroxime)
- Infections

Celebrex (celecoxib)
- Pain
- Painful menstruation
- Osteoarthritis
- Rheumatoid arthritis

Celexa (citalopram)
- Depression

chlorpromazine (Thorazine)
- Mania
- Nausea
- Psychosis

chlorpropamide (Diabinese)
- Diabetes

cholestyramine (Questran)
- Cholesterol and triglyceride control

cimetidine (Tagamet)
- Ulcers

ciprofloxacin (Cipro)
- Infections

clarithromycin (Biaxin)
- Duodenal ulcers

clotrimazole betamethasone (Lotrisone, Mycelex Troches)
- Fungal skin infections

clozapine (Clozaril)
- Schizophrenia

codeine (Promethazine with Codeine, Soma Compound with Codeine, Tussi-Organidin, Tylenol with Codeine)
- Congestion
- Cough
- Pain

Combivir (lamivudine and zidovudine)
- Human immunodeficiency virus (HIV) infections

Corgard (nadolol)
- Angina
- Hypertension

Coumadin (warfarin sodium)
- Blood thinner

Cozaar (losartan potassium)
- Diabetes
- Hypertension

Crestor (rosuvastatin)
- Cholesterol reduction

cromolyn sodium (Crolom, Intal, Nasalcrom)
- Asthma
- Conjunctivis
- Nasal allergies

Cymbalta (duloxetine)
- Chronic pain
- Depression
- Diabetic pain

Darvocet (acetaminophen and propoxyphene)
- Fever
- Pain

Demerol (meperidine)
- Moderate to severe pain

Depakote (divalproex sodium)
- Bipolar disorders
- Mania
- Migraine headaches
- Seizure disorders

Depo-Provera (medroxyprogesterone acetate)
- Injectable contraception

dexamethasone (Ciprodex, Decadron, TobraDex)
- Ear infections
- Eye infections
- Steroid-responsive disorders

Diabeta (glyburide)
- Diabetes

Diabinese (chloropropamide)
- Diabetes

diazepam (Valium)
- Anxiety
- Convulsive disorders
- Muscle spasms

diclofenac potassium (Cambia)
- Migraine headaches

Diflucan (flucanazole)
- Infections of esophagus, pharnyx

digoxin (Lanoxin)
- Heart failure

Dilantin (phenytoin sodium)
- Seizures

diltazem (Cardizem LA, Dilacor XR, Tiazac)
- Angina
- Hypertension

diphenhydramine (Benadryl Allergy, Nytol, Sominex)
- Colds or upper respiratory allergies (Benadryl)
- Insomnia (Nytol, Sominex)

docosanal (Abreva)
- Facial herpes
- Oral herpes
- Skin infections

Donnatal (belladonna alkaloids/phenobarbital)
- Intestinal inflammation
- Irritable bowel syndrome

Dovonex (calcipotriene)
- Plaque psoriasis

doxycycline (Doryx, Monodox, Vibramycin)
- Acne
- Infections

Dumyrox (fluvoxamine)
- Obsessive-compulsive disorder (OCD)

E.E.S. (erythromycin ethylsuccinate)
- Infections

Ecotrin (aspirin salicylate)
- Arthritis
- Coagulation disorders
- Juvenile rheumatoid arthritis
- Rheumatoid arthritis

Effexor XR (venlafaxine)
- Anxiety
- Depression
- Panic disorder

Elavil (amitriptyline)
- Bulimia
- Chronic pain
- Depression

Eldepryl (selegiline)
- Parkinson's disease

Embeda (morphine and naltrexone)
- Chronic pain

Enbrel (etanercept)
- Arthritis
- Inflammation of the vertebrae
- Juvenile rheumatoid arthritis
- Psoriasis
- Rheumatoid arthritis

Epipen (epinephrine)
- Emergency treatment of allergic reactions

Epivir HBV (lamivudine)
- Chronic hepatitis B

Epzicom (abacavir sulfate and lamivudine)
- Human immunodeficiency virus (HIV) infections

erythromycin (Benzamycin, Ery-Tab, Eryc, PCE)
- Acne
- Infections

erythromycin ethylsuccinate (E.E.S., Pediazole)
- Ear infections in children (Pediazole)
- Infections (E.E.S.)

Estrace (estradiol)
- Menopausal disorders
- Osteoporosis

Estraderm (estradiol)
- Menopausal disorders
- Osteoporosis

estradiol (Combipatch, Estrace, Estraderm, Femring, Vivelle)
- Menopausal disorders
- Osteoporosis

estrogens (Premarin, Prempro)
- Menopausal disorders
- Osteoporosis

ethinyl estradiol (Alesse, Fem HRT, Lo/Ovral, Mircette, Seasonale, Tri-Levlen, Yasmin)
- Oral contraception

Evista (raloxifene)
- Bone disorders
- Osteoporosis

famotidine (Pepcid, Pepcid AC)
- Heartburn
- Indigestion
- Ulcers

Flomax (tamsulosin)
- Enlarged prostate

Flumadine (rimantadine)
- Influenza A

fluoxetine (Prozac)
- Bulimia
- Depression
- Obsessive-compulsive disorder (OCD)
- Panic disorder

fluvoxamine (Dumyrox, Faverin, Fevarin, Luvox)
- Obsessive-compulsive disorder (OCD)

Forteo (teriparitide)
- Postmenopausal osteoporosis

Fosamax (alendronate)
- Bone disorders
- Osteoporosis
- Paget's disease (bone disease)

furosemide (Lasix)
- Edema
- Hypertension

gabapentin (Gabarone, Neurontin)
- Epilepsy
- Fibromyalgia
- Neuropathic pain
- Restless legs syndrome
- Seizures

gemfibrozil (Lopid)
- Lipid control

glipizide (Glucotrol XL, Metaglip)
- Type 2 diabetes

Glucophage XR (metformin)
- Type 2 diabetes

Glucotrol XL. *See* **glipizide**

glyburide (Diabeta, Glucovance, Micronasse)
- Type 2 diabetes

H1N1 vaccine
- Influenza A

Heparin (heparin sodium)
- Anticoagulation therapy

hepatitis B vaccine (Comvax, Engerix B, Pediarix, Recombivax HB, Twinrix)
- Hepatitis immunization

Humulin (insulin isophane suspension)
- Diabetes

hydrochlorothiazide (Atacand HCT, Diovan HCT, Dyazide, Hyzaar, Lopressor HCT)
- Hypertension

hydrocortisone (various)
- Dermatosis (Westcort)
- Eye infections (Cortisporin Ophthalmic)
- Hemorrhoids (Anusol HC Suppositories)

ibuprofen (Advil)
- Menstrual cramps
- Minor arthritic pain

Imodium (loperamide)
- Diarrhea

Inderal (propranolol)
- Angina
- Congestive heart failure and arrhythmias
- Hypertension
- Migraine headaches

iron sulfate (Feosol, Fer-in-Sol, Fero-Folic 500, Slow Fe)
- Iron deficiency
- Iron-deficiency anemia

isosorbide dinitrate (Bidil, Dilatrate-SR, Isordil)
- Mild angina
- Heart failure

isosorbide mononitrate (Imdur, Ismo, Monoket)
- Mild angina

isotretinoin (Accutane)
- Severe acne

itraconazole (Sporanox)
- Fungal infections

Kadian (morphine sulfate)
- Severe pain

K-Dur (potassium chloride)
- Hypokalemia

ketoconazole (Nizoral)
- Fungal skin infections

Klonopin (clonazepam)
- Restless legs syndrome
- Seizures

lactase (Lactaid)
- Lactose intolerance

Lamasil (terbinafine)
- Skin infections

Lasix (furosemide)
- Edema
- Hypertension

Levaquin (levofloxacin)
- Infections

levodopa (Parcopa, Sinemet, Stalevo)
- Parkinson's disease

levoflaxin (Levaquin, Quixin)
- Bacterial conjunctivitis
- Infections

levonorgestrel (Alesse, Levlite, Seasonale, Tri-Levlen)
- Oral contraception

Levothroid (levothyroxine sodium)
- Hypothyroidism

levothyroxine sodium (Levothroid, Synthroid)
- Hypothyroidism

Lexapro (escitalopram)
- Anxiety
- Depression

Librium (chlordiazepoxide)
- Anxiety

lisinopril (Zestril)
- Heart failure
- Hypertension

lithium carbonate (Lithobid)
- Mania

Lithobid. *See* **lithium carbonate**

Livalo (pitavastatin)
- High cholesterol

Lopressor (metoprolol tartrate)
- Angina
- Congestive heart failure and arrhythmias
- Hypertension

Lotrisone (betamethasone)
- Fungal skin infections
- Skin infections

Lunelle (progestin plus estrogen)
- Injectable contraception

Lunesta (eszopicione)
- Insomnia

Luvox (fluvoxamine)
- Obsessive-compulsive disorder (OCD)

Lyrica (pregabalin)
- Diabetic pain
- Epilepsy
- Fibromyalgia
- Neuropathic pain
- Restless legs syndrome

Lysteda (tranexamic acid)
- Heavy menstrual bleeding

Maxair Autohaler (pirbuterol)
- Asthma
- Bronchial spasm

Metamucil (psyllium husk)
- Constipation

miconazole (Monistat 1, Monistat 3, Monistat 7)
- Vaginal candidiasis

Minipress (prazosin)
- Hypertension

Minocin (minocycline)
- Acne
- Bacterial infections

minocycline. *See* **Minocin**

Mirapex (pramipexole)
- Parkinson's disease
- Restless legs syndrome

Monistat. *See* **miconazole**

morphine. *See* **Embeda, Kadian, MS Contin**

Motrin (ibuprofen)
- Arthritis
- Fever
- Juvenile rheumatoid arthritis
- Menstrual cramps
- Pain
- Rheumatoid arthritis

MS Contin (morphine sulfate)
- Severe pain

Namenda (memantine)
- Moderate to severe Alzheimer's dementia

Naprosyn (naproxen)
- Arthritis
- Inflammation of the joints
- Juvenile rheumatoid arthritis
- Menstrual cramps
- Pain
- Rheumatoid arthritis

Neosporin Plus (neomycin)
- Infections

Neurontin (gabapentin)
- Epilepsy

- Fibromyalgia
- Neuropathic pain
- Restless legs syndrome
- Seizures

Nicorette (nicotine polacrilex)
- Aid in smoking cessation

Nicotrol (nicotine transdermal patch)
- Aid in smoking cessation

nitroglycerin (Nitro-Bid EXT, Nitrolingual, Nitrostat)
- Angina

Nizoral (ketoconazole)
- Skin infections

Nonsteroidal anti-inflammatory drugs (NSAIDs)
- Arthritis
- Inflammation
- Joint pain
- Rheumatism

Norvasc (amlodipine)
- Angina
- Hypertension

NSAIDs. *See* **Nonsteroidal anti-inflammatory drugs (NSAIDs)**

nystatin (Mycostatin, Mytrex with Nystatin and Triamcinolone Acetonide)
- Candidiasis

ofloxacin (Floxin, Floxin Otic, Ocuflox)
- Infections

omeprazole (Prilosec, Prilosec OTC, Zegerid)
- Frequent heartburn (Prilosec OTC)
- Ulcers (Prilosec, Zegerid)

Onglyza (saxagliptin)
- Type 2 diabetes

orlistat (Alli, Xenical)
- Obesity

Os-Cal (calcium)
- Calcium supplement

oxycodone (Combunox, Oxycontin, OxyIR, Percocet, Percodan, Tylox)
- Pain

paroxetine (Paxil CR)
- Anxiety
- Depression
- Obsessive-compulsive disorder (OCD)
- Panic disorder
- Premenstrual anxiety disorder
- Social anxiety disorder

Paxil CR. *See* **paroxetine**

penicillin V (Veetids)
- Penicillin-sensitive infections

Pepcid (famotidine)
- Acid reflux
- Ulcers

Percocet (oxycodone and acetaminophen)
- Pain

phenytoin (Dilantin)
- Seizures

Plan B One-Step (levonorgestrel)
- Oral contraception

Pneumovax 23 (pneumococcal vaccine polyvalent)
- Pneumococcal immunization

polycarbophil. *See* **calcium polycarbophil**

polymyxin b (Cortisporin, Cortisporin Ophthalmic, Neosporin Plus, Polysporin)
- Dermatosis
- Eye inflammation and infection
- Infection
- Minor pain

Polysporin (bacitracin and polymixin b)
- Infections

potassium chloride (K-Tab, Slow-K)
- Hyperkalemia

PrandiMet (repaglinide and metformin HCl)
- Type 2 diabetes

Pravachol (pravastatin sodium)
- Adjunct to diet for heart conditions

prednisolone (Blephamide)
- Eye inflammation and infection

Precose (acarbose)
- Type 2 diabetes

Prilosec (omeprazole)
- Chronic heartburn
- Gastroesophageal reflux disease (GERD)
- Ulcers

procainamide (Procanibid)
- Arrhythmias

Procardia XL (dihydropyridine)
- Angina
- Hypertension

propranolol (Inderal)
- Angina
- Arrhythmias
- Hypertension
- Migraine headaches

Proventil (albuterol)
- Bronchial asthma

Provera (medroxyprogesterone acetate)
- Amenorrhea
- Menopausal disorders

Provigil (modafinil)
- Chronic fatigue
- Cognitive enhancement
- Narcolepsy
- Sleep apnea

Prozac (fluoxetine)
- Bulimia
- Depression
- Obsessive-compulsive disorder (OCD)
- Panic disorder

pseudoephedrine (Allegra-D, Clarinex-D, Dimetapp, Sudafed, Zytrec-D)
- Allergies
- Cough
- Nasal congestion

psyllium (Konsyl, Metamucil, Semmaprompt)
- Constipation

Questran (cholestyramine resin)
- Cholesterol or triglyceride level reduction

quinapril (Accupril)
- Heart failure
- Hypertension

Quinidex (quinidine sulfate)
- Arrhythmias

raloxifene (Evista)
- Bone disorders
- Osteoporosis

ranitidine (Zantac)
- Gastric reflux
- Ulcers

Reglan (metoclopramide)
- Gastrointestinal disorders
- Nausea

Remicade (infliximab)
- Arthritis
- Colorectal disorders
- Crohn's disease
- Inflammation of the joints
- Ulcerative colitis

Renova (tretinoin)
- Acne
- Skin discoloration
- Wrinkles

Risperdal (benzisoxazole)
- Bipolar disorders
- Mania
- Psychosis
- Schizophrenia

ropinirole hydrochloride (Requip)
- Parkinson's disease
- Restless legs syndrome

rosiglitazone (Avandia)
- Diabetes

Sarafem (fluoxetine)
- Premenstrual disorder

Savella (milnacipran)
- Fibromyalgia

Seasonale (levonorgestrel)
- Oral contraception

senna (Senokot)
- Constipation

Septra (sulfamethoxazole)
- Infections

Seroquel (dibenzothiazepine)
- Bipolar disorders
- Mania
- Psychosis
- Schizophrenia

sertraline (Zoloft)
- Depression
- Obsessive-compulsive disorder (OCD)
- Panic disorder
- Post-traumatic stress disorder (PTSD)
- Premenstrual disorder
- Social anxiety disorder

Sinemet (carbidopa)
- Parkinson's disease

Sinequan (doxepin)
- Anxiety
- Depression

Singulair (montelukast sodium)
- Asthma

Slow-K (potassium chloride)
- Hypokalemia

Stelazine (trifluoperazine)
- Anxiety
- Psychosis

Sudafed (pseudoephedrine HCl)
- Nasal congestion

sulfamethoxazole (Bactrim, Septra)
- Infections

Sumavel DosePro (sumatriptan injection)
- Cluster headaches
- Migraine headaches

sympathomimetic appetite suppressant (Adipex, Atti-Plex P, Bontril, Didrex, Fastin, Ionamin, Melfiat, Meridia, Phentercot, Tenuate, Tenuate Dospan)
- Appetite suppressant

Tagamet (cimetidine)
- Ulcers

Tamiflu (oseltamivir)
- Influenza in infants

tamoxifen (Nolvadex)
- Breast cancer

Tegetrol (carbamazepine)
- Neuralgia
- Seizure disorders

testosterone (Androgel)
- Low testosterone

Tranxene (clorazapate dipotassium)
- Anxiety

trifluoperazine (Stelazine)
- Anxiety
- Psychosis

Tums (calcium carbonate)
- Calcium supplement
- Hyperacidity

Tylenol (acetaminophen)
- Fever
- Minor aches and pains

Tylenol with Codeine (acetaminophen plus codeine)
- Mild to moderately severe pain

Valium (diazepam)
- Anxiety
- Seizure disorders
- Spasms

valproic acid (Depakene)
- Absence seizures

verapamil (Calan)
- Angina
- Arrhythmias
- Hypertension

Viagra (sildenafil citrate)
- Erectile dysfunction

Vicodin (acetaminophen and hydrocodone)
- Pain

Vytorin (ezetimibe and simvastatin)
- Cholesterol control

warfarin sodium (Coumadin)
- Blood thinner

Wellbutrin XL (buproprion HCl)
- Depression

Xenical (orlistat)
- Obesity

Yasmin (drospirenone)
- Oral contraception

Zantac (ranitidine)
- Ulcers

Zerit (stavudine)
- Human immunodeficiency virus (HIV)-1 infection

Zestril (lisinopril)
- Arrhythmias
- Hypertension

Zithromax (azithromycin)
- Infections

Zmax (azithromycin)
- Pneumonia
- Sinusitis

Zocor (simvastatin)
- Cholesterol control

Zoloft (sertraline)
- Anxiety
- Depression
- Obsessive-compulsive disorder (OCD)
- Panic disorder
- Premenstrual disorder

Zovirax (acyclovir)
- Chickenpox
- Herpes

Zyloprim (allopurinol)
- Gout
- Hyperuricemia

Zyprexa (olanzapine)
- Bipolar disorders
- Mania
- Psychosis
- Schizophrenia

—Mel Siegel, M.A.,
and Connie Rizzo, M.D., Ph.D. (consultant);
updated by Desiree Dreeuws

Types of Health Care Providers

ACUPUNCTURISTS

Training and Degrees: Program in acupuncture or Chinese medicine, preferably one approved by the Accreditation Commission for Acupuncture and Oriental Medicine (ACAOM)

—Diplomate in Acupuncture (Dipl.Ac.) or Master of Science (M.S.)

Duties: Pain reduction and health balance in the body through the use of thin needles inserted at specific points

Specializations: None

BIOTECHNOLOGISTS

Training and Degrees: Undergraduate degree program; graduate degree recommended

—Bachelor of Science (B.S.), Master of Science (M.S.)

Duties: The performance of research or application studies in the field of biology

Specializations: All medical fields

CHIROPRACTORS

Training and Degrees: Two years of premedical studies (minimum), followed by four years of chiropractic school

—Doctor of Chiropractic (D.C.)

Duties: The mechanical manipulation of the spinal column for the maintenance of health

Specializations: The use of radiology or physiotherapy to supplement manipulation

COUNSELORS

Training and Degrees: Varies; may range from personal experience to specialized training

—Bachelor of Arts (B.A.) or Bachelor of Science (B.S.), with possible advanced degree

Duties: One-on-one work with a patient to deal with specific emotional problems

Specializations: All areas of health care

CYTOLOGISTS

Training and Degrees: Undergraduate degree program, followed by graduate program and postgraduate training

—Doctor of Philosophy (Ph.D.) or Doctor of Medicine (M.D.)

Duties: The microscopic study of cells or tissue

Specializations:
- Hematology (the observation and study of blood cells or tissues associated with blood cell formation)
- Histology (the observation and study of tissue)

DENTISTS

Training and Degrees: Two years of undergraduate studies (minimum), followed by three to four years of dental college

—Doctor of Dental Surgery (D.D.S.) or Doctor of Dental Medicine (D.M.D.)

Duties: The repair, restoration, and cleaning of teeth

Specializations:
- Endodontics (the diagnosis and treatment of diseases of dental pulp and tissue)
- Oral pathology or surgery (the diagnosis and surgical repair of oral disorders)
- Orthodontics (the diagnosis and treatment of tooth irregularities)
- Pedodontics (the diagnosis and treatment of the dental problems of children)
- Periodontics (the diagnosis and treatment of disorders in tissue surrounding teeth)
- Prosthodontics (the production of artificial devices for tooth replacement)

DIETETIC TECHNICIANS

Training and Degrees: A two-year dietetic program

—Associate degree in a program approved by the American Dietetic Association

Duties: The assessment, design, and implementation of nutritional programs

Specializations:
- Dietitian (a person trained in nutritional care)
- Geriatric dietician (a person trained in the nutritional care of the elderly)
- Pediatric dietician (a person trained in the nutritional care of children)

IMMUNOLOGISTS

Training and Degrees: Undergraduate degree program; graduate or professional program

—Master of Science (M.S.); Doctor of Philosophy (Ph.D.)

Duties: The observation and study of the body's immune system

Specializations: None

INTERNS

Training and Degrees: The completion of a postgraduate program in the field of health care

—Master of Science (M.S.) or doctoral degree

Duties: The learning of medical procedures under the supervision of residents or other physicians

Specializations: All areas of health care

LABORATORY TECHNICIANS

Training and Degrees: A two-year or four-year school

—Associate degree, Bachelor of Science (B.S.) or Master of Science (M.S.)

Duties: The collection, preparation, and testing of tissues or fluids for diagnostic purposes; the carrying out of medical procedures under the direction of physicians

Specializations: Many medical fields

MEDICAL DOCTORS

Training and Degrees: Undergraduate degree program followed by medical school; specializations are generally based on training that begins during the years as a resident —Doctor of Medicine (M.D.)

Duties: The assessment and diagnosis of medical problems; the administration of procedures or drugs for treatment

Specializations:
- Anesthesiology (the administration of anesthetics for the relief or prevention of pain)
- Cardiology (the diagnosis and treatment of disorders of the heart)
- Dermatology (the diagnosis and treatment of skin disorders)
- Family practice (the diagnosis and treatment of disorders among all individuals, rather than specialization based on age or sex)
- Gastroenterology (the study of disorders of the stomach and intestinal tract)
- Geriatrics (the treatment of disorders of the elderly)
- Gynecology (the diagnosis and treatment of disorders of the female reproductive system)
- Internal medicine (the diagnosis and treatment of disorders affecting internal organs)
- Nephrology (the diagnosis and treatment of disorders associated with the kidneys)
- Obstetrics (the diagnosis and treatment of disorders dealing with pregnancy and childbirth)
- Oncology (the diagnosis and treatment of tumors)
- Ophthalmology (the diagnosis and treatment of disorders associated with the eyes)
- Pediatrics (the diagnosis and treatment of disorders of children)
- Plastic surgery (the surgical repair or restoration of visible areas of the body)
- Proctology (the diagnosis and treatment of disorders affecting the anus, colon, or rectum)
- Psychiatry (the diagnosis and treatment of mental disorders)
- Pulmonology (the diagnosis and treatment of disorders of the lungs or respiratory system)
- Rheumatology (the diagnosis and treatment of disorders affecting connective tissue)
- Urology (the diagnosis and treatment of disorders affecting the urinary tract)
- Vascular medicine (the diagnosis and treatment of disorders associated with the circulatory system)

MICROBIOLOGISTS

Training and Degrees: Undergraduate degree program; graduate degree recommended —Bachelor of Science (B.S.), Master of Science (M.S.)

Duties: The research, maintenance, or identification of microorganisms

Specializations:
- Bacteriology (the identification and study of bacteria)
- Mycology (the identification and study of molds)
- Virology (the identification and study of viruses)

MIDWIVES

Training and Degrees: Program in midwifery; registration and license to practice

Duties: The supervision of pregnancy, labor, delivery, and the postpartum period, in addition to counseling and family planning

Specialization: Certified nurse midwife (a person who is certified as both a nurse and a midwife)

NURSES

Training and Degrees: Undergraduate degree program, followed by study at an approved school of nursing; passage of the National Council Licensure Examination (NCLEX-RN) is required to become a Registered Nurse —Associate Degree in Nursing (A.D.N.), Bachelor of Science in Nursing (B.S.N.) (four-year program), Master of Science in Nursing (M.S.N.), Registered Nurse (R.N.)

Duties: The administration of medical treatments recommended by physicians; the monitoring and facilitation of medical care

Specializations:
- Clinical nurse specialist (R.N. with experience in dealing with overall health care; requires M.S.N.)
- Nurse educator (R.N. trained in the teaching of nurses)
- Nurse practitioner (R.N. with advanced training and experience in a particular branch of nursing)
- Obstetric nurse (R.N. specializing in pregnancy and childbirth)
- Pediatric nurse (R.N. trained in the nursing care of children)
- Surgical nurse (R.N. trained to assist during surgical procedures)

OPTOMETRISTS

Training and Degrees: Two years of undergraduate studies (minimum), followed by four years of optometry college; state license —Doctor of Optometry (D.O.)

Duties: Testing of the eyes for visual acuity; the prescription of corrective lenses

Specialization: Optician (a person who makes or sells corrective lenses)

OSTEOPATHS

Training and Degrees: Undergraduate degree program, followed by medical school and an internship, or graduation from a college of osteopathy —Doctor of Medicine (M.D.), Doctor of Osteopathy (D.O.)

Duties: The manipulation of body structures as supplemental treatment for disease

Specialization: Doctor of Medicine (M.D.)

PATHOLOGISTS

Training and Degrees: Undergraduate degree program, followed by medical school

—Doctor of Medicine (M.D.)

Duties: The observation of the effects of disease on the body

Specializations:

- Autopsy (the determination of the cause of death)
- Clinical pathology (the assessment of disease states as reflected in changes within the body)

PHARMACISTS

Training and Degrees: A two-year undergraduate program, followed by a two-year to three-year program in an approved school of pharmacy; state license

—Doctor of Pharmacology (Pharm.D.)

Duties: The formulation and dispensation of medications

Specializations: None

PHARMACOLOGISTS

Training and Degrees: Undergraduate degree program; graduate program

—Master of Science (M.S.); Doctor of Philosophy (Ph.D.)

Duties: The study of the properties and use of drugs or other pharmacologic agents

Specializations: None

PHYSICAL THERAPISTS

Training and Degrees: Undergraduate program in physical therapy, or a one-year certified course in conjunction with a degree program in a related field

Duties: The testing and treatment of persons who are physically handicapped, either temporarily or permanently

Specializations: None

PHYSICIAN ASSISTANTS

Training and Degrees: A two-year program for national certification by the American Association of Physician Assistants (AAPA)

Duties: The provision of assistance as requested by supervising physicians

Specializations:

- Radiology (providing aid during X-ray and related procedures)
- Surgery (assisting surgeons during operations)

PODIATRISTS

Training and Degrees: Two years of premedical studies (minimum), followed by four years of podiatry school; state license

—Doctor of Podiatric Medicine (D.P.M.)

Duties: The treatment of foot disorders

Specializations: None

PSYCHOLOGICAL ASSISTANTS

Training and Degrees: Undergraduate degree program, graduate degree, and an internship

—Master's degree or higher

Duties: The administration of psychological tests or their assessment under the supervision of psychologists

Specializations:

- Child psychology (the assessment of children)
- Clinical psychology (the assessment of behavioral disorders)
- Educational psychology (the preparation and administration of tests)

PSYCHOLOGISTS

Training and Degrees: Undergraduate degree program, graduate degree, an internship, and postdoctoral experience

—Doctor of Philosophy (Ph.D.), Doctor of Psychology (Psy.D.), Doctor of Education (Ed.D.)

Duties: The assessment, diagnosis, and administration of psychological tests and treatments for mental disorders and physical conditions that are affected by mental conditions

Specializations:

- Child psychology (the diagnosis and treatment of emotional disorders in children)
- Clinical psychology (the diagnosis and treatment of personality or behavioral disorders)
- Educational psychology (the application of psychology to education or testing procedures)

RADIOLOGISTS

Training and Degrees: Undergraduate degree program, followed by medical school and generally a residency in radiology

—Doctor of Medicine (M.D.)

Duties: The use of radioactive materials for the diagnosis and treatment of disease

Specializations:

- Diagnostic radiology (the use of radioactive materials for imaging)
- Nuclear medicine (the performance of diagnostic procedures and imaging involving the internal use of radiochemicals)
- Therapeutic radiology (the use of radiochemicals for the treatment of disorders)

RESIDENTS

Training and Degrees: Undergraduate degree program, followed by medical school and one year of internship

—Doctor of Medicine (M.D.)

Duties: Clinical duties in hospitals in any of several specialties

Specializations: All medical fields

RESPIRATORY THERAPISTS

Training and Degrees: Undergraduate degree from a school approved by American Medical Association, with training appropriate for passing the registry examination

—Associate degree or Bachelor of Science (B.S.)

Duties: The carrying out of treatments designed to improve or correct functions of the respiratory tract, under the direction of physicians

Specialization: Registered respiratory therapist (the graduate of an advanced program from the National Board of Respiratory Care)

Toxicologists

Training and Degrees: Undergraduate degree program; graduate program

—Master of Science (M.S.), Doctor of Philosophy (Ph.D.)

Duties: The study of poisonous compounds

Specializations: None

GENERAL BIBLIOGRAPHY

ACQUIRED IMMUNODEFICIENCY SYNDROME (AIDS). *See also* SEXUALLY TRANSMITTED DISEASES (STDs)

Bartlett, John G. *The Johns Hopkins Hospital 2005-6 Guide to Medical Care of Patients with HIV Infection.* 12th ed. Philadelphia: Lippincott Williams & Wilkins, 2005.

Bartlett, John G., and Ann K. Finkbeiner. *The Guide to Living with HIV Infection: Developed at the Johns Hopkins AIDS Clinic.* 6th ed. Baltimore: Johns Hopkins University Press, 2007.

Buckley, R. Michael, and Stephen J. Gluckman, eds. *HIV Infection in Primary Care.* Philadelphia: W. B. Saunders, 2002.

Cichocki, Mark. *Living with HIV: A Patient's Guide.* Jefferson, N.C.: McFarland, 2009.

Clark, Rebecca A., Robert T. Maupin, Jr., and Jill Hayes Hammer. *A Woman's Guide to Living with HIV Infection.* Baltimore: Johns Hopkins University Press, 2004.

Fan, Hung Y., Ross F. Conner, and Luis P. Villarreal. *AIDS: Science and Society.* 5th ed. Sudbury, Mass.: Jones and Bartlett, 2007.

Hubley, John. *The AIDS Handbook: A Guide to the Prevention of AIDS and HIV.* 3d ed. New York: Macmillan, 2002.

Jessen, Heiko, and Hans Jaeger, eds. *Primary HIV Infection: Pathology, Diagnosis, Management.* New York: Georg Thieme, 2005.

Masci, Joseph R. *Outpatient Management of HIV Infection.* 3d ed. Boca Raton, Fla.: CRC Press, 2001.

Matthews, Dawn D., ed. *AIDS Sourcebook.* 3d ed. Detroit: Omnigraphics, 2003.

Princeton, Douglas C. *Manual of HIV/AIDS Therapy.* Rev. ed. Laguna Hills, Calif.: Current Clinical Strategies, 2002.

Shearer, William T., and I. Celine Hansen, eds. *Medical Management of AIDS in Children.* Philadelphia: W. B. Saunders, 2003.

Stine, Gerald J. *AIDS Update 2010.* New York: McGraw-Hill Higher Education, 2010.

World Bank. *Education and HIV/AIDS: A Window of Hope.* Washington, D.C.: Author, 2002.

ALLERGY

Adkinson, N. Franklin, Jr., Bruce S. Bochner, A. Wesley Burks, William W. Busse, Stephen T. Holgate, Robert F. Lemanske, Jr., and Robyn E. O'Hehir. *Middleton's Allergy: Principles and Practice.* 8th ed. Philadelphia: Saunders, 2014.

Akim, Cem. *Mast Cells and Mastocytosis: An Issue of Immunology and Allergy Clinics.* Philadelphia: Elsevier, 2014.

Joo, Shirley, and Andrew Kau. *The Washington Manual of Allergy, Asthma, and Immunology Subspecialty Consult.* 2d ed. Philadelphia: Lippincott Williams & Wilkins, 2012.

Mahmoudi, Massoud. *Allergy and Asthma: Practical Diagnosis and Management.* New York: McGraw-Hill Professional, 2007.

Murphy, Kenneth. *Janeway's Immunobiology: The Immune System.* New York: Garland Science, 2011.

Nowak-Wegrzyn, Anna. *Food Allergies, An Issue of Immunology and Allergy Clinics.* Philadelphia: Saunders, 2012.

ALTERNATIVE/COMPLEMENTARY MEDICINE

Castleman, Michael. *Blended Medicine: How to Integrate the Best Mainstream and Alternative Remedies for Maximum Health and Healing.* Emmaus, Pa.: Rodale Press, 2002.

Ditchek, Stuart, Andrew Weil, and Russell H. Greenfield. *Healthy Child, Whole Child: Integrating the Best of Conventional and Alternative Medicine to Keep Your Kids Healthy.* New York: HarperCollins, 2002.

Freeman, Lyn. *Mosby's Complementary and Alternative Medicine: A Research-Based Approach.* 2d ed. St. Louis, Mo.: Mosby, 2004.

Goldberg, Burton, comp. *Alternative Medicine: The Definitive Guide.* 2d ed. Tiburon, Calif.: Future Medicine, 2002.

Kemper, Kathi J. *The Holistic Pediatrician: A Pediatrician's Comprehensive Guide to Safe and Effective Therapies for the Twenty-five Most Common Ailments of Infants, Children, and Adolescents.* Rev. ed. New York: Quill, 2002.

Mackenzie, Elizabeth R., and Birgit Rakel, eds. *Complementary and Alternative Medicine for Older Adults: A Guide to Holistic Approaches to Healthy Aging.* New York: Springer, 2006.

Micozzi, Marc S., ed. *Fundamentals of Complementary and Integrative Medicine.* 3d ed. St. Louis, Mo.: Saunders/Elsevier, 2006.

Murray, Michael T. *Pill Book Guide to Alternative Medicines.* New York: Bantam, 2002.

Pelletier, Kenneth. *The Best Alternative Medicine.* New York: Fireside, 2002.

Trivieri, Larry, Jr., and John W. Anderson, eds. *Alternative Medicine: The Definitive Guide.* 2d ed. Berkeley, Calif.: Ten Speed Press, 2002.

Weil, Andrew. *Healthy Aging: A Lifelong Guide to Your Physical and Spiritual Well-Being.* New York: Anchor Books, 2007.

White, B. Linda, and Steven Foster. *The Herbal Drugstore.* Emmaus, Pa.: Rodale Press, 2003.

AMBULATORY CARE

Barkin, Roger M., and Peter Rosen, eds. *Emergency Pediatrics: A Guide to Ambulatory Care.* 6th ed. New York: Elsevier, 2003.

Colyar, Margaret R., and Cynthia R. Ehrhardt. *Ambulatory Care Procedures for the Nurse Practitioner.* 2d ed. Philadelphia: F. A. Davis, 2004.

Fiebach, Nicholas H., et al., eds. *Principles of Ambulatory Medicine.* 7th ed. Philadelphia: Lippincott Williams & Wilkins, 2007.

Lewis, Marcia A., and Carol D. Tamparo. *Medical Law, Ethics, and Bioethics for Ambulatory Care*. 5th ed. Philadelphia: F. A. Davis, 2002.

Mengel, Mark B., and L. Peter Schwiebert, eds. *Family Medicine: Ambulatory Care and Medicine*. 4th ed. New York: Lange Medical Books/McGraw-Hill, 2005.

Wachtel, Tom J., and Michael D. Stein, eds. *Practical Guide to the Care of the Ambulatory Patient*. 2d ed. St. Louis, Mo.: Mosby, 2000.

ANATOMY

Abrahams, Peter H., Sandy C. Marks, Jr., and Ralph Hutchings. *McMinn's Color Atlas of Human Anatomy*. 6th ed. St. Louis, Mo.: Mosby/Elsevier, 2008.

Agur, Anne M. R., and Arthur F. Dalley. *Grant's Atlas of Anatomy*. 12th ed. Philadelphia: Wolters Kluwer Health/Lippincott Williams & Wilkins, 2009.

Bo, Walter J., et al. *Basic Atlas of Sectional Anatomy with Correlated Imaging*. 4th ed. Philadelphia: Saunders/Elsevier, 2007.

Eroschenko, Victor P. *Di Fiore's Atlas of Histology with Functional Correlations*. 10th ed. Philadelphia: Lippincott Williams & Wilkins, 2005.

Junqueira, Luis C., et al. *Basic Histology*. 10th ed. New York: McGraw-Hill, 2002.

Marieb, Elaine N. *Essentials of Human Anatomy and Physiology*. 9th ed. San Francisco: Pearson/Benjamin Cummings, 2009.

Moore, Keith L., and Anne M. R. Agur. *Essential Clinical Anatomy*. 4th ed. Philadelphia: Lippincott Williams & Wilkins, 2010.

Moore, Keith L., and T. V. N. Persaud. *The Developing Human*. 8th ed. Philadelphia: Saunders/Elsevier, 2008.

Rohen, Johannes W., Chihiro Yokochi, and Elke Lütjen-Drecoll. *Color Atlas of Anatomy: A Photographic Study of the Human Body*. 6th ed. Philadelphia: Lippincott Williams & Wilkins, 2006.

Scanlon, Valerie, and Tina Sanders. *Essentials of Anatomy and Physiology*. 5th ed. Philadelphia: F. A. Davis, 2007.

Snell, Richard S. *Clinical Neuroanatomy*. 6th ed. Philadelphia: Lippincott Williams & Wilkins, 2006.

Standring, Susan, et al., eds. *Gray's Anatomy*. 40th ed. New York: Churchill Livingstone/Elsevier, 2008.

Tortora, Gerard J., and Bryan Derrickson. *Principles of Anatomy and Physiology*. 12th ed. Hoboken, N.J.: John Wiley & Sons, 2009.

Van De Graaff, Kent M. *Human Anatomy*. 6th ed. Boston: McGraw-Hill, 2002.

ANESTHESIOLOGY

Barash, Paul, Bruce F. Cullen, Robert Stoelting, Michael Cahalan, M. Christine Stock, and Rafeal Ortega. *Clinical Anesthesia*. 7th ed. Philadelphia: Lippincott, Williams & Wilkins, 2013.

Butterworth, John, David C. Mackey, and John Wasnick. *Morgan and Mikhail's Clinical Anesthesiology*. 5th ed.

New York: McGraw-Hill Medical, 2013.

Hines, Roberta L., and Katherine Marschall. *Stoelting's Anesthesia and Co-existing Disease: Expert Consult*. 6th ed. Philadelphia: Saunders, 2012.

Jaffe, Richard A. *Anesthesiologist's Manual of Surgical Procedures*. Philadelphia: Lippincott Williams & Wilkins, 2009.

Loeser, John D., ed. *Bonica's Management of Pain*. 4th ed. Philadelphia: Lippincott Williams & Wilkins, 2010.

Miller, Ronald D., ed. *Miller's Anesthesia*. 7th ed. Philadelphia: Churchill Livingstone/Elsevier, 2010.

Nagelhout, John J., and Karen Plaus. *Nurse Anesthesia*. 5th ed. Philadelphia: Saunders, 2013.

BIOCHEMISTRY

Berg, Jeremy M., John L. Tymoczko, and Lubert Stryer. *Biochemistry*. 7th ed. New York: W.H. Freeman, 2010.

Cox, Michael M., Jennifer Doudna, and Michael O'Donnell. *Molecular Biology: Principles and Practice*. New York: W.H. Freeman, 2011.

Devlin, Thomas M. *Textbook of Biochemistry with Clinical Applications*. 7th ed. New York: John Wiley and Sons, 2010.

Lodish, Harvey, Arnold Berk, Chris Kaiser, and Monty Krieger. *Molecular Cell Biology*. 9th ed. New York: W. H. Freeman, 2012.

Nelson, David L., and Michael M. Cox. *Lehninger Principles of Biochemistry*. 6th ed. New York: W. H. Freeman 2012.

CARDIOVASCULAR SYSTEM

Blumenthal, Roger, JoAnne Foody, and Nathan D. Wong. *Preventative Cardiology: Companion to Braunwald's Heart Disease*. Philadelphia: Saunders, 2011.

Bonow, Robert O., Douglas L. Mann, Douglas P. Zipes, and Peter Libby. *Braunwald's Heart Disease: A Textbook of Cardiovascular Medicine*. Philadelphia: Saunders, 2011.

Chatterjee, Kanu, Mark Anderson, Donald Heistad, and Richard Kerber. *Cardiology: An Illustrated Textbook*. New Delhi, India: Jaypee Brothers Medical Publications, 2012.

Chizner, Michael. *Clinical Cardiology Made Ridiculously Simple*. Miami, FL: Medmaster, 2013.

Eisen, Howard J. *Heart Failure, An Issue of Cardiology Clinics*. Philadelphia: Elsevier, 2014.

Murphy, Joseph G. and Margaret A. Lloyd. *Mayo Clinic Cardiology: Concise Textbook*. New York: Oxford University Press, 2012.

Park, Myung K. *Park's Pediatric Cardiology for Practitioners*. 6th ed. Philadelphia: Mosby, 2014.

Topol, Eric J., and Paul S. Teirstein. *Textbook of International Cardiology*. 6th ed. Philadelphia: Saunders, 2012.

CRITICAL CARE

Albert, Richard K., et al., eds. *Clinical Critical Care Medicine*. Philadelphia: Mosby/Elsevier, 2006.

Bongard, Frederick, and Darryl Y. Sue, eds. *Current Critical Care Diagnosis and Treatment*. 3d ed. New York:

McGraw-Hill Medical, 2008.

Fink, Mitchell P., et al. *Textbook of Critical Care*. 5th ed. Philadelphia: Saunders/Elsevier, 2005.

Fuhrman, Bradley P., and Jerry J. Zimmerman, eds. *Pediatric Critical Care*. 3d ed. Philadelphia: Mosby/Elsevier, 2006.

Hogan, David E., and Jonathan L. Burstein. *Disaster Medicine*. 2d ed. Philadelphia: Lippincott Williams & Wilkins, 2007.

Irwin, Richard S., et al., eds. *Procedures and Techniques in Intensive Care Medicine*. 3d ed. Philadelphia: Lippincott Williams & Wilkins, 2003.

Irwin, Richard S., and James M. Rippe, eds. *Irwin and Rippe's Intensive Care Medicine*. 5th ed. Philadelphia: Lippincott Williams & Wilkins, 2003.

Lanken, Paul N., et al., eds. *The Intensive Care Unit Manual*. Philadelphia: W. B. Saunders, 2001.

Marini, John J., and Arthur P. Wheeler. *Critical Care Medicine: The Essentials*. 3d ed. Philadelphia: Lippincott Williams & Wilkins, 2006.

Marino, Paul L. *The ICU Book*. 3d ed. Philadelphia: Lippincott Williams & Wilkins, 2007.

Merenstein, Gerald B., and Sandra L. Gardner, eds. *Merenstein and Gardner's Handbook of Neonatal Intensive Care*. 7th ed. Maryland Heights, Mo.: Mosby/Elsevier, 2010.

Murray, Michael J., et al., eds. *Critical Care Medicine: Perioperative Management*. 2d ed. Philadelphia: Lippincott Williams & Wilkins, 2002.

Osborne, Molly L., ed. *Geriatric Critical Care*. Philadelphia: W. B. Saunders, 2003.

Slonim, Anthony D., and Murray M. Pollack, eds. *Pediatric Critical Care Medicine*. Philadelphia: Lippincott Williams & Wilkins, 2006.

Sue, Darryl Y., and Janine R. E. Vintch, eds. *Current Essentials of Critical Care*. New York: Lange Medical Books/McGraw-Hill, 2005.

Udwadia, Farokh Erach. *Principles of Critical Care*. 2d ed. New York: Oxford University Press, 2005.

DENTISTRY

Ash, Major M., Jr., and Stanley J. Nelson. *Wheeler's Dental Anatomy, Physiology, and Occlusion*. 9th ed. St. Louis, Mo.: Saunders/Elsevier, 2010.

Burt, Brian A., and Steven A. Eklund. *Dentistry, Dental Practice, and the Community*. 6th ed. St. Louis, Mo.: Saunders/Elsevier, 2005.

Cohen, Stephen, and Kenneth M. Hargreaves, eds. *Pathways of the Pulp*. 9th ed. St. Louis, Mo.: Mosby/Elsevier, 2006.

Diamond, Richard. *Dental First Aid for Families*. Ravensdale, Wash.: Idyll Arbor, 2000.

Gluck, George M., and William M. Morganstein. *Jong's Community Dental Health*. 5th ed. St. Louis, Mo.: Mosby, 2003.

Langlais, Robert P., and Craig S. Miller. *Color Atlas of Common Oral Diseases*. 4th ed. Philadelphia: Lippincott Williams & Wilkins, 2009.

Mitchell, David A. *An Introduction to Oral and Maxillofacial Surgery*. New York: Oxford University Press, 2006.

Parker, James N., and Philip M. Parker, eds. *The Official Patient Sourcebook on Tooth Decay*. San Diego, Calif.: Icon Health, 2002.

Peterson, Larry J., et al. *Contemporary Oral and Maxillofacial Surgery*. 4th ed. St. Louis, Mo.: Mosby, 2003.

Scully, Crispian, and Athanasios Kalantzis. *Oxford Handbook of Dental Patient Care*. 2d ed. New York: Oxford University Press, 2005.

Weiss, Charles M., and Adam Weiss. *Principles and Practice of Implant Dentistry*. St. Louis, Mo.: Mosby, 2001.

DERMATOLOGY

Bolognia, Jean L., Julie V. Schaffer, Karynne O. Duncan, and Christine Ko. *Dermatology Essentials*. Philadelphia: Saunders, 2014.

Habif, Thomas P. *Clinical Dermatology*. 5th ed. Philadelphia: Mosby, 2010.

Hall, John C., and Gordon C. Sauer. *Sauer's Manual of Skin Diseases*. 10th ed. Philadelphia: Lippincott Williams & Wilkins, 2010.

Robinson, June K., C. William Hanke, Daniel Mark Siegel, and Alina Fratila. *Surgery of the Skin*. 2d ed. Philadelphia: Mosby, 2010.

Schachner, Lawrence A., and Ronald C. Hansen. *Pediatric Dermatology*. 4th ed. Philadelphia: Mosby, 2011.

Turkington, Carol, and Jeffrey S. Dover. *The Encyclopedia of Skin and Skin Disorders*. 3d ed. New York: Facts On File, 2007.

Webster, Guy F., and Anthony V. Rawlings, eds. *Acne and Its Therapy*. New York: Informa Healthcare, 2007.

Weedon, David. *Skin Pathology*. 3d ed. Philadelphia: Churchill Livingstone/Elsevier, 2010.

Weston, William L., et al. *Color Textbook of Pediatric Dermatology*. 4th ed. St. Louis, Mo.: Mosby/Elsevier, 2007.

Wolff, Klaus, Richard Allen Johnson, and Dick Suurmond. *Fitzpatrick's Color Atlas and Synopsis of Clinical Dermatology*. 6th ed. New York: McGraw-Hill Medical, 2009.

DIAGNOSIS

Ferri, Fred F. *Ferri's Differential Diagnosis: A Practical Guide to the Differential Diagnosis of Symptoms, Signs, and Clinical Disorders*. 2d ed. Philadelphia: Mosby/Elsevier, 2011.

Pagana, Kathleen Deska, and Timothy J. Pagana. *Mosby's Diagnostic and Laboratory Test Reference*. 9th ed. St. Louis, Mo.: Mosby/Elsevier, 2009.

Raftery, Andrew, Eric KS Lim, Andrew J K Östör. *Churchill's Pocketbook of Differential Diagnosis*. 4th ed. London: Churchill Livingstone, 2014.

Swartz, Mark H. *Textbook of Physical Diagnosis*. 7th ed. Philadelphia: Saunders, 2014.

DICTIONARIES AND DIRECTORIES

Dorland, W. A. Newman, ed. *Dorland's Illustrated Medical Dictionary.* 32d ed. Philadelphia: Saunders/Elsevier, 2011.

Marcovitch, Harvey, ed. *Black's Medical Dictionary.* 42d ed. Lanham, Md.: Scarecrow Press, 2010.

Mosby's Medical Dictionary. 9th ed. St. Louis, Mo.: Mosby/Elsevier, 2012.

PDR for Nonprescription Drugs, Dietary Supplements, and Herbs. 31st ed. Montvale, N.J.: PDR Network, 2010.

Physicians' Desk Reference. 66th ed. Montvale, N.J.: PDR Network, 2011.

Professional Guide to Diseases. 10th ed. Philadelphia: Lippincott Williams & Wilkins, 2012.

Porter, Robert S., et al., eds. *The Merck Manual Home Health Handbook.* 3d ed. Whitehouse Station, N.J.: Merck Research Laboratories, 2009.

Stedman's Medical Dictionary for the Health Professions and Nursing. 7th ed. Philadelphia: Lippincott Williams & Wilkins, 2011.

Venes, Donald, ed. *Taber's Cyclopedic Medical Dictionary.* 22st ed. Philadelphia: F. A. Davis, 2013.

EMERGENCY MEDICINE

Adams, James G. *Emergency Medicine.* 2d ed. Philadelphia: Saunders, 2014.

American Medical Association. *Handbook of First Aid and Emergency Care.* Rev. and updated ed. New York: Random House Reference, 2009.

Anwar, Asif. *Concise Review of Critical Care, Trauma and Emergency Medicine: A Quick Reference Guide of ICU and ER Topics.* Philadelphia: Saunders, 2013.

Auerbach, Paul S. *Wilderness Medicine.* 6th ed. Philadelphia: Mosby, 2012.

Broder, Joshua. *Diagnostic Imaging for the Emergency Physician.* Philadelphia: Saunders, 2011.

Caroline, Nancy L. *Nancy Caroline's Emergency Care in the Streets.* 6th ed. Sudbury, Mass.: Jones and Bartlett, 2010.

Cline, David, D. John Ma, Rita Cydulka, Garth Meckler, Stephen Thomas, Dan Handel. *Tintinalli's Emergency Medicine Manual.* 7th ed. Philadelphia: Saunders, 2012.

Henry, Mark C., and Edward R. Stapleton. *EMT: Prehospital Care.* 4th ed. St. Louis, Mo.: Mosby/Elsevier, 2010.

Knoop, Kevin J., et al., eds. *The Atlas of Emergency Medicine.* 3d ed. New York: McGraw-Hill Medical, 2010.

Limmer, Daniel, et al. *Emergency Care.* 11th ed. Upper Saddle River, N.J.: Pearson/Prentice Hall Health, 2009.

Marx, John A., et al., eds. *Rosen's Emergency Medicine: Concepts and Clinical Practice.* 7th ed. Philadelphia: Mosby/Elsevier, 2010.

Roberts, James R. *Roberts and Hedges' Clinical Procedures in Emergency Medicine.* 6th ed. Philadelphia: Saunders, 2013.

Trott, Alexander T. *Wounds and Lacerations: Emergency and Closure.* 4th ed. Philadelphia: Saunders, 2012.

ENDOCRINOLOGY AND METABOLISM

Gardner, David, and Dolores Shoback. *Greenspan's Basic and Clinical Endocrinology.* 9th ed. New York: McGraw-Hill Medical, 2011.

Goodman, H. Maurice. *Basic Medical Endocrinology.* 4th ed. Boston: Academic Press/Elsevier, 2009.

Lebovitz, Harold E., ed. *Therapy for Diabetes Mellitus and Related Disorders.* 5th ed. Alexandria, Va.: American Diabetes Association, 2009.

Jameson, J. Larry. *Harrison's Endocrinology.* 3d ed. New York: McGraw-Hill Professional, 2013.

Jameson, J. Larry, and Leslie De Groot. *Endocrinology: Adult and Pediatric.* 6th ed. Philadelphia: Saunders, 2010.

Jameson, J. Larry, David M. de Kretser, John C. Marshall and Leslie J. De Groot. *Endocrinology Adult and Pediatric: Reproductive Endocrinology.* 6th ed. Philadelphia: Saunders, 2013.

Melmed, Shlomo, Kenneth S. Polonsky, P. Reed Larsen, and Henry M. Kronenberg. *Williams Textbook of Endocrinology.* 12th ed. Philadelphia: Saunders, 2012.

Weber, C. G. *Clinical Endocrinology.* 12th ed. Seattle: Primary Care Software, 2013.

Weir, Gordon C, J. Larry Jameson, and Leslie J. De Groot. *Endocrinology Adult and Pediatric: Diabetes Mellitus and Obesity.* 6th ed. Philadelphia: Saunders, 2013.

ETHICS

American Medical Association. *Code of Medical Ethics: Current Opinions with Annotations, 2012-2013.* Chicago: Author, 2012-2013.

Beauchamp, Tom L., and James F. Childress. *Principles of Biomedical Ethics.* 7th ed. New York: Oxford University Press, 2012.

Beauchamp, Tom L., and LeRoy Walters, eds. *Contemporary Issues in Bioethics.* 7th ed. Belmont, Calif.: Thomson/Wadsworth, 2008.

Beauchamp, Tom L., LeRoy Walters, Jeffrey P. Kahn, and Anna C. Mastroianni. *Contemporary Issues in Bioethics.* Stamford, Conn.: Cengage Learning, 2013.

Caplan, Arthur, L., and Robert Arp, eds. *Contemporary Debates in Bioethics.* New York: Wiley-Blackwell, 2013.

Farah, Martha J., ed., *Neuroethics: An Introduction with Readings.* Cambridge: The MIT Press, 2010.

Garrett, Thomas M., Harold W. Baillie, and Rosellen M. Garrett. *Health Care Ethics: Principles and Problems.* 5th ed. Upper Saddle River, N.J.: Prentice Hall, 2010.

Rae, Scott. *Moral Choices: An Introduction to Ethics.* Grand Rapids, Mich.: Zondervan, 2009.

Steinbock, Bonnie, ed. *The Oxford Handbook of Bioethics.* New York: Oxford University Press, 2009.

EVIDENCE-BASED MEDICINE

Greenhalgh, Trisha. *How to Read a Paper: The Basics of Evidence-Based Medicine.* 4th ed. Malden, Mass.: BMJ Books/Blackwell, 2010.

Hochman, Michael E. *50 Studies Every Doctor Should Know: The Key Studies that Form the Foundation of Evidence-Based Medicine.* New York: Oxford University

Press, 2013.

McGee, Steven. *Evidence-Based Physical Diagnosis*. 3d ed. Philadelphia: Saunders, 2012.

Straus, Sharon E., Paul Glasziou, W. Scott Richardson, and R. Brian Haynes. *Evidence-Based Medicine: How to Practice and Teach It*. 4th ed. London: Churchilll Livingstone, 2010.

FAMILY MEDICINE

Chan, Paul D., et al. *Family Medicine*. Blue Jay, Calif.: Current Clinical Strategies, 2010.

Moore, Stephen W. *Griffith's Instructions for Patients*. 8th ed. Philadelphia: Saunders, 2011.

Pfenninger, John L., and Grant C. Fowler. *Pfenninger and Fowler's Procedures for Primary Care*. 3d ed. Philadelphia: Saunders, 2011.

Rakel, Robert E., and David Rakel. *Textbook of Family Medicine*. 8th ed. Philadelphia: Saunders, 2011.

Tallia, Alfred F., Joseph E. Scherger, and Nancy Dickey. *Swanson's Family Medicine Review*. 7th ed. Philadelphia: Saunders, 2013.

GASTROENTEROLOGY

Feldman, Mark, Lawrence S. Friedman, and Lawrence J. Brandt, eds. *Sleisenger and Fordtran's Gastrointestinal and Liver Disease: Pathophysiology, Diagnosis, Management*. New ed. 2 vols. Philadelphia: Saunders/Elsevier, 2010.

Hawkey, C. J. Jaime Bosch, Joel E. Richter and Guadalupe Garcia-Tsao. *Textbook of Clinical Gastroenterology and Hepatology*. New York: Wiley-Blackwell, 2012.

Longo, Dan, and Anthony Fauci. *Harrison's Gastroenterology and Hepatology*. 2d ed. New York: McGraw-Hill, 2013.

Wyllie, Robert, and Jeffery S. Hyams. *Pediatric Gastrointestinal and Liver Disease*. 4th ed. Philadelphia: Saunders, 2011.

GENETICS AND HEREDITY

Davis, Dena S. *Genetic Dilemmas: Reproductive Technology, Parental Choices, and Children's Futures*. 2d ed. New York: Routledge, 2010.

Jorde, Lynn B., John C. Carey, and Michael J. Bamshad. *Medical Genetics*. 4th ed. Philadelphia: Mosby, 2010.

Pritchard, Dorian J., and Bruce R. Korf. *Medical Genetics at a Glance*. New York: Wiley-Blackwell, 2013.

Rimoin, David L., Reed E. Pyeritz and Bruce Korf. *Emery and Rimoin's Essential Medical Genetics*. Waltham, Mass.: Academic Press, 2013.

Saul, Robert A., ed. *Medical Genetics in Pediatric Practice*. Washington, D.C.: American Academy of Pediatrics, 2013.

Schaefer, G. Bradley, and James N. Thompson. *Medical Genetics*. New York: McGraw-Hill Professional, 2013.

Turnpenny, Peter D. *Emery's Elements of Medical Genetics*. 14th ed. London: Churchill Livingstone, 2012.

GERIATRICS

Beerman, Susan, and Judith Rappaport-Musson. *Eldercare 911: The Caregiver's Complete Handbook for Making Decisions*. Rev. ed. Amherst, N.Y.: Prometheus Books, 2008.

Beers, Mark H., and Robert Berkow, eds. *The Merck Manual of Geriatrics*. 3d ed. Whitehouse Station, N.J.: Merck Research Laboratories, 2000.

Birren, James E., and K. Warner Schaie, eds. *Handbook of the Psychology of Aging*. 6th ed. Boston: Academic Press/Elsevier, 2007.

Cassel, Christine K., et al., eds. *Geriatric Medicine*. 4th ed. New York: Springer, 2003.

Ferri, Fred F., Marsha Fretwell, and Tom J. Wachtel. *Practical Guide to the Care of the Geriatric Patient*. 3d ed. St. Louis, Mo.: Mosby/Elsevier, 2007.

Gauthier, Serge, ed. *Clinical Diagnosis and Management of Alzheimer's Disease*. 3d ed. Abingdon, Oxfordshire, England: Informa Healthcare, 2006.

Ham, Richard, et al., eds. *Primary Care Geriatrics: A Case-Based Approach*. 5th ed. St. Louis, Mo.: Mosby/Elsevier, 2007.

Hazzard, William R., et al., eds. *Principles of Geriatric Medicine and Gerontology*. 5th ed. New York: McGraw-Hill, 2003.

Herdt, Gilbert, and Brian de Vries, eds. *Gay and Lesbian Aging: Research and Future Directions*. New York: Springer, 2004.

Hill, Robert D. *Positive Aging: A Guide for Mental Health Professionals and Consumers*. New York: W. W. Norton, 2006.

Hooyman, Nancy, and H. Asuman Kiyak. *Social Gerontology: A Multidisciplinary Perspective*. New York: Prentice Hall, 2010.

Hoyer, William J., and Paul A. Roodin. *Adult Development and Aging*. 6th ed. Boston: McGraw-Hill, 2009.

Mace, Nancy L., and Peter V. Rabins. *The Thirty-Six-Hour Day: A Family Guide to Caring for Persons with Alzheimer Disease, Related Dementing Illnesses, and Memory Loss in Later Life*. 4th ed. Baltimore: Johns Hopkins University Press, 2006.

Masoro, Edward J., and Steven N. Austad, eds. *Handbook of the Biology of Aging*. 6th ed. Boston: Academic Press/Elsevier, 2007.

Weisstub, David N. *Aging: Caring for Our Elders*. Boston: Kluwer Academic, 2001.

GYNECOLOGY AND OBSTETRICS

Baskett, Thomas F., Andrew A. Calder, and Sabaratnam Arulkumaran. *Munro Kerr's Operative Obstetrics*. 12th ed. Philadelphia: Saunders, 2014.

Beckmann, Charles R. B., William Herbert, Douglas Laube, and Frank Ling. *Obstetrics and Gynecology*. 7th ed. Philadelphia: Lippincott Williams & Wilkins, 2013.

Cunningham, F. Gary, et al., eds. *Williams Obstetrics*. 23d ed. New York: McGraw-Hill, 2010.

Gabbe, Steven G., Jennifer R. Niebyl, Henry L. Galan, Eric R.

M. Jauniaux, Mark B Landon, Joe Leigh Simpson, and Deborah A Driscoll. *Obstetrics: Normal and Problem Pregnancies*. 6th ed. Philadelphia: Saunders, 2012.

Hacker, Neville F., Joseph C. Gambone, and Calvin J. Hobel. *Hacker & Moore's Essentials of Obstetrics and Gynecology*. 5th ed. Philadelphia: Saunders, 2010.

Hurt, K. Joseph, Matthew W. Guile, Jessica L. Bienstock, Harold E. Fox, Edward E. Wallach, eds. *The Johns Hopkins Manual of Gynecology and Obstetrics*. 4th ed. Philadelphia: Lippincott Williams & Wilkins, 2010.

James, David K., Philip J. Steer, Carl P. Weiner, and Bernard Gonik. *High Risk Pregnancy*. 4th ed. Philadelphia: Saunders, 2011.

Ogburn, Tony, and Betsy Taylor. *Procedures in the Office Setting, An Issue of Obstetric and Gynecology Clinics*. Philadelphia: Elsevier, 2013.

HEMATOLOGY

Ciesla, Betty. *Hematology in Practice*. 2d ed. Philadelphia: F. A. Davis, 2011.

Hoffman, Ronald, Edward J. Benz Jr., Leslie E. Silberstein, Helen Heslop, Jeffrey Weitz, and John Anastasi. *Hematology: Basic Principles and Practice*. 6th ed. London: Churchill Livingstone, 2012.

Jaffe, Elaine S., Nancy Lee Harris, James W. Vardiman, Elias Campo, and Daniel A. Arbe. *Hematopathology*. Philadelphia: Saunders, 2011.

Kaushansky, Kenneth, Marshall Lichtman, E. Beutler, Thomas Kipps, Josef Prchal, and Uri Seligsohn. *Williams Hematology*. 8th ed. New York: McGraw-Hill Professional, 2010.

Nathan, David G., and Stuart H. Orkin, eds. *Nathan and Oski's Hematology of Infancy and Childhood*. 7th ed. Philadelphia: Saunders/Elsevier, 2009.

Rodak, Bernadette F., George A. Fritsma, and Elaine Keohane. *Hematology: Clinical Principles and Applications*. 4th ed. Philadelphia: Saunders, 2011.

Treleaven, Jennifer G., and A. John Barrett. *Hematopoietic Stem Cell Transplantation in Clinical Practice*. London: Churchill Livingstone, 2009.

Weber, C. G. *Clinical Hematology-Oncology - 2014*. Seattle: Primary Care Software, 2013.

HOSPITALS AND ADMINISTRATION

American Hospital Association. *Hospital Statistics: The Comprehensive Reference Source for Analysis and Comparison of Hospital Trends*. Chicago: Health Forum, 2008.

Birenbaum, Aaron. *Wounded Profession: American Medicine Enters the Age of Managed Care*. Westport, Conn.: Greenwood Press, 2002.

Bodenheimer, Thomas S., and Kevin Grumbach. *Understanding Health Policy: A Clinical Approach*. 4th ed. New York: McGraw-Hill, 2005.

Cleverley, William O., and Andrew E. Cameron. *Essentials of Health Care Finance*. 6th ed. Sudbury, Mass.: Jones and Bartlett, 2007.

Dranove, David. *The Economic Evolution of American Health Care: From Marcus Welby to Managed Care*. Princeton, N.J.: Princeton University Press, 2002.

Joint Commission on Accreditation of Healthcare Organizations. *2010 Comprehensive Accreditation Manual for Hospitals: The Official Handbook*. Oakbrook Terrace, Ill.: Author, 2009.

Kavaler, Florence, and Allen D. Spiegel. *Risk Management in Health Care Institutions: A Strategic Approach*. 2d ed. Boston: Jones and Bartlett, 2003.

Kovner, Anthony R., and James R. Knickman, eds. *Jonas and Kovner's Health Care Delivery in the United States*. 8th ed. New York: Springer, 2005.

McConnell, Charles R. *The Effective Health Care Supervisor*. 6th ed. Sudbury, Mass.: Jones and Bartlett, 2007.

Shi, Leiyu, and Douglas A. Singh. *Delivering Health Care in America: A Systems Approach*. 3d ed. Boston: Jones and Bartlett, 2004.

Sultz, Harry A., and Kristina M. Young. *Health Care USA: Understanding Its Organization and Delivery*. 5th ed. Sudbury, Mass.: Jones and Bartlett, 2006.

Wolper, Lawrence F., ed. *Health Care Administration: Planning, Implementing, and Managing Organized Delivery Systems*. 4th ed. Boston: Jones and Bartlett, 2004.

IMMUNOLOGY

Abbas, Abul K., Andrew H. Lichtman, and Shiv Pillai. *Basic Immunology*. 4th ed. Philadelphia: Saunders, 2014.

Abbas, Abul K., Andrew H. Lichtman, and Shiv Pillai. *Cellular and Molecular Immunology*. 7th ed. Philadelphia: Saunders, 2012.

Erridge, Clett. *Undergraduate Immunology*. Seattle: Amazon Digital Services, 2013.

Male, David, Jonathan Brostoff, David Roth, and Ivan Roitt. *Immunology*. 8th ed. Philadelphia: Saunders, 2013.

Murphy, Kenneth. *Janeaway's Immunology*. 8th ed. Hoboken, N.J.: Garland Scientific, 2011.

Owen, Judy, Jenni Punt, and Sharon Stranford. *Kuby Immunology*. 7th ed. New York: W.H. Freeman, 2013.

Parkham, Peter. *The Immune System*. 3d ed. New York: Garland Science, 2000.

Sompayrac, Lauren M. *How the Immune System Works*. New York: Wiley-Blackwell, 2012.

INFECTIOUS DISEASES

Cherry, James, Gail J. Demmler-Harrison, Sheldon L. Kaplan, and William J. Steinbach. *Feigin and Cherry's Textbook of Pediatric Infectious Diseases*. 7th ed. Philadelphia: Saunders, 2013.

Cohen, Jonathan, William G. Powderly, and Steven Opal. *Infectious Diseases*. Philadelphia: Mosby, 2010.

Finch, Roger G., David Greenwood, Richard J. Whitley, and S. Ragnar Norrby. *Antibiotic and Chemotherapy*. 9th ed. Philadelphia: Saunders, 2011.

Long, Sarah S., Larry K. Pickering, and Charles G. Prober. *Principles and Practice of Pediatric Infectious Diseases*.

4th ed. Philadelphia: Saunders, 2012.

Magill, Alan J., Edward T. Ryan, and Tom Solomon. *Hunter's Tropical Medicine and Emerging Infectious Disease*. 9th ed. Philadelphia: Saunders, 2012.

Mandell, Gerald L., John E. Bennett, and Raphael Dolin. *Mandell, Douglas, and Bennett's Principles and Practice of Infectious Diseases*. 7th ed. London: Churchill Livingstone, 2013.

Palmer, S. R., Lord Soulsby, Paul Torgerson, and David W. G. Brown. *Oxford Textbook of Zoonoses: Biology, Clinical Practice, and Public Health Control*. New York: Oxford University Press, 2014.

Remington, Jack S., Jerome O. Klein, Christopher B. Wilson, Victor Nizel, and Yvonne Maldonado. *Infectious Diseases of the Fetus and Newborn*. Philadelphia: Saunders, 2010.

INTERNAL MEDICINE

Andreoli, Thomas E., et al., eds. *Andreoli and Carpenter's Cecil Essentials of Medicine*. 8th ed. Philadelphia: Saunders/Elsevier, 2010.

Ashar, Bimal, Redonda Miller, Stephen Sisson, and Johns Hopkins Hospital. *The Johns Hopkins Internal Medicine Board Review*. 4th ed. Philadelphia: Saunders, 2012.

Dan Longo, Anthony Fauci, Dennis Kasper and Stephen Hauser. *Harrison's Principles of Internal Medicine*. 18th ed. New York: McGraw-Hill Professional, 2011.

Ferri, Fred F. *Ferri's Practical Guide: Fast Facts for Patient Care*. 9th ed. Philadelphia: Mosby, 2014.

Goldman, Lee, and Andrew I. Schafer. *Goldman's Cecil Medicine*. 24th ed. Philadelphia: Saunders, 2012.

Qureshi, Zeshan. *The Unofficial Guide to Prescribing*. London: Churchill Livingstone, 2014.

Sabatine, Marc S. *Pocket Medicine: The Massachusetts General Hospital Handbook of Internal Medicine*. Philadelphia: Lippincott Williams & Wilkins, 2013.

Swartz, Mark H. *Textbook of Physical Examination*. 7th ed. Philadelphia: Saunders, 2014.

Talley, Nicholas J., and Simon O'Connor. *Examination Medicine*. 7th ed. London: Churchill Livingstone, 2014.

Walker, Brian R., Nicki R Colledge, Stuart H. Ralston, and Ian Penman. *Davidson's Principles and Practice of Medicine*. 22d ed. London: Churchill Livingstone, 2014.

LABORATORY METHODS

Chernecky, Cynthia C., and Barbara J. Berger. *Laboratory Tests and Diagnostic Procedures*. 6th ed. Philadelphia: Saunders, 2012.

Harr, Robert R. *Medical Laboratory Science Review*. 4th ed. Philadelphia: F. A. Davis, 2012.

Kee, Joyce LaFever. *Laboratory and Diagnostic Tests with Nursing Implications*. 9th ed. Upper Saddle River: New Jersey: Prentice Hall, 2013.

Laposata, Michael. *Laboratory Medicine: The Diagnosis of Disease in the Clinical Laboratory*. New York: McGraw-Hill Medical, 2010.

Lorsch, Jon. *Laboratory Methods in Enzymology: Cell, Lipid, and Carbohydrate*. Vol 533. New York: Academic Press, 2013.

McPherson, Richard A., and Matthew R. Pincus. *Henry's Clinical Diagnosis and Management by Laboratory Methods*. 22d ed. Philadelphia: Saunders, 2012.

Pagana, Kathleen Deska, and Timothy J. Pagana. *Mosby's Manual of Diagnostic and Laboratory Tests*. 5th ed. Philadelphia: Mosby, 2013.

Van Leeuwen, Anne M., Debra J. Poelhuis-Leth, and Mickey L. Bladh. *Davis's Comprehensive Handbook of Laboratory and Diagnostic Tests With Nursing Implications*. 5th ed. Philadelphia: F. A. Davis, 2013.

LEGAL MEDICINE

American College of Legal Medicine. *Legal Medicine*. 6th ed. Philadelphia: Mosby, 2004.

Boumil, Marcia M., Clifford E. Elias, and Diane Bissonnette Moes. *Medical Liability in a Nutshell*. 2d ed. St. Paul, Minn.: Thomson/West, 2003.

Fremgen, Bonnie F. *Medical Law and Ethics*. 2d ed. Upper Saddle River, N.J.: Pearson/Prentice Hall, 2006.

Furrow, Barry R., et al. *Health Law: Cases, Materials, and Problems*. 5th ed. St. Paul, Minn.: West, 2004.

Garner, Bryan A., ed. *Black's Law Dictionary*. 9th ed. St. Paul, Minn.: Thomson/West, 2008.

Hall, Mark A., Mary Anne Bobinski, and David Orentlicher. *Health Care Law and Ethics*. 6th ed. New York: Aspen, 2003.

Jonsen, Albert R., Mark Siegler, and William J. Winslade. *Clinical Ethics: A Practical Approach to Ethical Decisions in Clinical Medicine*. 6th ed. New York: McGraw-Hill, 2006.

Miller, Robert D. *Problems in Health Care Law*. 9th ed. Sudbury, Mass.: Jones and Bartlett, 2006.

Montgomery, Jonathan. *Health Care Law*. 2d ed. New York: Oxford University Press, 2003.

Pence, Gregory E. *Classic Cases in Medical Ethics: Accounts of Cases That Have Shaped Medical Ethics, with Philosophical, Legal, and Historical Backgrounds*. 4th ed. New York: McGraw-Hill, 2004.

Pozgar, George D. *Legal Aspects of Health Care Administration*. 10th ed. Sudbury, Mass.: Jones and Bartlett, 2006.

MANAGED CARE

Birenbaum, Aaron. *Wounded Profession: American Medicine Enters the Age of Managed Care*. Westport, Conn.: Greenwood Press, 2002.

Bondeson, William B., and James W. Jones, eds. *The Ethics of Managed Care: Professional Integrity and Patient Rights*. Boston: Kluwer Academic, 2002.

Dranove, David. *The Economic Evolution of American Health Care: From Marcus Welby to Managed Care*. Princeton, N.J.: Princeton University Press, 2002.

Fauman, Michael A. *Negotiating Managed Care: A Manual for Clinicians*. Washington, D.C.: American Psychiatric Publishing, 2002.

Freeborn, Donald K., and Clyde R. Pope. *Promise and Performance in Managed Care: The Prepaid Group Practice Model.* Rev. ed. Baltimore: Johns Hopkins University Press, 2000.

Kongstvedt, Peter R. *Managed Care: What It Is and How It Works.* 3d ed. Sudbury, Mass.: Jones and Bartlett, 2009.

_____, ed. *Essentials of Managed Health Care.* 5th ed. Sudbury, Mass.: Jones and Bartlett, 2007.

Marcinko, David Edward, ed. *Dictionary of Health Insurance and Managed Care.* New York: Springer, 2006.

Stanley, Kay B., ed. *Managing Managed Care in the Medical Practice.* 2d ed. Chicago: AMA Press, 2004.

MEDICAL INFORMATICS

Chen, Hsinchun, Sherrilynne S. Fuller, Carol Friedman, and William Hersh. *Medical Informatics: Knowledge Management and Data Mining in Biomedicine.* New York: Springer, 2010.

Hoyt, Robert E., Nora Bailey, and Ann Yoshihashi, eds. *Health Informatics: Practical Guide For Healthcare And Information Technology Professionals.* 5th ed. Raleigh, N.C: lulu.com, 2012.

Hoyt, Robert E., and Ann Yoshihashi. *Medical Informatics: Practical Guide for Healthcare and Information Technology Professionals.* 4th ed. Chicago: lulu.com, 2010.

Kudyba, Stephan P., ed. *Healthcare Informatics: Improving Efficiency and Productivity.* New York: CRC Press, 2010.

Nelson, Ramona, and Nancy Staggers. *Health Informatics: An Interprofessional Approach.* Philadelphia: Mosby, 2013.

Ong, Kenneth R., ed. *Medical Informatics: An Executive Primer.* Chicago: HIMSS, 2011.

Shortliffe, Edward II., and James J. Cimino, eds. *Biomedical Informatics: Computer Applications in Health Care and Biomedicine.* New York: Springer, 2013.

MICROBIOLOGY

Goering, Richard, Hazel Dockrell, Mark Zuckerman, Ivan Roitt, and Peter L. Chiodini. *Mims' Medical Microbiology.* 5th ed. Philadelphia: Saunders, 2013.

Greenwood, David, Richard C. B. Black, Michael Barer, and W. L. Irving. *Medical Microbiology.* 18th ed. London: Churchill Livingstone, 2012.

Guyot, Andrea, Silke Schelenz, and Steven H. Myint. *The Flesh and Bones of Medical Microbiology.* Philadelphia: Mosby, 2011.

Korsman, Stephen N. J., Gert Van Zyl, Wolfgang Preiser, Louise Nutt, and Monique I. Andersson. *Virology.* London: Churchill Livingstone, 2012.

Murray, Patrick. *Medical Microbiology.* 7th ed. Philadelphia: Mosby, 2013.

Pommerville, Jeffrey C. *Alcamo's Fundamentals of Microbiology.* 9th ed. Sudbury, Mass.: Jones and Bartlett, 2010.

Wiser, Mark F. *Protozoa and Human Disease.* Hoboken, N.J.: Garland Scientific, 2010.

NEUROLOGY

Budson, Andrew E., and Paul R. Solomon. *Memory Loss.* Philadelphia: Saunders, 2011.

Greenberg, David, Michael Aminoff, and Roger Simon. *Clinical Neurology.* 8th ed. New York: McGraw-Hill Professional, 2012.

Horton Jr., Arthur MacNeill and Danny Wedding. *The Neuropsychology Handbook.* 3rd ed. New York: Springer Publishing Company, 2008.

Howard, Jonathan. *Neurology Video Textbook.* New York: Demos Medical, 2013.

Kalat, James W. *Biological Psychology.* 11th ed. Belmont, CA: Wadsworth, 2013.

Kolb, B. ad I.Q. Whishaw. *Fundamentals of Human Neuropsychology.* 6th ed. New York, NY: Worth Publishers, 2009.

Lambert, K.G. and C.H Kinsley. *Clinical Neuroscience: Psychopathology and the Brain.* 2nd ed. New York, NY: Oxford University Press, 2011.

Morris, John G., and Padraic J. Grattan-Smith. *Manual of Neurological Signs.* New York: Oxford University Press, 2014.

O'Brien, Michael. *Aids to the Examination of the Peripheral Nervous System.* 5th ed. Philadelphia: Saunders, 2010.

Perkin, G. David, Douglas C. Miller, Russell Lane, Maneesh C. Patel and Fred H. Hochberg. *Atlas of Clinical Neurology.* 3d ed. Philadelphia: Saunders, 2010.

Preston, David C., and Barbara E. Shapiro. *Electromyography and Neuromuscular Disorders.* 3d ed. Philadelphia: Saunders, 2013.

Weber, C. G. *Clinical Neurology.* 14th ed. Pacific Primary Care Software, 2013.

Weiner, William J., Christopher G. Goetz, Robert K. Shin, and Steven L. Lewis. *Neurology for the Non-Neurologist.* 6th ed. Philadelphia: Lippincott Williams & Wilkins, 2010.

Werz, Mary Ann, and Ignacio L. Pita Garcia. *Epilepsy Syndromes.* Philadelphia: Saunders, 2011.

Zillmer, E.A., M.V. Spiers and W.C. Culbertson. *Principles of Neuropsychology.* 2nd ed. Thomson Wadsworth, 2008.

NURSING

Berman, Audrey, et al. *Kozier and Erb's Fundamentals of Nursing: Concepts, Process, and Practice.* 8th ed. Upper Saddle River, N.J.: Pearson/Prentice Hall, 2008.

Delaune, Sue C., and Patricia K. Ladner, eds. *Fundamentals of Nursing: Standards and Practices.* 4th ed. Clifton Park, N.Y.: Cengage Learning, 2010.

Ignatavicius, Donna D., and M. Linda Workman, eds. *Medical-Surgical Nursing: Critical Thinking for Collaborative Care.* 5th ed. Philadelphia: Saunders/Elsevier, 2006.

Nettina, Sandra M., ed. *The Lippincott Manual of Nursing Practice.* 8th ed. Philadelphia: Lippincott Williams & Wilkins, 2006.

Wilkinson, Judith M., and Karen Van Leuven. *Fundamentals of Nursing: Theory, Concepts, and Applications.* Philadelphia: F. A. Davis, 2007.

NUTRITION

Escott-Stump, Sylvia. *Nutrition and Diagnosis-Related Care*. 7th ed. Philadelphia: Lippincott Williams & Wilkins, 2011.

Geissler, Catherine A., and Hilary J. Powers, eds. *Human Nutrition*. 12th ed. New York: Churchill Livingstone/Elsevier, 2010.

Grodner, Michele, Sara Long Roth, and Bonnie C. Walkingshaw. *Nutritional Foundations and Clinical Applications: A Nursing Approach*. 5th ed. Philadelphia: Mosby, 2011.

Hornick, Betsy, Roberta Larson Duyff, and Alma Flor Ada. *American Dietetic Association Complete Food and Nutrition Guide*. 4th ed. Houghton Mifflin Harcourt, 2012.

Marinos, Elia, Olle Ljungqvist, Rebecca Stratton, and Susan A. Lanham-New, eds. *Clinical Nutrition*. 2d ed. New York: Wiley-Blackwell, 2013.

Nelms, Marcia, Kathryn P. Sucher, Karen Lacey, and Sara Long Roth. *Nutrition Therapy and Pathophysiology*. 2d ed. Stamford, Conn.: Cengage Learning, 2010.

Rolfes, Sharon Rady, Kathryn Pinna, and Ellie Whitney. *Understanding Normal and Clinical Nutrition*. 9th ed. Stamford, Conn.: Cengage Learning, 2011.

Whitney, Ellie, and Sharon Rady Rolfes. *Understanding Nutrition*. 12th ed. Belmont, Calif.: Wadsworth, 2009.

ONCOLOGY

Bragalone, Diedra L., ed. *Drug Information Handbook for Oncology*. 11th ed. Philadelphia: Lexi-Comp, 2013.

DeVita, Vincent T., Jr., Theodore S. Lawrence, Steven A. Rosenberg, Ronald A. DePinho, and Robert A. Weinberg, eds. *DeVita, Hellman, and Rosenberg's Cancer: Principles and Practice of Oncology*. 9th ed. Philadelphia: Lippincott Williams & Wilkins, 2011.

Casciato, Dennis A., ed. *Manual of Clinical Oncology*. 7th ed. Philadelphia: Lippincott Williams & Wilkins, 2012.

Cashen, Amanda F., and Brian Van Tine. *The Washington Manual of Hematology and Oncology Subspecialty Consult*. Philadelphia: Lippincott Williams & Wilkins, 2012.

Dark, Graham G. *Oncology at a Glance*. New York: Wiley, 2013.

Kantarjian, Hagop M., Robert A. Wolff, and Charles A. Koller. *The MD Anderson Manual of Medical Oncology*. 2d ed. New York: McGraw-Hill Professional, 2011.

Mendelsohn, John, Peter M. Howley, Mark A. Israel, Joe W. Gray, and Craig B. Thompson. *The Molecular Basis of Cancer*. 4th ed. Philadelphia: Saunders, 2015.

Niederhuber, John E., James O. Armitage, James H Doroshow, Michael B. Kastan, and Joel E. Tepper. *Abeloff's Clinical Oncology*. 5th ed. Philadelphia: Saunders, 2014.

OPHTHALMOLOGY

Agarwal, Anita. *Gass' Atlas of Macular Diseases*. 5th ed. Philadelphia: Saunders, 2012.

Fineman, Mitchell S., and Allen C. Ho. *Color Atlas and Synopsis of Clinical Ophthalmology - Willis Eye Institute - Retina*. Philadelphia: Lippincott Williams & Wilkins, 2012.

Gerstenblith, Adam T., and Michael P. Rabinowitz. *The Wills Eye Manual: Office and Emergency Room Diagnosis and Treatment of Eye Disease*. Philadelphia: Lippincott Williams & Wilkins, 2012.

Goldberg, Stephen, and William Trattler. *Ophthalmology Made Ridiculously Simple*. 5th ed. Miami, Fla.: MedMaster Inc, 2012.

Harper, Richard A. *Basic Ophthalmology*. 9th ed. San Francisco, Calif.: American Academy of Ophthalmology, 2010.

Kaiser, Peter K., Neil J. Friedman, and Roberto Pineda. *The Massachusetts Eye and Ear Infirmary Illustrated Manual of Ophthalmology*. 4th ed. Philadelphia: Saunders, 2014.

Kanski, Jack J., and Brad Bowling. *Clinical Ophthalmology: A Systematic Approach*. 7th ed. Philadelphia: Saunder, 2011.

Levin, Leonard A., Siv F. E. Nilsson, James Ver Hoeve, Samuel Wu, Paul L. Kaufman, and Albert Alm. *Adler's Physiology of the Eye*. 11th ed. Philadelphia: Saunders, 2011.

Rapano, Christopher J. *Willis Eye Institute - Cornea*. Philadelphia: Lippincott Williams & Wilkins, 2011.

Yannuzzi, Lawrence A. *The Retinal Atlas*. Philadelphia: Saunders, 2010.

ORTHOPEDICS

Brotzman, S. Brent, and Robert C. Manske. *Clinical Orthopaedic Rehabilitation: An Evidence-Based Approach*. 3d ed. Philadelphia: Mosby, 2011.

Brukner, Peter, and Karim Khan. *Brukner & Khan's Clinical Sports Medicine*. New York: McGraw-Hill, 2011.

Chung, Kevin C. *Reconstruction of the Traumatized Upper Extremity, An Issue of Hand Clinics*. Philadelphia: Elsevier, 2014.

Cohen, Bruce. *Tendon Transfers and Treatment Strategies in Foot and Ankle Surgery, An Issue of Foot and Ankle Clinics of North America*. Philadelphia: Elsevier, 2014.

Cook, Chad, and Eric Hegedus. *Orthopedic Physical Examination Tests: An Evidence-Based Approach*. 2d ed. Upper Saddle River, N.J: Prentice Hall, 2012.

Herring, John A. *Tachdjian's Pediatric Orthopaedics E-Book*. 5th ed. Philadelphia: Saunders, 2013.

Lee, Donald, and Robert J. Neviaser. *Operative Techniques: Shoulder and Elbow Surgery*. Philadelphia: Saunders, 2011.

Magee, David J. *Orthopedic Physical Assessment*. 6th ed. Philadelphia: Saunders, 2013.

Miller, Mark D., Stephen R. Thompson, and Jennifer Hart. *Review of Orthopaedics*. 6th ed. Philadelphia: Saunders, 2012.

Rouzier, Pierre A. *The Sports Medicine Patient Advisor*. 3d ed. Amherst, Mass.: SportsMed Press, 2010.

Skinner, Harry. *Current Diagnosis & Treatment in Orthopedics*. 5th ed. New York: McGraw-Hill Professional, 2013.

Skirven, Terri M., A. Lee Osterman, Jane Fedorczyk, and Peter C. Amadio. *Rehabilitation of the Hand and Upper Extremity*. 6th ed. Philadelphia: Mosby, 2011.

Weinstein, Stuart L., and John M. Flynn. *Lovell & Winter's Pediatric Orthopaedics*. 7th ed. Philadelphia: Lippincott Williams & Wilkins, 2013.

Wolfe, Scott W., Robert N. Hotchkiss, William C. Pederson, and Scott H. Kozin. *Green's Operative Hand Surgery*. 6th ed. Philadelphia: Churchill Livingstone, 2011.

OTOLARYNGOLOGY

Anniko, Matti, Manuel Bernal-Sprekelsen, Victor Bonkowsky, Patrick Bradley, and Salvatore Iurato. *Otolaryngology, Head and Neck Surgery*. New York: Springer, 2010.

Flint, Paul W., Bruce H. Haughey, Valerie J. Lund, John K. Niparko, Mark A. Richardson, K. Thomas Robbins, and J. Regan Thomas. *Cummings Otolaryngology - Head and Neck Surgery*. 5th ed. Philadelphia: Mosby, 2010.

Lee, K. J. *Essential Otolaryngology: Head and Neck Surgery*. 10th ed. New York: McGraw-Hill, 2012.

Licameli, Greg R., and David E. Tunkel, eds. *Pediatric Otorhinolaryngology: Diagnosis and Treatment*. New York: Thieme, 2012.

Logan, Bari M., Patricia Reynolds, and Ralph T. Hutchings. *McMinn's Color Atlas of Head and Neck Anatomy*. 4th ed. Philadelphia: Mosby, 2010.

Sahoo, G. C. *Emergencies in Otolaryngology*. New Delhi, India: Jaypee Brothers Medical Publishers, 2014.

Warnakulasuriya, Saman, and W. M. Tilakaratna. *Oral Medicine & Pathology: A Guide to Diagnosis and Management*. New Delhi, India: Jaypee Brothers Medical Pub, 2013.

PALLIATIVE CARE

Dunn, Geoffrey, Sugantha Ganapathy, and Vincent W. S. Chan. *Surgical Palliative Care and Pain Management, An Issue of Anesthesiology Clinics*. Philadelphia: Saunders, 2012.

Emanuel, Linda L., and S. Lawrence Librach. *Palliative Care*. 2d ed. Philadelphia: Saunders, 2011.

Goldstein, Nathan E., and R. Sean Morrison. *Evidence-Based Practice of Palliative Medicine*. Philadelphia: Saunders, 2013.

Howard, Penny, and Becky Chady. *Placement Learning in Cancer & Palliative Care Nursing*. Philadelphia: Bailliere Tindall, 2012.

Karakas, Serife Eti. *Palliative Care, An Issue of Primary Care Clinics in Office Practice*. Philadelphia: Saunders, 2011.

Mahon, Mimi. *Palliative and End of Life Care, An Issue of Nursing Clinics*. Philadelphia: Saunders, 2010.

PATHOLOGY

Buja, L. Maximilian, and Gerhard R. F. Krueger. *Netter's Illustrated Human Pathology Updated Edition*. Philadelphia: Saunders, 2014.

Cross, Simon. *Underwood's Pathology E-Book*. 6th ed. London: Churchill Livingstone, 2013.

Crowley, Leonard V. *Introduction to Human Disease: Pathology and Pathophysiology Correlations*. 8th ed. Sudbury, Mass.: Jones and Bartlett, 2010.

Dabbs, David J. *Diagnostic Immunohistochemistry*. 4th ed. Philadelphia: Saunders, 2014.

Fenderson, Bruce A., Raphael Rubin, David S. Strayer, and Emanuel Rubin. *Lippincott's Illustrated Q&A Review of Rubin's Pathology*. Philadelphia: Lippincott Williams & Wilkins, 2010.

Goldblum, John R., Sharon W. Weiss, and Andrew L. Folpe. *Enzinger and Weiss's Soft Tissue Tumors*. 6th ed. Philadelphia: Saunders, 2014.

Hornick, Jason L. *Practical Soft Tissue Pathology: A Diagnostic Approach*. Philadelphia: Saunders, 2013.

Kocjan, Gabrijela, Winifred Gray, Tanya Levine, Ika Kardum-Skelin, and Philippe Vielh. *Diagnostic Cytopathology Essentials*. London: Churchill Livingstone, 2013.

Kumar, Vinay, Abul K. Abbas, and Nelson Fausto, eds. *Robbins and Cotran Pathologic Basis of Disease*. 8th ed. Philadelphia: Saunders/Elsevier, 2010.

Mutter, George L., and Jamie Prat. *Pathology of the Female Reproductive Tract*. 3d ed. London: Churchill Livingstone, 2014.

Weedon, David. *Weedon's Skin Pathology*. 3d ed. London: Churchill Livingstone, 2010.

PATIENT EDUCATION

American Medical Association. *American Medical Association Family Medical Guide*. 4th rev. ed. Hoboken, N.J.: John Wiley & Sons, 2004.

Bartlett, John G., and Ann K. Finkbeiner. *The Guide to Living with HIV Infection: Developed at the Johns Hopkins AIDS Clinic*. 6th ed. Baltimore: Johns Hopkins University Press, 2007.

Blaivas, Jerry G. *Conquering Bladder and Prostate Problems: The Authoritative Guide for Men and Women*. Rev. ed. Cambridge, Mass.: Da Capo Press, 2001.

Bloom, Floyd E., M. Flint Beal, and David J. Kupfer, eds. *The Dana Guide to Brain Health*. New York: Dana Press, 2006.

Carlson, Karen J., Stephanie A. Eisenstat, and Terra Ziporyn. *The New Harvard Guide to Women's Health*. Cambridge, Mass.: Harvard University Press, 2004.

Conlon, Patrick. *The Essential Hospital Handbook: How to Be an Effective Partner in a Loved One's Care*. New Haven, Conn.: Yale University Press, 2009.

Dollinger, Malin, et al. *Everyone's Guide to Cancer Therapy*. 5th ed. Kansas City, Mo.: Andrews McMeel, 2008.

Duvoisin, Roger C., and Jacob Sage. *Parkinson's Disease: A Guide for Patient and Family*. 5th ed. Philadelphia: Lippincott Williams & Wilkins, 2001.

Foltz-Gray, Dorothy. *The Arthritis Foundation's Guide to Good Living with Rheumatoid Arthritis*. 3d ed. Atlanta: Arthritis Foundation, 2006.

Jackson, Marilynn. *Pocket Guide for Patient Education*. Sudbury, Mass.: Jones and Bartlett, 2009.

Keene, Nancy. *Childhood Leukemia: A Guide for Families, Friends, and Caregivers*. 4th ed. Sebastopol, Calif.: O'Reilly, 2010.

Komaroff, Anthony, ed. *Harvard Medical School Family Health Guide*. New York: Free Press, 2005.

Kushner, Thomasine Kimbrough. *Surviving Healthcare: A Manual for Patients and Their Families*. New York: Cambridge University Press, 2010.

Lorig, Kate, et al. *Patient Education: A Practical Approach*. 3d ed. Thousand Oaks, Calif.: Sage, 2000.

Moore, Stephen W. *Griffith's Instructions for Patients*. 7th ed. Philadelphia: Saunders/Elsevier, 2005.

Porter, Robert S., et al., eds. *The Merck Manual Home Health Handbook*. Whitehouse Station, N.J.: Merck Research Laboratories, 2009.

Saudek, Christopher D., Richard R. Rubin, and Cynthia S. Shump. *The Johns Hopkins Guide to Diabetes: For Today and Tomorrow*. Baltimore: Johns Hopkins University Press, 2001.

Woolf, Alan D., et al., eds. *The Children's Hospital Guide to Your Child's Health and Development*. Cambridge, Mass.: Perseus, 2002.

PEDIATRICS

Cherry, James, Gail J. Demmler-Harrison, Sheldon L. Kaplan, William J. Steinbach, and Peter Hotez. *Feigin and Cherry's Textbook of Pediatric Infectious Diseases*. 7th ed. Philadelphia: Saunders, 2014.

Greydanus, Donald E., Dilip R. Patel, and Helen D. Pratt, eds. *Behavioral Pediatrics*. 3d ed. 2 vols. New York: Nova Biomedical, 2009.

Hay, William, Myron Levin, Robin Deterding, and Mark Abzug. *Current Diagnosis and Treatment Pediatrics*. 21st ed. New York: McGraw-Hill Professional, 2012.

Lichtenstein, Richard, and Getachew Teshome. *Pediatric Emergencies*. Philadelphia: Elsevier, 2013.

Long, Sarah S., Larry K. Pickering, and Charles G. Prober, eds. *Principles and Practice of Pediatric Infectious Diseases*. 3d ed. Philadelphia: Churchill Livingstone/Elsevier, 2008.

Marcdante, Karen, and Robert M. Kliegman. *Nelson Essentials of Pediatrics*. 7th ed. Philadelphia: Saunders, 2015.

Martin, Richard J., Avroy A. Fanaroff, and Michele C. Walsh. *Fanaroff and Martin's Neonatal-Perinatal Medicine*. 9th ed. Philadelphia: Mosby, 2011.

McMillan, Julia, Carlton K. Lee, George K. Siberry, and Karen Carroll. *The Harriet Lane Handbook of Pediatric Antimicrobial Therapy*. 2d ed. Philadelphia: Saunders, 2014.

Park, Myung K. *Park's Pediatric Cardiology for Practitioners*. 6th ed. Philadelphia: Mosby, 2014.

Polin, Richard A., William W. Fox, and Steven H. Abman. *Fetal and Neonatal Physiology*. 4th ed. Philadelphia: Saunders, 2011.

Shah, Kara N. *Pediatric Dermatology*. Philadelphia: Elsevier, 2014.

Sperling, Mark A. *Pediatric Endocrinology*. 4th ed. Philadelphia: Saunders, 2014.

Zitelli, Basil J., Sara C. McIntire, and Andrew J. Nowalk. *Zitelli and Davis' Atlas of Pediatric Physical Diagnosis*. 6th ed. Philadelphia: Saunders, 2012.

PHARMACOLOGY AND THERAPEUTICS

Bardal, Stan, Jason Waechter, and Doug Martin. *Applied Pharmacology*. Philadelphia: Saunders, 2011.

Brenner, George M., and Craig Stevens. *Pharmacology*. 4th ed. Philadelphia: Saunders, 2012.

Golan, David E., Armen H. Tashjian Jr. Ehrin J. Armstrong, and April W. Armstrong. *Principles of Pharmacology: The Pathophysiologic Basis of Drug Therapy*. Philadelphia: Lippincott Williams & Wilkins, 2011.

Griffith, H. Winter. *Complete Guide to Prescription and Nonprescription Drugs*. Revised and updated by Stephen Moore. New York: Penguin Group, 2010.

Hart, Carl L., and Charles Ksir. *Drugs, Society & Human Behavior*. 15th ed. New York: McGraw-Hill, 2013.

Harvey, Richard A., Michelle A Clark, Richard Finkel, Jose A. Rey, and Karen Whalen. *Pharmacology*. Philadelphia: Lippincott Williams & Wilkins, 2011.

Katzung, Bertram, Susan Masters, and Anthony Trevor. *Basic and Clinical Pharmacology*. 12th ed. New York: McGraw-Hill, 2011.

Lehne, Richard A. *Pharmacology for Nursing Care*. 8th ed. Philadelphia: Saunders, 2012.

PDR for Nonprescription Drugs, Dietary Supplements, and Herbs. 31st ed. Montvale, N.J.: PDR Network, 2010.

Rees, Judith A., Ian Smith, and Jennie Watson. *Pharmaceutical Practice*. 5th ed. London: Churchill Livingstone, 2014.

Sobel, Stephen V. *Successful Psychopharmacology: Evidence-Based Treatment Solutions for Achieving Remission*. New York: W. W. Norton & Company, 2012.

Wecker, Lynn, Lynn Crespo, George Dunaway, Carl Faingold and Stephanie Watts. *Brody's Human Pharmacology*. 5th ed. Philadelphia: Mosby, 2010.

PHYSICAL MEDICINE AND REHABILITATION

Braddom, Randall L. *Physical Medicine and Rehabilitation*. 4th ed. Philadelphia: Saunders, 2011.

Cameron, Michelle H. *Physical Agents in Rehabilitation: From Research to Practice*. 3d ed. St. Louis, Mo.: Saunders/Elsevier, 2009.

Lennard, Ted A., David G Vivian, Stevan A. Walkowski, and Aneesh K. Singla. *Pain Procedures in Clinical Practice*. 3d ed. Philadelphia: Saunders, 2011.

Lusardi, Michelle M., Millee Jorge, and Caroline C. Nielsen. *Orthotics and Prosthetics in Rehabilitation*. 3d ed. Philadelphia: Saunders, 2012.

Magee, David J. *Orthopedic Physical Assessment*. 6th ed. Philadelphia: Saunders, 2013.

Neumann, Donald A. *Kinesiology of the Musculoskeletal System: Foundations for Rehabilitation*. 2d ed. St. Louis, Mo.: Mosby/Elsevier, 2010.

O'Sullivan, Susan B., Thomas J. Schmitz, and George Fulk. *Physical Rehabilitation*. Philadelphia: F.A. Davis, 2013.

Walker, Francis, and Michael S. Cartwright. *Neuromuscular Ultrasound*. Philadelphia: Saunders, 2011.

PHYSIOLOGY

Fox, Stuart. *Human Physiology*. 13th ed. New York: McGraw-Hill Science, 2012.

Hall, John E. *Guyton and Hall Textbook of Medical Physiology*. 12th ed. Philadelphia: Saunders, 2011.

Marieb, Elaine N., and Katia Hoehn. *Human Anatomy & Physiology*. 9th ed. London: Pearson, 2012.

Mulroney, Susan, and Adam Myers. *Netter's Essential Physiology*. Philadelphia: Saunders, 2009.

Sherwood, Lauralee. *Human Physiology: From Cells to Systems*. 8th ed. Stamford, Conn.: Cengage Learning, 2012.

Shier, David, Jackie Butler, and Ricki Lewis. *Hole's Human Anatomy & Physiology*. 13th ed. New York: McGraw-Hill Science, 2012.

Silverthorn, Dee Unglaub. *Human Physiology: An Integrated Approach*. 6th ed. London: Pearson, 2012.

Widmaier, Eric, Hershel Raff, and Kevin Strang. *Vander's Human Physiology: The Mechanisms of Body Function*. 13th ed. New York: McGraw-Hill Science, 2013.

PREVENTIVE MEDICINE AND PUBLIC HEALTH

Hales, Dianne. *An Invitation to Health Brief*. Updated ed. Belmont, Calif.: Wadsworth/Cengage Learning, 2010.

Koren, Herman. *Illustrated Dictionary and Resource Directory of Environmental and Occupational Health*. 2d ed. Boca Raton, Fla.: CRC Press, 2005.

Lee, Philip R., and Carroll L. Estes, eds. *The Nation's Health*. 7th ed. Sudbury, Mass.: Jones and Bartlett, 2003.

Levy, Barry S., et al., eds. *Occupational Health: Recognizing and Preventing Disease and Injury*. 5th ed. Philadelphia: Lippincott Williams & Wilkins, 2006.

Moeller, Dade W. *Environmental Health*. 3d ed. Cambridge, Mass.: Harvard University Press, 2005.

Rom, William N., ed. *Environmental and Occupational Medicine*. 4th ed. Philadelphia: Wolters Kluwer/Lippincott Williams & Wilkins, 2007.

Wallace, Robert B., ed. *Maxcy-Rosenau-Last Public Health and Preventive Medicine*. 15th ed. New York: McGraw-Hill, 2008.

PRIMARY HEALTH CARE. *See* FAMILY MEDICINE; INTERNAL MEDICINE

PSYCHIATRY

American Psychiatric Association. *Diagnostic and Statistical Manual of Mental Disorders: DSM-5*. 5th ed. Washington, D.C.: Author, 2013.

Andreasen, Nancy C., and Donald W. Black. *Introductory Textbook of Psychiatry*. 5th ed. Washington, D.C.: American Psychiatric Press, 2010.

Blazer, Dan G., David C. Steffens, and Ewald W. Busse, eds. *The American Psychiatric Publishing Textbook of Geriatric Psychiatry*. 4th ed. Washington, D.C.: American Psychiatric Publishing, 2009.

Kring, Ann M., et al. *Abnormal Psychology*. 12th ed. Hoboken, N.J.: John Wiley & Sons, 2013.

Lewis, Melvin, ed. *Child and Adolescent Psychiatry: A Comprehensive Textbook*. 4th ed. Philadelphia: Lippincott Williams & Wilkins, 2007.

RADIOLOGY AND IMAGING

Adam, Andy, Adrian K. Dixon, Jonathan Gillard, Cornelia Schaefer-Prokop, Ronald G. Grainger, and David J. Allison. *Grainger & Allison's Diagnostic Radiology*. 6th ed. London: Churchill Livingstone, 2014.

Bontrager, Kenneth L., and John Lampignano. *Textbook of Radiographic Positioning and Related Anatomy*. 8th ed. Philadelphia: Mosby, 2013.

Brant, William E., and Clyde Helms. *Fundamentals of Diagnostic Radiology*. Philadelphia: Lippincott Williams & Wilkins, 2012.

Kaufman, John A., and Michael J. Lee. *Vascular and Interventional Radiology: The Requisites*. 2d ed. Philadelphia: Saunders, 2013.

Rumack, Carol M., Stephanie R. Wilson, J. William Charboneau, and Deborah Levin. *Diagnostic Ultrasound*. 4th ed. Philadelphia: Mosby, 2011.

Som, Peter M., and Hugh D. Curtin. *Head and Neck Imaging - 2 Volume Set*. 5th Edition. Philadelphia: Mosby, 2011.

Weissleder, Ralph, Jack Wittenberg, Mukesh G. Harisinghani, and John W. Chen. *Primer of Diagnostic Imaging*. 5th ed. Philadelphia: Mosby, 2011.

RESPIRATORY SYSTEM

Cleveland, Robert H., ed. *Imaging in Pediatric Pulmonology*. New York: Springer, 2012.

Colt, Henri, and Septimiu Murgu. *Bronchoscopy and Central Airway Disorders*. Philadelphia: Saunders, 2012.

Ernst, Armin, and Felix J. F. Herth, eds. *Principles and Practice of Interventional Pulmonology*. New York: Springer, 2013.

Lewis, Michael I., and Robert J. McKenna. *Medical Management of the Thoracic Surgery Patient*. Philadelphia: Saunders, 2010.

Light, Michael J., Carol J. Blaisdell, Douglas N. Homnick, Michael S. Schechter, and Miles M. Weinberger, eds. *Pediatric Pulmonology*. Elk Grove Village, Ill.: American Academy of Pediatrics, 2011.

Mason, Robert J., et al., eds. *Murray and Nadel's Textbook of Respiratory Medicine*. 5th ed. Philadelphia: Saunders/Elsevier, 2010.

Mason, Robert J., V. Courtney Broaddus, Thomas Martin, Talmadge King, Jr., Dean Schraufnagel, and Jay A. Nadel. *Murray & Nadel's Image-Guided Thoracic Case Studies*. 5th ed. Philadelphia: Saunders, 2013.

Musani, Ali I. *Interventional Pulmonology, An Issue of Clinics in Chest Medicine*. Philadelphia: Elsevier, 2013.

Niederman, Michael. *Respiratory Tract Infections: Advances in Diagnosis, Management, and Prevention*. Philadelphia: Saunders, 2011.

Spiro, Stephen G., Gerard A Silvestri, Gerard A. Silvestri and Alvar Agustí. *Alvar Agustí Clinical Respiratory Medicine*.

4th ed. Philadelphia: Saunders, 2012.

Tanoue, Lynn, and Richard A. Matthay. *Lung Cancer*. Philadelphia: Saunders, 2011.

Turcios, Nelson L., and Robert J. Fink. *Pulmonary Manifestations of Pediatric Diseases*. Philadelphia: Saunders, 2009.

Weinberger, Steven E., Barbara A. Cockrill, and Jess Mandel. *Principles of Pulmonary Medicine*. 6th ed. Philadelphia: Saunders, 2013.

Wilmott, Robert W., Thomas F. Boat, Andrew Bush, Victor Chernick, Robin R. Deterding, and Felix Ratjen. *Kendig and Chernick's Disorders of the Respiratory Tract in Children*. 8th ed. Philadelphia: Saunders, 2012.

RHEUMATOLOGY

Cassidy, James T., Ross E. Petty, Ronald Laxer, and Carol Lindsley. *Textbook of Pediatric Rheumatology*. 6th ed. Philadelphia: Saunders, 2011.

Firestein, Gary S., Ralph C. Budd, Sherine E. Gabriel, Iain B. McInnes, and James R O'Dell. *Kelley's Textbook of Rheumatology*. 9th ed. Philadelphia: Saunders, 2013.

Hochberg, Marc C., Alan J. Silman, Josef S. Smolen, Michael E. Weinblatt, and Michael H. Weisman. *Rheumatology*. 5th ed. Philadelphia: Mosby, 2011.

Imboden, John, David Hellmann, and John Stone. *Current Diagnosis & Treatment in Rheumatology*. 3d ed. New York: McGraw-Hill, 2013.

Lawry, George V., Hans J. Kreder, Gillian Hawker, and Dana Jerome. *Fam's Musculoskeletal Examination and Joint Injection Techniques*. 2d ed. Philadelphia: Mosby, 2010.

Wakefield, Richard J., and Maria Antonietta D'Agostino. *Essential Applications of Musculoskeletal Ultrasound in Rheumatology*. Philadelphia: Saunders, 2010.

Watts, Richard A., Philip Conaghan, Chris Denton, Helen Foster, John Issacs, and Ulf Muller-Ladner. *Oxford Textbook of Rheumatology*. 4th ed. New York: Oxford University Press, 2013.

SEXUALLY TRANSMITTED DISEASES (STDs). *See also* ACQUIRED IMMUNODEFICIENCY SYNDROME (AIDS)

Beigi, Richard H., ed. *Sexually Transmitted Diseases*. New York: Wiley-Blackwell, 2012.

Larsen, Laura. *Sexually Transmitted Diseases Sourcebook*. Detroit: Omnigraphics, 2009.

Marrazzo, Jeanne. *Update in Sexually Transmitted Infections*. Philadelphia: Elsevier, 2013.

Stine, Gerald J. *AIDS Update 2010*. New York: McGraw-Hill Higher Education, 2010.

Taylor-Robinson, D., ed. *Clinical Problems in Sexually Transmitted Diseases*. New York: Springer, 2013.

Volberding, Paul, Warner Greene, Joep M. A. Lange, Joel E. Gallant, and Nelson Sewankambo. *Sande's HIV/AIDS Medicine*. 2d ed. Philadelphia: Saunders, 2012.

SPORTS MEDICINE

Altchek, David W. *Foot and Ankle Sports Medicine*. Philadelphia: Lippincott Williams & Wilkins, 2012.

American College of Sports Medicine. *ACSM's Guidelines for Exercise Testing and Prescription*. 8th ed. Philadelphia: Lippincott Williams & Wilkins, 2010.

Cole, Brian J., and Jon K. Sekiya. *Surgical Techniques of the Shoulder, Elbow, and Knee in Sports Medicine*. 2d ed. Philadelphia: Saunders, 2013.

France, Robert C. *Introduction to Sports Medicine and Athletic Training*. Stamford, Conn.: Cengage Learning, 2010.

Kenney, W. Larry, Jack H. Wilmore, and David L. Costill. *Physiology of Sport and Exercise with Web Study Guide*. 5th ed. Champaign, Ill.: Human Kinetics, 2011.

Meehan, William P., and Lyle J. Micheli. *Concussion in Sports*. Philadelphia: Saunders, 2011.

McArdle, William, Frank I. Katch, and Victor L. Katch. *Exercise Physiology: Energy, Nutrition, and Human Performance*. 7th ed. Boston: Lippincott Williams & Wilkins, 2010.

National Academy of Sports Medicine. *NASM Essentials Of Personal Fitness Training*. 4th ed. Sudbury, Mass.: Jones & Bartlett Learning, 2013.

Phelps, Kerryn, and Craig Hassed. *Sports Medicine*. London: Churchill Livingstone, 2010.

Sanders, Timothy G. *MRI in Sports Medicine*. Philadelphia: Elsevier, 2013.

Starkey, Chad. *Athletic Training And Sports Medicine: An Integrated Approach*. 5th ed. Sudbury, Mass; Jones & Bartlett Learning, 2012.

Toth, Cory. *Sports Neurology*. Philadelphia: Saunders, 2009.

STATISTICS

Chernick, Michael R., and Robert H. Friis. *Introductory Biostatistics for the Health Sciences: Modern Applications Including Bootstrap*. Hoboken, N.J.: Wiley-Interscience, 2003.

D'Agostino, Ralph B., Sr., Lisa M. Sullivan, and Alexa S. Beiser. *Introductory Applied Biostatistics*. Belmont, Calif.: Thomson/Brooks/Cole, 2005.

Daniel, Wayne W. *Biostatistics: A Foundation for Analysis in the Health Sciences*. 9th ed. Hoboken, N.J.: John Wiley & Sons, 2009.

Glantz, Stanton A. *Primer of Biostatistics*. 6th ed. New York: McGraw-Hill, 2005.

Hebel, J. Richard, and Robert J. McCarter. *A Study Guide to Epidemiology and Biostatistics*. 6th ed. Sudbury, Mass.: Jones and Bartlett, 2006.

Le, Chap T. *Health and Numbers: Problems-Based Introduction to Biostatistics*. Malden, Mass.: Blackwell, 2009.

Wassertheil-Smoller, Sylvia. *Biostatistics and Epidemiology: A Primer for Health and Biomedical Professionals*. 3d ed. New York: Springer, 2004.

SUBSTANCE ABUSE

Gahlinger, Paul M. *Illegal Drugs: A Complete Guide to Their History, Chemistry, Use, and Abuse*. Updated and rev. ed. New York: Plume, 2004.

Galanter, Marc, and Herbert D. Kleber, eds. *The American*

Psychiatric Publishing Textbook of Substance Abuse Treatment. 3d ed. Washington, D.C.: American Psychiatric Publishing, 2004.

Kuhn, Cynthia, et al. *Buzzed: The Straight Facts About the Most Used and Abused Drugs from Alcohol to Ecstasy.* 3d ed. New York: W. W. Norton, 2008.

Liddle, Howard A., and Cynthia L. Rowe, eds. *Adolescent Substance Abuse: Research and Clinical Advances.* New York: Cambridge University Press, 2006.

Lowinson, Joyce H., et al., eds. *Substance Abuse: A Comprehensive Textbook.* 4th ed. Philadelphia: Lippincott Williams & Wilkins, 2005.

Maisto, Stephen A., Mark Galizio, and Gerard J. Connors. *Drug Use and Abuse.* 4th ed. Belmont, Calif.: Thomson/Wadsworth, 2004.

Rogers, Peter D., and Richard B. Heyman, eds. *Addiction Medicine: Adolescent Substance Abuse.* Philadelphia: W. B. Saunders, 2002.

Weil, Andrew, and Winifred Rosen. *From Chocolate to Morphine: Everything You Need to Know About Mind-Altering Drugs.* Rev. and updated ed. New York: Houghton Mifflin, 2004.

SURGERY

Cameron, John L., and Andrew M. Cameron. *Current Surgical Therapy.* 11th ed. Philadelphia: Saunders, 2014.

Chaikof, Elliot L., and Richard P. Cambria. *Atlas of Vascular Surgery and Endovascular Therapy.* Philadelphia: Saunders, 2014.

Cioffi, William, and Juan A. Asensio. *Atlas of Trauma/Emergency Surgical Techniques.* Philadelphia: Saunders, 2014.

Fischer, Josef E., Daniel B. Jones, Frank B. Pomposelli, and Gilbert R. Upchurch Jr., eds. *Fischer's Mastery of Surgery.* 6th ed. Philadelphia: Lippincott Williams & Wilkins, 2011.

Forsythe, John L. R. *Transplantation.* 5th ed. Philadelphia: Saunders, 2013.

Holcomb, George W., III, J. Patrick Murphy, and Daniel J Ostlie. *Ashcraft's Pediatric Surgery.* 6th ed. Philadelphia: Saunders, 2014.

Lawrence, Peter F., Richard M. Bell, Merril T. Dayton, and James C. Hebert. *Essentials of General Surgery.* Philadelphia: Lippincott Williams & Wilkins, 2012.

Lennard, Thomas W. J. *Endocrine Surgery.* 5th ed. Philadelphia: Saunders, 2013.

Minter, Rebecca, and Gerard Doherty. *Current Procedures Surgery.* New York: McGraw-Hill Professional, 2010.

Morris, Peter, and Stuart J. Knechtle. *Kidney Transplantation - Principles and Practice.* 7th ed. Philadelphia: Sanders, 2014.

Mulholland, Michael W., Keith D. Lillemoe, Gerard M. Doherty, Ronald V. Maier, Diane M. Simeone, and Gilbert R. Upchurch Jr., eds. *Greenfield's Surgery: Scientific Principles & Practice.* Philadelphia: Lippincott Williams & Wilkins, 2011.

Novell, Richard, Daryll Baker, and Nicholas Goddard. *Kirk's General Surgical Operations.* 6th ed. London: Churchill Livingstone, 2013.

Quick, Clive R. G., Joanna B. Reed, Simon J. F. Harper, Kourosh Saeb-Parsy, and Philip J. Deakin. *Essential Surgery.* 5th ed. London: Churchill Livingstone, 2014.

Sellke, Frank, and Marc Ruel. *Atlas of Cardiac Surgical Techniques.* Philadelphia: Saunders, 2009.

Sellke, Frank, Pedro J. del Nido, and Scott Swanson. *Sabiston and Spencer's Surgery of the Chest.* 8th ed. Philadelphia: Saunders, 2010.

Townsend, Courtney M., Jr., R. Daniel Beauchamp, B. Mark Evers, and Kenneth L. Mattox. *Sabiston Textbook of Surgery: The Biological Basis of Modern Surgical Practice.* 19th ed. Philadelphia: Saunders, 2012.

Thorne, Charles H. *Grabb and Smith's Plastic Surgery.* Philadelphia: Lippincott Williams & Wilkins, 2013.

Velasco, Jose M. *Rush University Medical Center Review of Surgery.* 5th ed. Philadelphia: Saunders, 2011.

Young, Christopher J., and Marc A. Gladman. *Examination Surgery.* London: Churchill Livingstone, 2013.

Zollinger, Robert, Jr., and E. Ellison. *Zollinger's Atlas of Surgical Operations.* 9th ed. New York: McGraw-Hill Professional, 2010.

Zwischenberger, Joseph B. *Atlas of Thoracic Surgical Techniques.* Philadelphia: Saunders, 2011.

TOXICOLOGY

Bissell, Michael G. *Toxicology Testing.* Philadelphia: Saunders, 2012.

Hodgson, Ernest. *A Textbook of Modern Toxicology.* 4th ed. New York: Wiley, 2010.

Kruse, James. *Toxicology.* Philadelphia: Saunders, 2012.

Klaassen, Curtis. *Casarett & Doull's Toxicology: The Basic Science of Poisons.* 8th ed. New York: McGraw-Hill Professional, 2013.

Lugassy, Daniel M. *Clinical Toxicology.* Philadelphia: Elsevier, 2014.

Murray, Lindsay, Frank Daly, David McCoubrie, Jessamine Soderstrom, Ovidu Pascu, Jason Armstrong, and Mike Cadogan. *Toxicology Handbook.* 2d ed. London: Churchill Livingstone, 2010.

Pani, Balram. *Textbook of Toxicology.* New Delhi, India: I K International, 2010.

Püssa, Tõnu. *Principles of Food Toxicology.* 2d ed. New York: CRC Press, 2013.

TROPICAL MEDICINE

Farrar, Jeremy, Peter Hotez, Thomas Junghanss, Gagandeep Kang, David Lalloo, and Nicholas J. White. *Manson's Tropical Diseases.* 23d ed. Philadelphia: Saunders, 2014.

Guerrant, Richard L., David H. Walker, and Peter F. Weller. *Tropical Infectious Diseases: Principles, Pathogens and Practice.* 3d ed. Philadelphia: Saunders, 2011.

Keystone, Jay S., David O. Freedman, Phyllis Kozarsky, Hans D. Nothdurft, and Bradley A. Connor. *Travel Medicine.* 3d ed. Philadelphia: Saunders, 2013.

Magill, Alan J., Edward T. Ryan, Tom Solomon, and David

R. Hill. *Hunter's Tropical Medicine and Emerging Infectious Disease*. 9th ed. Philadelphia: Saunders, 2012.

UROLOGY

Docimo, Steven G., Douglas Canning, and Antoine Khoury, eds. *The Kelalis-King-Belman Textbook of Clinical Pediatric Urology*. 6th ed. New York: CRC Press, 2014.

Gearhart, John G., Richard C. Rink, and Pierre D. E. Mouriquand. *Pediatric Urology*. 2d ed. Philadelphia: Saunders, 2010.

Gebhart, John B. *Urologic Surgery for the Gynecologist and Urogynecologist*. Philadelphia: Saunders, 2010.

Hanno, Philip M., Thomas J. Guzzo, S. Bruce Malkowicz, and Alan J. Wein. *Penn Clinical Manual of Urology*. 2d ed. Philadelphia: Saunders, 2014.

MacLennan, Greg T. *Hinman's Atlas of UroSurgical Anatomy*. 3d ed. Philadelphia: Saunders, 2012.

McAninch, Jack, and Tom F. Lue. *Smith and Tanagho's General Urology*. 18th ed. New York: McGraw-Hill Professional, 2012.

Mitch, William E., and Saulo Klahr, eds. *Handbook of Nutrition and the Kidney*. 6th ed. Philadelphia: Lippincott Williams & Wilkins, 2010.

Scardino, Peter T., W. Marston Linehan, Michael J. Zelefsky, Nicholas J. Vogelzang, Brian I. Rini, Bernard H. Bochner, and Joel Sheinfeld, eds. *Comprehensive Textbook of Genitourinary Oncology*. Philadelphia: Lippincott Williams & Wilkins, 2011.

Smith, Joseph A., Jr., Stuart S. Howards, and Glenn M. Preminger. *Hinman's Atlas of Urologic Surgery E-Book*. 3d ed. Philadelphia: Saunders, 2012.

Wein, Alan J., Louis R. Kavoussi, Andrew C. Novick, Alan W. Partin, and Craig A. Peters. *Campbell-Walsh Urology*. 10th ed. Philadelphia: Saunders, 2012.

—Peter B. Heller, Ph.D.;
updated by Bryan Auday, Ph.D., Desiree Dreeuws,
and Michael A. Buratovich, Ph.D.

RESOURCES

ABORTION. *See* **REPRODUCTIVE ISSUES**

ACQUIRED IMMUNODEFICIENCY SYNDROME (AIDS)

AIDS Info
P.O. Box 6303
Rockville, MD 20849-6303
800-HIV-0440
TTY: 888-480-3739
Fax: 301-315-2818
E-mail: ContactUs@aidsinfo.nih.gov
Web site: http://www.aidsinfo.nih.gov
This federal Public Health Service project maintains a database on AIDS clinical trials. Provides information on the location of AIDS trials, criteria for inclusion or exclusion, and related assistance.

Centers for Disease Control and Prevention (CDC)
HIV/AIDS
800-CDC-INFO
TTY: 888-232-6348
E-mail: cdcinfo@cdc.gov
Web site: http://www.cdc.gov/hiv
This federal program offers information on AIDS and AIDS-related issues. Provides referrals to physicians, support groups, self-help groups, legal organizations, housing agencies, hospices, and home care services.

Gay Men's Health Crisis
446 West 33rd Street
New York, NY 10001-2601
800-AIDS-NYC
212-367-1000
Web site: http://www.gmhc.org
Provides support and therapy groups for persons with AIDS and their families. Offers volunteer crisis counselors, a buddy program for assistance with tasks, and an HIV-AIDS prevention program.

Good Samaritan Project
3030 Walnut
Kansas City, MO 64108
816-561-8784
Fax: 816-531-7199
Web site: http://www.gsp-kc.org
The mission of this organization is to provide supportive and responsive care for a diverse community of individuals affected by HIV-AIDS and to raise awareness through education and advocacy.

Project Inform
273 Ninth Street
San Francisco, CA 94103
800-822-7422
415-558-8669
Fax: 415-558-0684
Web site: http://www.projectinform.org
This clearinghouse and hotline provides AIDS and HIV treatment information and advocacy as well as information on current drugs and where they can be obtained.

WORLD: An Information and Support Network by, for, and About Women with HIV-AIDS
449 15th Street
Suite 303
Oakland, CA 94612
510-986-0340
Fax: 510-986-0341
Web site: http://www.womenhiv.org
Offers support and information for women infected with or affected by AIDS or HIV. Sponsors retreats and classes.

ADDICTION-ALCOHOL, DRUGS, AND SMOKING

Al-Anon/Alateen
1600 Corporate Landing Parkway
Virginia Beach, VA 23454-5617
888-4AL-ANON
757-563-1600
Fax: 757-563-1655
E-mail: wso@al-anon.org
Web site: http://www.al-anon.org
Provides a free self-help program of recovery from the family disease of alcoholism, based on the Twelve Steps and Twelve Traditions of Alcoholics Anonymous. Includes Alateen, a program for younger family members affected by another person's drinking.

Alcoholics Anonymous (AA)
P.O. Box 459
New York, NY 10163
212-870-3400
Web site: http://www.aa.org
This is a free self-help program for recovery from alcoholism. Members work to recover from alcoholism and help others to achieve sobriety through a Twelve-Step program, in which members share experiences, strength, and hope with one another. Web site provides information on local chapters of AA in the United States and Canada.

Cocaine Anonymous World Services
P.O. Box 492000
Los Angeles, CA 90049-8000

800-347-8998 (referral service)
310-559-5833
Fax: 310-559-2554
E-mail: cawso@ca.org
Web site: http://www.ca.org
Refers callers to local self-help Twelve-Step groups for persons addicted to cocaine and other mind-altering drugs.

Dual Recovery Anonymous
P.O. Box 8107
Prairie Village, KS 66208
913-991-2703
E-mail: draws@draonline.org
Web site: http://www.draonline.org
This self-help support group is based on the Twelve-Step program; for persons who have alcohol or drug addictions along with mental or emotional disorders.

Families Anonymous
P.O. Box 3475
Culver City, CA 90231-3475
847-294-5877
E-mail: famanon@FamiliesAnonymous.org
Web site: http://www.familiesanonymous.org
This Twelve-Step support group is for persons dealing with drug abuse or related behavior problems of a family member or friend. Refers callers to the nearest meetings, which are held throughout the world. Also provides referrals to other Twelve-Step programs and other resources and organizations.

Jewish Alcoholics, Chemically Dependent Persons, and Significant Others (JACS)
120 West 57th Street
New York, NY 10019
212-632-4600
Fax: 212-399-3525
E-mail: jacs@jacswcb.org
Web site: http://www.jbfcs.org/jacs
Promotes and assists recovery from chemical dependency for Jewish alcoholics and addicts, their families, and their friends.

National Center for Chronic Disease Prevention and Health Promotion
Office on Smoking and Health
800-CDC-INFO
TTY: 888-232-6348
E-mail: tobaccoinfo@cdc.gov
Web site: http://www.cdc.gov/tobacco
This site from the Centers for Disease Control and Prevention provides information on smoking cessation, smoking and teens, smoking during pregnancy, and passive smoking, among other resources. Also offers a comprehensive collection of Web links.

National Institute on Alcohol Abuse and Alcoholism (NIAAA)
5635 Fishers Lane, MSC 9304
Bethesda, MD 20892-9304
301-443-3860
E-mail: niaaaweb-r@exchange.nih.gov
Web site: http://www.niaaa.nih.gov
Provides information on clinical trials, intramural research, and publications and answers frequently asked questions, among other services.

Phoenix Center on Addiction and the Family
888-286-5027
E-mail: coaf@phoenixhouse.org
Web site: http://www.coaf.org
Provides information on the effects of parental abuse of alcohol and other substances on children. Looks for solutions to the problems of children of alcoholics.

Pride Institute
800-54-PRIDE
E-mail: support@pride-institute.com
Web site: http://www.pride-institute.com
Helps lesbian, gay, and bisexual individuals with chemical dependency and mental health problems.

Rational Recovery
P.O. Box 800
Lotus, CA 95651
530-621-2667, 530-621-4374
Web site: http://www.rational.org
Nonspiritual self-help program for recovery from substance addictions and overeating.

Women for Sobriety, Inc.
P.O. Box 618
Quakertown, PA 18951-0618
215-536-8026
Fax: 215-538-9026
Web site: http://www.womenforsobriety.org
Self-help group specifically for female alcoholics based on the Thirteen Acceptance Statements.

AGENT ORANGE

National Veterans Service Fund, Inc.
P.O. Box 2465
Darien, CT 06820-0465
800-521-0198
E-mail: philvet@nvsf.org
Web site: http://www.nvsf.org
Offers case-managed social services and limited medical assistance to Vietnam and Persian Gulf War veterans. Provides information on Agent Orange and works to see that affected veterans receive proper treatment. Helps veterans' children with birth defects.

AGING AND ELDER CARE

Eldercare Locator
800-677-1116
E-mail: eldercarelocator@n4a.org
Web site: http://www.eldercare.gov
A federal service that provides information on state and local resources for community-based services for the elderly.

Little Brothers-Friends of the Elderly
255 North Ashland Avenue
Chicago, IL 60607-1019
312-455-1000
Fax: 312-455-9674
E-mail: general@littlebrotherschicago.org
Web site: http://www.littlebrothers.org
Provides friendship and assistance to persons over seventy years of age who live alone and do not have emotional and physical help from families. Sponsors visitation programs and provides transportation, information, and referrals.

National Council on the Aging (NCOA)
1901 L Street NW
4th Floor
Washington, DC 20036
202-479-1200
TDD: 202-479-6674
Fax: 202-479-0735
Web site: http://www.ncoa.org
Answers questions on services available to seniors. Sponsors groups relating to such topics as employment for seniors, rural aging, adult day care, senior housing, and volunteer programs for seniors.

ALBINISM

National Organization for Albinism and Hypopigmentation (NOAH)
P.O. Box 959
East Hampstead, NH 03826-0959
800-473-2310
603-887-2310
Fax: 800-648-2310
Web site: http://www.albinism.org
Provides information on albinism and coordinates and promotes support groups for persons with albinism.

ALLERGIES

American Academy of Allergy, Asthma, and Immunology
555 East Wells Street
Suite 1100
Milwaukee, WI 53202-3823
414-272-6071
E-mail: info@aaaai.org
Web site: http://www.aaaai.org
An organization that provides consumers, professionals, and media with comprehensive information on allergies and related conditions and diseases.

ALZHEIMER'S DISEASE

Alzheimer's Association
225 North Michigan Avenue
Suite 1700
Chicago, IL 60601-7633
800-272-3900
TDD: 312-403-3073
Fax: 866-699-1246
E-mail: info@alz.org
Web site: http://www.alz.org
Promotes family support systems for relatives of persons with Alzheimer's disease.

Alzheimer's Disease Education and Referral Center
P.O. Box 8250
Silver Spring, MD 20907-8250
800-438-4380
Fax: 301-495-3334
E-mail: adear@nia.nih.gov
Web site: http://www.nia.nih.gov/alzheimers
Federal service through the National Institute on Aging that provides information on Alzheimer's disease, including symptoms and current research, and makes referrals to other organizations.

AMPUTATION

National Amputation Foundation
40 Church Street
Malverne, NY 11565
516-887-3600
Fax: 516-887-3667
E-mail: amps76@aol.com
Web site: http://www.nationalamputation.org
Assists veterans and other amputees in employment and social and mental rehabilitation. Sponsors a program in which amputees who have returned to normal life visit new amputees.

AMYOTROPHIC LATERAL SCLEROSIS (ALS)

ALS Association
1275 K Street NW, Suite 250
Washington, DC 20005
202-407-8580
202-289-6801
Fax: 818-880-9006
Web site: http://www.alsa.org
Provides research and information on ALS and patient care.

ANOREXIA NERVOSA. *See* EATING DISORDERS

APNEA

American Sleep Apnea Association
6856 Eastern Avenue NW
Suite 203
Washington, DC 20012
202-293-3650
Web site: http://www.sleepapnea.org
Offers educational programs and support groups through the Awake Network.

ARTHRITIS

Arthritis Foundation
1330 W. Peachtree Street
Suite 100
Atlanta, GA 30357-0669
800-283-7800
404-872-7100
Web site: http://www.arthritis.org
Provides information on arthritis support groups, exercise classes, and other resources for persons with arthritis. Also offers information, education, and publications specific to juvenile arthritis.

ASTHMA. *See* LUNG DISORDERS

ATAXIA

National Ataxia Foundation
2600 Fernbrook Lane
Suite 119
Minneapolis, MN 55447-4752
763-553-0020
Fax: 763-553-0167
E-mail: naf@ataxia.org
Web site: http://www.ataxia.org
Provides services and information to victims of ataxia and their families.

ATTENTION-DEFICIT DISORDER (ADD)

Attention Deficit Disorder Association
P.O. Box 7557
Wilmington, DE 19803-9997
800-939-1019
E-mail: info@add.org
Web site: http://www.add.org
Offers support to persons with attention-deficit disorder and their families. Maintains a database of support groups.

Children and Adults with Attention Deficit/ Hyperactivity Disorder
4601 Presidents Drive
Suite 300
Lanham, MD 20706

800-233-4050
301-306-7070
Fax: 301-306-7090
Web site: http://www.chadd.org
Local groups provide information and support for families affected by ADD.

AUTISM

Autism Society of America
4330 East-West Highway, Suite 350
Bethesda, MD 20814
800-3-AUTISM
301-657-0881
Web site: http://www.autism-society.org
Provides information, education, and publications about autism, as well as online services and referrals.

AUTOIMMUNE DISORDERS

American Autoimmune Related Diseases Association
22100 Gratiot Avenue
Eastpointe, MI 48021
586-776-3900
Fax: 586-776-3903
Web site: http://www.aarda.org
Provides education and information on autoimmunity, which causes several serious chronic diseases.

BATTEN'S DISEASE

Batten Disease Support and Research Association
1175 Dublin Road
Columbus, OH 43215
800-448-4570
E-mail: bdsra1@bdsra.org
Web site: http://www.bdsra.org
Provides support group activities, referrals, and information for families of children with Batten's disease.

BED-WETTING. *See* INCONTINENCE

BIRTH DEFECTS. *See also* SPECIFIC DEFECTS

Birth Defect Research for Children, Inc.
976 Lake Baldwin Lane
Suite 104
Orlando, FL 32814
407-566-8403
E-mail: staff@birthdefects.org
Web site: http://www.birthdefects.org
A nonprofit organization that provides parents and expectant parents with information about birth defects and support services for their children.

March of Dimes
1275 Mamaroneck Avenue
White Plains, NY 10605
914-997-4488
Web site: http://www.marchofdimes.com
An organization that supports research into the prevention of birth defects and offers consumers a range of excellent information on myriad birth defects, prenatal testing, and pregnancy health.

BLINDNESS. *See* VISION DISORDERS

BRAIN DISORDERS

American Brain Tumor Association
8550 W. Bryn Mawr Ave.
Suite 550
Chicago, IL 60631
800-886-2282
Fax: 773-577-8738
E-mail: info@abta.org
Web site: http://hope.abta.org
Provides educational materials and resource information to patients, families, and medical professionals. Mentors support group leaders and offers a database of support groups and a pen-pal program.

Brain Injury Association of America
1608 Spring Hill Road
Suite 110
Vienna, VA 22182
800-444-6443
703-761-0750
Fax: 703-761-0755
Web site: http://www.biausa.org
Provides services to persons with brain injuries and their families as well as information about traumatic brain injury. Links callers with support groups and local resources.

Brain Tumor Society
55 Chapel Street
Suite 200
Newton, MA 02458
617-924-9997
Fax: 617-924-9998
E-mail: info@braintumor.org
Web site: http://www.braintumor.org
Support for brain tumor patients and their families.

BULIMIA. *See* EATING DISORDERS

BURNS

Phoenix Society for Burn Survivors, Inc.
1835 R W Berends Drive SW
Grand Rapids, MI 49519-4955

800-888-2876
616-458-2773
Fax: 616-458-2831
E-mail: info@phoenixsociety.org
Web site: http://www.phoenix-society.org
This is a self-help service organization for burn survivors and their families. Offers seminars and school and job reentry programs.

CANADIAN ORGANIZATIONS

Canadian Centre for Occupational Health and Safety (CCOHS)/Le Centre canadien d'hygiène et de sécurité au travail (CCHST)
135 Hunter Street East
Hamilton, Ontario, Canada L8N 1M5
905-572-2981
Fax: 905-572-2206
Web site: http://www.ccohs.ca (English);
http://www.cchst.ca (French)
A not-for-profit federal department corporation that seeks the elimination of work-related illnesses and injuries.

Canadian Public Health Association (CPHA)
400-1565 Carling Avenue
Ottawa, Ontario, Canada K1Z 8R1
613-725-3769
Fax: 613-725-9826
E-mail: info@cpha.ca
Web site: http://www.cpha.ca/en/default.aspx
A national, independent, not-for-profit, and voluntary association representing public health in Canada, with links to the international public health community.

Health Canada/Santé Canada
Address Locator 0900C2
Ottawa, Ontario, Canada K1A 0K9
866-225-0709
613-957-2991
TTY: 800-465-7735
Fax: 613-941-5366
E-mail: Info@hc-sc.gc.ca
Web site: http://www.hc-sc.gc.ca/index-eng.php (English);
http://www.hc-sc.gc.ca/index-fra.php (French)
The federal department responsible for helping Canadians maintain and improve their health. Offers consumer safety information and information about First Nations, Inuit, and Aboriginal health.

Public Health Agency of Canada (PHAC)/L'Agence de la santé publique du Canada (ASPC)
Ontario office:
130 Colonnade Road
Address Locator 6501H
Ottawa, Ontario, Canada K1A 0K9
Manitoba office:
1015 Arlington Street

Winnipeg, Manitoba, Canada R3E 3R2
204-789-2000
Fax: 204-789-7878
Web site: http://www.phac-aspc.gc.ca/index-eng.php
(English); http://www.phac-aspc.gc.ca/index-fra.php
(French)
This government agency, formed in 2004, was created in response to growing concerns about the capacity of Canada's public health system to anticipate and respond effectively to public health threats.

CANCER

American Cancer Society
250 Williams Street NW
Atlanta, GA 30303
800-ACS-2345
TTY: 866-228-4327
Web site: http://www.cancer.org
Provides general information on cancer and information on the group's programs and services. Offers Look Good, Feel Better, a free, nonmedical program to help women overcome the appearance-related side effects of radiation and chemotherapy treatment.

American Childhood Cancer Organization
P.O. Box 498
Kensington, MD 20895
855-858-2226
Fax: 301-962-3521
Web site: http://www.acco.org
Provides information, support, and advocacy to families of children and adolescents with cancer, survivors of childhood cancer, and professionals who work with them.

National Cancer Institute
BG 9609 MSC 9760
9609 Medical Center Drive
Bethesda, MD 20892-8322
800-4-CANCER
TTY: 800-332-8615
Web site: http://www.cancer.gov
A component of the National Institutes of Health (NIH), the NCI is the federal government's principal agency for cancer research and training. Offers information on cancer treatment and diagnosis, clinical trials, rehabilitation, home care, financial aid, palliative care, supportive care for the side effects of treatment, quitting smoking, and cancer prevention.

National Coalition for Cancer Survivorship
1010 Wayne Avenue
Suite 315
Silver Spring, MD 20910
877-622-7937
Fax: 301-565-9670
E-mail: info@canceradvocacy.org
Web site: http://www.canceradvocacy.org

Provides support to cancer survivors and their families and friends. Facilitates peer support and maintains a list of organizations that are concerned with survivorship.

R. A. Bloch Cancer Foundation, Inc.
1 H&R Block Way
Kansas City, MO 64105
800-433-0464
816-854-5050
Fax: 816-854-8024
E-mail: hotline@blochcancer.org
Web site: http://www.blochcancer.org
Matches patients with volunteers who have had the same type of cancer. Provides resources, information, and free "Fighting Cancer" booklet.

Susan G. Komen for the Cure
5005 LBJ Freeway
Suite 250
Dallas, TX 75244
877-GO-KOMEN
Web site: http://www.komen.org
Trained volunteers provide information and resources to individuals concerned about breast health or breast cancer.

After Breast Cancer Diagnosis
5775 N Glen Park Road
Suite 201
Glendale, WI 53209
800-977-2141
414-977-1780
Fax: 414-977-1781
Web site: http://www.abcdbreastcancersupport.org
Provides information, referrals, and emotional support to women concerned about or diagnosed with breast cancer. National toll-free hotline is staffed by trained personnel and volunteers who have experienced breast cancer. Publications include information tailored for single women with breast cancer, teens, and partners of women with breast cancer.

CAREGIVERS. *See* AGING AND ELDER CARE; CHRONIC ILLNESSES

CELIAC SPRUE

Celiac Sprue Association (CSA)
P.O. Box 31700
Omaha, NE 68131-0700
877-CSA-4CSA
402-558-0600
Fax: 402-643-4108
E-mail: celiacs@csaceliacs.org
Web site: http://www.csaceliacs.org
Support and information on maintaining a gluten-free diet for persons affected by celiac sprue. Publications include a cookbook for gluten-free cooking.

CEREBRAL PALSY

United Cerebral Palsy
1825 K Street NW
Suite 600
Washington, DC 20006
800-872-5827
202-776-0406
E-mail: info@ucp.org
Web site: http://www.ucp.org
Provides information and referrals. Local affiliates provide family and individual support, early intervention programs, personal assistance and assistive technology services, and community-integrated living arrangements.

CHILDBIRTH. *See* REPRODUCTIVE ISSUES

CHRONIC ILLNESSES

Parents Helping Parents
1400 Parkmoor Avenue
Suite 100
San Jose, CA 95126
408-727-5775
Fax: 408-286-1116
Web site: http://www.php.com
Offer support for parents of children with special needs, including those with chronic or terminal illnesses. Assists new and ongoing parent support groups and resource centers.

Well Spouse Foundation
63 West Main Street, Suite H
Freehold, NJ 07728
800-838-0879
Fax: 732-577-8644
E-mail: info@wellspouse.org
Web site: http://www.wellspouse.org
Provides emotional support network for the spouse or partner of a chronically ill patient. Establishes local groups and provides information and materials.

CLEFT LIP AND PALATE

Children's Craniofacial Association (CAA)
13140 Coit Road
Suite 517
Dallas, TX 75240
800-535-3643
214-570-9099
Fax: 214-570-8811
E-mail: contactCCA@ccakids.com
Web site: http://www.ccakids.org
Refers callers to support groups for persons and families affected by craniofacial anomalies. Provides referrals to doctors and explains how to get financial assistance for food, travel, and lodging related to these conditions.

Cleft Palate Foundation
1504 East Franklin Street, Suite 102
Chapel Hill, NC 27514-2820
800-24-CLEFT
919-933-9044
Fax: 919-933-9604
Web site: http://www.cleftline.org
Provides general information on cleft lip, cleft palate, and craniofacial anomalies to affected persons and their families as well as information about health care teams and support groups for these conditions.

FACES: The National Craniofacial Association
P.O. Box 11082
Chattanooga, TN 37401
800-3FACES3
E-mail: faces@faces-cranio.org
Web site: http://www.faces-cranio.org
Provides information on related support groups and financial assistance for expenses while traveling for reconstructive surgery, based on financial and medical need. Provides referrals to other resources and organizations, support networks, and a speakers' bureau.

National Foundation for Facial Reconstruction
333 East 30th Street
Lobby Unit
New York, NY 10016
212-263-6656
Fax: 212-263-7534
Web site: http://www.nffr.org
Works to help children and others with craniofacial conditions to lead productive lives.

COLITIS. *See* CROHN'S DISEASE

COLOSTOMY. *See* ILEOSTOMY AND COLOSTOMY

CORNELIA DE LANGE SYNDROME

Cornelia de Lange Syndrome-USA Foundation
302 West Main Street
Suite 100
Avon, CT 06001
800-223-8355, 800-753-2357
860-676-8166, 860-676-8255
Fax: 860-676-8337
E-mail: info@cdlsusa.org
Web site: http://www.cdlsusa.org
Provides information and support for families, friends, and professionals dealing with Cornelia de Lange syndrome.

CROHN'S DISEASE

Crohn's and Colitis Foundation of America (CCFA)
733 Third Avenue

Suite 510
New York, NY 10016
800-932-2423
E-mail: info@ccfa.org
Web site: http://www.ccfa.org
Provides support groups, educational publications, and programs on Crohn's disease and ulcerative colitis.

CYSTIC FIBROSIS

Cystic Fibrosis Foundation
6931 Arlington Road
Bethesda, MD 20814
800-FIGHT-CF
301-951-4422
Fax: 301-951-6378
E-mail: info@cff.org
Web site: http://www.cff.org
Supports more than one hundred specialized care centers for people with cystic fibrosis.

DEATH AND DYING

American Association of Retired Persons (AARP)
Grief and Loss Program
601 E Street NW
Washington, DC 20049
888-OUR-AARP
Web site: http://www.aarp.org/families/grief_loss
This national outreach group consists of widowed volunteers who visit, support, and offer referrals to new widows and widowers. Includes a link to information in Spanish.

Center for Loss in Multiple Birth (CLIMB)
P.O. Box 91377
Anchorage, AK 99509
907-222-5321
E-mail: climb@pobox.alaska.net
Web site: http://www.climb-support.org
Provides peer support for parents who have lost a multiple birth child during pregnancy or after birth. Newsletter includes resources for dealing with multiple birth loss and names of parents willing to share experiences. Includes a link to information in Spanish.

Children's Hospice International
1101 King Street
Suite 360
Alexandria, VA 22314
703-684-0330
E-mail: info@chionline.org
Web site: http://www.chionline.org
Provides information on children's hospices, referrals to local hospices, and education for affected children and their families.

Compassionate Friends
P.O. Box 3696
Oak Brook, IL 60522-3696
877-969-0010
630-990-0010
Fax: 630-990-0246
Web site: http://www.compassionatefriends.org
This is a self-help organization for parents and siblings of a child who has died, with chapters throughout the United States. Includes a link to information in Spanish.

Helping Other Parents in Normal Grieving (HOPING)
P.O. Box 27452
Lansing, MI 48909-7452
888-288-0967
E-mail: info@lansingbabyloss.org
Web site: http://lansingbabyloss.org
Provides support for parents who have lost an infant to miscarriage, stillbirth, or infant death, from trained parents who have had a similar experience.

National Hospice and Palliative Care Organization (NHPCO)
1731 King Street
Suite 100
Alexandria, VA 22314
703-837-1500
Fax: 703-837-1233
E-mail: nhpco_info@nhpco.org
Web site: http://www.nhpco.org
Provides information on caring for terminally ill patients and their families. Gives referrals to hospices throughout the United States. Includes a link to information in Spanish.

Parents of Murdered Children, Inc.
4960 Ridge Avenue
Suite 2
Cincinnati, OH 45209
888-818-POMC
513-721-5683
Fax: 513-345-4489
Web site: http://www.pomc.org
This self-help organization offers support for anyone who has had a family member or friend murdered. Provides information about grief and the criminal justice system. Establishes self-help groups that meet regularly. Works on violence prevention programs.

SHARE: Pregnancy and Infant Loss Support
402 Jackson Street
St. Charles, MO 63301
800-821-6819
Web site: http://www.nationalshare.org
Provides support, information, and referrals for parents who have suffered miscarriage, stillbirth, or infant death. Assists local groups in organizing.

DEPRESSION. *See* **MENTAL HEALTH**

DIABETES

American Diabetes Association
1701 North Beauregard Street
Alexandria, VA 22311
800-DIABETES
E-mail: AskADA@diabetes.org
Web site: http://www.diabetes.org
Provides training, guidance, and education on diabetes. Includes a link to information in Spanish.

Juvenile Diabetes Research Foundation International
26 Broadway, 14th Floor
New York, NY 10004
800-533-CURE
Fax: 212-785-9595
E-mail: info@jdrf.org
Web site: http://www.jdrf.org
Regional groups offer support and activities for families affected by diabetes. Provides information on specific diabetes needs. Includes a link to information in Spanish.

National Diabetes Information Clearinghouse (NDIC)
1 Information Way
Bethesda, MD 20892-3560
800-860-8747
TTY: 866-569-1162
Fax: 703-738-4929
E-mail: ndic@info.niddk.nih.gov
Web site: http://diabetes.niddk.nih.gov
This clearinghouse offers information and publications on diabetes. Gives referrals to support groups and other relevant organizations. Includes a link to information in Spanish.

DIGESTIVE DISORDERS

National Digestive Diseases Information Clearinghouse (NDDIC)
2 Information Way
Bethesda, MD 20892-3570
800-891-5389
TTY: 866-569-1162
Fax: 703-738-4929
E-mail: nddic@info.niddk.nih.gov
Web site: http://digestive.niddk.nih.gov
Provides information on the prevention and management of digestive diseases and referrals to relevant support groups and other organizations. Offers publications on many digestive disorders.

DISABILITIES, GENERAL

American Network of Community Options and Resources (ANCOR)
101 King Street

Suite 380
Alexandria, VA 22314
703-535-7850
Fax: 703-535-7860
E-mail: ancor@ancor.org
Web site: http://www.ancor.org
This umbrella group for several hundred agencies provides services and support to persons with disabilities.

Americans with Disabilities Act
U.S. Department of Justice
950 Pennsylvania Avenue NW
Civil Rights Division
Disability Rights Section-NYA
Washington, DC 20530
800-514-0301
TTY: 800-514-0383
Fax: 202-307-1198
Web site: http://www.usdoj.gov/crt/ada
This government service provides information on Titles II and III of the Americans with Disabilities Act. Information is available over the phone from specialists, or documents may be ordered by fax or mail.

Association for the Help of Retarded Children
83 Maiden Lane
New York, NY 10038
212-780-2500
TTY: 800-662-1220
Web site: http://www.ahrcnyc.org
Provides support, training, clinics, and residential facilities for the mentally retarded and disabled and their families.

Easter Seals
233 South Wacker Drive
Suite 2400
Chicago, IL 60606
800-221-6827
E-mail: info@easterseals.org
Web site: http://www.easterseals.com
Provides information and referrals for people with disabilities and special needs, and their families. Includes a link to information in Spanish.

Federation for Children with Special Needs
529 Main Street
Suite 1M3
Boston, MA 02120
617-236-7210
Fax: 617-241-0330
E-mail: fcsninfo@fcsn.org
Web site: http://www.fcsn.org
Coalition of groups concerned with children and adults with disabilities. Provides information on resources, basic rights, and obtaining services. Works for parent involvement in the care of children with disabilities and chronic illnesses and supports parent training and information. Includes a link to information in Spanish.

HEATH Resource Center
George Washington University
2134 G Street NW
Suite 308
Washington, DC 20052-0001
800-449-7343
E-mail: askheath@gwu.edu
Web site: http://www.heath.gwu.edu
This national clearinghouse for people with disabilities who are seeking education or training after high school provides information about access, accommodations, program modifications, and national organizations. Gives referrals to local resources.

DISEASES, RARE. *See* RARE DISEASES

DONORS, MARROW AND ORGANS

Center for Organ Recovery and Education (CORE)
204 Sigma Drive
RIDC Park
Pittsburgh, PA 15238
800-DONORS-7
Fax: 412-963-3563
E-mail: mchristenson@core.org
Web site: http://www.core.org
Provides general information on becoming an organ donor. Accepts referrals for potential donors.

Living Bank
P.O. Box 6725
Houston, TX 77265-6725
800-528-2971
Fax: 713-961-0979
E-mail: info@livingbank.org
Web site: http://www.livingbank.org
Maintains a registry of organ donors. Provides educational materials and registration forms for organ donation.

National Marrow Donor Program
3001 Broadway Street Northeast
Suite 100
Minneapolis, MN 55413-1753
800-MARROW-2
612-627-5800 (outside the United States)
E-mail: patientinfo@nmdp.org
Web site: http://www.marrow.org
This central registry of unrelated potential volunteer marrow donors provides transplant information for patients with leukemia, aplastic anemia, and other life-threatening diseases.

DOWN SYNDROME

ACDS
4 Fern Place
Plainview, NY 11803
516-933-4700

Fax: 516-933-9524
Web site: http://www.acds.org
This is a resource and information source for parents of children with Down syndrome. Provides referrals and offers programs in New York State for preschool-age children and their siblings and recreational programs and support groups for older children.

National Down Syndrome Congress
30 Mansell Court
Suite 108
Roswell, GA 30076
800-232-NDSC
770-604-9500
Fax: 770-604-9898
E-mail: info@ndsccenter.org
Web site: http://www.ndsccenter.org
Assists parents in finding ways to meet children's needs, coordinates local parents' groups, and provides a clearinghouse for information on Down syndrome. Includes a link to information in Spanish.

National Down Syndrome Society
666 Broadway
8th Floor
New York, NY 10012
800-221-4602
Fax: 212-979-2873
E-mail: info@ndss.org
Web site: http://www.ndss.org
Provides information and referral services to families, local support groups, and community programs. Includes a link to information in Spanish.

DWARFISM

Little People of America, Inc.
250 El Camino Real
Suite 201
Tustin, CA 92780
888-LPA-2001
714-368-3689
Fax: 714-368-3367
E-mail: info@lpaonline.org
Web site: http://www.lpaonline.org
Provides support, publications, and information for dwarfs and other persons of short stature.

DYSLEXIA

International Dyslexia Association
40 York Road
4th Floor
Baltimore, MD 21204-5202
410-296-0232
Fax: 410-321-5069
Web site: http://www.interdys.org

Provides information, publications, and a computer database on dyslexia. Makes referrals for diagnosis and treatment.

EATING DISORDERS

National Eating Disorders Organization
165 West 46th Street
Suite 402
New York, NY 10036
212-575-6200
Fax: 212-575-1650
E-mail: info@NationalEatingDisorders.org
Web site: http://www.nationaleatingdisorders.org
Offers a referral service, support group packet, prevention video, and general information on eating disorders. Includes a link to information in Spanish.

ELDER CARE. *See* AGING AND ELDER CARE

ENDOMETRIOSIS. *See* WOMEN'S HEALTH

EPILEPSY

Epilepsy Foundation
8301 Professional Place
Landover, MD 20785
800-332-1000
Web site: http://www.epilepsyfoundation.org
Provides referrals and basic information on epilepsy for patients, families, physicians, and others. Includes a link to information in Spanish.

FATTY ACID OXIDATION DISORDERS

FOD: All in This Together
P.O. Box 54
Okemos, MI 48805-0054
517-381-1940
Fax: 866-290-5206
E-mail: deb@fodsupport.org
Web site: http://www.fodsupport.org
Provides information to families affected by fatty oxidation disorders.

FIBROMYALGIA. *See* CHRONIC FATIGUE SYNDROME AND FIBROMYALGIA

FRAGILE X SYNDROME

National Fragile X Foundation
1615 Bonanza St.
Suite 202
Walnut Creek, CA 94596
800-688-8765
925-938-9300
Fax: 925-938-9315
Web site: http://www.fragilex.org
Provides information about fragile X syndrome and gives referrals to specialists and support groups. Includes a link to information in Spanish.

GALACTOSEMIA

Parents of Galactosemic Children, Inc.
P.O. Box 2401
Mandeville, LA 70470-2401
866-900-PGC1
Web site: http://www.galactosemia.org
Provides support and information for parents of children with galactosemia.

GAUCHER'S DISEASE

National Gaucher Foundation
2227 Idlewood Road
Suite 6
Tucker, GA 30084
800-504-3189
Fax: 770-934-2911
E-mail: ngf@gaucherdisease.org
Web site: http://www.gaucherdisease.org
Provides support and information for persons with Gaucher's disease.

GENDER REASSIGNMENT SURGERY

Renaissance Transgender Association, Inc.
987 Old Eagle School Road
Suite 719
Wayne, PA 19087
610-636-1990
E-mail: info@ren.org
Web site: http://www.ren.org
Offers support and resources for transgender persons, including those who have had or wish to have gender reassignment surgery.

GENERAL

Angel Flight America
1515 East 71st Street
Suite 312
Tulsa, OK 74136
918-749-8992
Fax: 918-745-0879
E-mail: angel@angelflight.com
Web site: http://www.angelflight.com
Offers free air transportation to ambulatory patients who are traveling to and from specialized medical treatment and are in financial need.

Centers for Disease Control and Prevention (CDC)
National Center for Injury Prevention and Control (NCIPC)
Mailstop K-65
4770 Buford Highway NE
Atlanta, GA 30341-3717
800-CDC-INFO
TTY: 888-232-6348
Fax: 770-488-4760
E-mail: cdcinfo@cdc.gov
Web site: http://www.cdc.gov/injury
Offers a number of documents related to injury prevention and control. Both nontechnical information for patients and technical information for health care providers can be obtained.

MedicAlert Foundation International
2323 Colorado Avenue
Turlock, CA 95382
888-633-4298
209-668-3333 (from outside the United States)
Fax: 209-669-2450
Web site: http://www.medicalert.org
Provides medical facts pertaining to the MedicAlert emblem worn on bracelets or neck chains, with an emergency hotline number for medical professionals to call for further details. Operators available in many languages. Also gives information on obtaining a MedicAlert emblem.

National Patient Travel Center
c/o Mercy Medical Airlift
4620 Haygood Road
Suite 1
Virginia Beach, VA 23455
800-296-1217
757-318-9174
Fax: 757-318-9107
E-mail: info@mercymedical.org
Web site: http://www.mercymedical.org
Provides information on and referral to airline, charitable, and commercial service options for patients needing transport to specialized treatment facilities or places of continuing care.

National Rehabilitation Information Center
8201 Corporate Drive
Suite 600
Landover, MD 20785
800-346-2742
TTY: 301-459-5984
Web site: http://www.naric.com
This is a national disability and rehabilitation library and information center. Provides information on assistive devices and products. Also does document searches and takes orders for publications.

Office of Minority Health Resource Center
P.O. Box 37337
Washington, DC 20013-7337

800-444-6472
E-mail: info@minorityhealth.hhs.gov
Web site: http://www.minorityhealth.hhs.gov
This government agency is primarily for health professionals but gives information and referrals on minority health-related topics to the general public. Also offers resource lists and publications. Provides information to Latinos and Asians in their native languages.

Research! America
1101 King Street
Suite 520
Alexandria, VA 22314-2960
703-739-2577
Fax: 703-739-2372
E-mail: info@researchamerica.org
Web site: http://www.researchamerica.org
Offers resource referrals, data, and contact names for organizations nationwide that offer support and information on a wide range of diseases and disorders.

St. Jude Children's Research Hospital
262 Danny Thomas Place
Memphis, TN 38105
901-595-3300
E-mail: donors@stjude.org
Web site: http://www.stjude.org
Provides information on referrals to St. Jude Children's Research Hospital, which serves children who have not received extensive treatment for a disease being studied. Includes a link to information in Spanish.

Visiting Nurse Associations of America (VNAA)
601 13th Street NW
Suite 610N
Washington, DC 20006
202-384-1420
Fax: 202-384-1444
E-mail: vnaa@vnaa.org
Web site: http://www.vnaa.org
Gives referrals to callers' nearest Visiting Nurse Association. Services include general nursing; physical, occupational, and speech therapy; medical social services; case management; personal care; advanced therapies; adult day care; parent aid; care for the dying; nutritional counseling; friendly visit services; AIDS education and treatment; Meals on Wheels; and specialized nursing services.

GENETIC DISEASES. *See also* SPECIFIC DISEASES

Genetic Alliance
4301 Connecticut Avenue NW, Suite 404
Washington, DC 20008-2369
202-966-5557
Fax: 202-966-8553
E-mail: info@geneticalliance.org
Web site: http://www.geneticalliance.org

Provides information and support to persons and families affected by genetic disorders. Offers referrals to appropriate genetic support groups and professionals.

GLYCOGEN STORAGE DISEASES

Association for Glycogen Storage Disease
P.O. Box 896
Durant, IA 52747
563-514-4022
E-mail: info@agsdus.org
Web site: http://www.agsdus.org
Facilitates communication between patients and families of patients with glycogen storage diseases (GSDs) and provides information to families, patients, and health care professionals. Provides referrals for treatment and helps members get equipment needed to care for GSD patients.

GRIEF. *See* DEATH AND DYING

GROWTH DISORDERS

Human Growth Foundation
997 Glen Cove Avenue
Suite 5
Glen Head, NY 11545
800-451-6434
Fax: 516-671-4055
E-mail: hgf1@hgfound.org
Web site: http://www.hgfound.org
Provides information and support for individuals suffering from physical growth problems and their families. Includes a link to information in Spanish.

GUILLAIN-BARRÉ SYNDROME

GBS/CIDP Foundation International
The Holly Building
1041/2 Forrest Avenue
Narberth, PA 19072
866-224-3301
610-667-0131
Fax: 610-667-7036
Web site: http://www.gbs-cidp.org
Develops support groups for persons suffering from Guillain-Barré syndrome (GBS) and chronic inflammatory demyelinating polyneuropathy (CIDP), as well as their families.

HANSEN'S DISEASE. *See* LEPROSY

HEADACHE

National Headache Foundation
820 N. Orleans
Suite 217

Chicago, IL 60610
888-NHF-5552
312-274-2650
E-mail: info@headaches.org
Web site: http://www.headaches.org
Operates local support groups and provides information for headache sufferers, their families, and physicians.

HEARING LOSS

International Hearing Dog, Inc. (IHDI)
5901 E. 89th Avenue
Henderson, CO 80640
303-287-3277
Fax: 303-287-3425
E-mail: info@hearingdog.org
Web site: http://www.ihdi.org
Trains and places hearing dogs, who alert their hearing-impaired owners to doorbells, crying children, smoke alarms, ringing telephones, and other sounds that require attention or could indicate danger.

Starkey Hearing Foundation
6700 Washington Avenue South
Eden Prairie, MN 55344
866-354-3254
Fax: 952-828-6900
Web site: http://www.sotheworldmayhear.org
This foundation gives away hearing instruments and batteries, promotes hearing health awareness, and conducts research and education.

HEART ATTACK, DISEASE, AND FAILURE

Mended Hearts, Inc.
8150 N. Central Expressway, M2248
Dallas, TX 75206
888-HEART-99
214-206-9259
Fax: 214-295-9552
E-mail: info@mendedhearts.org
Web site: http://www.mendedhearts.org
Local groups offer advice, encouragement, and support for patients and families affected by heart disease.

HEMOCHROMATOSIS

Iron Overload Diseases Association
525 Mayflower Road
West Palm Beach, FL 33405
561-586-8246
E-mail: iod@ironoverload.org
Web site: http://www.ironoverload.org
Works with patients, families, and doctors. Offers patient referrals by phone.

HEMOPHILIA

National Hemophilia Foundation
116 West 32d Street, 11th Floor
New York, NY 10001
212-328-3700
Fax: 212-328-3777
E-mail: handi@hemophilia.org
Web site: http://www.hemophilia.org
Support, education, and information for families affected by hemophilia.

HEPATITIS

Hepatitis Foundation International
504 Blick Drive
Silver Spring, MD 20904
800-891-0707
301-879-6891
Fax: 301-879-6890
E-mail: info@hepatitisfoundation.org
Web site: http://www.hepfi.org
Provides education and information about viral hepatitis. Maintains a database of support groups.

HERPES

American Social Health Association (ASHA)
Herpes Resource Center
P.O. Box 13827
Research Triangle Park, NC 27709
800-227-8922
919-361-8400
Fax: 919-361-8425
Web site: http://www.ashasexualhealth.org/std-sti/Herpes.html
Provides support and information for persons with recurring genital herpes infections and referrals to self-help groups in the United States and Canada.

HISTIOCYTOSIS

Histiocytosis Association of America
332 North Broadway
Pitman, NJ 08071
856-589-6606
Fax: 856-589-6614
E-mail: info@histio.org
Web site: http://www.histio.org
Provides peer counseling, information, physician referrals, and parent/patient networking.

HIV. *See* ACQUIRED IMMUNODEFICIENCY SYNDROME (AIDS)

HOSPICE. *See* DEATH AND DYING

HUNTINGTON'S DISEASE

Huntington's Disease Society of America
505 Eighth Avenue, Suite 902
New York, NY 10018
800-345-HDSA
212-242-1968
E-mail: hdsainfo@hdsa.org
Web site: http://www.hdsa.org
Provides information and referrals to local support groups, chapter social workers, physicians, nursing homes, and other resources. Crisis intervention and other support available.

HYDROCEPHALUS

Guardians of Hydrocephalus Research Foundation
2618 Avenue Z
Brooklyn, NY 11235
718-743-4473
Fax: 718-743-1171
E-mail: ghrf2618@aol.com
Web site: http://ghrforg.org
Provides information on hydrocephalus.

Hydrocephalus Association
4340 East West Highway
Suite 905
Bethesda, MD 20814
301-202-3811
888-598-3789
Fax: 301-202-3813
E-mail: info@hydroassoc.org
Web site: http://www.hydroassoc.org
Facilitates networking among families affected by hydrocephalus, creates training for families, and sponsors social gatherings. Provides information in English and Spanish.

ILEOSTOMY AND COLOSTOMY

United Ostomy Associations of America, Inc.
P.O. Box 512
Northfield, MN 55057-0512
800-826-0826
E-mail: info@uoaa.org
Web site: http://www.uoaa.org
Provides information and referrals to support groups for persons who have had a colostomy, ileostomy, or similar surgical operation.

ILLNESSES, CHRONIC. *See* CHRONIC ILLNESSES

IMMUNIZATION

Centers for Disease Control and Prevention (CDC)
National Immunization Program (NIP)
NIP Public Inquiries

Mailstop E-05
1600 Clifton Road, NE
Atlanta, GA 30333
800-CDC-INFO
TTY: 888-232-6348
Fax: 888-232-3299
E-mail: cdcinfo@cdc.gov
Web site: http://www.cdc.gov/vaccines
Offers a number of documents related to immunization. Includes information on immunization schedules and general information on vaccines, information on specific vaccines, and how to report adverse reactions to vaccines. Provides nontechnical information for patients and technical information for health care providers.

IMMUNODEFICIENCY DISORDERS

Immune Deficiency Foundation (IDF)
40 West Chesapeake Avenue, Suite 308
Towson, MD 21204
800-296-4433
E-mail: idf@primaryimmune.org
Web site: http://www.primaryimmune.org
Provides information for patients with inherited immunodeficiency diseases and their families and for medical professionals.

IMPOTENCE. *See* SEXUAL DISORDERS AND DYSFUNCTION

INCONTINENCE

National Association for Continence (NAFC)
P.O. Box 1019
Charleston, SC 29402-1019
800-BLADDER
843-377-0900
Fax: 843-377-0905
E-mail: memberservices@nafc.org
Web site: http://www.nafc.org
This is a clearinghouse for information and services related to incontinence and assistive devices. Provides education, advocacy, and support on the causes, prevention, diagnosis, treatment, and management alternatives for persons with incontinence. Includes a link to information in Spanish.

Simon Foundation for Continence
P.O. Box 815
Wilmette, IL 60091
800-23-SIMON
847-864-3913
Fax: 847-864-9758
Web site: http://www.simonfoundation.org
Provides peer support and a speaker's bureau. Manages educational and self-help support groups on urinary and bowel incontinence and organizes self-help groups.

INFERTILITY. *See* REPRODUCTIVE ISSUES

INTRAVENTRICULAR HEMORRHAGE

IVH Parents
P.O. Box 56-1111
Miami, FL 33256-1111
305-232-0381
Fax: 305-223-9890
Provides support and information for parents of children with intraventricular hemorrhage.

KIDNEY DISORDERS

American Association of Kidney Patients (AAKP)
2701 N. Rocky Point Dr.
Suite 150
Tampa, FL 33607
800-749-2257
Fax: 813-636-8122
E-mail: info@aakp.org
Web site: http://www.aakp.org
This is an advocacy organization for kidney patients, persons on dialysis, and those with kidney transplants. Includes a link to information in Spanish.

American Kidney Fund (AKF)
11921 Rockville Pike
Suite 300
Rockville, MD 20852
800-638-8299
E-mail: helpline@kidneyfund.org
Web site: http://www.kidneyfund.org
Provides financial assistance for individuals with chronic kidney failure.

Cystinosis Research Network
302 Whytegate Court
Lake Forest, IL 60045
866-276-3669
847-735-0471
Fax: 847-235-2773
E-mail: info@cystinosis.org
Web site: http://www.cystinosis.org
A volunteer, nonprofit organization dedicated to supporting and advocating research, providing family assistance, and educating the public and medical communities about cystinosis.

National Kidney Foundation
30 East 33d Street
New York, NY 10016
800-622-9010
Fax: 212-689-9261
Web site: http://www.kidney.org
Makes referrals to local agencies. Supports patient services such as transportation, drug banks, and educational projects.

KLINEFELTER SYNDROME

KS&A: Knowledge Support & Action
P.O. Box 872
Pine, CO 80470-0872
888-999-9428
Fax: 303-838-0753
E-mail: info@genetic.org
Web site: http://www.genetic.org
Offers support and information for persons and families affected by Klinefelter syndrome, trisomy X, mosaicism, and other conditions caused by an uncommon number of X and/or Y chromosomes. Facilitates networking and the exchange of information.

LEAD POISONING

U.S. Environmental Protection Agency (EPA)
US EPA / Lead Paint Program
Office of Pollution Prevention & Toxics
1200 Pennsylvania Avenue N.W.7404T
Washington, DC 20460
800-424-LEAD
Web site: http://www.epa.gov/lead
This is a government program providing information about lead poisoning and its prevention. Includes a link to information in Spanish.

LEARNING DISABILITIES

Learning Disabilities Association of America (LDA)
4156 Library Road
Pittsburgh, PA 15234-1349
412-341-1515
Fax: 412-344-0224
Web site: http://www.ldanatl.org
Information, publications, and referral service concerning learning disabilities. State and local groups provide services to families, including camps and recreation programs.

LEPROSY

American Leprosy Missions (ALM)
1 ALM Way
Greenville, SC 29601
800-543-3135
Fax: 864-271-7062
E-mail: amlep@leprosy.org
Web site: http://leprosy.org
Provides medical, rehabilitation, and social care, as well as information about leprosy. Refers callers to treatment centers.

LEUKEMIA

Leukemia and Lymphoma Society
1311 Mamaroneck Avenue

White Plains, NY 10605
914-949-5213
Fax: 914-949-6691
Web site: http://www.leukemia.org
Provides callers with referrals in their area and offers educational materials and financial aid. Includes a link to information in Spanish.

LEUKODYSTROPHY

United Leukodystrophy Foundation (ULF)
224 North Second Street
Suite 2
DeKalb, IL 60115
800-728-5483
Fax: 815-748-0844
E-mail: office@ulf.org
Web site: http://www.ulf.org
Offers information and support to persons suffering from leukodystrophy and their families. Coordinates communication among families.

LIVER DISORDERS

American Liver Foundation
39 Broadway
Suite 2700
New York, NY 10006
212-668-1000
Fax: 212-483-8179
Web site: http://www.liverfoundation.org
Provides physician referrals and information on support groups for persons with liver disease and their families.

LUNG DISORDERS

American Lung Association
1301 Pennsylvania Avenue NW
Washington, DC 20004
800-LUNG-USA
Fax: 202-452-1805
Web site: http://www.lung.org
This organization seeks to prevent lung disease and promote lung health. The Web site includes in-depth information and recent research findings, a guide to local events and programs, and a section to share personal stories. Includes a link to information in Spanish.

Lung Line
National Jewish Medical and Research Center
1400 Jackson Street
Denver, CO 80206
800-225-5654
Web site: http://www.nationaljewish.org
Registered nurses provide information on the detection, treatment, and prevention of lung and immunological diseases and allergies, and give referrals to local doctors.

LUPUS

Lupus Foundation of America
2000 L Street NW
Suite 710
Washington, DC 20036
800-558-0121
202-349-1155
Fax: 202-349-1156
Web site: http://www.lupus.org
Provides information on lupus. Refers callers to local chapters, which provide support group details and physician referrals. Includes a link to information in Spanish.

LYME DISEASE

American Lyme Disease Foundation (ALDF)
P.O. Box 466
Lyme, CT 06371
Web site: http://www.aldf.com
Provides educational materials and information regarding Lyme disease and maintains a physician referral service. Includes a link to information in Spanish.

MARFAN SYNDROME

National Marfan Foundation
22 Manhasset Avenue
Port Washington, NY 11050
800-8-MARFAN
516-883-8712
Fax: 516-883-8040
E-mail: staff@marfan.org
Web site: http://www.marfan.org
Provides information on Marfan syndrome and a support network for patients and families.

MARROW DONORS. *See* DONORS, MARROW AND ORGANS

MÉNIÈRE'S DISEASE

Vestibular Disorders Association (VEDA)
5018 NE 15th Ave
Portland, OR 97211
800-837-8428
Fax: 503-229-8064
Web site: http://www.vestibular.org
A nonprofit organization that provides information to the public and health professionals about inner-ear balance disorders such as Ménière's disease, benign paroxysmal positional vertigo, and labyrinthitis. Includes a link to information in Spanish.

MENOPAUSE. *See* WOMEN'S HEALTH

MENTAL HEALTH

Depression and Bipolar Support Alliance (DBSA)
730 N. Franklin Street
Suite 501
Chicago, IL 60654-7225
800-826-3632
Fax: 312-642-7243
Web site: http://www.dbsalliance.org
Provides information on depressive and bipolar illnesses as medical diseases and promotes self-help for affected persons and their families.

Emotions Anonymous International
P.O. Box 4245
St. Paul, MN 55104-0245
651-647-9712
Fax: 651-647-1593
E-mail: info2gh99jsd@emotionsanonymous.org
Web site: http://www.emotionsanonymous.org
This is a self-help group using a 12-step program for recovery from emotional illnesses. Provides publications, information, and referrals to local groups. Includes a link to information in Spanish.

International Foundation for Research and Education on Depression (iFred)
P.O. Box 17598
Baltimore, MD 12197-1598
410-268-0044
Fax: 443-782-0739
E-mail: info@ifred.org
Web site: http://www.ifred.org
Provides referrals to doctors who specialize in treating depression and a list of local support groups.

Mental Health America
2000 North Beauregard Street
6th Floor
Alexandria, VA 22311
800-969-6642
703-684-7722
TTY: 800-433-5959
Fax: 703-684-5968
Web site: http://www.nmha.org
Offers regional support groups, information and referral programs, and other patient advocacy services.

National Alliance on Mental Illness (NAMI)
3803 North Fairfax Drive
Suite 100
Arlington, VA 22203
703-524-7600
Fax: 703-524-9094
Web site: http://www.nami.org
Provides emotional support and practical guidance for the mentally ill and their families. Offers referrals to local groups. Includes a link to information in Spanish.

National Institute of Mental Health (NIMH)
6001 Executive Boulevard
Room 8184, MSC 9663
Bethesda, MD 20892-9663
866-615-6464
301-443-4513
TTY: 301-443-8431
Fax: 301-443-4279
E-mail: nimhinfo@nih.gov
Web site: http://www.nimh.nih.gov
This government organization tries to help people better understand mental health and mental disorders. Provides the fax-on-demand service Mental Health FAX4U, with four hundred documents on mental illnesses such as Alzheimer's disease, bipolar disorder, depression, and seasonal affective disorder.

National Mental Health Consumers' Self-Help
  Clearinghouse
1211 Chestnut Street
Suite 1100
Philadelphia, PA 19107
800-553-4539
215-751-1810
Fax: 215-636-6312
E-mail: info@mhselfhelp.org
Web site: http://www.mhselfhelp.org
Provides technical assistance in the development of self-help projects, information referrals, publications, and consulting services.

National Resource and Training Center on
  Homelessness and Mental Illness
E-mail: generalinquiry@center4si.com
Web site: http://www.nrchmi.samhsa.gov
Provides technical assistance and comprehensive information on the treatment, services, and housing needs of homeless persons with severe mental illnesses.

Pride Institute
14400 Martin Drive
Eden Prairie, MN 55344
800-54-PRIDE
E-mail: support@pride-institute.com
Web site: http://www.pride-institute.com
Helps lesbian, gay, and bisexual individuals with chemical dependency and mental health problems.

MENTAL RETARDATION

Best Buddies
100 SE Second Street
Suite 2200
Miami, FL 33131
800-89-BUDDY
305-374-2233
Fax: 305-374-5305

Web site: http://www.bestbuddies.org
Facilitates friendships between people with mental retardation and others in the community.

MISCARRIAGE. *See* DEATH AND DYING; REPRODUCTIVE ISSUES

MUCOPOLYSACCHARIDOSIS (MPS)

National MPS Society
P.O. Box 14686
Durham, NC 27709-4686
877-MPS-1001
919-806-0101
Fax: 919-806-2055
E-mail: info@mpssociety.org
Web site: http://www.mpssociety.org
Refers parents whose children have been diagnosed with MPS or mucolipidosis (ML) to other families dealing with these diseases.

MULTIPLE BIRTHS. *See also* REPRODUCTIVE ISSUES

Multiples of America
2000 Mallory Lane
Suite 130-600
Franklin, TE 37067-8231
248-231-4480
E-mail: multiplesofamerica@aol.com
Web site: http://www.nomotc.org
Local groups provide information on multiples and their care.

Triplet Connection
P.O. Box 429
Spring City, UT 84662
Email: tc@tripletconnection.org
Web site: http://www.tripletconnection.org
Helps parents of triplets and larger multiple births prepare for and deal with high-risk multiple births. Provides supports and facilitates networking. Offers information on such topics as breast-feeding, medical services, preventing premature births, and clothing and equipment exchanges. Also provides support for mothers who have lost one or more babies of a multiple birth.

Twinless Twins Support Group International
P.O. Box 980481
Ypsilanti, MI 48198-0481
888-205-8962
E-mail: contact@twinlesstwins.org
Web site: http://www.twinlesstwins.org
Provides support to persons who have lost a multiple-birth sibling through death or disappearance and others dealing with multiple-birth losses. Also works to reunite multiple-birth siblings who were separated through adoption or for other reasons.

MULTIPLE SCLEROSIS

National Multiple Sclerosis Society
733 Third Avenue
New York, NY 10017
800-344-486
Web site: http://www.nationalmssociety.org
Provides services to persons with multiple sclerosis through local chapters.

MUSCULAR DYSTROPHY

Muscular Dystrophy Association (MDA)
National Headquarters
3300 E. Sunrise Drive
Tucson, AZ 85718
800-572-1717
Web site: http://www.mdausa.org
Combats neuromuscular diseases through research programs, medical and community services, and professional and public health education. Provides referrals to local groups for information about support groups, clinics, and summer camps. Includes a link to information in Spanish.

MYASTHENIA GRAVIS

Myasthenia Gravis Foundation of America, Inc.
355 Lexington Avenue
15th Floor
New York, NY 10017
800-541-5454
Fax: 212-3700-9047
E-mail: mgfa@myasthenia.org
Web site: http://www.myasthenia.org
Provides publications and information on myasthenia gravis.

NARCOLEPSY

Narcolepsy Network, Inc.
129 Waterwheel Lane
North Kingstown, RI 02852
888-292-6522
401-667-2523
Fax: 401-633-6567
Web site: http://www.narcolepsynetwork.org
Provides referral service, support group meetings, and communication among members.

NEUROFIBROMATOSIS

Children's Tumor Foundation
95 Pine Street
16th Floor
New York, NY 10005
800-323-7938
212-344-6633

Fax: 212-747-0004
E-mail: info@ctf.org
Web site: http://www.ctf.org
Provides information, peer counseling, and referral services.

Neurofibromatosis, Inc.
213 S. Wheaton Avenue
Wheaton, IL 60187
800-942-6825
630-510-1115
Fax: 630-510-8508
Web site: http://www.nfinc.org
Offers support, peer counseling, and information for patients and families affected by neurofibromatosis. Provides referrals to medical resources.

NIEMANN-PICK DISEASE

National Niemann-Pick Disease Foundation
P.O. Box 49
401 Madison Avenue, Suite B
Ft. Atkinson, WI 53538
877-287-3672
920-563-0930
Fax: 920-563-0931
E-mail: nnpdf@nnpdf.org
Web site: http://www.nnpdf.org
Support and phone referrals for parents of children with Niemann-Pick disease. Provides information on genetic counseling.

NUTRITION

American Dietetic Association (ADA)
120 South Riverside Plaza
Suite 2000
Chicago, IL 60606-6995
800-877-1600
Web site: http://www.eatright.org
The largest organization of food and nutrition professionals in the United States. Provides referrals to local registered dieticians and answers questions on food and nutrition.

OBESITY AND WEIGHT LOSS

Overeaters Anonymous (OA)
P.O. Box 44020
Rio Rancho, NM 87174-4020
505-891-2664
Fax: 505-891-4320
Web site: http://www.oa.org
This is a Twelve-Step support group for persons who want to stop their compulsive overeating.

Take Off Pounds Sensibly (TOPS)
4575 South Fifth Street
Milwaukee, WI 53207-0360

414-482-4620
E-mail: wondering@tops.org
Web site: http://www.tops.org
This is a self-help weight loss support group using group dynamics, competition, and recognition. Participants are required to consult with a doctor about weight loss goals and diets. Includes a link to information in Spanish.

OBSESSIVE-COMPULSIVE DISORDER. *See* MENTAL HEALTH

ORGAN DONORS. *See* DONORS, MARROW AND ORGANS

OSTEOPOROSIS

National Osteoporosis Foundation (NOF)
1150 17th Street NW
Suite 850
Washington, DC 20036
800-231-4222
202-223-2226
Web site: http://www.nof.org
Provides information about osteoporosis.

PAGET'S DISEASE

Paget Foundation
P.O. Box 24432
Brooklyn, NY 11202
800-23-PAGET
E-mail: PagetFdn@aol.com
Web site: http://www.paget.org
Provides information, patient assistance, and referrals to medical specialists for persons with Paget's disease, primary hyperparathyroidism, fibrous dysplasia, and osteopetrosis.

PAIN MANAGEMENT

American Chronic Pain Association (ACPA)
P.O. Box 850
Rocklin, CA 95677
800-533-3231
Fax: 916-632-3208
E-mail: acpa@theacpa.org
Web site: http://www.theacpa.org
Offers mutual support groups for sufferers of pain lasting more than six months. Provides information on pain management. Includes a link to information in Spanish.

PARALYSIS

National Spinal Cord Injury Association (NSCIA)
75-20 Astoria Blvd
Jackson Heights, NY 11370

718-803-3782
E-mail: info@spinalcord.org
Web site: http://www.spinalcord.org
Assists persons with spinal cord injuries or diseases. Facilitates networking for parents of children with spinal cord injuries or related diseases.

PARKINSON'S DISEASE

American Parkinson Disease Association, Inc. (ADPA)
135 Parkinson Avenue
Staten Island, NY 10305
800-223-2732
718-981-8001
Fax: 1-718-981-4399
E-mail: apda@apdaparkinson.org
Web site: http://www.apdaparkinson.org
Maintains information and referral centers and more than eight hundred support groups for patients and families.

National Parkinson Foundation, Inc.
200 SE 1st Street
Miami, FL 33131
800-473-4636
Fax: 305-537-9901
E-mail: contact@parkinson.org
Web site: http://www.parkinson.org
Provides information and referrals to local medical facilities. Offers evaluations at the National Parkinson Foundation Center and sponsors regional support groups.

Parkinson's Disease Foundation (PDF)
1359 Broadway
Suite 1509
New York, NY 10018
800-457-6676
212-923-4700
Fax: 212-923-4778
E-mail: info@pdf.org
Web site: http://www.pdf.org
Provides information about Parkinson's disease and referrals to physicians and hospitals.

PHENYLKETONURIA (PKU)

Children's PKU Network
3306 Bumann Rd
Encinitas, CA 92024
858-756-0079
Fax: 858-756-1059
E-mail: pkunetwork@aol.com
Web site: http://www.pkunetwork.org
Provides support groups, crisis intervention, financial assistance, and discount dietary aids for families affected by PKU.

PHOBIAS. *See* MENTAL HEALTH

POLIOMYELITIS

Post-Polio Health International (PHI)
4207 Lindell Boulevard
Suite 110
St. Louis, MO 63108-2915
314-534-0475
Fax: 314-534-5070
E-mail: info@post-polio.org
Web site: http://www.post-polio.org
Facilitates networking among persons who have had polio. Provides information and encourages research into the long-term effects of polio.

PORPHYRIA

American Porphyria Foundation
4900 Woodway
Suite 780
Houston, TX 77056-1837
866-APF-3635
713-266-9617
Fax: 713-840-9552
Web site: http://www.porphyriafoundation.com
Provides information on porphyria to affected persons, parents, and physicians.

PRADER-WILLI SYNDROME

Prader-Willi Syndrome Association (USA)
8588 Potter Park Drive
Suite 500
Sarasota, FL 34238
800-926-4797
941-312-0400
Fax: 941-312-0142
E-mail: info@pwsausa.org
Web site: http://www.pwsausa.org
Provides information, referrals, and publications on Prader-Willi syndrome.

PREGNANCY. *See* REPRODUCTIVE ISSUES

PURINE METABOLIC DISORDERS

Purine Research Society
5424 Beech Avenue
Bethesda, MD 20814-1730
301-530-0354
Fax: 301-564-9597
E-mail: purineresearchsociety@verizon.net
Web site: http://www.purineresearchsociety.org
Provides information on purine metabolic disorders, including gout, purine autism, Lesch-Nyban syndrome, and ADA deficiency.

RARE DISEASES

National Organization for Rare Disorders (NORD)
55 Kenosia Avenue
Danbury, CT 06813-1968
203-744-0100
Fax: 203-798-2291
Web site: http://www.rarediseases.org
Gathers and disseminates information on more than three thousand rare diseases. Facilitates networking between patients with the same disorder.

REPRODUCTIVE ISSUES. *See also* SURROGATE PARENTING

American Academy of Husband-Coached Childbirth
P.O. Box 5224
Sherman Oaks, CA 91413-5224
818-788-6662
800-4-A-BIRTH
Web site: http://www.bradleybirth.com
Refers callers to local teachers of the Bradley method of natural childbirth.

Couple to Couple League International, Inc.
4290 Delhi Avenue
Cincinnati, OH 45238-5829
800-745-8252
513-471-2000
Fax: 513-557-2449
Web site: http://www.ccli.org
Sponsors local groups for couples who wish to space pregnancies by timing intercourse in accordance with a woman's natural cycle of fertility, rather than by using contraceptives. Educational publications available in English, Polish, and Spanish.

La Leche League International
957 N. Plum Grove Road
Schaumburg, IL 60173
800-LA-LECHE
847-519-7730
Fax: 847-969-0460
Web site: http://www.lalecheleague.org
Provides help, education, and encouragement for mothers who want to breast-feed or who are breast-feeding. Offers informal discussion groups, telephone support, and publications. Includes a link to information in Spanish.

Lamaze International
2025 M Street NW
Suite 800
Washington, DC 20036-3309
800-368-4404
202-367-1128
Fax: 202-367-2128
Web site: http://www.lamaze.org

Provides information about the Lamaze method of prepared childbirth and how to locate a local certified childbirth educator.

Liberty Godparent Foundation
124 Liberty Mountain Drive
Lynchburg, VA 24502
800-542-4453
434-845-3466
Fax: 434-845-1751
Web site: http://www.godparent.org
A Christian maternity home that provides housing, education, medical care, and counseling for single, pregnant young women who wish to keep their child or place their child up for adoption. Offers a twenty-four-hour help line.

National Abortion Federation (NAF)
1660 L Street NW
Suite 450
Washington, DC 20036
800-772-9100
202-667-5881
Fax: 202-667-5890
E-mail: naf@prochoice.org
Web site: http://www.prochoice.org
Provides information and referrals to local abortion providers and information on pregnancy and abortion procedures.

National Infertility Network Exchange (NINE)
P.O. Box 204
East Meadow, NY 11554
516-794-5772
Fax: 516-794-0008
E-mail: info@nine-infertility.org
Web site: http://www.nine-infertility.org
Provides peer support group, education, and referrals for persons who are infertile.

National Life Center
686 North Broad Street
Woodbury, NJ 08096
800-848-LOVE
856-848-1819
Web site: http://www.nationallifecenter.com
Provides free pregnancy tests and medical, legal, and professional counseling referrals. Shelter, adoption, maternity care, and baby clothing are available through local affiliates. The toll-free number directs callers to the nearest pro-life pregnancy service.

Planned Parenthood Federation of America
434 West 33d Street
New York, NY 10001
800-230-PLAN
212-541-7800
Fax: 212-245-1845
Web site: http://www.plannedparenthood.org
Offers information on human sexuality and reproductive health. The toll-free number automatically connects callers to a local Planned Parenthood health center.

Postpartum Support International (PSI)
6706 SW 54th Avenue
Portland, Oregon 97219
800-944-4PPD
503-894-9453
Fax: 503-894-9452
E-mail: PSIOffice@postpartum.net
Web site: http://www.postpartum.net
Clearinghouse for information on postpartum depression, providing referrals, educational materials, and support for affected women and their families. Includes a link to information in Spanish.

REYE'S SYNDROME

National Reye's Syndrome Foundation, Inc.
P.O. Box 829
Bryan, OH 43506
800-233-7393
Fax: 419-924-9999
E-mail: nrsf@reyessyndrome.org
Web site: http://www.reyessyndrome.org
Provides a resource clearinghouse and support groups for patients with Reye's syndrome and their families. Gives referrals to treatment centers across the United States.

RUBINSTEIN-TAYBI SYNDROME

Rubinstein-Taybi Parent Group
158 S. Hassett Cir
Mesa, AZ 85208
480-432-3154
Web site: http://www.rubinstein-taybi.org
Provides support and information for parents of children with Rubinstein-Taybi syndrome.

SCHIZOPHRENIA. *See* MENTAL HEALTH

SCLERODERMA

Scleroderma Foundation
300 Rosewood Drive
Suite 105
Danvers, MA 01923
800-722-HOPE
978-463-5843
Fax: 978-463-5809
E-mail: sfinfo@scleroderma.org
Web site: http://www.scleroderma.org
Provides education and emotional support for persons and families affected by scleroderma.

Scleroderma Research Foundation
220 Montgomery Street
Suite 1411
San Francisco, CA 94104
800-441-CURE
Web site: http://www.srfcure.org
Provides support for parents and families and offers doctor referrals on scleroderma, a rare autoimmune disorder in which the body's immune system attacks its own tissues.

SELF-HELP ORGANIZATIONS, GENERAL

American Self-Help Clearinghouse
St. Clare's Health Services
25 Pocono Road
Denville, NJ 07834-2995
973-989-1122
Web site: http://www.mentalhelp.net/selfhelp
Publishes *The Self-Help Sourcebook*, which lists several hundred state and local self-help groups and self-help clearinghouses and gives information on how to start a self-help group. The publication is inexpensive and updated every other year.

SEXUAL DISORDERS AND DYSFUNCTION

Sex Addicts Anonymous
P.O. Box 70949
Houston, TX 77270
800-477-8191
E-mail: info@saa-recovery.org
Web site: http://www.saa-recovery.org
This is a Twelve-Step support group for persons who compulsively repeat sexual behavior that is detrimental to their lives.

Sexaholics Anonymous
P.O. Box 3565
Brentwood, TN 37024
866-424-8777
615-370-6062
Fax: 615-370-0882
E-mail: saico@sa.org
Web site: http://www.sa.org
This Twelve-Step self-help group is for persons who want to stop self-destructive thinking and behavior, such as the use of pornography, adultery, incest, or criminal sexual activity.

Survivors of Incest Anonymous
World Service Office
P.O. Box 190
Benson, MD 21018-9998
410-893-3322
Web site: http://www.siawso.org
This nonprofit organization for victims of incest and other sexual abuse is based on the Twelve Steps and Twelve Traditions of Alcoholics Anonymous.

Urology Care Foundation
1000 Corporate Boulevard
Linthicum, MD 21090
800-828-7866
410-689-3700
Fax: 410-689-3998
E-mail: auafoundation@auafoundation.org
Web site: http://www.urologyhealth.org
Educates patients, the public, and health care providers on sexual health issues, including erectile dysfunction. Includes a link to information in Spanish.

SEXUALLY TRANSMITTED DISEASES (STDs). *See also* ACQUIRED IMMUNODEFICIENCY SYNDROME (AIDS); HERPES

Centers for Disease Control and Prevention (CDC)
STD Prevention Fax Information Service
Fax: 888-CDC-FAXX
A number of documents related to STDs and other health issues are available from the CDC Fax Information Service as well as from its Web site. Both nontechnical information for patients and technical information for health care providers can be obtained.

SICKLE CELL DISEASE

Sickle Cell Disease Association of America
231 East Baltimore Street
Suite 800
Baltimore, MD 21202
800-421-8453
410-528-1555
Fax: 410-528-1495
E-mail: scdaa@sicklecelldisease.org
Web site: http://www.sicklecelldisease.org
Provides referrals to local chapters for educational materials and medical help.

SJÖGREN'S SYNDROME

Sjögren's Syndrome Foundation, Inc.
6707 Democracy Boulevard, Suite 325
Bethesda, MD 20817
800-475-6473
301-530-4420
Fax: 301-530-4415
E-mail: tms@sjogrens.org
Web site: http://www.sjogrens.org
This is a clearinghouse for information about Sjögren's syndrome.

SLEEP DISORDERS. *See also* APNEA

National Sleep Foundation
1010 N. Glebe Road

Suite 310
Arlington, VA 22201
703-243-1697
E-mail: nsf@sleepfoundation.org
Web site: http://www.sleepfoundation.org
A nonprofit organization dedicated to improving public health and safety by achieving understanding of sleep and sleep disorders and by supporting education, sleep-related research, and advocacy.

SMOKING. *See* ADDICTION-ALCOHOL, DRUGS, AND SMOKING

SPINA BIFIDA

Spina Bifida Association
4590 MacArthur Boulevard NW
Suite 250
Washington, DC 20007-4226
800-621-3141
202-944-3285
Fax: 202-944-3295
E-mail: sbaa@sbaa.org
Web site: http://www.sbaa.org
Provides support and information for families affected by spina bifida. Refers callers to local chapters. Includes a link to information in Spanish.

SPONDYLITIS

Spondylitis Association of America
P.O. Box 5872
Sherman Oaks, CA 91413
800-777-8189
818-892-1616
Fax: 818-892-1611
E-mail: info@spondylitis.org
Web site: http://www.spondylitis.org
Provides information and support for persons and families of persons suffering from ankylosing spondylitis, psoriatic arthritis, and Reiter's syndrome.

STRESS. *See* MENTAL HEALTH

STROKES

American Stroke Association
National Center
7272 Greenville Avenue
Dallas, TX 75231-4596
888-4-STROKE
Web site: http://www.strokeassociation.org
A division of the American Heart Association that focuses on reducing disability and death from stroke through research, education, fund-raising, and advocacy.

National Institute of Neurological Disorders and Stroke (NINDS)
NIH Neurological Institute
P.O. Box 5801
Bethesda, MD 20824
800-352-9424
301-496-5751
TTY: 301-468-5981
Web site: http://www.ninds.nih.gov
A government agency that conducts, fosters, coordinates, and guides research on the causes, prevention, diagnosis, and treatment of strokes and other neurological disorders. Includes a link to information in Spanish.

National Stroke Association
9707 East Easter Lane
Suite B
Centennial, CO 80112
800-STROKES
Fax: 303-649-1328
E-mail: info@stroke.org
Web site: http://www.stroke.org
An organization committed to fighting strokes in the United States. Provides education, services, and community-based activities in prevention, treatment, rehabilitation, and recovery. Includes a link to information in Spanish.

STURGE-WEBER SYNDROME

Sturge-Weber Foundation
P.O. Box 418
Mount Freedom, NJ 07970-0418
800-627-5482
973-895-4445
Fax: 973-895-4846
Web site: http://www.sturge-weber.org
Provides information and support for persons suffering from Sturge-Weber syndrome, Klippel-Trenaunay syndrome, and port-wine stains, as well as for their families.

STUTTERING

Stuttering Foundation of America
P.O. Box 11749
Memphis, TN 38111-0749
800-992-9392
901-761-0343
Fax: 901-761-0484
E-mail: info@stutteringhelp.org
Web site: http://www.stuttersfa.org
Provides referrals to speech pathologists, a nationwide resource list, and free brochures.

SUDDEN INFANT DEATH SYNDROME (SIDS)

First Candle/SIDS Alliance
2105 Laurel Bush Road

Suite 201
Bel Air, MD 21015
443-640-1049
E-mail: info@firstcandle.org
Web site: http://www.firstcandle.org
This organization seeks to advance infant health and survival in the fight against infant mortality resulting from SIDS, still-birth, and miscarriage. Offers support and information for affected families.

SUICIDE. *See* DEATH AND DYING

SURROGATE PARENTING. *See also* REPRODUCTIVE ISSUES

Center for Surrogate Parenting, Inc. (CSP)
9 State Circle
Suite 302
Annapolis, MD 21401
410-990-9860
Fax: 410-990-9862
Web site: http://www.creatingfamilies.com
Provide support for surrogate parents, enabling them to share experiences and information. Offer information about egg donation.

E-mail: bzager@msn.com
Web site: http://www.opts.com
Provides support for families created through surrogate parenting, including phone and e-mail support for members. Also provides information and referrals to infertile couples.

TAY-SACHS DISEASE

National Tay-Sachs and Allied Diseases Association, Inc.
2001 Beacon Street
Suite 204
Boston, MA 02135
617-277-4463
Fax: 617-277-0134
E-mail: info@ntsad.org
Web site: http://www.ntsad.org
Offers support groups for parents of children with Tay-Sachs and related diseases. Also acts as a clearinghouse of information for families and professionals.

TERMINAL ILLNESSES. *See* AGING AND ELDER CARE; DEATH AND DYING

TERMINAL ILLNESSES, WISHES FOR CHILDREN WITH

Children's Wish Foundation International, Inc.
8615 Roswell Road
Atlanta, GA 30350-7526

800-323-WISH
770-393-WISH
Fax: 770-393-0683
Web site: http://www.childrenswish.org
Seeks to fulfill the wishes of terminally ill children.

Dream Factory, Inc.
National Headquarters
200 West Broadway
Suite 504
Louisville, KY 40202
800-456-7556
502-561-3001
Fax: 502-561-3004
Web site: http://www.dreamfactoryinc.org
Seeks to fulfill the wishes of chronically or critically ill children and works to promote a more positive family atmosphere in the face of a prolonged illness.

Make-a-Wish Foundation of America
4742 North 24th Street
Suite 400
Phoenix, AZ 85016-4862
800-722-WISH
602-279-WISH
Fax: 602-279-0855
Web site: http://www.wish.org
Seeks to fulfill the wishes of children with terminal illnesses or other life-threatening conditions.

TORTICOLLIS

National Spasmodic Torticollis Association (NTSA)
9920 Talbert Avenue
Fountain Valley, CA 92708
800-487-8385
E-mail: NSTAmail@aol.com
Web site: http://www.torticollis.org
Provides support for persons with spasmodic torticollis.

TOURETTE'S SYNDROME

Tourette's Syndrome Association (TSA), Inc.
42-40 Bell Boulevard
Suite 205
Bayside, NY 11361
718-224-2999
Fax: 718-279-9596
Web site: http://tsa-usa.org
Offers physician referrals and provides access to support groups and other services for persons with Tourette's syndrome and their families. Helps people identify and understand Tourette's syndrome. Includes a link to information in Spanish.

TUBERCULOSIS. *See* LUNG DISORDERS

TURNER SYNDROME

Turner Syndrome Society of the United States
11250 West Road, Suite G
Houston, TX 77065
800-365-9944
Fax: 832-912-6446
Web site: http://www.turnersyndrome.org
Provides support and information for families affected by Turner syndrome.

URINARY DISORDERS. *See* INCONTINENCE; KIDNEY DISORDERS

VISION DISORDERS

American Council of the Blind
2200 Wilson Boulevard
Suite 650
Arlington, VA 22201
800-424-8666
202-467-5081
Fax: 703-465-5085
Web site: http://www.acb.org
Promotes the independence and dignity of blind and visually impaired persons. Includes the Council of Citizens with Low Vision International, which offers outreach programs, advocacy, and educational services for partially sighted and low-vision persons.

American Foundation for the Blind
2 Penn Plaza
Suite 1102
New York, NY 10121
212-502-7600
Fax: 888-545-8331
E-mail: afbinfo@afb.net
Web site: http://www.afb.org
This is an information and referral service for organizations for the blind. Includes a reference directory of services in the United States.

Blinded Veterans Association
477 H Street NW
Washington, DC 20001-2694
800-669-7079
202-371-8880
Fax: 202-371-8258
E-mail: bva@bva.org
Web site: http://www.bva.org
Provides information on benefits and services for blinded veterans.

Guide Dog Foundation for the Blind
371 East Jericho Turnpike
Smithtown, NY 11787-2976
800-548-4337

Fax: 631-930-9009
E-mail: info@guidedog.org
Web site: http://www.guidedog.org
Provides trained guide dogs to the visually impaired. Provides a training program, a dog, all necessary equipment, and airfare within the United States at no charge to students accepted by the program.

Lighthouse International
The Sol and Lillian Goldman Building
111 East 59th Street
New York, NY 10022-1202
800-829-0500
212-821-9200
TTY: 212-821-9713
Fax: 212-821-9707
E-mail: info@lighthouse.org
Web site: http://www.lighthouse.org
Provides educational material on vision and childhood development, vision and aging, and low vision. Gives referrals to vision rehabilitation agencies, low-vision resources, and support groups nationwide. Includes a link to information in Spanish.

National Library Service for the Blind and Physically Handicapped (NLS)
Library of Congress
1291 Taylor Street NW
Washington, DC 20542
888-NLS-READ
202-707-5100
TDD: 202-707-0744
Fax: 202-707-0712
E-mail: nls@loc.gov
Web site: http://www.loc.gov/nls
Provides Braille and audio books and free loans to persons with vision problems or other physical disabilities that prevent the person from reading. Makes referrals to state and local libraries.

WILSON'S DISEASE

Wilson's Disease Association International
5572 North Diversey Blvd.
Milwaukee, WI 53217
866-961-0533
414-961-0533
E-mail: info@wilsonsdisease.org
Web site: http://www.wilsonsdisease.org
Provides support and financial aid to needy families, information, and coordination among members and related organizations.

WOMEN'S HEALTH

Endometriosis Association
8585 N. 76th Place

Milwaukee, WI 53223
414-355-2200
Fax: 414-355-6065
Web site: http://www.endometriosisassn.org
Sponsors self-help support and informational meetings. Provides brochures in twenty-three languages and publications specifically for teens. Includes a link to information in Spanish.

North American Menopause Society (NAMS)
5900 Landerbrooke Drive, Suite 390
Mayfield Heights, OH 44124
440-442-7550
Fax: 440-442-2660
E-mail: info@menopause.org
Web site: http://www.menopause.org

Provides information on midlife medical issues. Maintains a database of menopause care providers and support groups.

Older Women's League (OWL)
1625 K Street NW
Suite 1275
Washington, DC 20036
202-567-2606
E-mail: info@owl-national.org
Web site: http://www.owl-national.org
Information on and support for issues affecting middle-aged and older women, such as health care and insurance, maintaining independence, and support for family caregivers.

—Irene Struthers Rush;
updated by Connie Pollock

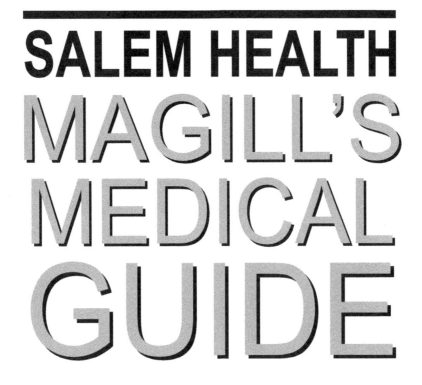

SALEM HEALTH

MAGILL'S MEDICAL GUIDE

ENTRIES BY ANATOMY OR SYSTEM AFFECTED

ALL
Abscesses
Abuse of the elderly
Accidents
Acupuncture
Adrenal glands
Aging
Aging: Extended care
Alternative medicine
Anatomy
Antibiotic resistance
Antibiotics
Antihypertensives
Anti-inflammatory drugs
Antioxidants
Autoimmune disorders
Autopsy
Bionics and biotechnology
Birth defects
Burkitt's lymphoma
Cancer
Carcinogens
Carcinoma
Chemotherapy
Chronic granulomatous disease
Clinical trials
Club drugs
Coccidioidomycosis
Cockayne Disease
Collagen
Congenital disorders
Critical care
Cryosurgery
Cysts
Death and dying
Diagnosis
Dietary reference intakes (DRIs)
Disease
Embryology
Emergency medicine
Emergency rooms
Emerging infectious diseases
Environmental diseases
Enzyme therapy
Epidemics and pandemics
Epidemiology
Epidermal nevus syndromes
Family medicine
Fascia
Fatigue
Fever
First aid

First responder
Food guide plate
Forensic pathology
Genetic diseases
Genetic engineering
Genetic Imprinting
Genetics and inheritance
Genomics
Geriatric assessment
Geriatrics and gerontology
Grafts and grafting
Growth
Healing
Herbal medicine
Histology
Homeopathy
Hydrotherapy
Hyperadiposis
Hyperthermia and hypothermia
Hypertrophy
Hypochondriasis
Iatrogenic disorders
Imaging and radiology
Immunopathology
Infection
Inflammation
Insect-borne diseases
Internet medicine
Interpartner violence
Invasive tests
Leptin
Lesions
Longevity
Macronutrients
Magnetic resonance imaging (MRI)
Malignancy and metastasis
Malnutrition
Massage
Medical home
Meditation
Men's health
Metabolic disorders
Metabolic syndrome
Mucopolysaccharidosis (MPS)
Multiple births
Münchausen syndrome by proxy
Neonatology
Noninvasive tests
Nursing
Nutrition
Occupational health
Oncology

Opportunistic infections
Ovaries
Over-the-counter medications
Pain
Pain management
Palliative care
Palliative medicine
Paramedics
Parasitic diseases
Pathology
Pediatrics
Perinatology
Physical examination
Physician assistants
Physiology
Phytochemicals
Plastic surgery
Positron emission tomography (PET) scanning
Preventive medicine
Progeria
Prognosis
Prostheses
Protein
Proteomics
Psychiatry
Psychosomatic disorders
Puberty and adolescence
Radiation therapy
Radiopharmaceuticals
Retroviruses
Safety issues for children
Safety issues for the elderly
Screening
Self-medication
Shock
Signs and symptoms
Stem cells
Stress
Stress reduction
Substance abuse
Sudden infant death syndrome (SIDS)
Suicide
Supplements
Surgical procedures
Surgical technologists
Syndrome
Systemic lupus erythematosus (SLE)
Systemic sclerosis
Systems and organs
Teratogens
Terminally ill: Extended care

Toxic shock syndrome
Toxicology
Transitional care
Tumor removal
Tumors
Viral hemorrhagic fevers
Viral infections
Vitamin D deficiency
Vitamins and minerals
Well-baby examinations
Wounds
Xenotransplantation
Zoonoses

ABDOMEN
Abdominal disorders
Adrenalectomy
Amebiasis
Amniocentesis
Aneurysmectomy
Appendectomy
Appendicitis
Back pain
Bariatric surgery
Bladder removal
Bypass surgery
Campylobacter infections
Candidiasis
Cesarean section
Cholecystectomy
Cholecystitis
Colitis
Colon
Colon therapy
Colorectal cancer
Colorectal polyp removal
Colorectal surgery
Constipation
Culdocentesis
Cushing's syndrome
Diabetes mellitus
Dialysis
Diarrhea and dysentery
Digestion
Diverticulitis and diverticulosis
Eating disorders
Endoscopic retrograde
    cholangiopancreatography (ERCP)
Endoscopy
Enemas
Fistula repair
Gallbladder
Gallbladder diseases
Gastrectomy
Gastroenteritis
Gastroenterology
Gastrointestinal disorders

Gastrointestinal system
Gastrostomy
Gaucher's disease
Hernia
Hernia repair
Ileostomy and colostomy
Incontinence
Internal medicine
Intestinal disorders
Intestines
Irritable bowel syndrome (IBS)
Kidney transplantation
Kidneys
Laparoscopy
Liposuction
Lithotripsy
Liver
Liver transplantation
Mesothelioma
Nephrectomy
Nephrology
Obesity
Pancreas
Pancreatitis
Peristalsis
Peritonitis
Polyps
Pregnancy and gestation
Prostate cancer
Reproductive system
Roseola
Shunts
Small intestine
Splenectomy
Stents
Sterilization
Stevens-Johnson syndrome
Stone removal
Stones
Tubal ligation
Tularemia
Ulcerative colitis
Ultrasonography
Urinary disorders
Urinary system
Urology
Vasculitis

ANUS
Amebiasis
Anal cancer
Colon therapy
Colorectal cancer
Colorectal polyp removal
Colorectal surgery
Endoscopy
Enemas

Episiotomy
Fistula repair
Hemorrhoid banding and removal
Hemorrhoids
Hirschsprung's disease
Human papillomavirus (HPV)
Intestinal disorders
Intestines
Irritable bowel syndrome (IBS)
Polyps
Rape and sexual assault
Rectum
Soiling
Sphincterectomy
Syphilis
Ulcerative colitis

ARMS
Amputation
Arthroplasty
Auras
Carpal tunnel syndrome
Casts and splints
Charcot-Marie-Tooth Disease
Cornelia de Lange syndrome
Cutis marmorata telangiectatica
    congenita
Dyskinesia
Fracture and dislocation
Fracture repair
Gigantism
Hemiplegia
Liposuction
Mesenchymal stem cells
Muscles
Neonatal brachial plexus palsy
Phlebotomy
Pityriasis alba
Quadriplegia
Roseola
Rotator cuff surgery
Sarcoma
Skin lesion removal
Slipped disk
Spinocerebellar ataxia
Streptococcal infections
Tendinitis
Thalidomide
Tremors
Upper extremities

BACK
Ankylosing spondylitis
Back pain
Bone disorders
Bone marrow transplantation
Bones and the skeleton

Chiropractic
Cushing's syndrome
Disk removal
Dwarfism
Juvenile rheumatoid arthritis
Kyphosis
Laminectomy and spinal fusion
Neuroimaging
Osteoporosis
Pityriasis alba
Pityriasis rosea
Sarcoma
Sciatica
Scoliosis
Slipped disk
Stevens-Johnson syndrome
Streptococcal infections
Sympathectomy
Tendon disorders

BLADDER
Abdomen
Abdominal disorders
Bed-wetting
Bladder cancer
Bladder removal
Candidiasis
Catheterization
Cystitis
Cystoscopy
Diuretics
Endoscopy
Fetal surgery
Fistula repair
Hematuria
Incontinence
Internal medicine
Lithotripsy
Polyps
Pyelonephritis
Schistosomiasis
Smoking
Sphincterectomy
Stone removal
Stones
Toilet training
Ultrasonography
Uremia
Urethritis
Urinalysis
Urinary disorders
Urinary system
Urology
Williams syndrome

BLOOD
Acquired immunodeficiency

syndrome (AIDS)
Anemia
Angiography
Antibodies
Aspergillosis
Avian influenza
Babesiosis
Biological therapies
Bleeding
Blood pressure
Blood testing
Blood vessels
Bone marrow transplantation
Bulimia
Candidiasis
Carbohydrates
Circulation
Cold agglutinin disease
Connective tissue
Cushing's syndrome
Cyanosis
Cytomegalovirus (CMV)
Deep vein thrombosis
Defibrillation
Dialysis
Disseminated intravascular
    coagulation (DIC)
Diuretics
E. coli infection
Ebola virus
End-stage renal disease
Epstein-Barr virus
Ergogenic aids
Fetal surgery
Fetal tissue transplantation
Fistula repair
Fluids and electrolytes
Glycolysis
Gulf War syndrome
Heart
Hematology
Hematomas
Hematuria
Hemolytic disease of the newborn
Hemolytic uremic syndrome
Hemophilia
Histiocytosis
Host-defense mechanisms
Hyperbaric oxygen therapy
Hypercholesterolemia
Hyperlipidemia
Hypoglycemia
Immune system
Immunization and vaccination
Jaundice
Laboratory tests
Leukemia

Liver
Lymph
Malaria
Menorrhagia
Methicillin-resistant staphylococcus
    aureus (MRSA) infection
Nephrology
Pharmacology
Phenylketonuria (PKU)
Phlebotomy
Plasma
Pulse rate
Rh factor
Salmonella infection
Schistosomiasis
Septicemia
Serology
Sickle cell disease
Single photon emission computed
    tomography (SPECT)
Snakebites
Staphylococcal infections
Sturge-Weber syndrome
Subdural hematoma
Thalassemia
Thrombocytopenia
Thrombolytic therapy and TPA
Thrombosis and thrombus
Thymus gland
Transfusion
Transplantation
Ultrasonography
Uremia
Von Willebrand's disease
Wiskott-Aldrich syndrome
Yellow fever

BLOOD VESSELS
Aneurysms
Angiography
Angioplasty
Arteriosclerosis
Avian influenza
Bedsores
Bile
Bleeding
Blood and blood disorders
Blood pressure
Blood testing
Blood vessels
Bruises
Bypass surgery
Caffeine
Carotid arteries
Catheterization
Cholesterol
Circulation

Claudication
Cluster headaches
Cold agglutinin disease
Cutis marmorata telangiectatica
  congenita
Deep vein thrombosis
Defibrillation
Diabetes mellitus
Disseminated intravascular
  coagulation (DIC)
Diuretics
Dizziness and fainting
Edema
Electrocauterization
Embolism
Embolization
End-stage renal disease
Endarterectomy
Erectile dysfunction
Eye infections and disorders
Facial transplantation
Hammertoe correction
Heart
Heart disease
Heat exhaustion and heatstroke
Hematomas
Hemorrhoid banding and removal
Hemorrhoids
Hormone therapy
Hypercholesterolemia
Hypertension
Hypotension
Infarction
Intravenous (IV) therapy
Ischemia
Kawasaki disease
Klippel-Trenaunay syndrome
Leptospirosis
Methicillin-resistant staphylococcus
  aureus (MRSA) infection
Necrotizing fasciitis
Nephritis
Neuroimaging
Obesity
Phlebitis
Phlebotomy
Plasma
Polycystic kidney disease
Polydactyly and syndactyly
Pulse rate
Raynaud's phenomenon
Rocky Mountain spotted fever
Roundworms
Schistosomiasis
Scleroderma
Scurvy
Single photon emission computed

tomography (SPECT)
Stenosis
Stents
Strokes
Sturge-Weber syndrome
Temporal arteritis
Thalidomide
Thrombolytic therapy and TPA
Thrombosis and thrombus
Toxemia
Transient ischemic attacks (TIAs)
Umbilical cord
Varicose vein removal
Varicose veins
Vascular medicine
Vascular system
Vasculitis
Venous insufficiency
Von Willebrand's disease

BONES
Amputation
Ankylosing spondylitis
Arthritis
Arthroplasty
Aspergillosis
Back pain
Bone cancer
Bone disorders
Bone grafting
Bone marrow transplantation
Bowlegs
Bunions
Cartilage
Casts and splints
Cells
Chiropractic
Cleft lip and palate
Cleft lip and palate repair
Connective tissue
Craniosynostosis
Cushing's syndrome
Dengue fever
Disk removal
Dwarfism
Ear surgery
Ears
Eating disorders
Ewing's sarcoma
Facial transplantation
Failure to thrive
Feet
Foot disorders
Fracture and dislocation
Fracture repair
Gaucher's disease
Gigantism

Hammertoe correction
Head and neck disorders
Hearing
Heel spur removal
Hip fracture repair
Hip replacement
Histiocytosis
Hormone therapy
Jaw wiring
Joints
Kneecap removal
Kyphosis
Laminectomy and spinal fusion
Leishmaniasis
Lower extremities
Marfan syndrome
Mesenchymal stem cells
Methicillin-resistant staphylococcus
  aureus (MRSA) infection
Motor skill development
Necrosis
Neurofibromatosis
Neurosurgery
Niemann-Pick disease
Nuclear medicine
Nuclear radiology
Orthopedic surgery
Orthopedics
Osteochondritis juvenilis
Osteogenesis imperfecta
Osteomyelitis
Osteonecrosis
Osteopathic medicine
Osteoporosis
Paget's disease
Periodontitis
Physical rehabilitation
Pigeon toes
Podiatry
Polydactyly and syndactyly
Prader-Willi syndrome
Rheumatology
Rickets
Rubinstein-Taybi syndrome
Sarcoma
Scoliosis
Spina bifida
Spinal cord disorders
Sports medicine
Syphilis
Teeth
Temporomandibular joint (TMJ)
  syndrome
Tendon disorders
Tendon repair
Upper extremities

BRAIN

Abscess drainage
Acidosis
Acquired immunodeficiency
  syndrome (AIDS)
Addiction
Adrenoleukodystrophy
Agnosia
Alcoholism
Altitude sickness
Alzheimer's disease
Amnesia
Anesthesia
Anesthesiology
Aneurysmectomy
Aneurysms
Angelman syndrome
Angiography
Anorexia nervosa
Anosmia
Antianxiety drugs
Antidepressants
Aortic stenosis
Aphasia and dysphasia
Apnea
Aromatherapy
Aspergillosis
Ataxia
Attention-deficit disorder (ADD)
Auras
Autism
Batten's disease
Biofeedback
Body dysmorphic disorder
Brain damage
Brain disorders
Brain tumors
Brucellosis
Bulimia
Caffeine
Carbohydrates
Carotid arteries
Cerebral palsy
Chiari malformations
Chronic wasting disease (CWD)
Cluster headaches
Cognitive development
Cognitive enhancement
Concussion
Cornelia de Lange syndrome
Craniotomy
Creutzfeldt-Jakob disease (CJD)
Cutis marmorata telangiectatica
  congenita
Cytomegalovirus (CMV)
Defibrillation
Dehydration

Dementias
Depression
Developmental stages
Dizziness and fainting
Down syndrome
Drowning
Dwarfism
Dyskinesia
Dyslexia
Electroencephalography (EEG)
Embolism
Embolization
Encephalitis
Endocrine glands
Endocrinology
Enteroviruses
Epilepsy
Ergogenic aids
Eye infections and disorders
Failure to thrive
Fetal alcohol syndrome
Fetal surgery
Fetal tissue transplantation
Fibromyalgia
Fragile X syndrome
Frontal lobe syndrome
Frontotemporal dementia (FTD)
Gigantism
Glioma
Gulf War syndrome
Head and neck disorders
Headaches
Hearing
Hearing loss
Hemiplegia
Hemolytic disease of the newborn
Hormone therapy
Huntington's disease
Hydrocephalus
Hypertension
Hypnosis
Hypotension
Hypothalamus
Infarction
Intraventricular hemorrhage
Ischemia
Kawasaki disease
Kinesiology
Kluver-Bucy syndrome
Korsakoff's syndrome
Lead poisoning
Learning disabilities
Leptospirosis
Leukodystrophy
Light therapy
Listeria infections
Lumbar puncture

Melatonin
Memory loss
Meningitis
Mental retardation
Mental status exam
Mirror neurons
Narcolepsy
Narcotics
Nausea and vomiting
Neuroimaging
Neurology
Neuropsychology
Neuroscience
Neurosis
Neurosurgery
Niemann-Pick disease
Nuclear radiology
Pharmacology
Phenylketonuria (PKU)
Phrenology
Pick's disease
Pituitary gland
Poliomyelitis
Polycystic kidney disease
Prader-Willi syndrome
Prion diseases
Psychiatric disorders
Rabies
Restless legs syndrome
Resuscitation
Reye's syndrome
Rocky Mountain spotted fever
Roseola
Sarcoidosis
Schizophrenia
Seizures
Shock therapy
Shunts
Single photon emission computed
  tomography (SPECT)
Sleep
Sleep disorders
Sleeping sickness
Sleepwalking
Spina bifida
Spinocerebellar ataxia
Split-brain
Strokes
Sturge-Weber syndrome
Subdural hematoma
Synesthesia
Syphilis
Teeth
Tetanus
Thrombosis and thrombus
Tics
Tinnitus

Tourette's syndrome
Transient ischemic attacks (TIAs)
Traumatic brain injury
Vagus nerve
Vertigo
Weight loss medications
Wernicke's aphasia
West Nile virus
Williams syndrome
Wilson's disease

BREASTS
Abscess drainage
Breast cancer
Breast disorders
Breast-feeding
Breast surgery
Cyst removal
Fibrocystic breast condition
Gender reassignment surgery
Glands
Gynecology
Gynecomastia
Hormone therapy
Klinefelter syndrome
Mammography
Mastectomy and lumpectomy
Mastitis
Premenstrual syndrome (PMS)
Raynaud's phenomenon
Stevens-Johnson syndrome
Tumor removal

CELLS
Acid-base chemistry
Alzheimer's disease
Antibodies
Bacteriology
Batten's disease
Biological therapies
Biopsy
Breast cancer
Cholesterol
Cloning
Conception
Cytology
Cytomegalovirus (CMV)
Cytopathology
Defibrillation
Dehydration
Diuretics
Electrocauterization
Epstein-Barr virus
Erectile dysfunction
Ergogenic aids
Eye infections and disorders
Fluids and electrolytes

Food biochemistry
Gaucher's disease
Gene therapy
Genetic counseling
Glycolysis
Gram staining
Gulf War syndrome
Hearing
Host-defense mechanisms
Hyperplasia
Immune system
Immunization and vaccination
In vitro fertilization
Karyotyping
Kinesiology
Laboratory tests
Lipids
Magnetic field therapy
Mesenchymal stem cells
Microbiology
Microscopy
Mutation
Necrosis
Parkinson's disease
Pharmacology
Phlebotomy
Plasma
Rhinoviruses
Sarcoma
Sickle cell disease
Sleep
Thymus gland
Turner syndrome

CENTRAL NERVOUS SYSTEM
Delirium
Minimally conscious state

CHEST
Achalasia
Aneurysmectomy
Antihistamines
Asthma
Bacillus Calmette-Guérin (BCG)
Bronchiolitis
Bronchitis
Bypass surgery
Cardiac rehabilitation
Cardiology
Choking
Cold agglutinin disease
Common cold
Congenital heart disease
Coughing
Cystic fibrosis
Defibrillation
Diaphragm

Electrocardiography (ECG or EKG)
Emphysema
Gulf War syndrome
Gynecomastia
Heart
Heart transplantation
Heart valve replacement
Heimlich maneuver
Hiccups
Legionnaires' disease
Lung cancer
Lungs
Oxygen therapy
Pacemaker implantation
Palpitations
Pityriasis rosea
Pleurisy
Pneumocystis jirovecii
Pneumothorax
Pulmonary diseases
Pulmonary medicine
Respiration
Resuscitation
Rhinoviruses
Sarcoidosis
Streptococcal infections
Thoracic surgery
Trachea
Tuberculosis
Vasculitis
Whooping cough

CIRCULATORY SYSTEM
Acute respiratory distress syndrome
  (ARDS)
Aneurysms
Angina
Angiography
Angioplasty
Antibodies
Antihistamines
Apgar score
Arteriosclerosis
Avian influenza
Biofeedback
Bleeding
Blood and blood disorders
Blood pressure
Blood testing
Blood vessels
Blue baby syndrome
Bypass surgery
Cardiac arrest
Cardiac rehabilitation
Cardiac surgery
Cardiology
Cardiopulmonary resuscitation (CPR)

Carotid arteries
Catheterization
Chest
Cholera
Cholesterol
Circulation
Claudication
Cold agglutinin disease
Computed tomography (CT) scanning
Congenital heart disease
Coronary artery bypass graft
Cutis marmorata telangiectatica
    congenita
Decongestants
Deep vein thrombosis
Defibrillation
Dehydration
Diabetes mellitus
Dialysis
Disseminated intravascular
    coagulation (DIC)
Diuretics
Dizziness and fainting
Drowning
Ebola virus
Echocardiography
Edema
Electrocardiography (ECG or EKG)
Electrocauterization
Embolism
Encephalitis
End-stage renal disease
Endarterectomy
Endocarditis
Ergogenic aids
Exercise physiology
Facial transplantation
Food allergies
Gigantism
Heart
Heart attack
Heart disease
Heart failure
Heart transplantation
Heart valve replacement
Heat exhaustion and heatstroke
Hematology
Hemolytic uremic syndrome
Hemorrhoid banding and removal
Hemorrhoids
Hormone therapy
Hormones
Hyperbaric oxygen therapy
Hypercholesterolemia
Hypertension
Hypotension
Immune system

Intravenous (IV) therapy
Ischemia
Juvenile rheumatoid arthritis
Kawasaki disease
Kidneys
Kinesiology
Klippel-Trenaunay syndrome
Lead poisoning
Liver
Lymph
Lymphatic system
Mesenchymal stem cells
Methicillin-resistant staphylococcus
    aureus (MRSA) infection
Mitral valve prolapse
Motor skill development
Obesity
Osteochondritis juvenilis
Oxygen therapy
Pacemaker implantation
Palpitations
Phlebitis
Phlebotomy
Placenta
Plasma
Preeclampsia and eclampsia
Pulmonary edema
Pulse rate
Resuscitation
Reye's syndrome
Rocky Mountain spotted fever
Roundworms
Sarcoidosis
Schistosomiasis
Scleroderma
Septicemia
Shunts
Single photon emission computed
    tomography (SPECT)
Smoking
Snakebites
Sports medicine
Staphylococcal infections
Stenosis
Stents
Steroid abuse
Streptococcal infections
Strokes
Sturge-Weber syndrome
Temporal arteritis
Testicular torsion
Thrombocytopenia
Thrombolytic therapy and TPA
Thrombosis and thrombus
Toxemia
Transfusion
Transient ischemic attacks (TIAs)

Transplantation
Typhoid fever
Typhus
Uremia
Varicose vein removal
Varicose veins
Vascular medicine
Vascular system
Vasculitis
Venous insufficiency
Yellow fever

EARS
Adenoids
Adrenoleukodystrophy
Agnosia
Altitude sickness
Antihistamines
Aspergillosis
Audiology
Auras
Bell's palsy
Cartilage
Charcot-Marie-Tooth Disease
Cold agglutinin disease
Cornelia de Lange syndrome
Cytomegalovirus (CMV)
Deafness
Decongestants
Dyslexia
Ear infections and disorders
Ear surgery
Earwax
Facial transplantation
Fetal alcohol syndrome
Fragile X syndrome
Hearing
Hearing aids
Hearing loss
Hearing tests
Histiocytosis
Leukodystrophy
Measles
Ménière's disease
Motion sickness
Myringotomy
Nervous system
Neurology
Osteogenesis imperfecta
Otoplasty
Otorhinolaryngology
Pharynx
Raynaud's phenomenon
Rubinstein-Taybi syndrome
Sense organs
Speech disorders
Streptococcal infections

Tinnitus
Tonsillitis
Vasculitis
Vertigo
Williams syndrome
Wiskott-Aldrich syndrome

ENDOCRINE SYSTEM
Addison's disease
Adrenalectomy
Adrenoleukodystrophy
Amenorrhea
Anorexia nervosa
Assisted reproductive technologies
Bariatric surgery
Biofeedback
Carbohydrates
Computed tomography (CT) scanning
Congenital adrenal hyperplasia
Congenital hypothyroidism
Corticosteroids
Cushing's syndrome
Diabetes mellitus
Dwarfism
End-stage renal disease
Endocrine disorders
Endocrine glands
Endocrinology
Ergogenic aids
Failure to thrive
Fibrocystic breast condition
Gender reassignment surgery
Gestational diabetes
Gigantism
Glands
Goiter
Gynecomastia
Hashimoto's thyroiditis
Hormones
Hyperparathyroidism and
    hypoparathyroidism
Hypoglycemia
Hypothalamus
Klinefelter syndrome
Lead poisoning
Liver
Melatonin
Nonalcoholic steatohepatitis (NASH)
Obesity
Overtraining syndrome
Pancreas
Pancreatitis
Parathyroidectomy
Pituitary gland
Placenta
Plasma
Polycystic ovary syndrome

Postpartum depression
Prader-Willi syndrome
Preeclampsia and eclampsia
Prostate gland
Prostate gland removal
Sexual differentiation
Small intestine
Steroid abuse
Steroids
Testicular cancer
Testicular surgery
Thymus gland
Thyroid disorders
Thyroid gland
Thyroidectomy
Turner syndrome
Weight loss medications
Williams syndrome

EYES
Acquired immunodeficiency
    syndrome (AIDS)
Adenoviruses
Adrenoleukodystrophy
Agnosia
Angelman syndrome
Ankylosing spondylitis
Antihistamines
Aspergillosis
Astigmatism
Auras
Batten's disease
Behçet's disease
Bell's palsy
Blindness
Blurred vision
Botox
Cataract surgery
Cataracts
Chlamydia
Color blindness
Conjunctivitis
Corneal transplantation
Cornelia de Lange syndrome
Cutis marmorata telangiectatica
    congenita
Cytomegalovirus (CMV)
Dengue fever
Diabetes mellitus
Dry eye
Dyslexia
Enteroviruses
Eye infections and disorders
Eye surgery
Face lift and blepharoplasty
Facial transplantation
Fetal alcohol syndrome

Fetal tissue transplantation
Galactosemia
Gigantism
Glaucoma
Gonorrhea
Gulf War syndrome
Hay fever
Juvenile rheumatoid arthritis
Keratitis
Kluver-Bucy syndrome
Laser use in surgery
Leptospirosis
Leukodystrophy
Lyme disease
Macular degeneration
Marfan syndrome
Motor skill development
Multiple chemical sensitivity
    syndrome
Myopia
Ophthalmology
Optometry
Pigmentation
Pterygium/Pinguecula
Ptosis
Refractive eye surgery
Reiter's syndrome
Rubinstein-Taybi syndrome
Sarcoidosis
Scurvy
Sense organs
Sjögren's syndrome
Sphincterectomy
Spinocerebellar ataxia
Stevens-Johnson syndrome
Strabismus
Sturge-Weber syndrome
Styes
Syphilis
Tears and tear ducts
Trachoma
Transplantation
Vasculitis
Vision
Vision disorders
Williams syndrome

FEET
Athlete's foot
Bones and the skeleton
Bowlegs
Bunions
Charcot-Marie-Tooth Disease
Cold agglutinin disease
Cornelia de Lange syndrome
Corns and calluses
Dyskinesia

Flat feet
Foot disorders
Fragile X syndrome
Frostbite
Ganglion removal
Gout
Hammertoe correction
Hammertoes
Heel spur removal
Lower extremities
Mesenchymal stem cells
Methicillin-resistant staphylococcus
    aureus (MRSA) infection
Nail removal
Nails
Orthopedic surgery
Orthopedics
Pigeon toes
Podiatry
Polydactyly and syndactyly
Raynaud's phenomenon
Rubinstein-Taybi syndrome
Spinocerebellar ataxia
Sports medicine
Stevens-Johnson syndrome
Streptococcal infections
Tendinitis
Tendon repair
Thalidomide
Tremors

GALLBLADDER

Abscess drainage
Bariatric surgery
Bile
Cholecystectomy
Cholecystitis
Chyme
Endoscopic retrograde
    cholangiopancreatography (ERCP)
Fistula repair
Gallbladder cancer
Gallbladder diseases
Gastroenterology
Gastrointestinal system
Internal medicine
Laparoscopy
Liver transplantation
Malabsorption
Nuclear medicine
Polyps
Stone removal
Stones
Typhoid fever
Ultrasonography

GASTROINTESTINAL SYSTEM

Abdomen
Abdominal disorders
Achalasia
Acid reflux disease
Acidosis
Acquired immunodeficiency
    syndrome (AIDS)
Adenoviruses
Allergies
Amebiasis
Anal cancer
Angelman syndrome
Ankylosing spondylitis
Anorexia nervosa
Anthrax
Anus
Appendectomy
Appendicitis
Asbestos exposure
Avian influenza
Bacterial infections
Bariatric surgery
Beriberi
Bulimia
Bypass surgery
Campylobacter infections
Candidiasis
Carbohydrates
Childhood infectious diseases
Cholecystectomy
Cholecystitis
Cholera
Cholesterol
Chyme
Clostridium difficile infection
Colic
Colitis
Colon
Colon therapy
Colonoscopy and sigmoidoscopy
Colorectal cancer
Colorectal polyp removal
Colorectal surgery
Computed tomography (CT) scanning
Constipation
Crohn's disease
Cytomegalovirus (CMV)
Diabetes mellitus
Diarrhea and dysentery
Digestion
Diverticulitis and diverticulosis
E. coli infection
Eating disorders
Ebola virus
Embolization
Endoscopic retrograde

cholangiopancreatography (ERCP)
Endoscopy
Enemas
Enterocolitis
Esophagus
Fiber
Fistula repair
Food allergies
Food biochemistry
Food poisoning
Fructosemia
Gallbladder
Gallbladder cancer
Gallbladder diseases
Gastrectomy
Gastroenteritis
Gastroenterology
Gastrointestinal disorders
Gastrostomy
Giardiasis
Glands
Gluten intolerance
Gulf War syndrome
Hand-foot-and-mouth disease
Hemolytic uremic syndrome
Hemorrhoid banding and removal
Hemorrhoids
Hernia
Hernia repair
Histiocytosis
Host-defense mechanisms
Ileostomy and colostomy
Incontinence
Internal medicine
Intestinal disorders
Intestines
Irritable bowel syndrome (IBS)
Klippel-Trenaunay syndrome
Kwashiorkor
Lactose intolerance
Laparoscopy
Lipids
Liver
Malabsorption
Malnutrition
Meckel's diverticulum
Metabolism
Motion sickness
Muscles
Nausea and vomiting
Nonalcoholic steatohepatitis (NASH)
Noroviruses
Obesity
Pancreas
Pancreatitis
Peristalsis
Peritonitis

Pharynx
Pinworms
Poisoning
Polycystic kidney disease
Polyps
Proctology
Protozoan diseases
Pyloric stenosis
Radiation sickness
Rectum
Reiter's syndrome
Rotavirus
Roundworms
Salmonella infection
Scleroderma
Sense organs
Shigellosis
Shunts
Small intestine
Smallpox
Smoking
Soiling
Staphylococcal infections
Stenosis
Stevens-Johnson syndrome
Tapeworms
Taste
Teeth
Toilet training
Toxoplasmosis
Trichinosis
Tumor removal
Typhoid fever
Ulcer surgery
Ulcerative colitis
Ulcers
Vagotomy
Vasculitis
Weaning
Weight loss and gain

GENITALS

Adrenoleukodystrophy
Aphrodisiacs
Assisted reproductive technologies
Behçet's disease
Candidiasis
Catheterization
Cervical procedures
Chlamydia
Congenital adrenal hyperplasia
Contraception
Cyst removal
Embolization
Endometrial biopsy
Episiotomy
Erectile dysfunction

Ergogenic aids
Fragile X syndrome
Gender identity disorder
Gender reassignment surgery
Glands
Gonorrhea
Gynecology
Hemochromatosis
Hermaphroditism and
     pseudohermaphroditism
Herpes
Hormone therapy
Human papillomavirus (HPV)
Hydroceles
Hyperplasia
Hypospadias repair and urethroplasty
Klinefelter syndrome
Kluver-Bucy syndrome
Masturbation
Mumps
Orchitis
Pap test
Pelvic inflammatory disease (PID)
Penile implant surgery
Prader-Willi syndrome
Rape and sexual assault
Reproductive system
Rubinstein-Taybi syndrome
Semen
Sexual differentiation
Sexual dysfunction
Sexuality
Sexually transmitted diseases (STDs)
Sperm banks
Sterilization
Stevens-Johnson syndrome
Streptococcal infections
Syphilis
Testicular cancer
Testicular surgery
Testicular torsion
Toilet training
Trichomoniasis
Urethritis
Urology
Uterus
Vas deferens
Vasectomy

GLANDS

Abscess drainage
Addison's disease
Adrenalectomy
Adrenoleukodystrophy
Assisted reproductive technologies
Biofeedback
Breast cancer

Breast disorders
Breast-feeding
Breast surgery
Cushing's syndrome
Cyst removal
Dengue fever
Diabetes mellitus
DiGeorge syndrome
Dwarfism
Endocrine disorders
Endocrine glands
Endocrinology
Epstein-Barr virus
Ergogenic aids
Eye infections and disorders
Gender reassignment surgery
Goiter
Gynecomastia
Hashimoto's thyroiditis
Hormones
Hyperhidrosis
Hyperparathyroidism and
     hypoparathyroidism
Hypoglycemia
Hypothalamus
Immune system
Internal medicine
Liver
Mastitis
Melatonin
Mumps
Neurosurgery
Nuclear medicine
Nuclear radiology
Pancreas
Parathyroidectomy
Pituitary gland
Prader-Willi syndrome
Prostate gland
Prostate gland removal
Quinsy
Semen
Sexual differentiation
Sleep
Steroids
Sweating
Testicular cancer
Testicular surgery
Thymus gland
Thyroid disorders
Thyroid gland
Thyroidectomy

GUMS

Abscess drainage
Bulimia
Cavities

Cleft lip and palate repair
Dengue fever
Dental diseases
Dentistry
Dentures
Fluoride treatments
Gingivitis
Gulf War syndrome
Gum disease
Jaw wiring
Mouth and throat cancer
Oral and maxillofacial surgery
Orthodontics
Periodontal surgery
Periodontitis
Root canal treatment
Scurvy
Teeth
Teething
Tooth extraction
Wisdom teeth

HAIR
Alopecia
Angelman syndrome
Anorexia nervosa
Collodion baby
Cornelia de Lange syndrome
Cushing's syndrome
Dermatitis
Dermatology
Gigantism
Gulf War syndrome
Hair
Hair transplantation
Klinefelter syndrome
Pigmentation
Radiation sickness

HANDS
Amputation
Arthritis
Arthroplasty
Bursitis
Carpal tunnel syndrome
Casts and splints
Charcot-Marie-Tooth Disease
Cold agglutinin disease
Cornelia de Lange syndrome
Corns and calluses
Dyskinesia
Fetal alcohol syndrome
Fracture and dislocation
Fragile X syndrome
Frostbite
Ganglion removal
Gigantism

Mesenchymal stem cells
Methicillin-resistant staphylococcus
    aureus (MRSA) infection
Nail removal
Nails
Neurology
Orthopedic surgery
Orthopedics
Polydactyly and syndactyly
Raynaud's phenomenon
Rheumatology
Rubinstein-Taybi syndrome
Scleroderma
Skin lesion removal
Spinocerebellar ataxia
Sports medicine
Stevens-Johnson syndrome
Streptococcal infections
Tendinitis
Tendon repair
Thalidomide
Tremors
Upper extremities
Vasculitis

HEAD
Alopecia
Altitude sickness
Aneurysms
Angelman syndrome
Angiography
Antihistamines
Bell's palsy
Botox
Brain
Brain disorders
Brain tumors
Cluster headaches
Concussion
Cornelia de Lange syndrome
Craniosynostosis
Craniotomy
Dengue fever
Dizziness and fainting
Dyskinesia
Electroencephalography (EEG)
Epilepsy
Eye infections and disorders
Facial transplantation
Fetal alcohol syndrome
Fibromyalgia
Hair transplantation
Head and neck disorders
Headaches
Hemiplegia
Hydrocephalus
Meningitis

Motion sickness
Nasal polyp removal
Neuroimaging
Neurology
Neurosurgery
Oral and maxillofacial surgery
Paget's disease
Pharynx
Rubinstein-Taybi syndrome
Seizures
Shunts
Single photon emission computed
    tomography (SPECT)
Spinocerebellar ataxia
Sports medicine
Stevens-Johnson syndrome
Strokes
Sturge-Weber syndrome
Tears and tear ducts
Temporomandibular joint (TMJ)
    syndrome
Thrombosis and thrombus
Tinnitus
Tremors
Whiplash

HEART
Acidosis
Anemia
Aneurysmectomy
Aneurysms
Angina
Angiography
Angioplasty
Anorexia nervosa
Anxiety
Aortic stenosis
Apgar score
Arrhythmias
Arteriosclerosis
Aspergillosis
Atrial fibrillation
Avian influenza
Beriberi
Biofeedback
Bites and stings
Blood pressure
Blood vessels
Blue baby syndrome
Brucellosis
Bulimia
Bypass surgery
Caffeine
Cardiac arrest
Cardiac rehabilitation
Cardiac surgery
Cardiology

Cardiopulmonary resuscitation (CPR)
Carotid arteries
Catheterization
Congenital heart disease
Cornelia de Lange syndrome
Coronary artery bypass graft
Defibrillation
Depression
Diabetes mellitus
DiGeorge syndrome
Diphtheria
Diuretics
Drowning
Echocardiography
Electrical shock
Electrocardiography (ECG or EKG)
End-stage renal disease
Endocarditis
Enteroviruses
Ergogenic aids
Exercise physiology
Fatty acid oxidation disorders
Fetal alcohol syndrome
Gangrene
Glycogen storage diseases
Heart attack
Heart disease
Heart failure
Heart transplantation
Heart valve replacement
Hemochromatosis
Hormone therapy
Hypercholesterolemia
Hypertension
Hypotension
Infarction
Internal medicine
Interstitial pulmonary fibrosis (IPF)
Intravenous (IV) therapy
Juvenile rheumatoid arthritis
Kawasaki disease
Kinesiology
Lyme disease
Marfan syndrome
Methicillin-resistant staphylococcus
  aureus (MRSA) infection
Mitral valve prolapse
Mononucleosis
Obesity
Oxygen therapy
Pacemaker implantation
Palpitations
Plasma
Prader-Willi syndrome
Pulmonary edema
Pulse rate
Renal failure

Respiratory distress syndrome
Resuscitation
Reye's syndrome
Rheumatic fever
Rheumatoid arthritis
Rubinstein-Taybi syndrome
Sarcoidosis
Scleroderma
Single photon emission computed
  tomography (SPECT)
Sleeping sickness
Sports medicine
Stenosis
Stents
Steroid abuse
Streptococcal infections
Strokes
Syphilis
Teeth
Thoracic surgery
Thrombolytic therapy and TPA
Thrombosis and thrombus
Transplantation
Ultrasonography
Uremia
Whooping cough
Williams syndrome

HIPS
Ankylosing spondylitis
Arthritis
Arthroplasty
Arthroscopy
Back pain
Bones and the skeleton
Bowlegs
Chiropractic
Dwarfism
Fracture and dislocation
Fracture repair
Hip fracture repair
Hip replacement
Liposuction
Lower extremities
Orthopedic surgery
Orthopedics
Osteochondritis juvenilis
Osteonecrosis
Osteoporosis
Paget's disease
Physical rehabilitation
Pigeon toes
Rheumatology
Sciatica

IMMUNE SYSTEM
Acquired immunodeficiency

syndrome (AIDS)
Adenoids
Adenoviruses
Allergies
Ankylosing spondylitis
Anorexia nervosa
Anthrax
Antibodies
Antihistamines
Arthritis
Asthma
Bacillus Calmette-Guérin (BCG)
Bacterial infections
Bacteriology
Bedsores
Bile
Biological therapies
Bites and stings
Blood and blood disorders
Bone grafting
Bone marrow transplantation
Candidiasis
Cells
Chagas' disease
Childhood infectious diseases
Chronic fatigue syndrome
Cold agglutinin disease
Conjunctivitis
Cornelia de Lange syndrome
Coronaviruses
Corticosteroids
Coughing
Cytology
Cytomegalovirus (CMV)
Cytopathology
Dermatology
Dermatopathology
DiGeorge syndrome
Disseminated intravascular
  coagulation (DIC)
Ehrlichiosis
Endocrinology
Epstein-Barr virus
Facial transplantation
Fetal tissue transplantation
Food allergies
Fungal infections
Gluten intolerance
Gram staining
Guillain-Barré syndrome
Gulf War syndrome
Hashimoto's thyroiditis
Hay fever
Hematology
Histiocytosis
Hives
Host-defense mechanisms

Human immunodeficiency virus (HIV)
Immunization and vaccination
Immunodeficiency disorders
Impetigo
Juvenile rheumatoid arthritis
Kawasaki disease
Leishmaniasis
Leprosy
Lymph
Lymphatic system
Magnetic field therapy
Malaria
Marburg virus
Mesenchymal stem cells
Microbiology
Mold and mildew
Monkeypox
Multiple chemical sensitivity syndrome
Mutation
Myasthenia gravis
Nephritis
Noroviruses
Pancreas
Pharmacology
Pharynx
Plasma
Poisoning
Polymyalgia rheumatica
Pulmonary diseases
Pulmonary medicine
Renal failure
Rh factor
Rheumatoid arthritis
Rheumatology
Roseola
Sarcoidosis
Scarlet fever
Scleroderma
Serology
Severe acute respiratory syndrome (SARS)
Severe combined immunodeficiency syndrome (SCID)
Sjögren's syndrome
Small intestine
Stevens-Johnson syndrome
Temporal arteritis
Thalidomide
Thymus gland
Tonsils
Toxoplasmosis
Transfusion
Transplantation
Ulcerative colitis
Vasculitis

Vitiligo
Wiskott-Aldrich syndrome

INTESTINES
Abdomen
Abdominal disorders
Acidosis
Acquired immunodeficiency syndrome (AIDS)
Adenoviruses
Amebiasis
Anus
Appendectomy
Appendicitis
Avian influenza
Bacterial infections
Bariatric surgery
Bulimia
Bypass surgery
Campylobacter infections
Carbohydrates
Celiac sprue
Cholera
Chyme
Colic
Colitis
Colon
Colon therapy
Colonoscopy and sigmoidoscopy
Colorectal cancer
Colorectal polyp removal
Colorectal surgery
Constipation
Crohn's disease
Diarrhea and dysentery
Digestion
Diverticulitis and diverticulosis
E. coli infection
Eating disorders
Endoscopy
Enemas
Enterocolitis
Fiber
Fistula repair
Food poisoning
Fructosemia
Gastroenteritis
Gastroenterology
Gastrointestinal disorders
Gastrointestinal system
Hemorrhoid banding and removal
Hemorrhoids
Hernia
Hernia repair
Hirschsprung's disease
Ileostomy and colostomy
Infarction

Internal medicine
Intestinal disorders
Irritable bowel syndrome (IBS)
Kaposi's sarcoma
Lactose intolerance
Laparoscopy
Malabsorption
Malnutrition
Meckel's diverticulum
Metabolism
Obesity
Peristalsis
Peritonitis
Pinworms
Polyps
Proctology
Rectum
Roundworms
Small intestine
Soiling
Sphincterectomy
Tapeworms
Toilet training
Trichinosis
Tumor removal
Typhoid fever
Ulcer surgery
Ulcerative colitis
Vasculitis

JOINTS
Amputation
Angelman syndrome
Ankylosing spondylitis
Arthritis
Arthroplasty
Arthroscopy
Back pain
Bowlegs
Brucellosis
Bursitis
Carpal tunnel syndrome
Cartilage
Casts and splints
Celiac sprue
Charcot-Marie-Tooth Disease
Cyst removal
Electrocauterization
Endoscopy
Ergogenic aids
Exercise physiology
Fracture and dislocation
Fragile X syndrome
Gout
Gulf War syndrome
Hemiplegia
Hip fracture repair

Juvenile rheumatoid arthritis
Klippel-Trenaunay syndrome
Kneecap removal
Ligaments
Lyme disease
Mesenchymal stem cells
Methicillin-resistant staphylococcus
    aureus (MRSA) infection
Motor skill development
Obesity
Orthopedic surgery
Orthopedics
Osteoarthritis
Osteochondritis juvenilis
Osteomyelitis
Osteonecrosis
Physical rehabilitation
Pigeon toes
Polymyalgia rheumatica
Reiter's syndrome
Rheumatology
Rotator cuff surgery
Rubella
Sarcoidosis
Sarcoma
Scleroderma
Spondylitis
Sports medicine
Streptococcal infections
Syphilis
Temporomandibular joint (TMJ)
    syndrome
Tendinitis
Tendon repair
Tularemia
Von Willebrand's disease

KIDNEYS
Abdomen
Abdominal disorders
Abscess drainage
Addison's disease
Adrenalectomy
Anemia
Anorexia nervosa
Aspergillosis
Avian influenza
Babesiosis
Carbohydrates
Cholera
Diabetes mellitus
Dialysis
Diuretics
Drowning
End-stage renal disease
Ergogenic aids
Fructosemia

Hantavirus
Hematuria
Hemolytic uremic syndrome
Hypertension
Hypotension
Infarction
Internal medicine
Intravenous (IV) therapy
Kidney cancer
Kidney disorders
Kidney transplantation
Laparoscopy
Leptospirosis
Lithotripsy
Metabolism
Methicillin-resistant staphylococcus
    aureus (MRSA) infection
Nephrectomy
Nephritis
Nephrology
Nuclear medicine
Nuclear radiology
Polycystic kidney disease
Polyps
Preeclampsia and eclampsia
Proteinuria
Pyelonephritis
Renal failure
Reye's syndrome
Rocky Mountain spotted fever
Sarcoidosis
Scleroderma
Scurvy
Sickle cell disease
Stone removal
Stones
Syphilis
Toilet training
Transplantation
Typhoid fever
Typhus
Ultrasonography
Uremia
Urinalysis
Urinary disorders
Urinary system
Urology
Vasculitis
Williams syndrome

KNEES
Amputation
Angelman syndrome
Arthritis
Arthroplasty
Arthroscopy
Bowlegs

Bursitis
Cartilage
Casts and splints
Endoscopy
Exercise physiology
Fracture and dislocation
Joints
Kneecap removal
Liposuction
Lower extremities
Lyme disease
Mesenchymal stem cells
Orthopedic surgery
Orthopedics
Osgood-Schlatter disease
Osteonecrosis
Physical rehabilitation
Pigeon toes
Rheumatology
Sports medicine
Stevens-Johnson syndrome
Tendinitis
Tendon repair

LEGS
Amputation
Arthritis
Arthroscopy
Auras
Back pain
Bone disorders
Bones and the skeleton
Bowlegs
Bursitis
Bypass surgery
Casts and splints
Charcot-Marie-Tooth Disease
Claudication
Cornelia de Lange syndrome
Cutis marmorata telangiectatica
    congenita
Deep vein thrombosis
Dwarfism
Dyskinesia
Fracture and dislocation
Fracture repair
Gigantism
Hemiplegia
Hip fracture repair
Kneecap removal
Liposuction
Lower extremities
Mesenchymal stem cells
Methicillin-resistant staphylococcus
    aureus (MRSA) infection
Muscles
Muscular dystrophy

Numbness and tingling
Orthopedic surgery
Orthopedics
Osteoporosis
Paget's disease
Paralysis
Paraplegia
Physical rehabilitation
Pigeon toes
Poliomyelitis
Quadriplegia
Rheumatology
Roseola
Sarcoma
Sciatica
Slipped disk
Spinocerebellar ataxia
Sports medicine
Stevens-Johnson syndrome
Streptococcal infections
Tendinitis
Tendon disorders
Tendon repair
Thalidomide
Tremors
Varicose vein removal
Vascular system
Vasculitis
Venous insufficiency

LIGAMENTS
Ankylosing spondylitis
Back pain
Bowlegs
Casts and splints
Collagen
Connective tissue
Electrocauterization
Eye infections and disorders
Flat feet
Joints
Mesenchymal stem cells
Muscles
Orthopedic surgery
Orthopedics
Osteogenesis imperfecta
Physical rehabilitation
Pigeon toes
Sports medicine
Tendon disorders
Tendon repair
Whiplash

LIVER
Abdomen
Abdominal disorders
Abscess drainage

Acquired immunodeficiency
    syndrome (AIDS)
Alcoholism
Amebiasis
Aspergillosis
Babesiosis
Bile
Blood and blood disorders
Brucellosis
Cholecystitis
Chyme
Circulation
Cirrhosis
Cold agglutinin disease
Cytomegalovirus (CMV)
Edema
Embolization
Endoscopic retrograde
    cholangiopancreatography (ERCP)
Ergogenic aids
Fatty acid oxidation disorders
Fetal surgery
Fructosemia
Galactosemia
Gastroenterology
Gastrointestinal system
Gaucher's disease
Glycogen storage diseases
Hematology
Hemochromatosis
Hemolytic disease of the newborn
Hepatitis
Histiocytosis
Hypercholesterolemia
Immune system
Internal medicine
Jaundice
Kaposi's sarcoma
Leptospirosis
Liver cancer
Liver disorders
Liver transplantation
Malabsorption
Malaria
Metabolism
Methicillin-resistant staphylococcus
    aureus (MRSA) infection
Niemann-Pick disease
Nonalcoholic steatohepatitis (NASH)
Phenylketonuria (PKU)
Polycystic kidney disease
Reye's syndrome
Shunts
Thrombocytopenia
Transplantation
Typhoid fever
Wilson's disease

Yellow fever

LUNGS
Abscess drainage
Acquired immunodeficiency
    syndrome (AIDS)
Acute respiratory distress syndrome
    (ARDS)
Adenoviruses
Allergies
Altitude sickness
Antihistamines
Apgar score
Apnea
Asbestos exposure
Aspergillosis
Asphyxiation
Asthma
Avian influenza
Bacterial infections
Bronchi
Bronchiolitis
Bronchitis
Cardiopulmonary resuscitation (CPR)
Chest
Childhood infectious diseases
Chlamydia
Choking
Chronic obstructive pulmonary
    disease (COPD)
Cold agglutinin disease
Common cold
Coronaviruses
Coughing
Croup
Cystic fibrosis
Cytomegalovirus (CMV)
Diaphragm
Drowning
Edema
Embolism
Emphysema
Endoscopy
Exercise physiology
Fetal surgery
Hantavirus
Hay fever
Heart transplantation
Heimlich maneuver
Hiccups
Histiocytosis
H1N1 influenza
Hyperbaric oxygen therapy
Hyperventilation
Hypoxia
Infarction
Influenza

Internal medicine
Interstitial pulmonary fibrosis (IPF)
Intravenous (IV) therapy
Kaposi's sarcoma
Kinesiology
Legionnaires' disease
Leptospirosis
Lung cancer
Lung surgery
Measles
Mesothelioma
Mold and mildew
Multiple chemical sensitivity
    syndrome
Niemann-Pick disease
Oxygen therapy
Plague
Pleurisy
Pneumocystis jirovecii
Pneumonia
Pneumothorax
Pulmonary diseases
Pulmonary edema
Pulmonary hypertension
Pulmonary medicine
Quinsy
Respiration
Respiratory distress syndrome
Resuscitation
Rhinoviruses
Roundworms
Sarcoidosis
Schistosomiasis
Scleroderma
Severe acute respiratory syndrome
    (SARS)
Sickle cell disease
Stevens-Johnson syndrome
Thoracic surgery
Thrombolytic therapy and TPA
Thrombosis and thrombus
Transplantation
Tuberculosis
Tumor removal
Vasculitis
Wiskott-Aldrich syndrome

LYMPHATIC SYSTEM
Acquired immunodeficiency
    syndrome (AIDS)
Adenoids
Antibodies
Bacillus Calmette-Guérin (BCG)
Bacterial infections
Biological therapies
Blood and blood disorders
Blood vessels

Breast cancer
Breast disorders
Bruises
Chlamydia
Cold agglutinin disease
Colorectal cancer
Coronaviruses
DiGeorge syndrome
Edema
Elephantiasis
Embolism
Epstein-Barr virus
Gaucher's disease
Hay fever
Hodgkin's disease
Immune system
Kawasaki disease
Klippel-Trenaunay syndrome
Leishmaniasis
Leptospirosis
Lower extremities
Lung cancer
Lymph
Lymphadenopathy and lymphoma
Mononucleosis
Overtraining syndrome
Prostate cancer
Roundworms
Rubella
Sarcoidosis
Skin cancer
Sleeping sickness
Small intestine
Splenectomy
Thymus gland
Tonsillectomy and adenoid removal
Tonsillitis
Tonsils
Tularemia
Upper extremities
Vascular medicine

MOUTH
Acid reflux disease
Acquired immunodeficiency
    syndrome (AIDS)
Adenoids
Angelman syndrome
Auras
Behçet's disease
Bell's palsy
Candidiasis
Canker sores
Chickenpox
Cleft lip and palate repair
Cold sores
Cornelia de Lange syndrome

Crowns and bridges
Dengue fever
Dental diseases
Dentistry
Dentures
DiGeorge syndrome
Dyskinesia
Eating disorders
Endodontic disease
Epstein-Barr virus
Esophagus
Facial transplantation
Fetal alcohol syndrome
Fluoride treatments
Gingivitis
Gum disease
Hand-foot-and-mouth disease
Heimlich maneuver
Herpes
Jaw wiring
Kawasaki disease
Lisping
Measles
Mouth and throat cancer
Oral and maxillofacial surgery
Orthodontics
Periodontal surgery
Pharynx
Quinsy
Rape and sexual assault
Raynaud's phenomenon
Reiter's syndrome
Root canal treatment
Rubinstein-Taybi syndrome
Sense organs
Sjögren's syndrome
Taste
Teething
Temporomandibular joint (TMJ)
    syndrome
Thumb sucking
Tooth extraction
Ulcers
Wisdom teeth

MUSCLES
Acidosis
Acupressure
Amputation
Anesthesia
Anesthesiology
Apgar score
Avian influenza
Back pain
Bed-wetting
Bedsores
Bell's palsy

Beriberi
Bile
Biofeedback
Botox
Bowlegs
Carbohydrates
Charcot-Marie-Tooth Disease
Chest
Chiari malformations
Childhood infectious diseases
Chronic fatigue syndrome
Cushing's syndrome
Diaphragm
Ebola virus
Electrocauterization
Electromyography
Epstein-Barr virus
Exercise physiology
Eye infections and disorders
Facial transplantation
Fatty acid oxidation disorders
Fibromyalgia
Flat feet
Foot disorders
Gangrene
Glycogen storage diseases
Glycolysis
Guillain-Barré syndrome
Gulf War syndrome
Head and neck disorders
Hemiplegia
Hiccups
Kinesiology
Kwashiorkor
Leukodystrophy
Mesenchymal stem cells
Methicillin-resistant staphylococcus
    aureus (MRSA) infection
Motor neuron diseases
Motor skill development
Multiple chemical sensitivity
    syndrome
Multiple sclerosis
Muscular dystrophy
Necrotizing fasciitis
Neurology
Numbness and tingling
Orthopedic surgery
Orthopedics
Osteopathic medicine
Overtraining syndrome
Palpitations
Palsy
Paralysis
Parkinson's disease
Physical rehabilitation
Pigeon toes

Poisoning
Poliomyelitis
Ptosis
Rabies
Respiration
Restless legs syndrome
Rotator cuff surgery
Sarcoma
Scurvy
Seizures
Smallpox
Speech disorders
Sphincterectomy
Spinocerebellar ataxia
Sports medicine
Steroid abuse
Strabismus
Streptococcal infections
Tattoos and body piercing
Temporomandibular joint (TMJ)
    syndrome
Tendon disorders
Tendon repair
Tetanus
Tics
Torticollis
Tourette's syndrome
Tremors
Trichinosis
Tularemia
Upper extremities
Weight loss and gain
Williams syndrome
Yoga

MUSCULOSKELETAL SYSTEM
Acupressure
Amputation
Amyotrophic lateral sclerosis
Anesthesia
Anesthesiology
Ankylosing spondylitis
Anorexia nervosa
Arthritis
Ataxia
Atrophy
Avian influenza
Back pain
Bed-wetting
Biofeedback
Bone cancer
Bone disorders
Bone grafting
Bone marrow transplantation
Bones and the skeleton
Brucellosis
Bulimia

Cartilage
Casts and splints
Cells
Charcot-Marie-Tooth Disease
Chest
Childhood infectious diseases
Chiropractic
Chronic fatigue syndrome
Cleft lip and palate
Cleft lip and palate repair
Collagen
Computed tomography (CT) scanning
Congenital hypothyroidism
Connective tissue
Dengue fever
Depression
Diaphragm
Dwarfism
Ear surgery
Ears
Ehrlichiosis
Ergogenic aids
Ewing's sarcoma
Exercise physiology
Feet
Fibromyalgia
Flat feet
Foot disorders
Fracture and dislocation
Fracture repair
Gigantism
Glycolysis
Guillain-Barré syndrome
Hammertoe correction
Head and neck disorders
Heel spur removal
Hematology
Hematomas
Hemiplegia
Hip fracture repair
Hyperparathyroidism and
    hypoparathyroidism
Jaw wiring
Joints
Juvenile rheumatoid arthritis
Kinesiology
Kneecap removal
Lead poisoning
Ligaments
Lower extremities
Marfan syndrome
Mesenchymal stem cells
Methicillin-resistant staphylococcus
    aureus (MRSA) infection
Motor neuron diseases
Motor skill development
Multiple sclerosis

Muscles
Muscular dystrophy
Myasthenia gravis
Neurology
Nuclear medicine
Nuclear radiology
Numbness and tingling
Orthopedic surgery
Orthopedics
Osgood-Schlatter disease
Osteoarthritis
Osteochondritis juvenilis
Osteogenesis imperfecta
Osteomyelitis
Osteonecrosis
Osteopathic medicine
Paget's disease
Palsy
Paralysis
Parkinson's disease
Physical rehabilitation
Poisoning
Poliomyelitis
Prader-Willi syndrome
Precocious puberty
Rabies
Radiculopathy
Respiration
Restless legs syndrome
Rheumatoid arthritis
Rheumatology
Rickets
Scoliosis
Seizures
Sleepwalking
Slipped disk
Speech disorders
Sphincterectomy
Spinal cord disorders
Spinocerebellar ataxia
Sports medicine
Staphylococcal infections
Teeth
Tendinitis
Tendon disorders
Tendon repair
Tetanus
Tics
Tourette's syndrome
Trichinosis
Upper extremities
Weight loss and gain

NAILS
Anorexia nervosa
Athlete's foot
Collodion baby

Dermatology
Fungal infections
Malnutrition
Nail removal
Podiatry

NECK
Botox
Carotid arteries
Casts and splints
Chiari malformations
Choking
Congenital hypothyroidism
Dyskinesia
Encephalitis
Endarterectomy
Facial transplantation
Goiter
Hashimoto's thyroiditis
Head and neck disorders
Heimlich maneuver
Hyperparathyroidism and
    hypoparathyroidism
Mouth and throat cancer
Neuroimaging
Paralysis
Parathyroidectomy
Pharynx
Pityriasis alba
Slipped disk
Stevens-Johnson syndrome
Streptococcal infections
Sympathectomy
Thyroid disorders
Thyroid gland
Thyroidectomy
Torticollis
Trachea
Tracheostomy
Vagus nerve
Whiplash
Whooping cough

NERVES
Agnosia
Alzheimer's disease
Anesthesia
Anesthesiology
Angelman syndrome
Avian influenza
Back pain
Bell's palsy
Biofeedback
Brain
Bulimia
Carpal tunnel syndrome
Cells

Cluster headaches
Concussion
Dyskinesia
Electromyography
Encephalitis
Epilepsy
Eye infections and disorders
Facial transplantation
Fibromyalgia
Guillain-Barré syndrome
Hearing
Herpes
Hirschsprung's disease
Huntington's disease
Leprosy
Leukodystrophy
Listeria infections
Local anesthesia
Lower extremities
Lumbar puncture
Lyme disease
Motor neuron diseases
Motor skill development
Multiple chemical sensitivity
    syndrome
Multiple sclerosis
Neonatal brachial plexus palsy
Nervous system
Neuroimaging
Neurology
Neurosis
Neurosurgery
Numbness and tingling
Palsy
Paralysis
Parkinson's disease
Physical rehabilitation
Poliomyelitis
Postherpetic neuralgia
Ptosis
Radiculopathy
Sarcoidosis
Sciatica
Seizures
Sense organs
Shock therapy
Skin
Slipped disk
Spinal cord disorders
Spinocerebellar ataxia
Sturge-Weber syndrome
Sympathectomy
Tics
Tinnitus
Touch
Tourette's syndrome
Tremors

Upper extremities
Vagotomy
Vasculitis

NERVOUS SYSTEM
Abscess drainage
Acupressure
Addiction
Adenoviruses
Adrenoleukodystrophy
Agnosia
Alcoholism
Altitude sickness
Alzheimer's disease
Amnesia
Amputation
Amyotrophic lateral sclerosis
Anesthesia
Anesthesiology
Aneurysms
Angelman syndrome
Anorexia nervosa
Anosmia
Anthrax
Antidepressants
Anxiety
Apgar score
Aphasia and dysphasia
Apnea
Aromatherapy
Ataxia
Atrophy
Attention-deficit disorder (ADD)
Auras
Avian influenza
Back pain
Balance disorders
Batten's disease
Behçet's disease
Beriberi
Biofeedback
Botulism
Brain
Brain damage
Brain disorders
Brain tumors
Brucellosis
Caffeine
Cells
Chagas' disease
Charcot-Marie-Tooth Disease
Chiari malformations
Chiropractic
Chronic wasting disease (CWD)
Cluster headaches
Cognitive development
Colon

Computed tomography (CT) scanning
Concussion
Congenital hypothyroidism
Creutzfeldt-Jakob disease (CJD)
Cutis marmorata telangiectatica
     congenita
Deafness
Defibrillation
Dementias
Developmental disorders
Developmental stages
Diabetes mellitus
Diphtheria
Disk removal
Dizziness and fainting
Down syndrome
Drowning
Dwarfism
Dyskinesia
Dyslexia
E. coli infection
Ear surgery
Ears
Ehrlichiosis
Electrical shock
Electroencephalography (EEG)
Electromyography
Encephalitis
Endocrinology
Enteroviruses
Epilepsy
Eyes
Facial transplantation
Fetal tissue transplantation
Fibromyalgia
Frontotemporal dementia (FTD)
Glands
Glasgow coma scale
Guillain-Barré syndrome
Hammertoe correction
Head and neck disorders
Headaches
Hearing tests
Heart transplantation
Hemiplegia
Hemolytic uremic syndrome
Histiocytosis
Huntington's disease
Hydrocephalus
Hypnosis
Hypothalamus
Intraventricular hemorrhage
Irritable bowel syndrome (IBS)
Kinesiology
Lead poisoning
Learning disabilities
Leprosy

Leptospirosis
Light therapy
Listeria infections
Local anesthesia
Lower extremities
Lumbar puncture
Lyme disease
Maple syrup urine disease (MSUD)
Measles
Memory loss
Ménière's disease
Meningitis
Mental retardation
Mental status exam
Mercury poisoning
Motion sickness
Motor neuron diseases
Motor skill development
Multiple chemical sensitivity
     syndrome
Multiple sclerosis
Mumps
Myasthenia gravis
Narcolepsy
Nausea and vomiting
Neurofibromatosis
Neuroimaging
Neurology
Neurosis
Neurosurgery
Niemann-Pick disease
Nuclear radiology
Numbness and tingling
Orthopedic surgery
Orthopedics
Overtraining syndrome
Palsy
Paralysis
Paraplegia
Parkinson's disease
Pharmacology
Phenylketonuria (PKU)
Physical rehabilitation
Pick's disease
Poisoning
Poliomyelitis
Porphyria
Precocious puberty
Preeclampsia and eclampsia
Prion diseases
Quadriplegia
Rabies
Radiculopathy
Restless legs syndrome
Reye's syndrome
Rocky Mountain spotted fever
Rubella

Sarcoidosis
Sciatica
Seasonal affective disorder
Seizures
Sense organs
Shingles
Shock therapy
Shunts
Skin
Sleep
Sleep disorders
Sleeping sickness
Sleepwalking
Slipped disk
Small intestine
Smell
Snakebites
Spina bifida
Spinal cord disorders
Spinocerebellar ataxia
Sports medicine
Staphylococcal infections
Strokes
Sturge-Weber syndrome
Stuttering
Sympathectomy
Synesthesia
Syphilis
Tardive dyskinesia
Taste
Tay-Sachs disease
Teeth
Tetanus
Thrombolytic therapy and TPA
Tics
Tinnitus
Touch
Tourette's syndrome
Toxoplasmosis
Tremors
Typhus
Upper extremities
Vagotomy
Vertigo
Vision
West Nile virus
Wilson's disease
Yoga

NOSE
Adenoids
Allergies
Anosmia
Antihistamines
Aromatherapy
Auras
Avian influenza

Cartilage
Casts and splints
Chickenpox
Childhood infectious diseases
Cold agglutinin disease
Common cold
Cornelia de Lange syndrome
Decongestants
Dengue fever
Epstein-Barr virus
Facial transplantation
Fifth disease
Hay fever
H1N1 influenza
Influenza
Methicillin-resistant staphylococcus
    aureus (MRSA) infection
Mold and mildew
Nasal polyp removal
Nasopharyngeal disorders
Otorhinolaryngology
Pharynx
Polyps
Pulmonary medicine
Respiration
Rhinitis
Rhinoplasty and submucous resection
Rhinoviruses
Rosacea
Rubinstein-Taybi syndrome
Sense organs
Sinusitis
Skin lesion removal
Smell
Sore throat
Stevens-Johnson syndrome
Taste
Tears and tear ducts
Vasculitis

PANCREAS
Abscess drainage
Alcoholism
Carbohydrates
Cholecystitis
Chyme
Diabetes mellitus
Digestion
Endocrine glands
Endocrinology
Endoscopic retrograde
    cholangiopancreatography (ERCP)
Fetal tissue transplantation
Food biochemistry
Gastroenterology
Gastrointestinal system
Glands

Hemochromatosis
Internal medicine
Malabsorption
Metabolism
Mumps
Pancreatitis
Polycystic kidney disease
Polycystic ovary syndrome
Transplantation

**PSYCHIC-EMOTIONAL
SYSTEM**
Acquired immunodeficiency
    syndrome (AIDS)
Addiction
Adrenoleukodystrophy
Alcoholism
Alzheimer's disease
Amnesia
Anesthesia
Anesthesiology
Angelman syndrome
Anorexia nervosa
Antianxiety drugs
Antidepressants
Antihistamines
Anxiety
Aphrodisiacs
Aromatherapy
Asperger's syndrome
Attention-deficit disorder (ADD)
Auras
Autism
Bariatric surgery
Biofeedback
Bipolar disorders
Body dysmorphic disorder
Bonding
Brain
Brain disorders
Bulimia
Chronic fatigue syndrome
Cognitive development
Colic
Death and dying
Dementias
Depression
Developmental disorders
Developmental stages
Dizziness and fainting
Down syndrome
Dyskinesia
Dyslexia
Eating disorders
Electroencephalography (EEG)
Encephalitis
Endocrinology

Factitious disorders
Failure to thrive
Fibromyalgia
Frontotemporal dementia (FTD)
Gender identity disorder
Gulf War syndrome
Headaches
Hormone therapy
Hormones
Hydrocephalus
Hypnosis
Hypochondriasis
Hypothalamus
Interpartner violence
Kinesiology
Klinefelter syndrome
Learning disabilities
Light therapy
Memory loss
Menopause
Mental retardation
Miscarriage
Morgellons disease
Motor skill development
Narcolepsy
Neurology
Neurosis
Neurosurgery
Obesity
Obsessive-compulsive disorder
Overtraining syndrome
Paranoia
Pharmacology
Phobias
Pick's disease
Postpartum depression
Post-traumatic stress disorder
Prader-Willi syndrome
Precocious puberty
Premenstrual syndrome (PMS)
Psychiatric disorders
Psychoanalysis
Psychosis
Rabies
Rape and sexual assault
Restless legs syndrome
Schizophrenia
Seasonal affective disorder
Separation anxiety
Sexual dysfunction
Sexuality
Shock therapy
Sleep
Sleep disorders
Sleeping sickness
Sleepwalking
Soiling

Speech disorders
Sperm banks
Steroid abuse
Strokes
Suicide
Synesthesia
Tics
Tinnitus
Toilet training
Tourette's syndrome
Weight loss and gain
West Nile virus
Wilson's disease
Yoga

REPRODUCTIVE SYSTEM
Abdomen
Abortion
Acquired immunodeficiency
    syndrome (AIDS)
Adrenoleukodystrophy
Amenorrhea
Amniocentesis
Anorexia nervosa
Assisted reproductive technologies
Avian influenza
Breast-feeding
Brucellosis
Candidiasis
Catheterization
Cervical procedures
Cesarean section
Childbirth
Childbirth complications
Chlamydia
Chorionic villus sampling
Computed tomography (CT) scanning
Conception
Congenital adrenal hyperplasia
Contraception
Culdocentesis
Cyst removal
Cystoscopy
Dysmenorrhea
Eating disorders
Ectopic pregnancy
Endocrine glands
Endocrinology
Endometrial biopsy
Endometriosis
Episiotomy
Erectile dysfunction
Fistula repair
Gamete intrafallopian transfer (GIFT)
Gender reassignment surgery
Genetic counseling
Gestational diabetes

Gigantism
Glands
Gonorrhea
Gynecology
Hermaphroditism and
    pseudohermaphroditism
Hernia
Herpes
Hormone therapy
Human papillomavirus (HPV)
Hydroceles
Hypospadias repair and urethroplasty
Hysterectomy
In vitro fertilization
Internal medicine
Klinefelter syndrome
Laparoscopy
Lead poisoning
Ligaments
Menopause
Menorrhagia
Menstruation
Miscarriage
Myomectomy
Obstetrics
Orchiectomy
Orchitis
Ovarian cysts
Pap test
Pelvic inflammatory disease (PID)
Penile implant surgery
Placenta
Polycystic ovary syndrome
Polyps
Precocious puberty
Preeclampsia and eclampsia
Pregnancy and gestation
Premature birth
Premenstrual syndrome (PMS)
Prostate cancer
Prostate enlargement
Prostate gland
Semen
Sexual differentiation
Sexual dysfunction
Sexuality
Sexually transmitted diseases (STDs)
Sperm banks
Sterilization
Steroid abuse
Stevens-Johnson syndrome
Stillbirth
Syphilis
Testicular surgery
Testicular torsion
Toxemia
Trichomoniasis

Tubal ligation
Turner syndrome
Ultrasonography
Urology
Uterus
Vas deferens
Vasectomy
Von Willebrand's disease

RESPIRATORY SYSTEM
Abscess drainage
Acidosis
Acquired immunodeficiency
  syndrome (AIDS)
Acute respiratory distress syndrome
  (ARDS)
Adenoviruses
Adrenoleukodystrophy
Altitude sickness
Amyotrophic lateral sclerosis
Anthrax
Antihistamines
Apgar score
Apnea
Asbestos exposure
Asphyxiation
Asthma
Avian influenza
Babesiosis
Bacterial infections
Bronchi
Bronchiolitis
Bronchitis
Cardiopulmonary resuscitation (CPR)
Chest
Childhood infectious diseases
Choking
Chronic obstructive pulmonary
  disease (COPD)
Cold agglutinin disease
Common cold
Computed tomography (CT) scanning
Coronaviruses
Coughing
Croup
Cystic fibrosis
Decongestants
Defibrillation
Diaphragm
Drowning
Dwarfism
Edema
Emphysema
Epiglottitis
Exercise physiology
Fetal surgery
Fluids and electrolytes

Food allergies
Fungal infections
Hantavirus
Hay fever
Head and neck disorders
Heart transplantation
Heimlich maneuver
Hiccups
H1N1 influenza
Hyperbaric oxygen therapy
Hyperventilation
Hypoxia
Influenza
Internal medicine
Kinesiology
Laryngectomy
Legionnaires' disease
Lung cancer
Lung surgery
Lungs
Measles
Mesothelioma
Methicillin-resistant staphylococcus
  aureus (MRSA) infection
Mold and mildew
Monkeypox
Multiple chemical sensitivity
  syndrome
Nasopharyngeal disorders
Niemann-Pick disease
Obesity
Otorhinolaryngology
Oxygen therapy
Pharynx
Plague
Plasma
Pneumocystis jirovecii
Pneumonia
Pneumothorax
Poisoning
Pulmonary diseases
Pulmonary edema
Pulmonary hypertension
Pulmonary medicine
Respiration
Resuscitation
Rheumatoid arthritis
Rhinitis
Rhinoviruses
Sarcoidosis
Severe acute respiratory syndrome
  (SARS)
Sinusitis
Sleep apnea
Smoking
Sore throat
Staphylococcal infections

Stevens-Johnson syndrome
Thoracic surgery
Thrombolytic therapy and TPA
Thrombosis and thrombus
Tonsillectomy and adenoid removal
Trachea
Tracheostomy
Transplantation
Tuberculosis
Tularemia
Tumor removal
Typhus
Vasculitis
Voice and vocal cord disorders
Whooping cough

SKIN
Abscess drainage
Acne
Acquired immunodeficiency
  syndrome (AIDS)
Acupressure
Adenoviruses
Adrenoleukodystrophy
Allergies
Amputation
Anesthesia
Anesthesiology
Angelman syndrome
Anorexia nervosa
Anthrax
Anxiety
Athlete's foot
Auras
Bacillus Calmette-Guérin (BCG)
Bariatric surgery
Batten's disease
Bedsores
Behçet's disease
Bites and stings
Blisters
Blood testing
Body dysmorphic disorder
Bruises
Burns and scalds
Candidiasis
Canker sores
Casts and splints
Cells
Chagas' disease
Chickenpox
Cleft lip and palate repair
Cold agglutinin disease
Cold sores
Collagen
Collodion baby
Corns and calluses

Cushing's syndrome
Cutis marmorata telangiectatica
    congenita
Cyanosis
Cyst removal
Dengue fever
Dermatitis
Dermatology
Dermatopathology
Ebola virus
Eczema
Edema
Electrical shock
Electrocauterization
Enteroviruses
Face lift and blepharoplasty
Facial transplantation
Fibrocystic breast condition
Fifth disease
Food allergies
Frostbite
Fungal infections
Gangrene
Glands
Gluten intolerance
Gulf War syndrome
Hair
Hair transplantation
Hand-foot-and-mouth disease
Heat exhaustion and heatstroke
Hematomas
Hemolytic disease of the newborn
Herpes
Histiocytosis
Hives
Hormone therapy
Host-defense mechanisms
Human papillomavirus (HPV)
Hyperhidrosis
Impetigo
Intravenous (IV) therapy
Jaundice
Kaposi's sarcoma
Kawasaki disease
Kwashiorkor
Laceration repair
Laser use in surgery
Leishmaniasis
Leprosy
Light therapy
Lower extremities
Lyme disease
Measles
Melanoma
Methicillin-resistant staphylococcus
    aureus (MRSA) infection
Mold and mildew

Moles
Monkeypox
Morgellons disease
Multiple chemical sensitivity
    syndrome
Nails
Necrotizing fasciitis
Neurofibromatosis
Numbness and tingling
Otoplasty
Pigmentation
Pinworms
Pityriasis alba
Pityriasis rosea
Polycystic ovary syndrome
Polydactyly and syndactyly
Porphyria
Psoriasis
Radiation sickness
Reiter's syndrome
Ringworm
Rocky Mountain spotted fever
Rosacea
Roseola
Rubella
Sarcoidosis
Scabies
Scarlet fever
Sense organs
Shingles
Skin cancer
Skin disorders
Skin lesion removal
Smallpox
Streptococcal infections
Sturge-Weber syndrome
Styes
Sweating
Tattoo removal
Tattoos and body piercing
Touch
Toxoplasmosis
Tularemia
Typhoid fever
Typhus
Umbilical cord
Upper extremities
Vasculitis
Vitiligo
Von Willebrand's disease
Williams syndrome
Wiskott-Aldrich syndrome

SPINE
Anesthesia
Anesthesiology
Ankylosing spondylitis

Atrophy
Back pain
Brain tumors
Brucellosis
Charcot-Marie-Tooth Disease
Chiari malformations
Chiropractic
Diaphragm
Disk removal
Fetal tissue transplantation
Head and neck disorders
Kinesiology
Laminectomy and spinal fusion
Lumbar puncture
Marfan syndrome
Meningitis
Mesenchymal stem cells
Methicillin-resistant staphylococcus
    aureus (MRSA) infection
Motor neuron diseases
Multiple sclerosis
Nervous system
Neuroimaging
Neurology
Neurosurgery
Orthopedic surgery
Orthopedics
Osteogenesis imperfecta
Osteoporosis
Paget's disease
Paralysis
Paraplegia
Physical rehabilitation
Poliomyelitis
Quadriplegia
Radiculopathy
Sciatica
Scoliosis
Slipped disk
Spina bifida
Spinal cord disorders
Spondylitis
Sports medicine
Stenosis
Sympathectomy
Whiplash
Williams syndrome

SPLEEN
Abscess drainage
Aspergillosis
Brucellosis
Cold agglutinin disease
Gaucher's disease
Hematology
Immune system
Internal medicine

Leptospirosis
Lymph
Lymphatic system
Malaria
Metabolism
Methicillin-resistant staphylococcus aureus (MRSA) infection
Mononucleosis
Niemann-Pick disease
Sarcoidosis
Sickle cell disease
Splenectomy
Thrombocytopenia
Transplantation
Typhoid fever

STOMACH
Abdomen
Abdominal disorders
Abscess drainage
Acid reflux disease
Adenoviruses
Allergies
Avian influenza
Bariatric surgery
Campylobacter infections
Chyme
Colitis
Digestion
Drowning
Eating disorders
Endoscopic retrograde cholangiopancreatography (ERCP)
Endoscopy
Esophagus
Food biochemistry
Food poisoning
Gastrectomy
Gastroenteritis
Gastroenterology
Gastrointestinal disorders
Gastrointestinal system
Gastrostomy
Hernia
Hernia repair
Internal medicine
Lactose intolerance
Malabsorption
Malnutrition
Metabolism
Motion sickness
Nausea and vomiting
Obesity
Peristalsis
Poisoning
Polyps
Pyloric stenosis

Radiation sickness
Ulcer surgery
Ulcers
Vagotomy
Weaning
Weight loss and gain

TEETH
Angelman syndrome
Bulimia
Cavities
Cornelia de Lange syndrome
Crowns and bridges
Dental diseases
Dentistry
Dentures
Eating disorders
Endodontic disease
Fluoride treatments
Fracture repair
Gastrointestinal system
Gingivitis
Gum disease
Jaw wiring
Lisping
Mouth and throat cancer
Oral and maxillofacial surgery
Orthodontics
Osteogenesis imperfecta
Periodontal surgery
Periodontitis
Prader-Willi syndrome
Rickets
Root canal treatment
Rubinstein-Taybi syndrome
Scurvy
Teething
Temporomandibular joint (TMJ) syndrome
Thumb sucking
Tooth extraction
Wisdom teeth

TENDONS
Ankylosing spondylitis
Carpal tunnel syndrome
Casts and splints
Collagen
Connective tissue
Exercise physiology
Ganglion removal
Hammertoe correction
Hemiplegia
Joints
Kneecap removal
Mesenchymal stem cells
Orthopedic surgery

Orthopedics
Osgood-Schlatter disease
Physical rehabilitation
Sports medicine
Tendinitis
Tendon disorders
Tendon repair

THROAT
Acid reflux disease
Acquired immunodeficiency syndrome (AIDS)
Adenoids
Antihistamines
Auras
Avian influenza
Catheterization
Choking
Croup
Decongestants
Diphtheria
Drowning
Eating disorders
Epiglottitis
Epstein-Barr virus
Esophagus
Fifth disease
Gastroenterology
Gastrointestinal system
Gonorrhea
Hay fever
Head and neck disorders
Heimlich maneuver
Hiccups
Histiocytosis
H1N1 influenza
Influenza
Laryngectomy
Laryngitis
Mononucleosis
Mouth and throat cancer
Nasopharyngeal disorders
Otorhinolaryngology
Pharyngitis
Pharynx
Polyps
Pulmonary medicine
Quinsy
Respiration
Rhinitis
Rhinoviruses
Smoking
Sore throat
Streptococcal infections
Tonsillectomy and adenoid removal
Tonsillitis
Tracheostomy

Tremors
Voice and vocal cord disorders
Whooping cough

URINARY SYSTEM
Abdomen
Abdominal disorders
Abscess drainage
Adenoviruses
Adrenalectomy
Avian influenza
Bed-wetting
Bladder cancer
Bladder removal
Candidiasis
Catheterization
Chlamydia
Cold agglutinin disease
Cystitis
Cystoscopy
Dialysis
Diuretics
E. coli infection
End-stage renal disease
Endoscopy
Fetal surgery
Fistula repair
Gonorrhea
Hematuria
Hemolytic uremic syndrome
Hermaphroditism and
    pseudohermaphroditism
Hormone therapy
Host-defense mechanisms
Hyperplasia
Hypertension
Incontinence
Internal medicine
Kidney cancer

Kidney disorders
Kidney transplantation
Kidneys
Laparoscopy
Leptospirosis
Lithotripsy
Nephrectomy
Nephrology
Plasma
Polyps
Prostate enlargement
Proteinuria
Pyelonephritis
Reiter's syndrome
Reye's syndrome
Schistosomiasis
Staphylococcal infections
Stevens-Johnson syndrome
Stone removal
Stones
Testicular cancer
Toilet training
Transplantation
Trichomoniasis
Ultrasonography
Uremia
Urethritis
Urinalysis
Urinary disorders
Urology

UTERUS
Abdomen
Abortion
Amniocentesis
Assisted reproductive technologies
Cervical procedures
Cesarean section
Childbirth

Childbirth complications
Chorionic villus sampling
Conception
Contraception
Dysmenorrhea
Electrocauterization
Embolization
Endocrinology
Endometrial biopsy
Endometriosis
Fistula repair
Gender reassignment surgery
Genetic counseling
Gynecology
Hormone therapy
Hyperplasia
Hysterectomy
In vitro fertilization
Internal medicine
Laparoscopy
Menopause
Menorrhagia
Menstruation
Miscarriage
Myomectomy
Obstetrics
Pap test
Pelvic inflammatory disease (PID)
Placenta
Polyps
Pregnancy and gestation
Premature birth
Reproductive system
Sexual differentiation
Sperm banks
Sterilization
Stillbirth
Tubal ligation
Ultrasonography

ENTRIES BY SPECIALTIES AND RELATED FIELDS

ALL
Abscesses
Accidents
Anatomy
Autoimmune disorders
Biostatistics
Carcinogens
Clinical trials
Cysts
Diagnosis
Disease
Emergency rooms
Emerging infectious diseases
Environmental diseases
Epidermal nevus syndromes
Fetal alcohol syndrome
First aid
Geriatrics and gerontology
Herbal medicine
Iatrogenic disorders
Internet medicine
Invasive tests
Medical home
Men's health
Neuroimaging
Physical examination
Physiology
Preventive medicine
Prognosis
Proteomics
Self-medication
Signs and symptoms
Substance abuse
Syndrome
Systemic sclerosis
Systems and organs
Terminally ill: Extended care
Toxicology
Transitional care

ALTERNATIVE MEDICINE
Acidosis
Acupressure
Acupuncture
Amyotrophic lateral sclerosis
Antioxidants
Aphrodisiacs
Aromatherapy
Back pain
Biofeedback
Biological therapies
Chemotherapy

Club drugs
Colon
Colon therapy
Enzyme therapy
Fiber
Genetic engineering
Healing
Hydrotherapy
Hypnosis
Irritable bowel syndrome (IBS)
Magnetic field therapy
Marijuana
Massage
Meditation
Melatonin
Pain management
Small intestine
Stress reduction
Supplements
Yoga

ANESTHESIOLOGY
Acidosis
Acupuncture
Anesthesia
Anesthesiology
Aneurysmectomy
Arthroplasty
Back pain
Catheterization
Cesarean section
Critical care
Defibrillation
Dentistry
Hyperbaric oxygen therapy
Hyperthermia and hypothermia
Hypnosis
Hypoxia
Intravenous (IV) therapy
Local anesthesia
Lumbar puncture
Mesenchymal stem cells
Oral and maxillofacial surgery
Oxygen therapy
Pain
Pain management
Palliative medicine
Pharmacology
Pulse rate
Surgical procedures
Surgical technologists

AUDIOLOGY
Adrenoleukodystrophy
Aging: Extended care
Charcot-Marie-Tooth Disease
Cockayne Disease
Deafness
Dyslexia
Ear infections and disorders
Ear surgery
Ears
Earwax
Hearing
Hearing aids
Hearing loss
Hearing tests
Ménière's disease
Neurology
Otoplasty
Otorhinolaryngology
Sense organs
Speech disorders
Tinnitus
Vertigo
Williams syndrome

BACTERIOLOGY
Acquired immunodeficiency
  syndrome (AIDS)
Amebiasis
Anthrax
Antibiotic resistance
Antibiotics
Antibodies
Bacillus Calmette-Guérin (BCG)
Bacterial infections
Botulism
Brucellosis
Campylobacter infections
Cells
Childhood infectious diseases
Chronic granulomatous disease
Cold agglutinin disease
Conjunctivitis
Cystitis
Cytology
Cytopathology
Diphtheria
E. coli infection
Encephalitis
Endocarditis
Epidemics and pandemics
Epiglottitis

Eye infections and disorders
Fluoride treatments
Gangrene
Gastroenteritis
Genomics
Gingivitis
Gram staining
Impetigo
Infection
Insect-borne diseases
Laboratory tests
Legionnaires' disease
Leprosy
Leptospirosis
Listeria infections
Lyme disease
Mastitis
Methicillin-resistant staphylococcus
   aureus (MRSA) infection
Microbiology
Microscopy
Necrotizing fasciitis
Opportunistic infections
Osteomyelitis
Peritonitis
Plague
Salmonella infection
Sarcoidosis
Scarlet fever
Serology
Shigellosis
Staphylococcal infections
Streptococcal infections
Styes
Syphilis
Tetanus
Tuberculosis
Tularemia
Typhoid fever
Typhus
Urethritis
Whooping cough
Zoonoses

BIOCHEMISTRY
Acid-base chemistry
Acidosis
Amyotrophic lateral sclerosis
Antibodies
Antidepressants
Autopsy
Avian influenza
Bacteriology
Bulimia
Caffeine
Carbohydrates
Cholesterol

Collagen
Colon
Connective tissue
Corticosteroids
Digestion
Endocrine glands
Endocrinology
Enzyme therapy
Ergogenic aids
Fatty acid oxidation disorders
Fluids and electrolytes
Fluoride treatments
Food biochemistry
Food guide plate
Fructosemia
Galactosemia
Gaucher's disease
Genetic engineering
Genomics
Gigantism
Gingivitis
Glands
Glycogen storage diseases
Glycolysis
Gram staining
Gulf War syndrome
Histology
Hormones
Hyperadiposis
Hypothalamus
Insect-borne diseases
Leptin
Leukodystrophy
Lipids
Lumbar puncture
Macronutrients
Malabsorption
Malaria
Metabolic disorders
Metabolism
Nephrology
Niemann-Pick disease
Nutrition
Osteogenesis imperfecta
Ovaries
Pathology
Pharmacology
Phenylketonuria (PKU)
Pituitary gland
Plasma
Protein
Respiration
Retroviruses
Rhinoviruses
Sleep
Small intestine
Stem cells

Steroids
Thymus gland
Tourette's syndrome
Urinalysis
Wilson's disease

BIOTECHNOLOGY
Antibodies
Assisted reproductive technologies
Biological therapies
Bionics and biotechnology
Cloning
Computed tomography (CT) scanning
Defibrillation
Dialysis
Electrocardiography (ECG or EKG)
Electroencephalography (EEG)
Fatty acid oxidation disorders
Gene therapy
Genetic engineering
Genomics
Glycogen storage diseases
Huntington's disease
Hyperbaric oxygen therapy
Insect-borne diseases
Magnetic resonance imaging (MRI)
Malabsorption
Mesenchymal stem cells
Nephrology
Pacemaker implantation
Positron emission tomography (PET)
   scanning
Prostheses
Rhinoviruses
Severe combined immunodeficiency
   syndrome (SCID)
Sperm banks
Stem cells
Xenotransplantation

CARDIOLOGY
Acute respiratory distress syndrome
   (ARDS)
Aging: Extended care
Anemia
Aneurysms
Angina
Angiography
Angioplasty
Antihypertensives
Anxiety
Aortic aneurysm
Aortic stenosis
Arrhythmias
Arteriosclerosis
Aspergillosis
Atrial fibrillation

Biofeedback
Blood pressure
Blood vessels
Blue baby syndrome
Brucellosis
Bypass surgery
Cardiac arrest
Cardiac rehabilitation
Cardiac surgery
Cardiopulmonary resuscitation (CPR)
Carotid arteries
Catheterization
Chest
Circulation
Computed tomography (CT) scanning
Congenital heart disease
Coronary artery bypass graft
Critical care
Defibrillation
DiGeorge syndrome
Diphtheria
Diuretics
Dizziness and fainting
Echocardiography
Electrocardiography (ECG or EKG)
Electrocauterization
Embolism
Emergency medicine
End-stage renal disease
Endocarditis
Enteroviruses
Exercise physiology
Fetal surgery
Gigantism
Heart
Heart attack
Heart disease
Heart failure
Heart transplantation
Heart valve replacement
Hematology
Hemochromatosis
Hormone therapy
Hypercholesterolemia
Hypertension
Hypotension
Infarction
Internal medicine
Ischemia
Kawasaki disease
Kinesiology
Leptin
Lesions
Lyme disease
Marfan syndrome
Metabolic syndrome
Methicillin-resistant staphylococcus

aureus (MRSA) infection
Mitral valve prolapse
Mucopolysaccharidosis (MPS)
Muscles
Neonatology
Noninvasive tests
Nuclear medicine
Oxygen therapy
Pacemaker implantation
Palliative care
Palpitations
Paramedics
Plasma
Polycystic kidney disease
Prader-Willi syndrome
Progeria
Prostheses
Pulmonary edema
Pulmonary hypertension
Pulse rate
Rheumatic fever
Rubinstein-Taybi syndrome
Sarcoidosis
Single photon emission computed
   tomography (SPECT)
Spondylitis
Sports medicine
Staphylococcal infections
Stem cells
Stenosis
Stents
Systemic lupus erythematosus (SLE)
Thoracic surgery
Thrombolytic therapy and TPA
Thrombosis and thrombus
Transplantation
Ultrasonography
Uremia
Varicose veins
Vascular medicine
Vascular system
Vasculitis
Venous insufficiency
Williams syndrome

CRITICAL CARE
Acidosis
Aging: Extended care
Amputation
Anesthesia
Anesthesiology
Aneurysmectomy
Anthrax
Apgar score
Botulism
Burns and scalds
Carotid arteries

Catheterization
Chronic granulomatous disease
Club drugs
Concussion
Craniotomy
Defibrillation
Diuretics
Drowning
Echocardiography
Electrical shock
Electrocardiography (ECG or EKG)
Electrocauterization
Electroencephalography (EEG)
Embolization
Emergency medicine
Epidemics and pandemics
Grafts and grafting
Hantavirus
Heart attack
Heart transplantation
Heat exhaustion and heatstroke
Hydrocephalus
Hyperbaric oxygen therapy
Hyperthermia and hypothermia
Hypotension
Hypoxia
Infarction
Insect-borne diseases
Intravenous (IV) therapy
Ischemia
Lumbar puncture
Methicillin-resistant staphylococcus
   aureus (MRSA) infection
Necrotizing fasciitis
Neonatology
Nursing
Oncology
Osteopathic medicine
Oxygen therapy
Pain management
Paramedics
Peritonitis
Psychiatry
Pulmonary medicine
Pulse rate
Radiation sickness
Resuscitation
Safety issues for children
Safety issues for the elderly
Severe acute respiratory syndrome
   (SARS)
Shock
Stevens-Johnson syndrome
Streptococcal infections
Thrombolytic therapy and TPA
Toxic shock syndrome
Tracheostomy

Transfusion
Whooping cough
Wounds

CYTOLOGY

Acid-base chemistry
Bionics and biotechnology
Biopsy
Blood testing
Breast disorders
Cancer
Carcinoma
Cells
Cholesterol
Cytopathology
Dermatology
Dermatopathology
Epstein-Barr virus
Eye infections and disorders
Fluids and electrolytes
Food biochemistry
Gaucher's disease
Gene therapy
Genetic counseling
Genomics
Glycolysis
Gram staining
Healing
Hematology
Hirschsprung's disease
Histology
Hyperplasia
Immune system
Karyotyping
Laboratory tests
Lipids
Metabolism
Microscopy
Mutation
Oncology
Pathology
Pharmacology
Plasma
Rhinoviruses
Sarcoma
Serology
Stem cells

DENTISTRY

Aging: Extended care
Anesthesia
Anesthesiology
Canker sores
Cavities
Cerebral palsy
Cockayne Disease
Crowns and bridges

Dental diseases
Dentures
Eating disorders
Endodontic disease
Fluoride treatments
Forensic pathology
Fracture repair
Gastrointestinal system
Gingivitis
Gum disease
Head and neck disorders
Jaw wiring
Lisping
Local anesthesia
Mouth and throat cancer
Oral and maxillofacial surgery
Orthodontics
Osteogenesis imperfecta
Periodontal surgery
Periodontitis
Prader-Willi syndrome
Prostheses
Root canal treatment
Rubinstein-Taybi syndrome
Sense organs
Sjögren's syndrome
Teeth
Teething
Temporomandibular joint (TMJ)
    syndrome
Thumb sucking
Tooth extraction
Von Willebrand's disease
Wisdom teeth

DERMATOLOGY

Abscess drainage
Acne
Acquired immunodeficiency
    syndrome (AIDS)
Adrenoleukodystrophy
Allergies
Alopecia
Angelman syndrome
Anthrax
Anti-inflammatory drugs
Athlete's foot
Bedsores
Bile
Biopsy
Blisters
Body dysmorphic disorder
Burns and scalds
Carcinoma
Chickenpox
Chronic granulomatous disease
Coccidioidomycosis

Cockayne Disease
Collodion baby
Corns and calluses
Cryosurgery
Cutis marmorata telangiectatica
    congenita
Cyst removal
Dermatitis
Dermatopathology
Eczema
Electrocauterization
Enteroviruses
Facial transplantation
Fungal infections
Ganglion removal
Gangrene
Genetic engineering
Glands
Gluten intolerance
Grafts and grafting
Hair
Hair transplantation
Hand-foot-and-mouth disease
Healing
Herpes
Histology
Hives
Hyperhidrosis
Immunopathology
Impetigo
Laser use in surgery
Lesions
Light therapy
Local anesthesia
Lyme disease
Melanoma
Methicillin-resistant staphylococcus
    aureus (MRSA) infection
Moles
Monkeypox
Morgellons disease
Multiple chemical sensitivity
    syndrome
Nails
Necrotizing fasciitis
Neurofibromatosis
Pigmentation
Pinworms
Pityriasis alba
Pityriasis rosea
Plastic surgery
Podiatry
Polycystic ovary syndrome
Postherpetic neuralgia
Prostheses
Psoriasis
Puberty and adolescence

Reiter's syndrome
Ringworm
Rocky Mountain spotted fever
Rosacea
Sarcoidosis
Scabies
Scleroderma
Sense organs
Shingles
Skin
Skin cancer
Skin disorders
Skin lesion removal
Smallpox
Staphylococcal infections
Stevens-Johnson syndrome
Streptococcal infections
Stress
Sturge-Weber syndrome
Styes
Sweating
Systemic lupus erythematosus (SLE)
Tattoo removal
Tattoos and body piercing
Touch
Vasculitis
Vitiligo
Von Willebrand's disease
Wiskott-Aldrich syndrome

EMBRYOLOGY
Amniocentesis
Assisted reproductive technologies
Birth defects
Blue baby syndrome
Brain disorders
Chorionic villus sampling
Cloning
Conception
Down syndrome
Ectopic pregnancy
Fetal tissue transplantation
Gamete intrafallopian transfer (GIFT)
Genetic counseling
Genetic diseases
Genetic engineering
Genetic Imprinting
Genetics and inheritance
Genomics
Growth
Hermaphroditism and
    pseudohermaphroditism
In vitro fertilization
Karyotyping
Klinefelter syndrome
Meckel's diverticulum
Miscarriage

Mucopolysaccharidosis (MPS)
Multiple births
Neonatology
Obstetrics
Ovaries
Perinatology
Phenylketonuria (PKU)
Placenta
Pregnancy and gestation
Premature birth
Reproductive system
Rh factor
Sexual differentiation
Spina bifida
Stem cells
Syphilis
Teratogens
Ultrasonography
Uterus

EMERGENCY MEDICINE
Abdominal disorders
Abscess drainage
Acidosis
Adrenoleukodystrophy
Advance directives
Altitude sickness
Amputation
Anesthesia
Anesthesiology
Aneurysmectomy
Aneurysms
Angiography
Anthrax
Appendectomy
Appendicitis
Asphyxiation
Atrial fibrillation
Back pain
Bites and stings
Bleeding
Blurred vision
Botulism
Bruises
Burns and scalds
Cardiac arrest
Cardiology
Cardiopulmonary resuscitation (CPR)
Carotid arteries
Casts and splints
Catheterization
Cesarean section
Choking
Cholecystitis
Chronic granulomatous disease
Club drugs
Cold agglutinin disease

Computed tomography (CT) scanning
Concussion
Critical care
Croup
Defibrillation
Dizziness and fainting
Drowning
Echocardiography
Electrical shock
Electrocardiography (ECG or EKG)
Electrocauterization
Electroencephalography (EEG)
Embolization
Epiglottitis
First responder
Fracture and dislocation
Frostbite
Gangrene
Grafts and grafting
Head and neck disorders
Heart attack
Heart transplantation
Heat exhaustion and heatstroke
Heimlich maneuver
H1N1 influenza
Hyperbaric oxygen therapy
Hyperthermia and hypothermia
Hyperventilation
Hypotension
Hypoxia
Impetigo
Infarction
Influenza
Interpartner violence
Interstitial pulmonary fibrosis (IPF)
Intravenous (IV) therapy
Jaw wiring
Laceration repair
Local anesthesia
Lung surgery
Meningitis
Mental status exam
Monkeypox
Nail removal
Necrotizing fasciitis
Noninvasive tests
Nursing
Osteopathic medicine
Oxygen therapy
Pain management
Palliative medicine
Paramedics
Peritonitis
Physician assistants
Plague
Plastic surgery
Pleurisy

Pneumonia
Pneumothorax
Poisoning
Pulmonary medicine
Pulse rate
Pyelonephritis
Radiation sickness
Rape and sexual assault
Resuscitation
Reye's syndrome
Rocky Mountain spotted fever
Safety issues for children
Safety issues for the elderly
Severe acute respiratory syndrome
    (SARS)
Shock
Snakebites
Spinal cord disorders
Splenectomy
Sports medicine
Stevens-Johnson syndrome
Streptococcal infections
Strokes
Surgical technologists
Thrombolytic therapy and TPA
Toxic shock syndrome
Tracheostomy
Transfusion
Transplantation
Tularemia
Wounds

ENDOCRINOLOGY
Addison's disease
Adrenalectomy
Adrenoleukodystrophy
Amenorrhea
Anti-inflammatory drugs
Assisted reproductive technologies
Bariatric surgery
Carbohydrates
Computed tomography (CT) scanning
Congenital adrenal hyperplasia
Congenital hypothyroidism
Corticosteroids
Cushing's syndrome
Diabetes mellitus
Dwarfism
End-stage renal disease
Endocrine disorders
Endocrine glands
Ergogenic aids
Failure to thrive
Gamete intrafallopian transfer (GIFT)
Gender identity disorder
Gender reassignment surgery
Gestational diabetes

Gigantism
Glands
Glioma
Goiter
Growth
Gynecology
Gynecomastia
Hashimoto's thyroiditis
Hemochromatosis
Hermaphroditism and
    pseudohermaphroditism
Hormone therapy
Hormones
Hyperadiposis
Hyperparathyroidism and
    hypoparathyroidism
Hyperplasia
Hypertrophy
Hypoglycemia
Hypothalamus
Hysterectomy
Internal medicine
Klinefelter syndrome
Laboratory tests
Laparoscopy
Leptin
Liver
Melatonin
Menopause
Menstruation
Metabolic disorders
Metabolic syndrome
Nephrology
Neurology
Niemann-Pick disease
Nonalcoholic steatohepatitis (NASH)
Nuclear medicine
Obesity
Ovaries
Pancreas
Pancreatitis
Parathyroidectomy
Pharmacology
Pituitary gland
Plasma
Polycystic ovary syndrome
Precocious puberty
Prostate enlargement
Prostate gland
Puberty and adolescence
Pulse rate
Radiopharmaceuticals
Sexual differentiation
Sexual dysfunction
Sleep
Small intestine
Stem cells

Steroids
Systemic lupus erythematosus (SLE)
Testicular cancer
Thymus gland
Thyroid disorders
Thyroid gland
Thyroidectomy
Tumors
Turner syndrome
Vitamins and minerals
Vitiligo
Weight loss and gain
Weight loss medications
Williams syndrome

ENVIRONMENTAL HEALTH
Acidosis
Asbestos exposure
Asthma
Babesiosis
Blurred vision
Cholera
Cognitive development
Coronaviruses
Creutzfeldt-Jakob disease (CJD)
Drowning
Elephantiasis
Enteroviruses
Food poisoning
Frostbite
Gastroenteritis
Gulf War syndrome
Hantavirus
Hyperthermia and hypothermia
Insect-borne diseases
Lead poisoning
Legionnaires' disease
Lung cancer
Lungs
Mercury poisoning
Microbiology
Mold and mildew
Multiple chemical sensitivity
    syndrome
Occupational health
Parasitic diseases
Pigmentation
Plague
Poisoning
Pulmonary diseases
Pulmonary medicine
Roundworms
Schistosomiasis
Skin cancer
Sleeping sickness
Smallpox
Stress

Stress reduction
Trachoma
Tularemia
Typhoid fever
Typhus
West Nile virus
Yellow fever

EPIDEMIOLOGY
Acquired immunodeficiency
  syndrome (AIDS)
Amebiasis
Avian influenza
Bacillus Calmette-Guérin (BCG)
Bacterial infections
Bacteriology
Brucellosis
Candidiasis
Cerebral palsy
Chickenpox
Childhood infectious diseases
Cholera
Coronaviruses
Creutzfeldt-Jakob disease (CJD)
Diphtheria
E. coli infection
Ebola virus
Elephantiasis
Encephalitis
Epidemics and pandemics
Food poisoning
Forensic pathology
Gulf War syndrome
Hantavirus
Hepatitis
H1N1 influenza
Human papillomavirus (HPV)
Influenza
Insect-borne diseases
Laboratory tests
Legionnaires' disease
Leprosy
Leptospirosis
Lyme disease
Marburg virus
Mercury poisoning
Methicillin-resistant staphylococcus
  aureus (MRSA) infection
Microbiology
Multiple chemical sensitivity
  syndrome
Necrotizing fasciitis
Occupational health
Parasitic diseases
Phenylketonuria (PKU)
Plague
Pneumonia

Poisoning
Poliomyelitis
Prion diseases
Pulmonary diseases
Rabies
Rhinoviruses
Rocky Mountain spotted fever
Rotavirus
Roundworms
Screening
Severe acute respiratory syndrome
  (SARS)
Sexually transmitted diseases (STDs)
Sleeping sickness
Smallpox
Staphylococcal infections
Stress
Syphilis
Trichomoniasis
Tularemia
Typhoid fever
Typhus
Viral hemorrhagic fevers
Viral infections
West Nile virus
Yellow fever
Zoonoses

ETHICS
Abortion
Advance directives
Assisted reproductive technologies
Cloning
Defibrillation
Ergogenic aids
Facial transplantation
Fetal surgery
Fetal tissue transplantation
Gender identity disorder
Genetic engineering
Genomics
Gulf War syndrome
Longevity
Marijuana
Münchausen syndrome by proxy
Neurosis
Sperm banks
Stem cells
Xenotransplantation

EXERCISE PHYSIOLOGY
Acidosis
Ataxia
Biofeedback
Blood pressure
Bones and the skeleton
Cardiac rehabilitation

Carotid arteries
Defibrillation
Dehydration
Electrocardiography (ECG or EKG)
Ergogenic aids
Fascia
Glycolysis
Heart
Hemiplegia
Hypotension
Hypoxia
Juvenile rheumatoid arthritis
Kinesiology
Ligaments
Lungs
Massage
Metabolism
Motor skill development
Muscles
Osteoarthritis
Overtraining syndrome
Physical rehabilitation
Pulmonary medicine
Pulse rate
Respiration
Slipped disk
Sports medicine
Stenosis
Steroid abuse
Sweating
Tendinitis
Vascular system

FAMILY MEDICINE
Abdominal disorders
Abscess drainage
Acne
Advance directives
Alcoholism
Allergies
Amenorrhea
Amyotrophic lateral sclerosis
Anemia
Angelman syndrome
Angina
Anorexia nervosa
Anosmia
Antianxiety drugs
Antidepressants
Antihistamines
Antihypertensives
Anti-inflammatory drugs
Antioxidants
Aspergillosis
Ataxia
Atrophy
Attention-deficit disorder (ADD)

Autism
Bed-wetting
Bell's palsy
Beriberi
Biofeedback
Bleeding
Blisters
Blood pressure
Blurred vision
Body dysmorphic disorder
Bronchiolitis
Bronchitis
Bruises
Bulimia
Bunions
Burkitt's lymphoma
Caffeine
Candidiasis
Canker sores
Carotid arteries
Casts and splints
Cerebral palsy
Chagas' disease
Chickenpox
Childhood infectious diseases
Cholecystitis
Cholesterol
Chronic fatigue syndrome
Chronic granulomatous disease
Cirrhosis
Clostridium difficile infection
Coccidioidomycosis
Cold sores
Common cold
Conjunctivitis
Constipation
Corticosteroids
Coughing
Cryosurgery
Cushing's syndrome
Cytomegalovirus (CMV)
Death and dying
Decongestants
Deep vein thrombosis
Defibrillation
Dehydration
Dengue fever
Depression
Diabetes mellitus
Diarrhea and dysentery
Digestion
Diphtheria
Dizziness and fainting
E. coli infection
Earwax
Eating disorders
Echocardiography

Ehrlichiosis
Electrocauterization
Enterocolitis
Epiglottitis
Ergogenic aids
Exercise physiology
Factitious disorders
Failure to thrive
Fatigue
Fever
Fiber
Fifth disease
Fungal infections
Ganglion removal
Geriatric assessment
Giardiasis
Gigantism
Gynecology
Headaches
Healing
Heart disease
Heat exhaustion and heatstroke
Hemiplegia
Hemolytic uremic syndrome
Hemorrhoid banding and removal
Hemorrhoids
Herpes
Hiccups
Hirschsprung's disease
Hives
H1N1 influenza
Hormone therapy
Hyperadiposis
Hyperlipidemia
Hypertension
Hypertrophy
Hypoglycemia
Hypoxia
Impetigo
Incontinence
Infarction
Infection
Inflammation
Influenza
Interpartner violence
Intestinal disorders
Juvenile rheumatoid arthritis
Kawasaki disease
Keratitis
Kluver-Bucy syndrome
Kwashiorkor
Leishmaniasis
Leukodystrophy
Malabsorption
Maple syrup urine disease (MSUD)
Mastitis
Measles

Methicillin-resistant staphylococcus aureus (MRSA) infection
Mitral valve prolapse
Moles
Mononucleosis
Motion sickness
Mumps
Münchausen syndrome by proxy
Myringotomy
Nail removal
Nasal polyp removal
Nasopharyngeal disorders
Neurosis
Niemann-Pick disease
Nonalcoholic steatohepatitis (NASH)
Obesity
Orchitis
Osteopathic medicine
Otoplasty
Over-the-counter medications
Palliative medicine
Parasitic diseases
Pediatrics
Pharmacology
Physician assistants
Pick's disease
Pinworms
Pituitary gland
Pityriasis alba
Pityriasis rosea
Pleurisy
Pneumonia
Polycystic ovary syndrome
Polyps
Prader-Willi syndrome
Precocious puberty
Premenstrual syndrome (PMS)
Psychiatry
Ptosis
Puberty and adolescence
Pulse rate
Pyelonephritis
Raynaud's phenomenon
Reiter's syndrome
Rheumatic fever
Rhinitis
Ringworm
Rocky Mountain spotted fever
Roseola
Rubella
Safety issues for children
Safety issues for the elderly
Salmonella infection
Scabies
Scarlet fever
Sciatica
Sexuality

Shingles
Shock
Sinusitis
Sjögren's syndrome
Skin disorders
Sleep
Slipped disk
Sore throat
Sports medicine
Sterilization
Stevens-Johnson syndrome
Streptococcal infections
Stress
Stuttering
Styes
Supplements
Systemic lupus erythematosus (SLE)
Temporomandibular joint (TMJ)
    syndrome
Tendinitis
Testicular torsion
Tetanus
Thalassemia
Tinnitus
Toilet training
Tonsillitis
Tonsils
Tourette's syndrome
Toxoplasmosis
Trachoma
Ulcers
Urethritis
Urology
Vascular medicine
Vasectomy
Viral infections
Vitamins and minerals
Von Willebrand's disease
Weaning
Weight loss medications
Whooping cough
Wounds

FORENSIC MEDICINE
Antianxiety drugs
Autopsy
Blood testing
Cytopathology
Defibrillation
Dermatopathology
Genetic engineering
Genetics and inheritance
Hematology
Laboratory tests
Pathology

GASTROENTEROLOGY
Abdomen
Abdominal disorders
Achalasia
Acid reflux disease
Acidosis
Acquired immunodeficiency
    syndrome (AIDS)
Adenoviruses
Amebiasis
Amyotrophic lateral sclerosis
Anal cancer
Anus
Appendicitis
Bariatric surgery
Bile
Bulimia
Bypass surgery
Campylobacter infections
Celiac sprue
Cholecystitis
Cholera
Chronic granulomatous disease
Chyme
Clostridium difficile infection
Colic
Colitis
Colon
Colonoscopy and sigmoidoscopy
Colorectal cancer
Colorectal polyp removal
Colorectal surgery
Computed tomography (CT) scanning
Constipation
Critical care
Crohn's disease
Cytomegalovirus (CMV)
Diarrhea and dysentery
Digestion
Diverticulitis and diverticulosis
E. coli infection
Emergency medicine
Endoscopic retrograde
    cholangiopancreatography (ERCP)
Endoscopy
Enemas
Enterocolitis
Epidemics and pandemics
Esophagus
Failure to thrive
Fiber
Fistula repair
Food allergies
Food biochemistry
Food poisoning
Gallbladder
Gallbladder cancer

Gallbladder diseases
Gastrectomy
Gastroenteritis
Gastrointestinal disorders
Gastrointestinal system
Gastrostomy
Giardiasis
Glands
Gluten intolerance
Hemochromatosis
Hemolytic uremic syndrome
Hemorrhoid banding and removal
Hemorrhoids
Hernia
Hernia repair
Hiccups
Ileostomy and colostomy
Infarction
Internal medicine
Intestinal disorders
Intestines
Irritable bowel syndrome (IBS)
Jaundice
Lactose intolerance
Laparoscopy
Lesions
Liver
Liver cancer
Liver disorders
Liver transplantation
Malabsorption
Malnutrition
Meckel's diverticulum
Metabolism
Nausea and vomiting
Nonalcoholic steatohepatitis (NASH)
Noroviruses
Pancreas
Pancreatitis
Peristalsis
Peritonitis
Polycystic kidney disease
Polyps
Proctology
Pyloric stenosis
Rectum
Rotavirus
Salmonella infection
Scleroderma
Shigellosis
Small intestine
Soiling
Stenosis
Stevens-Johnson syndrome
Stone removal
Stones
Tapeworms

Taste
Toilet training
Ulcer surgery
Ulcerative colitis
Ulcers
Vagotomy
Vagus nerve
Vasculitis
Von Willebrand's disease
Weight loss and gain
Wilson's disease

GENERAL SURGERY
Abscess drainage
Achalasia
Adenoids
Adrenalectomy
Amputation
Anesthesia
Anesthesiology
Aneurysms
Appendectomy
Arthroplasty
Bariatric surgery
Biopsy
Bladder removal
Bone marrow transplantation
Brain tumors
Breast biopsy
Breast cancer
Breast disorders
Breast surgery
Bunions
Bypass surgery
Casts and splints
Catheterization
Cesarean section
Cholecystectomy
Chronic granulomatous disease
Cleft lip and palate repair
Coccidioidomycosis
Colon
Colonoscopy and sigmoidoscopy
Colorectal polyp removal
Colorectal surgery
Corneal transplantation
Cryosurgery
Culdocentesis
Cyst removal
Disk removal
Ear surgery
Electrocauterization
Endarterectomy
Eye infections and disorders
Eye surgery
Face lift and blepharoplasty
Fistula repair

Gallbladder cancer
Ganglion removal
Gastrectomy
Gender identity disorder
Gender reassignment surgery
Gigantism
Grafts and grafting
Hair transplantation
Hammertoe correction
Heart transplantation
Heart valve replacement
Heel spur removal
Hemorrhoid banding and removal
Hernia repair
Hydroceles
Hydrocephalus
Hypospadias repair and urethroplasty
Hypoxia
Hysterectomy
Infarction
Intravenous (IV) therapy
Kidney transplantation
Kneecap removal
Laceration repair
Laminectomy and spinal fusion
Laparoscopy
Laryngectomy
Lesions
Liposuction
Liver transplantation
Lumbar puncture
Lung surgery
Mastectomy and lumpectomy
Meckel's diverticulum
Mesothelioma
Methicillin-resistant staphylococcus
    aureus (MRSA) infection
Mouth and throat cancer
Nasal polyp removal
Nephrectomy
Neurosurgery
Oncology
Ophthalmology
Orthopedic surgery
Otoplasty
Pain
Parathyroidectomy
Penile implant surgery
Periodontal surgery
Peritonitis
Phlebitis
Physician assistants
Plasma
Plastic surgery
Polydactyly and syndactyly
Polyps
Prostate gland removal

Prostheses
Pulse rate
Pyloric stenosis
Rhinoplasty and submucous resection
Rotator cuff surgery
Sarcoma
Shunts
Skin lesion removal
Small intestine
Sphincterectomy
Splenectomy
Staphylococcal infections
Sterilization
Stone removal
Streptococcal infections
Surgical procedures
Surgical technologists
Sympathectomy
Tattoo removal
Tendon repair
Testicular cancer
Testicular surgery
Thoracic surgery
Thyroidectomy
Tonsillectomy and adenoid removal
Tonsillitis
Toxic shock syndrome
Trachea
Tracheostomy
Transfusion
Transplantation
Tumor removal
Ulcer surgery
Ulcerative colitis
Vagotomy
Varicose vein removal
Vasectomy
Xenotransplantation

GENETICS
Adrenoleukodystrophy
Agnosia
Amniocentesis
Angelman syndrome
Antibiotic resistance
Assisted reproductive technologies
Attention-deficit disorder (ADD)
Autism
Batten's disease
Bioinformatics
Biological therapies
Bionics and biotechnology
Birth defects
Bone marrow transplantation
Breast cancer
Charcot-Marie-Tooth Disease
Chemotherapy

Chorionic villus sampling
Chronic granulomatous disease
Cloning
Cockayne Disease
Cognitive development
Colorectal cancer
Congenital adrenal hyperplasia
Congenital disorders
Cornelia de Lange syndrome
Cystic fibrosis
Diabetes mellitus
DiGeorge syndrome
Down syndrome
Dwarfism
Embryology
Endocrinology
Enzyme therapy
Failure to thrive
Fetal surgery
Fragile X syndrome
Fructosemia
Galactosemia
Gaucher's disease
Gender identity disorder
Gene therapy
Genetic counseling
Genetic diseases
Genetic engineering
Genetic Imprinting
Genetics and inheritance
Genomics
Grafts and grafting
Hematology
Hemophilia
Hermaphroditism and
   pseudohermaphroditism
Huntington's disease
Hyperadiposis
Immunodeficiency disorders
Immunopathology
In vitro fertilization
Karyotyping
Klinefelter syndrome
Klippel-Trenaunay syndrome
Laboratory tests
Leptin
Leukodystrophy
Malabsorption
Maple syrup urine disease (MSUD)
Marfan syndrome
Mental retardation
Metabolic disorders
Motor skill development
Mucopolysaccharidosis (MPS)
Multiple births
Muscular dystrophy
Mutation

Neonatology
Nephrology
Neurofibromatosis
Neurology
Niemann-Pick disease
Obstetrics
Oncology
Osteogenesis imperfecta
Ovaries
Paget's disease
Pain
Pediatrics
Phenylketonuria (PKU)
Polycystic kidney disease
Polydactyly and syndactyly
Polyps
Porphyria
Prader-Willi syndrome
Precocious puberty
Reproductive system
Retroviruses
Rh factor
Rhinoviruses
Rubinstein-Taybi syndrome
Sarcoidosis
Sarcoma
Severe combined immunodeficiency
   syndrome (SCID)
Sexual differentiation
Sexuality
Sickle cell disease
Sperm banks
Spinocerebellar ataxia
Stem cells
Synesthesia
Tay-Sachs disease
Thalassemia
Tourette's syndrome
Transplantation
Tremors
Turner syndrome
Williams syndrome
Wiskott-Aldrich syndrome

GERIATRICS AND GERONTOLOGY
Advance directives
Aging
Aging: Extended care
Alzheimer's disease
Arthroplasty
Assisted living facilities
Ataxia
Atrophy
Blindness
Blood pressure
Blurred vision

Bone disorders
Brain disorders
Cartilage
Cataracts
Chronic obstructive pulmonary
   disease (COPD)
Critical care
Deafness
Death and dying
Delirium
Dementias
Depression
Dyskinesia
Emergency medicine
End-stage renal disease
Eye infections and disorders
Eye surgery
Family medicine
Fatigue
Fiber
Frontal lobe syndrome
Geriatric assessment
Hip fracture repair
Hormone therapy
Hypotension
Incontinence
Interpartner violence
Joints
Light therapy
Longevity
Massage
Memory loss
Neuroscience
Nursing
Osteopathic medicine
Osteoporosis
Pain management
Palliative care
Paramedics
Parkinson's disease
Physician assistants
Pick's disease
Polymyalgia rheumatica
Psychiatry
Radiculopathy
Rheumatoid arthritis
Rheumatology
Safety issues for the elderly
Sleep disorders
Suicide
Temporal arteritis
Tremors
Vision disorders

GYNECOLOGY
Abdomen
Abortion

Acquired immunodeficiency syndrome (AIDS)
Amenorrhea
Assisted reproductive technologies
Biopsy
Bladder removal
Blurred vision
Breast biopsy
Breast cancer
Breast disorders
Breast-feeding
Cervical procedures
Cesarean section
Childbirth
Childbirth complications
Chlamydia
Conception
Contraception
Cryosurgery
Culdocentesis
Cyst removal
Cystitis
Cystoscopy
Dysmenorrhea
Ectopic pregnancy
Electrocauterization
Embolization
Endocrinology
Endometrial biopsy
Endometriosis
Endoscopy
Episiotomy
Fibrocystic breast condition
Gender reassignment surgery
Glands
Gonorrhea
Hermaphroditism and pseudohermaphroditism
Herpes
Hormone therapy
Human papillomavirus (HPV)
Hyperplasia
Hysterectomy
In vitro fertilization
Incontinence
Internal medicine
Laparoscopy
Leptin
Lesions
Mammography
Mastitis
Menopause
Menorrhagia
Menstruation
Miscarriage
Myomectomy
Obstetrics

Ovarian cysts
Ovaries
Pap test
Pelvic inflammatory disease (PID)
Polycystic ovary syndrome
Polyps
Postpartum depression
Preeclampsia and eclampsia
Pregnancy and gestation
Premenstrual syndrome (PMS)
Rape and sexual assault
Reiter's syndrome
Reproductive system
Sexual differentiation
Sexual dysfunction
Sexuality
Sexually transmitted diseases (STDs)
Sterilization
Syphilis
Toxic shock syndrome
Trichomoniasis
Tubal ligation
Turner syndrome
Ultrasonography
Urinary disorders
Urology
Uterus
Von Willebrand's disease

HEMATOLOGY
Acid-base chemistry
Acidosis
Acquired immunodeficiency syndrome (AIDS)
Anemia
Babesiosis
Biological therapies
Bleeding
Blood and blood disorders
Blood testing
Blood vessels
Bone grafting
Bone marrow transplantation
Bruises
Burkitt's lymphoma
Chronic fatigue syndrome
Circulation
Cold agglutinin disease
Connective tissue
Cyanosis
Cytology
Cytomegalovirus (CMV)
Cytopathology
Deep vein thrombosis
Dialysis
Disseminated intravascular coagulation (DIC)

Epidemics and pandemics
Epstein-Barr virus
Ergogenic aids
Fluids and electrolytes
Forensic pathology
Healing
Hemolytic disease of the newborn
Hemolytic uremic syndrome
Hemophilia
Histiocytosis
Histology
Hodgkin's disease
Hormone therapy
Host-defense mechanisms
Hypercholesterolemia
Hyperlipidemia
Hypoglycemia
Immune system
Immunopathology
Infection
Jaundice
Kidneys
Laboratory tests
Leukemia
Liver
Lymph
Lymphadenopathy and lymphoma
Lymphatic system
Nephrology
Niemann-Pick disease
Palliative care
Phlebotomy
Plasma
Rh factor
Septicemia
Serology
Sickle cell disease
Snakebites
Stem cells
Subdural hematoma
Thalassemia
Thrombocytopenia
Thrombolytic therapy and TPA
Thrombosis and thrombus
Transfusion
Uremia
Vascular medicine
Vascular system
Von Willebrand's disease

HISTOLOGY
Autopsy
Biopsy
Breast cancer
Breast disorders
Cancer
Carcinoma

Cells
Cold agglutinin disease
Colon
Cytology
Cytopathology
Dermatology
Dermatopathology
Endometrial biopsy
Eye infections and disorders
Fluids and electrolytes
Forensic pathology
Glioma
Healing
Laboratory tests
Microscopy
Nails
Necrotizing fasciitis
Pathology
Pityriasis alba
Rhinoviruses
Sarcoma
Small intestine
Smallpox
Tumor removal
Tumors

IMMUNOLOGY
Acquired immunodeficiency
    syndrome (AIDS)
Adenoids
Adenoviruses
Allergies
Ankylosing spondylitis
Antibiotics
Antibodies
Antihistamines
Aspergillosis
Asthma
Avian influenza
Bacillus Calmette-Guérin (BCG)
Bacterial infections
Biological therapies
Bionics and biotechnology
Bites and stings
Blood and blood disorders
Bone cancer
Bone grafting
Bone marrow transplantation
Cancer
Candidiasis
Carcinoma
Chickenpox
Childhood infectious diseases
Chronic fatigue syndrome
Chronic granulomatous disease
Cold agglutinin disease
Colorectal cancer

Coronaviruses
Corticosteroids
Crohn's disease
Cushing's syndrome
Cytology
Cytomegalovirus (CMV)
Dermatology
Dermatopathology
DiGeorge syndrome
Endocrinology
Epidemics and pandemics
Epstein-Barr virus
Fetal tissue transplantation
Food allergies
Fungal infections
Gluten intolerance
Grafts and grafting
Hay fever
Healing
Hematology
Histiocytosis
Hives
Homeopathy
Host-defense mechanisms
Human immunodeficiency virus
    (HIV)
Hypnosis
Immune system
Immunization and vaccination
Immunodeficiency disorders
Immunopathology
Juvenile rheumatoid arthritis
Kawasaki disease
Laboratory tests
Leprosy
Liver cancer
Lung cancer
Lymph
Lymphatic system
Malaria
Microbiology
Multiple chemical sensitivity
    syndrome
Multiple sclerosis
Myasthenia gravis
Nephritis
Noroviruses
Oncology
Opportunistic infections
Pancreas
Prostate cancer
Pulmonary diseases
Pulmonary medicine
Renal failure
Rheumatic fever
Rheumatoid arthritis
Rheumatology

Rhinitis
Rhinoviruses
Sarcoidosis
Scleroderma
Serology
Severe combined immunodeficiency
    syndrome (SCID)
Skin cancer
Small intestine
Smallpox
Stem cells
Stevens-Johnson syndrome
Stress
Stress reduction
Thalidomide
Thymus gland
Transfusion
Transplantation
Tularemia
Wiskott-Aldrich syndrome
Xenotransplantation

INTERNAL MEDICINE
Abdomen
Abdominal disorders
Acidosis
Acquired immunodeficiency
    syndrome (AIDS)
Adenoids
Alcoholism
Allergies
Alzheimer's disease
Amebiasis
Amyotrophic lateral sclerosis
Anemia
Angina
Anthrax
Antianxiety drugs
Antibodies
Anti-inflammatory drugs
Antioxidants
Anus
Anxiety
Aortic stenosis
Apnea
Arteriosclerosis
Arthritis
Aspergillosis
Ataxia
Auras
Babesiosis
Bacillus Calmette-Guérin (BCG)
Bacterial infections
Bariatric surgery
Bedsores
Behçet's disease
Bile

Biofeedback
Bleeding
Blood vessels
Blurred vision
Body dysmorphic disorder
Bronchiolitis
Bronchitis
Burkitt's lymphoma
Bursitis
Campylobacter infections
Candidiasis
Cardiac surgery
Carotid arteries
Casts and splints
Celiac sprue
Childhood infectious diseases
Cholecystitis
Cholera
Cholesterol
Chronic fatigue syndrome
Chronic granulomatous disease
Chyme
Cirrhosis
Coccidioidomycosis
Colitis
Colon
Common cold
Computed tomography (CT) scanning
Congenital hypothyroidism
Constipation
Coughing
Cushing's syndrome
Cyanosis
Delirium
Dengue fever
Diabetes mellitus
Dialysis
Diaphragm
Diarrhea and dysentery
Digestion
Disseminated intravascular
    coagulation (DIC)
Diuretics
Diverticulitis and diverticulosis
Dizziness and fainting
E. coli infection
Echocardiography
Edema
Electrocauterization
Embolism
Emphysema
Encephalitis
End-stage renal disease
Endocarditis
Endocrine glands
Endoscopic retrograde
    cholangiopancreatography (ERCP)

Enteroviruses
Epidemics and pandemics
Epiglottitis
Ergogenic aids
Factitious disorders
Family medicine
Fatigue
Fever
Fiber
Fungal infections
Gallbladder
Gallbladder diseases
Gastroenteritis
Gastroenterology
Gastrointestinal disorders
Gastrointestinal system
Gaucher's disease
Genetic diseases
Geriatric assessment
Gigantism
Gout
Guillain-Barré syndrome
Hantavirus
Headaches
Heart attack
Heart disease
Heart failure
Heat exhaustion and heatstroke
Hematuria
Hemochromatosis
Hepatitis
Hernia
Histology
Hives
Hodgkin's disease
H1N1 influenza
Hormone therapy
Hyperhidrosis
Hyperlipidemia
Hypertension
Hyperthermia and hypothermia
Hypertrophy
Hypoglycemia
Hypotension
Hypoxia
Impetigo
Incontinence
Infarction
Infection
Inflammation
Influenza
Interpartner violence
Interstitial pulmonary fibrosis (IPF)
Intestinal disorders
Intestines
Jaundice
Kaposi's sarcoma

Kidney disorders
Klippel-Trenaunay syndrome
Legionnaires' disease
Leprosy
Leptospirosis
Lesions
Leukemia
Liver
Liver disorders
Lymph
Lymphadenopathy and lymphoma
Malaria
Malignancy and metastasis
Measles
Melanoma
Metabolic syndrome
Methicillin-resistant staphylococcus
    aureus (MRSA) infection
Mitral valve prolapse
Monkeypox
Multiple sclerosis
Nail removal
Nephritis
Nephrology
Niemann-Pick disease
Nonalcoholic steatohepatitis (NASH)
Nuclear medicine
Obesity
Occupational health
Opportunistic infections
Osteopathic medicine
Pain
Palliative care
Palliative medicine
Pancreas
Pancreatitis
Parasitic diseases
Parkinson's disease
Peristalsis
Peritonitis
Pharynx
Phlebitis
Physician assistants
Pick's disease
Plasma
Pleurisy
Pneumonia
Polymyalgia rheumatica
Polyps
Proctology
Psoriasis
Puberty and adolescence
Pulmonary edema
Pulmonary medicine
Pulse rate
Pyelonephritis
Radiopharmaceuticals

Rectum
Renal failure
Reye's syndrome
Rocky Mountain spotted fever
Sarcoidosis
Scarlet fever
Schistosomiasis
Sciatica
Septicemia
Severe acute respiratory syndrome
  (SARS)
Sexuality
Sexually transmitted diseases (STDs)
Shingles
Shock
Sinusitis
Sleep
Sleeping sickness
Small intestine
Sports medicine
Staphylococcal infections
Stevens-Johnson syndrome
Stones
Stress
Supplements
Syphilis
Tetanus
Thrombosis and thrombus
Toxic shock syndrome
Tremors
Tumors
Typhoid fever
Typhus
Ulcers
Ultrasonography
Urethritis
Viral infections
Vitamins and minerals
Weight loss medications
Wilson's disease
Wounds

MICROBIOLOGY
Acquired immunodeficiency
  syndrome (AIDS)
Amebiasis
Anthrax
Antibiotic resistance
Antibiotics
Antibodies
Aspergillosis
Autopsy
Bacillus Calmette-Guérin (BCG)
Bacterial infections
Bacteriology
Bionics and biotechnology
Brucellosis

Campylobacter infections
Chemotherapy
Chlamydia
Cholera
Chronic granulomatous disease
Coccidioidomycosis
Conjunctivitis
Creutzfeldt-Jakob disease (CJD)
Dengue fever
Diphtheria
E. coli infection
Enteroviruses
Epidemics and pandemics
Epstein-Barr virus
Fluoride treatments
Fungal infections
Gastroenteritis
Gastroenterology
Gastrointestinal disorders
Genomics
Gonorrhea
Gram staining
Hematuria
Human immunodeficiency virus (HIV)
Immune system
Immunization and vaccination
Impetigo
Insect-borne diseases
Laboratory tests
Leptospirosis
Methicillin-resistant staphylococcus
  aureus (MRSA) infection
Microscopy
Mold and mildew
Opportunistic infections
Pathology
Pelvic inflammatory disease (PID)
Peritonitis
Pharmacology
Plasma
Pneumocystis jirovecii
Protozoan diseases
Serology
Severe acute respiratory syndrome
  (SARS)
Sleeping sickness
Staphylococcal infections
Streptococcal infections
Syphilis
Toxic shock syndrome
Trichinosis
Tuberculosis
Urinalysis
Urology

NEONATOLOGY
Angelman syndrome

Apgar score
Apnea
Birth defects
Blue baby syndrome
Bonding
Breast disorders
Cesarean section
Childbirth
Childbirth complications
Cleft lip and palate
Cleft lip and palate repair
Collodion baby
Congenital disorders
Congenital heart disease
Cutis marmorata telangiectatica
  congenita
Cystic fibrosis
Disseminated intravascular
  coagulation (DIC)
E. coli infection
Embryology
Failure to thrive
Fetal surgery
Genetic diseases
Hemolytic disease of the newborn
Hydrocephalus
Intraventricular hemorrhage
Karyotyping
Malabsorption
Maple syrup urine disease (MSUD)
Motor skill development
Multiple births
Neonatal brachial plexus palsy
Nursing
Obstetrics
Pediatrics
Perinatology
Phenylketonuria (PKU)
Physician assistants
Premature birth
Pulse rate
Respiratory distress syndrome
Rh factor
Shunts
Spina bifida
Sudden infant death syndrome (SIDS)
Syphilis
Tay-Sachs disease
Transfusion
Trichomoniasis
Umbilical cord
Well-baby examinations

NEPHROLOGY
Abdomen
Addison's disease
Anemia

Aspergillosis
Chronic granulomatous disease
Diabetes mellitus
Dialysis
Diuretics
E. coli infection
Edema
End-stage renal disease
Ergogenic aids
Hematuria
Hemolytic uremic syndrome
Internal medicine
Kidney cancer
Kidney disorders
Kidney transplantation
Kidneys
Leptospirosis
Lesions
Lithotripsy
Nephrectomy
Nephritis
Palliative care
Polycystic kidney disease
Polyps
Preeclampsia and eclampsia
Proteinuria
Pyelonephritis
Renal failure
Sarcoidosis
Stenosis
Stone removal
Stones
Transplantation
Uremia
Urinalysis
Urinary disorders
Urinary system
Urology
Vasculitis
Williams syndrome

NEUROLOGY
Acquired immunodeficiency
  syndrome (AIDS)
Adrenoleukodystrophy
Aging: Extended care
Agnosia
Altitude sickness
Alzheimer's disease
Amnesia
Amyotrophic lateral sclerosis
Anesthesia
Anesthesiology
Aneurysms
Angelman syndrome
Anorexia nervosa
Anosmia

Antidepressants
Aphasia and dysphasia
Apnea
Ataxia
Atrophy
Attention-deficit disorder (ADD)
Audiology
Auras
Balance disorders
Batten's disease
Bell's palsy
Biofeedback
Blindsight
Botox
Brain
Brain damage
Brain disorders
Brain tumors
Brucellosis
Caffeine
Capgras syndrome
Carotid arteries
Carpal tunnel syndrome
Cerebral palsy
Charcot-Marie-Tooth Disease
Chiari malformations
Chiropractic
Chronic wasting disease (CWD)
Cluster headaches
Cockayne Disease
Cognitive enhancement
Concussion
Cornelia de Lange syndrome
Craniotomy
Creutzfeldt-Jakob disease (CJD)
Critical care
Cryosurgery
Cutis marmorata telangiectatica
  congenita
Delirium
Dementias
Developmental stages
Diabetes mellitus
Disk removal
Dizziness and fainting
Dyskinesia
Dyslexia
Ear infections and disorders
Ears
Electrical shock
Electroencephalography (EEG)
Electromyography
Embolism
Emergency medicine
Encephalitis
Enteroviruses
Epilepsy

Eye infections and disorders
Fascia
Fetal tissue transplantation
Frontal lobe syndrome
Frontotemporal dementia (FTD)
Gigantism
Glasgow coma scale
Glioma
Grafts and grafting
Guillain-Barré syndrome
Head and neck disorders
Headaches
Hearing
Hearing tests
Hematomas
Hemiplegia
Hemolytic disease of the newborn
Hiccups
Huntington's disease
Hydrocephalus
Hyperhidrosis
Hypothalamus
Hypoxia
Infarction
Intraventricular hemorrhage
Ischemia
Korsakoff's syndrome
Learning disabilities
Lesions
Leukodystrophy
Lower extremities
Lumbar puncture
Lyme disease
Marijuana
Melatonin
Memory loss
Meningitis
Mercury poisoning
Minimally conscious state
Morgellons disease
Motion sickness
Motor neuron diseases
Motor skill development
Multiple chemical sensitivity
  syndrome
Multiple sclerosis
Myasthenia gravis
Narcolepsy
Neonatal brachial plexus palsy
Nervous system
Neurofibromatosis
Neuropsychology
Neuroscience
Neurosis
Neurosurgery
Niemann-Pick disease
Numbness and tingling

Otorhinolaryngology
Pain
Palsy
Paralysis
Paraplegia
Parkinson's disease
Phenylketonuria (PKU)
Phrenology
Pick's disease
Poliomyelitis
Porphyria
Postherpetic neuralgia
Prader-Willi syndrome
Precocious puberty
Preeclampsia and eclampsia
Prion diseases
Psychiatry
Quadriplegia
Rabies
Radiculopathy
Restless legs syndrome
Reye's syndrome
Rubinstein-Taybi syndrome
Sarcoidosis
Sciatica
Seizures
Sense organs
Shingles
Shock therapy
Skin
Sleep
Sleep disorders
Sleeping sickness
Sleepwalking
Smell
Spinal cord disorders
Split-brain
Stem cells
Stenosis
Strokes
Sturge-Weber syndrome
Stuttering
Subdural hematoma
Sympathectomy
Synesthesia
Syphilis
Tardive dyskinesia
Taste
Tay-Sachs disease
Tetanus
Tics
Tinnitus
Torticollis
Touch
Tourette's syndrome
Transient ischemic attacks (TIAs)
Traumatic brain injury

Tremors
Upper extremities
Vagotomy
Vagus nerve
Vasculitis
Vertigo
Vision
Wernicke's aphasia
West Nile virus
Williams syndrome
Wilson's disease

NEUROPSYCHOLOGY
Capgras syndrome
Frontal lobe syndrome
Minimally conscious state
Neuroscience
Traumatic brain injury
Wernicke's aphasia
Williams syndrome

NEUROSCIENCE
Blindsight
Frontal lobe syndrome
Glasgow coma scale
Mirror neurons
Neuroethics
Neuropsychology
Phrenology
Split-brain
Traumatic brain injury
Wernicke's aphasia

NEUROSURGERY
Chiari malformations
Minimally conscious state
Wernicke's aphasia

NUCLEAR MEDICINE
Chemotherapy
Imaging and radiology
Magnetic resonance imaging (MRI)
Noninvasive tests
Nuclear radiology
Pneumocystis jirovecii
Positron emission tomography (PET)
    scanning
Radiation therapy
Single photon emission computed
    tomography (SPECT)

NURSING
Acidosis
Aging: Extended care
Alzheimer's disease
Ataxia
Atrophy

Bedsores
Cardiac rehabilitation
Carotid arteries
Casts and splints
Critical care
Diuretics
Drowning
Emergency medicine
Epidemics and pandemics
Eye infections and disorders
Fiber
Home care
H1N1 influenza
Hypoxia
Infarction
Influenza
Intravenous (IV) therapy
Methicillin-resistant staphylococcus
    aureus (MRSA) infection
Minimally conscious state
Palliative care
Pediatrics
Physician assistants
Polycystic ovary syndrome
Pulse rate
Radiculopathy
Surgical procedures
Surgical technologists
Well-baby examinations

NUTRITION
Aging: Extended care
Anorexia nervosa
Antioxidants
Bariatric surgery
Bedsores
Bell's palsy
Bile
Breast-feeding
Bulimia
Carbohydrates
Cardiac rehabilitation
Celiac sprue
Cholesterol
Colon
Crohn's disease
Cushing's syndrome
Dietary reference intakes (DRIs)
Digestion
Exercise physiology
Eye infections and disorders
Fatty acid oxidation disorders
Fiber
Food allergies
Food biochemistry
Food guide plate
Fructosemia

Galactosemia
Gastroenterology
Gastrointestinal system
Gestational diabetes
Gluten intolerance
Glycogen storage diseases
Hemolytic uremic syndrome
Hyperadiposis
Hypercholesterolemia
Irritable bowel syndrome (IBS)
Jaw wiring
Korsakoff's syndrome
Kwashiorkor
Lactose intolerance
Leptin
Leukodystrophy
Lipids
Macronutrients
Malabsorption
Malnutrition
Mastitis
Metabolic disorders
Metabolic syndrome
Metabolism
Nursing
Obesity
Osteoporosis
Phenylketonuria (PKU)
Phytochemicals
Pituitary gland
Plasma
Polycystic ovary syndrome
Protein
Rickets
Scurvy
Small intestine
Sports medicine
Supplements
Taste
Ulcer surgery
Ulcers
Vagotomy
Vitamin D deficiency
Vitamins and minerals
Weaning
Weight loss and gain
Weight loss medications

OBSTETRICS
Amniocentesis
Apgar score
Assisted reproductive technologies
Birth defects
Breast-feeding
Cerebral palsy
Cesarean section
Childbirth

Childbirth complications
Chorionic villus sampling
Conception
Congenital disorders
Contraception
Critical care
Cytomegalovirus (CMV)
Disseminated intravascular
    coagulation (DIC)
Down syndrome
Embryology
Emergency medicine
Endometrial biopsy
Endoscopy
Episiotomy
Family medicine
Fetal surgery
Gamete intrafallopian transfer (GIFT)
Genetic counseling
Genetic diseases
Gestational diabetes
Growth
Gynecology
Hirschsprung's disease
Incontinence
Intravenous (IV) therapy
Karyotyping
Listeria infections
Mastitis
Miscarriage
Multiple births
Neonatal brachial plexus palsy
Neonatology
Noninvasive tests
Ovaries
Perinatology
Pituitary gland
Placenta
Polycystic ovary syndrome
Postpartum depression
Preeclampsia and eclampsia
Pregnancy and gestation
Premature birth
Pyelonephritis
Reproductive system
Rh factor
Sexuality
Sperm banks
Stillbirth
Streptococcal infections
Teratogens
Toxemia
Trichomoniasis
Tubal ligation
Turner syndrome
Ultrasonography
Urology

Uterus

OCCUPATIONAL HEALTH
Acidosis
Agnosia
Altitude sickness
Angelman syndrome
Asbestos exposure
Asphyxiation
Ataxia
Bacillus Calmette-Guérin (BCG)
Biofeedback
Blurred vision
Brucellosis
Cardiac rehabilitation
Carpal tunnel syndrome
Charcot-Marie-Tooth Disease
Gulf War syndrome
Hearing tests
Leptospirosis
Leukodystrophy
Lung cancer
Mercury poisoning
Mesothelioma
Multiple chemical sensitivity
    syndrome
Nasopharyngeal disorders
Pneumonia
Prostheses
Pulmonary diseases
Pulmonary medicine
Radiation sickness
Skin disorders
Slipped disk
Spinocerebellar ataxia
Stress reduction
Tendinitis
Tendon disorders
Tendon repair

OCCUPATIONAL THERAPY
Home care
Minimally conscious state
Williams syndrome

ONCOLOGY
Acquired immunodeficiency
    syndrome (AIDS)
Aging: Extended care
Amputation
Anal cancer
Anemia
Antibodies
Antioxidants
Anus
Asbestos exposure
Assisted suicide

Biological therapies
Biopsy
Bladder cancer
Bone cancer
Bone disorders
Bone marrow transplantation
Brain tumors
Breast cancer
Burkitt's lymphoma
Cancer
Carcinoma
Chemotherapy
Cold agglutinin disease
Colon
Colorectal cancer
Computed tomography (CT) scanning
Cryosurgery
Cystoscopy
Cytology
Cytopathology
Dermatology
Dermatopathology
Disseminated intravascular
    coagulation (DIC)
Embolization
Epstein-Barr virus
Ewing's sarcoma
Fibrocystic breast condition
Gallbladder cancer
Gastrectomy
Gastroenterology
Gastrointestinal system
Gastrostomy
Genetic Imprinting
Glioma
Gynecology
Hematology
Histology
Hodgkin's disease
Hormone therapy
Human papillomavirus (HPV)
Hysterectomy
Intravenous (IV) therapy
Kaposi's sarcoma
Karyotyping
Kidney cancer
Laboratory tests
Laryngectomy
Laser use in surgery
Lesions
Light therapy
Liver cancer
Lumbar puncture
Lung cancer
Lungs
Lymph
Lymphadenopathy and lymphoma

Malignancy and metastasis
Mammography
Massage
Mastectomy and lumpectomy
Meckel's diverticulum
Mesothelioma
Mouth and throat cancer
Necrosis
Nephrectomy
Oral and maxillofacial surgery
Pain
Pain management
Palliative care
Pap test
Pathology
Pharmacology
Plastic surgery
Proctology
Prostate cancer
Prostate gland
Prostate gland removal
Prostheses
Pulmonary diseases
Radiation sickness
Radiation therapy
Radiopharmaceuticals
Rectum
Retroviruses
Sarcoma
Serology
Skin
Skin cancer
Skin lesion removal
Small intestine
Smoking
Stem cells
Stenosis
Stress
Testicular cancer
Thalidomide
Thymus gland
Tonsils
Transplantation
Tumor removal
Tumors
Uterus
Wiskott-Aldrich syndrome

OPHTHALMOLOGY
Acquired immunodeficiency
    syndrome (AIDS)
Adrenoleukodystrophy
Aging: Extended care
Anesthesia
Anesthesiology
Anti-inflammatory drugs
Aspergillosis

Astigmatism
Batten's disease
Behçet's disease
Blindness
Blindsight
Blurred vision
Botox
Cataract surgery
Cataracts
Cockayne Disease
Conjunctivitis
Corneal transplantation
Cutis marmorata telangiectatica
    congenita
Dry eye
Eye infections and disorders
Eye surgery
Eyes
Glaucoma
Juvenile rheumatoid arthritis
Keratitis
Kluver-Bucy syndrome
Laser use in surgery
Lesions
Light therapy
Lyme disease
Macular degeneration
Marfan syndrome
Myopia
Optometry
Prostheses
Pterygium/Pinguecula
Ptosis
Refractive eye surgery
Reiter's syndrome
Rubinstein-Taybi syndrome
Sarcoidosis
Sense organs
Sphincterectomy
Spinocerebellar ataxia
Spondylitis
Stevens-Johnson syndrome
Strabismus
Sturge-Weber syndrome
Subdural hematoma
Tears and tear ducts
Trachoma
Vasculitis
Vision
Vision disorders
Williams syndrome

OPTOMETRY
Aging: Extended care
Astigmatism
Blindsight
Blurred vision

Cataract surgery
Cataracts
Cockayne Disease
Color blindness
Conjunctivitis
Eye infections and disorders
Eye surgery
Eyes
Glaucoma
Keratitis
Myopia
Ophthalmology
Pterygium/Pinguecula
Ptosis
Sarcoidosis
Sense organs
Spinocerebellar ataxia
Tears and tear ducts
Vision disorders
Williams syndrome

ORTHODONTICS

Bones and the skeleton
Dentistry
Jaw wiring
Periodontal surgery
Periodontitis
Teeth
Teething
Tooth extraction
Williams syndrome

ORTHOPEDICS

Amputation
Anti-inflammatory drugs
Arthritis
Arthroplasty
Arthroscopy
Ataxia
Atrophy
Bariatric surgery
Bone cancer
Bone disorders
Bone grafting
Bones and the skeleton
Bowlegs
Bunions
Cancer
Cartilage
Casts and splints
Cerebral palsy
Charcot-Marie-Tooth Disease
Chiropractic
Connective tissue
Craniosynostosis
Cutis marmorata telangiectatica
  congenita

Disk removal
Dwarfism
Endoscopy
Ergogenic aids
Ewing's sarcoma
Fascia
Feet
Flat feet
Foot disorders
Fracture and dislocation
Fracture repair
Growth
Hammertoe correction
Hammertoes
Heel spur removal
Hemiplegia
Hip fracture repair
Hip replacement
Hormone therapy
Joints
Juvenile rheumatoid arthritis
Kinesiology
Kneecap removal
Knock-knees
Kyphosis
Laminectomy and spinal fusion
Ligaments
Lower extremities
Marfan syndrome
Mesenchymal stem cells
Methicillin-resistant staphylococcus
  aureus (MRSA) infection
Motor skill development
Muscles
Necrosis
Neonatal brachial plexus palsy
Neurofibromatosis
Orthopedic surgery
Osgood-Schlatter disease
Osteoarthritis
Osteochondritis juvenilis
Osteogenesis imperfecta
Osteomyelitis
Osteonecrosis
Osteoporosis
Paget's disease
Physical rehabilitation
Pigeon toes
Podiatry
Prostheses
Radiculopathy
Reiter's syndrome
Rheumatology
Rickets
Rotator cuff surgery
Rubinstein-Taybi syndrome
Scoliosis

Slipped disk
Spondylitis
Sports medicine
Staphylococcal infections
Stenosis
Tendinitis
Tendon disorders
Tendon repair
Upper extremities
Whiplash

OSTEOPATHIC MEDICINE

Acidosis
Acquired immunodeficiency
  syndrome (AIDS)
Alternative medicine
Atrophy
Bones and the skeleton
Colon
Family medicine
Fascia
Ligaments
Muscles
Physical rehabilitation
Pituitary gland
Radiculopathy
Rickets
Slipped disk
Small intestine

OTOLARYNGOLOGY

Head and neck disorders
Ménière's disease
Vasculitis

OTORHINOLARYNGOLOGY

Acquired immunodeficiency
  syndrome (AIDS)
Adenoids
Allergies
Anosmia
Antihistamines
Anti-inflammatory drugs
Aromatherapy
Aspergillosis
Audiology
Cartilage
Cleft lip and palate
Cleft lip and palate repair
Cockayne Disease
Common cold
Croup
Cryosurgery
Decongestants
Ear infections and disorders
Ear surgery
Ears

Earwax
Epidemics and pandemics
Esophagus
Gastrointestinal system
Hay fever
Hearing aids
Hearing tests
Laryngectomy
Laryngitis
Lesions
Ménière's disease
Motion sickness
Myringotomy
Nasal polyp removal
Nasopharyngeal disorders
Nausea and vomiting
Oral and maxillofacial surgery
Pharyngitis
Pharynx
Polyps
Pulmonary medicine
Quinsy
Respiration
Rhinitis
Rhinoplasty and submucous resection
Rhinoviruses
Sense organs
Sinusitis
Sleep apnea
Smell
Sore throat
Taste
Tinnitus
Tonsillectomy and adenoid removal
Tonsillitis
Tonsils
Trachea
Vertigo
Voice and vocal cord disorders
Whooping cough

PATHOLOGY
Acquired immunodeficiency
    syndrome (AIDS)
Adrenoleukodystrophy
Anthrax
Antibodies
Atrophy
Autopsy
Avian influenza
Bacteriology
Biological therapies
Biopsy
Blood testing
Breast cancer
Cholecystitis
Chronic granulomatous disease

Cold agglutinin disease
Colon
Cytology
Cytopathology
Dermatopathology
Electroencephalography (EEG)
Embolization
Epidemics and pandemics
Epstein-Barr virus
Eye infections and disorders
Forensic pathology
Frontotemporal dementia (FTD)
Hematology
Histology
Homeopathy
Immunopathology
Inflammation
Karyotyping
Laboratory tests
Ligaments
Lumbar puncture
Malaria
Malignancy and metastasis
Mastectomy and lumpectomy
Melanoma
Mesothelioma
Microbiology
Microscopy
Motor skill development
Mutation
Niemann-Pick disease
Noninvasive tests
Oncology
Pityriasis rosea
Polycystic ovary syndrome
Prion diseases
Radiculopathy
Renal failure
Retroviruses
Rhinoviruses
Sarcoma
Serology
Small intestine
Smallpox
West Nile virus

PEDIATRICS
Acne
Adrenoleukodystrophy
Allergies
Angelman syndrome
Appendicitis
Ataxia
Attention-deficit disorder (ADD)
Autism
Batten's disease
Bed-wetting

Beriberi
Birth defects
Blisters
Blurred vision
Bowlegs
Bronchiolitis
Bruises
Burkitt's lymphoma
Casts and splints
Celiac sprue
Cerebral palsy
Charcot-Marie-Tooth Disease
Chickenpox
Childhood infectious diseases
Chronic granulomatous disease
Cleft lip and palate
Cleft lip and palate repair
Cockayne Disease
Cognitive development
Cold agglutinin disease
Colic
Collodion baby
Colon
Congenital disorders
Congenital heart disease
Cornelia de Lange syndrome
Crohn's disease
Croup
Cutis marmorata telangiectatica
    congenita
Cystic fibrosis
Cytomegalovirus (CMV)
Diabetes mellitus
Diarrhea and dysentery
DiGeorge syndrome
Diphtheria
Down syndrome
Dwarfism
E. coli infection
Eating disorders
Eczema
Ehrlichiosis
Emergency medicine
Enterocolitis
Epiglottitis
Epstein-Barr virus
Ewing's sarcoma
Eye infections and disorders
Failure to thrive
Family medicine
Fatty acid oxidation disorders
Fetal surgery
Fever
Fifth disease
Fistula repair
Fructosemia
Galactosemia

Gaucher's disease
Gender identity disorder
Genetic diseases
Genetics and inheritance
Giardiasis
Glycogen storage diseases
Growth
Hand-foot-and-mouth disease
Hearing tests
Hemolytic uremic syndrome
Hirschsprung's disease
Hives
H1N1 influenza
Impetigo
Incontinence
Influenza
Interpartner violence
Intravenous (IV) therapy
Juvenile rheumatoid arthritis
Kawasaki disease
Klippel-Trenaunay syndrome
Kluver-Bucy syndrome
Knock-knees
Kwashiorkor
Lead poisoning
Learning disabilities
Leukodystrophy
Listeria infections
Malabsorption
Malnutrition
Maple syrup urine disease (MSUD)
Massage
Measles
Menstruation
Mercury poisoning
Metabolic disorders
Methicillin-resistant staphylococcus
  aureus (MRSA) infection
Mold and mildew
Mononucleosis
Motor skill development
Mucopolysaccharidosis (MPS)
Multiple births
Multiple sclerosis
Mumps
Münchausen syndrome by proxy
Muscular dystrophy
Nail removal
Neonatal brachial plexus palsy
Neonatology
Neuroscience
Niemann-Pick disease
Nonalcoholic steatohepatitis (NASH)
Nursing
Osgood-Schlatter disease
Osteogenesis imperfecta
Otoplasty

Otorhinolaryngology
Palliative medicine
Perinatology
Phenylketonuria (PKU)
Pigeon toes
Pinworms
Pituitary gland
Pityriasis alba
Poliomyelitis
Polycystic ovary syndrome
Polydactyly and syndactyly
Porphyria
Prader-Willi syndrome
Precocious puberty
Premature birth
Progeria
Puberty and adolescence
Pulse rate
Pyloric stenosis
Respiratory distress syndrome
Reye's syndrome
Rheumatic fever
Rhinitis
Rickets
Roseola
Rotavirus
Rubella
Rubinstein-Taybi syndrome
Safety issues for children
Salmonella infection
Scarlet fever
Seizures
Severe combined immunodeficiency
  syndrome (SCID)
Sexuality
Small intestine
Soiling
Sore throat
Steroids
Stevens-Johnson syndrome
Streptococcal infections
Sturge-Weber syndrome
Stuttering
Sudden infant death syndrome (SIDS)
Syphilis
Tay-Sachs disease
Teething
Testicular torsion
Thalassemia
Thumb sucking
Toilet training
Tonsillectomy and adenoid removal
Tonsillitis
Tonsils
Toxoplasmosis
Trachoma
Weaning

Well-baby examinations
Whooping cough
Wiskott-Aldrich syndrome

PERINATOLOGY
Amniocentesis
Assisted reproductive technologies
Birth defects
Breast-feeding
Cesarean section
Childbirth
Chorionic villus sampling
Congenital hypothyroidism
Embryology
Fatty acid oxidation disorders
Glycogen storage diseases
Hydrocephalus
Karyotyping
Metabolic disorders
Miscarriage
Motor skill development
Neonatal brachial plexus palsy
Neonatology
Nursing
Obstetrics
Pediatrics
Premature birth
Shunts
Spina bifida
Trichomoniasis
Umbilical cord
Uterus
Well-baby examinations

PHARMACOLOGY
Acid-base chemistry
Acidosis
Acquired immunodeficiency
  syndrome (AIDS)
Aging: Extended care
Allergies
Antianxiety drugs
Antibiotic resistance
Antibiotics
Antibodies
Antihistamines
Antihypertensives
Assisted suicide
Autism
Bacteriology
Blurred vision
Chemotherapy
Chronic granulomatous disease
Club drugs
Colon
Critical care
Digestion

Diuretics
Dyskinesia
Emergency medicine
Epidemics and pandemics
Ergogenic aids
Fluids and electrolytes
Food biochemistry
Genetic engineering
Genomics
Glycolysis
Homeopathy
Hormones
Hypercholesterolemia
Hypotension
Laboratory tests
Marijuana
Melatonin
Mesothelioma
Metabolism
Methicillin-resistant staphylococcus
  aureus (MRSA) infection
Narcotics
Neuropsychology
Neuroscience
Oncology
Over-the-counter medications
Pain management
Polycystic ovary syndrome
Prader-Willi syndrome
Psychiatry
Rheumatology
Sleep
Small intestine
Sports medicine
Steroids
Tardive dyskinesia
Thrombolytic therapy and TPA
Tremors

PHYSICAL THERAPY
Aging: Extended care
Amputation
Amyotrophic lateral sclerosis
Angelman syndrome
Arthritis
Ataxia
Atrophy
Biofeedback
Bowlegs
Burns and scalds
Cardiac rehabilitation
Casts and splints
Cerebral palsy
Charcot-Marie-Tooth Disease
Cornelia de Lange syndrome
Disk removal
Dyskinesia

Electromyography
Exercise physiology
Facial transplantation
Fascia
Grafts and grafting
Hemiplegia
Home care
Hydrotherapy
Kinesiology
Knock-knees
Leukodystrophy
Ligaments
Lower extremities
Massage
Minimally conscious state
Motor skill development
Muscles
Muscular dystrophy
Neonatal brachial plexus palsy
Neurology
Numbness and tingling
Orthopedic surgery
Orthopedics
Osteopathic medicine
Osteoporosis
Pain
Pain management
Palsy
Paralysis
Parkinson's disease
Physical rehabilitation
Pigeon toes
Plastic surgery
Prostheses
Pulse rate
Radiculopathy
Scoliosis
Slipped disk
Spinal cord disorders
Spinocerebellar ataxia
Sports medicine
Tendinitis
Tendon disorders
Torticollis
Upper extremities
Whiplash
Williams syndrome

PLASTIC SURGERY
Amputation
Bariatric surgery
Body dysmorphic disorder
Botox
Breast surgery
Burns and scalds
Cleft lip and palate
Cleft lip and palate repair

Craniosynostosis
Cryosurgery
Cyst removal
DiGeorge syndrome
Face lift and blepharoplasty
Facial transplantation
Gender reassignment surgery
Grafts and grafting
Hair transplantation
Healing
Jaw wiring
Laceration repair
Liposuction
Malignancy and metastasis
Mastectomy and lumpectomy
Mesenchymal stem cells
Moles
Necrotizing fasciitis
Neonatal brachial plexus palsy
Neurofibromatosis
Oral and maxillofacial surgery
Otoplasty
Otorhinolaryngology
Prostheses
Ptosis
Rhinoplasty and submucous resection
Skin
Skin lesion removal
Spina bifida
Sturge-Weber syndrome
Surgical procedures
Tattoos and body piercing
Varicose vein removal
Varicose veins
Vision

PODIATRY
Athlete's foot
Bones and the skeleton
Bunions
Cartilage
Cerebral palsy
Corns and calluses
Feet
Flat feet
Foot disorders
Gout
Hammertoe correction
Hammertoes
Heel spur removal
Joints
Lesions
Lower extremities
Methicillin-resistant staphylococcus
  aureus (MRSA) infection
Nail removal
Orthopedic surgery

Orthopedics
Polydactyly and syndactyly
Tendon disorders
Tendon repair

PREVENTIVE MEDICINE
Acidosis
Acupressure
Acupuncture
Alternative medicine
Anemia
Aneurysmectomy
Antibodies
Antihistamines
Antihypertensives
Aromatherapy
Assisted living facilities
Bacillus Calmette-Guérin (BCG)
Biofeedback
Blurred vision
Breast cancer
Brucellosis
Caffeine
Cardiac surgery
Cardiology
Cerebral palsy
Chemotherapy
Chiropractic
Cholesterol
Club drugs
Computed tomography (CT) scanning
Congenital hypothyroidism
Croup
Electrocardiography (ECG or EKG)
Endometrial biopsy
Exercise physiology
Family medicine
Fiber
Food guide plate
Genetic counseling
Genetic engineering
Hormone therapy
Host-defense mechanisms
Immune system
Immunization and vaccination
Insect-borne diseases
Lead poisoning
Mammography
Massage
Meditation
Melatonin
Mesothelioma
Noninvasive tests
Nursing
Nutrition
Occupational health
Osteopathic medicine

Over-the-counter medications
Oxygen therapy
Pharmacology
Phytochemicals
Polycystic ovary syndrome
Psychiatry
Rhinoviruses
Screening
Scurvy
Serology
Sleep
Slipped disk
Smallpox
Sports medicine
Stress reduction
Tendinitis
Vitamin D deficiency
Yoga

PROCTOLOGY
Acquired immunodeficiency syndrome (AIDS)
Anal cancer
Anus
Bladder removal
Chronic granulomatous disease
Colorectal cancer
Colorectal polyp removal
Colorectal surgery
Diverticulitis and diverticulosis
Endoscopy
Fistula repair
Hemorrhoid banding and removal
Hemorrhoids
Hirschsprung's disease
Internal medicine
Polyps
Prostate gland removal
Rectum
Reproductive system
Urology

PSYCHIATRY
Acquired immunodeficiency syndrome (AIDS)
Addiction
Adrenoleukodystrophy
Aging: Extended care
Alcoholism
Alzheimer's disease
Amnesia
Amyotrophic lateral sclerosis
Angelman syndrome
Anorexia nervosa
Antianxiety drugs
Antidepressants
Anxiety

Asperger's syndrome
Attention-deficit disorder (ADD)
Auras
Autism
Bariatric surgery
Bipolar disorders
Body dysmorphic disorder
Bonding
Brain
Brain damage
Brain disorders
Breast surgery
Bulimia
Chronic fatigue syndrome
Club drugs
Cognitive enhancement
Computed tomography (CT) scanning
Dementias
Depression
Developmental disorders
Developmental stages
Dyskinesia
Eating disorders
Electroencephalography (EEG)
Emergency medicine
Factitious disorders
Failure to thrive
Family medicine
Fatigue
Frontotemporal dementia (FTD)
Gender identity disorder
Gender reassignment surgery
Gynecology
Havening touch
Huntington's disease
Hypnosis
Hypochondriasis
Hypothalamus
Incontinence
Interpartner violence
Kluver-Bucy syndrome
Korsakoff's syndrome
Light therapy
Marijuana
Masturbation
Memory loss
Mental retardation
Mental status exam
Morgellons disease
Münchausen syndrome by proxy
Neuropsychology
Neuroscience
Neurosis
Neurosurgery
Obesity
Obsessive-compulsive disorder
Pain

Pain management
Paranoia
Penile implant surgery
Phobias
Phrenology
Pick's disease
Postpartum depression
Post-traumatic stress disorder
Prader-Willi syndrome
Premenstrual syndrome (PMS)
Psychiatric disorders
Psychoanalysis
Psychosis
Psychosomatic disorders
Rape and sexual assault
Restless legs syndrome
Schizophrenia
Seasonal affective disorder
Separation anxiety
Sexual dysfunction
Sexuality
Shock therapy
Single photon emission computed
    tomography (SPECT)
Sleep
Sleep disorders
Speech disorders
Split-brain
Steroid abuse
Stress
Stress reduction
Sudden infant death syndrome (SIDS)
Suicide
Synesthesia
Tardive dyskinesia
Tinnitus
Toilet training
Tourette's syndrome
Traumatic brain injury
Tremors

PSYCHOLOGY
Abuse of the elderly
Addiction
Aging
Aging: Extended care
Alcoholism
Amnesia
Amyotrophic lateral sclerosis
Angelman syndrome
Anorexia nervosa
Antidepressants
Anxiety
Aromatherapy
Asperger's syndrome
Attention-deficit disorder (ADD)
Auras

Bariatric surgery
Bed-wetting
Biofeedback
Bipolar disorders
Blindsight
Bonding
Brain
Brain damage
Bulimia
Capgras syndrome
Cardiac rehabilitation
Cerebral palsy
Cirrhosis
Club drugs
Cognitive development
Death and dying
Depression
Developmental disorders
Developmental stages
Dyslexia
Eating disorders
Electroencephalography (EEG)
Ergogenic aids
Facial transplantation
Factitious disorders
Failure to thrive
Family medicine
Forensic pathology
Frontal lobe syndrome
Gender identity disorder
Gender reassignment surgery
Genetic counseling
Gulf War syndrome
Gynecology
Huntington's disease
Hypnosis
Hypochondriasis
Hypothalamus
Interpartner violence
Juvenile rheumatoid arthritis
Kinesiology
Klinefelter syndrome
Kluver-Bucy syndrome
Korsakoff's syndrome
Learning disabilities
Light therapy
Marijuana
Memory loss
Mental retardation
Mental status exam
Mirror neurons
Miscarriage
Motor skill development
Münchausen syndrome by proxy
Neonatal brachial plexus palsy
Neuropsychology
Neurosis

Obesity
Obsessive-compulsive disorder
Occupational health
Overtraining syndrome
Pain management
Palliative care
Palliative medicine
Paranoia
Phobias
Phrenology
Pick's disease
Plastic surgery
Polycystic ovary syndrome
Postpartum depression
Post-traumatic stress disorder
Premenstrual syndrome (PMS)
Psychosomatic disorders
Puberty and adolescence
Restless legs syndrome
Separation anxiety
Sexual dysfunction
Sexuality
Sleep
Sleep disorders
Sleepwalking
Speech disorders
Split-brain
Sports medicine
Steroid abuse
Stress
Stress reduction
Sturge-Weber syndrome
Sudden infant death syndrome (SIDS)
Suicide
Synesthesia
Temporomandibular joint (TMJ)
    syndrome
Tics
Toilet training
Tourette's syndrome
Traumatic brain injury
Weight loss and gain
Wernicke's aphasia
Williams syndrome

PUBLIC HEALTH
Acquired immunodeficiency
    syndrome (AIDS)
Acute respiratory distress syndrome
    (ARDS)
Adenoviruses
Advance directives
Aging: Extended care
Alternative medicine
Amebiasis
Antibiotic resistance
Antibodies

Assisted living facilities
Babesiosis
Bacillus Calmette-Guérin (BCG)
Bacteriology
Blood testing
Brucellosis
Cerebral palsy
Chagas' disease
Chickenpox
Childhood infectious diseases
Cholera
Chronic obstructive pulmonary
   disease (COPD)
Club drugs
Common cold
Coronaviruses
Creutzfeldt-Jakob disease (CJD)
Dengue fever
Dermatology
Diarrhea and dysentery
E. coli infection
Ebola virus
Elephantiasis
Emergency medicine
Encephalitis
Epidemics and pandemics
Epidemiology
Food guide plate
Food poisoning
Forensic pathology
Gulf War syndrome
Hantavirus
H1N1 influenza
Human papillomavirus (HPV)
Immunization and vaccination
Influenza
Insect-borne diseases
Interpartner violence
Legionnaires' disease
Leishmaniasis
Leprosy
Leptospirosis
Macronutrients
Malaria
Malnutrition
Managed care
Marijuana
Measles
Meningitis
Methicillin-resistant staphylococcus
   aureus (MRSA) infection
Microbiology
Monkeypox
Multiple chemical sensitivity
   syndrome
Neurosis
Niemann-Pick disease

Nursing
Nutrition
Obesity
Occupational health
Osteopathic medicine
Parasitic diseases
Pharmacology
Physician assistants
Pinworms
Plague
Pneumonia
Poliomyelitis
Polycystic ovary syndrome
Prion diseases
Protozoan diseases
Psychiatry
Rabies
Radiation sickness
Rape and sexual assault
Retroviruses
Rhinoviruses
Roundworms
Salmonella infection
Schistosomiasis
Screening
Serology
Severe acute respiratory syndrome
   (SARS)
Sexually transmitted diseases (STDs)
Shigellosis
Sleeping sickness
Smallpox
Syphilis
Tapeworms
Tattoos and body piercing
Tetanus
Trichinosis
Trichomoniasis
Tuberculosis
Tularemia
Typhoid fever
Typhus
West Nile virus
Yellow fever
Zoonoses

PULMONARY MEDICINE
Acquired immunodeficiency
   syndrome (AIDS)
Acute respiratory distress syndrome
   (ARDS)
Adrenoleukodystrophy
Amyotrophic lateral sclerosis
Antihistamines
Apnea
Aspergillosis
Asthma

Bronchi
Bronchiolitis
Bronchitis
Catheterization
Chest
Chronic granulomatous disease
Chronic obstructive pulmonary
   disease (COPD)
Coccidioidomycosis
Cold agglutinin disease
Coronaviruses
Coughing
Critical care
Cyanosis
Cystic fibrosis
Diaphragm
Drowning
Edema
Emergency medicine
Emphysema
Endoscopy
Epidemics and pandemics
Fluids and electrolytes
Forensic pathology
Fungal infections
Hantavirus
Hyperbaric oxygen therapy
Hyperventilation
Hypoxia
Internal medicine
Interstitial pulmonary fibrosis (IPF)
Leptospirosis
Lesions
Lung cancer
Lung surgery
Lungs
Mesothelioma
Methicillin-resistant staphylococcus
   aureus (MRSA) infection
Mold and mildew
Occupational health
Oxygen therapy
Palliative care
Paramedics
Pediatrics
Pharynx
Pleurisy
Pneumocystis jirovecii
Pneumonia
Pneumothorax
Polyps
Prader-Willi syndrome
Pulmonary diseases
Pulmonary edema
Pulmonary hypertension
Respiration
Respiratory distress syndrome

Sarcoidosis
Severe acute respiratory syndrome (SARS)
Single photon emission computed tomography (SPECT)
Sleep apnea
Smoking
Stem cells
Stevens-Johnson syndrome
Thoracic surgery
Thrombolytic therapy and TPA
Trachea
Tuberculosis
Tumors
Vasculitis

RADIOLOGY
Achalasia
Angiography
Aspergillosis
Atrophy
Biopsy
Bone cancer
Brain tumors
Breast cancer
Cancer
Cartilage
Catheterization
Chronic granulomatous disease
Cold agglutinin disease
Computed tomography (CT) scanning
Critical care
Cushing's syndrome
Embolization
Emergency medicine
Endoscopic retrograde cholangiopancreatography (ERCP)
Ewing's sarcoma
Eye infections and disorders
Gallbladder cancer
Imaging and radiology
Joints
Liver cancer
Lung cancer
Magnetic resonance imaging (MRI)
Mammography
Mastectomy and lumpectomy
Meckel's diverticulum
Mesothelioma
Methicillin-resistant staphylococcus aureus (MRSA) infection
Mouth and throat cancer
Neonatal brachial plexus palsy
Noninvasive tests
Nuclear medicine
Nuclear radiology
Oncology

Palliative care
Palliative medicine
Pneumocystis jirovecii
Positron emission tomography (PET) scanning
Prostate cancer
Radiation sickness
Radiation therapy
Radiculopathy
Radiopharmaceuticals
Sarcoidosis
Single photon emission computed tomography (SPECT)
Stents
Testicular cancer
Ultrasonography

REHABILITATION
Neuropsychology
Traumatic brain injury

RHEUMATOLOGY
Aging: Extended care
Ankylosing spondylitis
Anti-inflammatory drugs
Arthritis
Arthroplasty
Arthroscopy
Atrophy
Behçet's disease
Bone disorders
Brucellosis
Bursitis
Cartilage
Cold agglutinin disease
Collagen
Connective tissue
Fibromyalgia
Gout
Hip replacement
Hydrotherapy
Inflammation
Joints
Ligaments
Lyme disease
Mesenchymal stem cells
Methicillin-resistant staphylococcus aureus (MRSA) infection
Orthopedic surgery
Orthopedics
Osteonecrosis
Paget's disease
Pain
Polymyalgia rheumatica
Radiculopathy
Rheumatoid arthritis
Rotator cuff surgery

Sarcoidosis
Scleroderma
Sjögren's syndrome
Sports medicine
Syphilis
Temporal arteritis
Vasculitis

SEROLOGY
Babesiosis
Blood and blood disorders
Blood testing
Chronic granulomatous disease
Cold agglutinin disease
Cytology
Cytopathology
Dialysis
Epidemics and pandemics
Fluids and electrolytes
Forensic pathology
Hematology
Hemophilia
Hodgkin's disease
Host-defense mechanisms
Hyperbaric oxygen therapy
Hyperlipidemia
Hypoglycemia
Immune system
Immunopathology
Laboratory tests
Leukemia
Lymph
Plasma
Rh factor
Rhinoviruses
Sarcoidosis
Septicemia
Snakebites
Transfusion
Tremors

SPEECH PATHOLOGY
Adenoids
Agnosia
Amyotrophic lateral sclerosis
Angelman syndrome
Aphasia and dysphasia
Ataxia
Audiology
Autism
Cerebral palsy
Cleft lip and palate
Deafness
Dyslexia
Ear surgery
Ears
Electroencephalography (EEG)

Hearing loss
Hearing tests
Home care
Jaw wiring
Laryngitis
Lisping
Minimally conscious state
Pharynx
Rubinstein-Taybi syndrome
Speech disorders
Spinocerebellar ataxia
Strokes
Stuttering
Subdural hematoma
Thumb sucking
Voice and vocal cord disorders
Wernicke's aphasia

SPORTS MEDICINE
Acidosis
Acupressure
Arthroplasty
Atrophy
Biofeedback
Blurred vision
Bones and the skeleton
Cartilage
Casts and splints
Concussion
Critical care
Dehydration
Emergency medicine
Ergogenic aids
Exercise physiology
Fiber
Fracture and dislocation
Glycolysis
Head and neck disorders
Heat exhaustion and heatstroke
Hematomas
Hydrotherapy
Impetigo
Joints
Kinesiology
Ligaments
Macronutrients
Massage
Mesenchymal stem cells
Methicillin-resistant staphylococcus
    aureus (MRSA) infection
Motor skill development
Muscles
Nail removal
Orthopedic surgery
Orthopedics
Overtraining syndrome
Pain

Physical rehabilitation
Pigeon toes
Pulse rate
Radiculopathy
Rotator cuff surgery
Safety issues for children
Slipped disk
Steroid abuse
Steroids
Tendinitis
Tendon disorders
Tendon repair

TOXICOLOGY
Acidosis
Bites and stings
Blood testing
Chemotherapy
Club drugs
Critical care
Cyanosis
Diphtheria
Emergency medicine
Ergogenic aids
Food poisoning
Forensic pathology
Gaucher's disease
Hepatitis
Laboratory tests
Lead poisoning
Leukemia
Liver
Mold and mildew
Multiple chemical sensitivity
    syndrome
Neuroscience
Occupational health
Pharmacology
Poisoning
Sarcoidosis
Tremors
Urinalysis

UROLOGY
Abdomen
Adenoviruses
Bed-wetting
Bladder cancer
Bladder removal
Catheterization
Chronic granulomatous disease
Cold agglutinin disease
Congenital adrenal hyperplasia
Contraception
Cryosurgery
Cushing's syndrome
Cystitis

Cystoscopy
Dialysis
Diuretics
E. coli infection
Endoscopy
Erectile dysfunction
Fetal surgery
Fluids and electrolytes
Gender reassignment surgery
Hemolytic uremic syndrome
Hermaphroditism and
    pseudohermaphroditism
Herpes
Hydroceles
Hyperplasia
Hypospadias repair and urethroplasty
Incontinence
Kidney cancer
Kidney disorders
Kidneys
Laser use in surgery
Leptospirosis
Lesions
Lithotripsy
Nephrectomy
Nephrology
Orchiectomy
Pediatrics
Penile implant surgery
Polycystic kidney disease
Polyps
Prostate cancer
Prostate enlargement
Prostate gland
Prostate gland removal
Proteinuria
Pyelonephritis
Reiter's syndrome
Reproductive system
Semen
Sexual differentiation
Sexual dysfunction
Sexually transmitted diseases (STDs)
Sperm banks
Staphylococcal infections
Sterilization
Stevens-Johnson syndrome
Stone removal
Stones
Testicular cancer
Testicular surgery
Testicular torsion
Toilet training
Transplantation
Trichomoniasis
Ultrasonography
Uremia

Urethritis
Urinalysis
Urinary disorders
Urinary system
Vas deferens
Vasectomy

VASCULAR MEDICINE
Acidosis
Amputation
Aneurysms
Angiography
Angioplasty
Antihypertensives
Anti-inflammatory drugs
Aortic aneurysm
Arteriosclerosis
Biofeedback
Bleeding
Blood pressure
Blood vessels
Bruises
Cardiac surgery
Cardiology
Carotid arteries
Cholesterol
Circulation
Claudication
Cold agglutinin disease
Computed tomography (CT) scanning
Congenital heart disease
Cutis marmorata telangiectatica
    congenita
Dehydration
Diabetes mellitus
Electrocauterization
Embolism
Embolization
End-stage renal disease
Endarterectomy
Endocarditis
Glands
Healing
Heart failure
Hematology
Histology
Hormone therapy
Hypercholesterolemia

Hyperlipidemia
Infarction
Ischemia
Klippel-Trenaunay syndrome
Lesions
Lipids
Lungs
Lymphadenopathy and lymphoma
Lymphatic system
Mitral valve prolapse
Necrotizing fasciitis
Osteochondritis juvenilis
Phlebitis
Plasma
Podiatry
Preeclampsia and eclampsia
Progeria
Pulse rate
Raynaud's phenomenon
Respiration
Shunts
Smoking
Stem cells
Stents
Strokes
Sturge-Weber syndrome
Thrombolytic therapy and TPA
Thrombosis and thrombus
Transfusion
Transient ischemic attacks (TIAs)
Ultrasonography
Varicose vein removal
Varicose veins
Vascular system
Venous insufficiency
Von Willebrand's disease

VIROLOGY
Avian influenza
Chickenpox
Childhood infectious diseases
Cold agglutinin disease
Common cold
Conjunctivitis
Coronaviruses
Creutzfeldt-Jakob disease (CJD)
Croup
Cytomegalovirus (CMV)

Dengue fever
Ebola virus
Encephalitis
Enteroviruses
Epidemics and pandemics
Epstein-Barr virus
Eye infections and disorders
Fever
Gastroenteritis
Hand-foot-and-mouth disease
Hantavirus
Hepatitis
Herpes
H1N1 influenza
Human immunodeficiency virus (HIV)
Human papillomavirus (HPV)
Infection
Influenza
Laboratory tests
Marburg virus
Measles
Microbiology
Microscopy
Monkeypox
Mononucleosis
Noroviruses
Opportunistic infections
Orchitis
Paget's disease
Parasitic diseases
Poliomyelitis
Pulmonary diseases
Rabies
Retroviruses
Rhinoviruses
Rotavirus
Sarcoidosis
Serology
Severe acute respiratory syndrome
    (SARS)
Sexually transmitted diseases (STDs)
Shingles
Smallpox
Viral hemorrhagic fevers
Viral infections
West Nile virus
Yellow fever
Zoonoses

INDEX

A

ABCD1 gene, 52
Abdomen, 1-3, 104, 168, 1195, 1310-1311, 2311
Abdominal aortic aneurysm, 160
Abdominal disorders, 3-6, 168, 1105, 1754
Abdominal fluid, 572
Abdominal obesity, 1473
Abdominal pain, 507, 566, 972, 1270, 2141
Abdominoplasty, 1799
AbioCor artificial heart, 1070
ABO incompatibility, 1084
ABO system, 289, 297, 1948, 2015, 2273
Abortion, 7-10, 463, 848, 939, 1113-1114
    threatened, 1488
Abrasions, 1039
Abscess drainage, 11, 13, 862, 1908, 2155, 2331
Abscesses, 11-13, 344, 671, 763, 862, 1238, 1365, 1380, 1580, 1748, 1908, 1926, 2058, 2117, 2155, 2205, 2253, 2311, 2331
    brain, 165
Abstinence, 2035
Abuse, 2157-2158
Abuse of the elderly, 13-14
Accelerated aging, 499
Acceptance, 597
Accessible care, 1432
Accidents, 15-18, 238, 327, 532, 680, 826, 1154, 1449, 1725
    automobile, 2383
ACCOMPLISH trial, 1165
Accord trial, 642
Accutane, 29
Acetaminophen, 427, 1686, 1697, 1700, 1812
Acetyl group, 949
Acetylcholine, 89, 504, 1524, 1534, 1593, 2066
Acetylcholinesterase, 1534
Achalasia, 19, 1752
Achilles tendinitis, 1521, 2210, 2212
Achilles tendon, 841, 1372-1373, 2213
Achondroplasia, 397, 684-685, 953, 1010
Acid, 20, 22, 25
Acid-base chemistry, 20-22
Acid reflux disease, 23-24, 471, 919, 927, 1752, 2092
Acidosis, 22, 24-26
Acne, 26-30, 628, 1741, 1892, 2063
Acoustic reflex, 209
Acquired cystic kidney disease, 1819
Acquired immunodeficiency syndrome (AIDS), 30-34, 125-126, 257, 325, 373, 413, 477, 549, 592, 837, 903, 957,

1144-1146, 1170, 1213, 1281, 1306, 1387, 1647, 1737, 1803, 1805, 2034, 2272, 2291, 2357, 2375, 2392
Acrocyanosis, 505
Acromegaly, 761, 973, 1010
Acromioplasty, 1967
Acrosomal reaction, 1218
Action potential, 324, 1046
Action tremor, 2285
Activator, 949
Active transport, 865
Acupressure, 34-35, 80, 1497, 1697
Acupuncture, 34-39, 80, 1697, 1925
Acute eosinophilic pneumonia, 777
Acute hemorrhagic conjunctivitis, 775
Acute illness, 661
Acute lymphoblastic leukemia, 429
Acute pain, 1697
Acute promyelocytic leukemia, 430
Acute respiratory distress syndrome (ARDS), 39-40
Acyclovir, 438, 507, 2035
Adderall, 504
Addiction, 41-46, 366, 495, 752, 2130
Addison's disease, 46, 51-52, 556, 755, 1787, 2063, 2130
Adenocarcinoma, 517, 1377, 2134, 2297
Adenoid removal, 48, 705, 2251-2252
Adenoids, 47-48, 1392, 1759, 2251, 2253
Adenomas, 520
Adenomyosis, 1189, 1447, 2332
Adenosine, 366, 503, 2066
Adenosine deaminase (ADA) deficiency, 935, 1144, 1212, 2021
Adenosine triphosphate (ATP), 798, 809, 876, 990, 1292, 1477
Adenoviruses, 48-50, 1528
Adhesions, 766, 1191, 1798
Adipocyte, 1466
Adiponectin, 1629
Adipose tissue, 544, 834, 1117, 1354, 1629
Adjustment disorders, 157
Adjuvant therapy, 229, 431
Administration for Children and Families (ACF), 618
Adolescence, 636, 1890-1894, 2163
Adrenal cortex, 46, 556
Adrenal disorders *See* Addison's disease; Cushing's syndrome
Adrenal glands, 46, 50-51, 556, 573, 754, 757, 978, 2189
Adrenal insufficiency, 46, 52
Adrenal tumors, 573
Adrenalectomy, 51-52
Adrenaline, 51, 366, 2040, 2145, 2189
Adrenocorticotropic hormone (ACTH), 46, 50, 52, 556, 573, 759, 978, 1787,

1790, 2190
Adrenoleukodystrophy, 52-53, 1344
Adrenomyeloneuropathy, 52
Adult day care, 189
Advance beneficiary notice (ABN), 1434
Advance directives, 53-54
Adventitia, 159-160
Aerobic exercises, 994
Aerophobia, 1174
Aerospace medicine, 1845
Affect, 894
African American health, 296, 982
African sleeping sickness, 2075
Afterbirth, 1793
Age-related macular degeneration, 284
Agency for Healthcare Research and Quality (AHRQ), 618
Agency for Toxic Substances and Disease Registry (ATSDR), 619
Ageusia, 2197
Agglutination, 1948
Aging, 54-58, 125, 315, 401, 836, 927, 982, 1050, 1109, 1438, 1660, 1772, 1779, 1800, 1881, 2366
    extended care for the, 58-62, 189, 1881, 2215, 2259
    free radical theory of, 2366
    primary, 54
    secondary, 54
Agnosia, 62-63, 85, 1297, 2259
Agonist, 503, 1545-1547
Agoraphobia, 157, 1174, 1765
AIDS *See* Acquired immunodeficiency syndrome (AIDS)
Air pollutants, 558
Air pressure release ventilation (APRV), 40
Alastrim, 2080
Albinos, 954, 1788, 2063
Albright hereditary osteodystrophy, 951
Albumin, 718-719, 1573
Alcohol, 158, 607, 736, 836, 843, 899, 1168, 1184, 1361, 1363, 1365, 1504, 1669, 1714, 1747, 1812, 2005, 2162, 2308
Alcohol abuse, 894
Alcohol dependence, 1301
Alcoholism, 41-42, 63-66, 479, 843, 998, 1184, 1361, 1713, 1812, 2027, 2162, 2164, 2370
Aldosterone, 50, 556, 978, 1576, 2040, 2129, 2189
Aldrich syndrome, 2389
Alendronate, 1676
Alertness, 366
Alkaloids, 1098-1099
Alkalosis, 22
Alkylating agents, 430

Alleles, 127-129, 952-953

Allergens, 67-72, 869, 1031, 1958

Allergic reactions, 170, 187, 197, 274, 524, 624-625, 869, 1031, 1120, 2058, 2092

Allergies, 67-72, 147, 170, 196, 274, 466, 524, 543, 599, 624-625, 1031, 1215, 1551, 1735, 1896, 1958, 2053, 2058, 2092
    food, 869-871
    mold and, 1491
    peanut, 71

ALLHAT trial, 667

Allied health, 73-76, 1295, 1779

Allogeneic transplants, 2281

Allografts, 360, 1001-1002

Allopurinol, 999

Alopecia, 77-79, 1022, 1024, 2063, 2366
    cicatricial, 78
    mucinosa, 79
    nonscarring, 77-79

Alopecia areata, 1022

Alternating hemiplegia of childhood, 1083

Alternative medicine, 80-83, 1039, 1100

Altitude sickness, 84, 188, 662, 1174

Alveolar hypoventilation, 1899

Alveoli, 1803

Alveoli, 39, 745-746, 1380-1381, 1935, 1942

Alzheimer's disease, 57, 85-90, 325, 330-331, 606, 1002, 1119, 1349, 1440, 2087

Amaurosis fugax, 2150

Ambien, 2073

Amblyopia, 814, 816, 1890, 2360

Ambulatory phlebectomy, 2335

Ambulatory surgery centers, 487

Amebiasis, 90-91

Amebic dysentery, 90, 509, 653, 1728, 1871

Amenorrhea, 91-92, 129, 1457

American Anti-Vivisection Society, 124

American Association of Blood Banks, 294

American Cancer Society, 2298

American Medical Association (AMA), 8, 74, 92-93, 452, 807, 831, 1112, 1129, 1673

American Red Cross, 861

Amino acids, 1264, 1395, 1418, 1469, 1475, 1786, 1867

Aminoglycosides, 136-137

Aminoguanidine, 642

Amnesia, 93-94, 533, 1439-1440, 1596, 1599, 2283-2284

Amniocentesis, 95-98, 272, 537, 677, 845, 938, 942, 1268, 1304, 1637, 1839, 1950, 2311

Amnioinfusion, 9

Amniotic fluid, 95, 938, 1304

Amniotic membrane, 1889

Amniotic sac, 1838

Amphetamine salts, 504

Amphetamines, 158, 798

Amphotericin B, 187, 374, 498, 902-903

Amputation, 98-101, 306, 898-899, 1663, 1798, 1864, 2064, 2341, 2344

Amsterdam dwarfism, 551

Amygdala, 1029-1030, 1298

Amyloid fibrils, 85

Amyloidosis, 85, 123, 125

Amyotrophic lateral sclerosis, 101-103, 1012, 1375, 1498-1499, 1708, 2101-2102
    dementia and, 895

Anabolic steroids, 797, 1173, 2130-2131

Anaerobic bacteria, 2222

Anagen, 77-78

Anal cancer, 103-104

Anal fissures, 155, 1851, 2098

Anal intraepithelial neoplasia, 104

Analgesia, 1545, 1547

Analogues, 1147

Analysis of variance (ANOVA), 265

Anaphylaxis, 67-68, 71-72, 274, 1215, 2040
    first aid, 859

Anaplasmosis, 1346

Anastomosis, 1196

Anatomy, 104-107

Androgen insensitivity syndrome, 91

Androgens, 755, 978, 1820, 1861, 2129

Androstenedione, 797

Anemia, 108-111, 129, 505, 663, 674, 1078, 1137, 1410, 1412, 1447, 1455, 1839, 2048-2049, 2225, 2274
    aplastic, 110
    fetal, 97
    hemolytic, 109, 1078
    iron-deficiency, 108, 110, 1078, 1412
    macrocytic, 109
    megaloblastic, 1078
    microcytic, 108
    normocytic, 109
    sideroblastic, 109

Anemic anoxia, 188

Anencephaly, 330, 537, 735, 1460, 1839

Anesthesia, 37, 111-115, 125, 442, 886, 1177, 1559-1560, 1756
    epidural, 423, 442
    local, 111, 117, 1370-1371
    regional, 1370
    spinal, 112, 114, 442

Anesthesiology, 114-117, 2171-2172

Aneurysmectomy, 118

Aneurysms, 118-119, 123, 126, 173-174, 385, 386, 732-733, 893-894, 1080, 1376, 2151, 2228, 2231, 2340
    cerebral, 2150

Angelman syndrome, 119-120, 950

Anger, 596, 1179

Anger camera, 1200

Angina, 121, 161-162, 173, 387, 553, 1056, 1059, 1163, 2344

Angiogenesis, 253, 284, 2226-2227, 2343
    therapeutic, 2343

Angiography, 121-122, 175, 389, 669, 1061, 1064, 1201, 1269, 1397, 1589, 2152

Angiohemophilia, 2371

Angioplasty, 122-123, 390, 554, 1060, 1064, 1316, 2123

Angiosarcoma, 1985

Angiotensin, 149, 1576, 2040

Angiotensin-converting enzyme (ACE) inhibitors, 1165, 1474

Angora hair nevus syndrome, 786-787

Anhydrosis, 1563

Animal Liberation Front, 124

Animal rights vs. research, 123-126, 1818, 2396

Animals, 2402
    transplants from, 2396

Ankles, 321, 1770, 1955, 2210

Ankylosing spondylitis, 127-128, 178, 308, 2112

Anorexia nervosa, 129-131, 706, 708-709, 928, 1396, 1893, 2376
    genetic links, 708

Anosmia, 131-132, 560, 2011, 2082, 2084

Anoxia, 187-188, 662, 1325, 2005

Ansamycins, 136-137

Antacids, 24, 2303, 2307

Antagonist, 503, 1545-1547

Anterior, 893

Anterior cruciate ligament (ACL), 321

Anthrax, 132-134, 2402

Anti-angiogenics, 253

Antianxiety drugs, 134-135, 1831

Antibiotic resistance, 135-139

Antibiotics, 11, 135-136, 138-139, 140-144, 234-235, 352-353, 427, 431, 583-584, 653, 698, 747, 901, 1193, 1227, 1253, 1337-1339, 1482, 1757, 1805, 1901, 2014, 2093, 2118, 2291, 2323
    broad-spectrum, 141-142
    oral, 29
    topical, 28

Antibodies, 144, 224, 252, 288, 505-506, 1143, 1204, 1206, 1226, 1948, 2015-2016. 2305

Anticholinergic drugs, 1733

Anticoagulants, 600, 666, 1073, 2340

Antidepressants, 135, 145-146, 207, 215, 268, 622, 1634, 1734, 1831, 1877, 2162
    suicide and, 873

Antidiuretic hormone, 1790

Antidotes, 2265

Antiemetic drugs, 1560

Antiepileptic drugs, 427

Antiestrogens, 430

Antifungal agents, 187, 203, 374, 902, 904

Antigens, 224, 252, 291, 293, 505, 1203, 1948, 2016, 2280

Antihistamines, 71, 147-148, 438, 525, 599, 626, 1031, 1120, 1685, 1958, 2054

Antihypertensives, 148-151

Anti-inflammatory drugs, 152-153, 154

Antimetabolites, 136, 430
Anti-Mullerian hormone, 1685
Antioxidants, 154-155, 1438, 1622, 1783, 2166
Antiperspirants, 1157
Antipsychotic drugs, 1877, 2193
Antipyretic drugs, 852, 1167
Antiscarring drugs, 2186
Antisense technology, 258
Antisense therapy, 370
Antitoxins, 2224
Antivenin, 274
Antiviral drugs, 224, 1240
Anus, 155-156, 514, 773, 926, 1091, 1194, 1851, 1926, 2098
Anxiety, 59, 134, 156-158, 207, 302, 836, 1174, 1179, 1599, 1632, 1765, 1878, 2003, 2013, 2073
Aorta, 159-160, 299, 385, 539
Aortic aneurysm, 159-160
Aortic stenosis, 161-163
Aortic valve replacement, 163
Apathy, 894
Aperistalsis, 1752
Apgar score, 163-164
Aphasia, 164-166, 1596, 2094-2095, 2149, 2283-2284
Aphrodisiacs, 166
Aphthous ulcers, 244, 375
Apicoectomy, 1748
Aplasia cutis, 575
Apnea, 167, 836, 1543, 2067-2068, 2071, 2159
Apocrine glands, 976
Appendectomy, 167-168
Appendicitis, 6, 168-170, 514, 1261
Appendix, 168-170
Appetite, 1136, 1337
Apraxia, 85
Aqueous fluid, 401, 982, 1643, 2358
Arboviruses, 749, 2381
Arches, 840
Ariboflavinosis, 1410
Arnold-Chiari malformation, 437
Aromatase inhibitors, 337, 430
Aromatherapy, 82, 170, 1039
Arousal, 1485-1486
Arrhythmias, 171-172, 388, 390, 601, 674, 1063-1064, 1137, 1690, 1704, 1943, 2150
Arsenic, 430
Artefill, 1800
Arterial blood gas, 469
Arterial distension, 119
Arteries, 121, 172, 472, 1163, 1374, 1795, 2188, 2317, 2339, 2342
    chest, 433
    embolization, 732
Arteriosclerosis, 119, 172-176, 473, 480, 553, 641, 1056, 1059, 1062, 1119, 1157, 1163, 1352, 1450, 1622, 1626, 2005, 2026, 2149, 2152, 2231, 2339
Arteritis, 2208

Arthritis, 153, 176-180, 308-309, 352-353, 997, 1109, 1278, 1298, 1659, 1662, 1664, 1929, 1953, 1955, 2112, 2183, 2209
    juvenile rheumatoid, 1279-1280
    Lyme disease and, 1385
    septic, 996
Arthrodesis, 427
Arthroplasty, 181-182, 1109, 1278, 1957
Arthropod-borne diseases, 274
Arthroscopy, 17, 182-183, 772, 1278, 1661, 1968
Articulations, 314
Artificial heart, 1070
Artificial insemination, 192, 1232, 1234-1236, 2096
Artificial lens, 399, 403
Artificial respiration, 391
Artificial respirator, 1897
Artificial skin, 360
Asanas, 2399
Asbestos exposure, 183-184, 778, 1467-1468
Asbestosis, 184
Ascaris lumbricoides, 1969
Ascites, 480, 719, 922, 1365, 1367, 1573, 1754, 2311
Ascorbic acid, 2002
Aseptic techniques, 2168
Asherman's syndrome, 91
Ashkenazi Jews, 929
Asparaginase, 780
Asperger's syndrome, 185-186, 632-634, 2179
Aspergillosis, 186-187, 903, 1492
Asphyxiants, 17
Asphyxiation, 187-188, 680, 1075, 2223
    fetal, 2133
Aspiration, 39, 261, 333, 587, 680, 913, 1268, 1862, 2294
Aspirin, 153, 430, 1685, 1812, 1947, 2152, 2231-2232, 2303, 2307
Assessment, 644
Assisted living facilities, 189-191
Assisted reproductive technologies, 191-194, 912, 1218, 1489
    ethics and, 802
Assisted suicide, 195
Asthma, 187, 195-200, 350, 623, 1176, 1253, 1383, 1451, 1453, 1689, 1895-1896, 1902-1903, 1937
    first aid, 859
    mold and, 1491
Astigmatism, 200-201, 404, 814, 816, 822, 1928, 2011, 2360-2361
Astrocytes, 325, 985
Ataxia, 120, 201-202, 499, 2109
Atherectomy, 1060, 2123
Atherosclerosis, 123, 299-300
Atherosclerotic lesions, 126
Athlete's foot, 202-203, 842, 902, 1482, 1540
Athletes, 797, 1688
Atopic dermatitis, 623-624, 626, 716,

1791
Atresia, 1684
Atria, 1054
Atrial fibrillation, 173, 203-204, 385, 388, 607, 1057, 1063, 2231
Atrioventricular (A-V) node, 387, 1055, 1524, 1690
Atrioventricular defects, 540
Atrophic rhinitis, 1958
Atrophy, 204, 1172, 1375, 1498, 1524, 1707, 2317
    vaginal, 1445
Atropine, 1099
Attention-deficit disorder (ADD), 205-207
Audiology, 125-126, 208-211
Auditory brainstem potential (ABR) test, 1053
Auditory dyslexia, 689
Aural rehabilitation, 211
Auras, 211-212, 1033
Auscultation, 1767
Autism, 185-186, 212-215, 633, 1487, 2095
    mercury and, 1465
Autoantibody, 2183
Autografts, 360, 1001-1002
Autoimmune, 2208
Autoimmune disorders, 127, 216-219, 465-466, 663, 1010-1011, 1096, 1215, 1279, 1534, 1735, 1953, 2055, 2182, 2305
    endometriosis and, 767
Autoimmune hemolytic anemias, 505
Autoimmune response, 2186
Autologous transplants, 2281
Automated external defibrillators (AEDs), 602, 1945
Automated quantitative cytometry (AQC), 1379
Automatic external defibrillators (AEDs), 380
Automation, 1304
Automobile accidents, 2383
Autonomic nervous system, 248, 1055, 1164, 1579, 1756, 1781, 2178
    yoga and, 2399
Autonomy, 636
Autopsy, 220-223, 885, 1737
Autosomal dominant diseases, 941
Autosomal dominant trait, 2386
Autosomal recessive diseases, 499, 941
Autosome, 949
Avian influenza, 223-227, 1211, 2020
Avoidance, 1830
Avulsions, 1039
Awareness, 1485
Axons, 425-426, 1118, 1579, 1591, 1597, 1716
Azathioprine, 506
Azithromycin, 1330
Azotemia, 1552, 2186, 2318

B

B lymphocytes, 252, 1002, 1121, 1143, 1203-1204, 1206, 1212, 1387, 1392, 2389

B vitamins, 246, 471, 1622, 2365

Babesiosis, 228

Babinski reflex, 1927

Baby blues, 1829

Baby Fae, 2396

Bacilli, 132, 317, 1005-1006

Bacillus Calmette-Gu,rin (BCG), 228-229, 253, 276, 1207, 1335, 2291

Back, 663-664

Back disorders, 1302

Back pain, 230-231, 321, 664, 1310, 1674, 1696, 1992, 2078, 2108, 2112

Bacteremia, 1006, 1982

Bacteria, 11, 135-136, 138-139, 142, 231, 236, 366, 427, 587, 662, 695, 1003, 1142, 1252, 1356, 1480, 1757, 1981
anaerobic, 2222
flesh-eating, 1562
gram-positive, 1004
intestinal, 514

Bacterial chromosome, 135-136, 138

Bacterial endocarditis, 752

Bacterial infections, 5-6, 12, 231-234, 236, 366, 447, 493, 582, 662, 695, 720, 752, 763, 773, 788, 914, 917, 996, 1085, 1216, 1227, 1252, 1356, 1384, 1426, 1442, 1479, 1580, 1754, 2013, 2117, 2143, 2155, 2270, 2293, 2300-2301

Bacterial meningitis, 1442-1443

Bacteriology, 235-237, 1003

Bacteriophage, 135-136, 138, 490

Bacteriuria, 2322, 2324

Baker's cysts, 577

Balance, 2351

Balance disorders, 238-239, 2351

Balantidiasis, 1871

Baldness, 1022, 1024

Balloon angioplasty, 123, 405, 1060, 1064, 2152, 2340

Balloon catheter, 541

Balloon sinuplasty, 2054

Barbiturates, 117

Bargaining, 597

Bariatric surgery, 239, 1627

Barium, 1200

Barium swallow test, 19

Barley, 987

Baroreceptors, 673, 1780

Barrett's esophagus, 799, 2179

Bartholin's cysts, 577

Bartholin's glands, 577

Basal cell carcinoma, 572, 631, 2058, 2060, 2064-2065, 2297

Basal ganglia, 324, 692-694

Base, 20, 25

Basophils, 67-69, 71-72, 1203

Bats, 1910-1911

Batten's disease, 240-241

Battered elder syndrome, 13

Battle fatigue, 1831

Becker nevus syndrome, 786-787

Beckwith-Wiedemann syndrome, 951

Bed-wetting, 241-242

Bedsores, 100, 243-244, 1302, 2306

Bee stings, 663

Behçet's disease, 375

Behavior modification therapy, 214

Behavior therapy, 120

Behavioral observation audiometry, 1053

Behavioral studies, 125

Behavioral therapy, 43, 1633, 1784, 1878

Behçet's disease, 244

Beir blockade, 112

Bell's palsy, 245, 1705, 1708

Beneficence, 801

Benign cells, 369, 590

Benign forgetfulness, 605, 1439

Benign paroxysmal positional vertigo, 238

Benign prostatic hyperplasia (BPH), 967, 1082, 1161, 1451, 1453, 1855, 1857, 1863

Benign tumor, 986

Benzocaine, 1370

Benzodiazepines, 2068, 2072

Beriberi, 246, 876, 1410, 1412, 2367

Bernstein test, 24

Beta blockers, 149, 151

Beta carotene, 2365

Beta-lactamases, 136-137, 139

Bicarbonate, 1709

Bicuspids, 2204

Bifocals, 2358

Bile, 2, 246-247, 461, 471, 658, 862, 905, 907, 911, 918, 1360, 1364, 1366, 2129, 2188

Bile acids, 461

Bile duct, 455

Bile salts, 2, 579-580

Bilharziasis, 1987

Biliary colic, 909, 2138

Biliary system, 905

Bilirubin, 416, 1274, 1360, 1363, 1365-1367

Bimanual examination, 1018

Binding proteins, 1136

Binge eating, 356, 707
genetic links, 708

Bioengineering, 255

Bioethics, 800

Biofeedback, 81, 247-250, 255, 2147

Bioinformatics, 251-252, 963, 1869

Biologic disease response modifiers (BDRMs), 1954

Biological therapies, 252-254, 1677

Biological weapons, 133, 2081

Biomarkers, 1869

Biomechanics, 1295

Biomedical research, 123-125

Biomedicine, 123

Bionics, 254-259

Biopsy, 220, 259-262, 305, 335, 421, 589, 629, 631, 1268-1269, 1311, 1367, 1862, 2294, 2305
breast, 259, 333, 344
cone, 422
endometrial, 764-765
excisional, 261, 333
frozen section, 261
incisional, 261, 333
liver, 1604
needle, 261, 333, 1268, 1423, 1862, 2294

Biopsychology, 1597

Biostatistics, 263-265

Biotechnology, 254-259

Bioterrorism, 134, 783, 2081, 2353

Bioterrorist event, 353

Biotin, 2366

Biowarfare, 133

Bipolar disorders, 266-270, 620, 1598, 2003

Bird flu, 223, 1211, 2020

Birth See Childbirth; Childbirth complications

Birth control, 546, 2124, 2288, 2347

Birth control pills, 418, 547, 1017, 1137, 2124, 2130

Birth defects, 270-273, 463, 481, 539, 551, 579, 677, 735, 936, 1325, 1569, 1738, 1772, 1839, 1971, 2094, 2099, 2107, 2171, 2213, 2226
correction in utero, 844

Birthmarks, 628, 1296, 1316, 1492, 2060, 2153

Bisexuality, 2031

Bison, 352-354

Bisphosphonates, 1676

Bites, 274-275, 1120, 1909, 2402
first aid, 860

Black eye, 1032

Black mold, 1492

Black Plague, 782

Blackheads, 27, 628

Bladder, 2, 229, 256, 277, 583, 585, 772, 960, 1221, 1223, 1858, 1863, 2138, 2140, 2323, 2326, 2329

Bladder cancer, 229, 275-277

Bladder infections See Urinary disorders

Bladder removal, 276-277

Bladder stones, 2138, 2140, 2327

Blastocyst, 489-492, 733, 1684, 1836

Blastomere biopsy, 1219

Blastomycosis, 903

Bleeding, 278-282, 355, 665, 1037, 1077, 1079, 1087, 1308, 1316, 2229, 2371
abnormal, 1079
brain, 1267
first aid, 859
gum, 974
rectal, 669, 671, 1092
uterine, 764, 1447

Blepharitus, 682

Blepharoplasty, 825-826, 1799

Blepharospasm, 317, 682

Blind spot, 822

Blindness, 283-284, 641, 813, 982, 1284, 1397-1398, 1410, 1536, 2011, 2034-2035, 2150, 2270, 2362

Blindsight, 285-286

Blisters, 286-287, 625-626, 897-898, 1107, 2034, 2038, 2063, 2132
bedsores and, 243

Blood, 105, 287-290, 297, 545, 1076, 1117, 1203, 1304, 1359, 1797, 1943, 1948, 2015, 2168, 2188, 2271, 2329, 2342
collection of, 1764
urine, 1082

Blood banks, 1305

Blood banks, 291-295

Blood clotting, 600, 665, 711, 1037, 1087, 1191, 1273, 1447, 1761, 2041, 2229-2230, 2234, 2371

Blood disorders, 287-290, 665, 1078, 1084, 1086-1087, 2047, 2225, 2371

Blood donation, 2272

Blood doping, 798

Blood loss, 1190

Blood poisoning See Septicemia

Blood pressure, 295-296, 472, 672-673, 1055, 1059, 1162-1164, 1186, 1769, 1781, 1898, 1943, 2039-2040, 2189, 2342
diastolic, 1162
systolic, 1162

Blood substitutes, 2274

Blood testing, 289, 297-298, 1006, 1077, 1084, 1304, 1306, 1764, 1956, 2016, 2272
fecal occult, 2001

Blood transfusion, 2041

Blood transfusion reactions, 1215, 2276

Blood typing, 289, 297, 1305, 1948, 2016, 2273

Blood vessels, 299-300, 355, 512, 1080, 1374, 2312, 2317, 2342
growth, 2343
inflammation, 2345

Blount's disease, 318

Blue baby syndrome, 300-301, 576

Blue skin, 300, 576

Blurred vision, 301-302, 1397, 1536

Blushing, 2178

Body dysmorphic disorder, 302-303

Body mass index (BMI), 829, 878, 1625

Body piercing, 2200

Body temperature, 1073, 1167-1168, 2177
sleep and, 2066

Boils, 1479

Bolus, 471, 799

Bonding, 303-304, 342

Bone cancer, 305-308, 807, 1658

Bone densitometry, 1676

Bone disorders, 305-310, 314, 356, 558, 883, 1109, 1302, 1587, 1667, 1669, 1673, 1694, 1953, 1962

Bone fractures See Fracture and dislocation

Bone grafting, 310, 1670

Bone marrow, 305, 311, 369, 1078, 1204, 1214, 1340, 1342, 1466-1467, 2121, 2229

Bone marrow aspirate, 1466

Bone marrow stem cell, 1466-1467

Bone marrow transplantation, 310-312, 314, 1003, 1123, 1214, 1342, 1913, 2021, 2049

Bone matrix, 313

Bone scan, 305

Bones, 307, 310, 312-316, 558, 807, 840, 867, 891, 1038, 1117, 1275, 1277, 1523, 1658, 1660, 1798, 1920, 1954, 2314
broken, 398, 1038, 1109

Bortezomib, 506

Botox, 19-20, 316-317, 693, 1083, 1157, 1800

Botulism, 17, 233, 316-318, 880, 1482, 1800

Bouchard's nodes, 1664

Bovine spongiform encephalopathy, 470, 561

Bowel movements, 1115

Bowlegs, 318-319, 686, 1299, 1658

Bowman's capsule, 1291

Bowman's glands, 2084

Braces, orthodontic, 319-320, 614, 1657

Braces, orthopedic, 320-321, 1349, 1997

Brachial plexus, 1563-1566

Brachmann-de Lange syndrome, 551

Brachytherapy, 335

Bradycardia, 167, 171, 680, 1063, 1903

Bradykinesia, 1731-1732

Bradykinin, 1237

Braille, 284

Brain, 106, 322-325, 327, 499, 724-725, 1118, 1150, 1592, 1600, 1919, 2023, 2187
aging and, 55
anatomy of the, 322, 2188
bleeding in, 1267
implants, 256
mapping of, 1589
sleep and, 2065

Brain banks, 326-327

Brain connectivity, 1485

Brain damage, 16, 62, 327-328, 380, 681, 689, 789, 1460, 2259

Brain death, 330

Brain disorders, 87, 201, 324, 328-331, 437, 527, 689, 725, 748, 895, 1442, 2005

Brain doping, 1586

Brain hemispheres, 1601

Brain hemorrhage, 1376

Brain herniation, 2283-2284

Brain implants, 1587

Brain inflammation, 748

Brain injury, 1596-1597

Brain trauma, 980-981

Brain tumors, 165, 332-333, 726, 1581, 1717, 2005

Brain waves, 725, 2067

Brain, aging and, 56

Brain-machine interface, 1586-1587

Brainstem, 1545-1547

Branched-chain alpha-ketoacid dehydrogenase (BCKD), 1418

BRCA genes, 334, 338, 418, 429 1424-1425, 1684

Breast augmentation, 345, 1800

Breast biopsy, 259, 333, 344

Breast cancer, 333-338, 344, 348, 939, 1414, 1607, 1914
screening and, 2000

Breast cysts, 578, 586, 1423

Breast disorders, 338-340, 348, 436, 855, 1426

Breast-feeding, 340-343

Breast implants, 345, 1414, 1800

Breast milk, 341, 1426, 2374

Breast reduction, 345, 1800

Breast self-examination, 2000

Breast surgery, 344-346, 1799

Breasts, 435, 1413

Breasts, female, 333-334, 346-349, 855, 978, 1770, 1799, 1932

Breasts, male, 1020

Breathing, 167, 391, 557, 568, 1075, 1174, 1801

Breathing difficulty See Pulmonary diseases; Respiration; Respiratory distress syndrome.

Breathing exercises, 2399

Breech birth, 423, 442, 445

Bridges, 569-570, 617

Brief Abuse Screen for the Elderly, 13

Bright's disease, 1575

Broadmann's area 22, 2379

Broca's aphasia, 1597, 2284, 2380

Broca's area, 893

Broken bones, 1038, 1109

Bronchi, 350, 1381, 2268

Bronchiectasis, 1380

Bronchioles, 196, 350-351, 1381

Bronchiolitis, 350-351

Bronchitis, 350-352, 469, 558, 745, 747, 1378, 1382, 1450, 1453, 1689, 1895, 1900, 1902, 1937, 2370

Bronchodilators, 153, 198, 747, 1896

Bronchopneumonia, 1804

Bronchoscopy, 772, 1269, 1896

Bronze diabetes, 1083

Brucella, 352-354

Brucellosis, 352-354, 2402

Bruises, 355, 1032

Bruit, 174, 473, 2151

Bubble boy disease, 2020

Bubonic plague, 743, 1794, 2403

Buck teeth, 1656

Buerger's disease, 2346

Buffers, 21

Bulbourethral glands, 2008
Bulimia, 355-356, 928, 1396, 1893, 2376
  genetic links, 708
Bunions, 356-357, 842, 883, 1809
Bureau of Chemistry, 872
Burkitt's lymphoma, 357, 358, 794,
  1388-1389, 1482, 2297, 2357
Burns, 17-18, 358-361, 721, 1155, 2040,
  2059, 2258
  first aid, 860
Burns and scalds, 359, 361
Bursas, 356, 363, 577, 1660
Bursitis, 308, 362-363, 883, 1278, 1661,
  1967
Butterfly rash, 2183
Bypass surgery, 175-176, 363-365, 553,
  731, 1060, 1064, 2123, 2152, 2341
  gastric, 239

C

C-reactive protein (CRP), 1060
Caffeine, 158, 171, 343, 366, 490,
  503-504, 798, 836, 1174, 2066, 2071,
  2303, 2308
Calcaneus, 840, 1372
Calcification, 161
Calcinosis, 2186
Calcipotriol, 787
Calcitonin, 315, 967, 1137, 1676, 2189,
  2239
Calcitriol, 1677
Calcium, 312, 866, 977, 1159, 1161, 1410,
  1412, 1445, 1621, 1623, 1674, 1677,
  2239, 2366
Calcium-channel blockers, 149, 1165
Calcium deficiency, 867
Calculi See Stones
Calculus, 974
Calluses, 552-553, 883, 886-887, 889,
  1025, 1810
Calories, 1475, 1625-1626, 2375
Campylobacter infections, 366-367, 773,
  917
Canalith repositioning, 238
Cancer, 3, 106, 126, 253, 257, 335,
  367-371, 379, 410, 418, 428, 430-431,
  590, 593, 663, 779, 794, 955, 986, 993,
  1144, 1170, 1252, 1262, 1264, 1281,
  1306, 1312, 1317, 1362, 1406, 1554,
  1640, 1736, 1740, 1847, 1856, 1913,
  1985, 2166, 2294, 2297-2299, 2323,
  2357
  anal, 103-104
  bladder, 229, 275-277
  bone, 305-308, 807, 1658
  breast, 333-338, 344, 939, 1414,
    1607, 1914
  cervical, 417-421, 957-958, 1019,
    1147, 1715, 2332
  colon, 515-521, 923, 1092, 1196,
    1262, 1264, 1449, 1452, 1622,
    1852, 1926

Down syndrome and, 677
  endometrial, 418-420, 764, 957-958,
    2332
  esophageal, 799, 922
  gallbladder, 906-909
  gene therapy and, 935
  hyperthermia treatment for, 1169
  intestinal, 2134-2137
  kidney, 1285-1286
  liver, 923, 1361-1365, 1367
  lung, 1377-1380, 1382, 1449, 1452,
    1467, 1895, 1902
  men and, 1449
  mouth, 1504-1505
  nutrition and, 1622
  oral, 611-612, 2254
  ovarian, 417-421, 957-958
  pancreatic, 1711, 2134-2137
  prostate, 572, 961, 1449, 1452, 1654,
    1855-1857, 1861, 1863, 2130, 2349
  rectal, 517-519, 1926
  screening and, 2000
  skin, 571, 629, 1449, 1452, 1787,
    2060-2061, 2064-2065
  stomach, 915, 922, 2134-2137
  testicular, 961, 1449, 2218-2220
  throat, 1504-1505, 1759
  uterine, 417-421, 957-958, 1190
  vaginal, 957
  viruses and, 1946
Cancer growth inhibitors, 253
Cancer stem cells, 431
Candidiasis, 372-375, 584, 902-903, 957,
  1213, 1482
Canker sores, 375
Capacitation, 529
Capgras syndrome, 376-377
Capillaries, 575, 717, 2188, 2343
Capsids, 2354
Car accidents, 2383
Carbamazepine, 791
Carbapenems, 136-137
Carbidopa, 1733
Carbohydrates, 377, 657, 875, 1264, 1359,
  1395, 1470, 1621, 1623
  metabolism, 905, 989
Carbon dioxide, 21, 1055, 1174, 1381,
  1936, 1942
Carbon monoxide, 1155
Carcinogens, 378, 873
Carcinoma, 379, 2297
Cardiac arrest, 379-380, 391-392, 563,
  1250, 1693
Cardiac catheterization, 386, 405, 1269
Cardiac ischemia, 1273
Cardiac muscle, 106, 1054, 1118, 1523
Cardiac output, 148
Cardiac pacing, 1944
Cardiac rehabilitation, 380-384, 554, 812,
  1295
Cardiac surgery, 385-386
Cardiac tamponade, 2039, 2041
Cardiology, 291, 381, 385, 387-391, 1612

Cardiomyopathy, 123, 126, 389, 1450
Cardiopulmonary resuscitation (CPR),
  172, 380, 391-392, 563, 576, 602, 681,
  1250, 1720, 1897, 1943, 2041, 2214
Cardiovascular, 291
Cardiovascular disease, 1449
Cardiovascular medicine, 126
Caregiver Abuse Screen, 13
Caries, dental, 611
Carnitine, 839
Carotenoids, 1622, 1783
Carotid arteries, 393, 751, 2150, 2278,
  2334, 2339
Carpal tunnel syndrome, 178, 393-396,
  727, 834, 1583, 1615, 1638, 1718,
  2179, 2318
  yoga and, 2400
Cartilage, 17, 181, 396-397, 512, 544,
  1117, 1277, 1660, 1664, 1955, 2268
Case series, 783-785
Case-control study, 783-784
Castration, 1934
Casts, 321, 398-399, 891, 1997
CAT scans See Computed tomography
  (CT) scanning
Catabolism, 1475
Catagen, 77-78
Cataplexy, 1542-1543, 2068, 2071
Cataract surgery, 399-400, 817, 1316
Cataracts, 283-284, 399, 401-404, 624,
  813, 815, 817, 823, 1644, 2012,
  2360-2362
Catatonia, 2045
Catheterization, 404-405, 928, 1269
Catheters, 122-123, 405, 928, 1186, 1250,
  2233, 2323-2324
  balloon, 541, 2054
Cations, 865
Caudal block, 113
Cauliflower ear, 702, 1081
Cavities, 22, 406-407, 499, 610, 614, 926,
  1748, 2204, 2254
CDNA, 489
Cecum, 925, 1263
Celera Genomics, 964
Celiac disease, 922, 987, 2079
Celiac sprue, 407, 1401
Cell cycle, 368
Cell death, 1562
Cell development, 2120
Cell division, 428, 676
Cell injury, 589, 593, 661-662
Cell therapy, 82
Cells, 260, 408-411, 428, 458, 587, 592,
  1118, 1782, 2120
Cellulitis, 1479, 2143
Cellulose, 854
Centers for Disease Control and
  Prevention (CDC), 412-414, 618
Central nervous system, 106, 985,
  1545-1546, 1579, 1592, 1602, 1717,
  1732, 1781, 1843
Centrifugation, 2329

Cephalosporins, 136-138
Cerebellar tremor, 2285
Cerebellum, 322
Cerebral cortex, 324
Cerebral hemispheres, 2111
Cerebral palsy, 415-417, 1706-1708, 1739, 2317
Cerebrospinal fluid, 113, 330, 1012, 1150, 1268, 1304, 1376, 1442
  leaking of, 560
Cerebrovascular accident, 164, 173, 894, 1581, 2149, 2235, 2344
Cerebrovascular disease, 173, 2149
Cerebrum, 324, 2188
Certification, 75
Ceruloplasmin, 2387
Cerumen, 705, 1050
Cervarix, 1148
Cervical cancer, 417-421, 957-958, 1147, 1416, 1715, 2332
Cervical cap, 547
Cervical dilation, 441
Cervical os, 1018
Cervical procedures, 421-422
Cervical, ovarian, and uterine cancers, 418
Cervix, 421, 1018, 1189, 1230, 1714, 1932, 2332
  strawberry, 2287
Cesarean section, 423-424, 442, 444, 767, 1637
Chagas' disease, 19, 424-425, 1245, 1647, 1729, 1871, 2075
Chalazion, 586, 2155
Chancre, 2034, 2075, 2181
Charcoal, 2265
Charcot-Marie-Tooth Disease, 425-427
Charley horse, 1521
Checking behavior, 1631
Chelation, 778
Chemical burns, 360, 362
Chemical peeling, 825
Chemical warfare, 779
Chemicals, 797, 1511
Chemistry, 1305
Chemonucleolysis, 2078
Chemoreceptors, 673
Chemotherapy, 306, 336, 369, 427-431, 519, 1342, 1407, 1424, 1561, 1641, 2017, 2294
  regional, 1363
Chest, 104, 432-436, 1382, 2227
Chest compressions, 392
Chest pain, 23, 121, 381, 723, 752, 1163, 1174, 1225, 1378, 1752, 1801, 1896
Chewing tobacco, 1749
Chiari malformations, 436-437
Chickenpox, 286, 437-439, 447-448, 1107, 1828, 2038, 2355
Child abuse, 686, 1427, 1811, 2160
Child molester, 1923
CHILD syndrome, 786
Childbirth, 423, 439-443, 793, 1176, 1567, 1635, 1738, 1781, 2392

hydrotherapy and, 1152
Childbirth complications, 423, 443-445, 463, 475, 767, 862, 1747, 1841
Childhood disintegrative disorder, 632-633
Childhood infectious diseases, 438, 445-449, 659-660, 858, 1208, 1283, 1428, 1516-1517, 1739, 1966
Childhood obesity, 640-641
Chinese medicine, 34, 1039
Chinese restaurant syndrome, 2178
Chiropractic, 81, 242, 449-452, 835, 1039
Chlamydia, 452-453, 957, 996, 1743, 1929, 2034-2036, 2323
Chloracne, 779
Chlorambucil, 506
Chlorofluorocarbons (CFCs), 2061
Chloroform, 116
Choking, 454, 564, 1075
  first aid, 859
Cholangiography, 863
Cholangitis, 2305
Cholecystectomy, 454-455, 772, 906, 908, 910-911, 1311, 2138
Cholecystitis, 455-456, 909-910
Cholera, 233, 456-457, 776, 1848
Cholesteatoma, 703
Cholesterol, 458-462, 955, 1156-1158, 1352, 1359, 1450, 1603, 1795, 2128, 2131
  screening and, 2000
Cholinesterase inhibitors, 89
Chondrin, 544
Chondrocytes, 396, 1466
Chondroitin, 179, 1665
Chondrosarcoma, 1985
Chorea, 687-688, 1149
Chorionic villus sampling, 97, 272, 462-463, 537, 678, 938, 942, 1637, 1839
Chromatolysis, 1119
Chromomycosis, 902
Chromosomal abnormalities, 96, 735, 938, 1282, 1460
Chromosomes, 530, 580, 655, 676, 678, 680, 735, 937, 940-942, 949-951, 952-953, 1282, 1460, 1506, 1508-1509, 1531, 2386
Chronic disease, 127, 2363
Chronic fatigue syndrome, 463-466, 837-838
  endometriosis and, 767
  yoga and, 2400
Chronic granulomatous disease, 467-468
Chronic illness, 413, 661
Chronic myeloid leukemia, 430
Chronic obstructive pulmonary disease (COPD), 468-469, 576, 748, 1379, 1450, 1899, 1902, 1937, 2087, 2268
Chronic pain, 180, 1697
Chronic wasting disease (CWD), 470, 1849
Churg Strauss syndrome, 2346

Chyme, 471, 514, 657, 925, 1751, 2079, 2188
Chymopapain, 1099
Cialis, 796
Cidofovir, 1493
Cilia, 411, 2053
Circadian rhythms, 45, 81, 496, 2003, 2065, 2072-2073
Circle of Willis, 2149
Circulation, 98, 387, 471-474, 1054, 1359, 1374, 1943, 2149, 2259, 2342
Circulatory system, 717, 1058, 1062, 1065, 1086, 1393, 1762, 1942, 2039, 2188
  aging and, 55
Circumcision
  female, 474-476, 1934
  male, 476-479, 1934
Circumscribed, 376
Cirrhosis, 5-6, 63-64, 479-480, 1083, 1095, 1119, 1161, 1360, 1363, 1365, 1367-1368, 1451, 1604, 2027, 2047
Claudication, 174-175, 473, 480-481, 2107, 2340, 2344
Clawtoes, 1025
Cleavage, 733
Cleft lip repair, 484-485, 1799
Cleft palate, 481-485, 575, 1759, 2094, 2370
Cleft palate repair, 484-485, 1799
Clinical trials, 485-487, 872
Clinics, 487-489
Clitoridectomy, 475, 1934
Clitoris, 475, 1932
Clomiphene, 1219
Cloning, 194, 489-493, 948
Clostridia, 1481, 2222, 2224
Clostridium difficile infection, 493-494
Club drugs, 494-495
Clubbing, 1540
Clubfoot, 575, 841, 883
Cluster headaches, 495-497, 1034-1035
Coagulation, 278-280, 282, 600
Coagulation factors, 1087, 2371
Cobalamin, 109
Cobb angle measurement, 1996
Cocaine, 42, 45, 117, 158, 404, 537, 736, 836, 1098
  anesthesia, 1371
Cocci, 1005-1006
Coccidioidomycosis, 497-498
Cochlea, 594, 702, 1045, 2011
Cochlear implants, 256, 499, 595, 1047
Cockayne disease, 498-499, 686
Cocktail therapy, 33, 1147
Co-contraction, 692-693
Code situation, 1137
Codeine, 1099, 1546
Cognition, 604, 1463
Cognitive development, 56, 499-503, 635, 1009
Cognitive enhancement, 503-504
Cognitive rehabilitation, 1596

Cognitive therapy, 43
Cohort study, 783-785
Colchicine, 999, 1099
Cold agglutinin disease, 504-506
Cold sores, 506, 1107
Cold, therapeutic use of, 571, 1773
Colectomy, 521
Colic, 507-508
Colitis, 493, 509-512, 516, 521, 651, 653,
854, 919, 923, 927, 1196, 1261, 1852
Collagen, 396, 512, 544, 1038, 1117,
1348, 1787, 1800, 1993, 2186
Collection kits, 1307
Collodion baby, 513
Colon, 2, 82, 513-515, 521, 545, 658, 669,
772, 918, 923, 925, 1115, 1195, 1260,
1263, 1752, 1851, 1926, 2304-2305
irrigation of, 515
Colon cancer, 515-521, 923, 1092, 1196,
1262, 1264, 1449, 1452, 1622, 1852,
1926, 2001, 2305
Colon polyp removal, 516, 520, 1852
Colon polyps, 1824
Colon surgery, 520-522, 1850
Colon therapy, 82, 515
Colonoscopy, 515-516, 519-520, 669, 772,
920, 1269, 1852, 2001, 2305
Color blindness, 517, 536, 823, 941, 2011,
2358
Color synesthesia, 2180
Colorado tick fever, 1346
Colostomy, 521, 671, 1194-1197
Colostrum, 341, 1143
Colposcopy, 421
Coma, 330, 980-981, 1486, 1812-1813,
1909
Coma Recovery Scale-Revised, 1486
Combat neurosis, 1831
Comel-Netherton syndrome, 513
Commissure, 2111
Commissurectomy, 123, 125
Commissurotomy, 1601
Common cold, 351, 522-526, 1550-1551,
1681, 1804, 1900, 1961, 2020, 2084,
2198
Communication therapy, 120
Comparative genomics, 251, 964
Compartment syndrome, 398, 1081
Compensable injury, 1318
Competency, 1318-1319
Complement, 1213, 1215
Complement proteins, 505
Complement system, 1143, 1237, 1577
Complementary DNA, 489
Compression, breast, 1413
Compulsions, 157, 213, 1632
Computed tomography (CT) scanning,
160, 526-528, 760, 928, 967, 986,
1200-1201, 1367, 1379, 1589, 1606,
1641, 1915, 2152
Conception, 528-532, 1217, 1230, 1234,
1836
Concordance, 1506, 1508, 1510

Concrete operations stage, 501, 636
Concussion, 16, 532-534, 1032
Conditioning, 41, 1765
Condom, 546, 1453
female, 547
Conduction aphasia, 2380
Conductive hearing loss, 594, 702, 1047,
1050
Cone biopsy, 422
Conenose bug, 424
Cones, 517, 821, 2359
Confabulation, 1301
Confidentiality, 802
Congenital adrenal hyperplasia, 51,
534-535, 1161
Congenital disorders, 536-538
Congenital heart disease, 300, 388,
538-541, 684
Congenital hemidysplasia, 786
Congenital hypothyroidism, 314, 542-543,
684, 1411, 2242
Congenital megacolon, 1115
Congestion, 599
Congestive heart failure, 389-390, 541,
648, 1056, 1066, 1069, 1392, 1450,
1899, 2318
homocysteine and, 1068
Congo, 712
Conjugation, 136, 138-139, 695, 1274
Conjunctiva, 543, 682, 1888-1889
Conjunctival cell, 1888
Conjunctivitis, 543-544, 813, 815, 1643,
1929, 2034
acute hemorrhagic, 775
Connective tissue, 105, 396, 512, 544-545,
834, 1001, 1117, 1348-1349, 1985,
1993
tumors, 1985
Connexin 32, 426
Conotruncal defects, 539-540
Consciousness, 285, 1485-1486
Consent, 739, 800
Constant region, 144-145
Constipation, 514, 545-546, 658, 927,
1090, 1092-1093, 1115, 1222, 1270,
1926
Consumer protection, 871
Consumption coagulopathy, 665
Contact dermatitis, 624-626, 631, 716,
2058, 2317
Contact lenses, 201, 1649, 2362
Contact tracing, 453, 996, 1744
Continuous positive airflow pressure
(CPAP) machine, 2069
Contraception, 546-549, 1017, 1019,
1137, 2124, 2288, 2347
Contractions, 441
Contractures, 499, 1563, 1565
Contralateral, 2111
Convulsions, 2005
Co-occurring disorder, 2158
Cooley's anemia, 2225
Coordination, lack of, 201

Copper, 1470
Copper metabolism, 2387
Core decompression, 1670
Cornea, 401, 550, 813-814, 821, 982,
1284, 1643, 1649, 1888-1889, 2358
Corneal epithelium, 682
Corneal transplantation, 550-551, 816, 818
Corneal ulcers, 1644
Cornelia de Lange syndrome, 551-552
Corns, 552-553, 842, 883, 1025, 1810
Corona radiata, 530, 1218
Coronary artery bypass graft, 553-554
Coronary artery disease, 385, 387, 473,
1055, 1062, 1064, 1252, 1450, 1611,
1692, 1847
Coronary bypass surgery, 363, 385, 390,
1060, 1064
Coronary care unit (CCU), 1248
Coronaviruses, 523-524, 554-556, 781,
2019
Coroner, 885, 1737
Corpora cavernosa, 795
Corpus callosum, 2111
Corpus luteum, 1230, 1456, 1682, 1684,
1836
Corpus striatum, 1732
Corpuscle, 291
Corpuscles of Ruffini, 2009, 2258, 2260
Corrosives, 17
Corticosteroids, 40, 46, 153, 187, 198,
510, 556-557, 567, 626, 1213-1214,
1515, 1669, 1675, 1803, 1873, 1903,
1957, 1984, 2184, 2346
Corticosterone, 50
Corticotropin, 1514
Cortisol, 50, 535, 556, 573, 978, 1136,
2129, 2189
Cortisone, 1099, 1665, 1675, 2129
Cosmetic surgery, 345, 1653, 1681, 1799
Costochondritis, 397
Couching, 404
Coughing, 447, 454, 469, 526, 557-558,
568, 580, 746-747, 1550, 1804, 1896,
1961, 2384
Coumadin, 600, 1447
Cowpox, 1206, 1848
COX-2 inhibitors, 153, 430, 1665, 1697
Coxsackieviruses, 774, 1026
Craniosynostosis, 558
Craniotomy, 559-560, 1600, 2156
C-reactive protein, 1823
Creatine, 798
Creatine phosphate, 798, 992
Creatinine, 1575, 2318
Credentials, 75
CREST syndrome, 1993
Crestor, 461
Cretinism, 762, 1411-1412, 2242
Creutzfeldt-Jakob disease (CJD), 294,
560-561
Cri du chat syndrome, 271, 941
Critical care, 562-565, 681, 1248
Crohn's disease, 509, 514, 521, 566-568,

651, 653, 863, 919, 922-923, 1119, 1261, 1852, 2304-2305
Crossbite, 1656
Croup, 568-569, 1550, 1552, 2268
Crowns, 407, 569-570, 617
Cruise ships, illnesses on, 1608
Cryokinetics, 1774
Cryoprecipitate, 1087, 2276
Cryopreservation, 1235-1236, 2097
Cryoprobe, 403-404
Cryosurgery, 421, 570-572, 629, 1093
Cryotherapy, 570-571
  retinal detachment repair, 819
Cryptococcosis, 903, 1646
Cryptorchidism, 1932
CSA, 499
CSB, 499
CT scanning *See* Computed tomography (CT) scanning
Culdocentesis, 572-573
Culturing, 141, 372-373, 652, 1252, 1306, 1481, 1782
Curette, 2065
Cushing's syndrome, 51, 535, 557, 573-574, 755, 1626
Cuticle, hair, 1022
Cuticle, nail, 1539
Cutis marmorata, 575
Cutis marmorata telangiectatica congenita, 574-575
Cyanosis, 167, 540-541, 575-577, 1689, 1925
Cyberhand Project, 256
Cyclophosphamide, 506
Cyclosporine, 1012, 1874
Cyclothymia, 266, 621
Cyclotrons, 1921
Cyst removal, 577-578, 913, 1149
Cystectomy, 277
Cystic fibrosis, 187, 536, 578-582, 935, 941, 943, 955, 979, 1383, 1401, 1711, 1739, 1902, 1937, 2376
Cysticerci, 2192
Cysticercosis, 1728
Cystitis, 582-585, 2322, 2327
  interstitial, 229
Cystoscopy, 276, 585-586, 772
Cysts, 577, 586-587, 855, 913, 1149, 1292, 1861
  breast, 335, 344, 578, 586, 1423
  dermoid, 1682-1683
  kidney, 1819
  ovarian, 573, 577, 586, 957-958, 1682-1683, 1820
Cytokines, 252-253, 464, 1466, 2186
Cytology, 260, 408, 587-592
Cytomegalovirus (CMV), 591, 735, 1107, 1646, 1839, 2186
Cytopathology, 589, 592-593
Cytoplasm, 408
Cytoplasmic transfer, 194
Cytostatic therapies, 371
Cytotoxics, 2184

D

Dacrocystitis, 2202
Dairy products, 878, 1309
Dana Foundation, 1586
Danazol, 768, 958
Dandruff, 625, 628
Danger Assessment Tool, 1258
Dapsone, 987
Date rape, 1922-1923
De novo methyltransferase, 949
De Quervain's disease, 2210
Deacetylation, 949
Deafness, 594-595, 701, 1046, 1680
Death and dying, 566, 595-598, 804, 885, 1846, 2214
Debridement, 244, 1308
Decompression sickness, 662, 2236
Decompression surgery, 437
Decongestants, 147, 525, 599, 1552, 1685
Decubitus ulcers, 243, 966
Deductibles, 1417, 1434
Deep vein thrombosis, 600-601, 718, 1763, 2305, 2341
Defecation, 155, 1926
Defibrillation, 601-602
Defibrillators, 172, 380, 392, 1690, 1693, 1722, 1944-1945
Deformity, 887
Dehydration, 602-603, 607, 639, 650-652, 659, 675, 866, 1521, 1904, 1968, 2040, 2138, 2177, 2376
Delayed puberty, 1892-1893
Delirium, 604-605, 966
Delirium tremens, 63-64, 2006
Delusional misidentification, 376
Delusions, 1633, 1886, 1990
Dementias, 57, 60, 85, 94, 325, 329, 331, 604, 605-608, 894, 895, 966, 968, 1439, 1783, 2094-2095
  multiple infarct, 606, 1440
  vascular, 606
Democritus of Abdera, 2085
Demyelination, 52, 1011, 1513, 1581, 1584-1585
Dendrites, 1118, 1579, 1591, 1597, 1716, 2258
Dengue, 1243
Dengue fever, 608-610
Denial, 596
Dental caries, 499
Dental diseases, 483, 610-612, 614, 616, 763, 974, 2204
Dental pulp, 763, 2204
Dentin, 2203
Dentistry, 319, 613-615, 1176, 1651-1652, 1656, 2205, 2254
  history, 1653
Dentures, 615-617, 1275, 2205, 2388
Deoxyribonucleic acid (DNA), 298, 489-492, 498, 676, 940, 942, 949-951, 952, 962, 1209, 1532, 1922
Department of Health and Human

Services, 617-619, 871, 1433, 1553
Dependence, 1545, 2157-2158
Depolarization, 1716
Depression, 59, 129, 146, 266-267, 597, 607, 619-623, 836, 838, 894, 968, 1440, 1598, 1877, 1893, 2003, 2044, 2071, 2162-2164, 2364
  aging and, 57
  men and, 1451
  postpartum, 1829
Dermabrasion, 825
Dermatitis, 623-627, 716, 1791, 2058, 2063
Dermatitis herpetiformis, 407, 987
Dermatology, 627-630, 2059
Dermatome, 2038
Dermatopathology, 630-631
Dermatophytes, 202
Dermis, 2056, 2062
Dermoid cysts, 1682
Desensitization, 158, 1766, 1878
Designer drugs, 494
Desquamation, 513
Detached retina, 592, 819, 2361
Detoxification, 82, 515
Developmental disabilities, 843
Developmental disorders, 632-634
Developmental stages, 500, 634-638
Deviated septum, 1551-1553, 1959
Dexamethasone suppression test, 621
Dextrocardia, 540
Diabetes, gestational, 640
Diabetes insipidus, 560, 754, 955, 1116, 1137, 2327
Diabetes mellitus, 2-3, 6, 173, 283, 377, 607, 638-644, 648, 755, 757, 760, 814, 877, 945, 977, 993, 1025, 1185, 1253, 1306, 1449, 1452, 1470, 1473, 1584, 1626, 1711, 1739, 1742, 1747, 1752, 1839, 2026-2027, 2190, 2281
  bronze, 1083
  gestational, 970
  kidney disease and, 750
  nutrition and, 1623
  screening and, 2000
  type 1, 640-641, 760, 762, 849
  type 2, 642, 644, 971
Diabetic retinopathy, 814-815
Diagnosis, 644-645, 1252, 1767, 1854, 2050
Diagnostic and Statistical Manual of Mental Disorders, 645, 1876, 2026
Diagnostic transfer, 199
Dialysis, 3, 645-649, 750, 1086, 1288, 1574, 1930, 2190, 2327
Dialyzers, 646
Diaper rash, 373-374, 625
Diaphragm (contraceptive device), 547, 583
Diaphragm (muscle), 432, 435, 649-650, 1382, 2188
Diarrhea, 5, 90, 457, 471, 510, 514, 650-654, 658, 695, 773, 917, 922-923,

927, 1092, 1222, 1264, 1270, 1401, 1608, 1968, 2037, 2392
Diastole, 148
Diastolic blood pressure, 472, 1055, 1162
Diastolic pressure, 296
Diathermy, 1773
Diencephalon, 323
Diet *See* Nutrition
Diet pills, 2377
Dietary deficiencies *See* Malnutrition; Nutrition; Vitamins and minerals
Dietary Guidelines Advisory Committee, 878
Dietary Guidelines for Americans, 878-879
Dietary reference intakes (DRIs), 654-655
Diethylstilbestrol (DES), 1489
Dieting, 129, 1627-1628, 2375
Diffusion, 865, 1936
DiGeorge syndrome, 655-656, 850, 1212-1213, 1215
Digestion, 1, 471, 656-659, 854, 915, 918, 925, 1263, 1360, 1392, 1475, 1751, 2079, 2188, 2306
Digestive disorders, 579, 1264
Digestive system, 247, 799, 905, 1851 imaging, 770
Digital block, 1538
Digital mammography, 1414
Digital rectal examination, 1858, 1863
Digitalis, 541, 1067-1068, 1756, 1899
Dihydroepiandrosterone (DHEA), 797
Dihydrotestosterone, 77, 1857, 1934
Dilation and curettage (D&C), 9, 1448
Dilation and evacuation (D&E), 9
Diminished capacity, 1318
Dioscorides, 1100
Diosgenin, 1099
Diphteritic laryngitis, 1313
Diphtheria, 447-448, 659-660, 1207, 1313, 1902
Diplegia, 416
Disabilities, 1513
Disability insurance, 1042, 1044
Disarticulation, 99
Disasters, 565
Discs, 451
Disease, 222, 259, 412, 660-663, 1126, 1672, 1735, 2050
Disequilibrium, 2351
Disinhibition, 894
Disk diffusion test, 142
Disk removal, 663-664
Disks, 397, 664, 2078, 2104-2109
Dislocation, 307-308, 1658, 1661
Disorder of consciousness, 1485
Displacement, 157
Disseminated intravascular coagulation (DIC), 665-666, 711, 2133, 2229, 2276
Distillation, 63-64
Distress, 1746
Distributive justice, 801
Diuretics, 149, 666-668, 707, 719, 836,

1067, 1164, 1392, 1675, 1898
Diverticulitis, 514, 516, 521, 668-672, 927, 1196, 1261, 1431, 1852, 1926 and diverticulosis, 670-671
Diverticulosis, 521, 668-672, 1261
Diverticulum, 2330
Diving reflex, 680
Dizygotes, 1506, 1508
Dizziness, 238, 672-675, 1174, 1445, 2012, 2351
DNA analysis, 1922
DNA and RNA, 258, 409, 1640
DNA microarrays, 964
DNA sequencing, 962, 964
DNA testing, 1318-1319, 1321
Do Not Resuscitate order, 53-54
Disorder of consciousness, 1485-1486
Dominant diseases, 953
Dopamine, 503, 622, 759, 1707-1708, 1732-1733, 1941, 1991, 2246
Dopamine agonists, 1708, 1733
Doppler ultrasound scanning, 175, 540, 2151, 2312
Dose dense chemotherapy, 335
Double vision, 2358
Down syndrome, 95, 271, 536-537, 539, 663, 675-680, 940-941, 945, 1282, 1460, 1739, 1839, 2179
Doxycycline, 1964
DPT vaccine, 660, 1209, 2224
Dracunculiasis, 1970
Dreams, 1884
Driving and sleep-aids, 2073
Dronabinol, 1421
Drowning, 188, 564, 576, 680-681, 1168, 1174
Drowsiness, 147, 2065
Drug abuse, 894, 1741, 1811-1812, 2005, 2162
Drug addiction, 752
Drug interactions, 2007
Drug resistance, 143, 997, 1253, 2118, 2291
Drug Safety Oversight Board, 873
Drug screening, 1541
Drug testing, 264, 2328
Drugs, 872, 2007 therapeutic, 1755, 2391
Dry eyes, 682-683, 814, 816, 1928, 2055, 2202, 2360
Dry gangrene, 914
Dry mouth, 2055
DSM-5, 2193
DTaP vaccine, 448
Dual energy X-ray absorptionmetry (DEXA), 1675
Duchenne muscular dystrophy, 955, 1375, 1524, 1526-1528, 2318
Ductal carcinoma in situ, 335
Ductus arteriosus, 539
Dumping syndrome, 240, 916
Duodenum, 918, 925, 1360, 2303

Durable power of attorney, 53, 54
Dust mites, 1346
Dwarfism, 397, 683-686, 762, 1010, 1506
Dysarthria, 165, 2109
Dysdiadochokinesis, 786-787
Dysentery, 90, 650-654, 2037
Dysgraphia, 689
Dyskinesia, 324, 687-688, 693
Dyslexia, 688-691, 1324
Dysmenorrhea, 691-692, 765, 1457, 1535
Dyspareunia, 765-766, 1535
Dyspepsia, 471, 658, 923
Dysphagia
Dysphagia, 1752, 2186
Dysphasia, 85, 164-166
Dysphonia, 692-693
Dysplasia, 421, 1715
Dyspnea, 352, 505, 746, 752, 1259, 1803
Dysthymia, 266, 621, 968
Dystonias, 317, 1149, 1991, 2387
Dystrophin, 1528
Dysuria, 582, 2322

E

E. coli infection, 582-584, 651-652, 695-696, 917, 1006, 1085, 1482, 2331
Ear infections and disorders, 483, 696-700, 702, 1551, 2012
Ear surgery, 700-701, 704, 1799
Ear, nose, and throat medicine *See* Otorhinolaryngology
Earache, 1551
Eardrum, 594, 700, 702, 1045, 2010
Early-onset generalized dystonia, 693
Ears, 208, 594, 700-705, 1678-1679, 2010 anatomy of the, 696, 702, 1045, 2010
Earwax, 594, 697-698, 702, 705, 1050
Eating disorders, 129, 355-356, 706-709, 928, 1396, 1457, 1893, 2376
Eating while asleep, 2073
Ebola virus, 710-712, 781, 1418, 2352
Ecchymoses, 665, 886-887
ECG or EKG *See* Electrocardiography (ECG or EKG)
Echocardiography, 389, 713-714, 1063, 1606, 1705, 2311
Echoviruses, 774
Eclampsia, 1834-1836, 1839, 2262
Ecstasy, 494
Ectodermal dysplasia, 513
Ectopic pregnancy, 714-715, 1743, 1839, 2126
Ectropion, 513, 814, 816
Eczema, 623, 626, 715-716, 2063, 2389
Edema, 84, 631, 648, 716-719, 1027, 1063, 1066, 1119, 1226, 1409, 1573, 1717, 2283-2284, 2350
Education dental, 613
medical, 75-76, 92, 832, 1130, 1671, 1809
special, 1461, 2096

Edwards syndrome, 536
EEG *See* Electroencephalography (EEG)
Effusions, 1268
Eflornithine, 2075
Ego, 1883
Ehlers-Danlos syndrome, 512, 1349
Ehrlichiosis, 720
Ejaculation, 529, 1931
Elastic cartilage, 396
Elastin, 396, 544, 746, 1348
Elastin arteriopathy, 2386
Elastin gene, 2386
Elder Abuse Suspicion Index, 13
Elder mistreatment, 13
Elderly, 59, 1050, 1109, 1772, 1778, 1881
    bedsores and, 243
    eating disorders and, 707
Electric anesthesia, 117
Electrical burns, 360
Electrical shock, 362, 720-721
Electrocardiography (ECG or EKG), 380,
    389, 540, 722-723, 1060, 1063, 1606,
    1690, 1944
Electrocauterization, 422, 724
Electroconvulsive therapy, 2043
Electrodermal response, 248
Electroencephalogram, 981
Electroencephalograph, 1597-1598
Electroencephalography (EEG), 248, 324,
    724-726, 1589, 2006, 2067
Electrolysis, 1023
Electrolyte imbalance, 837, 866, 1930
Electrolytes, 602, 864-867, 1306, 1391,
    1621, 1797, 2328
Electromyograph, 248
Electromyography, 102, 426, 726-727,
    1525, 1773, 2147
Electrons, 1200
Electrophysiology, 1597
Elephantiasis, 728-730, 1386, 1393, 1728,
    1970
Elk, 352, 354
Embolism, 173, 329, 600, 718, 731, 751,
    894, 1191, 1762, 2149, 2231-2232,
    2234, 2339, 2344
    pulmonary, 2052
Embolization, 732-733
Embolus, 886, 890
Embryo, 733, 1219, 1506, 1508, 1510,
    1636, 1838, 2022
Embryo transfer, 1219
Embryology, 733-736
Embryonic development, 270, 481,
    538-539, 684, 733, 820, 1007, 1592,
    1838, 2022, 2102, 2107
Embryonic stem cells, 491-492, 2119
Emergency contraceptive pills, 548
Emergency medical technicians (EMTs),
    738, 1719, 1944
Emergency medicine, 390, 737-741, 1196,
    1719, 1943
    informed consent and, 800
Emergency room, 487, 737, 741-743

Emerging infectious diseases, 743-744
Emollients, 513
Emotional development, 635
Emotional distress, 1318
Emotional state, 1463
Emotions, biomedical causes and effects,
    1176, 2066
Emphysema, 188, 469, 744-747, 1119,
    1316, 1382, 1450, 1453, 1689,
    1895-1896, 1902-1903, 1937
    senile, 55
Enamel, 406, 2203
Encapsulated tumor, 986
Encephalitis, 165, 353, 438, 609, 748-749,
    775, 1580, 2402
    West Nile, 2381
Encephalocele, 537
Encephalopathy, 1365, 1367
Encephelotrigeminal angiomatosis, 2153
Encoscopy, 1852
End-stage renal disease, 749-750
Endarterectomy, 175, 751-752, 1453, 2152
Endocarditis, 123, 126, 373, 389, 714,
    752-753, 1061, 1071, 2206
    bacterial, 752
Endocrine disorders, 107, 753-757, 759,
    762, 995, 1222, 1306
Endocrine glands, 105, 756-758, 762, 976,
    1117, 1135, 1709, 2241
Endocrine system, 756, 762, 2189
    anatomy of, 753-754, 758
Endocrinology, 757-760, 979
    pediatric, 761-763
Endodontic disease, 763
Endodontics, 614, 1965
Endogenous, 1545
Endogenous opioid, 1546
Endogenous viruses, 2396
Endolymphatic hydrops, 1441
Endometrial biopsy, 764
Endometrial cancer, 418-420, 764,
    957-958, 2332
Endometrial hyperplasia, 1161
Endometriosis, 691, 714, 765-769,
    956-957, 1019, 1218, 1230, 1311, 1457,
    1933, 2332
Endometrium, 1932, 2332
Endoplasmic reticulum, 512
Endorphins, 35, 81, 1696, 1843-1844
Endoscopic retrograde
    cholangiopancreatography (ERCP),
    769-770, 906-907
Endoscopy, 19, 261, 520, 653, 669,
    770-772, 910, 920, 1268-1269, 1311,
    1357, 1680, 2169, 2173, 2308
Endospores, 2222
Endosteum, 313
Endothelial cell, 1338
Endotoxins, 851
Endotracheal tube, 116-117, 1721
Enemas, 82, 707, 773
Energy medicine, 83
Energy production, 990

Engorgement, 1426
Enhancer, 949
Enkephalins, 1843-1844
Entacapone, 1733
Entamoeba histolytica, 90
Enterocolitis, 773-774, 1115
Enterostomal therapists, 1197
Enteroviruses, 748, 774-775, 1026
Entropion, 814, 816
Enuresis *See* Bed-wetting
Environmental disasters, 565
Environmental diseases, 184, 271,
    775-778
Environmental health, 301, 776, 2265
Enzyme therapy, 83, 779, 839, 929, 935,
    990, 1472, 1603
Enzymes, 2, 21, 83, 579-580, 657, 779,
    839, 877, 925, 989, 1309, 1360, 1469,
    1475, 1506, 1710, 2201
Eosinophils, 1143, 1203
Ependymal cell, 985
Ephedra, 2166, 2377
Ephedrine, 798
Epidemics, 662, 712, 743, 780-783, 1210,
    1239, 1328, 1331, 1815, 1817, 1897,
    2391
Epidemiological triangle, 783, 785
Epidemiology, 776, 783-785, 1818, 1848
    genetic, 1869
Epidermal nevus syndromes, 786-788
Epidermis, 513, 1538, 1787, 2056, 2058,
    2062
Epididymis, 1931, 2338, 2349
Epididymitis, 1451, 1453, 1654, 2349
Epididymoorchitis, 1654-1655
Epidural anesthesia, 113, 423, 442
Epidural hematomas, 16
Epigenome, 951
Epiglottitis, 568, 788, 1550, 1552, 1759,
    2268
Epilepsy, 212, 324, 330-331, 726,
    789-792, 1581, 1613, 1706, 2005,
    2086, 2111
Epileptic focus, 2111
Epinephrine, 50, 870, 978
Epiphora, 819
Epiphysis, 886, 889
Episiotomy, 441, 767, 793
Epistaxis, 1668
Epithelial cells, 588
Epithelial placode, 77
Epithelial tissue, 105, 1001, 1117, 2297
Epithelium, 2305
Epstein-Barr virus, 793-795
Erb's palsy, 1563, 1565, 1707
ERCC6, 498
ERCC8, 498
Erectile dysfunction, 795-796
Erection, 795, 960, 1745, 1931,
    2026-2027
Ergogenic aids, 797-798
Ergonomics, 727, 2211
Ergot, 1492

Ergotism, 902
Erythema nodosum, 244, 2305
Erythrocyte sedimentation rate, 1823
Erythrocytes, 287, 291, 1077, 1292, 1340, 1576, 1797
Erythromycin, 1330, 1986
Erythropoietin, 797, 1137, 1292, 1576
Esophageal cancer, 799, 922
Esophageal spasm, 1752
Esophagomyotomy, 1752
Esophagus, 1, 19-2023, 657, 799, 918, 922, 925, 1752, 1759, 2268
Essential nutrients, 1475
Essential oils, 170
Essential tremor, 2285
Essure, 549
Estrogen, 347, 419, 440, 768, 978, 1133, 1173, 1424, 1444-1446, 1456, 1763, 1844, 2031, 2129
    autoimmune disorders and, 217
Estrogen replacement therapy See Hormone therapy (HT)
Ether, 115-116
Ethics, 92, 486, 799-804, 846-847, 872, 913, 1111, 1220, 2396
Etiology, 220, 661, 1005, 1735
Eukaryotic cells, 231, 489-490
Eustachian tubes, 599, 702, 1045, 1759
Euthanasia, 195, 566, 803-807, 1114, 1318-1319, 1321
Evista, 337, 1676
Evoked otoacoustic emissions (EOAE) test, 1053
Evoked response audiometry, 209
Ewing's sarcoma, 807-808, 1985
Examination, 487
Excitation, 1597
Executive function, 1463-1464
Exenatide, 643
Exercise, 315, 381, 602, 675, 723, 808, 842, 878, 992, 994, 1172, 1627, 1675, 1774, 1936, 2113, 2375
Exercise physiology, 382, 723, 808-812, 992, 1295, 1525
Exocrine glands, 105, 976, 1117, 1709, 2177
Exocytosis, 976
Exogenous, 1545
Exogenous opioid, 1546, 1547
Experimental treatments, 486
Extended care for the aging See Aging: Extended care
Extended care for the terminally ill See Terminally ill: Extended care
External cephalic version, 1637
Extracellular fluid, 865, 1780
Extracellular matrix, 396
Extracorporeal shock-wave lithotripsy, 1293, 1357, 2138, 2141, 2331
Extremities, 98, 1372, 1798, 2314, 2340
Eye
    aging and, 55
Eye disorders, 543, 2360

Eye examinations, 1397
Eye infections, 1284
Eye infections and disorders, 813-816, 1397, 1643, 2011, 2270
Eye movement desensitization and reprocessing (EMDR), 1831
Eye surgery, 201, 399, 550, 817-819, 1316, 1398
    refractive, 1928-1929
Eyeglasses, 200, 1649, 2362
Eyelashes, 1023
Eyelids, 814, 825, 2155, 2360
Eyes, 399, 517, 543, 550, 813, 817, 820-824, 1284, 1485, 1536, 1643, 1648, 2010, 2142, 2155, 2202
    anatomy of the, 401, 820, 1643, 2010, 2358
    dry, 814, 816, 2055
    watery, 814, 816

F

Fabry's disease, 780
Face lift, 825-826, 1799-1800
Facial palsy See Bell's palsy
Facial paralysis, 245
Facial prostheses, 1865-1866
Facial transplantation, 826-827, 1653
Factitious disorders, 828-829, 1887
Failure to thrive, 304, 499, 829-830
Fainting, 672-675, 1174, 1445, 2334
Fallen arches, 841, 864
Fallopian tubes, 549, 1018, 1189, 1684, 1932, 2125, 2288
Falls, 16, 18, 238, 327, 1302
Falls and immobility, 966
False aneurysm, 160
False negatives, 644
False positives, 645
Familial adenomatous polyposis (FAP), 520
Familial hypercholesterolemia, 955
Familial polyposis, 1196
Family medicine, 830-833
Fanconi syndrome, 2178
Fascia, 98, 544, 834-835, 1562-1563
Fasting, 2375
Fat, 544, 810, 1153, 1354, 1621, 1625, 1627, 1629, 2375
Fat cells, 1171, 1173
Fat necrosis, 339
Fatal familial insomnia, 1849
Fatigue, 464, 835-838, 1495
    fibromyalgia and, 857
Fats, 658, 875, 878, 1351, 1392
Fatty acid oxidation disorders, 839, 1470, 1472
Fatty acids, 514, 1264, 1351, 1395
Fatty liver, 1604
Fc-fusion proteins, 144-145
Fear, 1179, 1599, 1765, 1830, 2013
Febrile seizures, 1966
Fecal occult blood testing, 2001

Feces, 155, 471, 514, 545, 651, 658, 670, 773, 918, 923, 1222, 1751, 1926
    irrigation of, 515
Feedback, 1780, 2189
Feet, 202, 356, 840-843, 864, 1025, 1075, 1372-1373, 1785
    anatomy of the, 840, 1808
Female genital disorders, 418
Femoral hernias, 1103, 1105
Femur, 1372
Fenestration, 1681
Fenoterol, 198
Fermentation, 992, 994
Fertility drugs, 531, 1231
Fertilization, 530, 676, 953, 1217, 1230, 1635, 1836
Fertilization potential, 1861
Fetal alcohol syndrome, 537, 736, 843, 1838
Fetal death, 2133
Fetal distress, 423, 442, 445, 1746
Fetal fibronection, 1637
Fetal heart monitoring, 1637
Fetal macrosomia, 970
Fetal movement, 1746
Fetal surgery, 97, 844-846, 1637, 2100
Fetal tissue transplantation, 847-850, 1002, 1149
Fetus, 95, 462, 734, 848, 1636, 1747, 1793, 1838
Fever, 851-854, 1167, 1227, 1283, 1403
Fever blisters, 506
FGFR3 gene, 787
Fiber, 514, 546, 670, 672, 854-855, 1092, 1094, 1265, 1395, 1621-1622
Fiber optics, 928
Fibrillation, 1059, 1690
    atrial, 173, 607, 1057, 1063, 2231
    ventricular, 721, 1057, 1063, 1693
Fibrin, 278, 292, 2231, 2234
Fibrinolysis, 278
Fibrinolysis, 2231
Fibroadenoma, 339, 348
Fibroblast, 2186
Fibroblast growth factor, 787, 2343
Fibroblast Growth Factor Receptor 3, 786
Fibroblasts, 544, 2394
Fibrocartilage, 396
Fibrocystic breast condition, 339, 855-856
Fibrocystic breast disease, 344, 348, 1423
Fibroids
    uterine, 732, 957-958, 1019, 1189, 1447, 1535, 2332
Fibromyalgia, 464, 856-858, 1152
    endometriosis and, 767
Fibrosarcoma, 1985, 2297
Fibrosis, 1984, 1993, 2186
Fibrositis, 178
Fifth disease, 858-859
Fight-or-flight response, 1029, 2145-2146
Filariasis, 728, 730, 1386, 1970
Filgrastin, 335
Filiform papillae, 2195

Fillings, dental, 407, 614, 616, 1465
Filoviruses, 712, 781, 1418
Filtration, 865
Finasteride, 1022
Fingernail removal *See* Nail removal
Fingernails, 1538-1539
Fingers, 1538
First aid, 859-861, 1039, 1775
First responder, 861-862
Fish, 1623
Fistula repair, 862-863, 1191
Fistulas, 155, 671, 862, 1186, 1926
Fitness, 812
Fitz-Hugh Curtis syndrome, 1743
Flagellum, 1218
Flat feet, 841, 864, 883
Flatworms, 1728, 1987, 2192
Flaviviruses, 609, 2398
Flavonoids, 1783
Fleas, 1244, 1794
Flesh-eating bacteria, 1562
Flies, 1243, 2270
Floods, 1339
Flossing, 975
Flow defects, 539-540
Fluconazole, 374, 903
Fludarabine, 506
Fluid biopsy, 572
Fluids, 864-867, 1268, 1390, 1780
Flukes, 1728, 1987
Fluorescence in situ hybridization, 655
Fluorescent resection, 986
Fluoride, 22, 611, 1677, 1796
Fluoride treatments, 868-869
Fluorine, 1200
Fluoroquinolones, 137-138
Fluoroscope, 1466
Fluoroscopy, 1198, 1202
Foam cells, 1603
Focal dystonias, 317, 692-694
Focal motor deficits, 560
Focal motor seizure, 789
Foliate papillae, 2196
Folic acid, 109, 537, 736, 1068, 1078, 2100, 2365
Follicles, 1022, 1684
    ovarian, 1218-1219
Follicle-stimulating hormone (FSH), 1790
Folliculitis, 1479
Folliculostatin, 1685
Food, 366, 875, 925, 928, 1183, 1263, 1626-1627, 2197
Food additives, 872
Food allergies, 71, 869-871, 1120
Food and Drug Administration (FDA), 486, 618, 871-874, 882, 1127, 1757, 2166, 2265, 2367
Food biochemistry, 874-877, 1264, 1352
Food Guide Plate, 877-879
Food Guide Pyramid, 878
Food poisoning, 17, 234, 317, 654, 879-882, 917, 927, 1085, 1482, 2117, 2300

Foot disorders, 356, 552, 841, 864, 882-884, 1785, 1809
Forced-choice alternative paradigms, 285
Forceps, 442
Foregut, 1430
Foremilk, 341
Forensic, 1318
Forensic medicine, 1319-1321
Forensic medicine, 885, 2206, 2265
Forensic pathology, 221, 884-886, 1737
Foreskin, 477
Formal operations stage, 501, 636
Formalin, 326-327
Formula feeding, 343
Forteo, 1676
Fosamax, 1669, 1676
Foscarnet, 592
Fosfomycins, 137
Fovea, 821, 2359
Fracture and dislocation, 886-890
Fracture repair, 17, 398, 891-892, 1109, 1274, 2115
Fractures, 17, 307-308, 321, 398, 891, 1274, 1658, 1661, 1674, 1721, 1798, 2114
    compound, 886
    facial, 1274
    greenstick, 886
    simple, 886
    stress, 887
Fragile X syndrome, 893
Fragment antigen-binding, 144
Fragment crystallizable, 145
Framingham Heart Study, 1068
Freckles, 1787, 2062
Free association, 1884
Free radical theory of aging, 56
Free radicals, 56, 154, 2060, 2166
Freezing, 571
Frontal lobe, 894
Frontal lobe syndrome, 893-894
Frontotemporal dementia (FTD), 895-896, 1783
Frostbite, 576, 896-899, 1168, 1774
Frozen section biopsy, 261
Fructose, 900
Fructosemia, 900, 1361
Fruits, 878
Functional disease, 661, 923
Functional genomics, 251, 963
Functional magnetic resonance imaging (fMRI), 986, 1487, 1598
Fundoplication, 20
Fungal infections, 187, 202, 372, 497, 900-904, 1540, 1646, 1963
Fungi, 142, 901-902, 1481-1482, 1491
Fungiform papillae, 2196
Fusiform aneurysm, 160
Fusion inhibitors, 33
Future of Family Medicine (FMM) Project, 833

G

GABA, 2193
Gag reflex, 2334
Galactoceles, 339
Galactorrhea, 91, 1020
Galactose, 905
Galactosemia, 876, 905, 942, 1184, 1361
Galen of Pergamum, 328, 803, 1383, 2085
Gallbladder, 247, 455, 905-909, 919, 923, 1359, 2129, 2141, 2311
    imaging, 770
Gallbladder cancer, 906-909
Gallbladder diseases, 5, 455-456, 908-912
Gallbladder removal *See* Cholecystectomy
Gallstones, 247, 455, 770, 862, 906-907, 1274, 1311, 1713, 2129, 2138, 2140-2141
Galvanic skin response, 376
Gamete intrafallopian transfer (GIFT), 193, 912-913, 1232
Gamma-aminobutyric acid (GABA), 2066
Gamma camera, 1919, 2052
Gamma globulin, 1204, 1283
Gamma-hydroxybutyrate, 494
Gamma rays, 1200, 1919, 2051
Gamma-hydroxy butyrate, 1923
Ganciclovir, 592
Ganglion, 586
Ganglion removal, 587, 913
Gangliosides, 2201
Gangrene, 233, 641, 662, 897, 913-914, 1168, 1481, 1562, 1774, 2064, 2178
    dry, 914
García-Hafner-Happle syndrome, 786-787
Gardasil, 419, 1148, 1211
Garlic, 1100
Gas exchange, 1381-1382
Gasser syndrome, 1085
Gastrectomy, 915
Gastric banding, 239
Gastric bypass, 239
Gastric juice, 1, 657, 1264-1265, 1304
Gastric lavage, 2265
Gastritis, 6, 927
Gastroenteritis, 916-917, 927, 1085, 1608, 1968, 1982
Gastroenterology, 918-921, 927-928
Gastroesophageal reflux, 416
Gastroesophageal reflux disease (GERD), 19-20, 23, 799, 919, 927, 2186
Gastrointestinal disorders, 567, 658, 919, 921-924, 927
Gastrointestinal stromal tumors (GISTs), 1985
Gastrointestinal system, 2, 513-514, 566, 657, 918, 924-928, 2188
    aging and, 55
Gastrointestinal tract, 2, 155, 657, 669, 918, 925, 1750, 1926, 2304, 2306
Gastroparesis, 641, 1753, 2334
Gastroplasty, 239, 1153, 1627
Gastroscope, 772, 920

Gastrostomy, 920, 928-929
Gate control theory, 1696
Gaucher's disease, 513, 780, 929-930, 1353, 1472
Gender dysphoria, 931
Gender identity, 932, 2023
Gender identity disorder, 930-931
Gender reassignment surgery, 932-933, 1654
Gene expression, 949
Gene therapy, 253, 370, 933-937, 944, 946-947, 1144, 1286, 1472, 1528, 2021
General anesthesia, 111, 113, 889, 1756, 2172
General practice, 831
Generalized anxiety disorder, 156, 158
Generic drugs, 872, 1686
Genes, 255, 735, 936, 940, 952, 1530, 1735
Genetic counseling, 96, 272, 484, 581, 679, 936-939, 943, 1461, 1471, 1528, 1533
Genetic diseases, 255, 257, 270, 462, 578, 580-581, 663, 676, 735, 893, 933, 936, 940-943, 973, 1325, 1477, 1528, 1667, 1735, 1839, 2097, 2299
Genetic engineering, 255, 581, 934, 937, 943, 944-948, 980, 1114, 1478, 1533, 1946, 2356
    xenotransplantation and, 2396
Genetic imprinting, 948-951
Genetic predisposition, 955
Genetic sequencing See Genomics
Genetics, 580, 676, 680, 933, 937, 940, 943, 952-956, 962, 1530
Geniculostriate pathway, 285
Genital disorders, 1107
    female, 417-418, 956-959, 996, 2287
    male, 959-961, 996, 1855, 2287
Genital mutilation, 474-476, 1934
Genital warts, 571, 957-958, 1147-1148, 2034-2035
Genitals, 932, 1101, 2023
Genome, 490-491, 951
Genomes, 962
Genomics, 251, 962-965, 1869
Genu valgum, 1299
Genu varum, 318
Geriatric assessment, 965-966
Geriatrics and gerontology, 58, 966-969, 1881
Gestation, 1836-1840
Gestational diabetes, 640, 970-971
GHB, 494
Ghrelin, 1832
Giant cell arteritis, 1823, 2346
Giardiasis, 972, 1729, 1871
Gigantism, 314, 972-973, 1010
Gingiva, 974, 1015
Gingivectomy, 1748
Gingivitis, 406, 611-612, 974-975, 1015, 1748-1749, 1796, 2205
    menopause and, 974

pregnancy and, 974
    puberty and, 974
Ginkgo biloba, 503, 1925
Glands, 50, 105, 756, 976-980, 1117, 1156
Glasgow Coma Scale, 980-981, 2284
Glaucoma, 283-284, 814-815, 818, 823, 967, 969, 981-985, 1644, 2011, 2087, 2360-2362
Gleevec, 430, 1985
Glial cell, 985, 2111
Glioma, 985-986
Global warming, 1339
Glomerular filtration rate, 750, 1575, 1577
Glomeruli, 1291, 1573, 2325
Glomerulonephritis, 1286, 1288, 1293, 1573, 1577, 1819, 2093, 2327
Glucagon, 976
Glucocorticoids, 556, 1136, 1954, 2129, 2189
Glucosamine, 179, 1278, 1665
Glucose, 377, 639, 641-642, 675, 839, 876-877, 970, 990, 1182-1184, 1359, 1395, 1470, 1710, 2129
Glucose tolerance test, 970, 1184, 1306
Glutamate, 2066
Glutamine, 1149
Gluten, 407, 2079
Gluten intolerance, 986-988
Glycation, 1474
Glycogen, 377, 875, 992, 1359, 1395
    metabolism, 989
Glycogen storage diseases, 988-990, 1470
Glycolipids, 1351
Glycolysis, 876, 990-994
Glycopeptides, 136-137
Glycosides, 1098
Glycosylation, 1474
Glyclycyclines, 136-137
Goiter, 543, 663, 755, 979, 994-995, 1028, 1411-1412, 2240, 2243
Gonadotropin surge attenuating factor, 1685
Gonadotropin-releasing hormone, 1844
Gonadotropins, 1891
Gonads, 757
Goniometry, 1773
Gonioscope, 985
Gonorrhea, 233, 453, 957, 995-997, 1743, 2034, 2036
Gout, 177, 308-309, 842, 997-1000, 1278, 1471
Graft-versus-host disease (GVHD), 2021, 2281
Grafts and grafting, 310, 360, 827, 863, 1000-1003
    skin, 1799, 1801, 2258
Grains, 878
Gram staining, 232, 1003-1006, 1806
Grand mal seizure, 790, 2004
Granny battering, 13
Granulocytes, 288, 1203, 2276
Granulomas, 467, 468, 1984, 2126, 2349
Granulomatosis, 1213

Graves' disease, 218, 755, 757, 760, 979, 995, 2240, 2242
Gray hair, 2368
Gray matter, 322, 1118
Grief, 597, 2163
Groin pull, 2212
Group model HMO, 1042
Group therapy, 1831
Growth, 368, 683, 762, 1007-1010, 1171, 1173, 1660, 1740, 1769, 1890
Growth factors, 253
Growth fraction, 429
Growth hormone, 683-685, 759, 797, 973, 978-979, 1010, 1039, 1173, 1183, 1790, 2189
Growth hormone-releasing hormone (GHRH), 1790
GUARD trial, 1165
Guided imagery, 1435
Guillain-Barr, syndrome, 1010-1012
Guilt, 1179, 1632, 2161, 2163
Guinea worm, 1970
Gulf War syndrome, 777, 1013-1015
Gum bleeding, 974
Gum disease, 974, 1015-1017, 1748
Gums, 974, 1015, 1748, 2205
Gynecology, 1017-1020, 1635, 1770
Gynecomastia, 436, 797, 1020-1021

H

H1N1, 1211
Hair, 1022-1023, 1787, 2057, 2062, 2258
    aging and, 1134
Hair color, 1787
Hair follicle, 77-78, 80
Hair loss, 1022, 1024, 2063
Hair peg, 77
Hair removal, 1023
Hair transplantation, 1022, 1024
Halitosis, 1552-1553
Hallucinations, 1542, 1724, 1886, 2068
Hallucinogens, 42
Hamartoma, 786
Hammertoe correction, 1025, 1810
Hammertoes, 883, 1025-1026, 1810
Hamstring muscles, 1373
Hamstring pull, 2212
Hand-foot-and-mouth disease, 1026
Hantavirus, 1027
Hare lip See Cleft lip and palate
Harrington rod technique, 1997
Harvard Brain Tissue Resource Center, 326
Hashimoto's thyroiditis, 218, 979, 1028, 1136, 2240
Havening touch, 1028-1030
Hay fever, 147, 599, 1031
Hay-Well syndrome, 513
Head disorders, 1031-1032
Head Start, 618
Head trauma, 16-17, 131, 165, 533, 606, 1032, 1440, 1460, 1721, 2005, 2095,

2155, 2197

Headaches, 248, 495-496, 1033-1036, 1696

Healing, 398, 1036-1040, 1128, 1154, 1238, 1772, 2231

Health, 1672, 1775

Health care reform, 619, 1040-1042, 1778

Health care workers, 74, 2017

Health information, 412

Health insurance, 486, 1416, 1433
 ethics and, 802

Health maintenance organizations (HMOs), 1042-1044, 1043-1045, 1257, 1416, 1778

Health professions shortage areas (HPSAs), 833

Hearing, 208, 594, 697, 1045-1046, 2010

Hearing aids, 210, 595, 1047-1049, 1051

Hearing loss, 208, 483, 594, 697-698, 700, 702-703, 705, 1046, 1049-1052, 1551, 1681, 2095, 2248
 conductive, 700, 702, 1050
 sensorineural, 700, 702, 1050

Hearing tests, 1052-1054

Heart, 171, 296, 300, 380-381, 387, 432, 472, 601, 713, 723, 1054-1058, 1070-1071, 1523, 1606, 1690, 1704, 1920, 1943, 2188
 anatomy of the, 387, 432, 472, 539, 1054, 1058, 1062
 artificial, 1070

Heart attack, 173, 249, 380-381, 388, 390-391, 662, 713, 1056, 1058-1062, 1119, 1163, 1225, 1692, 1756, 1796, 1847, 1944, 2039, 2232, 2235, 2344

Heart block, 388, 1063, 1690

Heart defects, 388, 713

Heart disease, 122, 174, 381, 387, 539, 553, 753, 1061-1065, 1163, 1252, 1899, 2311
 congenital, 538
 men and, 1449
 nutrition and, 1622

Heart disorders, 171, 203, 1172, 1490, 1898

Heart failure, 161-162, 385, 540, 713, 718, 1056, 1063, 1065-1069, 1152, 1172, 1450, 1898, 2318

Heart murmurs, 388, 540-541, 752, 1072, 1768-1769, 2115

Heart rate, 171, 811, 1704

Heart transplantation, 385-386, 1057, 1068-1071, 2228

Heart valve replacement, 386, 1071-1073, 2228

Heart valves, 385, 1054, 1071, 1450

Heartbeat, 387, 1063

Heartburn, 23, 658, 922, 927

Heat exhaustion, 603, 1073-1074

Heat stroke, 603, 662, 1168, 2177

Heat therapy, 180

Heat, therapeutic use of, 1773

Heatstroke, 1073-1074

Heavy chain, 144

Heel spur removal, 1075

Heel spurs, 883, 1075

Heels, 840, 1075, 1372

Heimlich maneuver, 454, 859, 1075-1076, 1937

Helicobacter pylori, 919, 2308

HELLP syndrome, 1835

Hemagglutinin, 223

Hemangiomas, 575, 1296

Hemassist, 2274

Hematoceles, 2218

Hematochezia, 1431

Hematocrit levels, 2275

Hematology, 600, 1076-1079, 1305

Hematomas, 119, 560, 606, 702, 1080-1081, 1088, 1119, 1717, 2349, 2394
 epidural, 16
 subdural, 16, 1717, 2155-2157

Hematopoetic stem cells, 2121

Hematopoiesis, 108

Hematosis, 291

Hematoxylin and eosin (H & E), 260, 631

Hematuria, 582-583, 1081-1082, 1285, 2186, 2321, 2329

Hemifacial spasm, 317

Hemiparesis, 786-787

Hemiplegia, 416, 1082-1083, 1707, 2149
 spastic, 1082, 1707

Hemispheres of the brain, 1601

Hemochromatosis, 1083-1084, 1361, 1363, 1470, 1472, 2063

Hemodialysis, 646, 648, 750, 1288, 1574, 1930, 2266

Hemoglobin, 108, 287, 576, 937, 993, 1077, 1095, 1787, 1825, 1936, 2047, 2188, 2225, 2274

Hemoglobin-based oxygen carriers, 2274

Hemolysis, 505, 1274

Hemolytic disease of the newborn, 1084-1085, 1215, 1949

Hemolytic uremia, 2319

Hemolytic uremic syndrome, 1085-1086

Hemophilia, 31, 123, 125-126, 291, 601, 943, 955, 1086-1089, 1531, 1797, 2371

Hemoptysis, 1803

Hemorrhage, 609, 665, 711, 1088, 1267, 1403, 1419, 2040, 2229, 2352, 2371
 brain, 1376

Hemorrhagic fever, 609, 710-711, 781, 1027, 1418, 2352-2353

Hemorrhoid banding and removal, 521, 1089-1090, 1852

Hemorrhoidectomy, 1093

Hemorrhoids, 155, 521, 927, 1090-1094, 1851

Hemostasis, 278-280, 282, 1086, 2172

Henry Street Settlement, 1125

Heparin, 600, 1037, 1447, 2231-2232

Hepatitis, 3, 5-6, 126, 447, 919, 923, 1087, 1094-1097, 1208-1209, 1360-1361, 1363, 1365, 1367, 2034, 2354, 2392

immunization, 447

Hepatitis B, 1253, 1367, 2017, 2272

Hepatitis C, 1365, 1367

Hepatobiliary iminodiacetic acid, 456

Hepatocytes, 1360

Herald patch, 1792

Herbal ecstasy, 494

Herbal medicine, 83, 430, 1098-1100, 1272, 1858

Herberden's nodes, 1664

Herceptin, 253, 335, 337

Hermaphrodites, 535

Hermaphroditism, 1101, 1933, 2023, 2025

Hernia, 6, 835, 1102-1105
 femoral, 1103, 1105
 hiatal, 24, 927, 1105, 1201
 inguinal, 1103, 1105, 1933
 umbilical, 1105

Hernia repair, 1105-1106

Herniated disk, 397, 2077

Heroin, 42, 576, 1546

Herpangina, 774

Herpes, 286, 464, 506, 624, 628, 794, 957, 1107-1108, 1119, 1284, 1706, 1966, 2034-2035, 2355
 ocular, 813-814

Herpes zoster, 447, 628, 1107, 1583, 1644, 1706, 2038, 2356

Heterosexuality, 2030

Heterotopic tissue, 1430

Hiatal hernia, 24, 927, 1104, 1105, 1201

Hibernation, 1168

Hiccups, 1108

Highly active antiretroviral therapy (HAART), 33, 592, 1147, 1647

Hindgut, 1430

Hindmilk, 341

Hip fracture repair, 1109

Hip joint, 1109

Hip malformation, 575

Hip pain, 1109

Hip replacement, 181, 1109-1110, 1957

Hippocampus, 256

Hippocrates, 803, 1100

Hippocratic oath, 801, 1111-1114

Hips, 181, 1955

Hirschsprung's disease, 514, 1115

Hirsutism, 91, 1023, 1820

Histamine, 67-68, 71-72, 147, 869, 1031, 1038, 1120, 1237, 1958, 2066

Histamine blockers, 24

Histamine II blockers, 2308

Histiocytes, 1116, 1603

Histiocytosis, 1116

Histocompatibility, 1001

Histocompatibility leukocyte antigen (HLA), 297

Histology, 221, 259, 326, 630, 1001, 1116-1120

Histone, 949, 951-952

Histoplasmosis, 903

History taking, 644, 1768

Histotoxic anoxia, 188

HIV *See* Human immunodeficiency virus (HIV)
Hives, 1120
Hodgkin's disease, 1121-1123, 1387, 1389, 1393, 1482, 2297
Holistic medicine, 80, 450, 466, 1671
Holocrine glands, 976
Home care, 1124-1126, 1433, 2215
Home health aides, 1125
Home testing, 1307
Homeopathy, 83, 1126-1130
Homeostasis, 1144, 1672, 1735, 1780, 2145
Homocysteine, 1068
Homocysteinuria, 1471
Homonymous hemianopia, 285
Homosexuality, 2025, 2030
H1N1 influenza, 1130-1131
Hong Kong flu, 2396
Hookworms, 1727-1728, 1969
Hordeolum, 814, 2155
Hormesis, 778
Hormonal therapy, 430, 767, 1424
Hormone replacement therapy, 535
Hormone therapy, 1132-1134, 1135-1136, 1445
breast cancer and, 338
Hormones, 556, 754, 756, 759, 973, 976, 1135-1138, 1173, 1306, 1360, 1424, 1438, 1590, 1629, 1684, 1790, 1857, 1892, 2023, 2144, 2189
peptide, 1135
steroid, 1136
Hormonogenesis, 1684
Horner's syndrome, 1032, 1563, 1565
Hospice, 1125, 1138-1141, 1434, 1700, 1701, 2216
Hospital Insurance (HI), 1433
Hospitals, 76, 443, 487, 737, 741, 832, 1248, 1433, 2118
Host-defense mechanisms, 1141-1144
Hot flashes, 1133-1134, 1191, 1445
House calls, 832
HRAS gene, 787
Human chorionic gonadotropin, 1488, 1636, 1793
Human genome, 251, 935, 962, 964
Human Genome Project, 255, 962-964, 1529, 1870
Human growth hormone, 945
Human immunodeficiency virus (HIV), 30-31, 294, 325, 477, 537, 607, 743, 837, 903, 1087, 1144-1147, 1213, 1306, 1647, 1803, 1946, 2034, 2272, 2354, 2392
Human leukocyte antigen (HLA), 128-129, 1289
Human papillomavirus (HPV), 103, 253, 419, 1147-1148, 1211
Human Proteome Organization, 1870
Humerus, 2314
Humor, 501
Humoral response, 145

Humors, theory of, 222, 269, 290, 906, 1181
Hunter syndrome, 1505-1506
Huntington's disease, 325, 330, 536, 849, 937, 941, 945, 953, 1148-1149, 2261, 2317
Hurler's syndrome, 849, 1506
Hurricanes, 1338-1339
Hwalek-Sengstock Elder Abuse Screening Test, 13
Hyaline cartilage, 396
Hyaluronic acid, 1665
Hydatid disease, 1728
Hydrating solutions, 1266
Hydrocelectomy, 1149
Hydroceles, 961, 1149-1150, 2218
Hydrocephalus, 330-331, 606, 938, 1150-1151, 1267, 1376, 1460, 1739, 1741, 2046, 2102
fetal surgery and, 845
Hydrochloric acid, 657-658, 927, 2306, 2333, 2366
Hydrocortisone, 1099
Hydrogenation, 1351
Hydronephrosis, 2319
Hydrops fetalis, 2225
Hydrostatic pressure, 717-718, 1392
Hydrotherapy, 81, 1152, 1774
colon, 515
Hydroxymethylglutaryl coenzyme A, 459
Hygiene hypothesis, 199, 869
Hygienic Laboratory, 1555
Hyperactivity, 120, 205, 2246
Hyperadiposis, 1153-1154
Hyperandrogenism, 1820
Hyperbaric oxygen chamber, 1154
Hyperbaric oxygen therapy, 1154-1155
Hypercalcemia, 867, 2138, 2386
Hypercholesterolemia, 1156, 1450, 2131
familial, 955
Hypercoagulation, 601
Hyperglycemia, 1474
Hyperhidrosis, 317, 1156-1157, 2177
Hyperinsulinemia, 1820
Hyperkalemia, 148
Hyperkeratosis, 513
Hyperlipidemia, 173, 639, 941, 1157-1158, 1450, 1622, 1713
Hyperopia, 301, 814, 816, 822, 1928, 2011, 2360-2361
Hyperosmotic agent, 986
Hyperparathyroidism, 1159-1161, 1730, 2138
Hyperplasia, 764, 1161-1162, 1171, 1363, 1855, 1861
Hypersensitivity, 1215
Hypersplenism, 2110
Hypertension, 119, 174, 249, 296, 330, 607, 1055, 1062, 1162-1166, 1172, 1254, 1450, 1473, 1626, 1747, 2027, 2152, 2339
kidney disease and, 750
portal, 480, 2047

pregnancy and, 1834-1835, 2262
renal failure and, 1930
renovascular, 2339
screening and, 1999
Hyperthermia, 1166-1170, 2160
Hyperthyroidism, 757, 1157, 2240
Hypertrichosis, 786-787
Hypertrophic left ventricle, 161
Hypertrophy, 348, 1072, 1171-1173, 1527
Hyperuricemia, 998
Hyperventilation, 1174
Hyphae, 902
Hypnosis, 94, 1175-1178, 2148
Hypoadrenocorticism, 46
Hypocalcemia, 867
Hypochondriasis, 1178-1181
Hypocretins, 1545
Hypogammaglobulinemia, 1212-1213
Hypoglycemia, 674, 1182-1185, 2005, 2136
newborns and, 971
Hypogonadism, 1451, 1453
Hypogonadotropic hypogonadism, 1892
Hypokalemia, 148
Hypokalemic paralysis, 1718
Hypomania, 266, 894
Hypomanic episode, 267
Hyponychium, 1539
Hypoparathyroidism, 1159-1161
Hypophosphatemic rickets, 787
Hypophysectomy, 1600
Hypopituitarism, 1116, 1791
Hypoplasia, 786-787
Hypopnea, 2068
Hypospadias, 1185, 1932
Hypospadias repair, 1185-1186
Hypotension, 296, 1186-1187
Hypothalamus, 50, 323, 754, 756, 758, 978, 1074, 1187, 1626, 1790, 2084, 2239
Hypothermia, 648, 680, 851, 897, 1166-1170, 1774
Hypothyroidism, 91, 542, 755, 757, 978, 1028, 1183, 1626, 2240, 2242
congenital, 314, 542-543, 684, 1411, 2242
endometriosis and, 767
Hypovolemia, 674
Hypovolemic shock, 2040-2041
Hypoxemia, 40, 1689
Hypoxia, 164, 187, 329, 447, 589, 662, 897, 1154, 1188, 1689, 2160
Hypoxic anoxia, 188
Hysterectomy, 10, 419-420, 768, 1019, 1188-1192, 1444, 1448, 1933, 2125-2126
abdominal, 1190
vaginal, 1190-1191
Hysterosalpingography, 193, 1219
Hysteroscopy, 192, 1019, 1535
Hysterotomy, 10

I

Iatrogenic disorders, 1193-1194
Ichthyosis, 513, 2063
Id, 1883
Ileostomy, 511, 521, 1194-1197
Ileum, 918, 925, 1195
Illicit drugs, 604, 2007
Illness
  acute, 662
  chronic, 413, 662
Imaging, 527, 713, 920, 928, 1198-1202,
  1399, 1589, 1767, 1771, 1919, 2051,
  2311
Immobilization, 398, 891
Immune system, 196, 216, 233, 252, 274,
  311, 370, 373, 465-466, 663, 869, 1001,
  1142, 1176, 1202-1206, 1212, 1226,
  1289, 1391, 1735, 2016, 2021,
  2145-2146, 2238, 2280, 2355
Immunization, 257, 413, 1002, 1144,
  1206-1211, 1253, 1429, 1971, 2017
Immunoassay, 1306
Immunocompromised patients, 373-374,
  592, 903, 1214
Immunodeficiency disorders, 31, 1210,
  1212-1215, 1735, 2021, 2389
Immunogenicity, 1211
Immunoglobulin E (IgE), 67-68, 70-73,
  144, 197, 869, 1031
  antibodies, 197, 624
Immunoglobulins, 69, 72, 144, 342, 1210,
  2389
Immunologic stains, 260
Immunology, 126, 1205, 1215
Immunomodulators, 716
Immunopathology, 1215-1216
Immunosuppression, 1803
Immunosuppressive drugs, 219, 567,
  1088, 1205, 1290, 1362, 1368-1369,
  2280
Immunotherapy, 252
Impacted teeth, 1652, 2204, 2254
Impetigo, 286, 1216-1217, 2143
Impingement, 1967
Implanon, 548
Implantable cardioverter defibrillator,
  1693
Implants
  bladder, 256
  brain, 256
  breast, 345, 1414, 1800
  cochlear, 256, 595
  dental, 616
  larynx, 256
  penile, 1744
  retina, 256
Implicit processing, 285
Impotence, 960-961, 1744, 1862, 1864
In vitro fertilization, 192-194, 530-532,
  912, 1019, 1217-1221, 1232, 1840
  ethics and, 802
In vivo fertilization, 1218

Inattention, 604
Incest, 1922
Incidence, 783, 1563-1564, 1566
Incisors, 2204
Incontinence, 155, 242, 968, 1019, 1134,
  1221-1224, 1863
Incubation period, 2050
Incurably Ill for Animal Research, 125
Incus, 1045, 2011
Independent practice association, 1042,
  1043
Indicators of Abuse Screen, 13
Indigestion, 4, 471, 657-659, 909, 922,
  927, 1264
Indomethacin, 1267
Induction therapy, 1647
Infants, 635
Infarction, 1225
Infection, 11, 236, 662, 863, 1038, 1142,
  1225-1229, 1668, 1757
Infectious disease, 413
Infertility, 192, 531-532, 912, 1218, 1933
  female, 192, 531, 765-766,
    1229-1233, 1743
  male, 192, 531, 961, 1233-1236,
    1933, 2009, 2338
Infertility testing, 192, 764
Infibulation, 475, 1934
Inflammation, 78,153, 177, 308, 351, 363,
  670, 1038, 1226, 1237-1238, 1696,
  1803, 1823, 1955
  heart attacks and, 1060
Inflammatory bowel disease (IBD), 509,
  514, 521, 566, 1261, 2112, 2304
Influenza, 224, 743, 782, 879, 1130, 1210,
  1238-1241, 1253, 1451, 1453, 1585,
  1897, 2355, 2357
  avian, 223-227, 1211, 2020
  viral, 448
Influenza B, 446, 448, 1209
Informed consent, 739, 800, 1242
Infrared light, 1773
Ingrown nails, 1538
Ingrown toenails, 884, 1540
Inguinal hernias, 835, 1103, 1105, 1933
Inhalers, 198
Inheritance, 952-956
Inhibitions, 2247
Injuries, 15, 320, 355, 1696
  brain, 327
Inner cell mass, 489-491
Inner ear, 238, 2351
Inner ear disorder, 1441
Inotropic drugs, 1067
Insanity, 1318-1319
Insanity defense, 1319
Insect-borne diseases, 1242-1247, 1402
Insecticides, 1245
Insomnia, 1445, 2067, 2072
Instability, 886-887
Instincts, 1883
Institute for Genome Research, 964
Institute of Medicine, 1248

Institutional Review Board, 486, 739
Insulator, 949-950
Insulin, 2, 377, 639-641, 643, 754-755,
  760, 877, 970, 976, 993, 1136, 1138,
  1183-1184, 1533, 1710, 1820, 1839,
  2136, 2188, 2190
  fetal, 971
Insulin growth factor, 858
Insulin resistance, 1474
Insurance, 1041
Integra, 360
Intellectual disability, 893
Intelligence, 56
Intelligence quotient (IQ), 214, 1459
Intense pulsed light therapy, 2335
Intensive care See Critical care
Intensive care unit (ICU), 562, 1248-1251,
  1567
Intercourse, 529, 531, 546, 583-584, 1931,
  2026, 2322
Interferometry, 1283
Interferon, 253, 506, 2356
Intergenic regions, 963
Interleukin receptors, 2021
Interleukins, 73, 253, 2186
Intermittent claudication, 299-300, 480
Internal medicine, 1251-1254
International Agency for Research on
  Cancer, 378
International Classification of Diseases,
  645
Internet medicine, 1255-1257
Interpartner violence, 1258-1259
Interstitial compartment, 717
Interstitial cystitis, 229
Interstitial fluid, 1386
Interstitial nephritis, 1287
Interstitial pulmonary fibrosis (IPF),
  1259-1260
Intertrigo, 373, 625
Intestinal cancer, 2134-2137
Intestinal disorders, 509, 546, 567, 650,
  773, 1102, 1260-1262
Intestines, 2, 513-514, 1194, 1263-1265
Intima, 160
Intoxication See Alcoholism; Poisoning
Intracellular fluid, 865
Intracranial pressure, 2283-2284
Intracytoplasmic sperm injection, 194,
  912, 1219
Intraocular pressure, 981, 984
Intraperitoneal therapy, 419
Intrauterine devices (IUDs), 549, 714
Intrauterine growth retardation, 1793
Intravenous (IV) therapy, 1266-1267, 1721
Intravenous pyelogram (IVP), 1201, 1285
Intraventricular hemorrhage, 1267-1268
Intrinsic factor, 916
Intubation, 2268
Invasive tests, 1268-1269
Investigation, 784-785
Investigational new drugs, 872
Iodine, 542, 755, 760, 994, 1200,

1411-1412, 1920, 2240, 2242-2243
Iodine deficiency, 542, 1411, 2240
Ions, 865, 1709
Iontophoresis, 1157
Iraq War, 777
Iridectomy, 984
Iris, 401, 813, 1643, 2358
Iritis, 813, 815, 1929
Iron, 1078, 1083, 1360, 1470, 1622
Iron lung, 1816
Irritable bowel syndrome (IBS), 508, 651,
653, 919, 923, 1269-1272, 1753, 1852
fibromyalgia and, 857
Irritants, 17
Ischemia, 98, 173, 175, 329, 364, 387,
553, 662, 886-887, 1062, 1154, 1225,
1272-1273, 1562, 1774, 1796, 2150,
2231, 2339
Islets of Langerhans, 757, 976, 1709
Isoflavones, 1783
Isoimmunization, 97, 1636, 2133
Isoleucine, 1418
Isotopes, 1200
Isotypes, 144
Itching, 438, 624-626, 1120, 1345, 1789,
1963, 1986

J

Jansky-Bielchowsky disease, 240
Jarvik-7 artificial heart, 1070
Jaundice, 455, 909-910, 922, 1084, 1095,
1097, 1274, 1360, 1363, 1365-1366,
2013, 2138, 2141
Jaw, 319, 1274, 1652, 1656, 2204, 2209
Jaw wiring, 1274-1276
Jejunoileal bypass, 1153
Jejunum, 918, 925
Joint diseases, 177, 363, 998, 1664, 1669,
1953, 1955, 2209
Joint replacement, 181, 1659
Joints, 177, 182, 320, 396, 1025, 1109,
1268, 1277-1279, 1348-1349,
1658-1659, 1661, 1664, 1669, 1696,
1823, 1953-1955, 1967, 2183, 2209
*Journal of the American Medical
Association*, 92
Judgment, 1463-1464
Jumper's knee, 2210
Justice, 801

K

Kala-azar, 1332
Kaposi's sarcoma, 32, 1107, 1213, 1281,
1647, 1985, 2061
Karyotyping, 261, 678, 938, 942,
1282-1283, 1892
Katayama fever, 1987
Kawasaki disease, 1283-1284, 2346
Kefauver-Harris Amendment, 873
Keratin, 77, 552, 1022, 1538
Keratinocytes, 786-787, 1539, 2056

Keratitis, 813-814, 1284, 1644
Keratoconjuntivitis sicca, 682
Keratoconus, 814, 816
Keratomileusis, 2362
Keratoplasty, 550
Keratoses, 2065
Keratosis pilaris, 624
Ketamine, 494
Ketoacidosis, 877, 1552
Ketolides, 136-137, 139
Ketones, 971
Ketonuria, 639
Keyhole surgery, 364
Kidney cancer, 1285-1286
Kidney disorders, 3, 6, 582-583, 641, 684,
750, 953, 1086, 1164, 1285-1288, 1292,
1573, 1819, 1868, 1904, 1930
Kidney failure, 750, 1137
Kidney removal See Nephrectomy
Kidney stones, 1082, 1201, 1287-1288,
1293, 1311, 1358, 1905, 2140, 2327
Kidney transplantation, 3, 750,
1288-1290, 1572, 1574, 1930, 2190
Kidneys, 2, 22, 50, 667, 750, 1185, 1285,
1289, 1291-1294, 1571, 1575, 1611,
1904, 1920, 2140, 2189-2190, 2325,
2328
acidosis and, 25
Kinesiology, 83, 810, 1295, 1525
Kinesthetic imprinting, 690
Klinefelter syndrome, 436, 735, 1282,
1295-1296
Klippel-Trenaunay syndrome, 1296-1297
Klumpke's palsy, 1707
Kluver-Bucy syndrome, 1297-1298
Knee replacement, 181
Kneecap, 1298, 1373, 1663
Kneecap removal, 1298-1299
Knees, 16-17, 181, 321, 577, 1299, 1373,
1663, 1955
Knock-knees, 1299-1300, 1658
Kock pouch, 511, 1195
Korsakoff's Syndrome, 63-64, 94, 894,
1300-1301
Korsakow syndrome, 1298
Kufs' disease, 240
Kuru, 561, 1849
Kwashiorkor, 1301-1302, 1396, 1409,
1411-1412, 1867
Kyphoplasty, 886, 890
Kyphosis, 127-128, 1302-1303, 1674

L

Labor, 441, 1838
hydrotherapy and, 1152
induction of, 442, 1637
Laboratories, 1307
Laboratory tests, 141, 1252, 1304-1308,
2321, 2329
Labrum, 1466
Labyrinthitis, 673, 703, 2351
Laceration repair, 1308-1309

Lacerations, 1032, 1039, 1308
Lacrimal glands, 682, 976, 2202
Lacrimal puncti, 682
Lactase, 1309
Lactation, 347, 1790, 1932
Lactic acid, 1477
Lactose, 876, 905, 1005, 1309
Lactose intolerance, 876, 1302, 1309,
2079
Laetrile, 872
Lamellar ichthyosis, 513
Laminectomy, 437, 1310, 1600, 1725
Langerhans cell histiocytosis (LCH), 1116
Langerhans' cells, 2062
Language development, 501
Language disturbances, 164, 1773, 1784,
2094-2095
Lanugo, 1022
Laparoscopic surgery, 455
Laparoscopy, 51, 364, 455, 766, 772, 910,
1190, 1310-1312, 1431, 2125, 2288
diagnostic, 193, 1019
Laryngectomy, 1312, 1681
Laryngitis, 1313, 1550, 1552, 2369-2370
Laryngospasm, 576, 680
Larynx, 256, 1312-1313, 1381, 2268
Laser epithelial keratomileusis (LASEK),
1928
Lasers, 284, 768, 984, 1093, 1314, 1601
hair removal with, 1023
use in surgery, 201, 616, 818,
1314-1317, 1398, 1601, 2170,
2173, 2199, 2335, 2362
Laterality, 2111
Law and medicine, 221, 806, 885, 1114,
1318-1321
Law of Similars, 1127
Laxatives, 546, 651, 707
Lazy eye, 814, 2360
Lead poisoning, 108, 332, 662, 748, 777,
1322-1323, 1325, 1460, 1813, 2005
Leaky gut theory, 869
Learning disabilities, 689, 1324-1327
Learning theories, 502, 638
LeBoyer method, 443
Leg pain, 480
Legionnaires' disease, 233, 1328-1331,
1382, 1737
Legs, 318, 480, 1299, 1372, 1785, 2336
restlessness in, 1940
Leiomyosarcoma, 1985
Leishmaniasis, 1244, 1332, 1871
Lens, 399, 401, 821, 1643, 1649, 2358
artificial, 399, 403
Lentiviruses, 31, 1146
Leprosy, 233, 884, 1333-1336, 1584,
2063, 2226
Leptin, 1136, 1153, 1336-1337, 1629
Leptospirosis, 1337-1339
Lesch-Nyhan syndrome, 1471-1472
Lesions, 894, 1339-1340
acne, 27
biopsy, 261

brain, 62, 85, 165
breast, 348
cancer, 103
intestinal, 516
Kaposi's sarcoma, 32
lupus, 107
precancerous, 338
precursor, 104
skin, 286, 1495
Leucine, 1418
Leukemia, 332, 358, 429-430, 677, 779, 1002, 1078, 1215, 1340-1344, 1740, 2229, 2297
Leukocytes, 287, 291, 1002, 1077, 1203, 1237, 1340-1341, 1797, 2234
Leukocytosis, 2305
Leukodystrophy, 1344-1345
Leukoma, 816
Leukotrienes, 68-69, 71, 1959
Levitra, 796
Levodopa, 1733
Lewy bodies, 1734
Lhermitte-Duclos disease, 787
Li-Fraumeni syndrome, 1985
Libido, 1883
Lice, 1245, 1345-1348, 2301
Licensure, 76
Licofelone, 153
Lidocaine, 1370
Life expectancy, 1371
Life support, 563, 739
    termination of, 566, 805, 1114
Lifespan, 1371
Ligaments, 17, 321, 512, 544, 840, 1348-1349, 1660, 2106, 2114, 2383
Ligation, 1093
Light chain, 144
Light therapy, 81, 622, 1349-1350, 1877, 2003
Limb buds, 734
Limbic system, 748
LIMK1 gene, 2386
Lincosamides, 136, 137
Linear Cowden nevus, 787
Lines of Blaschko, 786
Lipid storage diseases, 929, 1352, 1602
Lipids, 875, 929, 1156-1157, 1344, 1350-1353, 1359, 1395, 1470, 1602, 2129, 2201
    metabolism, 929, 2201
Lipitor, 461
Lipopeptides, 137
Lipopigment, 240
Lipoproteins, 458, 1395
Liposarcoma, 1985
Liposomes, 934
Liposuction, 1153, 1354-1356
Lips, 485, 925, 1504
Liquid X, 494
Lisping, 1356, 2094
Listeria infections, 880, 1356-1357
Lithium, 267, 622, 1877
Lithotripsy, 911, 1293, 1357-1358, 2138,

2330
Liver, 2, 5, 247, 479, 918, 923, 1094, 1204, 1359-1362, 1364, 1368-1369, 1602, 1604, 1920, 2047, 2281
    glycogen storage diseases, 989
Liver cancer, 5, 923, 1361-1365, 1367
Liver disorders, 5, 479, 719, 1094-1095, 1184, 1274, 1360, 1362, 1364-1368, 1451, 1604, 2027, 2047, 2387
Liver failure, 360, 1368, 1552
Liver transplantation, 1362, 1368-1369, 1605, 2281
Livestock, 353-354
Living will, 53-54, 806, 1114, 1945
Lobular carcinoma in situ, 335
Local anesthesia, 111, 117, 889, 1370-1371, 2347
Local block, 112
Lockjaw See Tetanus
Locus, 949, 951
Longevity, 1371-1372
Long-term memory, 503-504, 1301
Lordosis, 2108
Lorenzo's oil, 53, 1344
Lotronex, 1271-1272
Lou Gehrig's disease See Amyotrophic lateral sclerosis
Lovastatin, 1344
Low-density lipoproteins (LDLs), 2131
Low estrogen, 968
Low testosterone, 968
Lower esophageal sphincter (LES), 23
Lower extremities, 99, 1372-1375, 2335, 2340
    prostheses for, 1865
LSD, 494
L-type calcium channel, 149
Lubricants, 546
Lujo fever, 2353
Lumbar puncture, 113, 1268, 1304, 1375-1376, 1443, 1725
Lumpectomy, 335, 344, 1422-1425, 2294
Lumps, breast See Breast cancer; Breast disorders; Breasts, female
Lung cancer, 1377-1380, 1382, 1449, 1452, 1467, 1895, 1902, 2086
Lung disease, 1259, 1450
Lung disorders, 1898
Lung reduction, 469
Lung surgery, 1379-1380
Lung transplantation, 469
Lungs, 350, 434, 745-746, 772, 1379, 1381-1384, 1801, 1807, 1895, 1900, 1920, 1935, 2188
    acidosis and, 25
    fetal, 96
Lunula, 1539
Lupus See Systemic lupus erythematosus (SLE)
Lupus erythematosus, 107, 218, 663, 884, 1119
    endometriosis and, 767
Luteal phase, 1843

Luteal phase defect, 764
Lutein, 1783
Luteinizing hormone (LH), 192, 531, 759, 978, 1790
Lyme disease, 274, 1346, 1384-1385, 2403
Lymph, 1117, 1203, 1385-1386, 1391
Lymph nodes, 1121-1122, 1203, 1386-1387, 1391, 1494
Lymphadenitis, 729
Lymphadenopathy, 1386-1390
Lymphadenopathy and lymphoma, 1387
Lymphangitis, 729
Lymphatic disorders See Lymphadenopathy and lymphoma
Lymphatic system, 353
Lymphatic system, 47, 728, 1203, 1386, 1390-1394, 2253
    anatomy of, 1121, 1203, 1386-1387, 1390
Lymphedema, 1386, 1392
Lymphocytes, 288, 373, 639, 869, 1121, 1143, 1203, 1212, 1341, 1386, 1391, 1393, 2016, 2238, 2280
Lymphogranuloma venereum, 453
Lymphoma, 357, 1107, 1121, 1386-1390, 1393, 2134, 2229
Lyric Hearing Aid, 1049
Lysosomal storage diseases, 929, 1353, 2201
Lysosomes, 410, 989, 1143
Lysosyme, 2202

M

Macrocephaly, 787
Macrolides, 136-138
Macronutrients, 1395-1396, 1621
Macrophages, 467, 1116, 1203, 1226-1227, 1382, 1984
Macrosomia, 970
Macula, 2359
Macular degeneration, 283-284, 814-815, 1397-1398, 2109, 2360-2361
Mad cow disease, 470, 561, 1849
Maduromycosis, 902
Magnesium, 1621, 2366
Magnetic field therapy, 83, 1399
Magnetic fields, 1399-1400
Magnetic resonance imaging (MRI), 102, 176, 305, 760, 928, 986, 1198, 1367, 1399-1401, 1589, 1606, 1915, 2152
Magnetoencephalography (MEG), 1589
Magnets, 1177, 1399-1400
Maillard reaction, 2361
Major histocompatibility complex, 953, 1001
Major histocompatibility proteins, 1205
Major League Baseball, 2128
Malabsorption, 239, 407, 916, 1401-1402, 1622
Malaria, 126, 274, 431, 743, 852, 1243, 1402-1405, 1482, 1533, 1729, 1871,

2403

Male genital disorders, 1856

Male pattern baldness, 1022

Malignancy, 335, 369, 418, 986, 1405-1409

Malignant cells, 590

Malignant hypertension, 2186

Malignant malnutrition, 1301-1302

Malignant melanoma, 629, 1436, 2058, 2065

Malleus, 1045, 2011

Malnutrition, 59, 246, 342, 650, 663, 684, 706, 719, 835, 876, 966, 1010, 1301-1302, 1396, 1409-1412, 1457, 1969

Malocclusion, 319, 611, 686, 1656, 2386

Malpractice, 1041, 1114, 2176

Mammary glands, 347, 435, 976

Mammography, 333, 335, 1413-1415, 1607, 1641, 2000

Managed care, 1043-1044, 1416-1417, 1435

Mandatory reporting requirements, 1258

Mandible, 1652

Mania, 266

Manic episode, 267

Manic-depressive disorder See Bipolar disorders

Manicure, 1539

Manometry, 1115, 1752

Mantoux test, 229

Maple syrup urine disease (MSUD), 1417-1418, 1469, 1471

Marasmus, 684, 1396, 1409, 1412

Marburg virus, 711, 1418-1419, 2352

March of Dimes, 1816

Marfan syndrome, 545, 953, 1419 1420

Marijuana, 42, 1421

Marinol, 1421

Mass spectrometry, 1870

Massage, 170, 1422, 1774

Mast cells, 67-69, 71, 1031, 1037

Mastectomy, 335-336, 344, 349, 1422-1425, 1914
  preventive, 939

Mastication, 2203

Mastitis, 339, 348, 1426

Mastoiditis, 705, 1551

Masturbation, 1427

Materia Medica, 1100, 1128

Maxilla, 1652

Maxillofacial surgery, 1651-1653

Maximally tolerated dose, 486

Mayo Clinic, 489

Maze procedure, 385-386

MDMA, 494

Measles, 446, 448, 1208, 1427-1430, 2017

Meckel's diverticulum, 1430-1432

Meconium ileus, 579

Media, 160

Median nerve, 394

Medicaid, 618, 1435

Medical home, 1432-1433

Medical schools, 443

Medicare, 618, 969, 1041, 1433-1435, 2217

Medigap policies, 1434

Meditation, 81, 1039, 1435-1436, 2147, 2399

Medulla oblongata, 322

Megacolon, 2305
  congenital, 1115

Meiosis, 489-490, 676, 952

Meissner's corpuscles, 2010, 2258, 2260

Melancholia, 269, 1990

Melanin, 1022, 1436, 1786-1787, 2056, 2062, 2368

Melanocytes, 1436, 1539, 1786-1787, 2056, 2060, 2062, 2368

Melanoma, 629, 1436-1437, 1449, 1492, 1788, 2058, 2060, 2064-2065, 2297

Melarsoprol, 2075

Melasmas, 2062

Melatonin, 754-755, 978, 1438-1439, 2003, 2065

Membranes, 1351, 1353

Memory, 1596

Memory cells, 1204

Memory loss, 93, 605, 1301, 1439-1440, 1543, 2044

Memory recall, 894

Menarche, 1455, 1891

Ménière's disease, 1441

Meninges, 1580

Meningitis, 353, 447-448, 775, 1376, 1442-1443, 1580, 2103, 2392
  bacterial, 1443
  West Nile, 2381

Meningoencephalitis, 1646

Meniscus, 1466

Menkes disease, 1470, 1472

Menopause, 1133, 1136, 1444-1447, 1674
  gingivitis and, 974
  hair growth, 1023
  premature, 1133
  surgical, 1133

Menorrhagia, 1447-1448, 1457, 1535, 2371

Men's health, 1448-1454

Menses, 1843

Menstrual extraction, 9

Menstrual pain, 691

Menstruation, 91, 342, 347, 530, 532, 691, 765, 957, 1133, 1136, 1230, 1446-1447, 1454-1458, 1836, 1932, 2124

Mental illness See Psychiatric disorders; specific diseases

Mental incompetence, 608

Mental retardation, 120, 542, 551, 1459-1462, 1741, 2095

Mental status, 604

Mental status exam, 1463-1464

Mercurochrome, 1465

Mercury poisoning, 777, 1460, 1464-1465

Meridians, 34-35

Merkel's disks, 2258, 2260

Merocrine glands, 976

Merozoites, 1403

Mesenchymal stem cells, 1465-1467

Mesenchyme, 1117, 1985

Mesothelioma, 184, 778, 1467-1468

Metabolic acidosis, 25

Metabolic disorders, 1469-1472

Metabolic syndrome, 1472-1474, 1629

Metabolism, 21, 63-65, 579, 810, 876, 942, 977, 993, 1167, 1184, 1359, 1469, 1475-1478, 1625
  amino acid, 1418
  carbohydrate, 905, 989
  copper, 2387
  errors in, 876, 1361
  fatty acid, 839
  fructose, 900
  glycogen, 989
  iron, 1083
  lipid, 929, 2201
  mucopolysaccharide, 1506

Metachromatic leukodystrophy, 1344

Metal exposure, 778

Metals, 1464

Metastasis, 335, 369, 418, 1363, 1405-1409, 2294

Metastasize, 986

Metatarsals, 840, 1372

Metformin, 370, 643, 1474, 1821

Methadone, 1861

Methamphetamine, 42, 1687

Methemoglobin, 576

Methicillin-resistant Staphylococcus aureus (MRSA) infections, 743, 1479-1480, 2118

Methotrexate, 1874

Methyl group, 949

Methylphenidate, 504

Methyltransferase, 949

Mevalonic acid, 459-460

Microbiology, 141, 143, 1004, 1305-1306, 1480-1483

Microbiome, 136, 139

Microbots, 258

Microbrachycephaly, 120

Microcephaly, 632, 1460

Microfilariae, 728-730

Microorganisms, 140, 1005, 1480

Microscopy, 107, 589, 1119, 1484
  electron, 589, 1353
  slitlamp, 823, 1485, 2387

Microsurgery, 2168, 2173

Midbrain, 323

Midges, 1244

Midgut, 1430

Midwives, 443

Migraine headaches, 212, 1033, 1035, 1696

Mildew, 1491-1492

Milk, 905, 1309

Milk ducts, 334, 341, 978

Milroy's disease, 1393

Mineralcorticoids, 556, 2129, 2189

Minerals, 663, 875, 1395, 1410, 1621, 1736, 2364-2368
Minimal inhibitory concentration, 142
Minimally conscious state, 981, 1485-1486
Ministrokes, 2278
Minoxidil, 1022
Miosis, 1563
Mirena (IUD), 549
Mirror neuron system, 215
Mirror neurons, 1487-1488
Miscarriage, 764, 1488-1489, 1838, 2025, 2133
Misdiagnosis, 645
Mites, 1345-1348, 1986
Mitochondria, 426, 410-411, 490-492, 809
Mitofusin 2, 426
Mitosis, 428, 676, 1282
Mitral valve disorders, 388
Mitral valve prolapse, 388, 1174, 1490
MLSK, 136-137
MMR vaccine, 214, 1518
Mnemonic, 503-504
Model organisms, 962
Molar pregnancy, 1488
Molars, 2204, 2388
Mold, 1491-1492
Molecular biology, 251
Moles, 1437, 1492-1493, 1787, 2058, 2060
Monkeypox, 1493-1494
Monoamine oxidase inhibitors (MAOIs), 146, 622, 1634, 1733, 1877
Monobactams, 136-137
Monoclonal antibodies, 144-145, 253, 256, 1612, 1921, 2017, 2305
Monocytes, 288, 1116, 1143, 1203
Monogamy, 2035
Mononucleosis, 464, 591, 794, 1107, 1494-1495, 1758, 2017, 2092
Monosaccharides, 875
Monosodium glutamate (MSG), 2178
Monothematic, 376
Monozygotes, 1506
Mood disorders, 59, 620, 2043
Morbidity and Mortality Weekly Report, 412
Morgellons disease, 1495-1496
Morning sickness, 1559-1560
Moro reflex, 1926
Morphea, 1993
Morphine, 576, 1099, 1546, 1861
Morphologic changes, 220
Morphology, 326
Morquio syndrome, 1506
Morton's neuroma, 883
Mosaicism, 676-677
Mosquitoes, 609, 728, 730, 749, 1243, 1402, 2381, 2398, 2403
Motion sickness, 1496-1498, 1559-1560, 2012
Motor activity, 692-693
Motor cortex, 692, 894

Motor disabilities, 415
Motor neuron, 692-693
Motor neuron diseases, 102, 1498-1500
Motor skill development, 1500-1504
Mouth, 925, 1142, 1504
  dry, 2055
Mouth cancer, 1504-1505
Movement disorder, 694
MRI *See* Magnetic resonance imaging (MRI)
Mucopolysaccharidosis (MPS), 1505-1506
Mucosae, 2305
Mucous glands, 976
Mucus, 976, 1142, 1381, 2084
Müllerian ducts, 2023
Multidisciplinary care, 1700, 1702-1704
Multiple births, 193, 1220, 1506-1510
Multiple chemical sensitivity syndrome, 1511-1512
Multiple infarct dementia, 606, 1440
Multiple sclerosis, 218, 1012, 1119, 1512-1516, 1581, 1717, 2027, 2050, 2102
  endometriosis and, 767
Multipotent, 1466
Mumps, 446, 926, 1516-1518, 1655
Münchausen syndrome by proxy, 1518-1519
Murmur, 161-162
Muscle cells, 588, 992, 1001
Muscle cramps, 1521
Muscle pain, 857, 1520
Muscle sprains, spasms, and disorders, 1011, 1375, 1498, 1520-1522, 1524, 1526, 2223, 2245, 2383
Muscle weakness, 1534
Muscles, 106, 321, 649, 809, 841, 992, 1171, 1498, 1520, 1522-1526, 1534, 1660, 1716, 1774, 2010, 2211, 2222
  aging and, 55
  atrophy, 204
  chest, 434
  glycogen storage diseases, 989
  lower extremities, 1372
  upper extremities, 2315
Muscular dystrophy, 107, 941, 943, 1173, 1375, 1520, 1524, 1526-1529, 1718, 2318
  Duchenne, 955, 1375, 1524, 1526-1528, 2318
Musician's dystoni, 693
Mutation, 271, 368, 410, 579-581, 676, 680, 684, 735, 937, 1529-1533, 1640, 1735, 2135, 2297
  recessive, 580
Mutations, 498-499
Myasthenia gravis, 218, 727, 1119, 1520-1521, 1524, 1533-1535, 1718, 2239
Mycobacteria, 229, 2290
Mycobacterium avium complex, 1646
Mycosis fungoides, 2061
Mycotoxins, 901, 1491

Myelin, 52, 1011-1012, 1118, 1513, 1515, 1580-1581, 1584, 2111
Myelin sheath, 425-427, 1344
Myelography, 1376
Myenteric plexus, 1750
Myocardial infarction *See* Heart attack
Myocardium, 389
Myoclonic dystonia, 693
Myoclonus, 2067
Myofibroblasts, 2186
Myomas, 2297
Myomectomy, 1019, 1189, 1448, 1535-1536
Myopathy, 1520
Myopia, 301, 814, 816, 822, 1536, 1928, 2011, 2360-2361
Myosarcoma, 2297
Myotomy, 20
MyPlate, 878-879
Myringotomy, 700, 704, 1537

N

Nail bed, 1539
Nail plate, 1539
Nail polish, 1540
Nail removal, 1538
Nails, 1538-1541, 2058
Naltrexone, 45
Namenda, 89
Nanobots, 258
Nanoparticles, 778
Nanorobotics, 258
Narcolepsy, 1541-1545, 2068, 2071, 2073
Narcotics, 17, 112, 1035, 1545-1548, 1697
Nasal cavity, 1549, 2083
Nasal polyp removal, 1548-1549, 1825
Nasal polyps, 131, 1549, 1552, 1824
Nasal surgery, 1959
Nasogastric tube, 915
Nasopharyngeal disorders, 794, 1549-1553
Nasopharyngeal tonsils, 47
National Cancer Institute (NCI), 486, 1553-1556
National Center for Environmental Health (NCEH), 412
National Center for Health Statistics (NCHS), 412
National Center for Infectious Diseases (NCID), 413
National Center for Injury Prevention and Control (NCIPC), 413
National Center on Elder Abuse, 14
National Collegiate Athletic Association, 2127
National Institute for Occupational Safety and Health (NIOSH), 414
National Institutes of Health (NIH), 618, 850, 1553, 1555-1557
National Registry of Evidence-Based Programs and Practices, 619
National Toxicology Program, 378

National Vaccine Plan, 413
Natural childbirth, 443
Natural killer cells, 252, 2021
Nausea, 922, 1558-1561
Nebulizers, 747
Neck, 321, 751, 1312
Neck disorders, 1031-1032, 2383
Neck injuries and disorders *See* Head and neck disorders
Neck pain, 2383
Necrosis, 590, 593, 914, 1118, 1225, 1562
Necrotizing enterocolitis, 774
Necrotizing fasciitis, 1562-1563, 2117, 2143, 2263
Needle biopsy, 261, 333, 1268, 1423, 2294
Negative feedback, 1780, 2189
Negligence, 2176
Nematodes, 1728, 1969, 2286
Neobladder, 276
Neonatal brachial plexus palsy, 1563-1566
Neonatology, 1566-1570, 1738, 2275
Nephrectomy, 1571-1572, 2331
Nephritis, 1287, 1573-1575, 1577, 1869, 2251, 2327
   interstitial, 1286
Nephrology, 1575-1578, 2329
Nephrons, 667, 1291, 2325, 2328
Nephrotic syndrome, 1287, 1573-1574, 1577
Nerve block, 112, 1370
Nerve cells, 106, 322, 588, 1001, 1118, 1171, 1344, 1579, 1583, 1590, 1716, 2104, 2257
Nerve conduction test, 727
Nerve disorders, 394
Nerve root compression, 1917
Nerves, 111, 394, 726, 1370, 2009, 2317, 2333-2334
   lower extremities, 1374
   pain, 1917
   pinched, 230
Nervous system, 178, 425, 451, 791, 1008, 1118, 1512, 1579-1583, 1590, 1594, 1600, 1715, 1717, 1732, 1781, 2103, 2178, 2187
   aging and, 55
Neural interface, 256
Neural therapy, 83
Neural tube, 734
Neuralgia, 1583-1586, 1653
Neuraminidase, 224
Neuritic plaques, 85
Neuritis, 123
Neuritis, 1583-1586
Neuroenhancement, 1586-1587
Neuroethicists, 1586
Neuroethics, 1586-1587
Neurofibrillary tangles, 85, 88
Neurofibromas, 1587, 2297
Neurofibromatosis, 953, 1587-1588, 1985, 2297
Neurofibrosarcoma, 1985
Neuroglia, 322, 1118, 1593

Neuroimaging, 1588-1589
Neuroleptics, 268, 2193-2194
Neurological abnormalities, 575
Neurology, 1590-1594
   pediatric, 1594-1595
Neuromas, 2297
Neuromodulator, 503
Neuromuscular electrical stimulation, 204
Neuron, 120, 425-426, 985, 1597, 1828
Neuronal ceroid lipofuscinoses, 240
Neuropathic pain, 427
Neuropathology, 326
Neuropathy, 426-427, 1583-1586
Neuropsychological tests, 1596
Neuropsychology, 1596-1597, 2283
Neuroscience, 1597-1598
Neurosis, 1598-1599
Neurosurgery, 559, 1599-1602, 1681
Neurotransmitters, 622, 791, 1524, 1534, 1545-1547, 1580, 1590, 1597, 1716, 1753, 2066, 2162, 2193
Neutral lipid storage disease, 513
Neutrophils, 288, 353, 1142, 1203, 1226-1227
Nevi, 1296, 1436
Nevus, 786-788
Nevus comedonicus, 787
Nevus flammeus, 575
Nevus sebaceous, 787
Nevus sebaceous syndrome, 786
Newborns, 163, 1567, 1746
Niacin, 461, 2166, 2365
Nicotine, 42, 158, 343, 504
Niemann-Pick disease, 1602-1603
Night blindness, 1410, 2002
Night terrors, 2068, 2072
Nightmares, 2067
Nipple discharge, 339
Nitrogen, 1396
Nitrogen mustard, 431
Nitrogen, liquid, 571
Nitroglycerin, 2028
Nitrosoureas, 430
Nitrous oxide, 115-116
Nociceptors, 1696
Nocturia, 582
Nodular prostatic hyperplasia, 1861, 1933
Nonalcoholic steatohepatitis (NASH), 1365, 1604-1605
Nonbullous congenital erythroderma, 513
Nondisjunction, 676-677, 679
Noninvasive tests, 1605-1607
Nonmaleficence, 801
Nonsteroidal anti-inflammatory drugs (NSAIDs), 152, 427, 519, 1665, 1697, 1954, 1957, 2184, 2303
Norepinephrine, 51, 503, 622, 2066
Norepinephrine and dopamine reuptake inhibitors (NDRIs), 622
Noroviruses, 916, 1608-1609
Norplant, 548
Norwalk-like viruses, 1608
Nose, 1381, 1678-1679, 1799, 1824, 1959,

2010, 2053, 2082
Nosebleeds, 724, 1551, 1553, 1668, 1958
Nosocomial infection, 136
Notochord, 733
Novocaine, 1370
NSDHL gene, 787
Nuclear medicine, 928, 1200, 1609-1612, 1614
Nuclear radiology, 1200, 1613-1615, 2051
Nucleic acid amplification tests, 294
Nucleoside, 1147
Nucleoside analogues, 507, 1147
Nucleotides, 952
Nucleus, 409
Numbness, 212, 897, 1011, 1174, 1370, 1445, 1615-1616, 2150, 2259
Nursing, 74, 1125, 1616-1620, 2176, 2215
   ICU, 1250
Nursing homes, 61, 189, 191, 832, 1433, 2216
   illnesses in, 1608
Nutraceuticals, 2165
Nutrients, 654, 875-876, 878, 1395, 1475, 1620, 2165
Nutrition, 654-655, 810, 876, 878-879, 1295, 1395, 1620-1624, 1782, 2165, 2393
Nuva Ring, 548

O

Oat cell carcinoma, 1377
Obesity, 131, 640, 643, 662, 707, 876, 878, 997, 1173, 1275, 1354, 1396, 1473, 1604, 1623, 1625-1628
   abdominal, 1473
   childhood, 640-641, 1628-1631
   genetic links, 708
   heart attacks and, 1060
   hormones and, 1136
   Prader-Willi syndrome and, 1832
   severe, 1153
   sleep apnea and, 2069
   weight loss medications and, 2377
Observational study, 783-784
Obsessions, 157
Obsessive-compulsive disorder, 1631-1634
Obstetrics, 1176, 1635-1637, 1746, 2311
Obstruction, 364, 398, 671, 1196, 1261, 1713, 2330
Obstructive sleep apnea (OSA), 2068
Obstructive urinopathy, 845
Obturator, 484
Occipital cortex, 285
Occlusion, 1656, 2149
Occupational health, 414, 1638-1639, 1775, 1845
Occupational injuries, 1846
Occupational Safety Health Administration (OSHA), 354
Occupational therapy, 416, 1125, 1525, 1596, 1772, 2109

Ocular herpes, 813-814
Ocular pneumoplethysmography, 2151
Office of Global Health, 414
Office of Public Health Genomics, 414
Oils, 1351
Old age abuse, 13
Older adults, 2363, 2364
Olfaction, 131, 2010, 2082
Oligodendrocyte, 985
Oligonucleotides, 258
Omega-3 fatty acids, 1623
Omphalomesenteric duct, 1432
Onchocerciasis, 1243
Oncogenes, 368, 410, 955, 1406, 1408,
    1640, 1736, 2299
Oncology, 1639-1642
Oncolytic virus therapy, 370
Oncovirus, 794
Onychomycosis, 1540
Oocyte, 1684
Oophorectomy, 1189, 1685
Open heart surgery, 363, 541, 1061, 2236
Operating room, 1619, 2174
Ophthalmology, 126, 682, 823, 1485,
    1642-1645, 1649
Ophthalmoscope, 823, 984
Opiates, 1545-1548
Opioid medications, 1702, 1703-1704
Opioids, 1545, 1546-1548
Opium, 1099
Opportunistic infections, 32, 903, 1142,
    1645-1648
Optic nerve, 822, 982, 2359
Optometry, 823, 1648-1650
Oral cancer, 2254
Oral contraceptives, 418, 547, 2130
Oral rehydration, 2393
Oral surgery, 614, 1651-1653, 2254
Orchiectomy, 1653-1654, 2218-2219
Orchiopexy, 2219
Orchitis, 446, 1654-1655, 2218
Orexins, 1545
Organ of Corti, 1045
Organ procurement, 327
Organ transplantation, 126
Organic disease, 661
Organs, 1780, 2187-2191
Ornithine transcarbamylase deficiency,
    935
Ortho Evra, 548
Orthodontics, 319, 614, 1655-1658, 2388
Orthognatic surgery, 1652
Orthologues, 964
Orthopedic braces *See* Braces, orthopedic
Orthopedic surgery, 183, 416, 1109, 1525,
    1658-1659, 1661, 1957
Orthopedics, 320, 1658-1663
Orthostatic hypotension, 148-149,
    151-152
Orthotic devices, 318, 1026, 1809
Osgood-Schlatter disease, 1663
Osmosis, 865
Osmotic pressure, 717, 866

Osseointegration, 1865
Ossicles, 594, 701-702, 2010
Osteitis deformans, 1694
Osteoarthritis, 177, 179, 181, 308-309,
    357, 397, 512, 884, 1109, 1278, 1310,
    1660, 1662, 1664-1666
Osteoblasts, 313, 545, 886, 889, 1466,
    1694
Osteochondritis juvenilis, 1666
Osteoclasts, 314, 1117, 1694
Osteocytes, 312, 886, 1117
Osteogenesis imperfecta, 512, 545,
    1666-1668
Osteomalacia, 308, 1410
Osteomas, 702
Osteomyelitis, 308, 398, 1154, 1479,
    1668-1669
Osteonecrosis, 1669-1670
Osteopathic medicine, 1670-1673
Osteopetrosis, 314
Osteoporosis,
Osteoporosis, 308, 315, 512, 545, 663,
    966-967, 1109, 1134, 1137, 1159, 1302,
    1410, 1412, 1445, 1660, 1673-1678,
    1824, 2087, 2105
    nutrition and, 1623
    screening and, 2001
Osteosarcoma, 305, 1985, 2297
Osteosclerosis, 703
Osteotomy, 425, 427, 1670
Ostomy, 1194
Othostatic hypotension, 1186
Otitis externa, 697-698, 702
Otitis media, 594, 599, 697, 699-700, 702,
    1050, 1053, 1537, 1551-1552, 2012
    acute, 1550
Otoacoustic emissions, 210
Otogram, 1053
Otoplasty, 1678, 1799
Otorhinolaryngology, 704, 1312,
    1678-1682
Otosclerosis, 697, 699-700, 1050, 1668
Otoscope, 704
Outpatient care, 487
Outpatient surgery, 487
Ovarian cancer, 417-421, 957-958, 1416,
    1684
Ovarian cysts, 573, 577, 586, 957-958,
    1682-1683, 1820
Ovarian failure, 91
Ovarian hyperstimulation syndrome, 1220
Ovarian medulla, 1684
Ovarian torsion, 577
Ovariectomy, 1685
Ovaries, 978, 1018, 1230, 1456,
    1682-1685, 1932, 2022
    polycystic, 1820
OvaSure, 420
Over-the-counter medications, 42,
    1685-1687, 2007-2008
Overbite, 319, 1656
Overdoses, 1811-1812
Overhydration, 866

Overtraining syndrome, 1688
Overweight, 878, 1625
Oviducts, 529-531, 1230, 1932
Ovulation, 529-531, 1218, 1229, 1456,
    1635, 1836, 2332
    induction of, 1219
Ovulation testing, 192
Ovum, 530, 532, 677, 1218, 1506, 1508,
    1684
    abnormal, 192
    harvesting, 193
Oxazolidionones, 136, 137
Oxidation-reduction, 25
Oximeter, 2069
Oxygen, 1055, 1188, 1381, 1936
Oxygen concentrator, 1689
Oxygen therapy, 81, 469, 1188, 1260,
    1689, 1900
    hyperbaric, 1154-1155
Oxygen transport, 2048
Oxygent, 2274
Oxytocin, 341, 759, 978, 1636, 1781,
    1790, 2189
Ozone layer, 1788, 2061

P

Pacemaker implantation, 1690-1694
Pacemakers, 172, 1064, 1452, 1690, 1944
Pacifiers, 2374
Pacinian corpuscles, 2009, 2258, 2260
Paget's disease, 1137, 1694-1695
Pain, 887, 1600-1601, 1696-1699, 1756
    abdominal, 507, 566, 972, 1270, 2141
    acute, 1697
    back, 230-231, 321, 664, 1303, 1310,
        1674, 1696, 1992, 2078, 2112
    chest, 23, 121, 381, 723, 752, 1163,
        1174, 1225, 1378, 1752, 1801,
        1896
    chronic, 180, 1697
    hip, 1109
    leg, 480
    menstrual, 691
    muscle, 857, 1520
    neck, 2383
    nerves, 1917
    referred, 1696
    stomach, 4
    types of, 1698
Pain management, 35, 37, 1152, 1176,
    1370, 1422, 1697, 1699-1700, 1701
Painful bladder syndrome, 229
Painkillers, 112, 442, 836, 1088, 1099,
    1685, 1697, 1699, 1714, 1756
Palatability, 2198
Palate, 481, 485, 925
Palliative, 986
Palliative care, 1125, 1138-1141,
    1700-1701
Palliative medicine, 1702-1704
Palpitations, 1445, 1704-1705, 1767
Palsy, 245, 1705-1708

Pancreas, 2, 471, 579, 639, 642, 657, 754, 757, 919, 923, 976, 1183, 1709-1712, 2135-2136, 2281, 2311
   imaging, 769
Pancreatic cancer, 1711, 2134-2137
Pancreatitis, 6, 446, 648, 923, 1710, 1712-1714
Pandemics, 223, 457, 743, 780-783, 1132
Panic attacks, 156, 158, 1174
Panic disorder, 156, 158
Pan-plexopathy, 1563, 1565
Pap test, 418, 420-421, 959, 1019-1020, 1147, 1269, 1714-1715, 1770
Papain, 780
Papaverine, 1099
Papillae, hair, 1022
Papillae, tongue, 2195
Papular nevus spilus, 787
Paracelsus, 2266
Paracentesis, 1268
Parafollicular cells, 1137
ParaGard (IUD), 549
Paralysis, 245, 317, 719, 886-887, 890, 1011, 1032, 1082, 1542, 1581, 1705, 1715-1718, 1815, 1907, 1909, 2102, 2317
   Botox and, 316
   facial, 245
   sleep, 1542, 2068, 2071
   spastic, 2223
Paralytic ileus, 1261
Paramedics, 738, 1719-1722, 1944
Paranoia, 59, 1723-1724, 1990
Paraphasias, 2380
Paraplegia, 1717, 1725
   bedsores and, 243
Parasitic diseases, 90, 228, 728, 917, 972, 1261, 1402, 1726-1729, 1789, 1871, 1969, 1987, 2075, 2192, 2286, 2301
Parasympathetic nervous system, 1055, 1580, 1781
Parathyroid glands, 756, 977, 1159, 1730, 2189, 2239, 2244
Parathyroid hormone, 977, 1159, 1730, 2189
Parathyroidectomy, 1730
Parkinson's disease, 606, 687, 848, 1581, 1600, 1707-1708, 1730-1734, 2027, 2285
Parkinsonism, 693, 1732
Parotid glands, 1517
Paroxysmal dystonia, 693
Paroxysmal localized hyperhidrosis, 1157
PARP inhibitors, 429
Parry's disease, 240, 241
Parthenogenesis, 489, 491
Partial dentures, 617
Pasteurization, 352, 354
Patanjali, 2399
Patch, birth control, 548
Patella, 1298, 1373
Patent ductus, 539-541
Patent ductus arteriosus, 576, 1899

Patents, 872
Paternalism, 801
Pathogen, 135-136, 139
Pathogenesis, 220, 661, 1252, 1735
Pathology, 220, 261, 589, 592, 630, 660, 1227, 1307, 1735-1738
PCBs, 343, 779
Peak flow meter, 198, 200, 469
Peanuts, 71
Pectin, 854
Pediarix, 1211
Pediatrics, 1738-1742, 1746, 2171
Pedicure, 1539
Pedodontics, 614
Pellagra, 1410, 1412
Pelvic examination, 1018
Pelvic fluid, 572
Pelvic inflammatory disease (PID), 453, 714, 957, 996, 1218, 1230, 1743-1744, 2034
Pena-Shokeir syndrome type II, 499
Penems, 137
Penicillin, 137-138, 143, 234-235, 428, 431, 901, 1004, 1491, 1757, 1986, 2014, 2035, 2093, 2182
Penile implant surgery, 796, 1744-1746
Penis, 477, 795, 932, 960, 1185, 1744, 1860, 1931
People for the Ethical Treatment of Animals (PETA), 124
Pepsin, 2, 657, 1264, 2306, 2333
Peptic ulcers *See* Ulcers
Peptide hormones, 1135
Percocet, 1700
Percussion, 1767
Percutaneous hepatic perfusion (PHP), 1363
Perfluorochemicals, 2274
Perforated eardrum, 697-698, 702, 1551
Pericarditis, 389
Perimenopause, 1133, 1444
Perinatal period, 1563, 1565
Perinatology, 1746-1747
Perineum, 793
Periodontal surgery, 1016, 1747-1748
Periodontitis, 406, 611, 614, 974-975, 1015, 1748-1749, 1796, 2205
Periosteum, 313
Peripheral artery disease, 2344
Peripheral Myelin Protein-22, 426
Peripheral nervous system, 425-426, 1579, 1602, 1717, 1781
Peripheral vascular disease, 1864
Peripheral vascular resistance, 148
Peripheral vision, 2358
Peristalsis, 19, 471, 514, 657, 773, 799, 918, 1196, 1261, 1263, 1270, 1749-1753, 1926, 2079, 2188, 2333
Peritoneal dialysis, 646, 648, 750, 1574
Peritonitis, 3, 170, 521, 671, 1105, 1754, 2303
Perpetrator, 1922-1924
Persistent vegetative state, 981

Personality disorders, 1723, 1784, 2163
Perspiration, 1074, 1156, 1167, 2057, 2062, 2177
Pertussis, 447-448
Pervasive developmental disorders, 185, 632
Pes cavus, 426-427
Pesticides, 777, 1245, 1511
PET scanning *See* Positron emission tomography (PET) scanning
Petechiae, 886, 890, 2229
Petit mal seizure, 790, 2005
Pets, 1911, 2402
Peyronie's disease, 2027
pH, 20, 22, 25, 1709, 2329
Phacoemulsification, 399, 817
Phacomatosis, 786, 788
Phacomatosis pigmentokeratotica, 786-788
Phagocytes, 288, 291-292, 467-468, 869, 1142
Phagocytosis, 373, 467, 851, 1142, 1203, 1226
Phalanges, 840, 1372
Phantom limb pain, 100, 1698, 2259
Pharmaceutical companies, 872
Pharmacodynamics, 41
Pharmacogenomics, 258
Pharmacokinetics, 41
Pharmacology, 256, 1754-1757
Pharyngeal tonsils, 47
Pharyngitis, 447, 1550, 1552, 1758-1759, 2092
Pharynx, 925, 1381, 1504, 1758-1759
Phenicols, 136-137
Phenobarbital, 324, 791
Phenylalanine, 1469
Phenylketonuria (PKU), 343, 537, 581, 876, 937, 954, 1460, 1469, 1533, 1737, 1759-1761, 2063
Phenytoin, 791
Pheromones, 1458, 2086
Phlebectasia, 575
Phlebitis, 600, 1761-1763, 2236, 2340, 2350
Phlebotomy, 291, 293, 1083, 1764
Phobias, 157-158, 1599, 1764-1766
Phocomelia, 2226
Phonemic error, 2380
Phospholipids, 875, 1351, 1359
Phosphorus, 1621, 2366
Phosphorylation, 459
Photocoagulation, 1398
Photodynamic therapy, 371, 1317, 1398
Photonutrients, 2165
Photopheresis, 2059
Photoreceptors, 517, 821, 2359
Photorefractive keratectomy (PRK), 819, 1316, 1928
Photosensitivity, 499
Phototherapy, 81, 1349, 1791, 1874, 2003
Phox, 467-468
Phrenic reflex, 242

Phrenology, 1766-1767
Physiatry, 1772
Physical deconditioning, 838
Physical examination, 1252, 1767-1771, 2113
Physical fitness, 812, 842
Physical rehabilitation, 100, 1525, 1771-1776, 2113
Physical therapy, 74, 100, 120, 416, 488, 1110, 1125, 1152, 1280, 1295, 1522, 1528, 1772, 2113
Physician assistants, 1776-1779
Physician-assisted suicide, 195
Physiology, 1779-1782
Phytochemicals, 1782-1783, 2166
Pica, 213
Pick's disease, 606, 1783-1785
PID See Pelvic inflammatory disease (PID)
Piebaldism, 2063
Pigeon toes, 1785-1786
Pigmentation, 1437, 1786-1789, 2062
disorders, 2368
Pigs, 2396
Pilocarpine, 983
Pimples, 26, 628, 2155
Pinched nerve, 230
Pineal gland, 754-755, 757, 978, 1438, 2065
Pingueculitis, 1889
Pinworms, 1728, 1789-1790, 1970
Pitocin, 1137, 1637
Pituitary gland, 314, 683-684, 754, 756, 758, 761, 973, 978, 1009, 1456, 1600, 1790-1791, 2085, 2189
Pituitary tumors, 573, 973
Pityriasis, 2063
Pityriasis alba, 1791
Pityriasis rosea, 1792
Placebo, 264, 1697
Placenta, 441-442, 462, 733, 1506, 1508-1509, 1636, 1747, 1793-1794, 1835, 1838
Placenta abruptio, 444, 1747, 1793, 1842, 2133
Placenta previa, 423, 1747, 1793, 1842
Placental insufficiency, 1793
Plague, 743, 782, 1244, 1794-1795, 2403
bubonic, 1794, 2403
pneumonic, 1795, 1897
Plantar fasciitis, 835
Plantar warts, 842, 884
Plants, 1098, 1782
Plaque, 406, 553
arterial, 174, 172, 387, 473, 751, 1056, 1059, 1062, 1157, 1163, 1795-1796, 2123, 2131, 2149, 2231, 2339
dental, 22, 610-611, 974, 1015, 1748, 1796-1797, 2204
Plasma, 278-279, 289, 1077, 1087, 1386, 1797, 2189, 2276
Plasma exchange, 1515, 1535, 2230

Plasmapheresis, 505-506, 1012, 1088, 1521, 2346
Plasmids, 136, 138, 695, 934
Plasmin, 2231
Plasminogen, 2231
Plastic surgery, 302, 825, 1354, 1681, 1798-1801
Plasticity, 1597
Platelet-derived growth factor, 2186
Platelets, 278-280, 282, 288, 1077, 1086, 1340, 1797, 2229, 2231, 2234, 2275, 2371, 2389
Pleura, 434, 1380, 1382, 1801
Pleurisy, 1801-1802, 1804
Pluripotent, 489, 491-493
Pneumocystis carinii pneumonitis, 32
Pneumocystis jirovecii , 1802-1803
Pneumocystis pneumonia, 1647, 1805
Pneumonia, 40, 233, 351, 467, 497, 523-524, 903, 1210, 1253, 1302, 1328, 1378, 1382, 1451, 1795, 1803-1806, 1895, 1902, 2110
Pneumonic plague, 1795, 1897
Pneumothorax, 1380, 1382, 1807-1808
Podiatry, 842, 1808-1810
Point-of-service plans, 1042, 1043
Poison control centers, 860
Poisoning, 17-18, 222, 662, 874, 1155, 1811-1814, 2011, 2265
first aid, 860
Poisons, 17, 222, 274, 589, 1736, 1812, 2012, 2264-2265
Poliomyelitis, 447-448, 774-775, 1119, 1207-1208, 1814-1818, 2103, 2354, 2356
Pollen, 1031
Pollution, 558, 1382
Polyarteritis, 2346
Polychondritis, 397
Polycystic kidney disease, 953, 1292, 1819-1820
Polycystic ovary syndrome, 91, 586, 1684, 1820-1821, 1933
Polycythemia, 576
Polydactyly, 271, 1821-1823
Polyhydramnios, 96
Polymerase, 949
Polymerase chain reaction, 261, 298, 945, 1138, 1240, 1506, 1803
Polymethylmethacrylate, 1800
Polymyalgia rheumatica, 1823-1824, 2208
Polyp removal See Colon polyp removal; Rectal polyp removal; Nasal polyp removal
Polypharmacy, 604, 966
Polyphenols, 1783
Polyposis, familial, 1196
Polyps, 516, 518-520, 1262, 1312-1313, 1549, 1552, 1824-1825, 1852, 2370
nasal, 1824
uterine, 1824
vocal cord, 1824
Polysaccharides, 875

Polysomnography, 167, 2069
Pons, 322
Pontiac fever, 1328
Porphyria, 1825-1826
Port-wine stains, 2060, 2153
Portacaval shunts, 2047
Positive end-expiratory pressure (PEEP), 40
Positive feedback, 1780
Positron emission tomography (PET) scanning, 1200, 1589, 1611, 1826-1828, 1920, 2052
Positrons, 1200
Postconcussive syndrome, 533
Postherpetic neuralgia, 1828-1829
Postmaturity, 445
Postmortem, 326-327
Postnasal drip, 1958
Postpartum depression, 1829-1830
Postpartum psychosis, 1829
Post-traumatic stress disorder, 1258, 1830-1831, 2067
Postural drainage, 747
Postural hypotension, 673-674
Posture, 230, 1302
Potassium, 1621, 2366
Prader-Willi syndrome, 950, 1832
Pramipexole, 1733
Precocious puberty, 1833-1834, 1892
Prediabetes, 641
Predisposition, 955
Prednisone, 245, 506
Prednisone eye drops, 1889
Preeclampsia, 1489, 1793, 1834-1836, 1839, 2133, 2184, 2262
Preferred provider, 1043, 1416
Preferred provider organizations (PPOs), 1044, 1416
Pregnancy, 95, 347, 462, 463, 529, 531, 1090, 1092, 1172, 1488, 1559-1560, 1747, 1781, 1793, 1836-1840, 2311, 2324
cervical cancer and, 419
complications of, 1835, 2262
diabetes during, 970
ectopic, 714-715, 1743, 1839, 2126
gingivitis and, 974
goiter and, 995
molar, 1488
teratogens and, 2213
Prehypertension, 296
Premature atrial contractions (PACs), 171
Premature birth, 445, 1568, 1637, 1738, 1747, 1840-1843
fetal surgery and, 846
toxemia and, 2262
Premature infants, 1938
Premature ovarian failure, 91
Premature ventricular contractions (PVCs), 171
Premenstrual dysphoric disorder (PMDD), 1843
Premenstrual syndrome (PMS), 1457,

1843-1844, 2179
Prenatal care, 1636
Prenatal diagnosis, 95, 97, 537, 679, 1219, 1282, 1637
Preoperational stage, 500, 635
Presbycusis, 594, 703, 1050
Presbyopia, 301, 814, 816, 822, 2012
Prescription drugs, 873
Presenilin, 86
Pressure sores, 243, 1302
Prevalence, 783
Preventive medicine, 381, 664, 812, 920, 939, 1041, 1060, 1064, 1434, 1671, 1772, 1777, 1779, 1845-1848, 1944, 2233
Priapism, 961, 2027
Primary aging, 54
Primary dystonia, 692
Primitive gut, 1430
Primitive reflexes, 1926-1927
Primitive streak, 733
Prion diseases, 470, 560, 778, 1848-1849
Prions, 470, 560, 1849
Privacy, 802
Proctitis, 1926
Proctology, 1850-1853
Progeria, 57, 1853
Progeroid appearance, 499
Progesterone, 347, 419-420, 440, 1133, 1137, 1173, 1230, 1456, 1843-1844
Progestins, 714, 768, 1133
Prognosis, 1854-1855, 2051
Progressive pigmentary retinopathy, 499
Prokaryotic cells, 231
Prolactin, 341, 347, 759-760, 1636, 1790
Prolactinomas, 760
Prolapse
  mitral valve, 388, 1490
  rectal, 923, 1851, 1926
  uterine, 957-958, 1189, 1191, 1933, 2332
Prolia, 1677
Prone, 886
Proof, 63-64
Propecia, 1022
Proprioception, 2351
Prostaglandins, 10, 68-69, 71, 180, 440, 529, 1237, 1456, 1843, 1925, 1957, 2008, 2307
Prostate, 967, 969
Prostate cancer, 572, 961, 1449, 1452, 1654, 1855-1857, 1861, 1863, 2130, 2349
  screening and, 2000
Prostate enlargement, 1451, 1453, 1855, 1857-1859, 1861, 1863, 2009
Prostate gland, 960, 1855, 1857, 1859-1863, 1931, 2008, 2130
Prostate gland removal, 1858, 1863-1864
Prostate-specific antigen (PSA), 2000, 2009
Prostatitis, 1451, 1453
Prostheses, 18, 99-101, 181, 1663, 1798,

1864-1867, 2170
Prostheses, penile, 1744
Protease inhibitors, 33, 1147
Proteins, 256, 409, 512, 657, 875, 878, 949, 951, 962, 1264, 1352, 1359, 1395, 1532, 1621, 1867-1869
  binding, 1136
  deficiency, 1301, 1867
  high levels in urine, 1868
Proteinuria, 750, 1578, 1835, 1868-1869, 2186, 2262
Proteomes, 1869
Proteomics, 251, 255, 963, 1869-1870
Proteus syndrome, 786
Proton-pump inhibitors, 20
Protozoa, 142, 1481, 1726, 1728, 1871
Protozoan diseases, 228, 424, 972, 1332, 1402, 1481, 1646, 1870-1871, 2075, 2287
Proviruses, 1146
Prozac, 146, 1925
Pruritus, 2186
Pseudohemophilia, 2371
Pseudohermaphroditism, 1101, 2024-2025
Pseudomembrane, 660
Pseudophedrine, 148
Psoralen, 1874, 2059
Psoriasis, 628, 1540, 1872-1875, 2058, 2063
Psychedelic drugs, 494
Psychiatric disorders, 185, 302, 565, 1875-1881, 1883, 2043, 2145, 2162
Psychiatry, 1879-1880
  geriatric, 1881-1882
Psychoanalysis, 709, 1178, 1882-1885
Psychobiology, 1597
Psychogenic dystonia, 693
Psychogenic tremor, 2285
Psychograph, 1767
Psychopathy, 1586
Psychophysiological disorders, 248
Psychosis, 63-64, 1301, 1598, 1885-1887
  postpartum, 1829
Psychosomatic disorders, 1496, 1887-1888, 2285
Psychostimulant, 503-504
Psychosurgery, 622, 1600, 1634
Psychotherapy, 268, 622, 1599, 1633, 1831, 1878, 2147
  behavioral, 623
  cognitive, 623
Psychotropic drug, 2158
PTEN, 787
Pterygium/pinguecula, 818, 1888-1889
Ptosis, 345, 814-815, 1563, 1889-1890
Puberty, 26, 347, 978, 1009, 1337, 1741, 1833, 1860, 1890-1894, 2085
  gingivitis and, 974
Pubic hair, 1022
Public health, 93, 412, 1556, 2264, 2391
Public Health Service, 1555
Pulled muscles, 1521, 1524
Pulmonary artery, 539-540

Pulmonary diseases, 184, 187, 197, 352, 469, 746, 1027, 1377, 1380, 1382, 1450, 1802, 1805, 1894-1897, 1899-1900, 1937, 2289
Pulmonary edema, 390, 576, 718, 1063, 1119, 1392, 1898-1899
Pulmonary embolism, 527, 600, 731, 1191, 2052, 2337
Pulmonary function tests, 469, 1902
Pulmonary hypertension, 1899-1900, 2069, 2186
Pulmonary medicine, 126, 1900-1903
Pulse, 886
Pulse rate, 1769, 1903-1904
Puncture wounds, 1039
Pupil, 401-402, 1643, 1645, 2358
Pure Food and Drug Act, 872
Purging, 707
Purine nucleoside phosphorylase (PNP), 2021
Pus, 11-12, 1203, 1227
Pyelogram, 1201
Pyelonephritis, 582, 584, 1287, 1904-1905, 2324
Pyloric stenosis, 1905-1906, 2303
Pyoderma, 624
Pyonephrosis, 1287
Pyorrhea, 611-612, 614
Pyrogens, 851-852, 1227
Pyruvate, 991

Q

Qi gong, 81
Quadrantectomy, 1424
Quadriplegia, 416, 1706, 1717, 1907
  biofeedback and, 250
Quality of life, 1701
Questran, 461
Quickening, 7, 1746
Quinidine, 1099
Quinine, 431, 1098, 1403
Quinolones, 138
Quinsy, 1550, 1552, 1908, 2251

R

Rabies, 126, 274, 749, 1909-1912, 2403
Radial keratotomy (RK), 819
Radiation, 271, 306, 402, 662, 736, 776, 1201, 1413, 1614, 1826, 1912, 1914, 1916
Radiation sickness, 1912-1913
Radiation therapy, 306, 335, 369, 1155, 1389, 1407, 1437, 1641, 1913-1916, 2294
Radical mastectomy, 344, 1423, 1425
Radiculopathy, 1917-1918
Radio frequency ablation, 2335
Radioactive isotopes, 335, 1200
Radioallergosorbent test (RAST), 71-72, 870
Radioimmunoassay, 761, 979, 1921

Radioisotopes, 253, 2051
Radiology, 126, 1198-1202, 1614
Radionucleotide scanning, 899
Radionuclides, 1610, 1826, 1919
Radiopharmaceuticals, 1610, 1614, 1826, 1914, 1918-1921
Radius, 2315
Raloxifene, 1676
Raloxifene hydrochloride, 337
Range of motion, 1564-1565
Rape, 1258, 1922-1924
Rapid eye movement (REM) sleep, 2067
Rapid-onset dystonia parkinsonism, 693
Rashes, 202, 438, 446, 774, 858, 987, 1107, 1283, 1384, 1428, 1493, 1791-1792, 1966, 1970, 1986, 2013, 2038, 2063, 2080, 2132, 2183, 2355, 2366
Rat infestations, 1339
Raynaud's phenomenon, 505, 576, 1774, 1925, 1993, 2178, 2186-2187
RayVa, 1925
Reaction time, 503
Reactive oxygen species, 467
Reading disorders, 688
Reading glasses, 2358
Rebound congestion, 599
Recessive diseases, 954
Recessive mutations, 580
Recombinant DNA, 944-945
Recommended daily (or dietary) allowances (RDAs), 654, 877, 2367
Reconstructive surgery, 345, 826, 1652, 1681, 1798
Rectal cancer, 517-519, 1926
Rectal polyp removal, 520, 1852
Rectal polyps, 1824
Rectal prolapse, 923, 1851, 1926
Rectal surgery, 520-522, 1850
Rectum, 514, 773, 918, 923, 926, 1090, 1195, 1851, 1925-1926
Recurrent infections, 468
Red blood cells, 108, 287, 937, 993, 1077, 1292, 1576, 1797, 2015, 2274
Red Cross, 861
Reduction, 398, 891
Redux, 2377
Reexperiencing, 1830
Refeeding, 130
Referred pain, 1696, 1698
Reflexes, 1708, 2101, 2222
primitive, 1926-1927
Reflux, 23, 416, 919, 927, 1752, 2092
Refractive errors, 823, 1649, 2360
Refractive eye surgery, 819, 1928-1929
Refsum disease, 1472
Regional anesthesia, 112-113, 1370
Registered dietitians, 1125
Registry, 76
Regression, 1884
Reiter's syndrome, 1929-1930, 2112
Rejection, 1003, 1070, 1289, 1369, 2280, 2396

Relapse, 1337-1338
Relaxation training, 2148, 2399
Remote monitoring, 60
Renal failure, 360, 373, 648, 684, 750, 1027, 1161, 1172, 1287-1289, 1392, 1577, 1819, 1930, 2027, 2138, 2190, 2280, 2327
Renal hypoplasia, 575
Renal osteodystrophy, 750
Renal pelvis, 2140
Renal tubules, 1291-1292, 2325, 2328
Renin, 149, 1576, 2040
Renovascular hypertension, 2339
Repertory, 1128
Report on Carcinogens, 378
Repression, 1883
Reproductive biology, 126
Reproductive surgery
male, 1744
Reproductive system, 1008, 1931-1934, 2022
female, 417-418, 529, 1018, 1134, 1770, 1931, 2124, 2288
male, 960, 1149, 1185, 1857, 1860, 1931, 2008, 2219, 2338, 2347
Research, 739
Research vs. animal rights *See* Animal rights vs. research
Resectoscope, 1863
Reserpine, 1099
Resistance, 143, 997, 1253, 1479, 2118, 2291
Respiration, 167, 187, 196, 434, 649, 745, 994, 1174, 1380-1382, 1801, 1899, 1935-1938, 1942, 2160, 2188, 2269
artificial, 391
Respirator, 1896, 1937
Respiratory acidosis, 25
Respiratory diseases, 233, 351, 469, 522, 580, 1253, 1382
Respiratory distress syndrome, 97, 576, 1027, 1383, 1938-1939
acute, 39
Respiratory system, 558, 745, 1253, 1381, 1720, 1895, 1935, 1942, 2188
aging and, 55
Rest tremor, 2285
Restless legs syndrome, 1939-1941, 2067, 2179
Resuscitation, 563, 680, 1250, 1942-1944
Retainers, 1657
Reticulocytes, 1077
Retina, 256, 517, 819, 821, 1397, 1536, 1643, 2359, 2361
Retinitis, 592, 2183
Retinoids, 1622
Retinopathy, 814-815
Retinotopic map, 285
Retroviruses, 31, 1145, 1408, 1945-1946, 2355
Rett's syndrome, 632-633
Revascularization, 2028
Reverse transcriptase, 1145, 1946

Reye's syndrome, 749, 1947, 2179
Rh factor, 97, 289, 1636, 1947-1951, 2016, 2273
Rh incompatibility, 1084, 1747, 1839, 1949, 2016
Rhabdomyosarcoma, 1985
Rheumatic fever, 388, 884, 1065, 1071, 1550, 1951-1952, 2017, 2093, 2143, 2251
Rheumatoid arthritis, 177, 179, 218, 308-309, 512, 545, 835, 884, 1109, 1278, 1349, 1662, 1774, 1952-1955, 2017, 2209
endometriosis and, 767
juvenile, 1279-1280
Rheumatology, 1662, 1954-1958
Rhinitis, 147, 523-524, 1958-1959
Rhinitis medicamentosa, 599
Rhinoplasty, 1799, 1801, 1959-1960
Rhinoviruses, 523-524, 1958, 1960-1961
Rhodopsin, 822
Rhonchi, 1803
Rib cage, 432
Riboflavin, 1410, 2365
Ribonucleic acid (RNA), 223, 711
viruses, 1946
Ribonucleic acid (RNA) interference, 258
Ribosomes, 409
Ribs, 321
Rickets, 308, 318, 1410, 1662, 1962-1963, 2365
Rickettsial diseases, 1962, 2301
Ricksettsial diseases, 1964
Ringworm, 902, 1963, 2403
Risk factor, 128
Ritalin, 207, 504
Ritualized behavior, 1632-1633
Rituxan, 253
Rituximab, 506
RNA, 949, 951
RNA polymerase, 949
Robots, 258
Rocky Mountain spotted fever, 1346, 1964, 2403
Rods, 517, 821, 2359
Roe v. Wade, 8, 1113
Rogaine, 1022
Rohypnol, 494, 1923
Rolfing, 835
Root canal treatment, 407, 569, 614, 763, 1748, 1964-1965
Root planing, 1749
Rosacea, 1965-1966
Roseola, 1107, 1966-1967
Rotator cuff, 1967, 2210
Rotator cuff surgery, 1967-1968
Rotaviruses, 916, 1968-1969
Rounds, 1249
Roundworms, 728, 1969, 2286, 2404
Rubella, 402, 446, 537, 594, 735, 1459, 1839, 1970-1971
Rubinstein-Taybi syndrome, 1972
Rule of nines, 359-360

Runners' knee, 1521
Runny nose, 524, 1958
Ruptured disk, 2077, 2106
Rye, 987

S

Saccades, 2109
Saccharin, 873
Saccular aneurysm, 160
Sacrococcygeal tumors, 845
Safety issues, 871
    children and, 1973-1977
elderly and, 1978-1981
Saline, 345, 1266, 1800
Salinomycin, 370
Saliva, 317, 657, 926, 2055
Salivary glands, 657, 926, 976, 1517
Salmeterol, 198
Salmonella infection, 233, 774, 879, 881,
    1261, 1981-1983, 2403-2404
Salt, 1622
San Joaquin Valley fever, 497
Sandflies, 1332
Sanger sequencing, 964
Santavouri-Haltia disease, 240
Saponins, 1099
Sarcoidosis, 884, 1899, 1983-1984
Sarcoma, 379, 1281, 1985, 2134, 2297
SARS See Severe acute respiratory
    syndrome (SARS)
Saturated fats, 1397, 1621
Saxitoxin, 1371
Scabies, 1346, 1986
Scalded skin syndrome, 2117
Scalds, 358-361
Scaling, 1749
Scalp reduction, 1022
Scapula, 434, 2314
Scarlet fever, 1986-1987, 2143
Scars, 1038, 1800, 2186, 2258
Schauder syndrome, 786
Schimmelpenning syndrome, 787
Schistosomiasis, 1987-1989
Schizophrenia, 687, 1581, 1633, 1724,
    1989-1992, 2045
Sciatic nerves, 1992
Sciatica, 727, 1583, 1992-1993, 2078
SCID See Severe combined
    immunodeficiency syndrome (SCID)
Scientific method, 1779
Scintillation camera, 1610
Sclera, 544, 1643-1644, 1888-1889
Scleral icterus, 1274
Scleritis, 1644
Sclerodactyly, 1993
Scleroderma, 218, 884, 1899, 1993-1994,
    2063, 2185, 2187
Sclerotherapy, 1093, 2335, 2337
Scoliosis, 308, 426-427, 1310, 1994-1998,
    2108
Scrapie, 561, 1849
Screening, 294, 420, 520, 537, 644, 679,

920, 937, 1052-1053, 1306, 1414,
    1434, 1452, 1471, 1768-1769, 1847,
    1870, 1998-2002, 2097, 2115, 2299
Scrotum, 960, 1149, 1745, 1931,
    2218-2219, 2347
Scurvy, 512, 545, 1410, 1412, 2002, 2365
Seasonal affective disorder, 621-622, 755,
    1349, 1877, 2002-2004
Sebaceous cysts, 578, 586
Sebaceous dermatitis, 625-626
Sebaceous glands, 578, 625, 976, 1022,
    2063
Sebaceous hyperplasia, 1161
Seborrheic dermatitis, 628
Second impact syndrome, 533
Secondary aging, 54
Secondary dystonia, 692
Secondary visual pathways, 285-286
Secondhand smoke, 778
Secretory cells, 588
Sed test, 178
Sedentary, 878
Seizures, 120, 211, 215, 324, 330-331,
    726, 789, 791, 1589, 1613, 1812,
    2004-2007, 2043, 2045, 2109, 2223
    eclampsia and, 1835
    febrile, 1966
    first aid, 859
    focal motor, 789
    temporal lobe, 790
Selective estrogen receptor modulators
    (SERMs), 337, 1134, 1677
Selective serotonin reuptake inhibitors
    (SSRIs), 134, 146, 303, 622, 1298,
    1633, 1844
Selective toxicity, 141, 427
Self-medication, 2007-2008
Self-limiting, 1337
Self-limiting infection, 1338
Semen, 529, 960, 1218, 1234, 1860,
    2008-2009, 2096, 2348
Semen analysis, 1219
Seminal fluid, 2008
Seminal vesicles, 2008
Seminiferous tubules, 1931
Senile emphysema, 55
Sense organs, 1643, 2009-2012, 2082,
    2256
Senses, 2082, 2187, 2195, 2198, 2256,
    2358
    aging and, 55
    connections (synesthesia), 2180
    impairment of the, 59
Sensorimotor stage, 500, 635
Sensorineural hearing loss, 594, 700, 702,
    1046, 1050, 1441
Sensory neuron, 692
Separation anxiety, 2012-2013
Sepsis, 39, 914
Septal defects, 539, 541
Septic arthritis, 996
Septic shock, 2013, 2040
Septicemia, 17, 1337-1338, 2013-2015

Seroconversion, 31
Serology, 141, 291, 2015-2018
Serotonin, 68, 134, 496, 622, 708-709,
    1237, 1271, 1298, 1843-1844, 2066
Serous glands, 976
Sertoli cells, 1931
Set point, 1153
Severe acute respiratory syndrome
    (SARS), 294, 555, 781, 2018-2020
Severe combined immunodeficiency
    syndrome (SCID), 934, 1144,
    1212-1214, 1215, 2020-2022
Severe obesity, 1153
Sex determination, 530-531, 953
Sexual desire, 166
Sexual development, 636
Sexual differentiation, 734, 1860,
    2022-2025
Sexual dysfunction, 166, 2025-2027, 2029
Sexual harassment, 1922, 1924
Sexual impotence, 2087
Sexual orientation, 2030
Sexuality, 1427, 1741, 1892, 2029-2033
Sexually transmitted diseases (STDs), 31,
    233, 413, 452, 477, 549, 852, 957-959,
    961, 996, 1147, 1228, 1452, 1743,
    2033-2037, 2181, 2287, 2323, 2331
    urethritis and, 2319
Shaken baby syndrome, 2156
Shaking, 2285, 2317
Shell shock, 1831
Shiatsu, 34
Shigellosis, 1261, 2037-2038
Shin splints, 2212
Shingles, 447, 628, 1107, 1583, 1706,
    1828-1829, 2038, 2356
Shivering, 1168
Shock, 360, 675, 721, 1074, 1721, 2013,
    2039-2042, 2234
    hypovolemic, 2040-2041
Shock therapy, 268, 622, 1878, 2042-2046
Shoes, 553, 1025
Short-term memory, 1300
Shotgun sequencing, 964
Shoulder dystocia, 1564
Shoulders, 1967
Shunts, 437, 541, 1151, 2046-2047
Sialorrhea, 317
Sicca syndrome, 2055
Sick building syndrome, 1511
Sickle cell anemia, 945, 2048-2049
Sickle cell disease, 109-110, 536, 581,
    663, 937, 941-942, 954, 1533, 1739,
    2047-2050
SIDS See Sudden infant death syndrome
    (SIDS)
Sigmoidoscopy, 2305
Sigmoidoscopy, 515-516, 520, 2001
Signs, 2050-2051
Silencing, 949
Silica, 183
Silicone, 345, 1800
Silicosis, 184, 2289

Silver-Russell syndrome, 951
Simian immunodeficiency virus (SIV), 1146
Sinemet, 1733
Single photon emission computed tomography (SPECT), 1200, 1589, 1610, 2051-2053
Sinoatrial (S-A) node, 171, 387, 1055, 1690
Sinuplasty, 2054
Sinuses, 1550, 1824, 2053-2054
Sinusitis, 599, 1551-1552, 1758, 2053-2055, 2370
Sitagliptin, 643
Sitz bath, 1092
Sixth disease, 1966
Sjögren's syndrome, 1993, 2055-2056
  endometriosis and, 767
Sjögren-Larsson syndrome, 513
Skeletal disorders and diseases See Bone disorders
Skeletal muscle, 106, 809, 1118, 1523, 1534
Skeletal muscle cells, 1171, 1523
Skeleton, 312-316, 396, 1277, 1658, 1660, 2314
Skin, 105, 248, 355, 627, 630, 825, 1117, 1142, 1739, 1786, 1799, 1963, 2009, 2056-2060, 2258, 2314
  aging and, 1134, 1800
  anatomy of the, 105, 627, 2056, 2062
  artificial, 360, 2059
Skin cancer, 571, 629, 1436, 1449, 1452, 1787, 2060-2061, 2064-2065
Skin color, 1786-1787, 2057
Skin conductance response, 376
Skin disorders, 202, 243, 361, 623-624, 627, 631, 715, 779, 883, 914, 1216, 1495, 1739, 1791-1792, 1872, 1963, 2060-2064, 2368
Skin grafting, 361, 827, 1799, 1801, 2258
Skin lesion removal, 571, 2064-2065
Skin lesions, 627, 631, 1026, 1334, 1340, 1436, 1495, 1872
Skull, 558-559, 1600
Skull fractures, 17
Sleep, 120, 2065-2068
Sleep apnea, 167, 836, 1543, 1652, 2067-2071
Sleep cycle, 858, 2065, 2071
Sleep deprivation, 2074
Sleep disorders, 167, 267, 836, 966, 1438, 1445, 1541-1542, 2067-2068, 2070-2074, 2076, 2109
  fibromyalgia and, 858
Sleep paralysis, 1542, 2068, 2071
Sleep studies, 2069, 2074
Sleepdriving, 2073
Sleepeating, 2073
Sleepiness, 147, 1542, 2068, 2071, 2073
Sleeping pills, 2068, 2072-2073
Sleeping sickness, 1244, 1729, 1871, 2074-2076

Sleepwalking, 2068, 2072-2073, 2076-2077
Slipped disk, 308-309, 664, 1993, 2077-2078, 2106
Slitlamp microscope, 1485, 1649
Slow viruses, 1146
Small intestine, 2, 651, 657, 918, 922, 925, 1260, 1263, 1750, 2078-2080, 2135-2136
Smallpox, 624, 743, 1145, 1206, 1208, 1210, 1228, 1493, 1848, 2080-2082
Smegma, 477, 1934
Smell, 2010, 2082-2086, 2197
  loss of, 131
Smoking, 42-43, 173, 197, 276, 350, 352, 469, 714, 736, 745, 748, 899, 923, 1062, 1378, 1382, 1449, 1504, 1675, 1838, 1846, 1895, 1902, 2027, 2086-2088, 2307, 2370
  macular degeneration and, 1397
Smooth muscle, 106, 1117, 1523, 1750, 1753, 2188
Snakebites, 274, 2088-2089
  first aid, 860
Sneezing, 524, 1958, 1961
Snellen chart, 822
Snoring, 167, 837, 2068, 2071
Social development, 185, 635
Social inappropriateness, 894
Social Security, 617, 969, 1433
Social skills, 1487
Social workers, 1125
Sodium, 2366
Sodium pentothal, 117
Soiling, 2090-2092
Somatic cell therapy, 936
Somatoform disorders, 302
Somatosensory cortex, 692
Somnambulism, 2073, 2076
Sorbitol, 900
Sore throat, 523, 788, 1494, 1550, 1552, 1758-1759, 1951, 2092-2094
Sound therapy, 81
Southern blot, 947
Soy, 1446, 1783
Soy products, 338
Spastic hemiplegia, 1082, 1707
Spastic paralysis, 2223
Spasticity, 317, 1082, 1499
Special education, 1461, 2096
Specialization, 2169
Spectral karyotyping, 1283
Speculum, 1018, 1770
Speech disability, 120
Speech disorders, 164, 416, 483, 1773, 2094-2096, 2149, 2154
Speech pathology, 2109
Speech therapy, 1125, 1312, 1772
Speech threshold detection, 209
Sperm, 529-532, 961, 1218, 1233-1234, 1860, 1931, 2008, 2096, 2338, 2348
  testing, 192
Sperm banks, 192, 2096-2098

Spermicides, 547
Spherocytosis, 109-110, 953
Sphincter, 19, 155, 925, 1091, 1222, 1750, 2098, 2326
Sphincterectomy, 2098-2099
Sphingomyelin, 1603
Sphygmomanometry, 296, 2000
Spider bites, 2404
Spielmeyer-Vogt disease, 240
Spina bifida, 272, 437, 537, 736, 938, 1460, 1581, 1739, 1839, 2027, 2099-2102
  correction in utero, 845
Spinal anesthesia, 114, 442
Spinal cord, 664, 1581, 1592, 1600, 1716-1717, 1739, 1815, 2101-2102, 2106
Spinal cord disorders, 178, 308, 1310, 1717, 1725, 1907, 2101-2104
Spinal disorders, 1995, 2107, 2112
Spinal fusion, 890, 1310, 1600, 2078
Spinal muscular atrophy, 1499
Spinal nerves, 1917
Spinal stenosis, 1917, 2123
Spine, 432, 449, 451, 1310, 2077, 2104-2108
  anatomy of, 1716, 1995, 2105
  curvature of, 1995, 2108
Spinocerebellar ataxia, 2109
Spirochetes, 2181
Spirometry, 469
Spitting up, 416
Spleen, 993, 1203, 1404, 1602, 1920, 2110, 2115, 2311
Splenectomy, 110, 2109-2110, 2115
Splenomegaly, 505
Splints, 321, 398-399
Split-brain, 2110-2111
Spondylitis, 309, 353, 2112-2113
Spondylolisthesis, 1310, 2108
Spondylolysis, 2107
Spondylosis, 684
Spongiform encephalopathies, 85, 470, 560, 1849
Spores, 132, 187, 317, 1491, 2222
Sporotrichosis, 902, 2404
Sports injuries, 16, 327, 532, 842, 1109, 1375, 1521-1522, 1772, 1810, 1967, 2113, 2210-2213, 2384
Sports medicine, 18, 181, 249, 320, 812, 842, 1295, 1525, 1688, 2113-2117
Sports psychology, 249, 1176, 1295
Sprains, 1349, 1520, 1661, 1770, 2114-2115
Sputum, 558
Squamous cell carcinoma, 572, 1377, 2060, 2064-2065, 2297
Src gene, 1946
Stabilization, 740, 1275
Staff model HMO, 1043
Staging, 306, 519, 1388, 2294
Stagnant anoxia, 188
Stains, 260, 1003, 1480

Stalking, 1258
Stapedectomy, 701
Stapes, 1045, 2011
Staphylococcal infections, 12, 880, 1216, 1426, 1479, 2117-2118, 2155, 2263
Starch, 377, 875
Starvation, 1396
Statins, 461, 1474, 1796
Statistics, 263
Statutory rape, 1922
Stein-Leventhal syndrome, 1684
Stem cell transplantation, 2109, 2187
Stem cells, 489, 491-492, 551, 849-850, 935, 1002, 1465-1467, 2103, 2118-2122, 2281, 2313
    cancer, 370, 431
    ethics and, 803
Stenosis, 174, 473, 540, 1063, 1072, 1796, 2122-2123, 2149
    aortic, 388
    mitral, 388
    pulmonary, 388
    spinal, 1917
    urethral, 1932
Stents, 2123-2124
Stereo vision, 2358
Stereotaxic surgery, 1601
Stereotypies, 213
Sterilization, 549, 1311, 2124-2127, 2288, 2347
Steroid abuse, 2127-2128, 2130
Steroid hormones, 1136, 2129
Steroids, 187, 198, 369, 556, 626, 747, 797, 1098, 1351, 1514, 1823, 1957, 2128-2131, 2189, 2280
    anabolic, 1173, 2130-2131
Sterols, 875
Stethoscope, 389, 1771
Stevens-Johnson syndrome, 643, 2132-2133
Stillbirth, 2133-2134
Stimulants, 207, 215, 690, 798, 836, 1543, 1633, 1877
Stings, 274-275, 2402
    first aid, 860
Stomach, 1, 4, 657, 915, 918, 922, 925, 928, 1750, 2134, 2303
Stomach cancer, 915, 922, 2134-2137
Stomach pain, 4
Stomach pumping, 2265
Stomach removal See Gastrectomy
Stomas, 277, 364, 511, 522, 1194
Stone removal, 455, 1293, 1311, 1316, 1357, 2137-2140, 2330
Stones, 455, 906-907, 1082, 1201, 1287-1288, 1292, 1311, 1316, 1357, 1861, 1905, 2138, 2140-2142, 2327, 2330
Strabismus, 120, 317, 787, 814, 823, 2142-2143, 2360
Strains, 1521, 1524, 2114-2115
Strangulated hernias, 1105
Strangulation, 188

Strawberry cervix, 2287
Strawberry mark, 628, 2060
Street drugs, 494
Strep throat, 233, 662, 1758, 2092, 2143
Streptococcal infections, 884, 1210, 1216, 1550, 1562, 1573, 1758, 1986, 2092, 2143, 2251, 2263
    sickle cell disease and, 2048
Streptogramins, 136-137
Streptokinase, 2232
Stress, 60, 249, 464, 565, 620, 698, 834, 1179, 1271, 1436, 1457, 1642, 1696, 1887, 2143-2147, 2215, 2297, 2303
    nutrition and, 1621
    sleep and, 2067
Stress echocardiography, 713
Stress fractures, 2114
Stress incontinence, 1221
Stress reduction, 1422, 1436, 2146-2148
Stress tests, 713, 723, 1611
Stretching, 1774
Stridor, 167, 788
Strokes, 164-165, 173, 328, 330, 393, 606, 719, 752, 1082, 1119, 1440, 1450, 1453, 1581, 1613, 1717, 1772-1773, 1796, 1847, 2005, 2095, 2148-2153, 2233, 2235, 2278, 2339, 2344
    and TIAs, 2150
    ischemic, 1272
    sickle cell disease and, 2048
Stromal cells, 2121
Structural genomics, 251, 963
Struvite, 2140
Sturge-Weber syndrome, 2153-2154
Stuttering, 2094-2095, 2154-2155
Styes, 814-815, 2155
Subarachnoid block, 112
Subarachnoid hemorrhage, 1376
Subcutaneous mastectomy, 1424
Subcutaneous tissue, 834
Subdural hematoma, 16, 1080, 1717, 2155-2157
Submucous resection, 1959-1960
Substance abuse, 2157-2158
Substance Abuse and Mental Health Services Administration (SAMHSA), 619
Substance P, 180, 858, 1696
Substantia nigra, 1707, 1732
Sucrose, 900
Suction curettage, 9
Sudden infant death syndrome (SIDS), 1739, 2159-2161
Suffocation See Asphyxiation
Sugars, 377, 657, 875-876, 900, 905, 1264, 1309
Suicidal ideation, 1464
Suicide, 59, 157, 623, 805, 836, 1811, 1893, 2003, 2161-2165
    antidepressants and, 873
    men and, 1451
Suicide gene therapy, 370
Suicide gesture, 2163

Sulcus, 974-975
Sulfa drugs, 141, 431
Sulfasalazine, 510-511
Sulfhemoglobin, 576
Sulindac, 519
Sunburn, 1436, 2057
Sunscreens, 1788
Superego, 1883
Superstition, 1632
Supertracker, 878
Supplements, 154, 179, 779, 872, 2165-2167
Suprachiasmatic nuclei, 2065
Supravalvular aortic stenosis, 2386
Suramin, 2075
Surfactant, 1383
Surgery, 37, 117, 369, 1176, 1619, 1778, 2172, 2174, 2271
    fetal, 844-846
    general, 2167-2170
    oral and maxillofacial, 1651-1653
    outpatient, 487
    pediatric, 558, 2170-2172
Surgical procedures, 37, 117, 1619, 2168, 2172-2173, 2175
Surgical technologists, 1619, 2173-2177
Surrogate motherhood, 1232
Surveillance, 783-784
Sutures, 1308
Swallowing, 1381
Sweat glands, 976, 1156
Sweating, 317, 603, 1156, 2177-2178
Sweets, 878
Swelling, 887
Swimmers' ear, 697, 698, 702
Swimmers' itch, 1989
Swine flu, 1585
Sylvan yellow fever, 2398
Symbiosis, 1726
Sympathectomy, 898, 1601, 2177-2178
Sympathetic nervous system, 149, 1055, 1156, 1182, 1580, 1781, 2178
Symptoms, 1126, 1252, 2050-2051, 2178
Synapses, 322, 1597
Syncope, 161-162
Syndactyly, 575, 1821-1823
Syndrome, 1252, 2178-2179
Syndrome of inappropriate antidiuretic hormone, 560
Synergistic effects, 872
Synesthesia, 2180-2181
Synovial fluid, 1955-1956
Synovitis, 1277
Synteny, 964
Synthetically made neuron, 1545
Syphilis, 537, 607, 629, 662, 735, 957, 1313, 1460, 2017, 2034-2036, 2181-2182, 2272
Syphilitic laryngitis, 1313
Syringomyelia, 2103
Systemic lupus erythematosus, 545
Systemic lupus erythematosus (SLE), 2017, 2064, 2182-2185

Systemic sclerosis, 1993, 2185-2187
Systems, 104, 1252, 1671, 1780, 2187-2191
Systole, 148
Systolic blood pressure, 296, 472, 1055, 1162

T

T lymphocytes, 252, 640, 656, 1002, 1121, 1143, 1203-1204, 1206, 1212, 1387, 1391, 2021, 2238, 2280, 2389
Tabes dorsalis, 2103
Tachycardia, 388, 601, 1063, 1693, 1803, 1903, 2040
Tachypnea, 1803
Tai Chi Chuan, 81
Tamoxifen, 337, 430, 1425
Tampon use, 2263
Tapeworms, 1728, 2192-2193
Tardive dyskinesia, 1991, 2193-2194
Tarsal tunnel syndrome, 178, 883
Tarsals, 840, 1372
Tartar, 406, 1015, 1796, 2205
Task-specific focal dystonia, 692-693
Taste, 1960, 2010-2011, 2194-2198
Taste buds, 2010, 2195-2196
Taste disorders, 2197
Tattoo removal, 2199
Tattoos, 2200
Taxanes, 369
Taxol, 336, 430, 1099
Tay-Sachs disease, 945, 2201
Tear breaking point, 682
Tear breakup time, 682
Tear ducts, 819, 2202-2203
Tears, 976, 2055, 2202-2203, 2360
Technetium, 1200, 1431
Technetium-99m pertechnate, 1431
Teeth, 319, 406, 569, 614, 616, 925, 1007, 1015, 1652, 1656, 1748, 1796, 1965, 2203-2207, 2254, 2388
Teething, 2207-2208
Telangiectasia, 575
Telemedicine, 1255
Telogen, 77-78
Telomeres, 371, 492
Temporal arteritis, 2208-2209
Temporal lobe seizure, 790
Temporal lobectomy, 792
Temporomandibular joint (TMJ) syndrome, 1652, 2209
Tend-and-befriend response, 2145
Tender points, 857
Tendinitis, 835, 1521, 1967, 2115, 2209-2212
Tendinosis, 2210
Tendon disorders, 1663, 2211-2212
Tendon repair, 2212-2213
Tendons, 512, 544, 834, 840, 913, 1373, 1660, 1663, 2010, 2115, 2210-2212, 2316
Tenesmus, 2305

Tennis elbow, 1521, 2116, 2210-2211, 2318
Tenosynovitis, 1521, 2212
Teratogens, 271, 735, 843, 1838, 2213-2214
Teriparatide, 1676
Terminal hair, 77-78
Terminal illness, 595-596, 2162, 2164
Terminally ill
    extended care for the, 804, 2214-2217
Termites, 1726
Test kits, 1307
Testes, 960, 978, 1149, 1931, 2022, 2219
Testicles, 1451, 1654, 2221
    undescended, 2217-2218
Testicular cancer, 961, 1449, 1654, 2218-2220
Testicular surgery, 1149, 2219-2220
Testicular torsion, 1451, 1453, 2221
Testosterone, 77-78, 80, 797, 932, 960, 978, 1172, 1857, 2023, 2027, 2031, 2129
Tests See Invasive tests; Laboratory tests; Noninvasive tests
Tetanospasmin, 2222
Tetanus, 233, 447, 899, 1207, 1482, 2221-2225, 2239
Tetany, 1159, 1161, 2223
Tetracyclines, 136-138, 2270
Tetrahydrocannabinol, 1421
Tetralogy of Fallot, 300, 539-540
Thalamus, 323, 2066
Thalassemia, 108, 954, 2048, 2225-2226
Thalidomide, 244, 253, 273, 735, 873, 2213, 2226-2227
Thanotophoric dwarfism, 686
Theophylline, 747
Theory of localization, 1766-1767
Theory of mind, 1487
Therapeutic index, 429
Thermometers, 853
Thermometry, 854
Thermoregulation, 1167-1168, 2062, 2177
Thiamine, 246, 876, 1301, 1410, 1418, 1784, 2365
Thiamine deficiency, 1301
Thiazide diuretic, 152
Thimerosal, 1465
Thoracentesis, 1268
Thoracic aortic aneurysm, 160
Thoracic surgery, 385, 436, 2227-2228
Thoracotomy, 2228
Threadworms, 1789
Throat, 1312, 1381, 1504, 1678-1679, 2269
Throat cancer, 1504-1505, 1759
Throat, sore See Sore throat
Thrombin, 2231
Thrombocytopenia, 2229-2230, 2275, 2389
Thrombolytic, 299-300
Thrombolytic therapy, 731, 2230-2233
Thrombophlebitis, 2350

Thrombosis, 173, 473, 718, 1761, 1796, 2149, 2234-2237, 2344
    deep vein, 600-601
Thrombotic thrombocytopenia purpura, 2229
Thrombus, 473, 600, 718, 731, 1689, 1761, 2149, 2231, 2234-2237, 2350
Thrush, 373
Thumb sucking, 1656, 2237-2238
Thymectomy, 1534
Thymus, 656, 754, 1204, 1521, 1534, 2021
    removal, 1534
Thymus gland, 2238-2239
Thyroglossal cysts, 578
Thyroid disorders, 218, 757, 760, 978, 995, 1028, 1136, 2239-2240, 2242
Thyroid gland, 542, 754, 756, 759-760, 977, 994, 1028, 1411, 1611, 1920, 2189, 2239, 2241-2243
    imaging of, 1200
Thyroid hormone, 2244
Thyroidectomy, 760, 2243-2244
Thyroid-stimulating hormone (TSH), 1790
Thyrotropin-releasing hormone (TRH), 1791
Thyroxine, 977, 995, 1028, 2145, 2239-2240, 2242
TIAs See Transient ischemic attacks (TIAs)
Tibia, 1372-1373, 1663
Tibia vara, 318
Tic douloureux, 1601, 2245
Ticks, 228, 720, 749, 1345-1348, 1384, 1964, 2403
Tics, 688, 2095, 2244-2247, 2260
Timolol maleate, 983
Tincture, 1128
Tinea nigra, 902
Tinea pedis, 202
Tinea versicolor, 902, 1792
Tingling, 212, 897, 1011, 1445, 1615-1616, 2259
Tinnitus, 698-699, 1050, 1441, 2012, 2248-2249, 2352
Tiredness See Fatigue
Tissue plasminogen activator (TPA or tPA), 779, 1945, 2230-2233
Tissues, 105, 260, 1782, 2010
    damage, 1339
T-lymphocytes, 2305
Tobacco, 42, 778, 1504, 1749, 1846, 1895
Toddlers, 635
Toenail removal See Nail removal
Toenails, 1538-1539
    ingrown, 884, 1540
Toes, 840, 1372-1373, 1538, 1785
Toilet training, 636, 1223, 2249-2250
Tolerance, 41, 1545-1547
Tomograms, 527
Tongue, 925, 1504, 2010, 2195
Tongue thrusting, 1656
Tonometer, 984-985

Tonsillectomy, 48, 705, 1758, 1908, 2092, 2251-2253
Tonsillitis, 1392, 1550, 1552, 1759, 1908, 2251-2253
Tonsils, 1392, 1759, 2251-2254
  nasopharyngeal, 47
Tooth decay, 406, 763, 868, 1796 See Cavities
Tooth extraction, 614, 2205, 2254-2255, 2388
Tooth loss, 616, 1749
Toothache, 610, 612
Tophi, 998
Topical anesthesia, 112
Torsion, 2219
Tort, 1318, 1320
Torticollis, 317, 2255
Totipotent, 489, 492
Touch, 2009, 2256-2260
Tourette's syndrome, 1633, 2246-2247, 2260-2261
Tourniquet, 1764
Toxemia, 1842, 2262
Toxic epidermal necrolysis, 2132
Toxic shock syndrome, 233, 1456, 2117, 2143, 2178, 2263-2264
Toxicity, selective, 427
Toxicology, 222, 776, 1127, 2264-2266
Toxins, 82, 274, 316-317, 537, 1325, 1361, 1736, 1755, 1811, 2014, 2222, 2264
  metal, 778
Toxoplasmosis, 123, 125-126, 880, 1646, 1729, 1871, 2266-2267, 2402, 2404
Trabeculectomy, 575, 984
Trabeculoplasty, 818
Trachea, 350, 772, 1379, 1381, 1935, 2267-2269
Tracheal transplantation, 2268
Tracheomalacia, 2268
Tracheostomy, 563, 1076, 1250, 2224, 2268-2269
Trachoma, 284, 550, 813-814, 2270
Tracking, 1256
Traction, 398, 891
Trance, 1175
Tranquilizers, 1634, 2068
Transcranial direct current stimulation, 503-504
Transcription, 949-950
Transcutaneous electrical nerve stimulation (TENS), 1699
TransCyte, 360
Transduction, 136, 138, 489
Transection, 886, 890
Transesophageal echocardiography (TEE), 713
Transfats, 1621
Transformation, 136, 138
Transforming growth factor-á1, 2186
Transfusion, 110, 1190, 1305, 1949, 2042, 2271-2277
Transgenic, 489

Transient ischemic attacks (TIAs), 165, 173, 174, 329-330, 894, 2149, 2278, 2344
Transitional care, 2279
Translation, 949
Translocation, 676, 679, 1985
Transplantation, 310, 592, 953, 1070, 1205, 1289, 2121, 2173, 2279-2283
  bone marrow, 310-312, 314, 1003, 1123, 1214, 1342, 1913, 2021, 2049
  corneal, 550-551, 816, 818
  ethics and, 802
  facial, 826-827, 1653
  hair, 1022, 1024
  heart, 1057, 1068-1071, 2228
  kidney, 750, 1288-1290, 1572, 1574
  liver, 1362, 1368-1369, 1605, 2281
  lung, 469
  tracheal, 2268
Transposition of the great arteries, 540-541
Transposons, 136, 138
Transsexualism, 932, 2025
Transthoracic echocardiography (TTE), 713
Trauma, 94, 565, 662, 1031, 1109, 1721, 1736, 1772, 2102
Trauma centers, 742
Trauma, emotional, 94, 1830
Traumatic brain injury, 894, 1596, 2283-2285
Travelers' diarrhea, 90, 651, 653, 927
Trembling, 2285
Tremors, 1731, 2285-2286
Trench fever, 1245
Trench mouth, 974
Trephination, 1602
Triage, 739, 742
Trichiasis, 2270
Trichinellosis, 2286
Trichinosis, 1728, 1970, 2286
Trichomonas vaginalis, 957
Trichomoniasis, 957-958, 2034, 2036, 2287-2288
Trichothyodystrophy, 513
Trichotillomania, 78-79
Tricyclic antidepressants, 135, 146, 427
Trigeminal nerve, 495-496, 1653, 2153
Triglycerides, 875, 1264, 1351-1352, 1359, 1395, 1450, 2000
Triiodothyronine, 977
Trimethoprim/sulfamethoxazole, 137
Trismus, 1908, 2388
Trophectoderm, 490
Tropical diseases, 730, 1402, 1728, 2398
Tropical medicine, 1987
True aneurysm, 160
Trust, 635, 637
Trypanosomes, 424, 2075
Trypanosomiasis, 1647, 2075
Tubal ligation, 549, 1311, 2125, 2288-2289, 2349

Tubal pregnancy, 714
Tubercles, 2289
Tuberculin skin test, 2291
Tuberculosis, 187, 228, 233, 413, 607, 743, 1207, 1383, 1895, 1901-1902, 2289-2292, 2403
Tuberculous laryngitis, 1313
Tubulointerstitial nephritis, 1573
Tularemia, 1346, 2293
Tumor immunity, 986
Tumor necrosis factor-alpha, 2305
Tumor removal, 1392, 2293-2296
Tumor suppressor genes, 955, 1406
Tumor vaccines, 1286
Tumors, 123, 126, 275, 332, 369, 518-519, 590, 760, 808, 886, 985-986, 1183, 1262, 1312, 1362, 1406, 1611, 1640, 1681, 1711, 1861, 1933, 2294, 2296-2299, 2311
  nerve, 1587
Tunnel vision, 816
Turbidity, 2321
Turbulence, 473
Turner syndrome, 91, 436, 536, 684, 735, 762, 1282, 2022, 2299-2300
Twins, 846, 938
  vanishing, 1489
Twin-twin transfusion, 1509
Tympanic membrane, 594, 700, 1045, 2010
Tympanoplasty, 701, 704
Type 2 segmental Cowden nevus, 786
Type A individuals, 2146
Type B individuals, 2146
Typhoid fever, 1982, 2300-2301
Typhus, 1245, 1346, 2301-2302
Tyrosine, 1786
Tyrosine kinase inhibitors, 253

U

UBE3A, 120-121
Ubiquitin, 120, 951
Ulcer surgery, 2303-2304
Ulcerative colitis, 514, 2304-2305
Ulcers, 6-7, 244, 471, 862, 915, 919, 922, 927, 1254, 1264, 1316, 2303, 2306-2309, 2333, 2350
  corneal, 1644
  decubitus, 243
  mouth, 244, 375
Ulna, 2314
Ultrasonography, 335, 919, 928, 938, 1198, 1357, 1506, 1509, 1606, 1637, 1746, 2138, 2309-2312
Ultrasound, 160, 175-176, 272, 713, 909, 1198, 1367, 1637, 2151-2152
Ultraviolet light, 1786, 1874, 2060
Ultraviolet radiation, 1787-1788, 1888
Umbilical cord, 1636, 1793, 1838, 2222, 2313
  entanglement, 2133
Umbilical cord stem cell, 2109

Umbilical hernias, 1105
Umbilical vesicle, 1430
Unconsciousness, 533, 1542, 1812
Uncontrollable movements, 2193
Underbite, 319
Upper extremities, 99, 2314-2318
  prostheses for, 1865
Uprima, 2028
Urea, 1575, 2318
Uremia, 750, 2318-2319
Ureters, 1190, 1904, 2140, 2326, 2329
Urethra, 585, 772, 960, 1185, 1855, 1860,
  1863, 1904, 1931, 2322, 2326, 2338
Urethral discharge, 2287, 2320
Urethritis, 1929, 2034, 2287, 2319-2320,
  2322, 2327, 2331
Urethroplasty, 1185-1186 See
  Hypospadias repair and urethroplasty
Urgent care, 487-488
Uric acid, 998, 2140
Uricosuric drugs, 999
Urinalysis, 1304, 1577, 2320-2321, 2329
Urinary disorders, 373, 582-583, 1221,
  1858, 2142, 2322-2324, 2327, 2329
Urinary incontinence, 966
Urinary system, 2, 585, 2325-2328
Urinary tract, 1904, 2142
Urinary tract infections, 275, 477, 695,
  1005, 1082, 1293, 1904, 2117, 2138,
  2319, 2327, 2331
Urination, 1858, 2327
Urine, 2, 667, 1304, 1904, 2140, 2189,
  2320, 2325, 2328
  blood in the, 1082, 2140
  high levels of protein in, 1868
Urology, 2328-2331
USDA Nutrition Evidence Library, 879
Uterine bleeding, 764, 1447
Uterine cancer, 417-421, 957-958, 1190,
  1416, 1446 See Cervical, ovarian, and
  uterine cancers
Uterine fibroids, 732, 957-958, 1189,
  1447, 1535, 2332
Uterine polyps, 1824
Uterine prolapse, 957-958, 1189, 1191,
  1933, 2332
Uterus, 440, 764-765, 1018, 1172-1173,
  1189, 1230, 1932, 2332
Uveitis, 124, 126, 128, 1644, 2305
Uvulopalatoplasty, 2070

V

Vaccination, 234-235, 257, 414, 447, 526,
  1144-1145, 1206-1211, 1228, 1429,
  1518, 1742, 1816-1817, 1910, 1971,
  2017, 2224, 2356, 2392
Vaccines, 224, 229, 253, 352, 354,
  1144-1145, 1148, 1206, 1240, 1337,
  1339, 1742, 2017, 2392
  autism and, 214
  mercury and, 1465
  tumor, 1286

Vacuum aspiration, 9
Vacuum tumescence therapy, 2028
Vagina, 793, 932, 1018, 1931
Vaginal cancer, 957
Vaginal discharge, 2287, 2320
Vaginal ring, 548
Vaginitis, 583, 957-958, 2034, 2287
  atrophic, 1445
Vagotomy, 2333-2334
Vagus nerve, 657, 919, 1032, 2333-2334
Valine, 1418
Vallate papillae, 2196
Valley fever, 497, 902
Valsalva maneuver, 674-675
Values History, 54
Valvuloplasty, 2123
Vancomycin, 2118
Vanishing twin syndrome, 1489
Variable region, 144
Varicella virus, 1828
Varicella-zoster virus, 2038
Varicoceles, 732, 961, 1234-1235, 1285,
  1933, 2220
Varicose vein removal, 2335-2336
Varicose veins, 473, 575, 718, 927, 1090,
  1296, 2232, 2335-2338, 2344, 2350
Varicosis, 2337
Variola, 2080
Vas deferens, 549, 960, 1219, 1860, 1931,
  2338, 2347
Vascular compartment, 717
Vascular dementia, 606-607
Vascular disease
  peripheral, 1864
Vascular endothelial growth factor
  (VEGF), 284, 1398, 1835, 2343
Vascular medicine, 2339-2341, 2344
Vascular system, 2311, 2339, 2342-2345
Vasculitis, 2345-2347
Vasectomy, 549, 2125, 2338, 2347-2350
Vasocclusion, 2048
Vasoconstriction, 148-149, 473, 673,
  1037, 1087, 1237, 1254, 2178, 2230
Vasodilation, 148-149, 473, 673-674,
  1037, 1067, 1074, 1237
Vasodilator drugs, 1067, 1165
Vasomotor instability, 1134
Vasopressin, 671, 758, 978, 1137, 1790,
  2040, 2189, 2326
Vasospasm, 1925, 2150
Vectors, 274, 489-490
  viral, 934
Vegans, 1410
Vegetables, 878
Vegetarians, 1410
Vegetations, 752-753
Veins, 472, 600, 1374, 1761, 1764, 2188,
  2317, 2335-2336, 2340, 2342, 2350
  chest, 434
Vellus, 77-78
Vellus hair, 1022
Vena cava, 299
Venipuncture, 1764

Venography, 1762
Venom, 274, 2089
Venous admixture, 576
Venous insufficiency, 2350-2351
Venous thrombosis, 718, 731, 1762, 2344
Ventilator, 40
Ventricles, 1054
Ventricular fibrillation, 171, 388, 601,
  721, 1057, 1063, 1693, 1944
Ventricular remodeling, 386
Ventricular tachycardia, 601
Ventriculoperitoneal shunts, 2046
Vertebrae, 432, 449, 451, 1302, 1600,
  2077, 2104-2109
Vertebroplasty, 886, 890
Vertigo, 238, 673, 698, 1441, 2011, 2150,
  2351-2352
Very long chain fatty acids, 52, 1344
Veterans, 1013, 1831
Viagra, 796, 1925
Vicodin, 1700
Vinca alkaloids, 430
Vincent's infection, 611-612
Vincristine, 506
Vioxx, 153, 873
Viral hemorrhagic fevers, 2352-2353
Viral infections, 5-6, 48, 223, 438, 447,
  523, 591, 710, 774, 794, 858, 916,
  1026-1027, 1095, 1107, 1146,
  1227-1228, 1238, 1252, 1360, 1418,
  1493, 1517, 1901, 1946-1947, 1961,
  1968, 2352, 2354-2357, 2398
Virions, 2354
Virology, 126
Virulence factors, 695
Viruses, 48, 135, 138-139, 142, 523-524,
  526, 662, 711, 774, 1238, 1428,
  1481-1482, 1495, 1901, 1909, 1946,
  1961, 2298, 2352, 2354
  endogenous, 2396
  use as vectors, 934
Vision, 285, 821, 1648, 2010, 2351,
  2358-2360
  blurred, 301-302, 1397, 1536
  color, 517
Vision correction, 201, 819, 2361
Vision disorders, 200, 201, 283, 301, 401,
  402, 813, 817-819, 983, 1397-1398,
  1536, 1928, 2011, 2142, 2361-2363
Visual dyslexia, 689
Visual reinforcement audiometry (VRA),
  1053
Vital signs, 2050
Vitamin A, 1622, 2365
Vitamin A acid, 28
Vitamin A deficiency, 1284, 1410, 1412
Vitamin B deficiency, 109, 916, 1410,
  1412, 2192, 2365
Vitamin C, 154, 545, 1622, 2002, 2365
Vitamin C deficiency, 2002
Vitamin D, 1622, 1677, 2057, 2363-2364,
  2365
Vitamin D deficiency, 1410, 1412, 1623,

1962, 2363-2365
Vitamin E, 1622, 2365
Vitamin K, 278, 282, 471, 2231
Vitamin K deficiency, 2276, 2366
Vitamins, 154, 247, 663, 875-876, 1360, 1395, 1410, 1412, 1622, 1736, 2002, 2165, 2364-2368
Vitelline duct, 1430, 1432
Vitiligo, 1792, 2063, 2368-2369
Vitravene, 258
Vitrectomy, 815
Vitreous, 2359
Vivisection, 124
Vocal cord disorders, 2369-2370
Vocal cord polyps, 1824
Vocal cords, 1313
Voice disorders, 1313, 2095, 2369-2370
Vomiting, 18, 707, 927, 1558-1561, 1608, 1752, 1905, 2012
Von Willebrand's disease, 1087-1088, 2371-2372
Vulva, 577, 1018, 1932

W

Waldemeyer's ring, 2251
Walking, 238, 1109
Wallerian degeneration, 425-426, 1565
Warburg effect, 993
Warfarin, 2232
Warts, 628, 884, 1147, 1312, 1406, 2298
    genital, 571, 957-958, 1147-1148, 2034-2035
    plantar, 842, 884
Watchful waiting, 1858
Water, 865, 1291
    therapy in, 1152
Water loss, 602
Watery eyes, 814, 816
Waxes, 1351
Weaning, 2373-2374
Websites, 1255
Wegener's granulomatosis, 2346
Weight gain, 1625, 1629, 2374-2376
Weight loss, 706, 1153, 1623, 2374-2377

Weight loss medications, 2377
Weight loss surgery, 239
Well-baby examinations, 2377-2378
Wernicke's aphasia, 2379-2380
Wernicke's encephalopathy, 1301
West Nile virus, 294, 609, 1243, 2380-2382
Western blot, 1307
Wheat, 407, 987
Whiplash, 1032, 2383-2384
Whipple's disease, 2079
Whipworms, 1728
Whirlpool therapy, 1152
White blood cells, 287, 467, 1077, 1116, 1203, 1282, 1797, 2016, 2276
White matter, 322, 1118
Whiteheads, 27
Whole blood, 2273
Whooping cough, 2384-2385
Wilderness first aid, 860
Wildlife, 352, 354
Williams syndrome, 2385-2387
Wilson's disease, 1361, 1365, 1470, 1478, 2387-2388
Windchill factor, 897
Winterbottom's sign, 2075
Wisdom teeth, 2204, 2388
Wiskott-Aldrich syndrome, 2389
Witches' milk, 347
Withdrawal, 42, 1545, 1547, 2005, 2051, 2157
Wolffian ducts, 2023
Woolsorter's disease, 132
World Health Organization (WHO), 138-139, 654, 880, 1208, 1335, 2225, 2390-2393
Worms, 728-729, 1727-1728, 1969, 2192, 2286
Wounds, 243, 565, 914, 1032, 1037, 1087, 1152, 1154, 1193, 1308, 1721, 1798, 2222, 2224, 2393-2395
    first aid, 860
Wrinkles, 317, 512, 825, 1653, 1799-1800
Wrists, 394, 1955, 2315
Writers' cramp, 1521, 1708

X

X-linked combined immunodeficiency (XCID), 2021
X chromosome, 953, 2022
X rays, 121, 369, 389, 450, 527, 540, 887, 920, 928, 1198, 1200, 1202, 1367, 1399, 1605, 1607, 1641, 1896, 1916
Xenograft, 360, 1001
Xenotransplantation, 2396-2397
Xerophthalmia, 2055
Xerostomia, 2055
XY chromosomes, 1509

Y

Y chromosome, 2022
Yaws, 2181
Yeast infections *See* Candidiasis
Yellow fever, 274, 609, 1243, 2398-2399
Yoga, 81, 1435, 2399-2401
Yolk sac, 1430-1431
Yuzpe method, 549

Z

Zellweger's syndrome, 1344
Zelnorm, 1271
Zetia, 461
Zidovudine, 1214
Zinc, 1398, 1861
Zinc deficiency, 1411
Zinc lozenges, 1961
Zocor, 461
Zona pellucida, 530, 1218
Zoonoses, 1909, 2286, 2352, 2402-2405
Zoonotic, 352, 1337
Zoster, 1828
Zygote, 530, 733, 1218, 1507-1508, 1510, 1635
Zygote intrafallopian transfer (ZIFT), 193, 912